Handbook of Cannabis

Handbooks in Psychopharmacology
Series Editor: Professor Les Iversen

Handbook of Cannabis

Edited by

Roger G. Pertwee
Institute of Medical Sciences
University of Aberdeen, UK

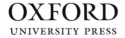

OXFORD

UNIVERSITY PRESS

Great Clarendon Street, Oxford, OX2 6DP,
United Kingdom

Oxford University Press is a department of the University of Oxford.
It furthers the University's objective of excellence in research, scholarship,
and education by publishing worldwide. Oxford is a registered trade mark of
Oxford University Press in the UK and in certain other countries

Chapters 1–38 and 40 © Oxford University Press 2014
Chapter 39 © European Monitoring Centre for Drugs and Drug Addiction 2010

The moral rights of the author have been asserted

First published 2014
First published in paperback 2016

Published in the United States of America by Oxford University Press
198 Madison Avenue, New York, NY 10016, United States of America

British Library Cataloguing in Publication Data
Data available

Library of Congress Cataloging in Publication Data
Data available

ISBN 978-0-19-966268-5 (Hbk.)
ISBN 978-0-19-879260-4 (Pbk.)

Dedication

for Teresa

Foreword: Beyond THC and Anandamide

One of the most appealing features of scientific research is the promise of discovery of unexpected new facets of our surroundings or even of our own world.

The original aim of cannabis research—like that of morphine, about a century earlier—was to identify the active principle and to make it available for biological and clinical investigations. Indeed, this type of research, which had started in the late nineteenth century, culminated in the 1960s and early 1970s with the elucidation of the chemistry of specific cannabis constituents, which were termed cannabinoids. Although many dozens of plant cannabinoids are now known, surprisingly, there is essentially only one compound, delta-9-tetrahydrocannabinol (THC), which causes the typical "marijuana" effects, although others, such as cannabidiol (CBD), modify its activity. Unexpectedly, the exciting saga of cannabinoid research did not end here, but led to further discoveries of wider importance. THC turned out to be an agonist to two major new receptors, which had their own endogenous agonists—anandamide and 2-arachidonoyl glycerol (2-AG). These endocannabinoids have complicated biosynthetic and degradation pathways. This elaborate new biochemical system, appropriately named the endocannabinoid system, has turned out to be of central importance in physiology. It has both direct biological effects, and effects due to modulation of other neurotransmitter systems. In fact the endocannabinoids are synthesized, when and where needed, in the postsynapse and move to the presynapse, where they affect the release of many of the major known neurotransmitters (Howlett et al. 2002; Pertwee et al. 2010).

The present book, edited by Roger Pertwee, one of the early pioneers in the area, presents a picture of our knowledge of the endocannabinoid field, with emphasis on the major biological systems in which the endocannabinoids are involved, with parts dealing with a wide spectrum of topics, stretching from history and international control, through chemistry and pharmacology, to clinical use and clinical promise. The roles of the endocannabinoid system in many central physiological mechanisms are emphasized. It gives us an almost complete picture of the present-day state of knowledge. But a final picture is never possible. There are already tiny slivers of published, unexplained facts, which will presumably open new vistas of which we are not fully aware today.

Just two examples:

Endocannabinoids and synthetic molecules acting through the type 2 cannabinoid receptor (CB_2) have been shown to affect a large number of pathological conditions—cardiovascular, neurodegenerative, reproductive, gastrointestinal, liver, lung, skeletal, and even psychiatric and cancer diseases. This receptor works in conjunction with the immune system and presumably with various other physiological systems. It seems that the CB_2 receptor is part of a major general protective entity. We are, of course, aware that the mammalian body has a highly developed immune system, whose main role is to guard against protein attack and prevent, reduce, or repair possible injury. It is inconceivable that through evolution analogous biological protective systems have not been developed against nonprotein attacks. Pál Pacher and I have previously posed the speculative question: "Are there mechanisms through which our body lowers the damage caused by various types of neuronal as well as non-neuronal insults? The answer is of course positive. Through evolution numerous protective mechanisms have evolved to prevent and limit tissue injury. We believe that lipid signaling through CB_2 receptors is a part of such a protective machinery and

CB_2 receptor stimulation leads mostly to sequences of activities of a protective nature" (Pacher and Mechoulam 2011).

In addition to anandamide and 2-AG there are many dozens, possibly hundreds, of chemically related compounds in the brain and possibly in the periphery. They are mostly fatty acid amides of amino acids (FAAAs) or of ethanol amines, or glycerol esters of fatty acids. More than 50 years ago Godel, in his philosophical work, suggested that everything in the world has meaning, which is analogous to the principle that everything has a cause, on which most of science rests. Along this line of thought: do these compounds play a physiological role? Those constituents that have been evaluated do not bind to the cannabinoid receptors, but possess various activities. Thus, arachidonoyl serine is a vasodilator and lowers brain damage; arachidonoyl glycine is antinociceptive; arachidonoyl dopamine affects synaptic transmission in dopaminergic neurons; oleoyl serine is antiosteoporotic; palmitoyl ethanolamide is anti-inflammatory etc., etc. Numerous papers have shown that in certain pathological conditions the levels of anandamide and 2-AG are modified and recently the levels of some of the FAAAs and related compounds of the types just mentioned have also been shown to change. Can we follow these changes to diagnose early neurological and other diseases? Does this cluster of compounds affect our physiological and psychological reactions, our moods, or even contribute to our personality? Linda Parker and I (Mechoulam and Parker 2013) have previously speculated that "It is tempting to assume that the huge possible variability of the levels and ratios of substances in such a cluster of compounds may allow an infinite number of individual differences, the raw substance which of course is sculpted by experience. The known variants of CB_1 and FAAH genes may also play a role in these differences. If this intellectual speculation is shown to have some factual basis, it may lead to major advances in molecular psychology."

I assume that the endocannabinoid system still holds quite a few surprises. I believe that we shall enjoy learning about them soon.

Institute for Drug Research   R. Mechoulam
Hebrew University, Medical Faculty
Jerusalem, Israel

References

Howlett, A.C., Barth, F., and Bonner, T.I., *et al.* (2002). International Union of Pharmacology. XXVII. Classification of cannabinoid receptors. *Pharmacological Reviews*, **54**, 161–202.

Mechoulam, R. and Parker, L. (2013). The endocannabinoid system and the brain. *Annual Review of Psychology*, **64**, 21–47.

Pacher, P. and Mechoulam, R. (2011) Is lipid signaling through cannabinoid 2 receptors part of a protective system? *Progress in Lipid Research*, **50**, 193–211.

Pertwee, R.G., Howlett, A.C., Abood, M.E., *et al.* (2010). International Union of Basic and Clinical Pharmacology. LXXIX. Cannabinoid receptors and their ligands: beyond CB_1 and CB_2. *Pharmacological Reviews*, **62**, 588–631.

Preface

The pharmacological effects of cannabis have been exploited for over 4800 years for recreational, medicinal, or religious purposes. However, it is less than 100 years since the chemicals in cannabis responsible for the production of some of its effects and the pharmacological actions of some of these chemicals were identified. Particularly noteworthy advances have been the discovery that cannabis is the source of a family of at least 104 compounds now known as phytocannabinoids, that one of these compounds is delta-9-tetrahydrocannabinol (THC), and that this is the main psychoactive constituent of cannabis. No less important was the elucidation of the chemical structure of THC, its chemical synthesis, its pharmacological characterization, and the discovery in the late 1980s that it produces many of its effects by activating a G protein-coupled receptor now known as the cannabinoid CB_1 receptor. Importantly, these major findings were followed by the discovery in the early 1990s first, that our tissues produce chemicals called endocannabinoids that activate this receptor, second that another cannabinoid receptor, the CB_2 receptor, is also activated by both THC and endocannabinoids, and third that this "endocannabinoid system" of cannabinoid receptors and endogenous agonists modulates the unwanted symptoms or even the progression of a number of disorders, often in an "autoprotective" manner. It is also noteworthy that two drugs subsequently found to activate the CB_1 receptor were first licensed as medicines a few years before the discovery of this receptor. These are nabilone (Cesamet®), a THC-like synthetic cannabinoid that is not present in cannabis, and synthetic THC, known as dronabinol (Marinol®). The discovery of the endocannabinoid system reinvigorated the interest of scientists, clinicians, research funders, and pharmaceutical companies in cannabis and cannabinoids. So too did a growing number of reports in the 1990s, for example, in the press, of the beneficial effects of self-medicating with cannabis, particularly for multiple sclerosis (Crowther et al. 2010).

This *Handbook of Cannabis* is divided into six parts, the first of which begins with a detailed description of the known chemical structures of many of the constituents of cannabis. Part 1 continues, first with a chapter that includes a historical account of how and why cannabis has been used over many centuries as a medicine, and then with a chapter that discusses the complex national and international regulations that confront those who wish to self-administer cannabis for recreational or medical purposes or to provide either cannabis or individual phytocannabinoids as medicines. This opening section concludes with two chapters about cannabis plants, one describing the complex morphology, cultivation, harvesting, and processing of these plants, and the other the extent to which their chemical composition can be manipulated by breeding particular genotypes.

Part 2 presents current knowledge about the main pharmacological actions and effects of cannabis constituents when these are administered acutely or repeatedly. The actions and effects that are described include the activation or blockade of cannabinoid receptors and/or of other important pharmacological targets, and the production of significant changes in the functioning of many major physiological systems and processes. This section ends with an account of the pharmacokinetics, metabolism, and forensic detection of phytocannabinoids.

Part 3 focuses on how cannabis, individual phytocannabinoids, and synthetic cannabinoids are currently being used to treat certain disorders, either as licensed medicines that in addition to Cesamet® and Marinol® now include the cannabis-based medicine Sativex®, or through self-medication with cannabis that is grown by patients or purchased by them, illegally from drug dealers or "legally" from "coffee shops" or dispensaries.

Part 4 describes the pharmacological actions and effects that seem to underlie the approved therapeutic uses of synthetic cannabinoid receptor agonists or of plant cannabinoids as licensed medicines: the amelioration by Cesamet® and Marinol® of nausea and vomiting, by Marinol® of anorexia and cachexia, and by Sativex® both of cancer pain and of the pain, spasms, and spasticity of multiple sclerosis.

Part 5 is made up of a group of chapters identifying an ever-growing number of potential, new, wide-ranging clinical applications for phytocannabinoids that are known to interact with cannabinoid receptors and/or with other pharmacological targets. These potential applications include the management of schizophrenia, of anxiety, mood and sleep disorders, of neurodegenerative disorders such as Parkinson's, Huntington's, and Alzheimer's diseases and amyotrophic lateral sclerosis, of some kinds of epilepsy, of cardiovascular, metabolic, hepatic, renal, and inflammatory disorders, of skin disorders such as psoriasis, of glaucoma, age-related macular degeneration, and uveoretinitis, of bone deficits, and of many kinds of cancer.

The final part, Part 6, turns to the complex issue of "recreational cannabis." Its first two chapters identify the sought-after effects of cannabis when it is taken recreationally, and indicate how cannabis can adversely affect mental health and mental performance, particularly in adolescents, for example, by increasing the risk of developing schizophrenia and by causing dependence/addiction. Also mentioned is the discovery that impairment of both mental health and mental performance by cannabis can be lessened by one of its nonpsychoactive phytocannabinoid constituents. The third chapter in Part 6 moves on to describe the main nonpsychological adverse effects of cannabis, including undesirable cardiovascular effects, and the risks associated with the smoking of cannabis; this chapter considers too, the extent to which cannabis prohibition is harming not only cannabis users, in particular, but also society in general. The next chapter in this section also describes the main harms resulting from taking cannabis recreationally, and from current policies directed at regulating cannabis use. It also considers how these harms might be minimized, and then goes on to list a set of questions, the answers to which would be expected to facilitate such harm minimization. The Handbook ends with a chapter about the emergence as recreational drugs of synthetic cannabinoid receptor agonists known as cannabinoid designer drugs, considers whether any of these drugs are more harmful than cannabis or THC, describes their forensic detection, and discusses the limitations of their current legal control.

It is clear from the contents of this Handbook that significant progress has already been made in our understanding both of how cannabis and some of its constituents produce beneficial or harmful effects in the brain or in other organs and tissues, and of how some of the beneficial effects can be exploited therapeutically with acceptable benefit-to-risk ratios. However, it is also clear that there are still numerous important needs that have yet to be met, just two of which being the need to characterize the pharmacology of the many phytocannabinoid and nonphytocannabinoid constituents of cannabis more completely, and the need to identify and then exploit the best new therapeutic applications for cannabis-based medicines.

Finally, this book would not be complete without an acknowledgement to the many eminent scientists, clinicians, and experts on drug regulation who contributed to it in the northern winter, spring, or summer months of 2013. It should also be noted that many cannabinoid scientists have stood on the shoulders of one particular giant in the field of cannabinoid research: Raphael Mechoulam, the author of the Foreword to this Handbook. It was he who first elucidated the structure of THC 50 years ago (Gaoni and Mechoulam 1964), and who, in addition to his many other achievements since then, led the research that resulted in the discovery of endocannabi-noids, initially in the form of anandamide (Devane et al. 1992), and hence in the discovery of the endocannabinoid system.

References

Crowther, S.M., Reynolds, L.A., and Tansey, E.M. (eds.). (2010). *The Medicalization of Cannabis.* Wellcome Witnesses to Twentieth Century Medicine. Vol. 40. London: Wellcome Trust Centre for the History of Medicine at UCL. Available at: http://www.history.qmul.ac.uk/research/modbiomed/Publications/wit_vols/44870.pdf.

Devane, W.A., Hanus, L., Breuer, A., *et al.* (1992). Isolation and structure of a brain constituent that binds to the cannabinoid receptor. *Science*, **258**, 1946–1949.

Gaoni, Y. and Mechoulam, R. (1964). Isolation, structure and partial synthesis of an active constituent of hashish. *Journal of the American Chemical Society*, **86**, 1646–1647.

Contents

Abbreviations

▼	Black Triangle medicine
11-OH-THC	11-hydroxy-THC
2-AG	2-arachidonoylglycerol
2D-GCMS	two dimensional gas chromatography mass spectrometry
4-AP	4-aminopyridine
5-HT	5-hydroxytryptamine
5-HT	5-hydroxytryptamine
5-HT_{1A}	5-hydroxytryptamine receptor type 1A
5-HT_3	5-hydroxytryptamine receptor type 3
8-OH-CBN	8-hydroxycannabinol
8-OH-DPAT	8-hydroxy-2-(di-n-propylamino) tetralin
AANAT	arylalkylamine N-acetyltransferase
abn	abnormal
abn-CBD	abnormal cannabidiol
ACEA	arachidonyl-2′-chloroethylamide
ACMD	Advisory Committee on the Misuse of Drugs
AD	Alzheimer's disease
ADHD	attention-deficit hyperactivity disorder
ADLs	activities of daily living
AEA	anandamide
AEA	arachidonoylethanolamide (anandamide)
AED	antiepileptic drug
AEE1	acyl-activating enzyme-1
AHPA	American Herbal Products Association
AIDS	acquired immunodeficiency syndrome
ALK	anaplastic lymphoma kinase
ALS	amyotrophic lateral sclerosis
AMD	age-related macular degeneration
AMP	adenosine monophosphate
AOM	azoxymethane
AP	area postrema
ARCI	Addiction Research Centre Inventory
ARCI MBG	Addiction Research Center Inventory – Morphine Benzedrine Scale
ARM	age-related maculopathy
ATF-4	activating transcription factor 4
AUC	area under the curve
b.i.d.	bis in die (twice a day)
BAC	blood alcohol content/concentration
BBB	blood–brain barrier
BCE	before common era
BCP	(E)-β-caryophyllene
BDNF	brain-derived neurotrophic factor
BDS	botanical drug substance
BMD	bone mineral density
BOLD	blood oxygen level-dependent
BPRS	Brief Psychiatric Rating Scale
BRM	botanical raw material
BSR	brain-stimulation reward
C	Celsius
Ca^{2+}	calcium
$[Ca^{2+}]$	calcium concentration
$[Ca^{2+}]_i$	intracellular calcium concentration
Caco	colorectal carcinoma
CADSS	Clinician Administered Dissociative States Scale
CAMS	Cannabis in Multiple Sclerosis
CB	cannabinoid
CB_1	cannabinoid receptor type 1
CB_1R	cannabinoid receptor type 1
CB_2	cannabinoid receptor type 2
CB_2R	cannabinoid receptor type 2
CBC	cannabichromene
CBCA	cannabichromenic acid
CBCV	cannabichromevarin
CBCVA	cannabichromevarinic acid
CBD	cannabidiol
CBDA	cannabidiolic acid
CBDM	cannabidiol monomethyl ether
CBDV	cannabidivarin
CBDVA	cannabidivarinic acid

CB_e	proposed endothelial cannabinoid receptor		COPD	chronic obstructive pulmonary disease
CBEA-C_5 A	cannabielsoic acid A		COS-7 cells	African green monkey kidney cells
CBEA-C_5 B	cannabielsoic acid B		COX	cyclooxygenase
CBE-C_5	cannabielsoin		COX-2	cyclooxygenase 2
CBG	cannabigerol		CPP	conditioned place preference
CBGA	cannabigerolic acid		CRH	corticotropin-releasing hormone
CBGAM	cannabigerolic acid monomethyl ether		CRT	choice reaction time
CBG-C_5	cannabigerol		CSA	Controlled Substances Act
CBGM	cannabigerol monomethyl ether		CSF	cerebral spinal fluid
CBGV	cannabigerovarin		CTA	Clinical Trial Application
CBGVA	cannabigerovarinic acid		CTD	Common Technical Document
CBGVAM	cannabigerovarinic acid monomethyl-ether		CTL	cytotoxic T lymphocyte
CBL	cannabicyclol		CYP2C9	cytochrome P450 2C9
CBL-C_3	cannabicyclovarin		D_2	dopamine receptor 2
CBLA	cannabicyclolic acid		DA	divarinolic acid (Chapter 5) or divided attention (Chapter 20) or dopamine
CBM	cannabinoid-based medicine		DAGL	diacylglycerol lipase
CBME	cannabis-based medicinal extract		DAGLα	diacylglycerol lipase alpha
CBN	cannabinol		DART	direct analysis in real time
CBND-C_3	cannabinodivarin		DEA	Drug Enforcement Administration
CBND-C_5	cannabinodiol		Δ^8-THC	delta-8-tetrahydrocannabinol
CCL2	chemokine C-C motif ligand 2		Δ^8-THC acid A	delta-8-tetrahydrocannabinolic acid A
CCR2	chemokine C-C motif receptor 2		Δ^9-THC	delta-9-tetrahydrocannabinol
CDER	Centre of Drug Evaluation and Research		Δ^9-THCA	delta-9-tetrahydrocannabinolic acid
CE	common era		Δ^9-THC acid A	delta-9-tetrahydrocannabinol carboxylic acid A
CFA	Freund's adjuvant-induced chronic arthritic pain		Δ^9-THC acid B	delta-9-tetrahydrocannabinol carboxylic acid B
CGRP	calcitonin gene-related peptide		Δ^9-THCV	delta-9-tetrahydrocannabivarin
CHO	Chinese hamster ovary		Δ^9-THCVA	delta-9-tetrahydrocannabivarinic acid
CHOP	C/EBP homologous protein			
CI	confidence interval		DH-CBD	dehydroxyl-cannabidiol (CBD minus one of its two hydroxyl groups)
CINV	chemotherapy-induced nausea and vomiting			
CMA	Canadian Medical Association		DL VAS	Drug Liking Visual Analogue Scale
C_{max}	maximum concentration		DMHP	dimethylheptylpyran
CME	crude marijuana extract		DNBS	dinitrobenzene sulfonic acid
CNB	carbon nutrient balance		DNFB	2,4-dinitrofluorobenzene
CNS	central nervous system		DOX	deoxyxylulose (pathway)
CoA	coenzyme A		DR	diabetic retinopathy
COMT	catechol-O-methyltransferase		DRN	dorsal raphe nucleus
ConA	concanavalin A			

DRUID	Driving under the Influence of Drugs Alcohol and Medicines (project)
DSHEA	Dietary Supplement Health and Education Act
DSM	*Diagnostic and Statistical Manual of Mental Disorders*
DTH	delayed-type hypersensitivity
DUID	driving under the influence of drugs
DVC	dorsal vagal complex
E2	estradiol
EAE	experimental allergic encephalomyelitis
EAU	experimental autoimmune uveoretinitis
(*E*)-BCP	(*E*)-β-caryophyllene
EBR	author Ethan B. Russo
EC	endocannabinoid
EC_{50}	half-maximal effective concentration
eCB	endocannabinoid
ECDD	WHO Expert Committee on Drug Dependence
ECoG	electrocorticography
ECS	endocannabinoid system
EDHF	endothelial-derived hyperpolarizing factor
EDSS	Expanded Disability Status Scale
EDTA	ethylenediaminetetraacetic acid
EEG	electroencephalography
EFS	electrical field stimulation
EGFR	epidermal growth factor receptor
EIU	endotoxin-induced uveitis
ELDD	European Legal Database on Drugs
ELISA	enzyme-linked immunosorbent assay
EMA	European Medicines Agency
EMCDDA	European Monitoring Centre for Drugs and Drug Addiction
EMG	electromyogram/electromyography
EOG	electrooculogram/electrooculography
EQ-5D	EuroQol 5-D
ER	endoplasmic reticulum
Erb	estrogen receptor beta
ERK	extracellular signal-regulated kinase
EU	European Union
FAAH	fatty acid amide hydrolase
FAQs	frequently asked questions
FDA	Food and Drug Administration

FGR	fetal growth restriction
FLV	friend leukemia virus
fMRI	functional magnetic resonance imaging
FSH	follicle-stimulating hormone
GABA	gamma-aminobutyric acid
GACP	Good Agricultural and Collection Practice
GAO	Government Accountability Office
GC	gas chromatography
GCDP	Global Commission on Drug Policy
GC-FID	gas chromatography-flame ionization detector
GCMS	gas chromatography mass spectrometry
GCMSMS	gas chromatography tandem mass spectrometry
GERD	gastroesophageal reflux disease
GH	growth hormone
GHB	gamma hydroxybutyric acid
GHRH	growth hormone-releasing hormone
GI	gastrointestinal
GM-CSF	granulocyte macrophage colony stimulation factor
GnRH	gonadotropin-releasing hormone
GOT	geranylpyrophosphate:olivetolate transferase
GPP	geranylpyrophosphate
GPR	G protein-coupled receptor
GPR55	G protein-coupled receptor 55
GW	GW Pharmaceuticals plc
ha	hectare
hCB_1	human cannabinoid receptor type 1
hCB_2	human cannabinoid receptor type 2
HD	Huntington's disease
HEK	human embryonic kidney
HFD	high-fat diet
HIV	human immunodeficiency virus
HL	human promyelocytic leukemia
HLA	human leukocyte antigen
HPA	hypothalamic–pituitary–adrenal
HPB-ALL	human peripheral blood acute lymphoid leukemia human T cell line
HPG	hypothalamic–pituitary–gonadal
HPLC	high-performance liquid chromatography

HPS	high-pressure sodium	iNOS	inducible nitric oxide synthase
HPT	hypothalamic–pituitary–thyroid	IOM	Institute of Medicine
HSV	herpes simplex virus	IOP	intraocular pressure
HU-211	dexanabinol	IPS	intermittent photic stimulation
HUD	Department of Housing and Urban Development	JWH-133	3-(1′,1′-dimethylbutyl)-1-deoxy-delta-8-tetrahydrocannabinol
huPBL-SCID	human peripheral blood lymphocytes implanted into severe combined immunodeficient mouse	JZL184	4-nitrophenyl-4-(dibenzo[d][1,3] dioxol-5-yl(hydroxy)methyl) piperidine-1-carboxylate
		LC	liquid chromatography
i.p.	intraperitoneal	LCMSMS	liquid chromatography tandem mass spectrometry
i.v.	intravenous		
I/R	ischemia-reperfusion *or* ischemic reperfusion	L-DOPA	L-3,4-dihydroxyphenylalanine
		LES	lower esophageal sphincter
IACM	International Association for Cannabinoid Medicines	LFP	local field potential
		LH	luteinizing hormone
IBD	inflammatory bowel disease	LiCl	lithium chloride
IBS	irritable bowel syndrome	LOB	lying on belly
IC	insular cortex	LOD	limit of detection
IC$_{50}$	half-maximal inhibitory concentration	LOQ	limit of quantification
		LPS	lipopolysaccharide
ICAM-1	intercellular adhesion molecule 1	LSD	lysergic acid diethylamide
ICH	International Conference on Harmonisation of Technical Requirements for registration of Pharmaceuticals for Human Use	MA	Marketing Authorisation
		MAA	Marketing Authorisation Application
ICNCP	International Code of Nomenclature for Cultivated Plants	MAGL	monoacylglycerol lipase
		MALDI-TOF	matrix-assisted laser desorption/ionization-time of flight
ICOS	inducible T-cell costimulator		
ICSD	International Classification of Sleep Disorders	MAPK	mitogen-activated protein kinase
		MCH	melanin-concentrating hormone
IFN-γ	interferon-gamma	MCP-1	monocyte chemoattractant protein-1
Ig	immunoglobulin	MDK	midkine
IHDC	Indian Hemp Drugs Commission	MEM	mineralized extracellular matrix
IL	interleukin	MES	maximal electroshock
IL-2	interleukin 2	MFB	medial forebrain bundle
IL-2R	interleukin-2 receptor	MHC-1	major histocompatibility complex
IL-4	interleukin 4	MHRA	Medicines and Healthcare products Regulatory Agency
ILAE	International League Against Epilepsy		
		MIP	macrophage inflammatory protein
IMP	investigational medicinal product	MMAR	Health Canada Marihuana Medical Access Regulations
IMPD	investigational medicinal product dossier		
		MRI	magnetic resonance imaging
IMMA	indomethacin morpholinylamide	MRM	multiple reaction monitoring
INCB	International Narcotics Control Board	MS	mass spectrometry (Chapter 40) *or* multiple sclerosis
		MSIS-29	Multiple Sclerosis Impact Scale
IND	investigational new drug		
INF	interferon	MTD	maximum tolerated dose

mTORC1	mammalian target of rapamycin complex 1	PAR	photosynthetically active radiation (Chapter 4) *or* Public Assessment Report (Chapter 19)
MVA	mevalonate (pathway)		
NAAA	*N*-acylethanolamine-hydrolyzing acid amidase	PBL	human peripheral blood leukocyte
		PBN	parabrachial nucleus
NAc	nucleus accumbens	PBQ	phenylbenzoquinone
NAPE-PLD	*N*-acyl phosphatidylethanolamine phospholipase D	PCA	principal component analysis
		pCB	phytocannabinoid
NCE	New Chemical Entity	PCP	phencyclidine
NCI	National Cancer Institute	PD	Parkinson's disease
NDA	new drug application	PDT	photodynamic therapy
NE	norepinephrine	PEA	*N*-palmitoylethanolamine
NF-κB	nuclear factor kappa B	PET	positron emission tomography
NFAT	nuclear factor of activated T cell	PF	parabolic flight maneuver
NIDA	US National Institute on Drug Abuse	PHA	phytohemagglutinin
		PII	posterior segment intraocular inflammation
NK	natural killer		
NK$_1$	neurokinin 1	PJC	prolonged juvenile chemotype
NMDA	*N*-methyl-D-aspartate	PK	pharmacokinetics
NMR	nuclear magnetic resonance	PMA	phorbol myristate acetate
NO	nitric oxide	PP	per protocol
NOS	nitric oxide synthase	PPAR	peroxisome proliferator-activated receptor
NP	normal phase		
NPP	nerylpyrophosphate	PPI	prepulse inhibition
NPY	neuropeptide Y	PPMS	primary progressive multiple sclerosis
Nrf-2	nuclear factor-erythroid 2-related factor 2	PPN	pedunculopontine tegmental nuclei
		PPR	panretinal photocoagulation
Nrg1	neuregulin-1	PTSD	posttraumatic stress disorder
Nrg1 TM HET	transmembrane domain Neuregulin-1 mutant	PTX	pertussis toxin
		PTZ	pentylenetetrazole
NRS	numeric rating scale	PVN	paraventricular nucleus
NTS	nucleus of the solitary tract	RANTES	regulated upon activation normal T-cell expressed and secreted
OA	olivetolic acid		
OAC	olivetolic acid cyclase	RBT	random roadside alcohol breath testing
OF	oral fluid	RCT	randomized controlled trial
OIG	Office of the Inspector General	RDT	roadside drug testing
OLS	olivetol synthase	REM	rapid eye movement sleep
OMC	Office of Medicinal Cannabis	Rf	retention factor
ONL	outer nuclear layer	ROS	reactive oxygen species
OR	odds ratio	ROSITA	Roadside Testing Assessment
OS	oleoyl serine	RPE	retinal pigment epithelium
OVA	ovalbumin	RRMS	relapsing-remitting multiple sclerosis
OVX	ovariectomy	RVM	rostral ventromedial medulla
OX1	orexin type 1	s.c.	subcutaneous
p.o.	oral	SAMHSA	Substance Abuse Mental Health Services Administration
PANSS	Positive and Negative Syndrome Scale		
		SAR	structure–activity relationship

SBA	Summary Basis of Approval	THCV	tetrahydrocannabivarin
SCA	spinocerebellar ataxia	THCVA	tetrahydrocannabivarinic acid
SCE	standardized cannabis extract	TKS	tetraketide synthase
SCS	skeletal cannabinoid system	TLC	thin layer chromatography
SD	standard deviation	TNBS	trinitrobenzene sulfonic acid
SDV	subjective drug value	TNF	tumor necrosis factor
SE	standard error	TNF-α	tumor necrosis factor alpha
SF CBC	San Francisco Cannabis Buyers Club	TRH	thyrotropin-releasing hormone
SGIC	Subject Global Impression of Change	TRIB3	tribbles-homologue 3
		TRP	transient receptor potential
SIM	single ion monitoring	TRPC 1	transient receptor potential 1
SIV	simian immunodeficiency virus	TRPV	transient receptor potential vanilloid receptor
SmPC	Summary of Product Characteristics		
SNP	single nucleotide polymorphism	TRPV1	transient receptor potential vanilloid type-1
SOD	superoxide dismutase		
SOD-1	superoxide dismutase-1	TRβ1	subtype β1 thyroid hormone receptor
SPARC	San Francisco Patients Resource Center		
		TSH	thyroid stimulating hormone (thyrotropin)
SPME	solid phase micro extraction		
SPMS	secondary progressive multiple sclerosis	UHR	ultra-high risk
		UN	United Nations
spp.	species	UNODC	United Nations Office on Drugs and Crime
sRBC	sheep red blood cell		
SRM	single reaction monitoring	v/w	volume per weight
STM	short-term memory	VA	visual acuity
STZ	streptozotocin	VAS	visual analogue scale
SWS	slow wave sleep	VASH	Visual Analogue Scale for Hunger
T	testosterone		
T$_3$	triiodothyrionine	V$_d$	volume of distribution
T$_4$	L-thyroxin	VEGF	vascular endothelial growth factor
Tat	trans-activating protein		
TBI	traumatic brain injury	VIC	visceral insular cortex
TCM	traditional Chinese medicine	VLC	vacuum liquid chromatography
TDP-43	TAR DNA-binding protein-43	vl-PAG	ventrolateral periaqueductal gray
TGF	transforming growth factor	VP	ventral pallidum
Th	T-helper	VPpc	parvicellular thalamic nucleus
Th1	type 1 T-helper cell	VTA	ventral tegmental area
Th2	type 2 T-helper cell	W	waking
THC	tetrahydrocannabinol	WAMM	Wo/men's Alliance for Medical Marijuana
THCA	tetrahydrocannabinolic acid		
THCCOOH	11-nor-9-carboxy-tetrahydrocannabinol	WHO	World Health Organization
		WN	author Willy Notcutt
		WT	wild type

Contributors

Lisa Aguilar-Turton
Laboratorio de Neurociencias Moleculares e Integrativas, Escuela de Medicina, División Ciencias de la Salud, Universidad Anáhuac Mayab, México

Oscar Arias-Carrión
Clinica de Trastornos de Sueño, Facultad de Medicina, Universidad Nacional Autónoma de México, México

Augusto Azuara-Blanco
Centre for Vision and Vascular Science, Queen's University Belfast, Institute of Clinical Science, UK

Itai Bab
Bone Laboratory, Hebrew University of Jerusalem, Israel

David Baker
Neuroinflammation and Trauma Group, UK

Sagnik Bhattacharyya
Institute of Psychiatry, King's College London, UK

Heather B. Bradshaw
Indiana University, USA

Maria Grazia Cascio
School of Medical Sciences, Institute of Medical Sciences, University of Aberdeen, UK

Guy A. Cabral
Virginia Commonwealth University, School of Medicine, USA

Emily L. Clarke
Medical School, University of East Anglia, UK

Francesca Comelli
Department of Biotechnology and Bioscience, University of Milano-Bicocca, Italy

Barbara Costa
Department of Biotechnology and Bioscience, University of Milano-Bicocca, Italy

Luigia Cristino
Endocannabinoid Research Group, Institute of Biomolecular Chemistry, Consiglio Nazionale delle Ricerche, Italy

H. Valerie Curran
Clinical Psychopharmacology Unit, Research Department of Clinical Psychology, University College London, UK

Eva de Lago
Department of Biochemistry and Molecular Biology, CIBERNED and IRYCIS, Faculty of Medicine, Complutense University, Spain

Etienne de Meijer
GW Pharmaceuticals, UK

Louisa Degenhardt
National Drug and Alcohol Research Centre, University of New South Wales, Australia

Vincenzo Di Marzo
Endocannabinoid Research Group, Institute of Biomolecular Chemistry, Consiglio Nazionale delle Ricerche, Italy

Marnie Duncan
GW Research Ltd, UK

Mahmoud ElSohly
The University of Mississippi, National Center for Natural Products Research, USA

Javier Fernández-Ruiz
Department of Biochemistry and Molecular Biology, CIBERNED and IRYCIS, Faculty of Medicine, Complutense University, Spain

Gabriela A. Ferreira
Virginia Commonwealth University, School of Medicine, USA

Concepción García
Department of Biochemistry and Molecular Biology, CIBERNED and IRYCIS, Faculty of Medicine, Complutense University, Spain

Moisés García-Arencibia
Department of Biochemistry and Molecular Biology, CIBERNED and IRYCIS, Faculty of Medicine, Complutense University, Spain

Eliot L. Gardner
Neuropsychopharmacology Section, Intramural Research Program, National Institute on Drug Abuse, US National Institutes of Health, USA

María Gómez-Ruiz
Department of Biochemistry and Molecular Biology, CIBERNED and IRYCIS, Faculty of Medicine, Complutense University, Spain

Megan Grabenauer
RTI International, USA

Franjo Grotenhermen
Nova-Institut, Huerth, Germany

Waseem Gul
ElSohly Laboratories, Inc., USA

Geoffrey Guy
GW Pharmaceuticals, UK

Manuel Guzmán
Department of Biochemistry and Molecular Biology I, Complutense University, Madrid, Spain

Wayne Hall
UQ Centre for Clinical Research, The University of Queensland, Australia

Arno Hazekamp
Bedrocan BV, The Netherlands

Matthew N. Hill
University of Calgary, Departments of Cell Biology and Anatomy & Psychiatry, The Hotchkiss Brain Institute, Canada

Cecilia J. Hillard
Neuroscience Research Center, Medical College of Wisconsin, USA

Marilyn A. Huestis
Chemistry and Drug Metabolism, IRP National Institute on Drug Abuse, National Institutes of Health, USA

Angelo A. Izzo
Department of Pharmacy, University of Naples Federico II, Italy

Nicholas A. Jones
GW Pharmaceuticals, UK

George Kunos
Laboratory of Physiologic Studies, Section on Neuroendocrinology, National Institute on Alcohol Abuse and Alcoholism, National Institutes of Health, USA

Verity Langfield
GW Pharmaceuticals, UK

Emma Leishman
Department of Psychological and Brain Sciences, Program in Neuroscience, Indiana University, USA

Mauro Maccarrone
Campus Bio-Medico University of Rome, Italy and European Center for Brain Research/ Santa Lucia Foundation, Italy

John M. McPartland
College of Medicine, University of Vermont, USA

Alice P. Mead
GW Pharmaceuticals, USA

Raphael Mechoulam
Hebrew University of Jerusalem, Medical Faculty, Institute for Drug Research, Israel

Stephanie Mijangos-Moreno
Laboratorio de Neurociencias Moleculares e Integrativas, Escuela de Medicina, División Ciencias de la Salud, Universidad Anáhuac Mayab, México

Celia J.A. Morgan
University College London, UK

Paul D. Morrison
Institute of Psychiatry, UK

Eric Murillo-Rodríguez
Laboratorio de Neurociencias Moleculares e Integrativas, Escuela de Medicina, División Ciencias de la Salud, Universidad Anáhuac Mayab, México

Robin M. Murray
Department of Psychosis Studies, Institute
of Psychiatry, King's College, London, UK

William Notcutt
Pain Management, James Paget University
Hospital, Great Yarmouth, UK

Sergio Oddi
University of Teramo, Italy and European
Center for Brain Research/Santa Lucia
Foundation, Italy

Saoirse E. O'Sullivan
School of Medicine, University of Nottingham
Royal Derby Hospital, UK

Pál Pacher
Laboratory of Physiologic Studies, Section on
Oxidative Stress and Tissue Injury, National
Institute on Alcohol Abuse and Alcoholism,
National Institutes of Health, USA

George Pappas
Bedrocan BV, The Netherlands

Linda A. Parker
Department of Psychology and Collaborative
Neuroscience Program, University of Guelph,
Canada

Daniela Parolaro
Department of Theoretical and Applied
Sciences, Biomedical Division, and Center
of Neuroscience, University of Insubria, Italy

Sachin Patel
Department of Psychiatry and Molecular
Physiology and Biophysics, Vanderbilt
University Medical Center, USA

Roger G. Pertwee
School of Medical Sciences, Institute of
Medical Sciences, University of Aberdeen, UK

Gerald T. Pollard
Howard Associates LLC, USA

David J. Potter
Director of Botanical Research and
Cultivation, GW Pharmaceuticals, UK

Gareth Pryce
Neuroinflammation and Trauma Group, UK

Erinn S. Raborn
Department of Microbiology & Immunology,
Virginia Commonwealth University School of
Medicine, USA

Amanda Reiman
School of Social Welfare, University of
California, Berkeley, USA

Erin M. Rock
Department of Psychology and Collaborative
Neuroscience Program, University of Guelph

Tiziana Rubino
Department of Theoretical
and Applied Sciences, Biomedical Division,
and Center of Neuroscience,
University of Insubria, Italy

Ethan B. Russo
GW Pharmaceuticals, USA

Onintza Sagredo
Department of Biochemistry and Molecular
Biology, CIBERNED and IRYCIS,
Faculty of Medicine, Complutense University,
Spain

Cristina Sánchez
Department of Biochemistry and Molecular
Biology I, Complutense University,
Madrid, Spain

Andrea Sarro-Ramírez
Clinica de Trastornos de Sueño, Facultad de
Medicina, Universidad Nacional Autónoma
de México, México

Michael L. Smith
US Army Forensic Toxicology Drug Testing
Laboratory Fort Meade, USA

Martin A. Sticht
Department of Psychology and Collaborative
Neuroscience Program, University of Guelph,
Canada

Jordyn M. Stuart
Indiana University, USA

Bela Szabo
Institut für Experimentelle und Klinische
Pharmakologie und Toxikologie Albert-
Ludwigs-Universität, Germany

Alison Thompson
GW Pharmaceuticals, UK

Brian F. Thomas
RTI International, USA

Guillermo Velasco
Department of Biochemistry and Molecular
Biology I, Complutense University, Spain

Mark A. Ware
Departments of Anesthesia and Family
Medicine, McGill University, Canada

Benjamin J. Whalley
University of Reading, UK

Jenny L. Wiley
RTI International, USA

Claire M. Williams
School of Psychology & Clinical
Language Sciences,
University of Reading, UK

Stephen Wright
GW Pharmaceuticals, UK

Heping Xu
Centre for Vision and Vascular Science,
Queen's University Belfast, UK

Erica Zamberletti
Department of Theoretical and Applied
Sciences, Biomedical Division, and
Center of Neuroscience,
University of Insubria, Italy

Part 1

Constituents, History, International Control, Cultivation, and Phenotypes of Cannabis

Ethan B. Russo

Part 1 Overview

This volume commences with an examination of cannabis constituents by ElSohly and Gull, presenting structures for the now over 100 agents that have come to be known as phytocannabinoids. Some of these may be artifacts of laboratory analysis, and perhaps only 12 have been investigated pharmacologically in any detail (Russo 2011).

Chapter 2 by Russo presents a pharmacological history of cannabis via a detailed chronology, followed by a discussion of four lesser-known indications for cannabis medicine: tinnitus, tetanus, burns, and its use in pediatrics through the ages, along with modern rationales for such usage.

In Chapter 3, Mead offers a clear and up-to-date dissection of current international law on medicinal cannabis usage that will be of great utility to anyone attempting to understand this difficult and changing topic.

Potter brings light in Chapter 4 to the heretofore clandestine topic of cannabis cultivation, explaining the process in great detail from vegetative propagation to subsequent harvest and processing for medical extraction.

Chapter 5 by de Meijer explains the fascinating topic of the process by which, through Mendelian genetics, it has been possible to selectively breed cannabis cultivars expressing high titers of specific phytocannabinoids for their formulation into new medicines.

Reference

Russo, E.B. (2011). Taming THC: potential cannabis synergy and phytocannabinoid-terpenoid entourage effects. *British Journal of Pharmacology*, **163**, 1344–1364.

Chapter 1

Constituents of *Cannabis Sativa*

Mahmoud ElSohly and Waseem Gul

1.1 Introduction

Cannabis is a widely distributed plant, found in a variety of habitats and altitudes (Merlin 2003). Its use by humans goes back for over 5000 years (Farnsworth 1969) and it is one of the oldest plant sources of food and textile fiber (Kriese 2004). The cultivation of *Cannabis sativa* (*C. sativa* L.) for textile fiber originated in Western Asia and Egypt, subsequently extended to Europe, and in 1606 hemp cultivation was introduced to North America (Port Royal, Canada) (Small and Marcus 2002). Under current federal laws, it is prohibited to cultivate cannabis in the United States.

Cannabis has been indicated for the treatment of pain, glaucoma, nausea, depression, and neuralgia (Guindon and Hohmann 2009; Jarvinen et al. 2002; Liang et al. 2004; Slatkin 2007; Viveros and Marco 2007). The therapeutic value of the phytocannabinoids has also been reported for HIV/AIDS symptom management and multiple sclerosis treatment (Abrams et al. 2007; Pryce and Baker 2005).

1.2 Constituents of *Cannabis sativa* L.

The total number of natural compounds identified or isolated from *C. sativa* L. has continued to increase over the last few decades. In 1980, 423 compounds were reported in cannabis (Turner et al. 1980). This number increased in 1995 to 483 (Ross and ElSohly 1995). Between 1995 and 2005 eight compounds were added (ElSohly and Slade 2005). The main focus of this chapter is to provide a chemical account of a total of 104 cannabinoids (isolated or reported to date) as well as of the 22 noncannabinoid constituents (isolated between 2005 and 2012) (Table 1.1). This brings the total number of constituents identified in cannabis to 545 compounds.

1.2.1 Cannabinoids (104)

Today, the term "cannabinoids" refers to not only the chemical substances isolated from *C. sativa* L. exhibiting the typical C_{21} terpenophenolic skeleton, but also to their derivatives and transformation products, with the term "phytocannabinoids" coined for those originating from the plant. A total of 104 phytocannabinoids have been isolated to date (Table 1.1), classified into 11 types, namely: (–)-delta-9-*trans*-tetrahydrocannabinol (Δ^9-THC), (–)-delta-8-*trans*-tetrahydrocannabinol (Δ^8-THC), cannabigerol (CBG), cannabichromene (CBC), cannabidiol (CBD), cannabinodiol (CBND), cannabielsoin (CBE), cannabicyclol (CBL), cannabinol (CBN), cannabitriol (CBT), and miscellaneous-type cannabinoids.

Table 1.1 Constituents of C. *sativa* L. by chemical class as of the end of 2012

Chemical class	Number of compounds
Δ^9-THC type	18
Δ^8-THC type	2
CBG type	17
CBC type	8
CBD type	8
CBND type	2
CBE type	5
CBL type	3
CBN type	10
CBT type	9
Misc type	22
Total cannabinoids	**104**
Total noncannabinoids	**441**
Total	**545**

1.2.1.1 (−)-Delta-9-*trans*-tetrahydrocannabinol (Δ^9-THC) type

The structure of Δ^9-THC (*1*) was first reported by Gaoni and Mechoulam (1964a) who not only determined its absolute configuration as *trans*-(6aR,10aR), but also discussed psychotropic properties of Δ^9-THC (Δ^1-THC according to the terpenoid numbering system). A hexane extract of hashish was chromatographed on florisil to yield an active fraction which was re-chromatographed on alumina to produce Δ^9-THC. Crystalline 3,5-dinitrophenyl urethane of Δ^9-THC was prepared and mild basic hydrolysis yielded pure Δ^9-THC. Archer et al. (1970) reported the detailed conformation of Δ^9-THC using X-ray and proton magnetic resonance analysis. Δ^9-Tetrahydrocannabinol carboxylic acid A (Δ^9-THC acid A, *2*) was first isolated by Korte et al. (1965a) from a hashish extract. Pure Δ^9-THC-acid A is sensitive to light and was not capable of crystallization. Mechoulam et al. (1969) isolated a second Δ^9-THC acid present in hashish (Δ^9-THC-acid B, *3*). Hashish sole (a flat form of illicit hashish that might be rectangular- or oval-shaped) was chromatographed on silicic acid by eluting with a 1:1 ether/petroleum ether solution. Δ^9-THC-acid B was shown to be more polar than Δ^9-THC-acid A on thin layer chromatography (TLC). Hashish soles that contained Δ^9-THC-acid B had little or no Δ^9-THC-acid A which could be caused by biochemical variation. The crystal structure of Δ^9-THC-acid B was determined by Rosenqvist and Ottersen (1975). Gill (1971) isolated Δ^9-tetrahydrocannabivarin (Δ^9-THCV, *4*) from hashish by eluting with 4:1 light petroleum/ether on a column containing deactivated alumina. Countercurrent distribution was used to separate the material after obtaining an orange oil from concentrating the column fractions. The distribution resulted in three fractions in which the second fraction went through another cycle to purify Δ^9-THCV. Fetterman and Turner (1972) reported spectral evidence for Δ^9-*trans*-tetrahydrocannabivarinic acid (Δ^9-THCVA, *5*) followed by mass spectral data (Turner et al. 1973). This report on C_3 homologs of cannabinoids was based on the evaluation of 51 samples from different geographical locations. Vree et al. (1972a) identified

Δ^9-tetrahydrocannabiorcol (*6*) from an extract of Brazilian cannabis as a homologue of Δ^9-THC that contained a methyl side chain. Electron voltage-mass fragment intensity graphs from gas chromatography/mass spectrometry (GCMS) provided a mass of 258 which was the only possible isomer of Δ^9-THC that contained 56 less mass units. The Δ^9-tetrahydrocannabiorcol concentration in hashish samples was very low and, therefore, was not expected to contribute much to the biological activity of the drug. Harvey (1976) discovered Δ^9-tetrahydrocannabinol-C_4 (*7*) and detected delta-9-*trans*-tetrahydrocannabinolic acid-C_4 (Δ^9-*trans*-THCA-C_4, *8*) by GCMS in samples of cannabis. He also detected Δ^9-*trans*-tetrahydrocannabiorcolic acid (*9*). Eight new tetrahydrocannabinol type compounds namely β-fenchyl-Δ^9-tetrahydrocannabinolate (*10*), α-fenchyl-Δ^9-tetrahydrocannabinolate (*11*), *epi*-bornyl-Δ^9-tetrahydrocannabinolate (*12*), bornyl-Δ^9-tetrahydrocannabinolate (*13*), α-terpenyl-Δ^9-tetrahydrocannabinolate (*14*), 4-terpenyl-Δ^9-tetrahydrocannabinolate (*15*), α-cadinyl-Δ^9-tetrahydrocannabinolate (*16*), and γ-eudesmyl-Δ^9-tetrahydrocannabinolate (*17*) were isolated by Ahmed et al. (2008a). Their structures (Fig. 1.1) were established on the basis of nuclear magnetic resonance (NMR) spectroscopic analysis and GCMS as mono- or sesquiterpenoid esters of Δ^9-tetrahydrocannabinolic acid A, the precursor of Δ^9-THC. Under the high temperature conditions of the GCMS analysis, these compounds fragment into their two components to yield Δ^9-THC and the mono- or sesquiterpene. These cannabinoid esters were isolated from a high-potency *C. sativa* variety using multiple chromatographic techniques, including vacuum liquid chromatography (VLC), C_{18} semipreparative high-performance liquid chromatography (HPLC), and semipreparative chiral HPLC (Ahmed et al. 2008a). Cannabisol (*18*, Fig. 1.1), a dimeric cannabinoid, was isolated employing flash silica gel column chromatography from a group of illicit cannabis samples with high CBG content (Zulfiqar et al. 2012).

1.2.1.2 (–)-Delta-8-*trans*-tetrahydrocannabinol (Δ^8-THC) type

There are only two Δ^8-THC–type cannabinoids in cannabis, namely delta-8-*trans*-tetrahydrocannabinol (Δ^8-THC, *19*) and delta-8-*trans*-tetrahydrocannabinolic acid A (Δ^8-THC acid, *20*, Fig. 1.2) (Hanuŝ and Krejčí 1975; Hively et al. 1966).

Hively et al. (1966) isolated Δ^8-THC (Δ^6-THC following the terpenoid numbering system) from a petroleum ether extract of the leaves and flowering tops of marijuana grown in Maryland. In 1970, Archer et al. (1970) published detailed NMR and X-ray data on Δ^8-THC.

Δ^8-THC acid was isolated from *Cannabis sativa* of Czechoslovakian origin (Hanuŝ and Krejčí 1975).

1.2.1.3 Cannabigerol (CBG) type

The first compound isolated from cannabis resin in a pure form was cannabigerol (CBG-C_5, *21*) (Fig. 1.3). Gaoni and Mechoulam (1964b) were the first to isolate CBG, and reported that it is produced by the condensation of geranyl pyrophosphate with olivetol. They also found cannabigerolic acid (CBGA, *22*), identified as its methyl ester from the acidic fraction of a hashish sole extract, being the most polar acid compound (Mechoulam and Gaoni 1965). Yamauchi et al. (1968) isolated cannabigerol monomethyl ether (CBGM, *23*) by heating the acid fraction of the benzene percolate of the leaves of Minamioshihara No. 1 variety (M-1) for 7 h to obtain a phenolic mixture. Using benzene to elute the compound by column chromatography, a pale yellow substance was obtained and purified by TLC. Mass spectra confirmed that this fraction was CBG monomethyl ether with a molecular weight of 330. Shoyama et al. (1970) isolated cannabigerolic acid monomethyl ether (CBGAM, *24*) by passing M-1 percolate (free of chlorophyll) through a silica gel column with 5:1 hexane/ethyl acetate. CBGAM eluted along with Δ^9-THC-acid. This

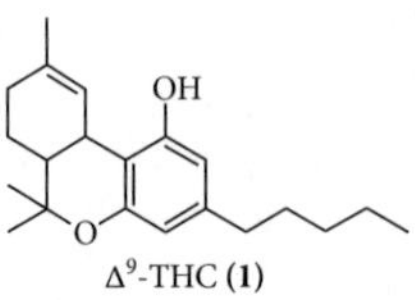

Δ⁹-THC (1)

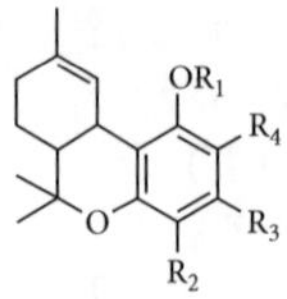

Δ⁹-THC acid A

Δ⁹-THC acid B

Δ⁹-THCV

Δ⁹-THCVA

Δ⁹-tetrahydrocannabiorcol

Δ⁹-tetrahydrocannbinol-C₄

Δ⁹-trans-THCA-C₄

Δ⁹-tetrahydrocannabiorcolic acid

(2) R_1 = H, R_2 = H, R_3 = C_5H_{11}, R_4 = COOH
(3) R_1 = H, R_2 = COOH, R_3 = C_5H_{11}, R_4 = H
(4) R_1 = H, R_2 = H, R_3 = C_3H_7, R_4 = H
(5) R_1 = H, R_2 = H, R_3 = C_3H_7, R_4 = COOH
(6) R_1 = H, R_2 = H, R_3 = CH_3, R_4 = H
(7) R_1 = H, R_2 = H, R_3 = C_4H_9, R_4 = H
(8) R_1 = H, R_2 = COOH or H, R_3 = C_4H_9, R_4 = COOH or H
(9) R_1 = H, R_2 = COOH or H, R_3 = CH_3, R_4 = COOH or H

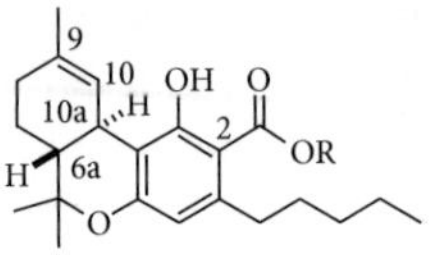

R =

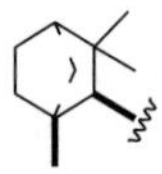

β-fenchyl-Δ⁹-tetrahydrocannabinolate (10)

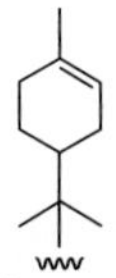

α-terpenyl-Δ⁹-tetrahydrocannabinolate (14)

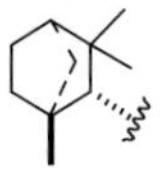

α-fenchyl-Δ⁹-tetrahydrocannabinolate (11)

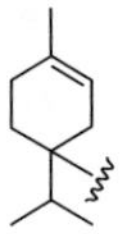

4-terpenyl-Δ⁹-tetrahydrocannabinolate (15)

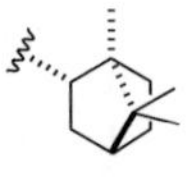

epi-bornyl-Δ⁹-tetrahydrocannabinolate (12)

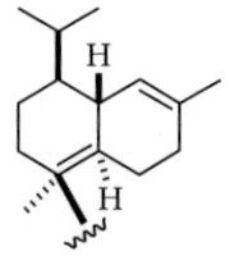

α-cadinyl-Δ⁹-tetrahydrocannabinolate (16)

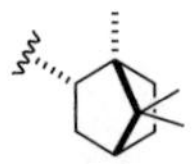

bornyl-Δ⁹-tetrahydrocannabinolate (13)

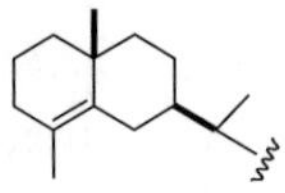

γ-eudesmyl-Δ⁹-tetrahydrocannabinolate (17)

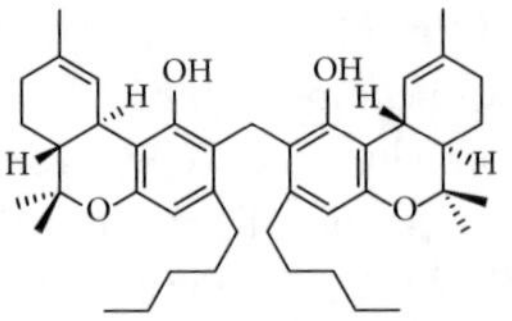

cannabisol (18)

Fig. 1.1 (–)-Δ⁹-*trans*-tetrahydrocannabinol (Δ⁹-THC) type cannabinoids.

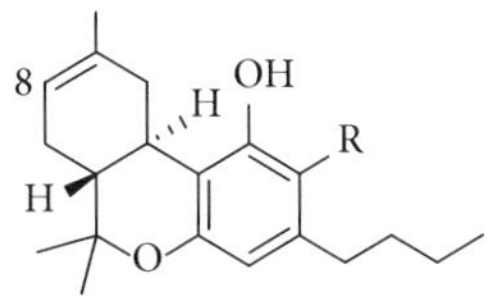

Δ8-THC   (**19**) R = H
Δ8-THC acid (**20**) R = COOH

Fig. 1.2 (−)-Δ8-*trans*-tetrahydrocannabinol (Δ8-THC) type cannabinoids.

mixture was purified on a second column filled with silver nitrate-silica gel which resulted in pure CBGAM. Cannabigerovarin (CBGV, *25*) was also isolated by Shoyama et al. (1975) by heating the benzene extract of cannabis at 160°C for 20 min to achieve decarboxylation. Neutral cannabinoid fractions were then eluted with benzene and a mixture of (20:10:1) benzene/hexane/diethyl amine from a silica gel column. CBGV was identified by comparison with synthetic CBGV prepared by Mechoulam and Yagen (1969). Cannabigerovarinic acid (CBGVA, *26*) was isolated by Shoyama et al. as a minor component of an extract of dried leaves of Thai *Cannabis* (Shoyama et al. 1977). The acid fraction from the dried leaves was purified by column chromatography on silica gel and eluted with a hexane/ethyl acetate mixture along with a 5:1 benzene-acetone mixture. The product appeared as clear needles after recrystallization from a hexane/chloroform solution. The spectral data showed that CBGVA is the major acid of CBGV and its structure was confirmed by comparison with synthetic CBGVA. Taura et al. (1995) isolated cannabinerolic acid (*27*) from a Mexican strain of C. *sativa* by extracting the air-dried leaves with benzene and evaporating to dryness. After dissolving the residue in Me$_2$CO and ridding of insoluble particles, the solution was dried and loaded on a silica gel column which was eluted with a 9:1 benzene/Me$_2$CO mixture. The fraction containing cannabigerolic acid was chromatographed again and eluted with 3:1 hexane/ethyl acetate to give pure cannabigerolic acid.

Ahmed et al. (2008a) isolated two cannabigerolic acid esters, γ-eudesmyl cannabigerolate (*28*) and α-cadinyl cannabigerolate (*29*), from C. *sativa* of high potency. The hexane extract of cannabis was purified on flash silica gel using VLC. Fractions that were shown to have compounds with higher retention factor (R_f) than that of Δ9-THC were mixed together and chromatographed on Sephadex® LH-20 and flash silica gel. Semipreparative reversed-phase (RP) and chiral HPLC were both used for further purification from which the two esters were isolated. The spectroscopic data of γ-eudesmyl cannabigerolate and α-cadinyl cannabigerolate proved that both compounds were esters of CBGA (Radwan et al. 2008a).

Radwan et al. (2008a, 2009) isolated six compounds (*30–35*), 5-acetyl-4-hydroxycannabigerol (*30*), 4-acetoxy-2-geranyl-5-hydroxy-3-*n*-pentylphenol (*31*) (±)-6,7-*trans*-epoxycannabigerolic acid (*32*), (±)-6,7-*cis*-epoxycannabigerolic acid (*33*), (±)-6,7-*cis*-epoxycannabigerol (*34*) and (±)-6,7-*trans*-epxoycannabigerol (*35*), from high-potency C. *sativa* (Fig. 1.3). Hexane extract was chromatographed on flash silica gel. Fractions close to the R_f of Δ9-THC were combined and purified by flash silica chromatography and Sephadex® LH-20, followed by preparative C$_{18}$ HPLC (Radwan et al. 2009). In their procedures, Appendino et al. (2008) fractionated cannabis extract on a RP C$_{18}$ silica gel column which was followed by silica gel column chromatography and subsequent use of normal phase (NP) HPLC to isolate a novel, polar dihydroxy cannabigerol derivative (carmagerol, *36*). Pollastro et al. (2011) isolated a lipophilic analogue of cannabigerol, sesquicannabigerol (*37*), from the waxy fraction of the variety Carma of fiber hemp. Methanolic KOH was used for the hydrolysis of the wax and purification was performed by gravity silica gel column chromatography which was followed by flash chromatography over neutral alumina.

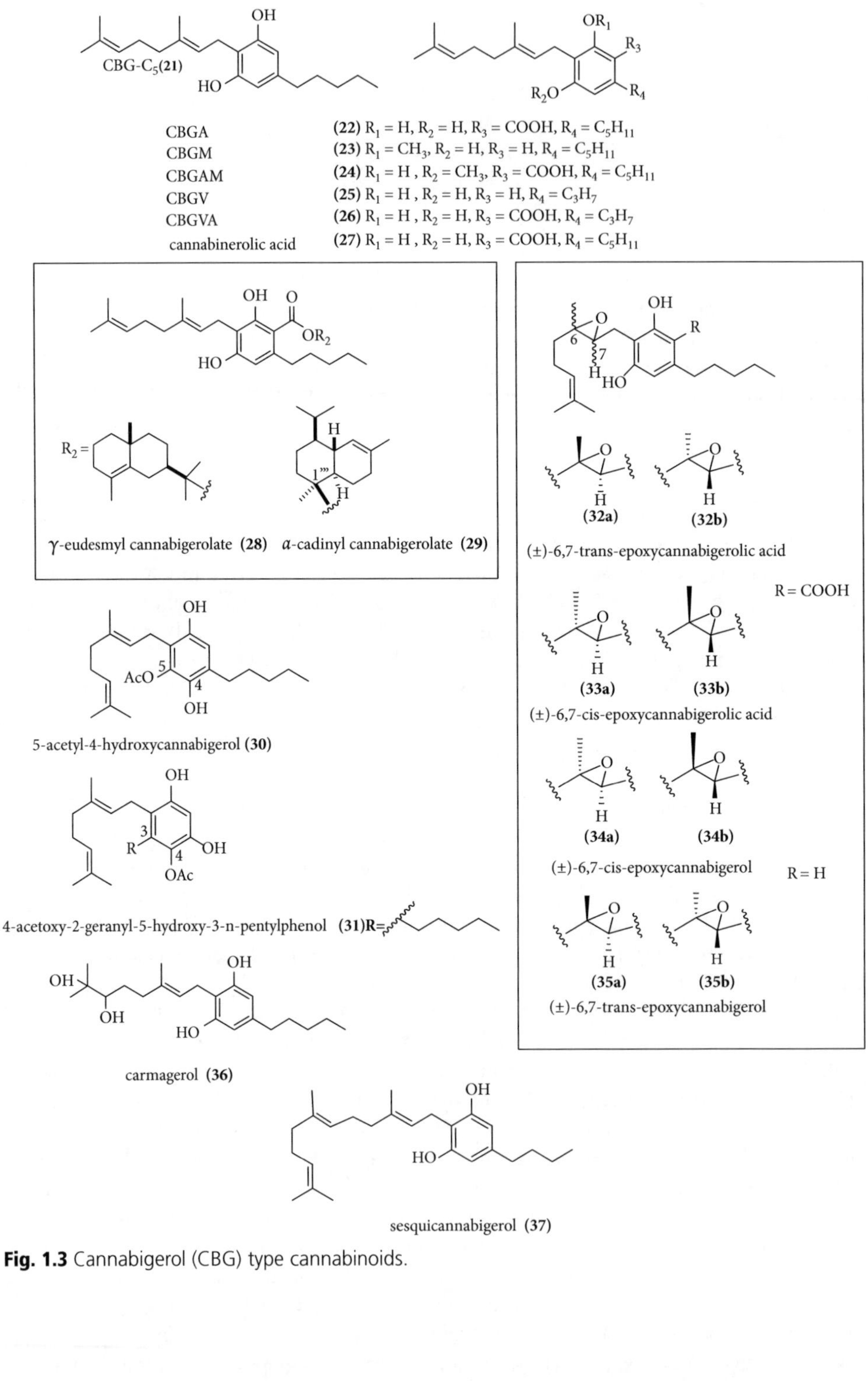

CBG-C$_5$(21)

CBGA
CBGM
CBGAM
CBGV
CBGVA
cannabinerolic acid

(**22**) R$_1$ = H, R$_2$ = H, R$_3$ = COOH, R$_4$ = C$_5$H$_{11}$
(**23**) R$_1$ = CH$_3$, R$_2$ = H, R$_3$ = H, R$_4$ = C$_5$H$_{11}$
(**24**) R$_1$ = H , R$_2$ = CH$_3$, R$_3$ = COOH, R$_4$ = C$_5$H$_{11}$
(**25**) R$_1$ = H , R$_2$ = H, R$_3$ = H, R$_4$ = C$_3$H$_7$
(**26**) R$_1$ = H, R$_2$ = H, R$_3$ = COOH, R$_4$ = C$_3$H$_7$
(**27**) R$_1$ = H , R$_2$ = H, R$_3$ = COOH, R$_4$ = C$_5$H$_{11}$

R$_2$ =

γ-eudesmyl cannabigerolate (**28**)   α-cadinyl cannabigerolate (**29**)

(**32a**)   (**32b**)
(±)-6,7-trans-epoxycannabigerolic acid

R = COOH

(**33a**)   (**33b**)
(±)-6,7-cis-epoxycannabigerolic acid

5-acetyl-4-hydroxycannabigerol (**30**)

(**34a**)   (**34b**)
(±)-6,7-cis-epoxycannabigerol

R = H

4-acetoxy-2-geranyl-5-hydroxy-3-n-pentylphenol (**31**)R=

(**35a**)   (**35b**)
(±)-6,7-trans-epoxycannabigerol

carmagerol (**36**)

sesquicannabigerol (**37**)

Fig. 1.3 Cannabigerol (CBG) type cannabinoids.

1.2.1.4 Cannabichromene (CBC) type

The research groups of Claussen et al. (1966) and Gaoni and Mechoulam (1966) independently disclosed cannabichromene (CBC-C$_5$, *38*). Gaoni and Mechoulam (1966) performed isolation from a hexane extract on Florisil that yielded 1.5% of CBC-C$_5$. Shoyama et al. (1968) isolated cannabichromenic acid (CBCA, *39*) from the benzene percolate of hemp via a procedure described by Shultz et al. (1960). A solvent system of 1:1 hexane/ethyl acetate yielded CBCA which was confirmed by NMR spectroscopy. The infrared (IR) spectra of CBCA displayed intermolecular hydrogen bonding between the carboxyl and hydroxyl groups and the structure showed similarities to that of THCA according to the location of the carboxyl group. Cannabichromevarin (CBCV, *40*) was isolated by Shoyama et al. (1975) as a brownish red cannabinoid by repeatedly passing the neutral cannabinoids from the benzene percolate of the leaves of Thai *Cannabis* through a silica gel column and eluting with benzene and 20:10:1 benzene-hexane-diethyl. Shoyama et al. (1977) also isolated cannabichromevarinic acid (CBCVA, *41*) as a minor fraction from young cannabis. The structure of natural CBCVA was confirmed by synthesis. A CBC-C$_3$ type compound with a 4-methyl-2-pentenyl side chain at C$_2$ (*42*) was separated and identified by Morita and Ando (1984).

Radwan et al. (2009) reported the isolation of three new cannabichromene type cannabinoids, namely (±)-4-acetoxycannabichromene (*43*), (±)-3″-hydroxy-Δ$^{4″}$-cannabichromene (*44*), and (−)-7-hydroxycannabichromane (*45*) from high-potency C. *sativa* by applying silica gel VLC, Si HPLC and C$_{18}$ HPLC (Fig. 1.4).

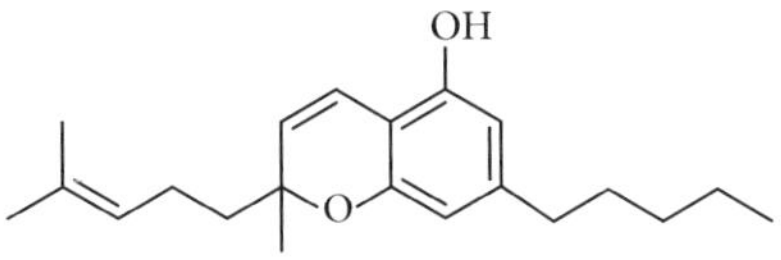

CBC-C$_5$ (**38**)

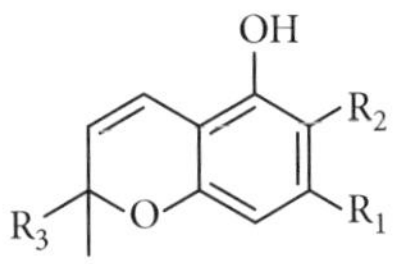

CBCA (**39**) R$_1$ = C$_5$H$_{11}$, R$_2$ = COOH, R$_3$ = (CH$_2$)$_2$CH = C(CH$_3$)$_2$
CBCV (**40**) R$_1$ = C$_3$H$_7$, R$_2$ = H, R$_3$ = (CH$_2$)$_2$CH = C(CH$_3$)$_2$
CBCVA (**41**) R$_1$ = C$_3$H$_7$, R$_2$ = COOH, R$_3$ = (CH$_2$)$_2$CH = C(CH$_3$)$_2$
CBC-C$_3$ (**42**) R$_1$ = C$_3$H$_7$, R$_2$ = H, R$_3$ = CH$_2$CH = CHCH(CH$_3$)$_2$

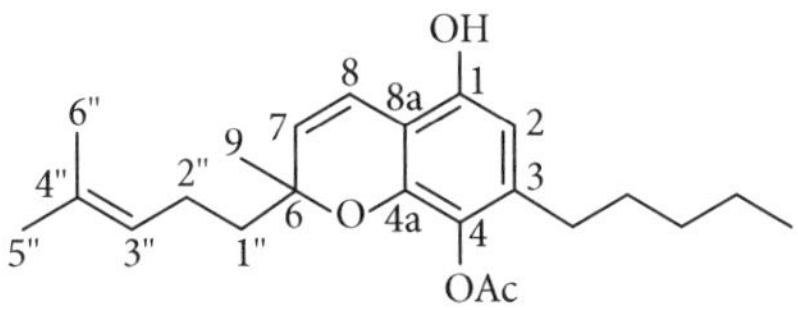

(±)-4-acetoxycannabichromene (**43**)

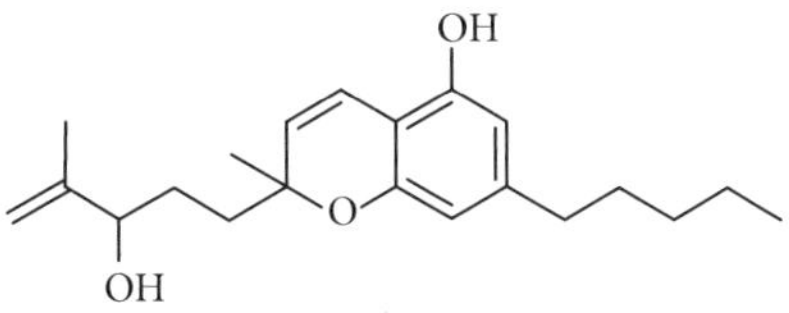

(±)-3″-hydroxy-Δ$^{4″}$-cannabichromene (**44**)

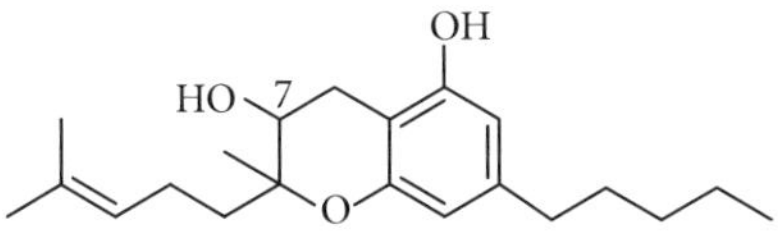

(−)-7-hydroxycannabichromane (**45**)

Fig. 1.4 Cannabichromene (CBC) type cannabinoids.

1.2.1.5 Cannabidiol (CBD) type

Cannabidiol (CBD, 46) and cannabidiolic acid (CBDA, 47) are the major metabolites of the nonpsychotropic (fiber-type) varieties of *C. sativa* (Fig. 1.5). Adams et al. (1940a) isolated cannabidiol (CBD) and after allowing the oily CBD to stand for several weeks CBD was crystallized, while, Petrzilka et al. (1969) reported its synthesis and absolute configuration as (−)-*trans*-(1R,6R). Krejčí and Šantavý (1955) isolated CBDA. Vollner et al. (1969) isolated cannabidivarin (CBDV, 48) when ligroin extract of hashish was chromatographed on silica gel. Shoyama et al. (1972a) isolated cannabidiol monomethyl ether (CBDM, 49) by obtaining neutral cannabinoids from the ethanol extract of the leaves from Minamioshihara No. 1 variety (M-1). The cannabinoids were then chromatographed on Florisil and eluted with benzene. The eluted fraction was rechromatographed on silica gel and eluted with 3:1 hexane/benzene to obtain CBDM. Cannabidiorcol (CBD-C_1, 50) was detected by Vree et al. (1972a) in an n-hexane extract of Lebanese hashish. In a similar extract of Brazilian marijuana, no cannabidiorcol was found. Harvey reported cannabidiol-C_4 (CBD-C_4, 51) in 1976. Crushed cannabis resin and leaves were percolated with ethyl acetate which upon filtration and concentration gave a residue. This residue was derivatized and analyzed on GCMS. Cannabidiol-C_4 was identified by its mass and methylene unit. From a benzene extract of Thailand cannabis, cannabidivarinic acid (CBDVA, 52) was isolated by Shoyama et al. (1977). Taglialatela-Scafati et al. (2010) recently isolated cannabimovone (53) as a polar cannabinoid from an acetone extract of *Cannabis sativa L.* that is nonpsychotropic.

1.2.1.6 Cannabinodiol (CBND) type

CBND-type cannabinoids are the aromatized derivatives of CBD. Cannabinodiol (CBND-C_5, 54) and cannabinodivarin (CBND-C_3, 55) (Fig. 1.6) are the only two compounds from this subclass that have been characterized from *C. sativa* (ElSohly and Slade 2005; Turner et al. 1980). Cannabinodiol was isolated from a hexane-ether extract of Lebanese hashish by Lousberg et al. (1977). The propyl homolog of cannabinodiol, cannabinodivarin, was detected by GCMS (Turner et al. 1980).

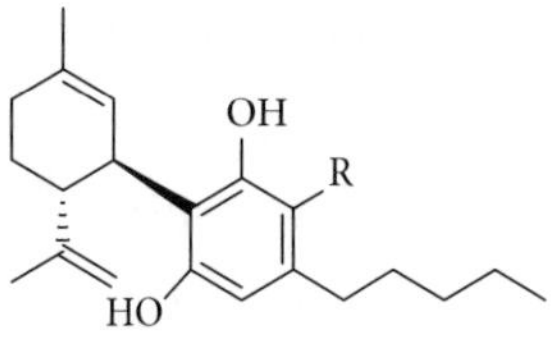

CBD   (46) R = H
CBDA (47) R = COOH

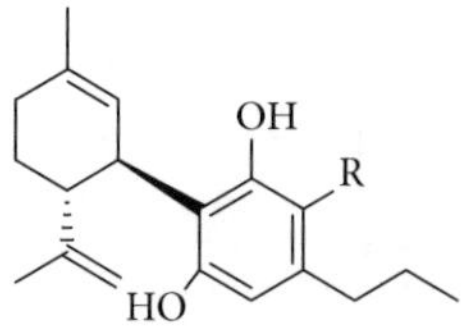

CBDVA (52) R = COOH
CBDV   (48) R = H

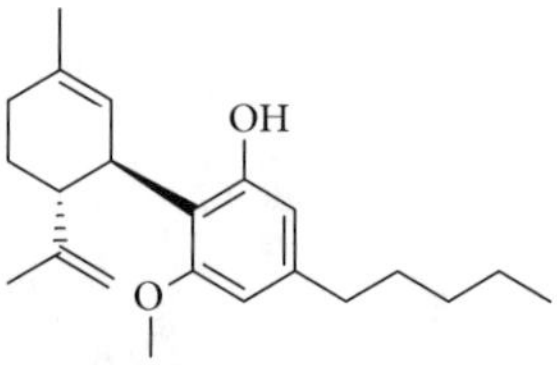

CBDM (49)

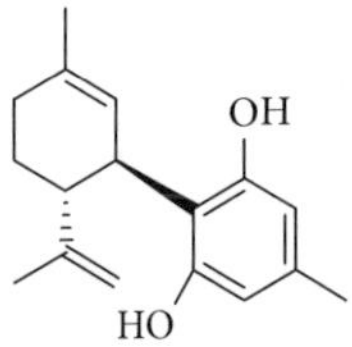

CBD-C_1 (50)

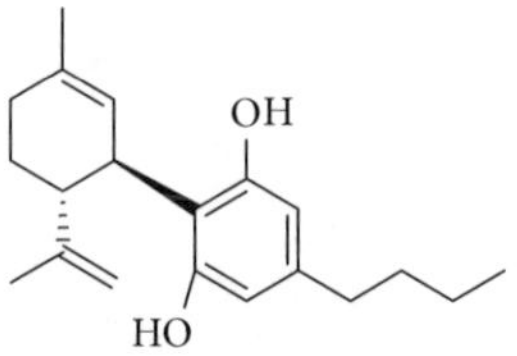

CBD-C_4 (51)

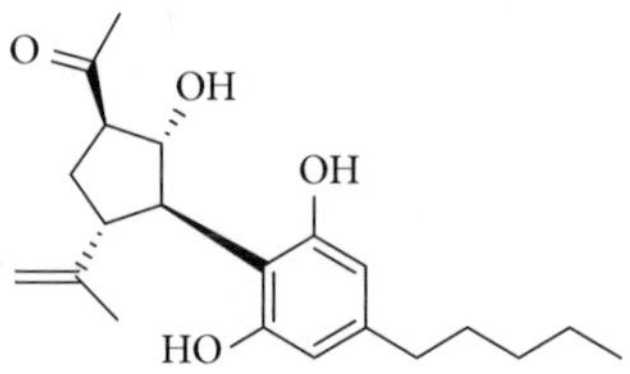

cannabimovone (53)

Fig. 1.5 Cannabidiol (CBD) type cannabinoids.

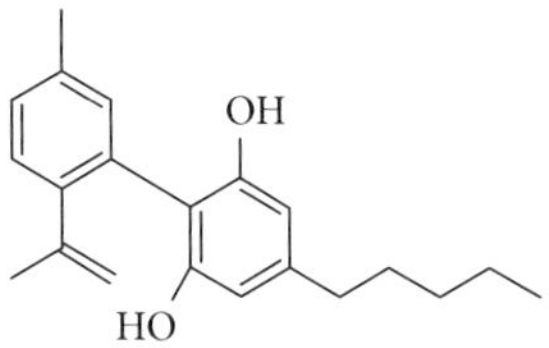

Fig. 1.6 Cannabinodiol (CBND) type cannabinoids.

CBND-C$_5$ (**54**)

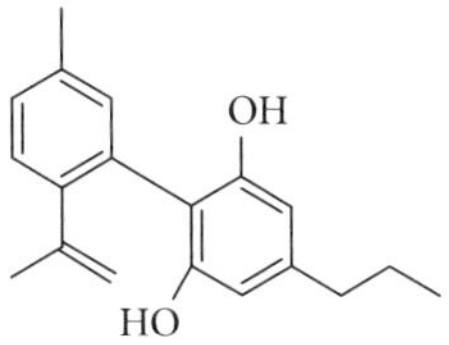

CBND-C$_3$ (**55**)

1.2.1.7 Cannabielsoin (CBE) type

Five cannabielsoin-type cannabinoids named as cannabielsoin (CBE-C$_5$, 56), cannabielsoic acid A (CBEA-C$_5$ A, 57), cannabielsoic acid B (CBEA-C$_5$ B, 58), cannabielsoin-C$_3$ (CBE-C$_3$, 59), and cannabielsoic-C$_3$ acid B (CBEA-C$_3$ B, 60) make up the cannabielsoin-type cannabinoids found in cannabis (Fig. 1.7). These cannabielsoin-type cannabinoids can be produced by photo-oxidation from naturally occurring CBD and CBD acids (Shani and Mechoulam 1974). Cannabielsion (CBE) was detected by Bercht et al. (1973) from an ethanolic extract of Lebanese hashish. This ethanolic extract was subjected to a 130-step counter current distribution. Uliss et al. (1974) established its structure by synthesis starting from cannabidiol diacetate. CBEA-C$_5$ A and CBEA-C$_5$ B were isolated from a benzene extract of Lebanese hashish (Shani and Mechoulam 1974). Furthermore, CBE-C$_5$ was also identified as a mammalian metabolite of CBD (Yamamoto et al. 1991).

1.2.1.8 Cannabicyclol (CBL) type

Cannabicyclol (CBL), cannabicyclolic acid (CBLA), and cannabicyclovarin (CBL-C$_3$) (Fig. 1.8) are the only compounds isolated from this subclass (Claussen et al., 1968; Korte and Sieper 1964; Mechoulam and Gaoni 1967; Shoyama et al. 1972b, 1981).

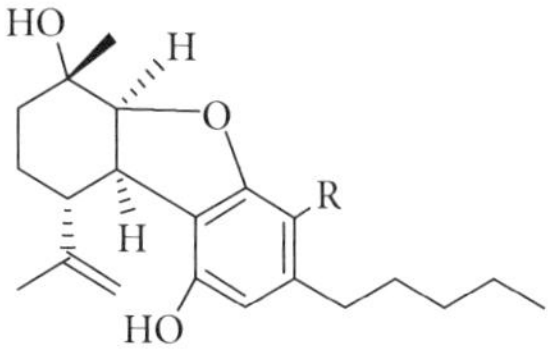

CBE-C$_5$ (**56**) R = H
CBEA-C$_5$ A (**57**) R = COOH

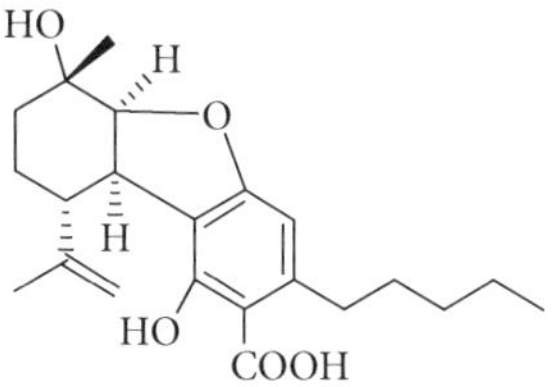

CBEA-C$_5$ B (**58**)

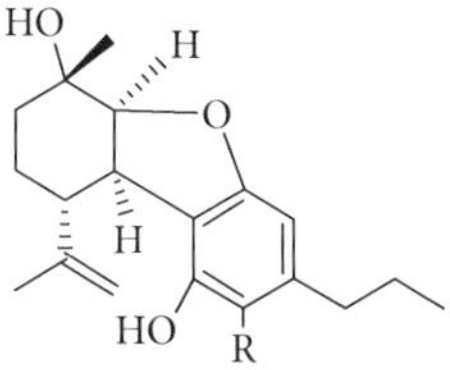

CBE-C$_3$ (**59**) R = H
CBEA-C$_3$ B (**60**) R = COOH

Fig. 1.7 Cannabielsoin (CBE) type cannabinoids.

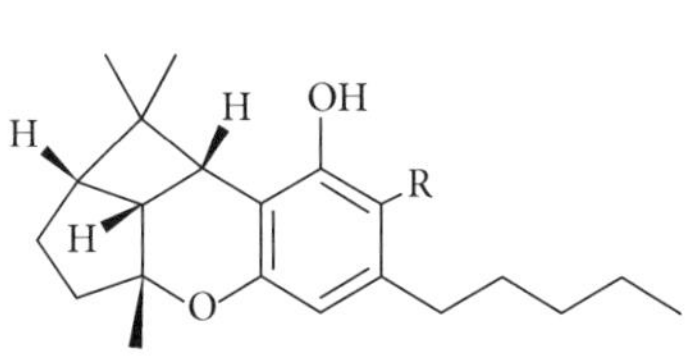

CBL (**61**) R = H
CBLA (**62**) R = COOH

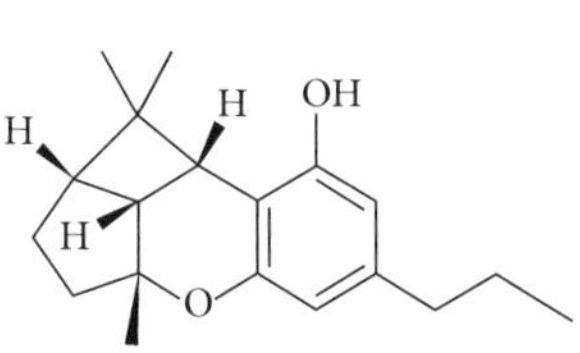

CBL-C$_3$ (**63**)

Fig. 1.8 Cannabicyclol (CBL) type cannabinoids.

CBL (*61*) was first detected by Korte and Sieper in 1964. Korte et al. (1965b) isolated CBL by TLC of various hashish and cannabis samples.

Cannabicyclolic acid (CBLA, *62*) was isolated from benzene extract of dried leaves of cannabis on a polyamide column (Shoyama et al. (1972b). Cannabicyclovarin (CBL-C$_3$, *63*) was identified in an ether extract of Congo marihuana by comparison of the electron voltage versus mass fragment graph for cannabicyclol and cannabicyclol-C$_3$ (Korte et al. 1965b).

1.2.1.9 Cannabinol (CBN) type

Cannabinol (CBN, *64*), was first named by Wood et al. in 1896. CBN was prepared as oil from exuded resin of Indian hemp. Later, Wood et al. (1899) acetylated this oil and obtained pure CBN as its acetate. Adams et al. (1940b) determined the correct structure of CBN. Cannabinolic acid A (CBNA, *65*) was isolated from a crude acidic fraction of hashish, which was esterified with dioazomethane and purified as its methyl ester on an acid-washed alumina column (Mechoulam and Gaoni 1965). Merkus isolated cannabivarin (CBN-C$_3$, *66*) from Nepalese hashish and confirmed the structure by mass spectral data (Merkus 1971a, 1971b). Cannabiorcol (*67*) was identified in the *n*-hexane extract of Brazilian marihuana and the structure was confirmed by electron voltage mass fragment intensity graphs (Vree et al. (1972a). Bercht et al. (1973) detected cannabinol methyl ether (*68*) from an ethanolic extract of Lebanese hashish. Cannabinol-C$_4$ (CBN-C$_4$, *69*) was detected by GCMS from an ethyl acetate extract of cannabis (Harvey 1976). Cannabinol-C$_2$ (CBN-C$_2$, *70*) was identified by Harvey from ethanolic extract of cannabis (Harvey 1985). Ahmed et al. (2008a) isolated 4-terpenyl cannabinolate (*71*, Fig. 1.9) from a high-potency variety of *C. sativa* through a semipreparative chiral HPLC method. When this compound was analyzed on GCMS, compound 71 fragmented to CBN and a monoterpenol. From the same variety of cannabis,

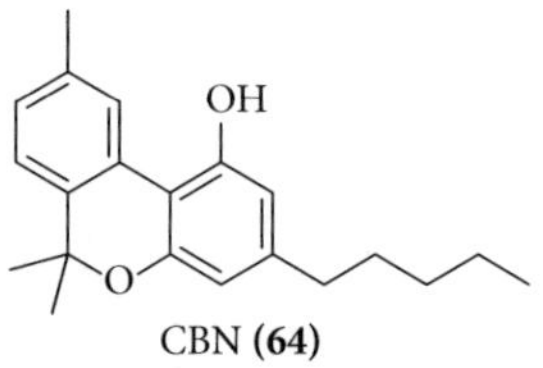

CBN (**64**)

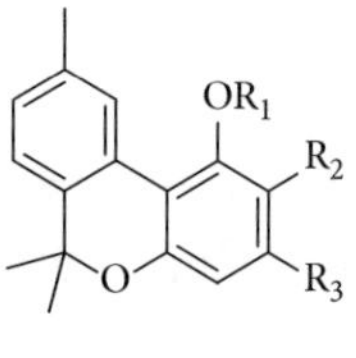

CBNA	(**65**) R$_1$ = H, R$_2$ = COOH, R$_3$ = C$_5$H$_{11}$
CBN-C$_3$	(**66**) R$_1$ = H, R$_2$ = H, R$_3$ = C$_3$H$_7$
cannabiorcol	(**67**) R$_1$ = H, R$_2$ = H, R$_3$ = CH$_3$
cannabinol methyl ether	(**68**) R$_1$ = CH$_3$, R$_2$ = H, R$_3$ = C$_5$H$_{11}$
CBN-C$_4$	(**69**) R$_1$ = H, R$_2$ = H, R$_3$ = C$_4$H$_9$
CBN-C$_2$	(**70**) R$_1$ = H, R$_2$ = H, R$_3$ = C$_2$H$_5$

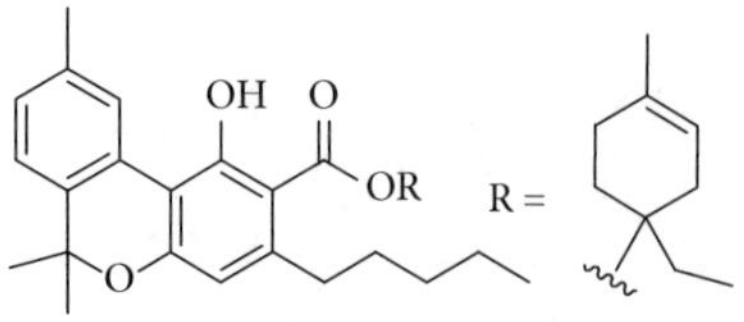

4-terpenyl cannabinolate (**71**)

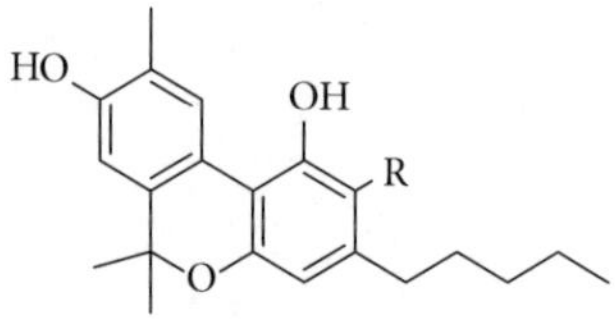

8-OH-CBN (**72**) R = H
8-OH-CBNA (**73**) R = COOH

Fig. 1.9 Cannabinol (CBN) type cannabinoids.

8-hydroxycannabinol (8-OH-CBN, *72*) and 8-hydroxy cannabinolic acid A (8-OH-CBNA, *73*) (Fig. 1.9) were isolated (Radwan et al. 2009). Compound 72, was isolated for the first time from a natural source using C_{18} solid phase extraction (SPE) although it was prepared earlier synthetically (Novak and Salemink 1983).

1.2.1.10 Cannabitriol (CBT) type

Obata and Ishikawa (1966) reported cannabitriol, but its chemical structure was elucidated by Chan et al. (1976) while its stereochemistry was determined by X-ray analysis (McPhail et al. 1984). A total of nine CBT-type cannabinoids, (−)-*trans*-cannabitriol ((−)-*trans*-CBT-C_5, *74*), (+)-*trans*-cannabitriol ((+)-*trans*-CBT-C_5, *75*), *cis*-cannabitriol ((±)-*cis*-CBT-C_5, *76*), (−)-*trans*-10-ethoxy-9-hydroxy-$\Delta^{6a(10a)}$-tetrahydrocannabinol ((−)-*trans*-CBT-OEt-C_5, *77*), *trans*-cannabitriol-C_3 ((±)-*trans*-CBT-C_3, *78*), CBT-C_3-homologue (*79*), *trans*-10-ethoxy-9-hydroxy-$\Delta^{6a(10a)}$-tetrahydrocannabivarin-C_3 ((−)-*trans*-CBT-OEt-C_3 80), 8,9-dihydroxy-$\Delta^{6a(10a)}$-tetrahydrocannabinol (8-OH-CBT-C_5, *81*), and cannabidiolic acid tetrahydrocannabitriol ester (CBDA-C_5 9-O-CBT-C_5 ester, *82*) (Fig. 1.10), were reported in cannabis (Ross and ElSohly 1995). Compounds 75 and 77 were isolated from an ethanolic extract of cannabis by ElSohly et al. in 1977. The ethanolic extract was chromatographed on silica gel 60 followed by TLC grade silica gel rechromatography. Chan et al. (1976) reported specific rotation of −107° for (−)-*trans*-CBT-C_5. (+)-*Trans*-CBT-C_5 had a rotation of +7° which indicated that the isolated (+)-*trans*-CBT-C_5 was a partially racemized mixture. Compounds 76 and 81 were obtained from a hexane extract of an Indian variant by silica gel chromatography (ElSohly et al. 1978). CBDA-C_5 9-O-CBT-C_5 ester (*82*) was isolated by Von Spulak et al. (1968) from a petroleum ether extract of hashish. As ethanol was used in the isolation of the two ethoxy cannabitriols (*77* and *80*), they are most likely artifacts (ElSohly et al. 1978; Harvey 1985), possibly resulting from the reaction of ethanol with the corresponding 9,10-epoxy-derivative.

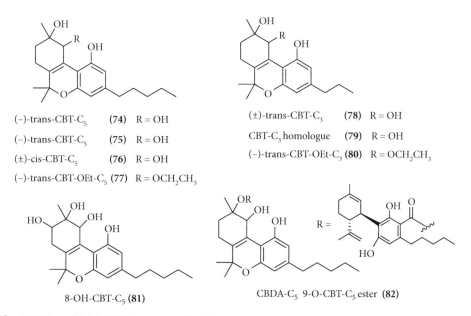

(−)-trans-CBT-C$_5$	**(74)**	R = OH
(−)-trans-CBT-C$_5$	**(75)**	R = OH
(±)-cis-CBT-C$_5$	**(76)**	R = OH
(−)-trans-CBT-OEt-C$_5$	**(77)**	R = OCH$_2$CH$_3$

(±)-trans-CBT-C$_3$	**(78)**	R = OH
CBT-C$_3$ homologue	**(79)**	R = OH
(−)-trans-CBT-OEt-C$_3$	**(80)**	R = OCH$_2$CH$_3$

8-OH-CBT-C$_5$ **(81)**

CBDA-C$_5$ 9-O-CBT-C$_5$ ester **(82)**

Fig. 1.10 Cannabitriol (CBT) type cannabinoids.

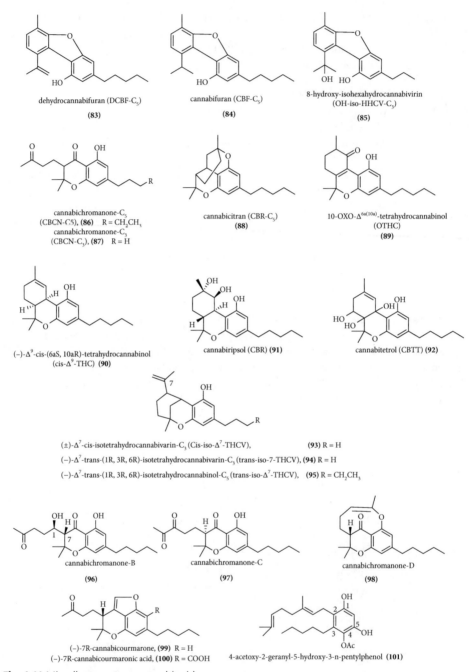

Fig. 1.11 Miscellaneous-type cannabinoids.

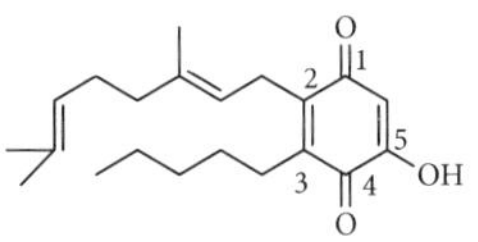

2-geranyl-5-hydroxy-3-n-pentyl-1,4-benzoquinone (**102**)

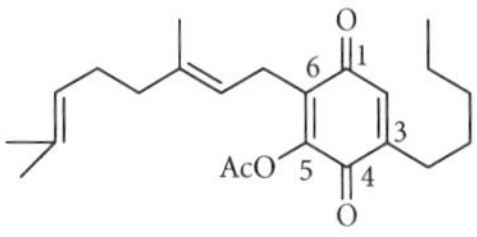

5-acetoxy-6-geranyl-3-n-pentyl-1,4-benzoquinone (**103**)

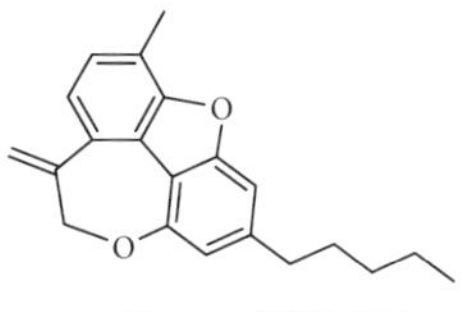

cannabioxepane (CBX) (**104**)

Fig. 1.11 (continued)

1.2.1.11 Miscellaneous-type cannabinoids

Miscellaneous-type cannabinoids discovered up to 2005 have been represented in a review by ElSohly and Slade (2005). These compounds are of diverse chemical structures. Fig. 1.11 shows the structure of these compounds as well as of additional compounds discovered after the ElSohly and Slade review (Ahmed et al. 2008b; Appendino et al. 2011; Pagani et al. 2011; Radwan et al. (2008b, 2009). Cannabichromanone-B (*96*), -C (*97*), and -D (*98*) were isolated by Ahmed et al. (2008b) from a high-potency cannabis variety, using C_{18} semipreparative HPLC. The absolute configuration was assigned on the basis of Mosher ester analysis and inspection of their circular dichroism spectra. (−)-7R-Cannabicoumarononic acid (*100*), 4-actoxy-2-geranyl-5-hydroxy-3-*n*-pentylphenol (*101*), and 2-geranyl-5-hydroxy-3-*n*-pentyl-1,4-benzoquinone (*102*) have been isolated from buds and leaves of the same variety of cannabis by application of several chromatographic techniques, including VLC over silica gel, solid phase extraction columns (C_{18} SPE) and NP HPLC (Radwan et al. 2009). The circular dichroism (CD) spectrum of 100 showed a positive cotton effect (CE) at 246 nm and negative CE at 295 nm, indicating a 7R absolute configuration. In addition, 5-acetoxy-6-geranyl-3-*n*-pentyl-1,4-benzoquinone (*103*) was isolated by employing silica gel column chromatography followed by NP HPLC (Radwan et al. 2008b). A tetracyclic cannabinoid (cannabioxepane, CBX, *104*) was recently isolated from *C. sativa*, variety carmagnole (Pagani et al. 2011).

1.2.2 Noncannabinoid constituents

Hundreds of noncannabinoid constituents belonging to a highly diverse chemical class have been identified in/isolated from cannabis (ElSohly and Slade 2005; Ross and ElSohly 1995; Turner et al. 1980). Twenty-two noncannabinoids (*105–126*) belonging to eight different chemical classes have been reported since 2005. These new constituents and their chemical classes are described in the following sections (sections 1.2.2.1–1.2.2.8).

1.2.2.1 Flavonoids

Since 2005, a total of four new flavonoids (*105–108*) have been reported (Fig. 1.12). Radwan et al. (2008b) isolated canflavin C (*105*), chrysoeriol (*106*), and 6-prenylapigenin (*107*) from a high-potency variety of cannabis using combinations of NP and RP chromatography. The flavonoid glycoside apigenin-6,8-di-C-β-D-glucopyranoside (*108*) was isolated from the *n*-butanol fraction of the methanol extract of hemp leaves and branches (Cheng et al. 2008).

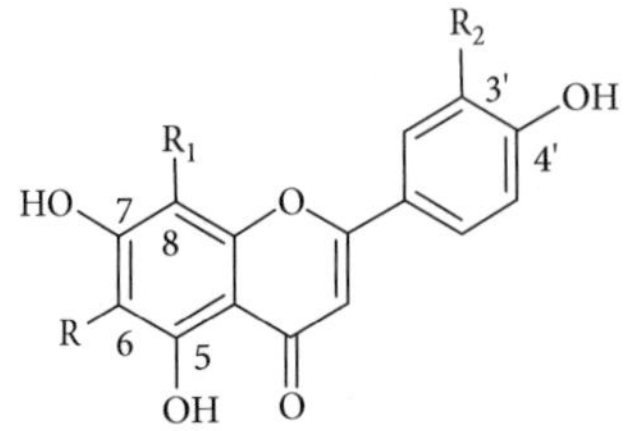

canflavin C   (**105**) R= H, R1= $\sim\sim$ R_2 = OMe

chrysoeriol   (**106**) R= R1 = H, R_2 = OMe

6-prenylapigenin (**107**) R= $\sim$ $R_1 = R_2 = H$

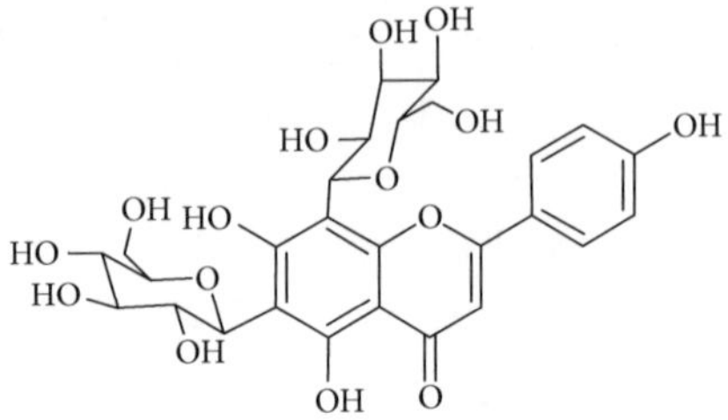

apigenin-6,8-di-C-β-D-glucopyranoside (**108**)

Fig. 1.12 Flavonoids.

1.2.2.2 Steroids

A total of four new steroids (*109–112*) have been reported since 2005 (Fig. 1.13). β-sitosteryl-3-O-β-D-glucopyranoside-2′-O-palmitate (*109*) was isolated from a high-potency variety of cannabis (Radwan et al. 2008b) using NP and RP chromatographic techniques. Cheng et al. (2008) isolated acetyl stigmasterol (*110*) and α-spinosterol (*111*) from the petroleum ether fraction of the methanol extract of the leaves and branches of hemp, while daucosterol (*112*) was isolated from the fruits of cannabis (Qian et al. 2009). Purification of the latter was carried out using silica gel column and Sephadex® LH-20 chromatography.

1.2.2.3 Phenanthrenes

Four phenanthrene derivatives (*113–116*) have been reported since 2005 (Fig. 1.14). Radwan et al. (2008b) isolated 4,5-dihydroxy-2,3,6-trimethoxy-9,10-dihydrophenanthrene (*113*), 4-hydroxy-2,3,6,7-tetramethoxy-9,10-dihydrophenanthrene (*114*) and 4,7-dimethoxy-1,2,5-trihydroxyphenanthrene (*115*) from the ethanolic extract of a high-potency cannabis variety

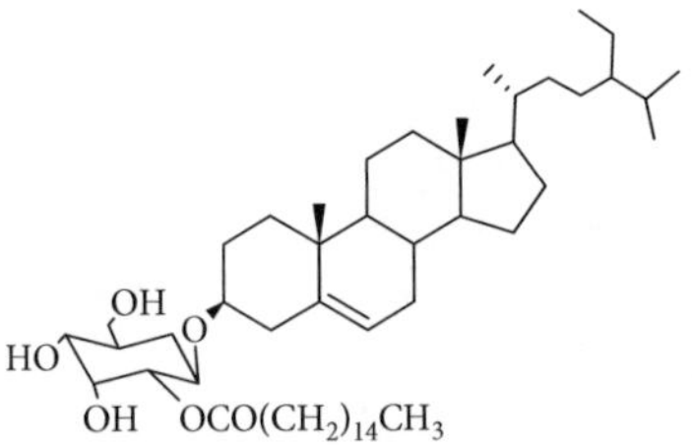

β-sitosteryl-3-O-β-D-glucopyranoside-2′-O-palamite (**109**)

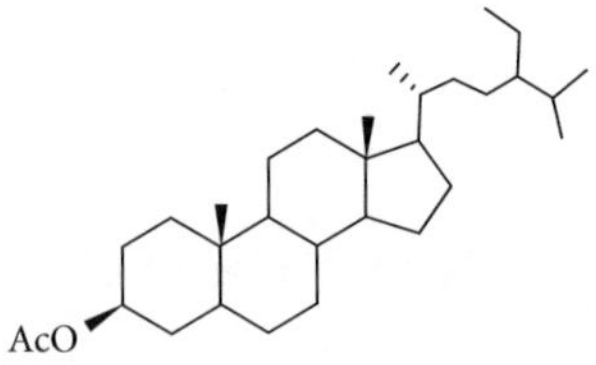

acetyl stigmasterol (**110**)

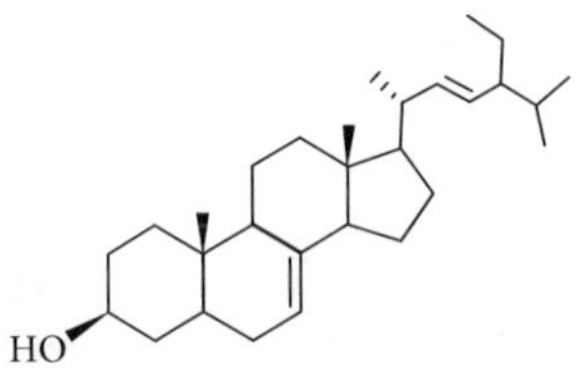

α-spinasterol (**111**)

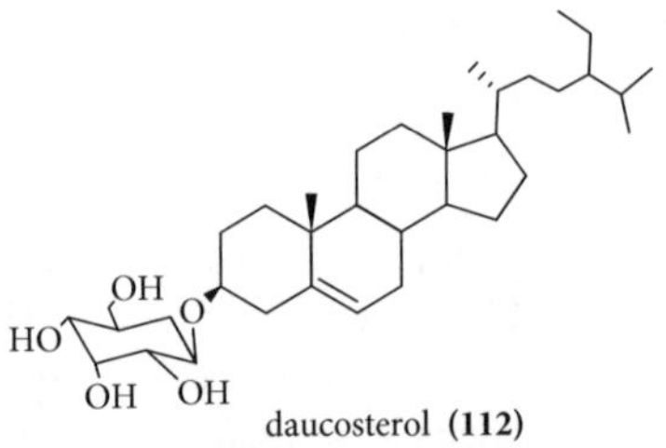

daucosterol (**112**)

Fig. 1.13 Steroids.

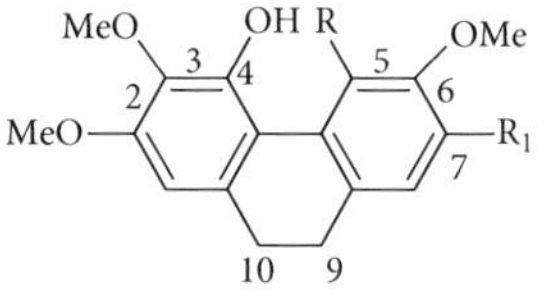

4,5-dihydroxy-2,3,6-trimethoxy-
9,10-dihydroxy-phenanthrene   **(113)** R=OH, R₁=H

4-hydroxy-2,3,6,7-tetramethoxy-
9,10-dihydrophenanthrene   **(114)** R=H, R₁=OMe

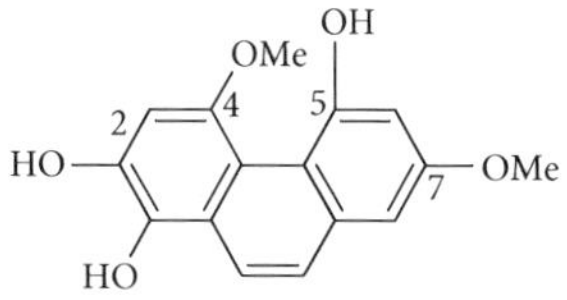

4,7-dimethoxy-1,2,5-trihydroxyphenanthrene **(115)**

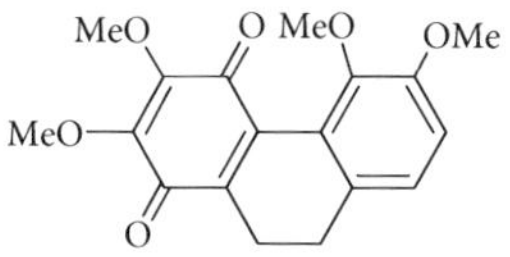

9,10-dihydro-2,3,5,6-tetramethoxyphenanthrene-1,4-dione **(116)**

Fig. 1.14 Phenanthrenes.

using combination of NP and RP chromatographic techniques. On the other hand, Cheng et al. (2010) isolated 9,10-dihydro-2,3,5,6-tetramethoxyphenanthrene-1,4-dione (*116*) from the leaves and branches of *C. sativa* L. by silica gel and Sephadex® LH-20 chromatography, followed by semi-preparative liquid chromatography.

1.2.2.4 Fatty acids

Four fatty acids were reported in cannabis since 2005 (*117–120*) (Fig. 1.15). Docosanoic acid methyl ester (*117*) was isolated from the petroleum ether fraction of the methanol extract of hemp leaves and branches (Cheng et al. 2008) and isoselachoceric acid (*118*) was isolated from the fruits of cannabis and purified by silica gel chromatography (Qian et al. 2009). In addition, two polyun-saturated hydroxyl-C18 fatty acids (*119–120*) were reported from a fiber cultivar of cannabis (vari-ety carmagnola) and purified by RP C$_{18}$ flash chromatography and NP HPLC (Pagani et al. 2011).

1.2.2.5 Spiroindans

Two spiroindans (*121, 122*) were isolated since 2005 (Fig. 1.16). Radwan et al. (2008a) isolated 7-methoxy-cannabispirone from the extract of a high-potency cannabis variety using NP chro-matography followed by C$_{18}$ HPLC, while Pagani (2011) isolated isocannabispiradienone (*122*) from the extract of a fiber cultivar.

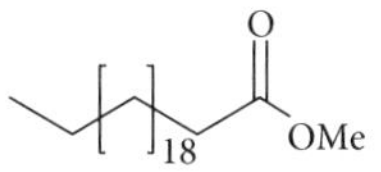

docosanoic acid methyl ester **(117)**

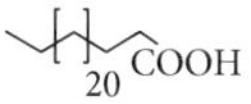

isoselachoceric acid **(118)**

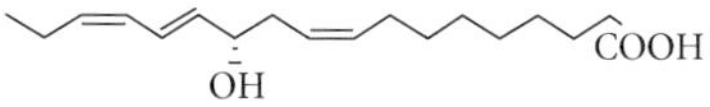

polyunsaturated hydroxy fatty acid **(119)**

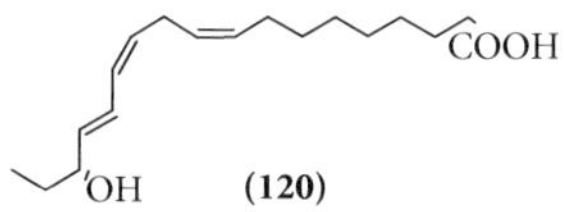

polyunsaturated hydroxy fatty acid **(120)**

Fig. 1.15 Fatty acids.

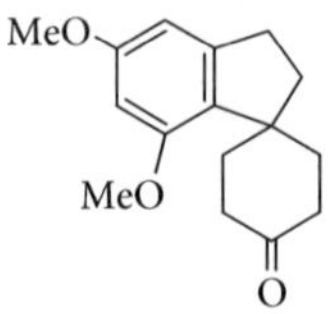

Fig. 1.16 Spiroindans.　　7-methoxy-cannabispirone **(121)** 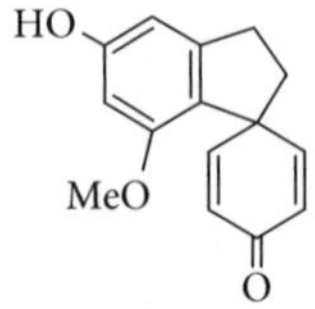　　Isocannabispiradienone **(122)**

1.2.2.6 Nitrogenous compounds

The two nitrogenous compounds isolated from cannabis since 2005 are uracil (*123*) and cannabsin (*124*) (Fig. 1.17). Uracil (*123*) was isolated from the *n*-butanol fraction of the methanolic extract of hemp leaves and branches (Cheng et al. 2008), while cannabsin (*124*) was isolated from the fruits of *C. sativa* and purified by silica gel column and Sephadex® LH-20 chromatography (Qian et al. 2009).

1.2.2.7 Xanthones

Only one xanthone derivative, 1,3,6,7-tetrahydroxy-2-C-β-D-gluco-pyranosylxanthone (*125*), was reported since 2005 (Fig. 1.18). The compound was isolated from the *n*-butanol fraction of a methanolic extract of hemp leaves and branches (Cheng et al. 2008).

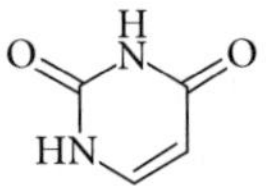

uracil **(123)**

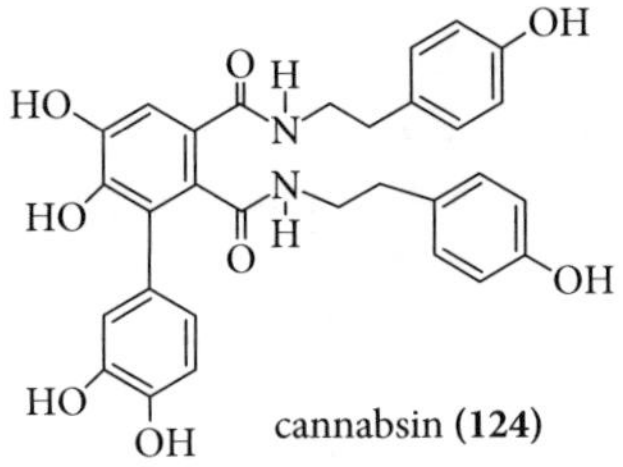

cannabsin **(124)**

Fig. 1.17 Nitrogenous compounds.

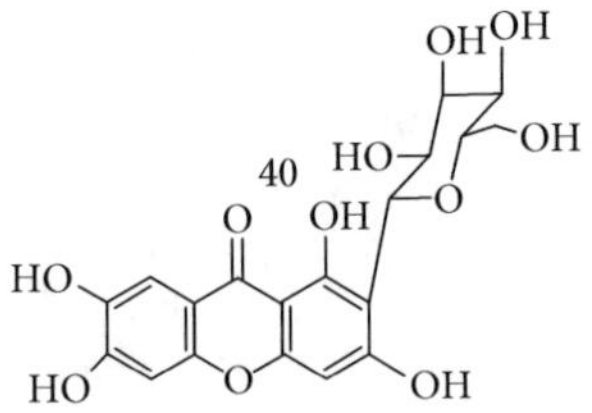

1,3,6,7-tetrahydroxy-2-C-β-D-glucopyranosyl xanthone
(125)

Fig. 1.18 Xanthones.

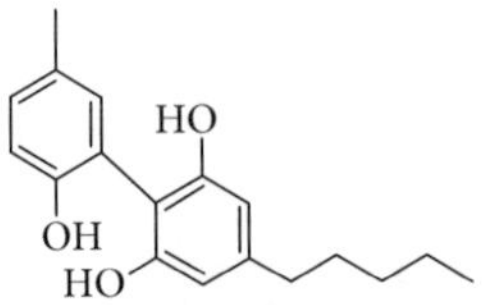

5'-methyl-4-pentylbiphenyl-2,6,2'-triol
(126)

Fig. 1.19 Biphenyls.

1.2.2.8 Biphenyls

The only biphenyl derivative reported in cannabis since 2005 is 5′-methyl-4-pentyl-2,6,2′-trihydroxybiphenyl (*126*) (Fig. 1.19), which was isolated from a high-potency cannabis variety and purified by a combination of NP chromatography and C_{18} HPLC (Radwan et al. 2008a).

Acknowledgments

Author's contribution to the Work was done as part of the Author's official duties as an NIH employee and is a Work of the United States Government. Therefore, copyright may not be established in the United States. The authors are indebted to Ms. Candice Tolbert for her technical assistance in the production of this chapter.

References

Abrams, D.I., Jay, C.A., Shade, S.B., *et al.* (2007). Cannabis in painful HIV-associated sensory neuropathy: a randomized placebo-controlled trial. *Neurology*, **68**, 515–521.

Adams, R., Baker, B.R., and Wearn, R.B. (1940b). Structure of cannabinol III. Synthesis of cannabinol, 1-hydroxy-3-n-amyl-6,6,9-trimethyl-6-dibenzopyran. *Journal of the American Chemical Society*, **62**, 2204–2207.

Adams, R., Hunt, M., and Clark, J.H. (1940a). Structure of cannabidiol, a product isolated from the marihuana extract of Minnesota wild hemp. I. *Journal of the American Chemical Society*, **62**, 196–200.

Ahmed, S.A., Ross, S.A., Slade, D., *et al.* (2008a). Cannabinoid ester constituents from high-potency *Cannabis sativa. Journal of Natural Products*, **71**, 536–542.

Ahmed, S.A., Ross, S.A., Slade, D., *et al.* (2008b). Structure determination and absolute configuration of cannabichromanone derivatives from high potency *Cannabis sativa. Tetrahedron Letters*, **49**, 6050–6053.

Appendino, G., Chianese, G., and Taglialatela-Scafati, O. (2011). Cannabinoids: occurrence and medicinal chemistry. *Current Medicinal Chemistry*, **18**, 1085–1099.

Appendino, G., Giana, A., Gibbons, S., *et al.* (2008). A polar cannabinoid from *Cannabis sativa* var. Carma. *Natural Product Communications*, **12**, 1977–1980.

Archer, R.A., Boyd, D.B., Demarco, P.V., Tyminski, I.J., and Allinger, N.L. (1970). Structural studies of cannabinoids. A theoretical and proton magnetic resource analysis. *Journal of the American Chemical Society*, **92**, 5200–5206.

Bercht, C.A.L., Lousberg, R.J.J.CH., Küppers, F.J.E.M., *et al.* (1973). Cannabis. VII. Identification of cannabinol methyl ether from hashish. *Journal of Chromatography*, **81**, 163–166.

Chan, W.R., Magnus, K.E., and Watson, H.A. (1976). The structure of cannabitriol. *Experientia* **32**, 283–284.

Cheng, L., Kong, D., and Hu, G. (2008). Study on hemp I. Chemical constituents from petroleum ether and *n*-butanol portions of the methanol extract. *Chinese Journal of Pharmaceutics*, **39**, 18–21.

Cheng, L., Kong, D., Hu, G., and Li, H. (2010). A new 9,10-dihydrophenanthrenedione from *Cannabis sativa. Chemistry of Natural Compounds*, **46**, 710–712.

Claussen, U., Von Spulak, F., and Korte, F. (1966). The chemical classification of plants –XXXI, Hashish-10. Cannabichromene, a new Hashish component. *Tetrahedron*, **22**, 1477–1479.

Claussen, U., Von Spulak, F., and Korte, F. (1968). Hashish. XIV. Components of hashish. *Tetrahedron* **24**, 1021–1023.

ElSohly, M.A., Boerenm, E.G., and Turner, C.E. (1978). (±)-9,10-Dihydroxy-$\Delta^{6a(10a)}$-tetrahydrocannabinol and (±)-8,9-dihydroxy-$\Delta^{6a(10a)}$-tetrahydrocannabinol: 2 new cannabinoids from *Cannabis sativa* L. *Experientia* **34**, 1127–1128.

ElSohly, M.A., El-Feraly, F.S., and Turner, C.E. (1977). Isolation and characterization of (−)-cannabitrol and (−)-10-ethoxy-9-hydroxy-$\Delta^{6a(10a)}$-tetrahydrocannabinol: two new cannabinoids form *Cannabis sativa* L. extract. *Lloydia*, **40**, 275–280.

ElSohly, M.A. and Slade, D. (2005). Chemical constituents of marijuana: the complex mixture of natural cannabinoids. *Life Sciences*, **78**, 539–548.

Farnsworth, N.R. (1969). Pharmacognosy and chemistry of *Cannabis sativa*. *Journal of American Pharmacists Association*, **N59**, 410.

Fetterman, P.S. and Turner, C.E. (1972). Constituents of *Cannabis sativa* L. I: propyl homologs of cannabinoids from an Indian variant. *Journal of Pharmaceutical Sciences*, **61**, 1476–1477.

Gaoni, Y. and Mechoulam, R. (1964a). Hashish. III. Isolation, structure, and partial synthesis of an active constituent of hashish. *Journal of the American Chemical Society*, **86**, 1646–1647.

Gaoni, Y. and Mechoulam, R. (1964b). Structure and synthesis of cannabigerol, a new hashish constituent. *Proceedings of the Chemical Society*, 82.

Gaoni, Y. and Mechoulam, R. (1966). Cannabichromene, a new active principle in hashish. *Chemical Communications*, **1**, 20–21.

Gill, E.W. (1971). Propyl homologue of terahydrocannabinol: its isolation from cannabis, properties, and synthesis. *Journal of the Chemical Society* C, 579–582.

Guindon, J. and Hohmann, A.G. (2009). The endocannabinoid system and pain. *CNS & Neurological Disorders: Drug Targets*, **8**, 403–421.

Hanuš, L. and Krejčí, Z. (1975). Isolation of two new cannabinoid acids from *Cannabis sativa* L. of Czechoslovakia origin. *Acta Universitatis Palackianae Olomucensis Facultatis Medicae*, **74**, 161.

Harvey, D.J. (1976). Characterization of the butyl homologues of Δ^1-tetrahydrocannabinol, cannabinol, and cannabidiol in samples of *Cannabis* by combined gas chromatography and mass spectrometry. *Journal of Pharmacy and Pharmacology*, **28**, 280–285.

Harvey, D.J. (1985). Examination of a 140 year old ethanolic extract of *Cannabis*: identification of new cannabitriol homologues and the ethyl homologue of cannabinol. In: D.J. Harvey, W. Paton, and G.G. Hahas (eds.). *Marihuana '84: Proceedings of the Oxford symposium on Cannabis: 9th International Congress of Pharmacology, 3rd Satellite Symposium on Cannabis*. Washington, DC: IRL, pp. 23–30.

Hively, R.L., Mosher, W.A., and Hoffman, F.W. (1966). Isolation of *trans*-Δ^6-tetrahydrocannabinol from marijuana. *Journal of the American Chemical Society*, **8**, 1832–1833.

Jarvinen, T., Pate, D.W., and Laine, K. (2002). Cannabinoids in the treatment of glaucoma *Pharmacology and Therapeutics*, **95**, 203–220.

Korte, F., Haag, M., and Claussen, U. (1965a). Tetrahydrocannabinolcarboxylic acid, a component of hashish. *Angewandte Chemie*, **77**, 862–867.

Korte, F. and Sieper, H. (1964). Chemical classification of plants. XXIV. Hashish constituents by thin-layer chromatography. *Journal of Chromatography*, **13**, 90–98.

Korte, F., Sieper, H., and Tira, S. (1965b). New results on hashish-specific constituents. *Bulletin on Narcotics*, **17**, 35.

Krejčí, Z. and Šantavý, F. (1955). The isolation of further substances from the leaves of Indian hemp (*Cannabis sativa* L., var. indica). *Acta Universitatis Palackianae Olomucensis, Faculty of Medicine*, **6**, 59–66.

Kriese, U., Schumann, E., Weber, W.E., *et al.* (2004). Oil content, tocopherol composition and fatty acid patterns of the seeds of 51 *C. sativa* L. genotypes. *Euphytica*, **137**, 339–351.

Liang, Y.C., Huang, C.C., and Hsu, K.S. (2004). Therapeutic potential of cannabinoids in trigeminal neuralgia. *Current Drug Targets: CNS & Neurological Disorders*, **3**, 507–514.

Lousberg, R.J.J.C., Bercht, C.A.L., van Ooyen, R., and Spronck, H.J.W. (1977). Cannabinodiol: conclusive identification and synthesis of a new cannabinoid from *Cannabis sativa*. *Phytochemistry*, **16**, 595–597.

McPhail, A.T., ElSohly, H.N., Turner, C.E., and ElSohly, M.A. (1984). Stereochemical assignments for the two enantiomeric pairs of 9,10-dihydroxy-$\Delta^{6a(10a)}$-tetrahydrocannabinols. X-ray crystal structure analysis of (±)-*trans*-cannabitriol. *Journal of Natural Products*, **47**, 138–142.

Mechoulam, R., Ben-Zvi, Z., Yagnitinsky, B., and Shani, A. (1969). A new tetrahydrocannabinolic acid. *Tetrahedron Letters*, **28**, 2339–2341.

Mechoulam, R. and Gaoni, Y. (1965). The isolation and structure of cannabinolic, cannabidiolic and cannabigerolic acids. *Tetrahedron*, **21**, 1223–1229.

Mechoulam, R. and Gaoni, Y. (1967). Recent advances in the chemistry of hashish. *Fortschritte der Chemie Organischer Naturstoffe*, **25**, 175–213.

Mechoulam, R. and Yagen, Y. (1969). Stereoselective cyclizations of cannabinoid 1,5 dienes. *Tetrahedron Letters*, **10**, 5349–5352.

Merkus, F.W.H.M. (1971a). Cannabivarin, een nieuw bestanddeel van haschisch. *Pharmaceutisch weekblad. Scientific edition*, **106**, 69.

Merkus, F.W.H.M. (1971b). Cannabivarin and tetrahydrocannabivarin, two new constituents of hashish. *Nature*, **232**, 579–580.

Merlin, M.D. (2003). Archaeological evidence for the tradition of psychoactive plant use in the old world. *Economic Botany*, **57**, 295–323.

Morita, M. and Ando, H. (1984). Analysis of hashish oil by gas chromatography/mass spectrometry. *Kagaku Keisatsu Kenkyujo Hokoku. Hokagaku-Hen*, **37**(2), 137–140.

Novak, J. and Salemink, C.A. (1983). Cannabis. XXVII: Synthesis of 8-, 10-, and 11-oxygenated cannabinols. *Journal of the Chemical Society, Perkin Trans*, **12**, 2867–2871.

Obata, Y. and Ishikawa, Y. (1966). Constituents of hemp plant (*Cannabis sativa*). III. Isolation of a Gibbs-positive compound from Japanese hemp. *Agricultural and Biological Chemistry*, **30**, 619–620.

Pagani, A., Scala, F., Chianese, G., *et al.* (2011). Cannabioxepane, a novel tetracyclic cannabinoid from hemp, *Cannabis sativa* L. *Tetrahedron*, **67**, 3369–3373.

Petrzilka, T., Haefliger, W., and Sikemeier, C. (1969). Synthesis of hashish components. IV. *Helvetica Chimica Acta*, **52**, 1102–1134.

Pollastro, F., Taglialatela-Scafati, O., Allarà, M., *et al.* (2011). Bioactive prenylogous cannabinoid from fiber hemp (*Cannabis sativa*). *Journal of Natural Products*, **74**, 2019–2022.

Pryce, G. and Baker, D. (2005). Emerging properties of cannabinoid medicines in management of multiple sclerosis. *Trends in Neuroscience*, **28**, 272–276.

Qian, S., Cai, G.-M., He, G.-X., and Du, F.L. (2009). Study of the chemical constituents of the fruits of *C. sativa* L. *Natural Product Research and Development*, **21**, 784–786.

Radwan, M.M., ElSohly, M.A., Slade, D., *et al.* (2008b). Non-cannabinoid constituents from a high potency *Cannabis sativa* variety. *Phytochemistry*, **69**, 2627–2633.

Radwan, M.M., ElSohly, M.A., Slade, D., Ahmed, S.A., Ross, S.A. (2009). Biologically active cannabinoids from high potency *Cannabis sativa*. *Journal of Natural Products*, **72**, 906–911.

Radwan, M.M., Ross, S.A., Slade, D., *et al.* (2008a). Isolation and characterization of new cannabis constituents from a high potency variety. *Planta Medica*, **74**, 267–272.

Rosenqvist, E. and Ottersen, T. (1975). The crystal and molecular structure of Δ^9-tetrahydrocannabinol acid B. *Acta Chemica Scandinavia B*, **29**(3), 379–384.

Ross, S.A. and ElSohly, M.A. (1995). Constituents of *Cannabis sativa* L. XXVIII. A review of the natural constituents: 1980–1994. *Zagazig Journal of Pharmaceutical Science*, **4**, 1–10.

Schultz, O.E. and Haffner, G. (1960). *Archives of Pharmaceutical Research*, **293**, 1.

Shani, A. and Mechoulam, R. (1974). Cannabielsoic acids. Isolation and synthesis by a novel oxidative cyclization. *Tetrahedron*, **30**, 2437–2446.

Shoyama, Y., Fujita, T., Yamauchi, T., and Nishioka, I. (1968). Cannabichromenic acid, a genuine substance of cannabichromene. *Chemical and Pharmaceutical Bulletin*, **10**(6), 1157–1158.

Shoyama, Y., Kuboe, K., Nishioka, I., and Yamauchi, T. (1972a). Cannabidiol monomethyl ether. A new neutral cannabinoid. *Chemical and Pharmaceutical Bulletin*, **20**(9), 2072.

Shoyama, Y., Oku, R., Yamauchi, T., and Nishioka, I. (1972b). Cannabis. VI. Cannabicyclolic acid. *Chemical and Pharmaceutical Bulletin*, **20**, 1927–1930.

Shoyama, Y., Hirano, H., Makino, H., Umekita, N., and Nishioka, I. (1977). Cannabis. X. The isolation and structures of four new propyl cannabinoid acids, terahydrocannabivarinic acid, cannabidivarinic acid, cannabichromevarinic acid and cannabigerovarinic acid from Thai cannabis, 'Meao Variant'. *Chemical and Pharmaceutical Bulletin*, **26**(9), 2306–2311.

Shoyama, Y., Hirano, H., Oda, M., Somehara, T., and Nishioka, I. (1975). Cannabichromevarin and cannabigerovarin, two new propyl homologues of cannabichromene and cannabigerol. *Chemical and Pharmaceutical Bulletin*, **23**(8), 1894–1895.

Shoyama, Y., Morimoto, S., and Nishioka, I. (1981). Cannabis. XIV. Two new propyl cannabinoids, cannabicyclovarin and Δ^7-*cis*-*iso*-tetrahydrocannabivarin, from Thai cannabis. *Chemical and Pharmaceutical Bulletin*, **29**, 3720–3723.

Shoyama, Y., Yamauchi, T., and Nishioka, I. (1970). Cannabis. V. Cannabigerolic acid monomethyl ether and cannabinolic acid. *Chemical and Pharmaceutical Bulletin*, **18**, 1327–1332.

Slatkin, N.E. (2007). Cannabinoids in the treatment of chemotherapy-induced nausea and vomiting: beyond prevention of acute emesis. *Journal of Supportive Oncology*, **5**, 1–9.

Small, E. and Marcus, D. (2002). Hemp: a new crop with new uses for North America. In: J. Janick and A. Whipkey (eds.). *Trends in New Crops and New Uses*. Alexandria, VA: ASHS, pp. 284–326.

Taglialatela-Scafati, O., Pagani, A., Scala, F., *et al.* (2010). Cannabimovione, a cannabinoid with a rear-ranged terpenoid skeleton from Hemp. *European Journal of Organic Chemistry*, **11**, 2067.

Taura, F., Morimoto, S., and Shoyama, Y. (1995). Cannabinerolic acid, a cannabinoid from *Cannabis sativa*. *Phytochemistry*, **39**(2), 457–458.

Turner, C.E., ElSohly, M.A., and Boeren, E.G. (1980). Constituents of *Cannabis sativa* L. XVII. A review of the natural constituents. *Journal of Natural Products*, **43**, 169–234.

Turner, C.E., Hadley, K., and Fetterman, P.S. (1973). Constituents of *Cannabis sativa* L. VI: propyl homologs in samples of known geographical origin. *Journal of Pharmaceutical Sciences*, **62**, 1739–1741.

Uliss, D.B., Razdan, R.K., and Dalzell, H.C. (1974). Stereospecific intramolecular epoxide cleavage by phe-nolate anion. Synthesis of novel and biologically active cannabinoids. *Journal of the American Chemical Society*, **96** (23), 7372–7374.

Viveros, M.P. and Marco, E.M. (2007). Cannabinoids, anxiety and depression. In: J.N. Govil, V.K. Singh, and N.T. Siddqui (eds.). *Natural Products II*. **Vol. 18**. New York: Studium Press, LLC, pp. 227–249.

Vollner, L., Bieniek, D., and Korte, F. (1969). Haschisch XX. Cannabidivarin, ein neuer Haschisch-inhaltsstoff. *Tetrahedron Letters*, **3**, 145–147.

Von Spulak, F., Claussen, U., Fehlhaber, H.W., and Korte, F. (1968). Haschisch-XIX. Cannabidiol carbonsaure-tetrahydrocannabitrol-ester ein neuer haschisch-inhaltsstoff. *Tetrahedron*, **24**, 5379–5383.

Vree, T.B., Breimer, D.D., Van Ginneken, C.A.M., and Van Rossum, J.M. (1972a). Identification in hash-ish of tetrahydrocannabinol, cannabidiol and cannabinol analogues with a methyl side-chain. *Journal of Pharmacy and Pharmacology*, **24**, 7–12.

Vree, T.B., Breimer, D.D., van Ginneken, C.A.M., and van Rossum, J.M. (1972b). Identification of can-nabicyclol with a pentyl or propyl side chain by means of combined gas chromatography-mass spec-trometry. *Journal of Chromatography*, **74**, 124–127.

Wood, T.B., Spivey, W.T., and Easterfield, T.H. (1896). XL-*Charas*. The resin of Indian hemp. *Journal of the Chemical Society*, **69**, 539–546.

Wood, T.B., Spivey, W.T., and Easterfield, T.H. (1899). III-Cannabinol. Part I. *Journal of the Chemical Society*, **75**, 20–36.

Yamauchi, T., Shoyama, Y., Matsuo, Y., and Nishioka, I. (1968) Cannabigerol monomethyl ether, a new component of hemp. *Chemical and Pharmaceutical Bulletin*, **16**(6), 1164–1165.

Yamamoto, I., Gohda, H., Narimatsu, S., Watanabe, K., and Yoshimura, H. (1991). Cannabielsoin as a new metabolite of cannabidiol in mammals. *Pharmacology Biochemistry and Behavior*, **40**, 541–546.

Zulfiqar, F., Ross, S.A., and Slade, D., *et al.* (2012). Cannabisol, a novel Δ^9-THC dimer possessing a unique methylene bridge, isolated from *Cannabis sativa*. *Tetrahedron Letters*, **53**, 3560–3562.

Chapter 2

The Pharmacological History of Cannabis

Ethan B. Russo

2.1 Introduction

The circumstances whereby cannabis was first used medicinally are lost in time and mystery. More than likely, it happened at many times and in many places with rediscoveries figuring prominently alongside the landscape of human peregrinations and conquests in a rapidly changing mosaic of Eurasian languages and cultures, a process this author has termed "cannabis interruptus" (Russo 2001b, 2004a, 2007). As a ubiquitous "camp follower," cannabis accompanied the early nomads around the Old World for millennia, as they deciphered that certain plants were better for fiber, others for edible seed, while certain chemovars were pharmacologically superior. Rarely does a triple-purpose plant appear in nature, such as that discovered in Nepal (Clarke 2007).

The breadth of cannabis history does not lend itself to comprehensive treatment in a brief chapter. Rather, this effort will focus on a chronology (Table 2.1), followed by some possible new therapeutic directions.

2.2 Pharmacology of cannabis chronology

Table 2.1 Cannabis chronology

2700 BCE	Oral tradition in *Shen Nong Ben Cao Jing* notes hallucinatory effects, appetite stimulation, tonic and antisenility effects	Shou-Zhong 1997
c. 2000 BCE	Cannabis seeds in Margiana, Proto-Zoroastrian site, part of religious rites	Sarianidi 1998
c. 1800 BCE	30 citations from Ancient Sumeria and Akkadia for grief, epilepsy, neuralgia, and pediculocide	Babylon and Thompson 1903; Russo 2007; Thompson 1924; 1949
1534 BCE	*Ebers Papyrus*, Egypt, for vaginal contractions, ophthalmological conditions, etc.	Manniche 1989; Russo 2007
c. 1500 BCE	*Atharva Veda* notes *bhanga* to "release us from anxiety"	Grierson 1894; Indian Hemp Drugs Commission 1894; Russo 2005
c. 750 BCE	*Kaneh bosem* (aromatic cane) part of holy anointing oil of Hebrews (*Exodus* 30:22-25)	Alter 2004; Russo 2007

Table 2.1 (continued) Cannabis chronology

700 BCE	Cannabis cache from Yanghai Tombs,Xinjiang; biochemical and genomic analysis demonstrate THC chemotype	Jiang et al. 2006; Russo et al. 2008
c.600 BCE	Persia: *Avesta* notes ritual use, and in combination to produce miscarriage	Darmesteter 1895
450 BCE	Intoxication in Central Asian funerary rites, subsequently documented in frozen tombs in Siberia	Artamonov 1965; Herodotus 1998; Rudenko 1970; Russo 2007
c.214 BCE	*Erh-Ya*, China describes dioecious status, superiority of males for fiber, females for intoxication	Carr 1979; Russo 2007
First century CE	"The juice extracted from it when green and instilled is appropriate for earaches"	Dioscorides and Beck 2011 (p. 248)
First century CE	Pliny the Elder notes *gelotophyllis* ("Leaves of laughter" from Bactria) producing hallucinations; also hemp infusion for looseness in beasts of burden, root for joint contractures and gout, herb for burns	Pliny 1951 (Book XX, Ch. 98, p. 298), 1980 (Book XXIV, Ch. 164, p. 117); Russo 2007
Second century CE	Galen notes leaves for flatus and seed juice for otalgia, chronic pain	Brunner 1973; Butrica 2002; Sethi 1868
Second century CE	Hua-Tho in China notes use in wine as surgical anesthetic/analgesic	Julien 1849
Late second century CE	Egyptian *Fayyum Medical Book* for tumors	Reymond 1976; Russo 2007
c.350 CE	Carbonized cannabis found in Israeli cave by remains of woman dying in childbirth	Zias 1995; Zias et al. 1993
c.550 CE	*The Syriac Book of Medicines*, for excess spittle, hemp plug for anal fissures	Budge 1913
570	Taoist incense	Needham and Gwei-Djen 1974
Eighth century	Psychoactivity noted, Jabir ibn Hayyan in Persia/Iraq	Lewis et al. 1971
c.850	In Persia, ibn Sahl uses compound medicine with flower juice intranasally for migraine, uterine pains to prevent miscarriage	Kahl 1994; Russo 2001b, 2002
875	In Iraq, muscle relaxant	Al-Kindi and Levey 1966; Russo 2007
Ninth century	*The Old English Herbarium* recommends pounded hemp or its sap for wounds, and for "pain of the innards"	Pollington 2000 (p. 301)
Ninth century	Ibn al-Baytar, Egypt, vermicidal, for neuralgia	Lozano 2001
c.900	Al-Razi, Persia, to stimulate hair growth	Lozano 2001
Tenth century	Hemp part of "holy salve" in Anglo-Saxon *Lacnunga*	Grattan and Singer 1952 (p. 123)
c.1000	al-Mayusi first mention in epilepsy, leaf juice intanasally	Al-Mayusi 1877; Lozano 2001

Table 2.1 (continued) Cannabis chronology

Eleventh century	Roots for fever, tumors, herb juice for ears, and leaves for dandruff	Ibn Sina (Avicenna), 1294
Eleventh century	*Olde English Herbarium*, hemp and fat applied to breast to disperse swelling and purge diseased matter; herb when drunk to relieve pain of the innards	Vriend 1984
Twelfth century	In Spain, Sheshet Benveniste recommends *theriaca* with cannabis as tonic, curing sterility, repairing the womb, stomach and head	Barkai 1998
1158	Hildegard von Bingen, for headache, stomach slime, and compress for sores, wounds	Fankhauser 2002; Hildegard and Throop 1998
1200	*Anandakanda*, India, increasing longevity	Russo 2005
Thirteenth century	Italy, *Codex Vindobonensis 93*, ointment for breast swelling, pain	Russo 2002; Zotter 1996
Thirteenth century	ibn Rasul, headache and ear pains	Lewis et al. 1971
1542	Latin binomial: *Cannabis sativa*; root boiled for gout, raw for burns, wild hemp boiled, wrapped for tumors	Fuchs 1999
1546	Boiled root for sore muscles, stiff joints, gout, rheumatism, herb juice for colicky horses, raw on burns	Rabelais 1990
1563	Indian hemp engenders laughter, allays anxiety, increases appetite, improves work	Da Orta 1913
1570	Feckenham cites "hemmp" as part of honey/wine mixture for wounds, fistulae	Macgill 1990
1596	Li Shi-Chen: flowers for menstrual disorders, root juice for retained placenta, post-partum hemorrhage	Stuart 1928; Russo 2002
1597	Hemp for jaundice and colic	Gerard and Johnson 1975; Crawford 2002
Seventeenth century	In Far East, benefits on mood, gonorrhea, pleurisy, hernia	Rumpf and Beekman 1981
1621	Indian hemp produces ecstasy, laughter	Burton 1907
Eighteenth century	In India, *Makhzan al-adwiya*, leaf snuff for "deterging the brain," to remove dandruff and vermin, treat diarrhea, gonorrhea, powder for wounds, sores, herb to prolong life	Russo 2005
1712	Psychotropic effects in Persia, India	Kaempfer 1996
1751	*Medicina Britannica*, hemp precipitates menses, "against Pissing the Bed"	Short 1751 (p. 138)
1772	Linneaus summarizes cannabis: "narcotica, phantastica, dementans, repellens"	Linné 1772
1784	In Scotland, hemp oil for urinary burning, incontinence and "restraining venereal appetites"	Lewis 1794

Table 2.1 (continued) Cannabis chronology

1830	Extract in wine for nervousness	Nees Von Esenbeck and Ebermaier 1830
1839	O'Shaughnessy studies Indian pharmacopoeia, tests dogs, then patients, for tetanus, rabies, epilepsy, rheumatoid disease	O'Shaughnessy 1838–1840
1843	Indian hemp treats cough in tuberculosis, pertussis, migraine, rheumatic joint pain, gout, morphine withdrawal	Clendinning 1843; Russo 2001b
1843	Treatment success in convulsions	Pereira 1843
1843	Hashish treats bubonic plague	Aubert-Roche 1843
1843	Testing in psychiatry	Moreau 1845
1845	In Ireland, Donovan treats migraine, neuralgia and musculoskeletal pain	Donovan 1845, 1851; Russo 2001b
1848	For neuralgia and sleep	Christison 1848
1849	Uterine hemorrhage	Churchill 1849; Russo 2002
1851	Enhances uterine contractions in labor	Christison 1851
1857	Tolerance and reverse tolerance described	Ludlow 1857
1860	Case report in bipolar disease	McMeens 1860
1860	Restores natural sleep in 1000 patients	Fronmüller 1860
1862	Life-saving in *hyperemesis gravidarum*	Russo 2002; Wright 1863, 1862
1860s	American Civil War, employed for war injuries, with opium for dysentery	United States. Dept. Of the Army. Office of the Surgeon General et al. 1990
1867	Delirium tremens treated with tincture	Tyrell 1867
1870	Melancholia, obsession and anxiety	Polli 1870; Russo 2001a
1883	Mental depression with insomnia	Strange 1883
1886	Ringer endorses for migraine prophylaxis, dysuria, urinary retention and dysmenorrhea	Ringer 1886
1887	Advantages over opiates, distancing from pain	Hare 1887; Russo 2001b
1887	For chronic daily headache	Mackenzie 1887a, 1887b, 1894
1888	Superiority in migraine, tremor of parkinsonism	Gowers 1888
1889	Suppositories for menopause	Farlow 1889; Russo 2002
1890	Touted for migraine, senility, dysmenorrhea, childhood convulsions, teething	Reynolds 1890; Russo 2001b, 2002
1890	Gastrointestinal pain	Sée 1890
1890	Delirium tremens and cyclic vomiting	Aulde 1890
1891	Cocaine, chloral hydrate and opiate addiction and "it calms the pain of clap"	Mattison 1891; Russo 2001a
1894	Migraine, syphilitic and functional gastrointestinal pain	Mackenzie 1894

Table 2.1 (continued) Cannabis chronology

1897	Oromucosal activity	Marshall 1897; Russo 2007
1899	Pain, including herpes zoster	Shoemaker 1899
1900	Dysmenorrhea, malarial symptoms	Lewis 1900
1915	Most satisfactory remedy for migraine	Osler and Mccrae 1915; Russo 2001b
1934	Psychiatric sequelae reviewed, finding little lasting harm	Bromberg 1934
1942	Menstrual migraine	Fishbein 1942
1944	Loewe reviews cannabinoid pharmacology, structure-activity relationships	New York (N.Y.). Mayor's Committee on Marihuana. et al. 1944
1947	Duodenal ulcers	Douthwaite 1947
1964	Isolation, synthesis of tetrahydrocannabinol	Gaoni and Mechoulam 1964
1968	Landmark clinical investigation	Weil et al. 1968
1971	Cannabis decreases intraocular pressure	Hepler and Frank 1971
1975	THC antineoplastic in lung adenocarcinoma	Munson et al. 1975
1975	THC antiemetic, cancer chemotherapy	Sallan et al. 1975
1975	THC equi-analgesic to codeine	Noyes et al. 1975
1976	THC equals salbutamol as bronchodilatator	Williams et al. 1976
1981	CBD anticonvulsant in humans	Carlini and Cunha 1981
1981	THC reduces spasticity	Petro and Ellenberger 1981
1982	CBD reduces anxiety after THC	Zuardi et al. 1982
1985	Anti-inflammatory component, cannflavin A, discovered	Barrett et al. 1985
1985	Marinol®, synthetic THC, approved for chemotherapy nausea, US	
1988	Discovery of cannabinoid receptor, CB_1	Devane et al. 1988
1989	CB_1 a G-protein-coupled receptor	Matsuda et al. 1990
1991	Cannabis improves night vision in Jamaica and Morocco, subsequently experimentally demonstrated	Merzouki and Molero Mesa 1999; Russo et al. 2004a; West 1991
1991	THC has 20 times anti-inflammatory power of aspirin, twice that of hydrocortisone	Evans 1991
1992	Discovery of endogenous cannabinoid, arachidonoylethanolamide (anandamide, AEA)	Devane et al. 1992
1993	CB_2 receptor identified	Munro et al. 1993
1993	CBD reduces anxiety	Zuardi et al. 1993
1993	Anandamide active in cannabinoid tetrad	Fride and Mechoulam 1993
1994	(Supra)normal development in infants born to mothers smoking in pregnancy	Dreher et al. 1994

Table 2.1 (continued) Cannabis chronology

1995	Endogenous cannabinoid, 2-arachidonoylglycerol	Mechoulam et al. 1995; Sugiura et al. 1995
1995	Δ^8-THC safe, effective in nausea and vomiting in children on chemotherapy	Abrahamov and Mechoulam 1995
1995	CBD improves psychosis	Zuardi et al. 1995
1997	THC reduces agitation in dementia	Volicer et al. 1997
1998	GW Pharmaceuticals begins cultivation, UK	Guy and Stott 2005
1998	"Endocannabinoids" described: "relax, eat, sleep, forget, and protect"	Di Marzo 1998
1998	Endocannabinoid "entourage effect"	Ben-Shabat et al. 1998; Mechoulam and Ben-Shabat 1999
1998	THC, CBD, neuroprotective antioxidants	Hampson et al. 1998
1998	THC produces apoptosis in glioma	Sanchez et al. 1998
2000	CBD antagonizes tumor necrosis factor-alpha in rheumatoid model	Malfait et al. 2000
2001	CBD is a TRPV1 agonist, fatty acid amide hydrolase-inhibitor, stimulator of AEA synthesis	Bisogno et al. 2001
2001	Clinical endocannabinoid deficiency syndrome hypothesized	Russo 2001a, 2001b, 2004b
2002	CBD antinausea effects	Parker et al. 2002
2003	First trial of Sativex® in multiple sclerosis symptoms	Wade et al. 2003
2003	Smoked cannabis in HIV/AIDS immunologically safe	Abrams et al. 2003
2003	THC, cannabis extract benefit mobility, subjective spasticity in MS	Zajicek et al. 2003
2003	THC improves Tourette symptoms without neuropsychological sequelae	Müller-Vahl et al. 2003a, 2003b
2004	Sativex® benefits pain	Notcutt et al. 2004
2004	Cannabis extracts reduce urological symptoms in MS	Brady et al. 2004
2004	Sativex®, high-THC extracts effective in brachial plexus avulsion pain	Berman et al. 2004
2004	THC reduces MS pain	Svendsen et al. 2004
2004	CBD increases wakefulness, counteracts THC sedation	Nicholson et al. 2004
2005	Sativex® approved in Canada for neuropathic pain in MS	Rog et al. 2005
2005	THCV CB_1 antagonist	Thomas et al. 2005
2005	CBD agonist at serotonin-1A	Russo et al. 2005
2006	CBD, other phytocannabinoids cytotoxic in breast cancer	Ligresti et al. 2006
2006	Sativex reduces pain, disease activity in rheumatoid arthritis	Blake et al. 2006

Table 2.1 (continued) Cannabis chronology

2006	CBD enhances adenosine receptor A2A signaling	Carrier et al. 2006
2006	Efficacious in morning sickness	Westphall et al. 2006
2006	Hepatitis C patients using cannabis better adhere to treatment	Sylvestre et al. 2006
2006	Cannabis lowers lung cancer risk	Hashibe et al. 2006
2007	Sativex® in peripheral neuropathic pain	Nurmikko et al. 2007
2007	Sativex® approved in Canada in opioid-resistant cancer pain	Johnson et al. 2010
2007	Smoked cannabis in short-term trials of sensory neuropathy in HIV/AIDS	Abrams et al. 2007a
2007	Vaporization pharmacokinetics/pharmacodynamics comparable to smoking	Abrams et al. 2007b
2007	CBD antagonizes CB_1 in presence of THC	Thomas et al. 2007
2007	CBD reduces prions, toxicity	Dirikoc et al. 2007
2008	Benefit in short-term study of HIV neuropathy	Ellis et al. 2009
2008	CBD, CBG antibiotic for methicillin-resistant *Staphylococcus aureus*	Appendino et al. 2008
2008	β-caryophyllene, sesquiterpenoid, potent CB_2 agonist	Gertsch et al. 2008
2008	Cannabis effective in brief neuropathic pain trial	Wilsey et al. 2008
2009	Cannabichromene-predominant plant; concentrated as enriched trichome product	De Meijer et al. 2009; Potter 2009
2010	Sativex® approved UK, Spain for intractable spasticity in MS	Novotna et al. 2011
2010	Sativex® reduces pain in opioid-resistant cancer	Johnson et al. 2010
2010	THCV anticonvulsant	Hill et al. 2010
2010	Single inhalations reduce neuropathic pain	Ware et al. 2010
2010	Sativex® benefits urological MS symptoms	Kavia et al. 2010
2010	Cannabigerol a potent TRPM8 antagonist for prostate cancer	De Petrocellis and Di Marzo 2010
2010	THCV reduces hyperalgesia in animals	Bolognini et al. 2010
2010	Cannabidivarin, THCV anticonvulsant	Hill et al. 2010; Jones et al. 2010
2010	Sativex® improves intractable nausea of chemotherapy	Duran et al. 2010
2010	THC attenuates breast cancer	Caffarel et al. 2010
2010	*Cannabis* genome published	Medicinal Genomics 2012; Van Bakel et al. 2011
2011	THC, CBD synergize with temozolomide reducing glioma growth	Torres et al. 2011
2012	CBD equals standard antipsychotic	Leweke et al. 2012

2.3 **Selected topics**

2.3.1 **Cannabis and tinnitus**

In 1698, Nicholas Lémery wrote, "Hemp contains much oil, little salt, it is specific for burns, *for roaring in the ears*, to kill worms," (Lémery 1727, p. 109, translation EBR). Tinnitus is a nettlesome syndrome of myriad causes, notoriously recalcitrant to treatment. However, many attestations to the benefits of cannabis are posted online, and Grinspoon and Bakalar (1997) offered one case report, and another documents improvement in tinnitus associated with benign intracranial hypertension by tetrahydrocannabinol (THC) administration (Raby et al. 2006). These claims gain plausibility when it is considered that the cannabinoid receptor type 1 (CB_1) is expressed in cochlear nucleus cells, is downregulated in salicylate-treated rats (Zheng et al. 2007), and there is no epidemiological evidence of recreational cannabis usage increasing tinnitus (Han et al. 2010). Thus, there is preliminary evidence to support the contention that THC may be helpful, while Lémery's report suggests cannabidiol (CBD) may also be beneficial. The latter supposition is supported by indirect evidence. To whit, transient receptor potential vanilloid receptor (TRPV)-4 is expressed in inner ear hair cells (Lowry et al. 2009), wherein CBD is an agonist (Moran et al. 2011). Additionally, since CBD is also a TRPV1 agonist/desensitizer (Bisogno et al. 2001), and the expression of mouse RNA of TRPV1 is increased after kanamycin administration, while TRPV4 expression is diminished by this tinnitus-producing treatment, suggests that both vanilloid mechanisms may be operative. Therapeutic trials of cannabinoids in humans certainly seem warranted, particularly with a combination of THC and CBD.

2.3.2 **Cannabis and tetanus**

In 1838, in India when O'Shaughnessy began experiments, tetanus was virtually uniformly fatal, even in England (Cock and Wilks 1858). Gowers cited mortality of 90% decades later (Gowers 1888). Prior ethnobotanical use in India for this indication was not apparent in the literature (Ainslie 1813). O'Shaughnessy essayed it in three cases, all of whom survived the acute disorder, but with one succumbing to gangrene after refusing amputation (O'Shaughnessy 1838–1840). Frequent dosing relaxed spasmodic paroxysms, allowing nutrition/hydration until recovery ensued, sometimes weeks later. He described similar successes in colleagues' efforts, saving the lives of three of six affected people. One case report was detailed by his cousin (O'Shaughnessy 1842). Treatment failed in one case for another (Shaw 1843) in India, but in England, Miller saw success in a 7-year-old treated with cannabis tincture (Miller 1845), who tolerated well a dose that previously intoxicated an adult. Christison (1848) similarly endorsed for this and other spasmodic diseases. In South Carolina, Gaillard reported two survivors with *trismus nascentium*, the infantile form (Gaillard and Desaussure 1853). Another case in an 18-year-old required 110 doses before cure (Cock and Wilks 1858). Cannabis was utilized successfully in a 9-year-old girl in Honduras (Skues 1858). In 1863, a Union soldier survived a musket ball wound with compound radioulnar fractures, tetanus and gangrene after amputation, and cannabis tincture (United States. Dept. Of the Army. Office of the Surgeon General. et al. 1990, Vol. 12, p. 822). In India, another case was successfully treated with a combination of cannabis with smoked opium (Fayrer 1865). In a review article from St. Louis (Roemer 1873), it was observed, "As standard remedies, opium, cannabis indica and the calabar bean are entitled to the greatest confidence" (p. 377). In India, Khastagir documented five cures employing smoked cannabis for tetanus to avoid difficult oral administration, and to titrate effects to spasm severity (Khastagir 1878). Lucas suggested the same to the West (Lucas 1880). By the end of the century, it was stated, "The treatment of Tetanus by smoking GUNJAH (Indian Hemp) . . . promises to supersede all others in India" (Waring 1897, p. 252). As late as 1962 in India, *charas* (hashish) was still recommended (Dastur 1962).

Despite worldwide attempts at immunization, tetanus afflicts 100–200 Americans per year, and 1 million victims worldwide with a mortality exceeding 50% (Rowland 2000). Given these striking statistics, and the marked success of modern cannabinoid pharmacology in treating spasticity (Novotna et al. 2011), prospective treatment for tetanus with Sativex® certainly seems warranted, especially in developing countries where intensive care and mechanical ventilation for weeks at a time are unavailable.

2.3.3 Cannabis and burns

Pliny the Elder may have been first to write of the benefit of cannabis for this indication, "It is applied raw to burns, but it must be frequently changed, so as to not let it dry" (Pliny 1951, Book XX, Ch. 97, p. 298). Variations of this approach continued for many centuries, with occasional elaboration. Leonhart Fuchs noted, "The raw root, pounded and wrapped, is good for the burn" (translation courtesy of Franjo Grotenhermen) (Fuchs 1999). Rabelais advised, "If you want to cure a burn, no matter whether it be from boiling water or burning wood, just rub on raw Pantagruelion [hemp], just as it comes out of the earth, without doing anything else. But be careful to change the dressing when you see it drying out on the wound" (Rabelais 1990, Book III, Ch. 51, p. 371). Parkinson suggested, "Hempe . . . is good to be used, for any place that hath been burnt by fire, if the fresh juyce be mixed with a little oyle or butter" (Parkinson et al. 1640). Lémery noted hemp "specific for burns" (Lémery 1727). William Salmon described various preparations (Salmon 1710, p. 510):

> XVIII. *The Oil by Insolation, Infusion, or Decoction.* It is good to be applied to any place which is burn'd with Fire, and to remove inflammation in any part; so also if an Oil of Ointment is made, by mixing the fresh juice with Oil Olive, or Hogs Lard, or fresh Butter, it heals Burning of Scaldings after an admirable Manner.

Chomel (1782, pp. 369–370) preferred hemp seed for burns (and tumors), "This oil mixed with a little melted wax, is a good remedy for burns from which it appeases the pain" (translation EBR). Marcandier (1758, p. 41, translation EBR) recommended a mixture, "Crushed and ground fresh, with butter in a mortar, one applies to burns, which it soothes infinitely, provided it is often renewed." It is noteworthy that all these preparations save the roots employ European hemp, generally in its raw state. This suggests that further investigation of cannabidiolic acid be undertaken. If any is converted in processing to CBD, then certainly its activity as a TRPV1 agonist/ desensitizer is germane in decreasing both attendant pain and apoptotic cell death after burns (Radtke et al. 2011).

2.3.4 Cannabis in pediatrics

This author has addressed this topic previously (Russo 2003), but with subsequent advances in cannabis-based therapeutics, the need to re-examine the issue is clear, in spite of any attendant controversy. It is a simple truism that any pharmacological agent released to general usage eventually finds application in children, and in fact, regulatory bodies in the European Union and US now require pediatric clinical trials for all newly approved pharmaceuticals. The questions then become, not whether to employ cannabis in children, but rather, how to do so safely and for what indications.

Actually, as the chronology attests, cannabis has been employed in children probably as long as in any other age group. This is additionally supported by ethnobotanical evidence. In Nepal, cannabis has been mixed with sweets to calm children while their mothers worked the fields (Fisher 1975). Cannabis candy is employed in Uzbekistan as an analgesic for boys undergoing circumcision (Benet 1975). In Jamaica, cannabis is an essential item of the folk pharmacopoeia. *Ganja* compresses are utilized for pain and wounds, even in neonates (Comitas 1975). *Ganja* tea and tonics are administered for marasmus, infantile diarrhea, teething, and as all-purpose remedies (Dreher 1982). Even noncannabis smokers believe the tea "brainifies" and maintains the young healthy (Dreher 1982, p. 72). Among Rastafarians, cannabis smoke may be passively blown towards infants to "make dem smart" and provide "wisdom and health" (Dreher 1982, p. 73). In Costa Rica in two children with asthma, one treated the malady by smoking cannabis, while the other abstained, and succumbed to the disease (Carter 1980). In Morocco, cannabis is combined with mint tea to expel intestinal worms in infants, while infantile diarrhea calls for passive smoke administration (Merzouki and Molero Mesa 1999).

Powdered cannabis in sugar was used in Berlin to treat paroxysmal coughing in children with pertussis (Dierbach 1828). In Calcutta, O'Shaughnessy included children in his trials, among them a 40-day-old infant with convulsions. After 20 days, "The child is now in the enjoyment of robust health, and has regained her natural plump and happy appearance" (O'Shaughnessy 1838–1840). Notice quickly spread throughout the British Empire and beyond. Ley followed upon this success by similarly treating a 9-month-old infant (Ley 1842). In England, Clendinning observed benefit of cannabis extract in cough of tuberculosis, and pertussis in a 9-week-old with reduced paroxysms and improved sleep.

Experimentation extended indications in children, including tetanus (*vide infra*). In Ireland, success was observed in Sydenham's (post-streptococcal) chorea (Corrigan 1845). Benefits on acute and chronic migraine were evident in children (Anstie 1871; Russo 2001b). Reynolds noted the same, plus benefit in spasmodic dysmenorrhea, infantile convulsions, the "temper disease of Marshall Hall," and even infant teething (Reynolds 1890), the latter also espoused in India contemporaneously (Dymock et al. 1890). Its popularity is highlighted by the presence of cannabis in numerous patent medicines sold for children.

In the twentieth century, Morris Fishbein, editor of the *Journal of the American Medical Association*, espoused cannabis in childbirth to aid in a painless labor with no attendant adverse events for the baby (Anonymous 1930).

More recently, the late Ester Fride pioneered exploration of the role of the endocannabinoid system in early development, demonstrating it essential to early initiation of feeding and maternal bonding (Fride 2002b), suggesting application in cystic fibrosis (Fride 2002a), neurotrauma, degenerative diseases, and "non-organic failure to thrive" (Fride 2004, pp. 24–25):

> Developmental observations suggest further that CB_1 receptors develop only gradually during the postnatal period, which correlates with an insensitivity to the psychoactive effects of cannabinoid treatment in the young organism.

This statement is further supported by histological studies in human brain development (Glass et al. 1997), the frequent mention in the nineteenth-century literature that children often tolerated perfectly well heroic doses of cannabis medicines that would engender prostration in an adult, and similar attestations in modern clinical use. One compelling example of the latter is the clinical trial in Israel with Δ^8-THC, up to 0.64 mg/kg/dose, administered onto the tongues of children to allay nausea in chemotherapy, in which it was virtually totally effective and free of side effects (Abrahamov and Mechoulam 1995).

Similarly, in Germany, Lorenz published detailed case reports employing Marinol® (synthetic THC) 0.04–0.12 mg/kg/d in eight children severely affected with degenerative diseases, epilepsy, posttraumatic, and hypoxic encephalopathy (Lorenz 2004). Prominent positive results included reduced seizures, spasms, improved social interaction, and palliation in terminal cases. Another case series provides support (Gottschling 2011). Dronabinol (average dose 0.2 mg/kg/d) was administered to 13 severely neurologically impaired children, aged 7 months to 17 years with uniform benefit on spasticity and pain, and improved sleep in ten. No tolerance or dose escalation was apparent in treatment, up to 5 years. More than 50 patients from the age of 3 months were treated for nausea and inanition from chemotherapy. Marked benefit was noted with no serious side effects aside from one self-limited case of tenfold accidental overdose, and no withdrawal effects were seen even after abrupt withdrawal following months of therapy.

An entire book was devoted to a case study of a youngster with severe behavioral abnormalities, controlled by oral cannabis confections (Jeffries and Jeffries 2003), allowing more normal socialization and mainstream education. Numerous anecdotal accounts claim benefit of cannabis in attention-deficit hyperactivity disorder (ADHD) (Grinspoon and Bakalar 1997). As counter-intuitive as this may seem, this author (EBR) saw many families and patients in clinical practice with independent attestation of benefits in ADHD. Support has been evident from animal models, wherein impulsive behavior was reduced by a CB_1 agonist (Adriani et al. 2003), or prenatal treatment of mothers with AM404 (inhibitor of cellular uptake of anandamide) to increase anandamide reduced hyperactivity in progeny (Viggiano et al. 2003). Clinical trials of both THC and cannabis (Müller-Vahl et al. 2003a, 2003b) have shown promise in treatment of tics and psychiatric symptoms in Tourette syndrome.

In animal experiments, high-dose THC attenuated induced insulitis and hyperglycemia in a diabetes model (Li et al. 2001), while CBD allowed a lower incidence of diabetes in mice (Weiss et al. 2006), was neuroprotective and retina-preserving in diabetic animals (El-Remessy et al. 2006), and attenuated myriad pathologies associated with diabetic cardiomyopathy (Rajesh et al. 2010). Clinical work in humans certainly seems indicated in type I diabetic children.

Application of cannabinoids for primary cancer treatment has been evident for centuries, and came to the fore once again after early experimental studies of THC in animals (Munson et al. 1975), and in treating human glioblastoma multiforme (Guzman et al. 2006). Recently, two detailed case studies with magnetic resonance imaging and histology have documented complete regression of pilocytic astrocytomas in children treated by their parents with cannabis (Foroughi et al. 2011). Certainly, if such treatment can be effected without psychoactive liability, whether with THC- or CBD-predominant preparations, future applications could be quite promising to achieve benefit with lower toxicity than with conventional chemotherapy. Additional possibilities are only limited by the imagination. Clinical cannabis will likely never be fully accepted in mainstream medicine until it can be proven safe and effective in serious disorders in children. To restate the issue, "If and when cannabis establishes its efficacy in pediatric diseases, it shall have achieved a fair measure of redemption from the derision it has elicited during the past century" (Russo 1998, p. 171).

References

Abrahamov, A. and Mechoulam, R. (1995). An efficient new cannabinoid antiemetic in pediatric oncology. *Life Sciences*, **56**, 2097–2102.

Abrams, D.I., Hilton, J.F., Leiser, R.J., *et al.* (2003). Short-term effects of cannabinoids in patients with HIV-1 infection. A randomized, placbo-controlled clinical trial. *Annals of Internal Medicine*, **139**, 258–266.

Abrams, D.I., Jay, C.A., Shade, S.B., *et al.* (2007a). Cannabis in painful HIV-associated sensory neuropathy: a randomized placebo-controlled trial. *Neurology*, **68**, 515–521.

Abrams, D.I., Vizoso, H.P., Shade, S.B., *et al.* (2007b). Vaporization as a smokeless cannabis delivery system: a pilot study. *Clinical Pharmacology and Therapeutics*, **82**, 572–578.

Adriani, W., Caprioli, A., Granstrem, O., Carli, M., and Laviola, G. (2003). The spontaneously hypertensive-rat as an animal model of ADHD: evidence for impulsive and non-impulsive subpopulations. *Neurosciene and Biobehavioral Reviews*, **27**, 639–651.

Ainslie, W. (1813). *Materia Medica of Hindoostan, and Artisan's and Agriculturist's Nomenclature*. Madras, India: Printed at the Government Press.

Al-Kindi and Levey, M. (1966). *The Medical Formulary, or Aqrabadhin of al-Kindi*. Madison, WI: University of Wisconsin Press.

Al-Mayusi. (1877). *Kamil al-sina 'a al-tibbiyya*. Bulaq.

Alter, R. (2004). *The Five Books of Moses: A Translation with Commentary*. New York: W.W. Norton & Co.

Anonymous. (1930). Effects of cannabis and alcohol during labor. *Journal of the American Medical Association*, **94**, 1165.

Anstie, F.E. (1871). *Neuralgia and the Diseases that Resemble It*. London: Macmillan.

Appendino, G., Gibbons, S., Giana, A., *et al.* (2008). Antibacterial cannabinoids from *Cannabis sativa*: a structure-activity study. *Journal of Natural Products*, **71**, 1427–1430.

Artamonov, M.I. (1965). Frozen tombs of the Scythians. *Scientific American*, **212**, 101–109.

Aubert-Roche, L.R. (1843). *De la peste, ou typhus d'Orient*. Paris: Just Rouvie.

Aulde, J. (1890). Studies in therapeutics – *Cannabis indica*. *Therapeutic Gazette*, **14**, 523–526.

Barkai, R. (1998). *A history of Jewish gynaecological texts in the Middle Ages*. Leiden: Boston, Brill.

Barrett, M. L., Gordon, D., and Evans, F. J. (1985). Isolation from *Cannabis sativa* L. of cannflavin – a novel inhibitor of prostaglandin production. *Biochemical Pharmacology*, **34**, 2019–2024.

Ben-Shabat, S., Fride, E., Sheskin, T., *et al.* (1998). An entourage effect: inactive endogenous fatty acid glycerol esters enhance 2-arachidonoyl-glycerol cannabinoid activity. *European Journal of Pharmacology*, **353**, 23–31.

Benet, S. (1975). Early diffusion and folk uses of hemp. In: V. Rubin (ed.). *Cannabis and Culture*. The Hague: Mouton.

Berman, J.S., Symonds, C., and Birch, R. (2004). Efficacy of two cannabis based medicinal extracts for relief of central neuropathic pain from brachial plexus avulsion: results of a randomised controlled trial. *Pain*, **112**, 299–306.

Bisogno, T., Hanus, L., De Petrocellis, L., *et al.* (2001). Molecular targets for cannabidiol and its synthetic analogues: effect on vanilloid VR1 receptors and on the cellular uptake and enzymatic hydrolysis of anandamide. *British Journal of Pharmacology*, **134**, 845–852.

Blake, D.R., Robson, P., Ho, M., Jubb, R.W., and McCabe, C.S. (2006). Preliminary assessment of the efficacy, tolerability and safety of a cannabis-based medicine (Sativex) in the treatment of pain caused by rheumatoid arthritis. *Rheumatology (Oxford)*, **45**, 50–52.

Bolognini, D., Costa, B., Maione, S., *et al.* (2010). The plant cannabinoid Delta9-tetrahydrocannabivarin can decrease signs of inflammation and inflammatory pain in mice. *British Journal of Pharmacology*, **160**, 677–687.

Brady, C. M., Dasgupta, R., Dalton, C., *et al.* (2004). An open-label pilot study of cannabis based extracts for bladder dysfunction in advanced multiple sclerosis. *Multiple Sclerosis*, **10**, 425–433.

Bromberg, W. (1934). Marihuana intoxication: a clinical study of *Cannabis sativa* intoxication. *American Journal of Psychiatry*, **91**, 303.

Brunner, T.F. (1973). Marijuana in ancient Greece and Rome? The literary evidence. *Bulletin of the History of Medicine*, **47**, 344–355.

Budge, E. A. W. (1913). *The Syriac Book of Medicines: Syrian Anatomy, Pathology and Therapeutics in the Early Middle Ages with Sections on Astrological and Native Medicine and Recipes*. London: Oxford University Press.

Burton, R. (1907). *The Anatomy of Melancholy.* London: Chatto and Windus.

Butrica, J.L. (2002). The medical use of cannabis among the Greeks and Romans. *Journal of Cannabis Therapeutics,* **2**, 51–70.

Caffarel, M.M., Andradas, C., Mira, E., *et al.* (2010). Cannabinoids reduce ErbB2-driven breast cancer progression through Akt inhibition. *Molecular Cancer,* **9**, 196.

Carlini, E.A. and Cunha, J.M. (1981). Hypnotic and antiepileptic effects of cannabidiol. *Journal of Clinical Pharmacology,* **21**, 417S–427S.

Carr, M.E. (1979). *A Linguistic Study of the Flora and Fuana Sections of the Erh-Ya.* Tucson, AZ: University of Arizona.

Carrier, E.J., Auchampach, J.A., and Hillard, C.J. (2006). Inhibition of an equilibrative nucleoside transporter by cannabidiol: a mechanism of cannabinoid immunosuppression. *Proceedings of the National Academy of Sciences of the United States of America,* **103**, 7895–7900.

Carter, W.E. (1980). *Cannabis in Costa Rica: A Study of Chronic Marihuana Use.* Philadelphia, PA: Institute for the Study of Human Issues.

Chomel, P.J.B. (1782). *Abrégé de l'histoire des plantes usuelles.* Paris: Libraires Associés.

Christison, A. (1851). On the natural history, action, and uses of Indian hemp. *Monthly Journal of Medical Science of Edinburgh, Scotland,* **13**, 26–45, 117–121.

Christison, R. (1848). *A Dispensatory or Commentary on the Pharmacopoeias of Great Britain and the United States.* Philadelphia, PA: Lea and Blanchard.

Churchill, F. (1849). *Essays on the Puerperal Fever and Other Diseases Peculiar to Women.* London: Sydenham Society.

Clarke, R.C. (2007). Traditional *Cannabis* cultivation in Darchula District, Nepal- seed, resin and textiles. *Journal of Industrial Hemp,* **12**, 19–42.

Clendinning, J. (1843). Observation on the medicinal properties of *Cannabis sativa* of India. *Medico-Chirurgical Transactions,* **26**, 188–210.

Cock, M. and Wilks, D. (1858). Case of recovery from acute and severe traumatic tetanus. *Medical Times and Gazette,* 8–9.

Comitas, L. (1975). The social nexus of ganja in Jamaica. In: V. Rubin (ed.) *Cannabis and Culture.* The Hague: Mouton Publishers.

Corrigan, O. (1845). Treatment of chorea by the use of Cannabis indica. *Medical Times,* **12**, 291–292.

Crawford, V. (2002). A homelie herbe: medicinal cannabis in early England. *Journal of Cannabis Therapeutics,* **2**, 71–79.

Da Orta, G. (1913). *Colloquies on the Simples and Drugs of India.* London: Henry Sotheran.

Darmesteter, J. (1895). *Zend-Avesta, Part I, The Vendidad.* London: Oxford University.

Dastur, J.F. (1962). *Medicinal Plants of India and Pakistan; A concise Work Describing Plants Used for Drugs and Remedies According to Ayurvedic, Unani and Tibbi Systems and Mentioned in British and American Pharmacopoeias.* Bombay: D.B. Taraporevala Sons.

De Meijer, E.P.M., Hammond, K.M., and Micheler, M. (2009). The inheritance of chemical phenotype in *Cannabis sativa* L. (III): variation in cannabichromene proportion. *Euphytica,* **165**, 293–311.

De Petrocellis, L. and Di Marzo, V. (2010). Non-CB$_1$, non-CB$_2$ receptors for endocannabinoids, plant cannabinoids, and synthetic cannabimimetics: focus on G-protein-coupled receptors and transient receptor potential channels. *Journal of Neuroimmune Pharmacology,* **5**, 103–121.

Devane, W.A., Dysarz, F.A., 3rd, Johnson, M.R., Melvin, L.S., and Howlett, A.C. (1988). Determination and characterization of a cannabinoid receptor in rat brain. *Molecular Pharmacology,* **34**, 605–613.

Devane, W. A., Hanus, L., Breuer, A., *et al.* (1992). Isolation and structure of a brain constituent that binds to the cannabinoid receptor. *Science,* **258**, 1946–1949.

Di Marzo, V. (1998). 'Endocannabinoids' and other fatty acid derivatives with cannabimimetic properties: biochemistry and possible physiopathological relevance. *Biochimica et Biophysica Acta,* **1392**, 153–175.

Dierbach, J.H. (1828). *De neusten Entdeckungen in der Materia Medica*. Heidelberg and Leipzig.

Dioscorides, P. and Beck, L.Y. (2011). *De Materia Medica*. Hildesheim: Olms-Weidmann.

Dirikoc, S., Priola, S.A., Marella, M., Zsurger, N., and Chabry, J. (2007). Nonpsychoactive cannabidiol prevents prion accumulation and protects neurons against prion toxicity. *J Neurosci*, **27**, 9537–9544.

Donovan, M. (1845). On the physical and medicinal qualities of Indian hemp *(Cannabis indica)*; with observations on the best mode of administration, and cases illustrative of its powers. *Dublin Journal of Medical Science*, **26**, 368–402, 459–461.

Donovan, M. (1851). Observations on the resin of Indian hemp. *Dublin Medical Press*, **25**, 182–183.

Douthwaite, A.H. (1947). Choice of drugs in the treatment of duodenal ulcer. *British Medical Journal*, **2**, 43–47.

Dreher, M.C. (1982). *Working Men and Ganja: Marihuana Use in Rural Jamaica*. Philadelphia, PA: Institute for the Study of Human Issues.

Dreher, M.C., Nugent, K., and Hudgins, R. (1994). Prenatal marijuana exposure and neonatal outcomes in Jamaica: an ethnographic study. *Pediatrics*, **93**, 254–260.

Duran, M., Perez, E., Abanades, S., *et al.* (2010). Preliminary efficacy and safety of an oromucosal standardized cannabis extract in chemotherapy-induced nausea and vomiting. *British Journal of Clinical Pharmacology*, **70**, 656–663.

Dymock, W., Warden, C.J.H., and Hooper, D. (1890). *Pharmacographia Indica. A History of the Principal Drugs of Vegetable Origin, Met With in British India*. London: K. Paul Trench Trübner & Co.

El-Remessy, A.B., Al-Shabrawey, M., Khalifa, Y., *et al.* (2006). Neuroprotective and blood-retinal barrier-preserving effects of cannabidiol in experimental diabetes. *American Journal of Pathology*, **168**, 235–244.

Ellis, R.J., Toperoff, W., Vaida, F., *et al.* (2009). Smoked medicinal cannabis for neuropathic pain in HIV: a randomized, crossover clinical trial. *Neuropsychopharmacology*, **34**, 672–680.

Evans, F.J. (1991). Cannabinoids: the separation of central from peripheral effects on a structural basis. *Planta Medica*, **57**, S60–S67.

Fankhauser, M. (2002). History of cannabis in Western medicine. In: F. Grotenhermen and E.B. Russo (eds.). *Cannabis and Cannabinoids: Pharmacology, Toxicology and Therapeutic Potential*. Binghamton, NY: Haworth Press.

Farlow, J.W. (1889). On the use of belladonna and *Cannabis indica* by the rectum in gynecological practice. *Boston Medical and Surgical Journal*, **120**, 507–509.

Fayrer, J. (1865). A case of traumatic tetanus treated by opium smoking and internal administration of chloroform and hemp. *Edinburgh Medical Journal*, **10**, 716–720.

Fishbein, M. (1942). Migraine associated with menstruation. *Journal of the American Medical Association*, **237**, 326.

Fisher, J. (1975). Cannabis in Nepal: an overview. In: V. Rubin (ed.). *Cannabis and Culture*. The Hague: Mouton Publishers.

Foroughi, M., Hendson, G., Sargent, M.A., and Steinbok, P. (2011). Spontaneous regression of septum pellucidum/forniceal pilocytic astrocytomas – possible role of Cannabis inhalation. *Child's Nervous System*, **27**, 671–679.

Fride, E. (2002a). Cannabinoids and cystic fibrosis:a novel approach. *Journal of Cannabis Therapeutics*, **2**, 59–71.

Fride, E. (2002b). Cannabinoids and feeding: the role of the endogenous cannabinoid system as a trigger for newborn suckling. *Journal of Cannabis Therapeutics*, **2**, 51–62.

Fride, E. (2004). The endocannabinoid-CB receptor system: importance for development and in pediatric disease. *Neuroendocrinology Letters*, **25**, 24–30.

Fride, E. and Mechoulam, R. (1993). Pharmacological activity of the cannabinoid receptor agonist, anandamide, a brain constituent. *European Journal of Pharmacology*, **231**, 313–314.

Fronmüller, B. (1860). *Cannabis indica* as a hypnotic. *Journal of Materia Medica*, **2**, 474.

Fuchs, L. (1999). *The great herbal of Leonhart Fuchs: De historia stirpium commentarii insignes, 1542 (notable commentaries on the history of plants).* Stanford, CA: Stanford University Press.

Gaillard, P.C. and Desaussure, W. (1853). Two cases of trismus nascentium, which recovered under the use of *Cannabis indica. Charleston Medical Journal and Review,* **8**, 808–811.

Gaoni, Y. and Mechoulam, R. (1964). Isolation, structure and partial synthesis of an active constituent of hashish. *Journal of the American Chemical Society,* **86**, 1646–1647.

Gerard, J. and Johnson, T. (1975). *The Herbal: or, General History of Plants.* New York: Dover Publications.

Gertsch, J., Leonti, M., Raduner, S., *et al.* (2008). Beta-caryophyllene is a dietary cannabinoid. *Proceedings of the National Academy of Sciences of the United States of America,* **105**, 9099–104.

Glass, M., Dragunow, M., and Faull, R. L. (1997). Cannabinoid receptors in the human brain: a detailed anatomical and quantitative autoradiographic study in the fetal, neonatal and adult human brain. *Neuroscience,* **77**, 299–318.

Gottschling, S. (2011). Cannbinoide bei Kindern. Gute Erfahrungen bei Schmerzen, Spastik und in der Onkologie. *Angewandte Schmerztherapie und Palliativmedizin,* 55–57.

Gowers, W.R. (1888). *A Manual of Diseases of the Nervous System.* Philadelphia, PA: P. Blakiston Son & Co.

Grattan, J.H.G. and Singer, C.J. (1952). *Anglo-Saxon Magic and Medicine. Illustrated Specially From the Semi-Pagan Text "Lacnunga."* London: Oxford University Press.

Grierson, G.A. (1894). The hemp plant in Sanskrit and Hindi literature. *Indian Antiquary,* 260–262.

Grinspoon, L. and Bakalar, J.B. (1997). *Marihuana, the Forbidden Medicine.* New Haven, CT: Yale University Press.

Guy, G.W. and Stott, C.G. (2005). The development of Sativex – a natural cannabis-based medicine. In: R. Mechoulam (ed.). *Cannabinoids as Therapeutics.* Basel: Birkhäuser Verlag, pp. 231–263.

Guzman, M., Duarte, M.J., Blazquez, C., *et al.* (2006). A pilot clinical study of Delta(9)-tetrahydrocannabinol in patients with recurrent glioblastoma multiforme. *British Journal of Cancer,* **95**, 197–203.

Hampson, A.J., Grimaldi, M., Axelrod, J., and Wink, D. (1998). Cannabidiol and (-)delta9-tetrahydrocannabinol are neuroprotective antioxidants. *Proceedings of the National Academy of Sciences of the United States of America,* **95**, 8268–8273.

Han, B., Gfroerer, J.C., and Colliver, J.D. (2010). Associations between duration of illicit drug use and health conditions: results from the 2005–2007 national surveys on drug use and health. *Annals of Epidemiology,* **20**, 289–297.

Hare, H.A. (1887). Clinical and physiological notes on the action of *Cannabis indica. Therapeutic Gazette,* **2**, 225–228.

Hashibe, M., Morgenstern, H., Cui, Y., *et al.* (2006). Marijuana use and the risk of lung and upper aerodigestive tract cancers: results of a population-based case-control study. *Cancer Epidemiology, Biomarkers and Prevention,* **15**, 1829–1834.

Hepler, R.S. and Frank, I.R. (1971). Marihuana smoking and intraocular pressure. *Journal of the American Medical Association,* **217**, 1392.

Herodotus. (1998). *The Histories.* Oxford: Oxford University Press.

Hildegard and Throop, P. (1998). *Hildegard von Bingen's Physica: the Complete English Translation of Her Classic Work on Health and Healing.* Rochester, VT: Healing Arts Press.

Hill, A.J., Weston, S.E., Jones, N.A., *et al.* (2010). Delta-Tetrahydrocannabivarin suppresses in vitro epileptiform and in vivo seizure activity in adult rats. *Epilepsia,* **51**, 1522–1532.

Ibn Sina (Avicenna) (1294). *Al-Qanun fi l-tibb (Canon of medicine).* Bulaq.

Indian Hemp Drugs Commission. (1894). *Report of the Indian Hemp Drugs Commission, 1893–94.* Simla: Govt. Central Print. Office.

Jeffries, D. and Jeffries, L. (2003). *Jeffrey's Journey: A Determined Mother's Battle for Medical Marijuana for Her Son.* Rocklin, CA: LP Chronicles.

Jiang, H.E., Li, X., Zhao, Y.X., *et al.* (2006). A new insight into *Cannabis sativa* (Cannabaceae) utilization from 2500-year-old Yanghai Tombs, Xinjiang, China. *Journal of Ethnopharmacology*, **108**, 414–422.

Johnson, J.R., Burnell-Nugent, M., Lossignol, D., *et al.* (2010). Multicenter, double-blind, randomized, placebo-controlled, parallel-group study of the efficacy, safety, and tolerability of THC:CBD extract and THC extract in patients with intractable cancer-related pain. *Journal of Pain and Symptom Management*, **39**, 167–179.

Jones, N.A., Hill, A.J., Smith, I., *et al.* (2010). Cannabidiol displays antiepileptiform and antiseizure properties in vitro and in vivo. *Journal of Pharmacology and Experimental Therapeutics*, **332**, 569–577.

Julien, M.S. (1849). Chirugie chinoise. Substance anesthétique employée en Chine, dans le commencement du III-ième siecle de notre ère, pour paralyser momentanement la sensibilité. *Comptes Rendus Hebdomadaires de l'Académie des Sciences*, **28**, 223–229.

Kaempfer, E. (1996). *Exotic pleasures*. Carbondale, IL: Southern Illinois University Press.

Kahl, O. (1994). *Sabur ibn Sahl: Dispensatorium parvum (al-Aqrabadhin al-Saghir)*. Leiden: E.J. Brill.

Kavia, R., De Ridder, D., Constantinescu, C., Stott, C., and Fowler, C. (2010). Randomized controlled trial of Sativex to treat detrusor overactivity in multiple sclerosis. *Multiple Sclerosis*, **16**, 1349–1359.

Khastagir, A.C. (1878). Hemp (ganja) smoking in tetanus on a new principle. *Indian Medical Gazette*, 210–211.

Lémery, N. (1727). *Dictionaire ou traité universel des drogues simples*. Rotterdam: Jean Hofhout.

Leweke, F.M., Piomelli, D., Pahlisch, F., *et al.* (2012). Cannabidiol enhances anandamide signaling and alleviates psychotic symptoms of schizophrenia. *Translational Psychiatry*, **2**, e94.

Lewis, B., Menage, V.L., Pellat, C.H., and Schacht, J. (1971). *The Encyclopedia of Islam*. Leiden: E.J. Brill.

Lewis, H. (1900). *Cannabis indica*: A study of its physiologic action, toxic effects and therapeutic indications. *Merck's Archives of Materia Medica and its Uses*, **2**, 247–251.

Lewis, W. (1794). *The Edinburgh New Dispensatory*. Edinburgh: Printed for W. Creech.

Ley, W. (1842). On the efficacy of Indian hemp in some convulsive disorders. *Provincial Medical and Surgical Journal*, **4**, 407–409.

Li, X., Kaminski, N.E., and Fischer, L.J. (2001). Examination of the immunosuppressive effect of delta9-tetrahydrocannabinol in streptozotocin-induced autoimmune diabetes. *International Immunopharmacology*, **1**, 699–712.

Ligresti, A., Moriello, A.S., Starowicz, K., *et al.* (2006). Antitumor activity of plant cannabinoids with emphasis on the effect of cannabidiol on human breast carcinoma. *Journal of Pharmacology and Experimental Therapeutics*, **318**, 1375–1387.

Linné, C.A. (1772). *Materia medica per regna tria naturae*. Lipsiae et Erlangae: Wolfgang Waltherum.

Lorenz, R. (2004). On the application of cannabis in paediatrics and epileptology. *Neuroendocrinology Letters*, **25**, 40–44.

Lowry, C.A., Lightman, S.L., and Nutt, D.J. (2009). That warm fuzzy feeling: brain serotonergic neurons and the regulation of emotion. *Journal of Psychopharmacology*, **23**, 392–400.

Lozano, I. (2001). The therapeutic use of *Cannabis sativa* L. in Arabic medicine. *Journal of Cannabis Therapeutics*, **1**, 63–70.

Lucas, J.C. (1880). Notes on tetanus; with remarks on the efficacy of *Cannabis indica* when administered through the lungs. *Medical Times and Gazette*, 202–204.

Ludlow, F.H. (1857). *The Hasheesh Eater: Being Passages From the Life of a Pythagorean*. New York: Harper.

Macgill, E.R. (ed.) (1990). *This Booke of Sovereigne Medicines*. Ann Arbor, MI: UMI.

Mackenzie, S. (1887a). Indian hemp in persistent headache. *Journal of the American Medical Association*, **9**, 732.

Mackenzie, S. (1887b). Remarks on the value of Indian hemp in the treatment of a certain type of headache. *British Medical Journal*, **1**, 97–98.

Mackenzie, S. (1894). Therapeutique médicale: De la valeur therapeutique speciale du chanvre indien dans certains états morbides. *Semaine Médicale*, **14**, 399–400.

Malfait, A.M., Gallily, R., Sumariwalla, P.F., *et al.* (2000). The nonpsychoactive cannabis constituent cannabidiol is an oral anti-arthritic therapeutic in murine collagen-induced arthritis. *Proceedings of the National Academy of Sciences of the United States of America*, **97**, 9561–9566.

Manniche, L. (1989). *An Ancient Egyptian Herbal*. Austin, TX: University of Texas.

Marcandier, M. (1758). *Traité du chanvre*. Paris: Chez Nyon.

Marshall, C.R. (1897). The active principle of Indian hemp: a preliminary communication. *Lancet*, **1**, 235–238.

Matsuda, L.A., Lolait, S.J., Brownstein, M.J., Young, A.C., and Bonner, T.I. (1990). Structure of a cannabinoid receptor and functional expression of the cloned cDNA. *Nature*, **346**, 561–564.

Mattison, J.B. (1891). *Cannabis indica* as an anodyne and hypnotic. *St. Louis Medical and Surgical Journal*, **61**, 265–271.

McMeens, R.R. (1860). Report of the Ohio State Medical Committee on *Cannabis indica*. White Sulphur Springs, OH: Ohio State Medical Society.

Mechoulam, R. and Ben-Shabat, S. (1999). From gan-zi-gun-nu to anandamide and 2-arachidonoylglycerol: The ongoing story of cannabis. *Natural Products Report*, **16**, 131–143.

Mechoulam, R., Ben-Shabat, S., Hanus, L., *et al.* (1995). Identification of an endogenous 2-monoglyceride, present in canine gut, that binds to cannabinoid receptors. *Biochemical Pharmacology*, **50**, 83–90.

Medicinal Genomics. (2012). *Medicinal Genomics Sequences the Cannabis Genome to Assemble the Largest Known Gene Collection of this Therapeutic Plant* [Online]. Available at: http://www.medicinalgenomics.com/medicinal-genomics-sequences-the-cannabis-genome-to-assemble-the-largest-known-gene-collection-of-this-therapeutic-plant/.

Merzouki, A. and Molero Mesa, J. (1999). La [sic] chanvre (*Cannabis sativa* L.) dans la pharmacopée traditionelle du Rif (nord du Maroc). *Ars Pharmaceutica*, **40**, 233–240.

Miller, J. (1845). Case of traumatic tetanus, following injury of the finger; treated by amputation of the injured part, the application of cold to the spine, and the internal use of the *Cannabis indica*. *Monthly Journal of Medical Science*, **5**, 22–30.

Moran, M.M., McAlexander, M.A., Biro, T. and Szallasi, A. (2011). Transient receptor potential channels as therapeutic targets. *Nature Reviews Drug Discovery*, **10**, 601–620.

Moreau, J.-J. (1845). *Du hachisch et de l'aliénation mentale: Études psychologiques*. Paris: Fortin Masson.

Müller-Vahl, K.R., Prevedel, H., Theloe, K., *et al.* (2003a). Treatment of Tourette syndrome with delta-9-tetrahydrocannabinol (delta 9-THC): no influence on neuropsychological performance. *Neuropsychopharmacology*, **28**, 384–388.

Müller-Vahl, K.R., Schneider, U., Prevedel, H., *et al.* (2003b). Delta9-tetrahydrocannabinol (THC) is effective in the treatment of tics in Tourette syndrome: a 6-week randomized trial. *Journal of Clinical Psychiatry*, **64**, 459–465.

Munro, S., Thomas, K.L., and Abu-Shaar, M. (1993). Molecular characterization of a peripheral receptor for cannabinoids. *Nature*, **365**, 61–65.

Munson, A.E., Harris, L.S., Friedman, M.A., Dewey, W.L., and Carchman, R.A. (1975). Antineoplastic activity of cannabinoids. *Journal of the National Cancer Institute*, **55**, 597–602.

Needham, J. and Gwei-Djen, L. (1974). *Science and Civilisation in China. Chemistry and Chemical Technology*. Cambridge: Cambridge University Press.

Nees Von Esenbeck, T.F.L. and Ebermaier, K.H. (1830). *Handbuch der medicinisch-pharmaceutischen botanik*. Düsseldorf: Arnz and Comp.

New York (N.Y.). Mayor's Committee on Marihuana, Wallace, G.B., and Cunningham, E.V. (1944). *The Marihuana Problem in the City of New York; Sociological, Medical, Psychological and Pharmacological Studies*. Lancaster, PA: The Jaques Cattell Press.

Nicholson, A.N., Turner, C., Stone, B.M., and Robson, P.J. (2004). Effect of delta-9-tetrahydrocannabinol and cannabidiol on nocturnal sleep and early-morning behavior in young adults. *Journal of Clinical Psychopharmacology*, **24**, 305–313.

Notcutt, W., Price, M., Miller, R., *et al.* (2004). Initial experiences with medicinal extracts of cannabis for chronic pain: results from 34 "N of 1" studies. *Anaesthesia*, **59**, 440–452.

Novotna, A., Mares, J., Ratcliffe, S., *et al.* (2011). A randomized, double-blind, placebo-controlled, parallel-group, enriched-design study of nabiximols* (Sativex®), as add-on therapy, in subjects with refractory spasticity caused by multiple sclerosis. *European Journal of Neurology*, **18**, 1122–1131.

Noyes, R., Jr., Brunk, S.F., Avery, D.A.H., and Canter, A.C. (1975). The analgesic properties of delta-9-tetrahydrocannabinol and codeine. *Clinical Pharmacology and Therapeutics*, **18**, 84–89.

Nurmikko, T.J., Serpell, M.G., Hoggart, B., *et al.* (2007). Sativex successfully treats neuropathic pain characterised by allodynia: a randomised, double-blind, placebo-controlled clinical trial. *Pain*, **133**, 210–220.

O'Shaughnessy, R. (1842). Case of tetanus, cured by a preparation of hemp (the *Cannabis indica.*). *Transactions of the Medical & Physical Society of Calcutta*, **8**, 462–469.

O'Shaughnessy, W.B. (1838–1840). On the preparations of the Indian hemp, or gunjah *(Cannabis indica)*; their effects on the animal system in health, and their utility in the treatment of tetanus and other convulsive diseases. *Transactions of the Medical and Physical Society of Bengal*, 71–102, 421–461.

Osler, W. and Mccrae, T. (1915). *The Principles and Practice of Medicine.* New York: Appleton and Company.

Parker, L.A., Mechoulam, R., and Schlievert, C. (2002). Cannabidiol, a non-psychoactive component of cannabis and its synthetic dimethylheptyl homolog suppress nausea in an experimental model with rats. *Neuroreport*, **13**, 567–70.

Parkinson, J., Bonham, T., and L'Obel, M.D. (1640). *Theatrum Botanicum: The Theater of Plants.* London: Tho. Cotes.

Pereira, P. (1843). *The Elements of Materia Medica and Therapeutics.* Philadelphia, PA: Lea & Blanchard.

Petro, D.J. and Ellenberger, C. (1981). Treatment of human spasticity with delta9-tetrahydrocannabinol. *Journal of Clinical Pharmacology*, **21**, 413S–416S.

Pliny. (1951). *Pliny: Natural History.* Cambridge, MA: Harvard University.

Pliny. (1980). *Natural History, Books XXIV–XXVII.* Cambridge, MA: Harvard University Press.

Polli, G. (1870). Further Observations On Haschish In Medicine. *St. Andrew's Medical Graduates Association Transactions*, **3**, 98–101.

Pollington, S. (2000). *Leechcraft: Early English Charms, Plant Lore, and Healing.* Hockwold-cum-Wilton: Anglo-Saxon Books.

Potter, D.J. (2009). *The Propagation, Characterisation and Optimisation of Cannabis sativa L. as a Phytopharmaceutical.* PhD thesis, King's College London.

Rabelais, F. (1990). *Gargantua and Pantagruel.* New York: Norton.

Raby, W.N., Modica, P.A., Wolintz, R.J., and Murtaugh, K. (2006). Dronabinol reduces signs and symptoms of idiopathic intracranial hypertension: a case report. *Journal of Ocular Pharmacology and Therapeutics*, **22**, 68–75.

Radtke, C., Sinis, N., Sauter, M., *et al.* (2011). TRPV channel expression in human skin and possible role in thermally induced cell death. *Journal of Burn Care and Research*, **32**, 150–159.

Rajesh, M., Mukhopadhyay, P., Batkai, S., *et al.* (2010). Cannabidiol attenuates cardiac dysfunction, oxidative stress, fibrosis, and inflammatory and cell death signaling pathways in diabetic cardiomyopathy. *Journal of the American College of Cardiology*, **56**, 2115–2125.

Reymond, E.A.E. (1976). *From the contents of the Libraries of the Suchos Temple in the Fayyum, Part I, a medical book from Crocodilopolis. Papyrus Vindobonensis D.* 6257. Vienna: Österreichische Nationalbibliothek.

Reynolds, J.R. (1890). Therapeutical uses and toxic effects of *Cannabis indica. Lancet*, **1**, 637–638.

Ringer, S. (1886). *A Handbook of Therapeutics*. New York: W. Wood.

Roemer, B. (1873). On tetanus and tetanoid affections, with cases. *St. Louis Medical & Surgical Journalq*, **10**, 363–378.

Rog, D.J., Nurmiko, T., Friede, T., and Young, C. (2005). Randomized controlled trial of cannabis based medicine in central neuropathic pain due to multiple sclerosis. *Neurology*, **65**, 812–819.

Rowland, L.P. (ed.). (2000). *Merritt's Neurology*. Philadelphia, PA: Lippincott, Williams and Wilkins.

Rudenko, S.I. (1970). *Frozen Tombs of Siberia; The Pazyryk Burials of Iron Age Horsemen*. Berkeley, CA: University of California Press.

Rumpf, G.E. and Beekman, E.M. (1981). *The Poison Tree: Selected Writings of Rumphius on the Natural History of the Indies*. Amherst, MA: University of Massachusetts Press.

Russo, E. (1998). Cannabis for migraine treatment: the once and future prescription? An historical and scientific review. *Pain*, **76**, 3–8.

Russo, E. (2002). Cannabis treatments in obstetrics and gynecology: a historical review. *Journal of Cannabis Therapeutics*, **2**, 5–35.

Russo, E.B. (2001a). *Handbook of Psychotropic Herbs: A Scientific Analysis of Herbal Remedies for Psychiatric Conditions*. Binghamton, NY: Haworth Press.

Russo, E.B. (2001b). Hemp for headache: an in-depth historical and scientific review of cannabis in migraine treatment. *Journal of Cannabis Therapeutics*, **1**, 21–92.

Russo, E.B. (2003). Future of cannabis and cannabinoids in therapeutics. *Journal of Cannabis Therapeutics*, **3**, 163–174.

Russo, E.B. (2004a). History of cannabis as medicine. In: G.W. Guy, B.A. Whittle, and P. Robson (eds.). *Medicinal Uses of Cannabis and Cannabinoids*. London: Pharmaceutical Press.

Russo, E.B. (2004b). Clinical endocannabinoid deficiency (CECD): Can this concept explain therapeutic benefits of cannabis in migraine, fibromyalgia, irritable bowel syndrome and other treatment-resistant conditions? *Neuroendocrinology Letters*, **25**, 31–39.

Russo, E.B. (2005). Cannabis in India: ancient lore and modern medicine. In: R. Mechoulam (ed.). *Cannabinoids as Therapeutics*. Basel: Birkhäuser Verlag.

Russo, E.B. (2007). History of cannabis and its preparations in saga, science and sobriquet. *Chemistry & Biodiversity*, **4**, 2624–2648.

Russo, E.B., Burnett, A., Hall, B., and Parker, K.K. (2005). Agonistic properties of cannabidiol at 5-HT-1a receptors. *Neurochemical Research*, **30**, 1037–1043.

Russo, E.B., Jiang, H.E., Li, X., *et al.* (2008). Phytochemical and genetic analyses of ancient cannabis from Central Asia. *Journal of Experimental Botany*, **59**, 4171–4182.

Russo, E.B., Merzouki, A., Molero Mesa, J., Frey, K.A., and Bach, P.J. (2004). Cannabis improves night vision: a pilot study of dark adaptometry and scotopic sensitivity in kif smokers of the Rif Mountains of Northern Morocco. *Journal of Ethnopharmacology*, **93**, 99–104.

Sallan, S.E., Zinberg, N.E. and Frei, E.D. (1975). Antiemetic effect of delta-9-tetrahydrocannabinol in patients receiving cancer chemotherapy. *New England Journal of Medicine*, **293**, 795–797.

Salmon, W. (1710). *Botanologia. The English herbal: or, History of Plants*. London: I. Dawkes.

Sanchez, C., Galve-Roperh, I., Canova, C., Brachet, P., and Guzman, M. (1998). Delta9-tetrahydrocannabinol induces apoptosis in C6 glioma cells. *FEBS Letters*, **436**, 6–10.

Sarianidi, V. (1998). *Margiana and Protozoroastrism*. Athens: Kapon Editions.

Sée, M.G. (1890). Usages du *Cannabis indica* dans le traitement des névroses et dyspepsies gastriques. *Bulletin de l'Academie Nationale de Medecine*, **3**, 158–193.

Sethi, S. (1868). *Syntagma de alimentorum facultatibus*. Leipzig: B.G. Teubner.

Shaw, J. (1843). On the use of the *Cannabis indica* (or Indian hemp)-1st-in tetanus-2nd-in hydrophobia-3rd-in cholera-with remarks on its effects. *Madras Quarterly Medical Journal*, **5**, 74–80.

Shoemaker, J.V. (1899). The therapeutic value of *Cannabis indica*. *Texas Medical News*, **8**, 477–488.

Short, T. (1751). *Medicina Britannica: Or a Treatise on Such Physical Plants*. Philadelphia, PA: Re-printed, and sold by B. Franklin and D. Hall.

Shou-Zhong, Y. (1997). *The Divine Farmer's Materia Medica: A Translation of the Shen Nong Ben Cao Jing*. Boulder, CO: Blue Poppy Press.

Skues, E.W. (1858). Tetanus treated with extract of Indian hemp: recovery. *Edinburgh Medical Journal*, **3**, 877–878.

Strange, W. (1883). *Cannabis indica*: as a medicine and as a poison. *British Medical Journal*, 14.

Stuart, G. (1928). *Chinese Materia Medica*. Shanghai: Presbyterian Mission.

Sugiura, T., Kondo, S., Sukagawa, A., *et al.* (1995). 2-Arachidonoylglycerol: a possible endogenous cannabinoid receptor ligand in brain. *Biochemical and Biophysical Research Communications*, **215**, 89–97.

Svendsen, K.B., Jensen, T.S., and Bach, F.W. (2004). Does the cannabinoid dronabinol reduce central pain in multiple sclerosis? Randomised double blind placebo controlled crossover trial. *British Medical Journal*, **329**, 253.

Sylvestre, D.L., Clements, B.J., and Malibu, Y. (2006). Cannabis use improves retention and virological outcomes in patients treated for hepatitis C. *European Journal of Gastroenterology and Hepatology*, **18**, 1057–1063.

Thomas, A., Baillie, G.L., Phillips, A.M., *et al.* (2007). Cannabidiol displays unexpectedly high potency as an antagonist of CB_1 and CB_2 receptor agonists in vitro. *British Journal of Pharmacology*, **150**, 613–623.

Thomas, A., Stevenson, L.A., Wease, K.N., *et al.* (2005). Evidence that the plant cannabinoid delta-9-tetrahydrocannabivarin is a cannabinoid CB_1 and CB_2 antagonist. *British Journal of Pharmacology*, **146**, 917–926.

Thompson, R.C. (trans.). (1903). *The Devils and Evil Spirits of Babylonia*. London: Luzac and Co.

Thompson, R.C. (1924). *The Assyrian Herbal*. London: Luzac and Co.

Thompson, R.C. (1949). *A Dictionary of Assyrian Botany*. London: British Academy.

Torres, S., Lorente, M., Rodriguez-Fornes, F., *et al.* (2011). A combined preclinical therapy of cannabinoids and temozolomide against glioma. *Molecular Cancer Therapy*, **10**, 90–103.

Tyrell, H.J. (1867). On the treatment of delirium tremens by Indian hemp. *Medical Press and Circular*, **17**, 243–244.

United States. Dept. Of the Army. Office of the Surgeon General, Barnes, J.K., Woodward, J.J., and Otis, G.A. (1990). *The Medical and Surgical History of the Civil War*. Wilmington, NC: Broadfoot Publishing Co.

Van Bakel, H., Stout, J.M., Cote, A.G., *et al.* (2011). The draft genome and transcriptome of *Cannabis sativa*. *Genome Biology*, **12**, R102.

Viggiano, D., Ruocco, L.A., Pignatelli, M., Grammatikopoulos, G., and Sadile, A. G. (2003). Prenatal elevation of endocannabinoids corrects the unbalance between dopamine systems and reduces activity in the Naples High Excitability rats. *Neuroscience and Biobehavior Reviews*, **27**, 129–139.

Volicer, L., Stelly, M., Morris, J., McLaughlin, J., and Volicer, B. J. (1997). Effects of dronabinol on anorexia and disturbed behavior in patients with Alzheimer's disease. *International Journal of Geriatric Psychiatry*, **12**, 913–919.

Vriend, H.J.D. (1984). *The Old English Herbarium and, Medicina de quadrupedibus*. London: Published for the Early English Text Society by the Oxford University Press.

Wade, D.T., Robson, P., House, H., Makela, P., and Aram, J. (2003). A preliminary controlled study to determine whether whole-plant cannabis extracts can improve intractable neurogenic symptoms. *Clinical Rehabilitation*, **17**, 18–26.

Ware, M.A., Wang, T., Shapiro, S., *et al.* (2010). Smoked cannabis for chronic neuropathic pain: a randomized controlled trial. *CMAJ*, **182**, E694–701.

Waring, E.J. (1897). *Remarks on the Uses of Some of the Bazaar Medicines and Common Medical Plants of India*. London: J. & A. Churchill.

Weil, A.T., Zinberg, N.E., and Nelsen, J.M. (1968). Clinical and psychological effects of marihuana in man. *Science*, **162**, 1234–1242.

Weiss, L., Zeira, M., Reich, S., *et al.* (2006). Cannabidiol lowers incidence of diabetes in non-obese diabetic mice. *Autoimmunity*, **39**, 143–151.

West, M.E. (1991). Cannabis and night vision. *Nature*, **351**, 703–704.

Westphall, R., Janssen, P., Lucas, P., and Capler, R. (2006). Survey of medicinal cannabis use among child-bearing women: patterns of its use in pregnancy and retroactive self-assessment of tis efficacy against 'morning sickness'. *Complementary Therapies in Clinical Practice*, **12**, 27–33.

Williams, S.J., Hartley, J.P., and Graham, J.D. (1976). Bronchodilator effect of delta1-tetrahydrocannabinol administered by aerosol of asthmatic patients. *Thorax*, **31**, 720–723.

Wilsey, B., Marcotte, T., Tsodikov, A., *et al.* (2008). A randomized, placebo-controlled, crossover trial of cannabis cigarettes in neuropathic pain. *Journal of Pain*, **9**, 506–521.

Wright, T.L. (1862). Correspondence. *Cincinnati Lancet and Observer*, **5**, 246–247.

Wright, T.L. (1863). Some therapeutic effects of *Cannabis indica*. *Cincinnati Lancet and Observer*, **6**, 73–75.

Zajicek, J., Fox, P., Sanders, H., *et al.* (2003). Cannabinoids for treatment of spasticity and other symptoms related to multiple sclerosis (CAMS study): multicentre randomised placebo-controlled trial. *Lancet*, **362**, 1517–1526.

Zheng, Y., Baek, J.H., Smith, P.F., and Darlington, C.L. (2007). Cannabinoid receptor down-regulation in the ventral cochlear nucleus in a salicylate model of tinnitus. *Hear Res*, **228**, 105–111.

Zias, J. (1995). *Cannabis sativa* (Hashish) as an effective medication in antiquity: the anthropological evidence. In: S. Campbell and A. Green (eds.). *The Archaeology of Death in the Ancient Near East*. Oxford: Oxbow Books, pp. 232–234.

Zias, J., Stark, H., Sellgman, J., *et al.* (1993). Early medical use of cannabis. *Nature*, **363**, 215.

Zotter, H. (1996). *Medicina antiqua: Codex Vindobonensis 93 der Österreichischen Nationalbibliothek: Kommentar*. Graz: Akademische Druck- u. Verlagsanstalt.

Zuardi, A.W., Cosme, R.A., Graeff, F.G., and Guimaraes, F.S. (1993). Effects of ipsapirone and cannabidiol on human experimental anxiety. *Journal of Psychopharmacology*, **7**, 82–88.

Zuardi, A.W., Morais, S.L., Guimaraes, F.S., and Mechoulam, R. (1995). Antipsychotic effect of cannabidiol [letter]. *Journal of Clinical Psychiatry*, **56**, 485–486.

Zuardi, A.W., Shirakawa, I., Finkelfarb, E., and Karniol, I. G. (1982). Action of cannabidiol on the anxiety and other effects produced by delta 9-THC in normal subjects. *Psychopharmacology*, **76**, 245–250.

Chapter 3

International Control of Cannabis

Alice P. Mead

3.1 Introduction

Over the centuries, many cultures have utilized preparations derived from the opium poppy (*Papaver somniferum*), cannabis plant (*Cannabis sativa*), and coca bush (*Erythroxylum coca*). These psychoactive substances were widely used in religious rituals, as indications of social status, as medications, and as intoxicants. Indeed, the lines between such uses were often blurred, particularly the line between medical and 'quasi-medical' (i.e., not prescribed by Western-trained physicians, such as home remedies, folk cures) use. For example, in India even into the twentieth century, the general population had little access to medical care provided by physicians, indigenous and traditional medical systems flourished, and home remedies and tonics were common. Treatment with herbal products was well accepted, and an organized, robust medical "profession" did not exist (I.C. Chopra and Chopra 1957; R.N. Chopra and Chopra 1955; UNODC 1953).

As Westernized technology, science, and medicine progressed and became dominant, these lines became better defined for opium, coca, and their manufactured derivatives. However, greater technological advances were needed to investigate and develop the properties/potential of the cannabis plant (Crowther et al. 2010). As a result, cannabis and its preparations occupied an uncertain status, enjoying a brief period of interest in Western medicine, but not gaining a wide and lasting acceptance as a valuable tool in the medical armamentarium. Only recently has science evolved to the point where modern cannabis-derived medications have been properly characterized and developed and their value recognized by the medical profession. Nevertheless, the criteria remain elusive for determining how, and whether, lines should be drawn between their various uses.

3.2 The role of Britain in early attitudes about cannabis and cannabis medicines

Britain has played an important role over time in several aspects of the cannabis issue. During the late eighteenth and nineteenth centuries, the East India Company and later the colonial government in India were confronted with the fact that both cannabis preparations and opium were widely employed for a variety of purposes: medical, "quasi/alternative," and nonmedical (Booth 2004; I.C. Chopra and Chopra 1957; Mills 2003).

At home in Britain, hemp was well known as an important and useful plant. Its fiber was manufactured into sails, cordage, and a variety of other textile and naval products which were essential to a maritime and imperial power. Until the studies of William B. O'Shaughnessy were published in the 1830s and 1840s (O'Shaughnessy 1839), physicians had much less knowledge of, or interest in, the use of tetrahydrocannabinol-containing strains of cannabis either as intoxicants or as medicines. However, in subsequent decades, cannabis preparations began to be utilized extensively as medications both in Europe and North America (Mills 2003).

3.2.1 **Britain and the Indian cannabis and opium commissions**

During this time, the British Parliament was under assault by anti-opium forces, and cannabis was swept into the campaign. In response, Parliament required the colonial Government of India to establish two commissions: a Royal Commission on opium to investigate whether the opium trade could be abolished and the economic impact of doing so, as well as the extent of consumption in India; and a commission to investigate the "ganja question": the Indian Hemp Drugs Commission (IHDC). Meeting almost concurrently in 1893–1894, these commissions enabled Parliament to divert attention away from the real question, i.e., the British India Government's supplying of vast quantities of opium to China in violation of Chinese law (Mills 2003).

The IHDC concluded that moderate use of cannabis drugs had no appreciable physical effects on the body, no harmful effect on the brain (except possibly for individuals predisposed to act abnormally), and no adverse influence on morality (Abel 1980; Booth 2004). Rather than attempt to prohibit production and use, the IHDC stated that the government should do nothing to promote moderate use or encourage smuggling, or force individuals to use more hazardous substances, and should actively discourage excessive use. In short, it recommended a system of taxation, control, and restriction (Mills 2003).

The Royal Opium Commission reached parallel conclusions. It determined that the use of smoking opium was rare in India; most use was oral, and misuse was a "negligible feature" in Indian life. Opium was taken for various disorders and as a general stimulant in those of "failing strength." It found "strong evidence" indicating moderation on the part of the consumer and "general immunity from any evident ill effects," even from habitual use. The Commission opined that it would be impractical to limit opium consumption to strictly medical purposes and that "alternative" medical and nonmedical uses were so entwined with medical uses that no distinct line could be drawn between the two (R.N. Chopra and Chopra 1955).

After the two commissions had issued their reports, cannabis faded from attention in Parliament.

3.3 **The impact of nineteenth-century scientific developments**

European medical journals paid little heed to the IHDC report (Mills 2003) but, as a result of several factors, the popularity of cannabis as a medicine peaked at the end of the nineteenth century and then gradually declined (Crowther et al. 2010). Various major developments were changing the way that Westerners viewed medical treatment, and therefore, "legitimate" scientific and medical products, purposes, and uses. This perspective was of pivotal importance during the development of international drug control measures and, therefore, in the control of the cannabis plant.

3.3.1 **Technology and single molecules**

Improved technology facilitated the study of pharmacology and organic chemistry and the isolation of active ingredients from natural products, as well as the synthesis of pure molecules (Anderson 2005). In 1805, morphine was identified and isolated by Freidrich Serturner, and soon thereafter, the development of the hypodermic needle permitted rapid production of its analgesic effect (Musto 1987). Later in the century, aspirin provided another source of pain relief. Other synthetic medicines, such as barbiturates and chloral hydrate, and certain vaccines, etc., were developed. A pharmaceutical industry appeared to manufacture and commercialize many of these products. Increasingly, complex, unrefined herbal medicines were eclipsed by manufactured medications containing only one isolated or synthetic primary active ingredient.

Cannabis proved to be a significant challenge for the current technology. Despite the efforts of researchers in Britain and across Europe to identify and isolate the active intoxicating ingredient of cannabis, it remained elusive (Crowther et al. 2010; Mechoulam 1973; Walton 1938). Preparations were unstandardized and unstable, and patient response was variable (Abel 1980; I.C. Chopra and Chopra 1957). In light of the proliferation of other more reliable options available to them, practicing physicians gradually lost interest in prescribing such preparations (Adams 1942/1973). Modern medicine gradually left cannabis behind, in both Europe and North America. Hence, when cannabis was swept into the controversy over drug control in the international arena, the medical profession did not rise up vigorously and consistently in its defense.

3.3.2 The ascendancy of professional pharmaceutical influence

The gradual ascendancy of pharmacy and other organized health professions in Europe and, later, North America further narrowed the concept of "medical use." The growth of these professions was an important factor in the implementation of domestic control over opium/opium preparations and cannabis. For example, the newly formed Pharmaceutical Society in Britain had a professional incentive to support legislation such as the Pharmacy Act of 1868. The Act gave registered pharmacists the responsibility for the identification and regulation/distribution of poisons and other dangerous drugs, including opium and cannabis (Anderson 2005). This authority gave them a competitive advantage over unregistered druggists, grocers, and others who tried to sell these substances to the public (Musto 1987). In Germany, the Pharmacy Ordinance of 1872 limited the sale of cannabis by pharmacies (Ballotta et al. 2008). Thus, the principle that psychoactive drugs should be used only for medical purposes (as defined by Western medicine) was gaining acceptance in European nations and would eventually become a foundational principle of international drug control conventions.

3.4 The development of international control mechanisms

In the first decades of the twentieth century, interest was growing in international cooperation on matters of mutual concern, and opium was one of the primary targets of attention.

3.4.1 The years 1900–1925

An international conference in Shanghai (1909), followed by a convention in The Hague (1912), resulted in early attempts to control international trade in opium. During the deliberations, the US sought to convince the colonial powers to adopt a narrow definition of "legitimate use" of opium, which would preclude any use not defined as medical or scientific according to Western standards. The colonial powers, however, advocated for a broader approach. These concepts would come to play an important role in the future control of cannabis (Abel 1980; Mills 2003; Sinha 2001).

The demands of World War I eclipsed international interest in drug control issues. However, following the end of hostilities, concerns over opium and manufactured drugs re-emerged. Two conferences were held in Geneva in 1924 and 1925. During the Second Opium Conference, cannabis was not on the agenda, but the Egyptian delegate objected that hashish was "at least as harmful as opium" and should be included in the same category as the other narcotics under discussion (Booth 2004; Bruun et al. 1975). He contended that hashish was the "principal cause of most of the cases of insanity occurring in Egypt" (Mills 2003; Sinha 2001). As a result, provisions requiring the imposition of import/export controls over trade in cannabis and the prevention of illicit traffic in cannabis and resin were incorporated into the treaty. Subsequently, cannabis extracts or tinctures were also brought within its purview (Bruun et al. 1975; UNODC 1962). For the first time, then, cannabis and cannabis preparations came under international control.

3.4.2 The years 1926–1961

Drugs continued to be smuggled through nonsignatory countries, and over the next 35+ years, two more treaties (1931 and 1936 Geneva Conventions) and several protocols were promulgated. The need for a single, consolidated treaty instrument became evident. Cannabis was a matter of increasing attention and concern. The World Health Organization (WHO) in 1954 reported that cannabis and cannabis preparations had become obsolete and were little used by the medical profession (Wayne 1968, Append. 2). Furthermore, most nations had gradually come to endorse the principle that the consumption of opium (and, by analogy, other psychoactive plants) should be restricted exclusively to medical and scientific needs (UNODC 1953). Even in non-Western countries, such as India, the use of cannabis preparations in modern medical practice declined and, by the late 1950s, they were "hardly used" (I.C. Chopra and Chopra 1957). Consequently, the future of cannabis as a medicine appeared bleak.

3.4.3 The 1961 United Nations (UN) Single Convention on Narcotic Drugs

The 1961 UN Single Convention on Narcotic Drugs maintained the requirements of prior conventions relating to licensing, reporting of national estimates of drug requirements and statistical returns, and establishing limits on production and manufacture, etc. Moreover, it extended control systems to the plants cultivated to provide the raw materials for narcotic drugs.

The Convention's Preamble established two, competing foundational principles: (1) drug abuse is a scourge and parties must limit exclusively to medical and scientific purposes the production, manufacture, export/import, distribution, trade, use, and possession of drugs; and (2) the use of psychoactive substances for medical and scientific purposes is indispensable and their availability for such purposes should not be unduly restricted.

Psychoactive substances, i.e., "drugs," were placed in one of four schedules. These controlled substance schedules were distinct from those established under the national laws of most Western countries, e.g., the US and the UK. The Single Convention's Schedule I was not the most restrictive of its Schedules; rather it set forth the restrictions and requirements that applied to many drugs.

The most restrictive level of control was imposed by Schedule IV, which contained drugs viewed as being particularly dangerous with regard to their abuse liability and as having extremely limited therapeutic value. All drugs listed in Schedule IV were also listed in Schedule I. Hence, it was this joint placement in Schedules IV and I that imposed the greatest degree of control under the Convention. With regard to Schedule IV drugs, under Article 2, paragraph 5, a Party was required to (1) adopt any *special measures of control* that *in its opinion* were necessary, taking into account the particularly dangerous properties of the drug; and (2) *if in its opinion* the prevailing conditions in its country rendered it the most appropriate means of protecting the public health and welfare, *prohibit* the production, manufacture, export and import of, trade in, possession or use of any such drugs *except for amounts which may be necessary to medical and scientific research only*. Therefore, parties were empowered, but not necessarily required, completely to prohibit Schedule IV substances. Subsequently, many countries chose to enact prohibitory legislation.

The Single Convention explicitly brought within its control the cannabis plant, resin, extracts, and tinctures. Cannabis and cannabis resin were placed in Schedules IV and I (Table 3.1).

Table 3.1 Scheduling of cannabis and cannabinoids under UK, US, and international treaty law

Material	Single Convention	Psychotropic Convention	UK Misuse of Drugs Regulations	UK Misuse of Drugs Act	US Controlled Substances Act
Cannabis/resin	Schedule I and IV	–	Schedule I	Schedule 2, Part II, Class B	Schedule I
Cannabis extracts/ tincture	Schedule I	–	Schedule I	Schedule 2, Part II, Class B	Schedule I
MHRA-approved extracts	Schedule I	–	Schedule 4.1	Schedule 2, Part II, Class B	Schedule I
Pure THC	–	Schedule I	Schedule 2	Schedule 2, Part II, Class B	Schedule I
Dronabinol/Δ^9-THC	–	Schedule II	Schedule 2	Schedule 2, Part II, Class B	Schedule III
Pure CBD	–	Not scheduled	Not scheduled	Not scheduled	Schedule I
Other non-THC pure cannabinoids	–	Not scheduled	Not scheduled	Not scheduled	Schedule I

However, cannabis extracts and tinctures were listed only in Schedule I; therefore, they were not governed by the more restrictive provisions of Schedule IV. Nevertheless, cannabis extracts and tinctures could only be used for "medical and scientific purposes." Since these substances had been abandoned by the medical profession, this criterion, at the time, appeared effectively to prohibit their use.

Under Articles 23, 26, and 28, countries that permitted cultivation (or importation) of the opium poppy, cannabis plant, or coca bush were required to establish a national monopoly that would take possession of and distribute the crops. Furthermore, if the "prevailing conditions" in the country were to render the prohibition of such cultivation the "most suitable measure, *in its opinion*, for protecting the public health and welfare and preventing diversion," Article 22, paragraph 1 *obligated* the party to prohibit cultivation.

Parties to the Single Convention were required (or empowered) to enact domestic legislation to enforce its requirements. Article 36, paragraph 1(a) mandated each signatory, subject to its constitutional limitations, to establish measures to ensure that activities (including cultivation, production, manufacture, extraction, preparation, possession, offering, offering for sale, distribution, purchase, sale, transport, importation, and exportation) contrary to the treaty would be punishable offences, and that serious offences would be liable to adequate punishment particularly by imprisonment or other penalties of deprivation of liberty. Following a 1972 amendment, the Single Convention, Article 36, paragraph 2(b), permitted parties to provide to drug abusers, as an alternative/in addition to conviction or punishment, treatment, or other nonpunitive options.

3.4.4 The 1971 UN Convention on Psychotropic Substances

The Single Convention did not encompass newer synthetic psychotropic substances, and use of these drugs was on the increase, thereby necessitating a new system of international control. The 1971 UN Convention on Psychotropic Substances was modelled after the Single Convention. The Psychotropic Convention also classified substances into four schedules, but the structure differed from the Single Convention. Schedule I was the most restrictive and Schedule IV the most lenient.

With regard to Schedule I substances, Article 7 required parties, among other things, to prohibit all use except for scientific and very limited medical purposes by duly authorized persons, in medical or scientific facilities that are directly under the control of, or specifically approved (and closely supervised) by, the government.

Tetrahydrocannabinol and its isomers were originally classified in Schedule I. In 1991, dronabinol (also known as delta-9-tetrahydrocannabinol) was moved to Schedule II (ECDD 2006). Other synthetic or otherwise pure cannabinoids, such as cannabidiol (CBD), were not controlled under the Psychotropic Convention (Table 3.1). Accordingly, many countries do not control such pure cannabinoids under their national laws, but other nations, such as the US, have chosen to do so.

Like the Single Convention, the 1971 Convention required a party, subject to its constitutional limitations, to enact legislation classifying an action contrary to the treaty as a punishable offence and ensuring that serious offences must be liable to adequate punishment, particularly by imprisonment or other deprivation of liberty. Nevertheless, Article 22, paragraph 1(b) offered a savings clause, allowing parties to provide treatment, education, aftercare, rehabilitation and social reintegration either as an *alternative* to conviction or punishment, or *in addition to* punishment, when dealing with an *individual* drug abuser.

3.4.5 1988 UN Convention against Illicit Traffic in Narcotic Drugs and Psychotropic Substances

As international drug trafficking escalated, it became apparent that additional control mechanisms were necessary. The 1988 UN Convention Against Illicit Traffic in Narcotic Drugs and Psychotropic Substances addressed a number of new matters, including money laundering, asset seizure, agreements on mutual legal assistance (in investigations, prosecutions and judicial proceedings), and the diversion of precursor chemicals.

The enforcement provisions of the 1988 Convention have been the source of considerable commentary and controversy. With regard to offences and sanctions, Article 3, paragraph 1, of the 1988 Convention required a party, among other things, to make the cultivation of the opium poppy, coca bush or cannabis plant, *in violation of the 1961 Convention*, a criminal offence. This requirement is *not* explicitly subject to a country's constitutional principles and the basic concepts of its legal system (but would be subject implicitly to many of the exceptions and qualifications of the 1961 treaty, such as the requirement that legitimate research be allowed). However, pursuant to paragraph 4(c), in appropriate cases of a minor nature in paragraph 1, the parties were permitted to provide, as alternatives to conviction or punishment, such options as education, rehabilitation, or social reintegration, as well as, when the offender is a drug abuser, treatment and aftercare. In nonminor offences, such alternatives could only be provided in addition to punishment.

Under Article 3, paragraph 2, possession of drugs for personal consumption was also to be made a criminal offence under national law, but the qualifying language does limit this obligation. Furthermore, under paragraph 4(d), a party may provide alternative options, either in addition to, or as an alternative to, conviction or punishment.

Accordingly, as one author has noted, "The 1988 Convention clearly offers alternative ways of dealing with persons possessing, purchasing or cultivating small amounts of drug for [their] own consumption" (Krajeski 2000, p. 335).

3.5 How absolute are the treaty obligations?

Out of respect for the autonomy of countries' domestic laws, all of the treaties contain qualifying ("loophole") language that can mitigate certain of their legal obligations. Under the Single

Convention, for example, a party must prohibit the production and use of Schedule IV substances (such as cannabis) *if in its opinion* the prevailing conditions render prohibition the most appropriate means of protecting the public health and welfare. Of course, such a qualifier is not completely open-ended. The Vienna Convention on the Law of Treaties of 1969 obliges parties to interpret treaties in good faith and to respect the object and purpose of all Conventions (Ballotta et al. 2008; Bewley-Taylor 2003).

Other obligations, particularly those relating to the duty to enact criminal and other penalties for certain acts, are often qualified by the following language: "Subject to its constitutional principles and the basic concepts of its legal system" (Bewley-Taylor and Jelsma 2012). This provision has come into play in a number of cases. For example, Canadian courts have ruled that, under the Canadian Charter, individuals with a bona fide need to use cannabis for medical purposes cannot be penalized or denied access to the substance (*Regina v Parker* 2000). The Constitutional Court of Colombia in 1994 invalidated a law criminalizing possession of cannabis for personal consumption (Krajeski 2000). A number of nations, particularly in Latin America, have been actively considering whether such qualifying language would permit them to revise their drug control laws.

This qualification is also relevant in a country with a federal structure, in which states or provinces have a significant degree of legislative and judicial autonomy, such as the US and Australia. In the US, federal law is the supreme law of the land. State laws that actively impede or conflict with federal law are invalid under Article VI, clause 2 (the Supremacy Clause) of the US Constitution (*Emerald Steel Fabricators, Inc. v Bureau of Labor and Industries* 2010). On the other hand, states are free to repeal their own laws, and, in addition, cannot criminalize conduct that is found to be protected by state courts under the state constitution, as is the case in Alaska (*Ravin v State* 1975). Furthermore, in the US, the courts have ruled that federal government cannot "commandeer" states to enact laws or otherwise take action to implement federal law (*New York v United States* 1992; *Printz v United States* 1997). The International Narcotics Control Board (INCB) has taken note of this complex problem (INCB 2012). However, it is uncertain how a nation should deal with such a situation, other than attempting to exert its influence over the states/provinces (perhaps through the exercise of other powers, such as the power to withhold federal funding for state programs) and/or utilizing its own resources to enforce national law (if there is a national law on the subject).

Finally, the concept of "expediency" or prosecutorial discretion may be considered to be one of the basic principles of a country's legal system. As a result of limited resources or other considerations, a country (or state/province or local subdivision therein) may de-prioritize certain types of prosecutions, either by formal guidance or on a case-by-case basis. The Dutch relied in part on the expediency principle in issuing national prosecutorial guidelines that, under certain circumstances, permit the retail sale of cannabis in "coffee houses." Nevertheless, this approach also must be applied with circumspection, and perhaps only to minor offences, since it could be employed to avoid any or perhaps all international obligations, thereby undermining the entire treaty system. "It would be enough to introduce certain provisions and at the same time to forget about them" (Krajeski 2000, p. 336).

3.6 How have nations interpreted and implemented their obligations?

Over the past two or more decades, many countries have, either by law or in practice, lessened the penalties that attach to certain cannabis-related conduct (MacCoun and Reuter 2001). For the most part, this greater leniency has been applied to possession of cannabis for personal consumption, although the scope of "personal use" may also be variously defined with regard to, e.g., quantities of, and locations where, cannabis that may be possessed, and whether cultivation of small amounts is allowed (EMCDDA 2012f). In many countries, it is increasingly unlikely that first-time cannabis offenders will face jail time for possession. However, significant criminal sanctions generally still apply to supply-type activities, such as larger-scale cultivation, possession of significant amounts with intent to sell, etc. (EMCDDA 2012e). These legal reforms have been instituted either *de jure* (in written law) or de facto (in practice). There is considerable discussion among scholars over the appropriate analytical framework for classifying such changes.

3.6.1 Depenalization

This concept has been described as legal changes that reduce the severity of penalties, whether criminal or civil (Pacula et al. 2004). Under many of these schemes, possession remains a criminal offence, but in most cases, offenders are cautioned or diverted to alternative resources, including education, treatment, etc. Depending on the jurisdiction, diversion can occur at various stages of the criminal prosecution. Offenders will still therefore often incur a criminal record of arrest or conviction (Room et al. 2010). Indeed, in many US states that reduced or eliminated criminal penalties for cannabis possession, arrests for such conduct actually rose (Pacula et al. 2004).

In some countries, the law states that the penalty for a certain activity, e.g., possessing a controlled drug, will depend on the type or classification of the drug in question. Cannabis may specifically be placed in a category or schedule that does not incur the most severe penalties. For example, cannabis is classified in Class B of the UK Misuse of Drugs Act, a class that incurs intermediate penalties (Table 3.1). In the Netherlands, cannabis products are listed in Schedule II of the Opium Act, whereas "hard" drugs are in Schedule I. In the US, sanctions under federal law generally depend on the schedule of the substance, although some specific penalties apply to cannabis.

In other countries, the law (at least as written) applies the same punishment for an activity, no matter which substance is involved. However, there often is a discrepancy between the formal legal texts and actual (de facto) practice. Courts do consider the nature of the substance, quantity and any aggravating or other factors when sentencing, either using their discretionary power or by applying a guideline, directive, or judicial precedent (EMCDDA 2012b).

In a federalized system, states or provinces may reduce criminal penalties under local law, even if a substance is restrictively scheduled at the national level. In the US over the past 40 years, a number of states have passed legislation reducing the status of the criminal offence of personal possession of cannabis from a felony to a misdemeanor, although cannabis remains in Schedule I of the federal Controlled Substances Act (MacCoun and Reuter 2001; Pacula et al. 2004; Room et al. 2010) (Table 3.1).

In some cases, the scheduling system determining criminal penalties may be different from the one governing the availability of drugs for medical use. In the UK, cannabis is a Class B substance under Schedule 2, Part II, of the Misuse of Drugs Act 1971 (the intermediate classification), but it is a Schedule 1 substance under the Misuse of Drugs Regulations 2001 (the most restrictive schedule), which determine access to a substance for research or for medical prescription or supply (Table 3.1).

3.6.2 Decriminalization

This widely used term may perhaps most accurately be applied to changes which retain the illegal status of cannabis possession/use, but which transform it from a criminal to a noncriminal or civil offence, making it a subcategory of depenalization (Pacula et al. 2004; Room et al. 2010). A non-criminal punishment may involve a fine, a citation, diversion to counselling or treatment, or some other administrative sanction, such as loss of a driver's license. This change in character or status may only apply to certain minor offences. An example of this is Portugal, which in 2001 removed from the criminal law all personal possession, use, and acquisition of drugs. Possession is still illegal, and offenders are channeled to "Commissions for the Dissuasion of Drug Addictions," which offer treatment, but can also impose other penalties. Personal possession amounts are defined (EMCDDA 2011; Room et al. 2010). Some Australian jurisdictions also employ this model, under which only civil penalties attach to minor possession cases and, in some jurisdictions, small-scale cultivation (Room et al. 2010). In some countries, such as Luxembourg, consumption of cannabis is not a criminal offence, unless it occurs in front of/with minors, in the workplace, or in schools (EMCDDA 2012). However, in most jurisdictions, possession/ cultivation of larger quantities and distribution/sale are still criminal offences (Commission of the European Communities 2009; EMCDDA 2012e).

Civil penalty schemes are not without problems. Because of the ease with which police may issue notices, a type of "net widening" may result, with a greater number of people being cited. Since a large percentage of individuals fail to pay their fines when due, the effect can be to "increase the numbers at risk of criminal sanction for nonpayment of fines, an outcome that can particularly disadvantage those with limited financial means" (Room et al. 2010, p. 115). Abuses of the system may also occur, such as criminal gangs aggregating small cultivation plots to avoid incurring the criminal penalties that would attach to cultivation for supply (Room et al. 2010).

Legal commentary is mixed on the extent to which various decriminalization or depenalization schemes comport with the Conventions. In general, scholars believe that depenalization or decriminalization of possession for personal consumption, particularly of cannabis, is permissible under the treaties, although depenalization, which retains the criminal character of an act, may be more defensible (Krajeski 2000).

3.6.3 Legalization

Various descriptions have also been applied to the concept of "legalization." In general, legalization denotes that an activity is not illegal and therefore incurs no sanctions, criminal or civil. The scope of legalization could be narrow or broad and could take place by means of legislation or judicial ruling. For example, individual possession and cultivation of small amounts of cannabis for personal use could be legalized in certain locations, such as small amounts in the home (*Ravin v State* 1975). Possession in other circumstances or involving large amounts, or larger scale cultivation and distribution might still be unlawful. Farther along the continuum, a system of commercial cultivation and manufacturing, wholesale distribution and retail sales could be permitted, with attendant taxation, licensure, and governmental regulation and oversight, including limits on advertising. At the farthest end of the continuum, cannabis could be produced, sold, and consumed like coffee, although even here there would likely be regulations pertaining to quality, safety, and content of the products and, no doubt, limits on distribution to minors.

At this moment, Uruguay is the only country in the world permitting full commercialization of a cannabis trade, from "seed to shelf" (Room et al. 2010, Serrano et al. 2014). Uruguay permits individuals to obtain cannabis in one (only) of three ways: purchase up to 40 grams/month from registered pharmacies; cultivate up to 6 plants at home, with an annual maximum of 480 grams; or join a cannabis club, which can cultivate up to 99 plants per group with the same annual cap per member. The law took effect on May 6, 2014. Legal scholars generally agree that such a system falls afoul of the Single Convention, because it would authorize the use of cannabis for nonmedical purposes (Bewley-Taylor 2003). Nevertheless, in the face of pressing international and domestic economic pressures, and escalating violence resulting from the drug trade in Mexico and elsewhere, discussion of legalization has become more visible and widespread (Kilmer et al. 2010).

In a few countries, such as Spain, certain regions have permitted "cannabis social clubs" to flourish. Such noncommercial organizations cultivate and sell limited amounts of cannabis, only enough for the personal needs of their members, who pay membership fees proportionate to their consumption. Members may be subject to certain restrictions, such as agreeing not to distribute the cannabis to others (Room et al. 2010). Some supporters of this model believe that it is preferable to outright legalization (Alonso 2011).

In November, 2012, two voter initiatives in the US (Colorado and Washington) were passed, each having two aspects: (1) removal of all penalties for possession by adults of one ounce or less of cannabis for personal use (and in Colorado, cultivation of six plants), and (2) legalization of commercial cultivation, production, distribution, and sale of cannabis to adults. These events garnered tremendous international publicity and interest. On August 29, 2013, the US Department of Justice issued a guidance memorandum to federal prosecutors, indicating that they should not at present take enforcement action against cannabis-related activities that are authorized under state law and that do not adversely impact eight specified areas of federal priority. The sheer volume of sales or the for-profit status of an operation will not alone be triggers for federal prosecution. States, however, must implement strong and effective regulatory and enforcement systems to mitigate against threats to federal enforcement interests (DOJ 2013). It remains to be seen how the rest of the world will respond to this development and to the new Uruguayan program. In 2016, the UN General Assembly will review current policies and strategies to confront the global drug problem.

3.6.3.1 The unique case of the Netherlands

The Netherlands offers a unique blend of approaches. Beginning in 1976, the country reduced penalties for cannabis possession for personal use and ultimately allowed retail outlets called "coffee shops" to sell small quantities of cannabis. Formal national guidelines govern the scheme. The guidelines do not authorize cultivation and supply, creating what has been called the "backdoor problem" (Room et al. 2010, p. 95). This system has been described as "prohibition with an expediency principle" or "de facto legalisation," because of the retail element (MacCoun and Reuter 2001, p. 246).

3.7 Is it possible to distinguish between medical and nonmedical use?

Both the Single Convention and the 1971 Psychotropic Convention obligate a country to take steps to ensure that cannabis and other psychoactive substances are manufactured, distributed, used, etc., exclusively for medical and scientific purposes. Therefore, with regard to cannabis, a nation must devise regulatory or other tools to distinguish medical from nonmedical and, perhaps, "alternative" medical applications. At one end of the continuum, it could be determined (as Dennis Peron, a prominent US cannabis advocate, famously claimed) that "all use [of cannabis] is medical" (Rendon 2012). At the other end, medical use could be limited solely to a product that is prescribed by a physician and dispensed by a pharmacy, and that has achieved marketing authorization from the national regulatory authority. As with their criminal and/or civil sanctioning schemes, governments have taken different approaches to this question.

3.7.1 Classification or scheduling as a tool

Under many domestic regulatory laws, a particular scheduling is often necessary, but not sufficient, for medical access. In most cases, the national pharmaceutical regulatory process, which governs the registration of new medications, also must be completed in order for a rescheduled/classified product containing a controlled drug to be prescribed and dispensed. In the UK, dronabinol (Marinol®) is in Schedule 2 of the Misuse of Drugs Regulations, but no dronabinol-containing product has been approved for marketing (although individual physicians may prescribe it on a "named patient" basis). In the US, opium and coca leaves are Schedule II substances, but all products containing, or derived from, those drugs have (or would need to secure) marketing approval from the US Food and Drug Administration (FDA) before they could be prescribed to patients.

If a country wishes to maintain an even stricter distinction between nonmedical and medical use of cannabis, it may place a registered cannabis-derived prescription medication into a different classification or schedule from unrefined herbal material (and other unapproved preparations) under its national controlled drugs legislation. This would be particularly appropriate for medications derived from cannabis extracts or tinctures, since these preparations are already less restrictively scheduled than herbal cannabis under the Single Convention. In Australia, the government rescheduled a specifically-described cannabis-derived medication (Sativex®) from Schedule 9 (prohibited drugs) to Schedule 8 (controlled but not prohibited), while cannabis remained in Schedule 9. Germany amended its narcotic law in May 2011 to permit the "use of cannabis preparations authorized in finished medicines." This change did not apply to herbal cannabis. The US took this approach in 1985, when the Drug Enforcement Administration (DEA) rescheduled a specific FDA-approved formulation of dronabinol (Marinol®) and placed it in Schedule II (and later III) of the US Controlled Substances Act (Table 3.1). All other tetrahydrocannabinol (THC) products remained in Schedule I. Such differential scheduling is not uncommon, and it is not limited to THC or cannabis. In the US, the illicit version of gamma hydroxybutyric acid (GHB) is a Schedule I substance. However, when formulated in an FDA-approved pharmaceutical product, it is classified in Schedule III (Neuman 2004).

3.7.2 Can "alternative" medical use be permitted?

The 1961 and 1971 Conventions appear to contemplate a fairly narrow concept of medical purpose and use. Accordingly, one could argue that a country's accepted medicinal product regulatory processes must be applied to cannabis and cannabis preparations; that is, no special exceptions should be afforded cannabis, without some convincing justification for the differential treatment.

3.7.2.1 Cannabis as an herb or dietary supplement?

Some cannabis advocates contend that cannabis is "a harmless herb," but such a claim may not accord with conventional regulatory criteria. First, potent psychoactive substances are generally not included within the class of herbs and dietary supplements. Second, in the US, UK, and the European Union overall, an item becomes a medical product or "drug" subject to rigorous regulation, in part if it is intended to be used in the treatment, diagnosis, prevention, or mitigation of a disease or condition (MHRA 2012a, 2012b). Thus, if the manufacturer or retailer makes medical claims for the item, those claims may transform the item into a medical product (FDA 2011, 2012). Ojai berries, vitamin C, and wheatgrass juice could, in theory, "become" medical products.

Such products may only be marketed after extensive preclinical studies and properly controlled clinical trials have developed robust proof of quality, safety, and efficacy. A quick survey of the Internet demonstrates that cannabis manufacturers and distributor-dispensaries often disseminate medical claims and patient testimonials, which would normally move their cannabis preparations into the category of products that must be registered as conventional medicines.

Many believe that the current regulatory schemes governing herbal products do not adequately protect consumers (Cohen 2005). For example, herbal practitioners may not be licensed or regulated (MHRA 2012). In the US, under the Dietary Supplement Health and Education Act, herbs are subject to a much lower degree of regulatory scrutiny. In many cases, manufacturers fail to adhere even to these lesser quality control standards and other requirements. As a result, contaminated, mislabeled, or otherwise inferior products can be placed on the market (FDA 2011; OIG 2012; Schneeman et al. 2005). There is a serious concern whether this regulatory path should be extended to cannabis-containing medicinal products.

3.7.2.2 Cannabis via compassionate access?

Another option might be a type of compassionate access scheme, monitored by physicians. However, if such a program does not require proper physician supervision, documentation, data collection, etc., the line between medical and alternative medical or nonmedical use may still be difficult to maintain. Several countries have implemented such programs. In some cases, this approach is viewed as only a temporary measure necessary to relieve suffering until properly characterized and standardized products can secure marketing registrations. The US Institute of Medicine (IOM) issued a report recommending, among other things, the short-term (less than 6 months) use of smoked cannabis for patients with debilitating symptoms under certain limited conditions (Joy et al. 1999). In the UK, the House of Lords Select Committee recommended that herbal cannabis be placed in Schedule 2 of the Misuse of Drugs Regulations so physicians could prescribe it on a named patient basis (House of Lords 1998). The UK government rejected that recommendation but several years later permitted a cannabis-derived pharmaceutical product (approved in Canada but not in the UK) to be made available to hundreds of patients by their physicians. The US briefly maintained a "Compassionate Access Investigational New Drug program," which provided cannabis to certain individual patients with various conditions who were monitored by their physicians (but this was closed to new patients in 1992) (Randall and O'Leary 1998).

In other cases, such programs are of much broader scope and duration, effectively constituting a completely separate system, which operates outside of standard regulatory processes. For example, in 2000, the Netherlands established the Office of Medicinal Cannabis (OMC). OMC licensed two cultivators to grow cannabis under controlled conditions (only one cultivator, Bedrocan®, is currently licensed), and in 2003, legislation was enacted to allow physicians to prescribe, and pharmacies to supply, such herbal cannabis to patients. The intention was ultimately to develop and register cannabis-based prescription medications. However, progress toward the development of a licensed medication has been slow. Furthermore, the program has been undermined because patients are free to purchase cannabis through "coffee shops" (Hazekamp 2006). Israel also has established a program to provide herbal cannabis to selected patients.

The INCB has criticized these alternative systems for accessing cannabis. It has opined that a country should not make or permit such extensive exceptions to its customary regulatory requirements, since the quality, safety, and efficacy of the materials and their dosage forms have not been properly determined (INCB 2003). Perhaps ironically, in the countries described earlier that maintain "alternative" medical access systems, a cannabis-derived pharmaceutical product is still required to pass through the standard, rigorous regulatory process in order to be registered as a prescription medication. This can be said to create a type of regulatory "cognitive dissonance."

Again, it can be argued that any compassionate access scheme should comport with other, similar programs already in place under national law. In Europe, several types of compassionate access are recognized. First, individual patients may access a medication on the initiative and responsibility of their treating physicians (who request the products directly from the manufacturer) on a "named-patient basis." Second, a government may permit access to a cohort of seriously ill patients, who have no conventional treatment options and cannot enroll in a clinical trial. Typically, the product is either the subject of a marketing application or is undergoing clinical trials (EMA 2007). Finally, patients who have previously participated in a clinical trial may be allowed to enter an expanded access or open-label extension study, which permits them to continue to use the investigational product. All of these access programs are limited in scope, involve products that have been manufactured to prescription quality and standards, and contrast sharply with the cannabis access programs described previously.

3.7.2.3 Maintaining the integrity of alternative cannabis access schemes

The challenges of maintaining the integrity of such alternative access systems can be significant. These challenges have become evident in the US, where 18 states and the District of Columbia have allowed the use of herbal cannabis for medical purposes with the "recommendation" of a physician or other type of healthcare provider (a Schedule I substance cannot be prescribed in the US). In the early days of these laws, physicians, fearful of possible federal law enforcement activity and lacking knowledge about the quality and composition of cannabis products, were reluctant to recommend these materials to their patients. In addition, the first laws permitted only patients and their actual caregivers to cultivate cannabis; dispensaries were rare. Subsequently, however, many physicians discovered that there was an economic opportunity in issuing recommendations, and a cottage industry developed (Lopez 2009; Rendon 2012). In addition, dispensaries opened, either because they were directly authorized under state law or because state law was interpreted to be ambiguous. As a result, the numbers of patients exploded, many having a self-diagnosis (Caplan 2012).

Other countries may face related challenges. Canada, as a result of a series of court rulings, has established a government-sponsored program to cultivate and provide cannabis for medical use. A national agency, the Office of Marihuana Medical Access, regulates the production and distribution of herbal cannabis; qualifying patients, with their physician's approval, may seek permission to grow their own, designate a surrogate cultivator, or obtain the government's cannabis through the Marihuana Medical Access Regulations (MMAR) (Health Canada 2001). Many individuals contend that the Health Canada system is cumbersome and that the government's cannabis is of lesser quality than that offered by such dispensaries (Lucas 2008). In addition to the government-regulated system, a parallel system of dispensaries or "compassion centers" exists outside the law. So long as such nonofficial sources of access flourish, it is difficult for a national government to ensure that cannabis is being used strictly for legitimate medical (or even "alternative" medical) purposes in accordance with the Single Convention.

Removing the government from the system altogether may not resolve the problem. Canada is now considering changes to the MMAR, which would effectively remove Health Canada's role in: (1) determining who may access cannabis and (2) providing a source of material. Individuals would submit a document from a physician, specifying the individual's authorized daily quantity, to one of a number of licensed cultivators. There would no longer be any limits on qualifying medical conditions (Health Canada 2012). Since little evidence supports the medical use of smoked or otherwise inhaled herbal cannabis in other than a few medical conditions, it is unlikely that this system would comport with the country's other alternative access systems, such as its Special Access Programme (Health Canada 2002, 2008).

3.8 What factors will affect future access?

Controversy over the medical, "alternative" medical, and/or nonmedical use of cannabis and cannabinoids continues to grow in intensity. Competing concerns and developments will affect the future accessibility of cannabis for any, or all, purposes.

3.8.1 The impact of the Internet

The Internet will continue to play a significant role. Previously, information gathering and distribution were difficult. Newspapers and television were the primary vehicles for broad public communication, and even those would reach a limited and often local audience. By contrast, the Internet has allowed information and advocacy to be disseminated instantly to an international audience. This has facilitated increased membership in, and fundraising by, advocacy groups, enabling them to organize effectively and expand their influence amongst, not only the public, but also government representatives and other policymakers and opinion leaders. Particularly in the US, their greater sophistication has allowed them to utilize a panoply of state and local vehicles for legal and social change that have a cumulative impact over time: organizing state and local initiative processes, pressuring local jurisdictions to de-prioritize cannabis law enforcement, etc. Internet communication has also allowed a "community" of individuals to develop. Chat rooms and list-serves enable the participants to share ideas, opinions, experiences (both positive and negative), and even drug "recipes." Individuals who might otherwise feel isolated instead experience support and obtain encouragement for their activities, ideas, and opinions. Improved coordination and increased influence may result in more liberalized cannabis policies.

3.8.2 Growing international influence of non-governmental organizations (NGOs)

The influence of drug reform NGOs and drug policy institutes/entities has expanded, and they have a consistent and conspicuous presence at the annual meetings of the Commission on Narcotic Drugs. Many of these groups, such as the Transnational Institute and the International Drug Policy Consortium, publish legal and policy analyses favorable to drug policy reform, testify during open sessions, and issue position papers and recommendations that garner considerable media attention. For example, in 2011, the Global Commission on Drug Policy (GCDP) issued a report entitled *War on Drugs* in which the members made a number of recommendations for changes to the international system of drug control (GCDP 2011). GCDP was convened in July 2010 and has been working to establish a road map for change in drug laws and policies around the world (GCDP 2012).

3.8.3 Increasing variety and sophistication of cannabis products

The proliferation of cannabis dispensaries, clubs, or other distribution sources, has spawned a cannabis industry, complete with a wide range of products. These products offer alternatives to smoking, such as vaporizers and e-cigarettes. This technology has made it possible to partake of cannabis inhalation in various environments that would not permit smoking. For those who do not wish conspicuously to consume cannabis in the presence of their children or in public spaces, a variety of "infused" products, such as beverages and edibles, are available. Some companies claim to have products (albeit often of variable composition and quality) that are high in CBD and low in THC, which purport to provide therapeutic relief without intoxication. This wider product choice may expand the numbers of cannabis consumers.

3.8.4 Improved technology permitting the development of complex cannabis-derived prescription medications

In the face of improved technological tools, national regulatory agencies, such as the UK Medicines and Healthcare products Regulatory Agency (MHRA) and the US FDA, have demanded increasingly sophisticated levels of manufacturing quality control, batch-to-batch consistency, extensive characterization, and pharmacological and other types of preclinical product testing to ensure the quality and safety (and, of course, efficacy) of prescription medications. These standards were developed primarily for new chemical entities (NCEs), for which the path to registration has become prolonged, arduous, and expensive, and pose a potentially formidable set of obstacles to products derived from complex botanical materials (Crowther et al. 2010). Nevertheless, recognition appears to be growing that such products, including those derived from cannabis, may be able to meet modern regulatory standards. Guidance from the US FDA sets forth the pathway for developing a botanical product into a prescription medicine (FDA 2004).

Furthermore, disillusionment with the "single molecule/single target" approach of the past 30 years may increase receptivity to the multifold activity of complex botanical extracts. The importance of micronutrients is well accepted in nutrition and agriculture. Modern medicine appears to be moving in the direction of multimodal cocktails of medications, such as the recent Gilead "4-in-1" AIDS treatment product (Stribild®); however, with NCEs, this approach is hugely difficult and expensive. The development of complex extracts (properly standardized and quality-controlled) may offer this synergy at a lower cost (Russo 2011).

3.8.5 Impact of legalization or decriminalization on "medical marijuana"

As indicated previously (section 3.6.3), it is too soon to tell if the legalization initiatives in the US states of Colorado and Washington will sweep the country and the world. If commercial production and supply of cannabis do become more commonplace, there may very well be an impact on programs that currently permit the sale and use of herbal cannabis for medical purposes. In the US, it is hard to imagine that individuals will seek and pay for a cannabis recommendation from a physician, who may not provide anything in the way of care (e.g., treatment plan, diagnostic tests, follow-up supervision, etc.). There may be little incentive for cannabis advocates to continue to expend time and resources to pass state "medical marijuana" initiatives or to convince state and federal legislatures to enact such legislation. Similarly, such groups, other than the few that are solely devoted to medical access, would have little reason to provide extensive information on the Internet, describing the results of new cannabinoid studies on medical uses. Since physicians would no longer be the gatekeepers to an individual's legal access to cannabis, they would no longer be under pressure to consider herbal cannabis as a treatment option, particularly since unregistered cannabis products cannot in most countries be prescribed and reimbursed by national health insurance. Unless consumer demand for CBD products were significant, the current publicity surrounding the development of high-CBD strains and products may take a back seat to promotion and further diversification of high-THC preparations. As one manufacturer of cannabis products opined, "Medical will be phased out; instead of 100,000 patients, we will have 1,000,000 customers" (Keber 2012).

On the other hand, if legalization or decriminalization provisions are limited in scope, e.g., permitting only the possession and exchange of small amounts of cannabis without remuneration, there will continue to be incentives to maintain and expand the number of jurisdictions that allow production and supply for medical use (Kampia 2012).

3.8.6 Growing interest in "alternative" medical products and services

Despite the potential pitfalls of loosely regulated dietary supplements, public interest in vitamins, minerals, and herbal medicines continues to grow. Even in countries with nationalized healthcare, cost pressures have often made it difficult for patients to access certain types of medical interventions in a timely way. In the US, patients spend a hasty few minutes with their physicians, with whom they are unlikely to have had a longstanding relationship; pharmaceutical companies are portrayed by the media as mercenary giants, willing to seduce physicians with gifts, to conceal negative safety information about their products, and to engage in inappropriate product promotion (Angell 2005). Product recalls have frightened patients who believed that their national regulatory systems were adequate to protect them against dangerous side effects or contaminated products (EMA 2008; GAO 2009). A return to home-grown remedies or sources outside "the system" has considerable public appeal. Such public pressure may increasingly revive the historical concept of "alternative" (or "quasi") medical use, and allow cannabis preparations increasingly to slip past conventional regulatory regimes.

On the other hand, the price of these "remedies" may deter users. Various sources indicate that the average individual using cannabis for medicinal purposes consumes 2.2 g per day. At many dispensaries, the average cost of herbal cannabis is about $13 per g. Therefore, the average (30-day) monthly cost is $858. Vernacular CBD preparations are also costly, especially considering that many patients use several hundred grams of CBD per day. For example, a daily dose of 300–800 mg of CBD (doses used in some clinical trials) may cost $2520–6720 per 30-day month (Dixie Botanicals 2013), which is not covered by health insurance since the product is not FDA approved. Furthermore, the quality and potency of such products may be uncertain and often unreliable.

3.8.7 Additional factors

Numerous other factors may also significantly impact the scope of permissible cannabis use. In the US and a number of other countries, antismoking provisions increasingly limit the locations in which smoking can occur, such as multiunit dwellings, beaches and parks, university campuses, etc. (Allday 2012; HUD 2011). It is likely that such provisions would apply to smoking cannabis (particularly if mixed with tobacco, as occurs in many parts of the world). Concern about the dangers of "drugged driving" and workplace safety are also on the rise around the world, and expanded drug testing technology may significantly affect when a person may smoke or ingest cannabis without imperiling his/her employment or driving privileges (ELDD 2003; EMCDDA 2012c; EMCDDA 2012d). Fears about the link of cannabis use with harm to mental health and cognitive capacity may result in more restrictive policies. By contrast, the growing prominence of civil libertarianism as a political movement may support greater liberalization.

3.9 Conclusion

Cannabis has accurately been described as a "curious boundary substance, capable of shifting between the categories of licit medicine and illicit drug, and back again, depending on the different scientific, cultural or political understandings of the day" (Crowther et al. 2010. p. 4). Today, as in India in the nineteenth century, the lines between medical, "alternative" medical, and nonmedical use are indistinct, particularly in the US, creating significant challenges for rational and evidence-based regulation. What does the future hold? It is likely that a variety of cannabis-derived prescription medications may enter the conventional medical armamentarium. Cannabis legalization for recreational purposes may become widespread around the US and ultimately the rest of the world. In either case, it is possible, but not certain, that these lines will become more clearly demarcated.

References

Abel, E.L. (1980). *Marihuana: The First Twelve Thousand Years*. New York: Plenum Press, pp. 126–131.

ACMD (Advisory Committee on the Misuse of Drugs), Hallucinogens Subcommittee (Wayne, E. Chairman). (1968). *Report on Cannabis*. London: Home Office.

Adams, R. (1973). Marihuana. In: T.H. Mikuriya (ed.). *Marihuana: Medical Papers 1839–1972*. Oakland, CA: Medi-Comp Press, pp. 345–374. (Work originally published in 1942.)

Allday, E. (2012). UC system banning smoking from all campuses. *San Francisco Chronicle*, January 13.

Alonso, M.B. (2011). *Cannabis Social Clubs in Spain*. Series on Legislative Reform of Drug Policies Nr. 9. Transnational Institute. Available at: http://www.tni.org/sites/www.tni.org/files/download/dlr9.pdf (accessed November 20, 2013).

Anderson, S. (ed.). (2005). *Making Medicines*. London: Pharmaceutical Press.

Angell, M. (2005). *The Truth About Drug Companies: How They Deceive Us and What to Do About It*. New York: Random House.

Ballotta, D., Bergeron H., and Hughes, B. (2008). Cannabis control in Europe. In: S. Rödner Sznitman, B. Olsson, and R. Room (eds.). *A Cannabis Reader: Global Issues and Local Experiences*. Lisbon: EMCDDA, pp. 97–117.

Bewley-Taylor, D. and Jelsma, M. (2012). *The Limits of Latitude*. Series on Legislative Reform of Drug Policies Nr. 18. Transnational Institute. Available at: http://www.tni.org/sites/www.tni.org/files/download/dlr18.pdf (accessed September 19, 2012).

Bewley-Taylor, D.R. (2003). Challenging the UN drug control convention: problems and possibilities. *International Journal of Drug Policy*, **14**, 171–179.

Booth, M. (2004). *Cannabis: A History*. New York: St. Martin's Press.

Bruun, K., Pan, L., and Rexed, I. (1975). *The Gentlemen's Club: International Control of Drugs and Alcohol*. Chicago, IL: University of Chicago Press.

Caplan, G. (2012). Medical marijuana: a study of unintended consequences. In: Symposium: the road to legitimizing marijuana: what benefit at what cost? *McGeorge Law Review* **43**, 127–146.

Chopra, I.C. and Chopra, R.N. (1957). The use of the cannabis drugs in India. *Bulletin on Narcotics*. Available at: http://www.unodc.org/unodc/en/data-and-analysis/bulletin/bulletin_1957-01-01_1_page003.html (accessed September 9, 2012).

Chopra, R.N. and Chopra, I.C. (1955). Quasi-medical use of opium in India and its effects. *Bulletin on Narcotics*. Available at: http://www.unodc.org/unodc/en/data-and-analysis/bulletin/bulletin_1955-01-01_3_page002.html (accessed September 9, 2012).

Cohen, P.J. (2005). Science, politics, and the regulation of dietary supplements: it's time to repeal DSHEA. *American Journal of Law and Medicine*, **31**, 175–214.

Commission of Inquiry into the Non-Medical Use of Drugs (Gerald Le Dain, Chairman). (1972). *Interim Report*. Ottawa: Commission of Inquiry into the Non-Medical Use of Drugs.

Commission of the European Communities (EC). (2009). *Report from the Commission on the implementation of Framework Decision 2004/757/JHA laying down minimum provisions on the constituent elements of criminal acts and penalties in the field of illicit drug trafficking*. SEC (2009) 1661. Brussels. Available at: http://eur-lex.europa.eu/LexUriServ/LexUriServ.do?uri=COM:2009:0669:FIN:EN:PDF (accessed September 16, 2012).

Crowther, S.M., Reynolds L.A., and Tansey, E.M. (eds.). (2010). *The Medicalization of Cannabis.* Wellcome Witnesses to Twentieth Century Medicine. Vol. 40. London: Wellcome Trust Centre for the History of Medicine at UCL.

Dixie Botanicals. (2013). *Dixie Botanicals Hemp Oil Supplement Capsules.* [Online] Available at: http:// dixiebotanicals.com/products/hemp-oil-capsules/ (accessed January 13, 2013).

DOJ (Department of Justice). (2013). *Memorandum for all United States Attorneys.* Available at: http:// www.justice.gov/iso/opa/resources/3052013829132756857467.pdf (accessed August 30, 2013).

ECDD (World Health Organization Expert Committee on Drug Dependence). (2003). *Thirty-Third Report.* Geneva: WHO.

ECDD. (2006a). *Critical Report: Assessment of Dronabinol and its Stereoisomers.* Geneva: WHO. Available at: http://www.who.int/medicines/areas/quality_safety/4.2DronabinolCritReview.pdf (accessed September 13, 2012).

ECDD. (2006b). *Thirty-Fourth Report.* Geneva: WHO.

***Emerald Steel Fabricators, Inc. v Bureau of Labor and Industries,* 348 Or. 157,** (2010).

ELDD (European Legal Database on Drugs). (2003). *Drugs and Driving.* Available at: http://www.emcdda. europa.eu/attachements.cfm/att_5737_EN_Drugs_and_driving.pdf (accessed September 15, 2012).

EMCDDA (European Monitoring Centre for Drugs and Drug Addiction) (2011). *Drug Policy Profiles: Portugal.* Lisbon: EMCDDA. Available at: http://www.emcdda.europa.eu/publications/drug-policy-profiles/portugal (accessed September 15, 2012).

EMCDDA. (2012a). *Country Legal Profiles: Luxembourg.* Lisbon: EMCDDA. http://www.emcdda.europa. eu/html.cfm/index5174EN.html# (accessed September 13, 2012).

EMCDDA. (2012b). *Legal Topic Overviews: Classification of Controlled Drugs.* Available at: http://www. emcdda.europa.eu/html.cfm/index146601EN.html (accessed September 13, 2012).

EMCDDA. (2012c). *Legal Topic Overviews: Legal Approaches to Drugs and Driving.* Available at: http:// www.emcdda.europa.eu/html.cfm/index19034EN.html (accessed September 14, 2012).

EMCDDA. (2012d). *Legal Topic Overviews: Legal Status of Drug Testing in the Workplace.* Available at: http://www.emcdda.europa.eu/html.cfm/index16901EN.html (accessed September 14, 2012).

EMCDDA. (2012e). *Legal Topic Overviews: Penalties for Illegal Drug Trafficking.* Available at: http://www. emcdda.europa.eu/html.cfm/index146646EN.html (accessed September 15, 2012).

EMCDDA. (2012f). *Legal Topic Overviews: Possession of Cannabis for Personal Use.* Lisbon: EMCDDA. Available at: http://www.emcdda.europa.eu/legal-topic-overviews/cannabis-possession-for-personal-use#countries (accessed September 15, 2012).

EMA (European Medicines Agency), Committee for Medicinal Products for Human Use (CHMP). (2007). *Guideline on Compassionate Use of Medicinal Products Pursuant to Article 83 of Regulation (EC) No 726/2004.* Lisbon: EMA. Available at: http://www.ema.europa.eu/docs/en_GB/document_library/ Regulatory_and_procedural_guideline/2009/10/WC500004075.pdf (accessed September 14, 2012).

EMA. (2008). *Press Release. The European Medicines Agency recommends suspension of the marketing authorization of Accomplia.* Available at: http://www.ema.europa.eu/docs/en_GB/document_library/ Press_release/2009/11/WC500014774.pdf (accessed September 13, 2012).

European Parliament and the Council of the European Union. (2001). *Directive 2001/83/EC: Community Code relating to Medicinal Products for Human Use.* Available at: http://eur-lex.europa.eu/LexUriServ/ LexUriServ.do?uri=CELEX:32001L0083:EN:NOT (accessed September 14, 2012).

FDA (Food and Drug Administration). (2004). *Guidance for Industry: Botanical Drug Products.* Available at: http://www.fda.gov/cder/guidance/index.htm (accessed September 19, 2012).

FDA. (2011a). *Recall: Firm Press Release. Globe All Wellness, LLC Issues a Voluntary Recall of Dietary Supplement Found to Contain an Undeclared Drug Ingredient.* Available at: http://www.fda.gov/Safety/ Recalls/ucm256649.htm (accessed September 10, 2012).

FDA. (2011b). *Warning Letter: Ancient Formulas.* Available at: http://www.fda.gov/ICECI/ EnforcementActions/WarningLetters/2011/ucm244190.htm (accessed September 10, 2012).

FDA. (2012). *News Release: FDA Issues Warning Letters to Dietary Supplement Firms in Colorado and Texas for Promoting Unapproved Products as Drugs.* Available at: http://www.fda.gov/NewsEvents/Newsroom/ PressAnnouncements/ucm318445.htm (accessed September 10, 2012).

GAO (Government Accountability Office). (2009). *Drug Safety: FDA Has Begun Efforts to Enhance Postmarket Safety, but Additional Actions Are Needed. Report to the Ranking Member, Committee on Finance, U.S. Senate.* Washington, DC: GAO. Available at: http://www.gao.gov/new.items/d1068.pdf (accessed September 10, 2012).

GCDP (Global Commission on Drug Policy). (2011). *War on Drugs.* Available at: http://www. globalcommissionondrugs.org/wp-content/themes/gcdp_v1/pdf/Global_Commission_Report_English. pdf (accessed September 16, 2012).

GCDP. (2012). *Global Commission on Drug Policy Meets in Poland and Takes the Debate to the East.* Available at: http://www.globalcommissionondrugs.org/global-commission-on-drug-policy-meets-in-poland-and-takes-the-debate-to-the-east/ (accessed September 16, 2012).

Hazekamp, A. (2006). An evaluation of the quality of medicinal grade cannabis in the Netherlands. *Cannabinoids* 1(1), 1–9.

Health Canada. (2001). *Marihuana Medical Access Regulations.* Available at: http://laws-lois.justice.gc.ca/ eng/regulations/SOR-2001-227/index.html (accessed November 15, 2012).

Health Canada. (2002). *Special Access Programme—Drugs.* Available at: http://www.hc-sc.gc.ca/dhp-mps/ acces/drugs-drogues/sapfs_pasfd_2002-eng.php (accessed November 15, 2012).

Health Canada. (2008). *Guidance Document for Industry and Practitioners.* Available at: http://www.hc-sc. gc.ca/dhp-mps/acces/drugs-drogues/sapg3_pasg3-eng.php (accessed November 15, 2012).

Health Canada. (2012a). *Brief History of Drug Regulation in Canada.* Available at: http://www.hc-sc.gc.ca/ dhp-mps/homologation-licensing/info-renseign/hist-eng.php (accessed November 4, 2012).

Health Canada. (2012b). *Marihuana for Medical Purposes Regulations (Proposed).* Available at: http:// gazette.gc.ca/rp-pr/p1/2012/2012-12-15/html/reg4-eng.html (accessed November 15, 2012).

House of Lords (House of Lords Select Committee on Science and Technology). (1998). *Cannabis: The Scientific and Medical Evidence.* The House of Lords Session 1997–8, 9th report. London: Stationery Office.

HUD (Department of Housing and Urban Development). (2011). *Medical Use of Marijuana and Reasonable Accommodation in Federal Public and Assisted Housing (Memorandum).* Washington, DC: HUD. Available at: http://www.scribd.com/doc/47657807/HUD-policy-Memo-on-Medical-Marijuana-in-Public-Housing

INCB (International Narcotics Control Board). (2003). *Report of the International Narcotics Control Board for 2002.* New York: United Nations.

INCB. (2008). *Report of the International Narcotics Control Board for 2007.* New York: United Nations.

INCB. (2012). *Report of the International Narcotics Control Board for 2011.* New York: United Nations.

Joy, J.E., Watson S.J., and Benson J.A. (eds.). (1999). *Marijuana and Medicine: Assessing the Science Base.* Washington, DC: National Academy Press, Institute of Medicine.

Kampia, R. (2012). *Election 2012: How National, State Results Affect Your MMJ Business.* Denver: National Marijuana Business Conference 2012.

Keber, T. (2012). *Infused Product Makers: How to Flourish in 2013.* Denver: National Marijuana Business Conference 2012.

Kilmer, B., Caulkins, J.P., Pacula, R.L., et al. (2010). *Altered State? Assessing How Marijuana Legalization in California Could Influence Marijuana Consumption and Public Budgets.* Santa Monica, CA: RAND Corporation.

Krajeski, K. (2000). How flexible are the United Nations drug conventions? *International Journal of Drug Policy,* 10 (4), 329–338.

Lopez, S. (2009). A visit to the medical marijuana doctor. *Los Angeles Times*, October 28. Available at: http://www.latimes.com/news/local/la-me-lopez28-2009oct28,0,874874.column (accessed September 20, 2013).

Loucas, P.G. (2008). Regulating compassion: an overview of Canada's federal medical cannabis policy and practice. *Harm Reduction Journal*, **5**, 5.

MacCoun, R.J. and Reuter, P. (2001). *Drug War Heresies: Learning from Other Vices, Times, & Places.* Cambridge: Cambridge University Press.

McAllister, W. (2000). *Drug Diplomacy in the Twentieth Century*. London: Routledge.

Mechoulam, R. (ed.). (1973). *Marijuana*. New York: Academic Press.

MHRA (Medicines and Healthcare products Regulatory Agency). (2012a). *A Guide to What is a Medicinal Product*. MHRA Guidance Note No. 8. Available at: http://www.mhra.gov.uk/home/groups/is-lic/documents/publication/con007544.pdf (accessed September 18, 2012).

MHRA. (2012b). *Borderline Products*. Available at: http://www.mhra.gov.uk/Howweregulate/Medicines/Doesmyproductneedalicence/Borderlineproducts/index.htm#l3 (accessed September 18, 2012).

MHRA. (2012c). *Herbal Medicines Regulation: Unlicensed Herbal Medicines Supplied by a Practitioner Following a One-to-One Consultation*. Available at: http://www.mhra.gov.uk/Howweregulate/Medicines/Herbalmedicinesregulation/Unlicensedherbalmedicinessuppliedbyapractitionerfollowingaonetooneconsultation/index.htm (accessed September 18, 2012).

Mills, J.H. (2003). *Cannabis Britannica: Empire, Trade, and Prohibition*. Oxford: Oxford University Press.

Musto, D.F. (1987). The History Of Legislative Control Over Opium, Cocaine, And Their Derivatives. In: R. Hamowy (ed.). *Dealing with Drugs: Consequences of Government Control*. Lexington MA: Lexington Books, pp. 37–71.

Musto, D.F. (1999). *The American Disease: Origins of Narcotic Control*. 3rd ed. New York: Oxford University Press.

Neuman, A. (2004) *GHB's Path to Legitimacy: An Administrative and Legislative History of Xyrem*. [Paper submitted for course requirement in Food and Drug Law, Winter Term 2004, Harvard Law School.] Available at: http://dash.harvard.edu/bitstream/handle/1/9795464/Neuman.html?sequence=2 (accessed September 20, 2013).

New York v United States. (1992) 505 U.S. 144.

OIG (Office of the Inspector General). (2012). Dietary supplements: companies may be difficult to locate in an emergency. October 2012 OEI-01-11-00211. Washington, DC: US Department of Health & Public Services.

O'Shaughnessy, W.B. (1839). On the preparations of the Indian hemp, or gunjah *(Cannabis indica)*; their effects on the animal system in health, and their utility in the treatment of tetanus and other convulsive diseases. *Transactions of the Medical and Physical Society of Bengal 1838–1840*, 71–102, 421–461.

Pacula, R.L., MacCoun, R.J., Reuter, P., *et al.* (2004). *What Does it Mean to Decriminalize Marijuana? A Cross-National Empirical Examination*. Center for the Study of Law and Society, Jurisprudence and Social Policy Program, U.C. Berkeley. Available at: http://www.escholarship.org/uc/item/9v76p00j (accessed September 20, 2013).

Printz v United States. (1997). 521 U.S. 898.

Ravin v State, **537 P.2d 494** (Ala. 1975).

Regina v Parker. (2000). CanLII 5762 (ON CA). Available at: http://www.canlii.org/en/on/onca/doc/2000/2000canlii5762/2000canlii5762.html (accessed November 10, 2013).

Rendon, J. (2012). *Super-Charged: How Outlaws, Hippies, and Scientists Reinvented Marijuana*. Portland, OR: Timber Press.

Room, R., Fischer, B., Hall, W., *et al.* (2010). *Cannabis Policy: Moving Beyond Stalemate*. Oxford: Beckley Foundation.

Ross v Ragingwire Telecommunications. (2008). 42 Cal.4th 920, 70 Cal.Rptr.3d 382.

Russo, E.B. (2011). Taming THC: potential cannabis synergy and phytocannabinoid-terpenoid entourage effects. *British Journal of Pharmacology*, **163**, 1344–1364.

Schneeman, B.O., Azarnoff, D.L., Christiansen, C.L., *et al.* (2005). *Dietary Supplements: A Framework for Evaluating Safety*. Washington, DC: National Academies Press, Institute of Medicine.

Serrano, A. Uruguay Unveils Marijuana Regulation Details, May 3, 2014. Aljazeera America. http://america.aljazeera.com/articles/2014/5/3/uruguay-unveils-marijuanaregulationdetails.html (accessed May 21, 2014).

Single, E. (1999). Options for cannabis reform. *International Journal of Drug Policy*, **10**(4), 281–290.

Sinha, J. (2001). *The History and Development of the Leading International Drug Control Conventions. Report Prepared for The Senate Special Committee On Illegal Drugs*. Ottawa: Canadian Library of Parliament.

Randall, R.C. and O'Leary, A.M. (1998). *Marijuana Rx: The Patients' Fight for Medicinal Pot*. New York: Thunder's Mouth Press.

UNODC. (United Nations Office on Drugs and Crime). (1953). Quasi-medical use of opium. *Bulletin on Narcotics*, 3, 19–23. Available at: http://www.unodc.org/unodc/en/data-and-analysis/bulletin/bulletin_1953-01-01_3_page008.html (accessed September 10, 2012).

UNODC. (1962). The Cannabis Problem: a note on the problem and the history of international action. *Bulletin on Narcotics*, 4, 27–31. Available at: http://www.unodc.org/unodc/en/data-and-analysis/bulletin/bulletin_1962-01-01_4_page005.html (accessed September 10, 2012).

Walton, R.P. (1938). *Marihuana: America's New Drug Problem*. Philadelphia, PA: J.B. Lippincott Co.

Chapter 4

Cannabis Horticulture

David J. Potter

4.1 **Introduction**

Cannabis is a drug romantically associated by many with peace and love, as exalted by the youth and countercultures that emerged in the 1960s. With the turn of the millennium, however, production of this soft drug became more commonly associated with hard crime, as organized gangs muscled in on the lucrative production market. Reported associations between cannabis use and distressful psychoses further tarnished the plant's image. This imbalanced reputation overshadows the fact that, when used responsibly, the cannabis plant has proved to be a botanical paragon of virtues, having supplied man with food, fiber, oil, and medicine for several millennia. It is indeed likely that its medicinal use predated any recreational consumption. Evidence suggests that the plant had a place in Ayurvedic (Russo 2004) and Chinese medicine (Mechoulam 1986) at least as early as 3000 years ago. Its medicinal qualities have since been widely used across the globe.

The World Health Organization has estimated that over 21,000 plant species are used for medicinal purposes around the world, but only about 100 of these will be specifically grown for the pharmaceutical industry (EUROPAM 2008). Cannabis is perhaps the only pharmaceutical feedstock that is grown indoors. This provides the extra security that this highly marketable drug requires. It also enables GW Pharmaceuticals to grow material with a higher level of control than any outdoor-grown pharmaceutical crop.

GW Pharmaceuticals' glasshouse facilities incorporate computerized horticultural management systems that deliver the temperatures, lighting levels, and day lengths required. The detailed growing conditions are recorded, thus enabling each batch of plants to be certified as correctly grown according to set parameters. Documentary control systems ensure the provenance and authenticity of each batch. This is a pharmaceutical industry requirement and, because cannabis is a Controlled Drug as defined by the Misuse of Drugs Act 1971, it is also a strict Home Office requirement.

Although experienced amateur cannabis producers often claim that cannabis growing is *more of an art than a science*, propagation of cannabis for the pharmaceutical market is the strict preserve of the scientist. High standards of quality, safety, and efficacy are demanded of the medicine, and this requires the starter material to be grown under rigorously controlled conditions. This is especially the case when producing a complex botanical drug such as GW Pharmaceuticals' first licensed medicine Sativex®. A botanical or herbal drug such as this can be defined as a well characterized, multicomponent standardized medicine extracted from plant sources. Some of these multicomponents in cannabis may act together synergistically (Russo 2011, Williamson 2001), and hence relatively small variations in the ratios can have potentially large effects on the overall activity. By growing the plants in tightly controlled uniform conditions, a consistent ratio of these ingredients can be achieved.

The producers of cannabis for Sativex® manufacture needed to develop growing systems that enabled the feedstock to be reliably and efficiently produced at all times of the year. It was also essential to gain an understanding of how variations in growing conditions might affect the concentrations and ratios of the active ingredients within the plant. With the knowledge gained, the horticultural team was better placed to agree a growing protocol that defined the tolerance levels in growing conditions. In addition to Sativex®, the company has a pipeline of other medicines derived from other cannabis genotypes in development. The optimum growing conditions and timings for these new plants required optimization.

Much of the horticultural and agricultural research performed at GW Pharmaceuticals has proved useful in the field of forensic science, and some of this is reported here. However, more specific details are given regarding the parameters applying to the propagation of phytopharmaceutical raw material for pharmaceutical use.

4.2 **Cannabis origins**

It is generally accepted that the genus *Cannabis* originated in Central Asia, but a more precise location is widely debated. The Himalayan foothills and Pamir Plain have been favored by some researchers. A more westerly origin, in what is now Azerbaijan, has been suggested (de Bunge 1860) with others pointing much further east to Northwest China (Bouquet 1950). Western China is the suggested source of Cannabis's only close relative—the hop (*Humulus* spp.) (Neve 1991, p. 1) implying perhaps that the entire Cannabaceae family evolved in this area. Because of its many qualities, over many millennia the cannabis plant became widely spread by man. With or without human intervention, the species adapted to survive and indeed flourish in widely contrasting climates and habitats. As a result, vastly different forms of the species now exist, some just 20 cm in height when fully grown while other cultivated forms attain 6 m or more, although 1–3 m is more common (UNODC 2009a, p. 7). It is estimated that approximately one-third of the earth's land mass would be suitable for outdoor cannabis cultivation in some form, the most southerly suggested location being 47°S in New Zealand (UNODC 2009b, p. 95). In the northern hemisphere, commercial oilseed hemp crops grow satisfactorily as far as 62°N in Finland (Calloway and Laakkonen 1996) and some cannabis plants have been observed as far north as 66° N in Russia (Grigoryev 1998).

4.3 **Morphology**

Although occasionally existing as a perennial in subtropical to tropical areas (Emboden 1974), *Cannabis sativa* L. is generally an annual, its growth pattern very much dictated by the seasons. It is typically a *short-day plant*, only commencing to flower late in summer, once the day length starts to fall. The species is naturally dioecious, by definition producing separate male and female plants. However, because the sexes produce fiber with differing characteristics, fiber hemp varieties have been specifically bred to be monoecious (hermaphrodite), thereby producing a more uniform crop (Small and Cronquist 1976).

The species is wind-pollinated. When mature, sepals on the male flowers open to expose the anthers, which hang freely on fine filaments. The exposed anthers soon split to shed pollen onto any passing air current. The males are typically taller than the females, giving them greater exposure to the passing breeze. The male and female plants continue to produce abundant inflorescences (clusters of flowers) for several days or weeks, and during this period, the females form an abundance of receptive white (or more rarely pink or orange) stigmas. Once a pollen grain is captured by the stigma, fertilization is enabled. With the cessation of flowering, and its role fulfilled, the male dies. The pollinated females from the same population also cease flowering, but survive for much longer as they set seed.

The female inflorescences are, by definition indeterminate. These flower clusters never produce a true terminal flower. If grown in the absence of pollen, the period of development of new flowers within the seed-free inflorescence is unnaturally extended. As new flowers continue to develop, unnaturally large inflorescences can form and the yield of floral material is increased. This all-female form of cannabis is almost ubiquitous in indoor illicit growing operations, and is widely referred to as *sinsemilla* (from Spanish, meaning without seeds).

4.4 **Secondary metabolite distribution**

The value of cannabis as a recreational or medicinal drug is attributable to the presence of a number of terpenophenolic secondary metabolites called cannabinoids. (Secondary metabolites are by definition organic compounds not directly involved in normal growth, development or reproduction of organisms.) Although it is often erroneously claimed that molecules of this type are only found in cannabis, some are detectable elsewhere in the plant kingdom, e.g., *Helichrysum* spp. (Bohlman and Hoffman 1979), albeit in extremely low levels. *Cannabis sativa* L. is certainly unique in producing cannabinoids in such high concentrations and indeed few plant species exceed such a concentration of any secondary metabolites.

The cannabinoids are not evenly distributed throughout the plant. They are totally absent from the roots and seeds. Dried stem material of a drug variety will typically contain around 0.3% or less tetrahydrocannabinol (THC) (Fritschi et al. 2006; Potter 2004, p. 28). The lower leaves contain less than 1% and mixed samples, which contain all the foliage including the uppermost leaves of female plants, will more typically contain 2–3% THC (Potter and Duncombe 2012; UNODC 2009a, p. 14). However, unpollinated, all-female floral material is by far the main source of THC and most other cannabinoids. A THC content of well over 20% can be found in some samples. It must be emphasized though that the cannabinoid content of floral material is extremely variable within a single plant (Potter 2013), and high content values in small samples are often not truly representative of the plants from which they came (EMCDDA 2004). The cannabinoids cannabichromene (CBC) and cannabichromevarin (CBCV) are more commonly associated with juvenile tissue and, except in specifically bred genotypes, these are typically more dominant in foliage.

The marked variation in concentration of cannabinoids in individual plant tissues is mainly due to the presence or absence of small structures called glandular or capitate trichomes. It is widely accepted that the cannabinoids are predominantly, or more likely entirely, synthesized and sequestered in these structures (Mahlberg et al. 1984). Most of the monoterpenes and sesquiterpenes in cannabis are also found here (Malingré et al. 1975; Turner et al. 1980). Being so important, when considering cannabinoid production, these structures are now described in some detail.

4.5 **Cannabis trichome form and function**

The general term *trichome,* when applied to plants, refers to a type of epidermal appendage. They exist throughout the plant kingdom in an extremely diverse number of forms, of which over 300 have been described (Payne 1978). Their diversity has attracted much attention since the earliest microscopists studied them and recorded their detail (Hooke 1665). Trichomes can be broadly segregated into nonglandular and glandular types, both of which are found on cannabis. Nonglandular trichomes, in the form of simple plant hairs, occur in the majority of vascular plants, but glandular trichomes are found in just 20–30% (Dell and McComb 1978). Fossilized remains of the fern *Blanzeopteris praedentata* reveal that glandular trichomes existed at least as long as 300 million years ago, in the Late Carboniferous period (Krings et al. 2003). The functions of trichomes are either guessed at or totally unknown, and many of the hypotheses have not been experimentally tested (Werker 2000). Suggestions include the deterrence of predators and protection against environmental stresses. Reviews by Werker (2000) and Wagner et al. (2004) described 17 different trichome functions, many of which could be applicable to cannabis.

Because of their importance, cannabis trichomes have been studied in depth for many years, a notable example being the detailed descriptive and illustrated work of Briosi and Tognini (1894), which is still regularly quoted. A sample of this work is shown in Fig. 4.2A. Two nonglandular types exist, neither of which is associated with cannabinoid and/or terpenoid production. Three types of glandular trichome have been described on female cannabis, viz., bulbous, capitate-sessile and capitate-stalked. Males have been found to exhibit a fourth type—the antherial glandular trichome (Fairbairn 1972). Detailed trichome studies have given a greater understanding of the biogenesis and distribution of the cannabinoids (Dayanandan and Kaufman 1976). Mahlberg et al. (1984) showed that capitate sessile and stalked trichomes differed in their distribution, as well as in their cannabinoid content and profile, and this was linked to the differing cannabinoid distribution in the plant.

The five trichomes associated with female cannabis plants include the nonglandular *simple unicellular trichomes* and the *cystolythic trichomes*. Simple trichomes, also known as covering trichomes, can first be seen on the surface of cotyledons immediately after germination. They continue to develop in abundance on the underside of leaves (and to a much lesser extent on the upper surface) throughout the plant's life. By covering the underside of the leaf with a layer of trapped air, a pubescence of trichomes reduces water loss and provides some insulation against extreme temperatures (Ehleringer 1984). Cystolythic trichomes are first observed on the upper surface of the initial pair of true leaves on a cannabis seedling and give the foliage a rough texture. At the base of each is a concretion of calcium carbonate crystals called a cystolyth (Dayanandan and Kaufman 1976). These tough trichomes would presumably reduce the palatability of the foliage to leaf-eating predators. Phytodermatitis and hives in cannabis growers have been linked to long-term exposure to cannabis herbage, and abrasive cystolythic trichomes are the suspected cause. The high concentrations of oxalic acid in cannabis foliage could exacerbate these effects.

Of greater significance to the pharmacologist is the existence and roles of the glandular trichomes, which are described in turn in sections 4.5.1–4.5.3.

4.5.1 Capitate sessile trichomes

Apart from on the cotyledons and the supporting hypocotyl, sessile trichomes are observed on all other aerial epidermal surfaces. The example shown in Fig. 4.1 was a rare find, being perfectly situated on a leaf edge and viewable in profile. The trichome can be seen to possess a somewhat flattened hemispherical structure, commonly referred to as the resin head, with a disc of secretory cells at its base. This resin head is connected to the green mesophyll cells of the leaf via a stalk, which is normally hidden from view. Within the mesophyll tissue, photosynthesis generates sugars, some of which are then channeled to the secretory cells where they fuel cannabinoid and terpene biosynthesis. Above the secretory cells, and below the trichome's outer membrane,

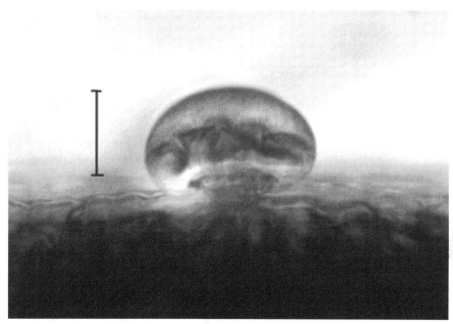

Fig. 4.1 (See also colour plate section.) A capitate sessile trichome observed on the edge of one of the first pair of true leaves of a cannabis seedling. (Scale bar = 25μm.)

is a chamber within which a resinous mixture of cannabinoids and essential oils is sequestered (Mahlberg et al. 1984). The trichome's function is not known, but across the plant kingdom its role is guessed to be the protection of the plant tissue against predators. Sessile trichomes on cannabis contain, amongst other things, bitter tasting sesquiterpenes that reduce palatability. This form of trichome is found in many other plant families and, due to its flattened shape and short stalk, is often referred to as a *peltate trichome*, the name being derived from the Latin word *pelta*—a short-handled, hand-held, round shield. This name is especially appropriate, considering its suggested defensive role.

The botanically unique combination of cystolythic hairs on the adaxial (upper) leaf surface and longer trichomes and sessile glands on the abaxial surface, enables positive forensic identification of *Cannabis sativa* L., even when restricted to fragmented material (UNODC 2009a).

4.5.2 **Capitate stalked trichomes**

These trichomes proliferate on the calyx, bracteoles, bracts, and accompanying petioles of female plants, but are much less common on males. Capitate stalked trichomes are the most complex type. They develop a resin head, similar to that of the sessile type, but in mature specimens this is surmounted on a multicellular stalk (Fig. 4.2B). This stalk incorporates an active channel of hypodermal cells, through which nutrients are transported to the resin head from the phloem. It is near impossible to distinguish between sessile and immature glandular stalked trichomes, where the stalk is yet to form. When fully developed the resin heads on capitate stalked trichomes typically reach 100 μm in diameter. This is approximately twice the breadth of, and consequently eight times the volume of, an average sessile trichome, thus enabling it to sequester a much greater quantity of cannabinoid.

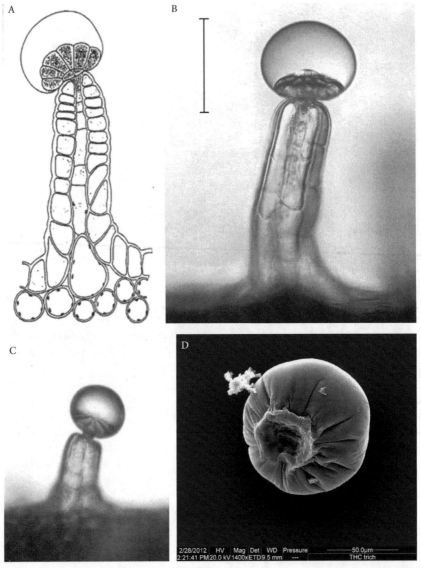

Fig. 4.2 (See also colour plate section.) (A) An illustration of a capitate stalked trichome on *Cannabis sativa* by Briosi and Tognini (1894).

Reproduced from Briosi, G. and Tognini, F., Intorna alla anatomia deila canapa *Cannabis sativa* L. Parte prima: Organi sessuali. Atti 1st Bot. *Pavia*, 2(3), pp. 91–209, 1894.

(B) A capitate stalked trichome, temporarily mounted in glycerol and viewed in transmitted light.

Reproduced from Potter, D. J. "The propagation, characterisation and optimisation of cannabis as a phytopharmaceutical" © 2009, The Author..

(C) A glandular trichome with partly abscised resin head.

Reproduced from Potter, D. J. "The propagation, characterisation and optimisation of cannabis as a phytopharmaceutical" © 2009, The Author..

(D) Like an undocked Apollo Landing Module, a detached capitate stalked trichome resin head floats into the void.(Electron microscope view, D.J. Potter and G. Vizcay, Centre for Ultrastructural Imaging, Kings College London.)

As in the sessile form, the resin head incorporates a disk of secretory cells at the base, its secretions being sequestered within the resin head. The contents of the resin head are crystal clear during the earlier stages of development, and in many cases remain so, right up to the fully mature harvest stage. However, it is common as the plant ages for these trichomes to become translucent or almost opaque white. Excessive ageing sometimes results in the resin heads turning brown. This coloration is often seen to commence within the disk of secretory cells, and is possibly due to necrosis of the by-now inactive tissues. This browning continues after plants had been harvested and dried.

Many guides in the gray literature advise that cannabis plants are at peak potency and ready for harvest only when the capitate stalked trichomes are at the milky white stage. However, a study of over 300 dry cannabis samples indicated minimal correlation between trichome color and potency, except in relation to darker brown samples, which are clearly past the peak of potency (Potter 2009, p.77).

One change in trichome morphology, that is sometimes associated with ageing, is the partial separation of the trichome resin head from the trichome stalk (Fig. 4.2C). Complete separation of the resin head from the stalk occurs during hashish manufacture. The highest potency preparations will contain almost nothing apart from the excised trichome resin heads (Fig. 4.2D).

On the female plant's calyx, bracteoles, bracts, and associated petioles the capitate stalked trichomes can be seen to form a dense pubescence (Fig. 4.3A), which would act as a physical barrier to small phytophagous insects. Like the covering of simple hairs on the underside of leaves, this pubescence would act as a garment, providing some protection against desiccating cold winds (Mahlberg et al. 1984). By reflecting infrared light, a dense trichome pubescence has cooling properties and, being effective across the complete light spectrum, it also reflects ultraviolet (UV) light (Roberecht and Caldwell 1980). Phenolic resins like the cannabinoids have also been shown to offer UV protection by absorbing the harmful radiation (Rhodes 1977). This is especially welcome in floral structures housing gametophytic tissues, which are susceptible to damage by UV-B radiation (Caldwell *et al.* 1983).

Struggling insects are frequently found trapped to the resin heads of these trichomes, thereby inhibiting them from further feeding and reproduction (Fig. 4.3B). This defensive insect

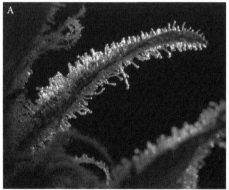 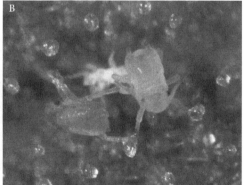

Fig. 4.3 (See also colour plate section.) (A) A dense pubescence of glandular stalked trichomes on a bract within a cannabis female inflorescence. The orange/brown structures are senesced stigmas. (B) Two young cotton-melon aphids (*Aphis gossypii*) irreversibly adhered to the resin heads of capitate stalked trichomes.

entrapment role of trichomes is observed in many other plant species, e.g., lucerne, *Medicago sativa* (Shade et al. 1975), *Pelargonium* spp. (Walters et al. 1991), and the wild potato (*Solanum berthaultii*) (Kowalski et al. 1992). A common insect pest on *Cannabis* in UK studies is the cotton melon aphid, *Aphis gossypii*. Usually found as a predator on the underside of younger leaves, this insect occasionally wanders onto the resinous inflorescence and is seen to struggle desperately as it becomes ensnared on the capitate stalked trichomes. When attacked by predators, *Aphis gossypii* can emit an alarm pheromone to warn others of danger (Byers 2005). It is possible that a trichome-ensnared aphid responds similarly during the tussle. One of the most common pests of cannabis, the tobacco thrip, *Thrips tobaci,* is often similarly trapped. It too is capable of emitting an alarm pheromone (Anathakrishnan 1993). If this theory is correct, the loss of a few trichomes to insects could discourage a more extensive attack on the floral tissue.

Restricted allocation of capitate stalked trichomes to floral tissue is widespread throughout the plant kingdom, where plants optimize investment in defense by allocating secondary metabolites to tissues in direct proportion to their value (Herms and Mattson 1992). It is notable that sessile trichomes play no part in insect entrapment, suggesting that these had a different function, likely relying more specifically on their bitter caryophyllene content to deter herbivorous attack. When separate, fresh capitate stalked and sessile trichomes have been removed from the same plant and analyzed, the capitate stalked samples exhibit a much higher proportion of volatile monoterpenes, which give the trichome contents a solvent-based adhesive quality (Potter 2009, pp. 96–97). The cannabinoids cannabigerolic acid and tetrahydrocannabinolic acid have been shown to cause apoptosis in insect cells, and it has been suggested that this is an important defensive role for cannabinoids in capitate stalked and sessile trichomes (Sirikantaramas et al. 2005). The different ratios of cannabinoids and terpenes, between floral-derived stalked trichomes and more foliar-derived sessile trichomes, emphasizes the importance of maintaining a consistent balance of leaf and flower material when the material is used to manufacture a complex botanical drug, such as Sativex®.

4.5.3 Bulbous trichomes

With a diameter of approximately 10–20 μm, these are the smallest of the glandular trichomes (Fig. 4.4). First seen on the stem and the lower leaves, these are widespread across the entire surface of the aerial part of the plant. Connected to the epidermis by two cells (the top one much

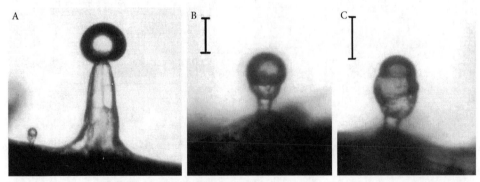

Fig. 4.4 (See also colour plate section.) (A) A small bulbous trichome alongside a fully developed glandular stalked trichome. The contrast in resin head diameter (10 μm vs. 100 μm) is clear. (B) A simple bulbous trichome and (C) a complex bulbous trichome. These are 10–15 μm in diameter.

larger than the lower) these produce a simple, spherical glandular head or a rarer, complex, multicompartmented glandular head (Fig. 4.4C). Their function is not known. Being so small, they potentially contribute little to the secondary metabolites of the plant.

Specifically bred cannabigerol (CBG)-rich chemotypes produce characteristically opaque white sessile and stalked trichome resin heads, due to the unnatural accumulation of CBG (de Meijer 2005). The bulbous trichomes on these chemotypes remain clear, suggesting a lack of cannabinoid in this trichome type. It is possible that a present or past role of the bulbous trichomes may be to alert the cannabis plant to insect movement on its surface, as has been observed to be the case in a small form of trichome in tomato (Tooker et al. 2010). In the latter's case, once ruptured by predatory insect movement, the resultant chemical release stimulates increased development of larger glandular trichome forms, thus boosting the plant's defense capabilities.

4.5.4 Nature's justification for phytocannabinoid biosynthesis

The specific roles of the cannabinoids within the glandular trichomes are much debated. Throughout the plant kingdom, trichomes biosynthesize a wide range of true terpenes, containing just carbon and hydrogen (e.g., myrcene $C_{10}H_{16}$), or more oxygenated relatives such as the terpene alcohols and ketones (e.g., menthol and menthone $C_{10}H_{20}O$ and $C_{10}H_{18}O$) along with various terpene aldehydes (e.g., geranial $C_{10}H_{16}O$) and esters (e.g., geranyl acetate $C_{12}H_{20}O_2$ (Croteau and Johnson 1984). It is notable that in cannabis at least 90% of the terpene family of chemicals found there are pure terpenes, devoid of oxygen (Mediavilla and Steinemann 1997). The cannabinoids are strong antioxidants, similar in performance to vitamin E. Perhaps they have a role in maintaining the reduced state of these terpenes, which for some reason the cannabis plant, through evolution, has found advantageous. As stated earlier, the cannabinoids' main function may be to absorb damaging UV light, and to act somewhat unromantically, as a vital ingredient in a simple solvent-based adhesive. Here the plant's preference for true monoterpenes, over more oxygenated counterparts like the terpene alcohols, may be down to the fact that they are the most readily volatalized, increasing the speed with which the ruptured trichome contents solidify.

Some of the suggested defensive functions of trichomes just described may seem tenuous. However, they are supported by the profound words of Charles Darwin, in his *On the Origin of Species* (Darwin 1859) that:

> Individuals having any advantage, however slight, over others, would have the best chance of surviving and procreating their kind.

4.5.5 Isolation of trichomes for pharmaceutical use

The *World Drug Report 2009* (UNODC 2009b, p. 12) estimated that between 2.2 and 9.9 million tons of cannabis resin (hashish) were produced a year. Most of this would be for recreational use.

Cannabis resin is principally made from capitate stalked glandular trichomes. These are removed from the plant, in a variety of cultural methods, and then compressed to make a solid mass. Indian hashish was the starter material used by Dr. William O'Shaughnessy in 1841 to make the first cannabis-based medicines introduced to Western medicine.

Modern methods have been developed in which brittle trichomes are first dislodged by agitating cannabis in iced water. The trichome laden liquid is then sieved to separate the resin heads from the remaining pulp. Jansen and Terris (2002) reported that, with a Dutch Government subsidy, this technique had been adapted to make hashish for pharmaceutical research purposes.

Although usually performed to collect capitate stalked trichome resin heads from floral tissue, it can also be used to produce sessile trichome-based hashish. This proved especially useful in the production of CBC-rich resin (Potter 2009, p. 93).

4.6 Plant development

4.6.1 Natural outdoor cultivation of cannabis

Cannabis is in most cases a short-day plant, flowering at the end of summer and setting seed before the arrival of winter. Prior to flowering, the plant diverts maximum energy into the production of stems and foliage. In a commercial hemp crop especially, this growth is vigorous enough to outcompete most weeds, and herbicide use is rarely needed. When the so-called *critical day length* is reached, floral development is stimulated. The plant is actually responding to changes in conformation of light-sensitive phytochrome protein dimers that occur during darkness (Halliday and Fankauser 2003). The critical day length for an individual variety is greatly affected by its geographical origin, and would generally be greatest in those plants derived well away from the equator (de Meijer and Keizer 1994). Exceptions to this response occur in plants adapted to grow in equatorial regions, where there is minimal variation in day length. Flowering in tropical cannabis plants is more closely related to plant age.

In short-day types, the ability to measure the night-length would appear to be remarkably accurate. Experimental outdoor crops of one variety, grown outdoors by GW Pharmaceuticals over 10 successive years in Southern England at latitude 51°N, always exhibited their first flowers within 4 days of August 26, irrespective of planting date and prevailing weather. Tests suggest that the *critical day length* for this variety, at which flowering is initiated, is 14 h 20 min. This variety was in fact bred from plants naturalized in Turkey at latitude 41°N, where a day length of 14 h 20 min occurs approximately 3 weeks earlier at the beginning of August. This illustrates that when growing any genotype outdoors, at a more extreme latitude than its original home, a delay in flowering is to be expected. As a consequence, there is a reduction in the number of days available for floral development before unfavorable winter conditions arrive. In Canada, most Western US states and Northern Europe, the climate is mostly unfavorable for floral development of most drug-type varieties, making indoor or glasshouse propagation the only reliable local option.

4.6.2 Indoor growth of cannabis

Since the 1970s, in those locations in the US and Canada where outdoor growing is possible, a law enforcement crackdown and large-scale eradication efforts may have inadvertently encouraged more growers indoors (UNODC 2008, p. 14). In recent decades the Western cannabis market has changed, with an increasing proportion preferring to consume only unfertilized floral parts of the female cannabis plant (*sinsemilla*), and most of it is grown indoors (Leggett 2006). In the more easily controlled indoor environment, the quality of this material is increasingly guaranteed (UNODC 2009b, p. 97). Quality is an even greater consideration in pharmaceutical cannabis production, and indoor growing makes it possible to provide the higher level of environmental control required to achieve this.

Within the indoor environment, to produce a high yielding crop of desirable quality, the grower has to create a favorable environment and manipulate the plants' natural flowering response to changing day length.

4.6.2.1 Selection of best genetic material

In the licensed and illicit arena, a grower can commence activity with either seeds or rooted clones from a reliable source. The latter, of course, should only be from female plants with proven genetics.

Growing batches of plants from clones guarantees that all the new plants produced are genetically identical to the source of propagation material. This greatly improves the uniformity of the final product. Even if grown from seeds derived from just two parents, there will always be a large degree of natural variation between sibling seedlings. It is common practice to initially plant seeds, and then take cuttings from the best performing candidates. This ultimately results in higher performing, as well as more uniform, plant populations. To achieve this, more than one cutting has to be taken from each seedling and at least one induced to flower, while another in maintained in vegetative growth (as described in section 4.6.2.2). When mature, the flowering plants are assessed for their agronomic performance (vigor, yield, resin gland density, etc.) and, then ideally analyzed for chemical content by one of several forms of chromatography. Having identified the best flowering plant, vegetative cuttings derived from the same seedling source are used for all ongoing propagation.

4.6.2.2 Encouraging vegetative growth

To maximize yields, indoor cannabis crops are initially grown in an artificial long-day length environment, to establish a good vegetative structure. This day length must exceed the critical day length (section 4.6.1) to avoid the initiation of the flowering process. Sufficient vegetative growth is most rapidly achieved by maintaining an artificial environment of 24 h day length, for approximately 3 weeks. However, some growers opt for a shorter day length of as little as 18 h. In 2006, Leggett reported that:

> The choice of an 18 hour day/6 hour night regime for the vegetative phase appeared to be returning to vogue because, while continual light can increase yields, this advantage is offset by the expense of additional lighting. (Leggett 2006, p. 17)

Recent observations at illicit cannabis crime scenes, set up by organized criminal gangs in the UK, suggests that an 18 h day length for the vegetative phase is popular even amongst growers who abstract (steal) their electrical energy.

A GW Pharmaceuticals study compared the growth rates of eight varieties in day lengths of 18 and 24 h. After 3 weeks the plants in the 18 h day length (mean height 32.3 cm, dry foliage weight 4.00 g) were shorter and lighter than those in a 24 h day length (mean 36.2 cm and 7.34 g). The reduction in height was not statistically significant (paired 2-tailed t-test, $p = 0.054$) but the weight decrease was highly so ($p = 2.53 \times 10^{-5}$).

Compared to plants grown in 24 h days for 21 days, plants grown more slowly in 18 h days were judged to have achieved a similar stage of development after 25 days. However, there were differences in morphology, which included a significantly greater mean height in the 18 h day length/25-day regime, plants (39.7 cm vs. 36.2 cm, $p = 0.033$). Although they had produced a similar weight of stem, the mean dry weight of foliage was significantly reduced (5.51 g vs. 4.38 g/ plant, $p = 0.0011$.) An increase in height without a concomitant increase in stem weight results in a less robust plant. To produce a similar mass of foliage to the plants in the 24 h day length/21-day regime, plants in 18 h would have required closer to 28 days, at which point the total quantity of light energy emitted would have been the same. The policy of using a 24 h day length during the vegetative period was hence vindicated by this study.

4.6.2.3 Thigmomorphogenesis

In a growth room environment, in the irradiance conditions typically used for an unlicensed crop, excessive height gain is rarely a problem. However, in a glasshouse setting this can be an issue, especially when growing specifically bred pharmaceutical crops with a high degree of hybrid vigor. The preference is to suppress the tendency of some glasshouse grown varieties to produce excessive height during this phase. Adapting a trick from the culinary herb industry, known as thigmomorphogenesis or mechanical perturbation, the stems are brushed almost flat on a daily basis for the first 2–3 weeks. Responding as they would if buffeted by wind, the plants produce stockier thicker stems, more able to support the coming canopy of heavy resinous flowers.

4.6.2.4 Mother plant stock

To initially guarantee adequate vegetative material for production of cuttings, and to avoid the carefully selected genetics being lost, a sufficient number of 'mother' plants have to be retained in long-day length. However, once production has stabilized, it is often possible to simply acquire cuttings by removing lower branches from the production crop. Minimal valuable growing space therefore needs be dedicated to mother plant propagation.

4.6.2.5 Induction and maintenance of floral development

It is an almost ubiquitous recommendation, in all indoor cannabis growing guides, that flowering should be induced and maintained by placing plants in a 12 h day length. Observations at illicit cannabis plantations support this widespread practice. Ironically, in a natural environment at many latitudes, a 12 h day length would herald the end of the flowering process, not its induction. Indeed Pliny the Elder, referring to crops in what is now the Aegean coastal area of Turkey, suggested a few days after the equinox as an ideal harvest time (Pliny c.60AD/1951). As stated earlier (section 4.6.1), one variety used by GW Pharmaceuticals was suggested to have a critical day length of 14 h 20 min. By inducing the plant to flower in a 12 h regime, the flowering plant is apparently being deprived of at least 2 h of potentially beneficial light energy. However, glasshouse-based studies support the belief that the 12 h day is the optimum. Tests showed that while consuming more energy, a 13 h day produced more biomass, and often taller plants, but no increase in total weight of cannabinoid. Conversely, a reduced day length of 11 h produced a proportional decrease in yield (Potter 2009, pp. 140–141). GW Pharmaceuticals continues therefore to use a 12 h day length for flowering period as this minimizes cost and environmental impact attributable to electrical consumption.

Once placed in a 12 h day length, stem and foliar development initially continue, but both slow down and eventually stop after 3–4 weeks. Floral development, however, remains vigorous for many weeks before slowing down. As a result, the ratio of floral to foliar material is continually increasing, as shown in Fig. 4.5. This is an important consideration for GW Pharmaceuticals, who use the flowers and leaves as a feedstock for their medicine. This leaf and flower mixture is referred to as botanical raw material (BRM). As the foliar and floral materials within the BRM differ in secondary metabolite concentration and profile, any alteration to harvest timing will potentially affect the leaf/flower ratio and the overall secondary metabolite content of this feedstock.

It is important to emphasize that the foliage weighed to obtain the data shown in Fig. 4.5 included the leaves from the stems and branches, plus the outer bracts of the inflorescence. Research by de Backer et al. (2012) showed that the overall THC concentration of inflorescence material increases rapidly during early floral development before finally stabilizing. However, the majority of *sinsemilla* cannabis supplied for recreational use consists of the innermost parts of the inflorescence only. The bracts that form the outer part of the inflorescence produce far fewer

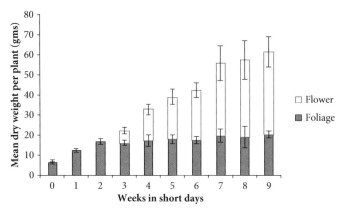

Fig. 4.5 The mean weight of foliar and floral material (± standard deviation, n = 4) in batches of plants (Sativex® THC chemotype) harvested between 0 and 9 weeks after placement in 12h day length.

glandular trichomes, and hence lack potency. These are removed in a process known colloquially as manicuring. The ratio of resinous floral tissue to less potent outer bract material increases as the inflorescence grows. With the outer bract tissue removed, the cannabinoid content of the manicured material produced within the inflorescence is much more consistent, as shown in Fig. 4.6. The plants used in this study were clones of the THC chemotype used for Sativex® production. This suggests that, throughout inflorescence development, if conditions are stable the plant will divert a steady proportion of available assimilates to trichome and cannabinoid formation. In effect the plant equally vigorously defends the oldest and youngest florets.

Additional studies showed that, within the range of irradiance levels typically used for indoor cannabis production, altering the irradiance levels had no effect on the THC concentration of the floral material. Increasing the light level, however, did increase the flower to foliage weight ratio (Potter and Duncombe 2012). This emphasizes the desirability of maintaining uniform light conditions, when producing BRM containing a mixture of leaf and flower material, each of which has slightly different secondary metabolite profiles.

The optimum period in short-day length before harvest varies according to the genotype. A survey of the recommended time for 200 commercially available cannabis varieties showed an average of 57 days with 88% of varieties having an optimum short-day requirement of between 7 and 9 weeks. The majority of the remainder were slower-growing varieties that are more likely to be of interest only to growers with specialized interests (EMCDDA 2012, p. 34).

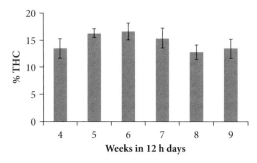

Fig. 4.6 The THC concentration (± standard deviation, n = 4) of manicured inflorescence material from plants (Sativex® THC chemotype) sampled at weekly intervals, 4–9 weeks after placement in short days.

Towards the end of the flowering process, plant growth slows and fewer new florets are formed within the inflorescence. The relative proportion of fertile and senesced stigmas is a guide to the slowing of growth. Recreational cannabis users would often harvest their plants when about 95% of the visible stigmas had senesced, but this would vary according to the variety and the grower's personal preference (Clarke 1981, p. 135). As well as considerations of yield and potency, harvest timing is suggested to affect the taste of the final product. However, in the case of a pharmaceutical crop, appropriate harvest timing can be important to ensure that the correct proportions of controlled secondary metabolites are present. A notable variation affected by early or late harvest is the ratio of THC or CBD to their precursor CBG. When the CBG:THC ratios were assessed in 25 cloned accessions, from a range of varieties, the average proportion of CBG in the CBG + THC total, assessed after 6, 8, and 10 weeks in short-day length, was 3.7%, 3.2%, and finally 2.7%. Both decreases in CBG proportion were highly significant ($p = 0.021$ and $p < 0.01$) (Potter 2009, p. 127). However, to put these variations into context, these maturity-related differences were small in relation to the differences observed between varieties, where CBG concentrations varied between 0.5 and 10% of the CBG + THC total.

Separate tests have compared the monoterpene and sesquiterpene profiles of the chemotypes used to produce THC and CBD for Sativex®. These were seen to vary little over this same period (Potter 2009, pp. 96–97).

4.6.2.6 Effect of irradiance level on plant and cannabinoid yield

During the first year of regular propagation at GW Pharmaceuticals, a large seasonal yield variation was observed, with winter yields down by half. The cannabinoid content (w/w) of BRM (flower and leaf) of winter crops was as little as half that of summer crops. As a consequence of the combined drop in crop-yield and potency the cannabinoid yield of winter crops was found to be roughly a quarter of that achieved in summer. This was despite the presence of a supplementary lighting system within the glasshouse, using mercury vapor lamps, that boosted winter irradiance levels by 17 W m^{-2} of photosynthetically active radiation [PAR]. This is typical of that installed in the well-equipped glasshouses producing salad crops. To achieve acceptable year-round uniformity of cannabis plants, a new extremely bright supplementary lighting system, using high-pressure sodium lamps, was introduced that produced 55 W m^{-2} [PAR]. As a result, only a small seasonal variation in yield remained. By boosting dull daylight levels throughout the year, yields of weekly harvested crops were significantly increased (paired t-test, $p < 0.001$ (Fig. 4.7).

The requirement for such high levels of supplementary lighting is understandable. At the temperate latitude 50° N in southern England, average solar radiation levels are approximately half

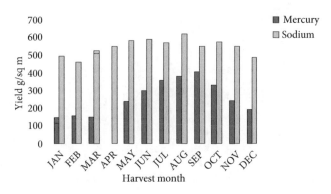

Fig. 4.7 The average yield of the THC chemovar before and after the replacement of mercury vapor lamps (17 W m^{-2}) with high pressure sodium lamps (55 W m^{-2}) of improved supplementary lighting (± standard deviation). The mean is typically for four crops per month. No crop was harvested in April of the first year.

those encountered at 30° N, in the semitropical environment existing at such important cannabis growing regions as Nepal, Pakistan, Afghanistan, and Mexico (Albuisson et al. 2006). Although *Cannabis sativa* L. grown for fiber or seed is often planted at the more northerly latitude, the THC chemotype grown outdoors for its cannabinoid content is more commonly found at latitudes of 30° or less (Small and Beckstead 1973a, 1973b). In addition to the suboptimal natural irradiance conditions falling on the GW Pharmaceuticals' glasshouse, due to latitude, the natural light levels reaching the plants is further weakened by the fact that transmission through a typical glass roof is reduced by at least 30% (Heuvelink et al. 1995). Supplementary lighting has been increasingly used in commercial glasshouses in the UK for salad crop production. Such installations provide up to 40 W m^{-2} [PAR], while commercial glasshouses growing some ornamental plants, such as *Dendrobium* orchids are recommended to use as much as 50 W m^{-2} [PAR]. The installation of a commercial scale glasshouse supplementary lighting system, delivering 55 W m^{-2} [PAR] over an area of 5000 m^{-2}, as used at GW Pharmaceuticals, is highly unusual in the UK. During the winter months, this lighting system remains permanently switched on, throughout the day. As summer approaches, fewer hours of supplementary lighting are required each day. Over the course of the whole year, approximately half the light energy falling on the crop is provided by electrical lamps.

Glasshouse growing is unusual amongst illicit cannabis growers, who correctly feel that their crops would be too easily detected. Therefore much more energy-intensive indoor growing is the norm. As an alternative to glasshouse growing, GW Pharmaceuticals has also produced cannabis in a totally solid building, where crops would not be exposed to seasonal changes in light levels. The irradiance levels of the installed lighting system initially delivered 75 W m^{-2} [PAR]. Crop yields achieved in the first full year of growth were monitored. Yields showed a slight downward trend, commensurate with the manufacturer's predicted age-related fall in irradiance from their lamps. The variation in mean monthly yield resulting from this fading lamp performance, was compared statistically to the small seasonal variation in yield that persisted after the installation of high pressure sodium (HPS) supplementary lighting. No significant difference in mean monthly yield was observed (F-test, $p > 0.05$) between the two growing environments.

It should be stressed that the irradiance level in the solid building (75 W m^{-2} [PAR]) is half that typically utilized by illicit and independent cannabis producers. The numerous printed and online growing guides repeatedly recommend a HPS lighting system, primarily using 600 W HPS lamps, consuming between 400 and 600 watts per square meter of crop (Potter and Duncombe 2012; Vanhove et al. 2011). A forensic study of the lighting installations, at illicit cannabis growth rooms in the Netherlands, reported a median electrical energy consumption per unit area of 510 W m^{-2} (Toonen et al. 2006). HPS lamps typically convert about 30% of the electricity consumed into PAR (Langton et al. 2001). This suggests therefore that the predicted median irradiance at Netherlands crime scenes would deliver an of irradiance level 150 W m^{-2} [PAR].

This highlights the typical illicit growers' desire for maximum yield. The potential cost of this light energy has been calculated to approximate to 1 g of dry floral material for every kW hour used by the lighting system during the growth of the crop (EMCDDA 2012, p. 35). However, it is extremely common for illicit growers to be using abstracted (stolen) electricity, where energy consumption and cost is often not a consideration. The police have estimated that the value of this stolen electricity at around £200 million per year in the UK alone (BBC 2012).

Cannabis growth is strongly correlated to light intensity (Chandra et al. 2008) and greater yields are achieved by consuming vast quantities of electrical energy. Light is vital for photosynthesis, which enables plants to produce the sugars and proteins necessary for structural development.

Biosynthesis of THC, and the accompanying essential oils in cannabis, demands especially high amounts of energy. The amount of energy required to biosynthesize terpenoid molecules has been calculated to be up to three times greater than that required to synthesize an equivalent weight of sugars (Gershenzon 1994). The amount of prevailing light energy therefore has a potential effect on cannabinoid content as well as yield. This possibility is supported by the much debated carbon nutrient balance (CNB) which predicts that, in an environment where the availability of nitrogen is limited (as is possible in the last weeks of cannabis growth), increasing availability of carbon from photosynthesis will result in plants producing greater proportions of carbon-based defense chemicals (Herms and Mattson 1992). A recent study has shown that, when light intensity is increased, the overall THC content of the cannabis plant is boosted, as predicted by the CNB hypothesis (Potter and Duncombe 2012). However, this is due to plants in brighter conditions producing proportionally more female flowers, which contain a greater concentration of THC than foliage. The same study, and additional research by Vanhove et al. (2011) have shown that within the range of light conditions typically used by indoor cannabis growers, light intensity does not affect the potency (THC concentration) of this floral material.

4.6.2.7 The emergence of *Autoflowering* cannabis

The requirement for a short day length for induction of flowering is not necessary in some genotypes. As stated earlier, those plants adapted to growing in equatorial locations experience minimal variation in natural day length, and flowering in tropical cannabis plants is more closely related to plant age. Similarly, commencement of flowering is not controlled by day length in plants adapted to survive in colder extreme latitudes with very brief growing seasons. These can commence flowering within days of germination, irrespective of the day length. The oilseed variety FIN-314, is an early cultivated example. This is derived from Russian accessions k-313 and k-315 from the Vavilov Institute. Adapted to growing in Finland, during extremely short summers, FIN-314 begins flowering within 3 weeks of germination, irrespective of day length (Grigoryev 1998). In around 2004, a recreational cannabis variety called Lowryder arrived in Europe. This demonstrated the same early-flowering trait (Rosenthal 2004, p. 80). This variety is very short, has a lower THC content than most recreational varieties, and is not high yielding. In addition, it is also almost impossible to duplicate it through cuttings (clones). However, it can be grown in confined spaces without the need for artificial day-length control. Several crops can be grown outdoors each year. A large number of so-called auto-flowering varieties are now entering the market, with much improved yields and increased THC content. Their impact on the seed market, and on organized illicit cannabis production, is yet to be seen but is potentially profound. They may influence the breeding of cannabis for pharmaceutical purposes.

Whereas conventional indoor varieties produce about 500 g m^{-2} of floral material (dry weight), commercially available auto-flowering varieties tested in growth rooms at GW Pharmaceuticals have routinely yielded 1100 g m^{-2} of combined flower and leaf material. Of this, 770 g m^{-2} was foliar material, containing 13% THC. The time taken from the transplanting of a small seedling to the harvesting of a fully mature plant is just 10 weeks. By flowering in a 24 h day length, as opposed to the conventional day, these plants receive twice as much light energy per day. Yields of floral material, produced by auto-flowering plants in continuous lighting, have been seen to equate to approximately 1 g per kW h of energy, consumed by the lighting system. This is the same as that typically achieved by conventional plants flowering in 12 h days. However, because of the more compact growing operation, less expenditure is required for heating and ventilation, making the economics of such plants increasingly attractive.

4.6.2.8 Setting the growing temperature

Photosynthesis and resultant growth is markedly affected by temperature. Cannabis varieties originating from different agro-climatic zones worldwide vary in their optimum temperature, ranging between 25°C and 35°C (Chandra et al. 2011). GW Pharmaceutical crops are generally grown at a controlled daily average temperature of 25°C. This temperature was considered the maximum possible while maintaining acceptable staff welfare. It also took into account the potential effect of warmer temperatures on the growth of insect pests and spider mites. Raising the growing temperature by 3°C is reported to halve the time for such pests as spider mites to complete their life cycle (McPartland et al. 2000, pp. 93–95).

Cooling a large glasshouse in summer requires carefully managed ventilation and shading. Growers can take some delight in the knowledge that the plants themselves make a substantial contribution. Just as in animal perspiration, when plants lose water to the surrounding atmosphere through the foliage (transpiration), the conversion of water from liquid to vapor is endothermic. The absorption of latent heat cools the surroundings.

4.6.2.9 Biocontrol

The application of pesticides to pharmaceutical crops is normal practice. However, Good Agricultural and Collection Practice (GACP) guidelines dictate that they should be avoided wherever possible. If absolutely necessary, they should be applied at the minimum effective level in accordance with recommendation of the manufacturers and authorities (EMA 2006, paragraph 9.3.2). If applied, stringent tests would be required to ensure that they did not leave an unacceptable residual presence in the final medicine.

GW Pharmaceuticals has avoided the application of pesticides. Disease and insect pest control is achieved by the dual approach of prevention and cure. In addition to controlling the temperature, humidity levels are managed where possible, to avoid extreme conditions. Very high humidity encourages fungi, while extreme arid conditions favor spider mite infestation, so a middle path is walked. Insect and mite infestations are controlled by the introduction of beneficial insects, which predate or parasitize the intruders.

4.6.2.10 Growth medium

Cannabis grown in the UK for pharmaceutical purposes is propagated in individual pots of a peat and perlite-based growth medium (Potter 2009). The bulk of seized illicit crops within Northern Europe are also found in a similar medium. Peat is widely used in horticulture, due to an unequalled range of favorable characteristics. Peat is naturally free from pests, diseases, and weeds. It has good water and air retention capabilities and it readily allows root penetration. The use of peat is widely criticized as being unfavorable to the environment. Natural renewal of peat is a very slow process. In anaerobic bog habitats, peat locks up carbon dioxide, but this is released to the atmosphere once peat is aerated in a horticultural setting. However, commercial growers of many crops contest that peat is the only suitable medium for reliable production of high-quality, reproducible plants. Although many cannabis varieties are easy-going, others are more exacting and show a clear preference for peat. Ongoing research is evaluating alternative media.

The production of cannabis has in the past been commonly associated with hydroponic (soil-free) growing systems, a perception being held that this produces more potent cannabis. Hydroponic systems are expensive and complicated to install. They do prevent the accumulation of used soil and peat, which aid the detection of illicit cannabis growing. However, some hydroponic systems still generate large quantities of fiberglass or other waste materials. Evidence suggests that yields and potency are not improved by hydroponic growing (UNODC 2006; Vanhove et al. 2012).

4.6.2.11 Plant nutrition

Cannabis requires a large number of inorganic nutrients to support growth. These are commonly divided into the macronutrients (nitrogen, potassium, phosphate, magnesium, calcium, and sulfur) which are required in relatively large quantities, and a range of similarly important but less heavily consumed micronutrients (McPartland et al. 2000). Once the minimum required dose of a nutrient has been made available to the plant, further additions will initially have minimal effect on plant development. However, a point is reached, the critical toxicity content, at which the nutrient reaches toxic levels. There is typically a very wide difference between the critical deficiency and the critical toxicity levels. Therefore, it is possible for large variations in nutrient content to occur with no serious penalty on plant growth, and this allows the grower a large degree of flexibility. As the plant depletes the nutrient content of the growth medium, appropriate feeding may be necessary to avoid deficiencies occurring.

Cannabis sativa L. has been planted by humans for thousands of years. Cultivated plants have generally been selected for desirable agricultural traits in soils with high fertility, where the availability of major nutrients is typically at least two orders of magnitude greater than those occupied by wild plants (Evans 1975). Cultivated plants generally respond most rapidly to increases in soil nutrients. Of these nutrients, nitrogen alters plant composition more than any other mineral nutrient (Marschner 2002). The nitrogen content of the growing medium therefore needs to be controlled with especial care. GW Pharmaceuticals generally maintains acceptable growth medium nutrition by incorporating a controlled release fertilizer that slowly releases nitrogen and other nutrients throughout the plant's life.

The degree to which soil nutrition affects the secondary metabolite content of plant material is majorly governed by whether or not the metabolite contains nitrogen. Plants have evolved to produce secondary metabolites by three main biosynthetic routes, i.e., the terpenoid, phenolic, and nitrogen pathways. Photosynthesis normally ensures a more than adequate supply of precursors for carbon compounds, such as the terpenoids and phenolics. By contrast, nitrogen uptake by the plant is limited, and the enzymes synthesizing secondary metabolites containing nitrogen (e.g., alkaloids) will compete with those requiring nitrogen for protein synthesis. The cost of the secondary metabolite has to be balanced against the cost of new plant growth. As expressed by Herms and Mattson (1992), the plant has a dilemma, whether to grow or to defend. The nitrogen pathway leads to nitrogen-containing secondary metabolites, such as the alkaloids (e.g., nicotine), cyanogens, mustard oils, and nonprotein amino acids (Harborne 1993, pp. 73–78). The quantity of this type of metabolite is affected by the quantity of nitrogen in the growth medium, or made available via nitrogen fixation. In a plant such as tobacco (*Nicotiana* spp.), which produces two types of trichome on the same plant—producing nitrogen-based nicotine or carbon-based phenylpropanoids—growth medium nitrogen content and/or photosynthetic rate will affect the ratio of these two compounds (Fritz et al. 2006).

Cannabis only produces carbon-based secondary metabolites. Of these the monoterpenes, and sesquiterpenes are made via the terpenoid route, while the flavonoids are made via the phenolic route. The cannabinoids are made from moieties derived from both routes. In marked contrast to a plant like tobacco, photosynthesis is normally able to supply enough carbon for secondary metabolite biosynthesis. The secondary metabolite profile of a plant like tobacco is thus sensitive to growing conditions, while cannabis is conveniently less so.

4.6.2.12 Harvest and drying

Once the crop is harvested, prompt drying is essential as a moist crop is vulnerable to fungal or bacterial spoilage. Numerous recommendations within the gray literature encourage a period of slow drying, or "curing." This is suggested to bring about a reduction in starch, sugar, and chlorophyll and a resultant improvement in flavor. In a pharmaceutical crop, emphasis centers on the secondary metabolite content and taste is less of a consideration.

The propagation and harvest process in summarized as a flow chart in Fig. 4.8.

4.6.2.13 Processing

Once harvested, it is a widespread cultural practice to remove (manicure) and discard the leaves and outer bract tissue, to leave the resinous floral tissue only. When producing cannabis as a feedstock for the manufacture of medicines, GW Pharmaceutical staff strip the flowers and leaves from the stem. The stems are discarded but the retained mixture of floral and foliar tissues constitutes their standardized BRM. The retained material is closely examined. Any substantial stem material is removed, as are any other potential contaminants, e.g., biocontrol packaging. This whole process is sometimes referred to as garbling. The material is then stored in a holding area with closely monitored temperature and humidity levels prior to onward processing. The stems, along with all plant waste from the glasshouse, are composted and used elsewhere as a soil conditioner.

4.6.3 Sativex® BRM quality control

As emphasized earlier, the feedstock for Sativex® is a BRM containing both floral and foliar material. The floral tissue is abundantly covered in capitate stalked trichomes, but these are absent on foliage. The more diminutive sessile trichomes on foliage produce a slightly different secondary metabolite profile. Any alterations to growing conditions that majorly affect the foliage to floral

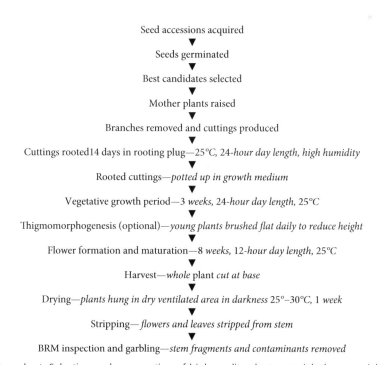

Fig. **4.8** Flow chart. Selection and propagation of high-quality plant material: the essential steps.

tissue ratio have the potential to alter the overall chemical content of the BRM. Guarding against this possibility, each batch of BRM is analyzed for its chemical content. The material is rejected if the analyses are not within agreed acceptance levels. A much more detailed analysis is performed on the BDS (botanical drug substance) made from this material.

4.6.4 Sativex® BDS manufacture

To produce a cannabis extract, batches of dried plant material are immersed in liquid carbon dioxide at extremely high pressure. The ingredients dissolving in this solvent are then separated and purified.

Sativex® is formulated by incorporating BDSs containing THC and CBD in an accurately measured ratio. The only incipients are ethanol, propylene glycol and peppermint oil, the latter being added to improve palatability. By blending two BDSs, a uniform THC:CBD ratio is assured.

4.7 Future research

This chapter has described how alterations to growing conditions and timings affect the cannabis plant, and the secondary metabolites produced within it. To grow cannabis in a glasshouse, for the production of a botanical medicine, it is vitally important that uniformly favorable conditions are maintained for 12 months a year. Cannabis yields are highly affected by temperature and light conditions, and keeping these parameters uniform throughout the year is especially challenging. The energy consumption required is possibly higher than in any other UK glasshouse crop. Ongoing research at GW Pharmaceuticals is further investigating how to maintain high yields, while reducing the environmental impact.

As potential new cannabinoid-based medicines are identified, new chemotypes are steadily arriving in the glasshouse and the growing requirements of each are ascertained.

This chapter emphasized the fundamental importance of the glandular trichome on *Cannabis sativa* L. By sieving cannabis material, preparations have been made that consist almost exclusively of detached trichome resin heads, a single specimen of which is shown in Fig. 4.2D. These have contained up to 67% THC. Such cannabinoid enriched trichome preparations may prove a useful alternative starter material to BRM for the future production of BDSs.

References

Albuisson, M., Lefevre, M., and Wald, L. (2006). *Averaged Solar Radiation 1990–2004*. Paris: Ecole des Mines de Paris/Armines. Available at: http://www.soda-is.com/eng/map/index.html#monde (accessed March 21, 2008).

Anathakrishnan, T.N. (1993). Bionomics of thrips. *Annual Review of Entomology*, **38**, 71–92.

BBC. (2012). *Cannabis Farms' £200m Stolen Electricity Cost 'Staggering'*. [Online] Available at: http://www.bbc.co.uk/news/uk-england-tyne-17898587 (accessed August 14, 2013).

Bohlmann, F. and Hoffmann, E. (1979). Cannabigerol-ähnliche Verbindungen aus Helichrysum umbraculigerum. *Phytochemistry*, **18**, 1371–1374.

Bouquet, R. (1950). Cannabis. *Bulletin on Narcotics*, 4, 14–30 Available at: http://www.unodc.org/unodc/en/data-and-analysis/bulletin/bulletin_1950-01-01_4_page003.html.

Briosi, G. and Tognini, F. (1894). Intorna alla anatomia deila canapa *Cannabis sativa* L. Parte prima: Organi sessuali. Atti 1st Bot. *Pavia*, **2**(3), 91–209.

Byers, J.A. (2005). The cost of alarm pheromone production in cotton aphids, *Aphis gossypii*. *Naturwissenschaften*, **92**, 69–72.

Caldwell, M.M., Robberecht, R., and Flint, S.D. (1983). Internal filters: prospects for UV-acclimation in higher plants. *Physiologia Plantarum*, **58**, 445–450.

Callaway, J.C. and Laakkonen, T.T. (1996). Cultivation of *Cannabis* oil seed varieties in Finland. *Journal of the International Hemp Association*, **3**(1), 32–34.

Chandra, S., Lata, H., Khan, I.A., and ElSohly, M.A. (2008), Photosynthetic response of *Cannabis sativa* L. to variations in photosynthetic photon flux densities, temperature and CO_2 conditions. *Physiology and Molecular Biology of Plants* **14**, 299–306.

Chandra, S., Lata, H., Khan, I.A., and ElSohly, M.A. (2011). Temperature response of photosynthesis in different drug and fiber varieties of *Cannabis sativa* L. *Physiology and Molecular Biology of Plants*, **17**, 297–303.

Clarke, R.C. (1981). *Marijuana Botany*. San Francisco, CA: Ronin Publishing.

Croteau, R. and Johnson, M.A. (1984). Biosynthesis of terpenoids in glandular trichomes. In: E.P. Rodriguez, L. Healey, and I. Mehta (eds.). *Biology and Chemistry of Plant Trichomes*. London: Plenum Press, pp. 133–185.

Darwin, C. (1859). *On the Origin of Species by Means of Natural Selection, or the Preservation of Favoured Races in the Struggle for Life*. Chapter IV, para 1. Available at: http://darwin-online.org.uk/contents.html#books.

Dayanandan, P. and Kaufman, P.B. (1976). Trichomes in *Cannabis sativa* L. (Cannabaceae). *American Journal of Botany*, **63**(5), 578–591.

de Backer, B.B., Maebe, K.K., Verstraete, A.G., and Charlier, C.C. (2012). Evolution of the content of THC and other major cannabinoids in drug-type cannabis cuttings and seedlings during growth of plants. *Journal of Forensic Sciences*, **57**(4), 918–922.

de Bunge, A. (1860). Lettre de M. Alex. de Bunge à M. Decaisne. *Botanique de France*, **7**, 29.

de Meijer, E.P.M. and Hammond, K.H. (2005). The inheritance of chemical phenotype in *Cannabis sativa* L. (II): Cannabigerol predominant plants. *Euphytica*, **145**, 189–198.

de Meijer, E.P.M. and Keizer, L.C.P. (1994). Variation of *Cannabis* for phenological development and stem elongation in relation to stem production. *Field Crops Research* **38**, 37–46.

Dell, B. and McComb, A.J. (1978). *Plant Resins – Their Formation, Secretion and Possible Functions. Advances in Botanical Research*. San Diego, CA: Academic Press.

Ehleringer, J. (1984). Ecology and ecophysiology of leaf pubescence in North American desert plants. In: E. Rodriguez, P.L. Healey, and I. Mehta (eds.). *Biology and Chemistry of Plant Trichomes*. New York: Plenum Press, pp. 113–132.

EMA (European Medicines Agency), Committee on Herbal Medicinal Products. (2006). *Guideline on Good Agricultural and Collection Practice (GACP) for Starting Materials of Herbal Origin*. Available at: http://www.ema.europa.eu/ema/pages/includes/document/open_document.jsp?webContentId=WC500003362 (accessed March 17, 2013).

Emboden, W.A. (1974). Cannabis – a polytypic genus. *Economic Botany*, **28**(3), 304–310.

EMCDDA (European Monitoring Centre on Drugs and Drug Addiction). (2004). *An Overview of Cannabis Potency in Europe*. EMCDDA Insights, no. 6. Lisbon: EMCDDA.

EMCDDA. (2012). *Cannabis Production and Markets in Europe*. EMCDDA Insights, no. 12. Lisbon: EMCDDA.

EUROPAM. (2008). *Guidelines for Good Wild Crafting Practice (GWP) of Medicinal and Aromatic Plants*. Available at: http://bpa.peru-v.com/documentos/Europam_GWP_Medicinal_Aromatic.pdf (accessed September 3, 2013).

Evans, L.T. (1975). The physiological basis of crop yield. In: L.T. Evans (ed.). *Crop Physiology*. London: Cambridge University Press, pp. 327–355.

Fairbairn, J.W. (1972). The trichomes and glands of *Cannabis sativa* L. Bulletin on Narcotics, **24**(4), 29–33.

Fritschi, G., Klein, B., and Szilluweit, W. (2006). Verteilung der THC-Gehalte in Marihuanapflanzen: Bestimmung der Gehalte in Wurzeln, Stängeln, Blättern und Blüten. *Toxichem+Krimtech*, **73**(2), 54–56.

Fritz, C., Palacios-Rojas N., Feil, R., and Stitt, M. (2006). Regulation of secondary metabolism by the carbon–nitrogen status in tobacco: nitrate inhibits large sectors of phenylpropanoid metabolism. *The Plant Journal*, **46**, 533–548.

Gershenzon, J. (1994). Metabolic costs of terpenoid accumulation in higher plants. *Journal of Chemical Ecology*, **20** (6), 1281–1328.

Grigoryev, S. (1998). Hemp (*Cannabis sativa* L.) genetic resources at the VIR: from the collection of seeds, through to the collection of sources, towards the collection of donors of traits. The history of cultivation of hemp in Russia. Online publications, N.I. Vavilov Research Institute of Plant Industry. Available at: http://www.vir.nw.ru/hemp/hemp1.htm (accessed on August 19, 2011).

Halliday, K.J. and Fankauser, C. (2003). Phytochrome-hormonal signalling networks. *New Phytologist*, **157**, 449–463.

Harborne, J.B. (1993). *Introduction to Ecological Biochemistry*. 4th ed. London: Academic Press.

Herms, D.A. and Mattson, W.J. (1992). The dilemma of plants: to grow or defend. *The Quarterly Review of Biology*, **67**(3), 283–335.

Heuvelinke, E., Batta, L.G.G., and Daqmen, T.H.J. (1995). Transmission of solar radiation by a multispan Venlo-type glasshouse: validation of a model. *Agricultural and Forest Meteorology*, **74**(1–2), 41–59.

Hooke, R. (1665). *Micrographia or Some Physiological Description of Minute Bodies Made by Magnifying Glasses with Observations and Enquiries Thereon*. Available at: http://www.gutenberg.org/ebooks/15491.

Jansen, M. and Terris, R. (2002). One woman's work in the use of hashish in a medical context. In: E. Russo, M. Dreher, and M.L. Mathre (eds.). *Women and Cannabis, Medicine, Science and Technology*. New York: Haworth Press, pp. 135–143.

Kowalski, S.P., Eannetta, N.T., Hirzel, A.T., and Steffens J.C. (1992) Purification and characterization of polyphenol oxidase from glandular trichomes of *Solanum berthaultii*. *Plant Physiology*, **100**, 677–684.

Krings, M., Kellog, D., Derek, W., Kerp, H., and Taylor, T.N. (2003). Trichomes of the seed fern *Blanzyopteris praedentata*: implications for plant-insect interactions in the Late Carboniferous. *Botanical Journal of the Linnean Society*, **141**(2), 133–149.

Langton, F.A, Fuller, D.P., and Abbott, J.D. (2001). *Supplementary Lighting of Pot Chrysanthemums – A Grower Guide*. Final report of Horticultural Development Council. PC 92e. East Malling: Horticultural Development Council.

Leggett, T. (2006). A review of the world cannabis situation. *Bulletin of Narcotics*, **58**, 1–36.

Mahlberg, P.G., Hammond, C.T., Turner, J.C., and Hemphill, J.K. (1984). Structure, development and composition of glandular trichomes of *Cannabis sativa* L. In: E.O. Rodriguez, L. Healey, and I. Mehta (eds.). *Biology and Chemistry of Plant Trichomes*. London: Plenum Press, pp. 23–51.

Malingré, T., Herndriks, H., Battermann, S., Bos, R., and Visser, J. (1975). The essential oil of *Cannabis sativa* L. *Planta Medica*, **28**, 56–61.

Marschner, H. (2002). Nitrogen supply, plant growth and plant composition. In: *Mineral Nutrition in Higher Plants*. London: Academic Press, pp. 250–254.

McPartland, J.M., Clarke, R.C., and Watson, D.P. (2000). *Hemp Diseases and Pests Management and Biological Control*. Oxford: CABI Publishing.

Mechoulam, R. (1986). The pharmacohistory of *Cannabis sativa*. In: R. Mechoulam (ed.). *Cannabinoids as Therapeutics Agents*. Boca Raton, FL: CRC Press, pp. 1–19.

Mediavilla, V. and Steinemann, S. (1997). Essential oil of *Cannabis sativa* L. strains. *Journal of the International Hemp Association*, **4**, 80–82.

Neve, R.A. (1991). *Hops*. London: Chapman and Hall.

Payne, W.W. (1978). A glossary of plant hair technology. *Brittonia*, **30**, 239–255.

Pliny. (c.60AD). *Natural History*. Vol. 6. Translated by W.H.S. Jones (1951). Cambridge, MA: Harvard University Press.

Potter, D.J. (2004). Growth and morphology of medicinal cannabis. In: G.W. Guy, B.A. Whittle, and P.J. Robson (eds.). *The Medicinal Uses of Cannabis and Cannabinoids*. London: Pharmaceutical Press, pp. 17–54.

Potter, D.J. (2009). *The Propagation, Characterisation and Optimisation of Cannabis as a Phytopharmaceutical*. PhD thesis, Kings College London. Available at: http://www.gwpharm.com/uploads/finalfullthesisdjpotter.pdf (accessed May 21, 2014).

Potter, D.J. (2013). A review of the cultivation and processing of cannabis *Cannabis sativa* L. for production of prescription medicines in the UK. *Drug Testing and Analysis*, **6**, 31–38.

Potter, D.J. and Duncombe, P. (2012). The effect of electrical lighting power and irradiance on indoor-grown cannabis potency and yield. *Journal of Forensic Sciences*, **57**, 618–622.

Roberecht, R. and Caldwell, M.M. (1980). Leaf ultraviolet optical properties along a latitudinal gradient in the arctic-alpine life zone. *Ecology*, **61**, 612–619.

Rhodes, D.F. (1977). Integrated antiherbivore, antidesiccant, and ultraviolet screening properties of creosote bush resin. *Biochemical Systematics and Ecology*, **5**, 281–290.

Rosenthal, E. (2004). *The Big Book of Buds*. Vol. 2. Oakland, CA: Quick American Archives.

Russo, E.B. (2004). History of cannabis as a medicine. In: G.W. Guy, B.A. Whittle, and P.J. Robson (eds.). *The Medicinal Uses of Cannabis and Cannabinoids*. London: Pharmaceutical Press, pp. 1–16.

Russo, E.B. (2011). Taming THC: potential cannabis synergy and phytocannabinoid-terpenoid entourage effects. *British Journal of Pharmacology*, **163**, 1344–1364.

Shade, R.R., Thompson, T.E., and Campbell, W.R. (1975). An alfalfa weevil larval resistance mechanism detected in *Medicago*. *Journal of Economic Entomology*, **68**, 399–404.

Sirikantaramas, S., Taura, F., Tanaka, F., Ishikawa, Y., Morimoto, S., and Shoyama, S. (2005). Tetrahydrocannabinolic acid synthase, the enzyme controlling marijuana psychoactivity is secreted into the storage cavity of the glandular trichomes. *Plant & Cell Physiology*, **46**(9), 1578–1582.

Small, E. and Beckstead, H.D. (1973a). Common cannabinoid phenotypes in 350 stocks of Cannabis. *Lloydia*, **36**, 144–165.

Small, E. and Beckstead, H.D. (1973b). Cannabinoid phenotypes in *Cannabis sativa* L. *Nature*, **245**, 147–148.

Small, E. and Cronquist, A. (1976). A practical and natural taxonomy for cannabis. *Taxon*, **25**, 405–435.

Toonen, M., Ribot, S., and Thissen, J. (2006). Yield of illicit indoor cannabis cultivation in the Netherlands. *Journal of Forensic Science*, **51**, 1050–1054.

Tooker, J.F., Peiffer, M., Luthe, D.S., and Felton, G.W. (2010). Trichomes as sensors: detecting activity on the leaf surface. *Plant Signaling & Behavior*, **5**, 73–75.

Turner, A.E., El Sohly, M.A., and Boeren, E.G. (1980). Constituents of *Cannabis sativa* L. XV11. A review of the natural constituents. *Journal of Natural Products*, **43**, 169–233.

UNODC (United Nations Office on Drugs and Crime). (2006). Cannabis: why we should care. In: *World Drug Report 2006*. Vienna: UNODC, pp. 188–189. Available at: http://www.unodc.org/pdf/WDR_2006/wdr2006_chap2_why.pdf (accessed July 30, 2007).

UNODC. (2008). *World Drug Report 2008*. Vienna: UNODC. Available at: http://www.unodc.org/documents/wdr/WDR_2008/WDR_2008_eng_web.pdf (accessed August 15, 2013).

UNODC. (2009a). *Recommended Methods for the Identification and Analysis of Cannabis and Cannabis Products. Manual for Use by National Drug Analysis Laboratories*, Laboratory and Scientific Section – UNODC. Vienna: UNODC. Available at: http://www.unodc.org/documents/scientific/ST-NAR-40-Ebook.pdf (accessed August 15, 2013).

UNODC. (2009b). *World Drug Report 2009*. New York: United Nations Publications. Available online at: http://www.unodc.org/documents/wdr/WDR_2009/WDR2009_eng_web.pdf (accessed August 15, 2013).

Vanhove, W., Surmont, T., Van Damme, P., and De Ruyver, B. (2012). Yield and turnover of illicit indoor cannabis (*Cannabis* spp.) plantations in Belgium. *Forensic Science International*, **220**, 265–270.

Vanhove, W., Van Damme, P., and Meert, N. (2011). Factors determining yield and quality of illicit indoor cannabis (*Cannabis* spp.) production. *Forensic Science International*, **212**, 158–163.

Wagner, G.J., Wang, E., and Shepherd, W. (2004). New approaches for studying and exploiting an old protuberance, the plant trichome. *Annals of Botany*, **93**, 3–11.

Walters, D.S., Harman, J., Craig, R., AND Mumma, R.O. (1991). Effect of temperature on glandular trichome exudate composition and pest resistance in geraniums. *Entomologia Experimentalis et Applicata*, **60**, 61–69.

Werker, E. (2000). Trichome diversity and development. In: D.L. Hallahan, J.C. Gray, and J.A. Callow (eds.). *Advances in Botanical Research incorporating Advances in Plant Pathology Plant Trichomes*. Vol. 31. London: Academic Press, pp. 1–35.

Williamson, E.M. (2001). Synergy and other interactions in phytomedicines. *Phytomedicine*, **8**(5), 401–409.

Chapter 5

The Chemical Phenotypes (Chemotypes) of *Cannabis*

Etienne de Meijer

5.1 Introduction

Cannabinoids belong to a class of terpenophenolic compounds that, with some reported exceptions in the plant kingdom (Bohlmann and Hoffmann 1979; Raederstorff et al. 2012; Toyota et al. 1994, 2002), is largely unique to the genus *Cannabis*. In a review, ElSohly and Slade (2005) estimated the total number of cannabinoids at 70, but this number is dynamic and subject to definitions and limitations. Since then, ElSohly's group has added about 35 new cannabinoid terpene esters, cannabigerol-, and cannabichromanone-related substances. In the GW Pharmaceuticals (GW) laboratories, a range of fatty acid esters, cannabitriol esters, cannabitriol ethers, terpene esters, dimers and prenylated products of cannabinoids have been identified. These, with the proven and expected existence of several cannabinoid alkyl homologues, would bring the total number of cannabinoid-related compounds significantly in excess of 130 (A. Sutton, personal communication). Only a few of them are considered major, in the sense that they commonly occupy substantial proportions of a plant's total cannabinoid fraction. The large majority of the cannabinoids occur in trace proportions. Many of them appear to, or are expected to, induce specific physiological effects in mammals and are therefore of potential pharmaceutical interest. Pharmaceutical research, and product development especially, requires an ample availability of the compounds of interest. Economic and efficient horticultural production of cannabinoids is realized by the cultivation of uniform female crops with high yields of botanical raw material (BRM, the combined fraction of stem leaves and floral bracts and bracteoles), high cannabinoid content, and well-defined cannabinoid profiles that are strongly dominated by a single compound. These criteria provide the rationale and targets for a medicinal *Cannabis* breeding program. The economic production of the naturally minor cannabinoids particularly would not have been possible without committed breeding work. The focus of this chapter is on the currently available range of chemotypes, as expressed by selected female clones obtained through conventional breeding methods. These are discussed in terms of underlying genotype, breeding history, production level, and, in some instances, highly characteristic trichome morphology. A genetic model for chemotype inheritance is presented. Finally, the increasing molecular biological interest in *Cannabis* is addressed as this development may result in advanced breeding approaches, novel cannabinoid variants, and chemotypes beyond the current range.

5.2 Chemical phenotype and *Cannabis* classification

The genus *Cannabis* L. is unambiguously recognizable by botanical criteria. Within the genus, the variability of chemotypical and other characteristics is impressive and there is a long history of taxonomic controversy on the number of species to be recognized. Cannabinoids belong to the more conspicuous and spectacular attributes of the genus and cannabinoid chemotypes have been employed to classify groups within the genus, both casually and in formal taxonomy. Informally many authors refer to plants with high tetrahydrocannabinol (THC) content and low cannabidiol (CBD) content as "drug-type" and those with low THC content and high CBD content as "fiber-type" (e.g., Kojoma et al. 2006; Lydon and Teramura 1987). Although this may sound logical, such terminology is problematic. There are no strict natural relationships between fiber characteristics and cannabinoid content or – composition; only artificial associations for which exceptions occur (de Meijer and Keizer 1996).

Small and Cronquist (1976) attributed taxonomic importance to chemotype and used the THC:CBD ratio as a criterion to discriminate within the single species *C. sativa* L., two subspecies *sativa* and *indica* and, per subspecies, two varieties: one domesticated and one wild. Hillig and Mahlberg (2004) discriminated *C. sativa* and *C. indica* as separate species. However, their definitions of the categories *sativa* and *indica* deviate significantly from Small's and other (e.g., Anderson 1980; Schultes et al. 1974) taxonomic systems. They used chemotype-related criteria such as the B_T- and B_D allele frequency (encoding tetrahydrocannabinolic acid and cannabidiolic acid synthase, respectively), THC content, and the level of propyl cannabinoids. The great difficulty with such criteria is that they have, directly or indirectly, been subjected to human selection for ages. Furthermore, cannabinoid ratios are governed by simple genetic mechanisms and in segregating populations, or even in single plant progenies, morphologically similar (sister) plants can be found with strongly contrasting chemotypes. This makes the cannabinoid chemotype unsuitable as a taxonomic criterion.

Agreement on *Cannabis* taxonomy has never been reached and none of the proposed systems appears practically applicable as, under investigation, actual plants usually end up as "intermediate" between categories. A monospecific concept, with no further subspecific division, has implicitly been adopted in virtually all, nontaxonomic, publications on *Cannabis*. Also, in this author's opinion, the genus should be considered as monospecific, i.e., comprising only the single species *C. sativa* L. The reasons for this view are simple. All groups of plants belonging to the genus are perfectly interfertile and the morphological diversity within the genus shows a diffuse and continuous pattern. Hence, neither biological nor morphological criteria are available for the discrimination of more than one species. However, the issue remains of how to adequately indicate the different groups of plants within this single species. The current pattern of *Cannabis* diversity is primarily due to intentional actions of humans and reflects a long, intense, and divergent process of domestication which has blurred any natural evolutionary pattern of diversity. It is even questionable if truly wild *Cannabis* still exists, therefore a characterization of groups within the genus/species in nontaxonomic terms appears most appropriate. For instance, groups could be defined by their type of utilization: ("crop-use groups": fiber hemp, drug strains, seed hemp), their (usually secondary) geographic provenance, their domestication status [landraces (locally adapted, traditional varieties), cultivars of diverse nature, weedy escapes] and key agronomic features (chemotype, fiber content, etc.). Without any formal taxonomic intention, this provides a coherent idea of a group phenotype, a complex of commonly associated features resulting from domestication. To avoid taxonomic impasse and confusion, the use of "cultonomic" rather than natural taxonomic criteria has been recommended for domesticated plants in general (van den Berg 1999, 2004). Cultonomic classification has been formalized in the International Code of Nomenclature for Cultivated Plants (ICNCP, Brickell et al. 2004) and provides two categories, "Group" and "cultivar." The Group is a category for assembling cultivars on the basis of some defined similarity and, along with other users' criteria, chemotype would be a suitable attribute to specify Groups. The implementation of a system according to the ICNCP would be useful to all who need to refer to *Cannabis* plant materials.

5.3 **Defining chemotype**

5.3.1 **Components of chemotype**

For a systematic approach, it is important to discriminate qualitative and quantitative aspects of chemotype. The cannabinoid composition, i.e., the mutual ratio of the different cannabinoids, represents the qualitative chemotype and is generally controlled by simple genetic mechanisms, shows discrete distribution patterns in progenies and populations, and is hardly affected by the environment (de Meijer et al. 2003). The quantitative aspects of chemotype are controlled by different, polygenic mechanisms, show Gaussian distributions in progenies and populations, and are greatly affected by environmental factors. The yield of a certain cannabinoid in a horticultural production system can be considered as a complex characteristic composed of four components:

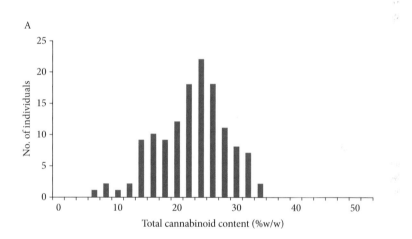

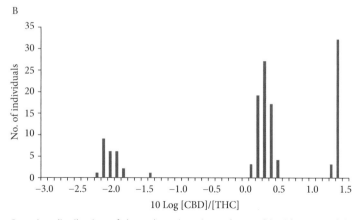

Fig. 5.1 The Gaussian distribution of the polygenic trait total cannabinoid content (A) and the discrete distribution of the monogenic trait cannabinoid profile (log [CBD]/[THC]) (B), in a segregating progeny of 130 sister-individuals.

the total above ground dry matter yield, the proportion of BRM (leaf and inflorescence), the total cannabinoid content in the homogenized BRM, and the proportion (purity) of the target cannabinoid in the total cannabinoid fraction. The first three components are quantitative in nature. The purity, or the mutual ratio of cannabinoids, has generally a monogenic background. Fig. 5.1 shows the differences in distribution patterns of the polygenic trait total cannabinoid content and the monogenic trait cannabinoid composition. For male and female *Cannabis* plants, the same principles for chemotype inheritance apply and the cannabinoid compositions (ratios) are similarly expressed. However, the dry matter yields, the BRM proportions, and the total cannabinoid contents reach lower values for the males than for the females. This is due to the typical male morphology: fewer floral bracts and bracteoles that carry the trichomes where the cannabinoid production takes place. Data presented in this chapter relate to mature female plants.

5.3.2 **Production procedures and conditions**

The plasticity of the quantitative components of chemotype requires some specification of the production environment. Data referred to in this chapter (e.g., Table 5.1) are based on the procedures and conditions in the GW glasshouse. For propagation of the production clones, shoot-cuttings are taken from mother plants. These are treated with a rooting hormone and incubated for 2 weeks under permanent light. Then, cuttings are transplanted to 5 L pots of compost and kept under permanent light (80 W/m^2 photosynthetically active radiation (PAR)) for a 3-week period of vegetative development. Crops are then spaced to 10 plants/m^2 under a 12 h photoperiod for flower induction, flowering, and maturation for a further 8–9 weeks. The average light intensity at crop level in the winter period is around 400 and in the summer period around 600 μmol.m^{-2}.s^{-1} (c.80 and 120 W/m^2 PAR, respectively). Temperature is kept at 25°C throughout the growing period. The compost used is an adjusted Begonia growth mix with a neutral pH. The structure is

Table 5.1 Achieved production levels of current clones representing nine different chemotypes. BRM indicates the total dry yield of leaf and floral tissue at maturity; C_{tot} is the total cannabinoid content in the BRM; purity is the proportion of the target cannabinoid in the total cannabinoid fraction; yield is the resulting quantity of the target cannabinoid produced. Performance of the propyl cannabinoid clones is still suboptimal and breeding aimed at yield improvement ongoing

Chemotype (main cannabinoid)	Clone (code)	BRM (g/m^2)	C_{tot} (%w/w)	Target cannabinoid	
				Purity (%w/w)	Yield (g/m^2)
CBG	M378	792	11.2	99.9	89
CBGV	M350	507	10.4	87.4	46
THC	M87	650	15.3	96.8	96
THCV	M264	609	14.5	81.7	72
CBD	M255	810	14.5	88.7	104
CBDV	M276	475	9.5	71.0	32
CBC	M394	731	2.9	93.4	20
CBCV	M206	283	1.8	52.6	3
Cannabinoid-free	M299	620	0.0		

medium-coarse with added perlite for aeration and free draining. After the generative period the above-ground plant material is collected, air dried, and the BRM separated from the stems and branches. Total cannabinoid contents (% w/w) are determined for the dry, homogenized (milled) BRM fraction. Compositions (ratios) and purities are expressed as the weight proportions (% w/w) of the individual cannabinoids in the total cannabinoid fraction.

5.4 **Genetic determination of chemotype**

5.4.1 **Cannabinoid biogenesis**

Cannabinoids are terpenophenolic products. The monoterpenoid precursors, predominantly geranylpyrophosphate (GPP) and to a lesser extent nerylpyrophosphate (NPP), originate from the deoxyxylulose (DOX) pathway (Fellermeier et al. 2001). The phenolic precursors (5-*n*-alkyl-resorcinolic acid homologues) are generated by the polyketide pathway (Raharjo et al. 2004). In the cannabinoid polyketide pathway, acyl-activating enzyme-1 (AAE1; Stout et al. 2012) binds coenzyme A (CoA) to different short-chain fatty acids. The most common phenolic precursor, 5-*n*-pentyl-resorcinolic acid (olivetolic acid, OA) results from the condensation of *n*-hexanoyl-CoA with three molecules of malonyl-CoA. In a two-step reaction, first a tetraketide intermediate is formed by olivetol synthase (OLS; sequenced by Taura et al. 2009), recently renamed as tetraketide synthase (TKS; Gagne et al. 2012). Subsequently, the tetraketide intermediate is cyclisized by the recently identified olivetolic acid cyclase (OAC; Gagne et al. 2012). Also the less common 5-*n*-propyl-resorcinolic acid homologue (divarinolic acid, DA) can be formed from *n*-butanoyl-CoA and three molecules of malonyl-CoA, probably by the same promiscuous enzyme system. Other resorcinolic acid alkyl homologues from C_1 through to C_7 are produced in minute quantities.

The phenolic and terpenoid moieties are subsequently condensed into terpenophenolics (cannabinoid acids) by the prenyltransferase enzyme geranylpyrophosphate:olivetolate transferase (GOT; Fellermeier and Zenk 1998). GOT was sequenced by Page and Boubakir (2011). Most commonly, geranylpyrophosphate (GPP) is condensed with OA to produce cannabigerolic acid (CBGA). With lower affinity, GOT condenses also NPP with OA to produce CBGA's optical isomer cannabinerolic acid (Taura et al. 1995a). Based on Shoyama et al. (1984) it can be deduced that GOT is promiscuous and also accepts resorcinolic acid homologues other than OA, but probably with lower affinity and/or turnover. Incorporation of these OA alkyl homologues results in the corresponding homologues of CBGA (i.e., CBGA-C_1 through to CBGA-C_7) and cannabinerolic acid.

The variability among cannabinoid structures is mainly attributable to the incorporation of different resorcinolic acid variants. Recently however, Pollastro et al. (2011) reported on a cannabinoid prenyl variant, a "sesqui-CBGA," which is apparently the condensation product of the sesquiterpene farnesylpyrophosphate and OA. According to Samuelsson (1999), unlike monoterpenes, these sesquiterpenes are not derived from the DOX pathway, but from the mevalonate pathway (MVA).

The various homologues of CBGA and cannabinerolic acid are the central intermediates in the cannabinoid pathway. Three different enzymatically catalyzed oxidative cyclizations lead to three categories of cannabinoid end products: the various alkyl homologues of tetrahydrocannabinolic acid (THCA-C_5), cannabidiolic acid (CBDA-C_5), and cannabichromenic acid (CBCA-C_5). Per enzymatic conversion, CBGA and cannabinerolic acid yield the same cyclization product (Morimoto et al. 1998; Taura et al. 1996). Kinetic parameters of THCA synthase were characterized by Taura et al. (1995b) and the gene was sequenced by Sirikantaramas et al.

(2004); Taura et al. (1996) characterized the kinetic parameters of CBDA synthase and the gene was sequenced by Taura et al. (2007); kinetic parameters of CBCA synthase were characterized by Morimoto et al. (1998) but it remains to be sequenced.

A hydroxy-methoxy substitution reaction of the CBGA type intermediates results in canna-bigerolic acid monomethyl ether (CBGAM; Shoyama et al. 1970). Most commonly occurring is the C_5 homologue CBGAM; the C_3 homologue cannabigerovarinic acid monomethyl ether (CBGVAM) is less common and other homologues occur as traces. Although obviously geneti-cally controlled, as yet a gene/enzyme combination for this methoxylation has not been identified.

Post harvest, under the influence of heat, a nonenzymatic decarboxylation reaction takes place which results in neutral cannabinoid molecules (e.g., THCA → THC). Under the influence of UV light and the presence of oxygen these neutral structures can further degrade. Alkyl homologues of cannabinol (CBN), cannabielsoin (CBS), and cannabicyclol (CBL) are the degradants of the corresponding alkyl homologues of THC, CBD, and CBC, respectively.

The large number of possible CBGA alkyl homologues, the various parallel pathways from CBGA type structures, and the various nonenzymatic conversions together lead to a large num-ber of compounds classified as cannabinoids. However, in wild-type *Cannabis* plants and their processed products only a few of these are found to occupy substantial proportions of the total cannabinoid fraction. These are: THCA-C_5 and its degradants THC-C_5 and CBN-C_5; THCA-C_3 (THCVA, tetrahydrocannabivarinic acid) and its degradant THC-C_3 (THCV, tetrahydrocanna-bivarin); CBDA-C_5 and its degradant CBD-C_5; CBCA-C_5 and its degradant CBC-C_5. All other cannabinoids are generally classified as minor.

5.4.2 **A model for chemotype inheritance**

The inheritance of chemotype has been investigated in the course of a long-term medicinal *Cannabis* breeding program, commenced at HortaPharm B.V. (The Netherlands) and continued at GW Pharmaceuticals (UK). A key technique in this program has been the self-fertilization of female plants after a chemically induced partial masculinization. In contrast to the natural out-breeding propagation system, this enables the creation of homozygous inbred lines, contrasting crosses between homozygous female plants and the systematic study of chemotypical segregation patterns in the cross progenies. Besides production clones of different chemotype (Table 5.1), the program has also resulted in a genetic model for the regulation and inheritance of chemotype (Fig. 5.2). Evidence for this model has been published by de Meijer et al. (2003, 2009a, 2009b) and de Meijer and Hammond (2005).

The formation of the phenolic moieties incorporated in cannabinoids (resorcinolic acids) can be obstructed by a monogenic factor. In the homozygous state, this factor induces a cannabinoid-free chemotype (de Meijer et al. 2009b). We postulated a single locus "O" with a mutant null allele *o* that blocks the resorcinol synthesis and a functional wild-type allele O that does not interfere. The null allele has a strong but incomplete dominance over the functional one. In segregating progenies, the O/o genotypes have only one-tenth of the cannabinoid content of O/O genotypes. The dominance of the knockout factor reflects the nature of a dominant repressor of a pathway gene rather than a fatal mutation in a structural pathway gene itself.

A postulated multiple locus "A" determines which of the resorcinolic acids is formed, olivetolic acid and/or divarinolic acid. Ongoing breeding experiments (unpublished) strongly suggest that this genetic factor is oligo- or polygenic with locus A carrying alleles $A_{pe}^{1\ to\ n}$ and $A_{pr}^{1\ to\ n}$. The $A_{pe}^{1\ to\ n}$ alleles encode for the more common olivetolic acid synthesis and the subsequent forma-tion of cannabinoids with a pentyl side chain. The $A_{pr}^{1\ to\ n}$ alleles encode for the less common

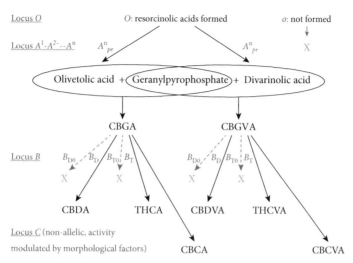

Fig. 5.2 A genetic model for chemotype regulation. Locus *O* determines if cannabinoids are formed. The multiple locus *A* determines the alkyl homologue ratio. Wild-type alleles at locus *B* control the ratios CBDA:THCA and/or CBDVA:THCVA whereas mutant alleles induce CBGA and/or CBGVA accumulation. Locus *C* is fixed but its chemotypical effect can be strongly modulated by morphological factors.

divarinolic acid synthesis and the subsequent formation of propyl cannabinoids. The codominant *A* alleles contribute additively but not equally to the chemotype (propyl:pentyl cannabinoid ratio); some having major, and others minor effects. Cannabinoid alkyl homologues other than the propyl- and pentyl ones do occur (C_1 through to C_7 homologues have been detected in *Cannabis* extracts). So far these homologues have only been detected in insignificant proportions and therefore the corresponding pathways are not covered by the model.

Olivetolic acid and divarinolic acid condense with geranylpyrophosphate into CBGA and cannabigerovarinic acid (CBGVA) respectively. There are no signs of allelism at this level, the enzyme GOT appears to be promiscuous and prenylates resorcinolic acids regardless of the alkyl side chain length. In spite of GOT's promiscuity for resorcinolic acid substrates, experiments by Shoyama et al. (1984) suggest that the enzyme's substrate affinity might be differential, with a preference for the C_5 homologue. CBGA and CBGVA are classified as true cannabinoids and form the substrates for a number of enzymatic conversions into cannabinoid end products: CBGA is converted into THCA, CBDA, CBCA, and CBGAM, respectively; CBGVA into THCVA, CBDVA (cannabidivarinic acid), CBCVA (cannabichromevarinic acid), and CBGVAM, respectively.

A monogenic locus "*B*" that controls the conversions of CBGA/CBGVA into THCA/THCVA (allele B_T) and CBDA/CBDVA (allele B_D) regardless of the alkyl side chain is postulated (de Meijer et al. 2003). Alleles B_T and B_D are codominant, i.e., heterozygous individuals (genotype B_T/B_D) express a chemotype composed of substantial proportions of both THCA/THCVA and CBDA/CBDVA. The ratios CBDA:THCA and CBDVA:THCVA are highly progeny specific and can deviate strongly from 1/1. This has been attributed to sequence variation in the B_T and B_D alleles, leading to synthases with differential catalytic properties. At the extremes of the locus *B* allelic range we find recessive, minimally functional, and nonfunctional alleles. In the homozygous state these induce a chemotype characterized by a high proportion of the accumulated precursor CBGA and/or CBGVA (de Meijer and Hammond 2005). Two of such alleles have been

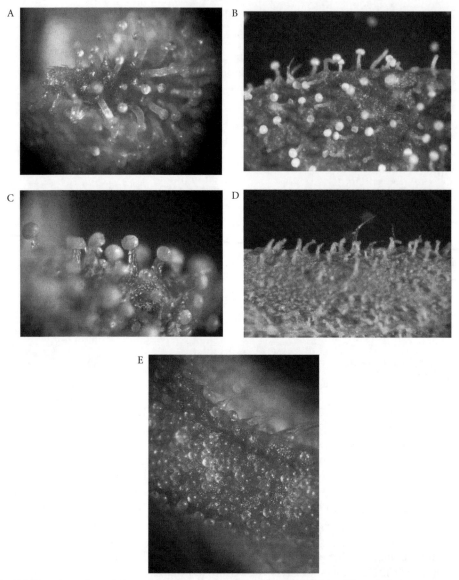

Fig. 5.3 (See also colour plate section.) Glandular trichomes associated to different chemotypes. (A) CBDA- and/or THCA-predominant plants carry stalked trichomes with large transparent heads. CBGA-predominant clones with underlying B_{D0}^2/B_{D0}^2 (B) and B_{T0}/B_{T0} (C) genotype both show white opaque trichome heads. (D) Cannabinoid-free chemotypes carry trichomes with shriveled heads. (E) Optimized CBCA-predominant clones lack stalked trichomes and show a high density of sessile trichomes.

© T.J. Wilkinson.

found in the form of B_D mutants and are indicated as $B_{D0}{}^1$ and $B_{D0}{}^2$. A B_T mutant, indicated as B_{T0}, has subsequently been found. It also induces a substantial CBGA and/or CBGVA accumulation along with a minimal THCA/THCVA production (unpublished data).

Independently of the THCA and CBDA synthase genes, a locus "*C*" regulates the conversion of CBGA/CBGVA into CBCA/CBCVA (de Meijer et al. 2009a). Locus *C* is fixed; it shows no allelism. Nevertheless, *Cannabis* chemotypes can vary greatly in the proportion of CBCA/CBCVA that they contain. The ontogenetic (developmental) variation in CBCA proportion has been commonly observed (e.g., Morimoto et al. 1997, 1998; Rowan and Fairbairn 1977; Shoyama et al. 1975). Apparently, CBCA synthase best competes with THCA synthase and CBDA synthase for the common CBGA/CBGVA substrate in the early juvenile stage. It would be problematic to exploit this feature for commercial CBCA or CBCVA production but, as an alternative strategy, we found different morphological mutations (reflecting underlying mono- and polygenic mechanisms) that enhance the activity of CBCA synthase throughout the life cycle of the plant. These mutations have in common the reduction of the presence of stalked glandular trichomes to the advantage of sessile trichomes (Fig. 5.3E) and are indicated as "PJC" genes (prolonged juvenile chemotype) in our model. The common "wild-type" status, not inducing this prolonged juvenile chemotype, is referred to as "pjc."

A fourth conversion, the methoxylation of CBGA and CBGVA results in the monomethyl ethers CBGAM and CBGVAM, respectively (Shoyama 1970). These compounds are not very prominent in the cannabinoid profile. Small and Beckstead (1973) reported the consistent presence of small amounts of CBGAM in plants from north-eastern Asia. We found that the presence of methoxylated cannabinoids is irregular but obviously inheritable. The methoxylation of CBGA and CBGVA does not appear to be controlled by the loci *B* and *C*. We found CBGAM and CBGVAM proportions up to 5% of the total cannabinoid fraction of certain lineages and hypothesized that such plants carry an active allele *M* in the homozygous state at a locus *M*, whereas plants devoid of these compounds carry the wild-type, inactive allele *m*. A breeding experiment aimed at the clarification and possible utilization of this mechanism has recently commenced and the role of CBGAM and CBGVAM in chemotypes will not be addressed further.

Obviously there is a gap between a genetic model that predicts and explains the outcome of breeding experiments and the actual events at the molecular level. Increasingly the different chemotypes are being investigated in transcriptome and gene expression studies which further clarify the mechanisms of chemotype regulation. For example, the powerful effect of the cannabinoid knockout factor at the monogenic locus *O* in heterozygous individuals was initially hard to explain. Recently it was found that the OLS (TKS) gene sequence of cannabinoid-free plants is identical to the wild-type sequence but that the gene is not expressed, probably due to a dominant monogenic repressor (unpublished data). In addition, the hypothesis that the accumulation of CBGA and CBGVA is due to normally expressed but minimally functional and nonfunctional alleles at locus *B*, is now supported by transcriptome analysis. Our CBGA/CBGVA-rich plants were found to express sequence variants of THCA and CBDA synthase, with radical amino acid substitutions in the conserved domains (unpublished data).

5.5 Results of chemotype breeding

5.5.1 Chemotype breeding

Chemotype manipulation is a target in the context of fiber/seed hemp breeding (suppression of THCA content), recreational drug breeding (high THCA content), and pharmaceutical drug breeding (various cannabinoid profiles). The most common chemotypes are CBDA and THCA predominant and can be encountered in all crop groups. Other, more specific chemotypes result from breeding programs such as the one initiated at HortaPharm and continued at GW, committed to increasing the purity and content of a range of different cannabinoids for commercial development. At an early stage in this program, a key technique allowing mass-scale self-fertilization and mutual crossing of female plants was developed. Source materials of various provenances and their first inbred generations were screened through gas chromatographic (GC) analyses. Selected progenitor genotypes, often with deviant profiles, were preserved in seed collections and clone libraries and used for line selection to obtain true-breeding (homozygous) inbred lines. Novel, recombinant cannabinoid profiles were established by crossing homozygous materials with different pure profiles, followed by self-fertilization. The newly inbred parental clones were then added to the library and, per chemotype, mutually crossed, in order to produce vigorous heterotic hybrids for production.

5.5.2 Currently available pure chemotypes

5.5.2.1 THCA-predominant chemotype

THCA predominance can be considered as a "wild-type" condition. In terms of the genetic model, it results from wild-type alleles at the loci O, A and B and a wild-type status (pjc) at the loci that induce the morphological features associated with prolonged CBCA catalysis: $O/O\text{-}A_{pe}^{1\ to\ n}/A_{pe}^{1\ to\ n}\text{-}B_T/B_T\text{-}pjc_{mono}/pjc_{mono}\text{-}pjc_{poly}$. THCA predominance is not exclusively associated with drug strains. Individuals of drug type landraces can be CBDA predominant or show a mixed CBDA/THCA profile, whereas certain fiber hemp strains of Far-Eastern provenance often comprise THCA-predominant individuals. Common relationships between cannabinoid chemotype and fiber yield or quality parameters are artificial and by no means natural. The purity of THCA, i.e., its proportion in % w/w in the total cannabinoid fraction reaches levels of 96–98%, with a residual fraction composed of traces of THCVA, CBCA, and CBGA. Modern, specifically bred THCA-predominant drug clones express total cannabinoid contents up to 25–30% w/w of the dry, "manicured" inflorescences. The total cannabinoid content of THCA-predominant drug landrace materials and fiber strains is much lower, 2–5% and <2%, respectively.

In marijuana strains, even landraces (e.g., from Thailand and South Africa), locus B has usually reached a fixed homozygous status (B_T/B_T) resulting in populations that are entirely composed of THCA-predominant individuals. In contrast, traditional hashish landraces (e.g., from Morocco, Pakistan, Afghanistan) are usually polymorphic at locus B and comprise THCA- and CBDA-predominant and -intermediate individuals. A plausible explanation for this difference is the fact that marijuana (dried inflorescences) is still an intact and recognizable tissue which allows seed retention. This enables generation from individuals selected for an appreciated smoking quality, i.e., high THCA purity. With a monogenic factor inducing a desirable phenotype, it is quite simple to select against the undesired allele (B_D) and create a fixed homozygous population. Hashish is traditionally collected in the field as a bulk crop extract and post harvest, when the overall quality is assessed, it is no longer possible to select the seeds from particular plants.

Numerous THCA-predominant clones and seed progenies circulate on the recreational market. Due to their illicit nature, these materials are not formally registered so their identity and stability are not guaranteed. The many different names (e.g., Haze, Skunk, Northern Lights, White Widow) cannot be considered as unequivocal cultivar names. They refer to more or less coherent groups, all THCA predominant, but with differences in the terpene entourage, morphology, phenological development, photoperiod requirements for flower induction, etc. A small number of THCA clones have been through the Plant Breeders Rights registration procedure and received European Breeders Rights. Examples are the cultivar "Medisins" (HortaPharm) and GW's clones used for the raw material production of Sativex®.

5.5.2.2 CBDA-predominant chemotype

As with THCA predominance, CBDA predominance is also a common wild-type condition. It results from wild-type alleles at the loci O, A, and B and a wild-type (pjc) status at the loci that induce the morphological features associated with prolonged CBCA catalysis: O/O-$A_{pe}^{1\ to\ n}/A_{pe}^{1\ to\ n}$-$B_D/B_D$-pjc$_{mono}$/pjc$_{mono}$-pjc$_{poly}$. CBDA predominance is common and usually fixed in modern hemp fiber and seed cultivars. It is common, but not usually fixed, in fiber and hashish landraces. The purity of CBDA, i.e., the proportion in % w/w in the total cannabinoid fraction reaches levels of 85–90%, with a residual fraction composed of CBDVA, CBCA, CBGAM, THCA, and CBGA. In specially bred CBDA drug clones the total cannabinoid content reaches levels as in THCA clones: up to 25–30% w/w of the dry, "manicured" inflorescences. In hashish landraces and fiber strains, individuals reach much lower levels of 1–5%. The consistent presence of a 4–5% w/w proportion of THCA in the total cannabinoid fraction of CBDA-predominant plants is intriguing but has rarely been addressed in the literature. Lydon and Teramura (1987) ruled out CBDA as photochemically converted into THCA. Possibly, besides the main cyclization of CBGA to CBDA, CBDA synthase might be able to perform a second minor conversion of CBGA to THCA. Evolutionarily this would indicate that the CBDA synthase gene has evolved from an ancestral THCA synthase gene (vice versa, THCA-predominant plants contain practically no CBDA). Alternatively, this THCA could be the product of "inactive" THCA synthase homologues that were reported by Kojoma et al. (2006) for CBDA-predominant and -intermediate CBDA/THCA chemotypes. However, these homologues were $c.40$ SNPs (single nucleotide polymorphisms) different from the active sequence published by Sirikantaramas et al. (2004), so it is questionable if they really have retained any catalytic ability. Furthermore, the small amount of THCA in CBDA plants occurs invariably in the form of both the cis and the trans isomer in a 1:3 ratio, whereas in true THCA-predominant plants solely the trans isomer is found (A. Sutton, personal communication). Although not a perfect 1:1 racemic ratio, this finding suggests as a third possibility that a nonenzymatic reaction occurs in these plants. A possible approach to clarify this issue could be an in vitro assay with each of the heterologously expressed proteins of the THCA and CBDA synthase sequence variants. Practically, the consistent presence of some THCA in CBDA-predominant chemotypes can be problematic in the case of fiber and seed cultivars with a relatively high overall cannabinoid content. For these, a limit of 0.2% THC is legally enforced in the European Union (EU). As THCA occupies 4–5% of the cannabinoid fraction of a CBDA-predominant chemotype this limit will be reached at a total cannabinoid content of 4% w/w. In CBD-rich pharmaceutical extracts too, the associated presence of psychoactive THC can be undesirable.

Around 60 fiber cultivars with a CBDA-predominant chemotype are registered in the EU. Plants Breeders Rights have also been obtained for GW's CBDA-rich clones used for the raw material production of Sativex®.

5.5.2.3 CBGA-predominant chemotypes

Fournier et al. (1987) were the first to report on a CBGA-rich plant in a normally CBDA-predominant French fiber hemp population. Accumulation of this otherwise minor compound is a mutant condition induced by an absence of sufficiently active THCA and/or CBDA synthase. According to the genetic model, CBGA predominance results from wild-type alleles at the loci O and A, mutant ("null") alleles at locus B (de Meijer and Hammond 2005) and a wild-type status (pjc) at the loci that induce the morphological features associated with prolonged CBCA catalysis: O/O-$A_{pe}^{1\ to\ n}/A_{pe}^{1\ to\ n}$-$B_0/B_0$-pjc$_{mono}$/pjc$_{mono}$-pjc$_{poly}$. We have obtained two different CBGA-predominant chemotypes with a residual presence of CBDA from fiber hemp source populations. The inbred generation of a marijuana clone revealed a second CBGA-rich chemotype with a residual presence of THCA. It was postulated that the first category is attributable to minimally functional CBDA synthase (alleles B_{D0}^1 and B_{D0}^2, which was subsequently found), and the second category to minimally functional THCA synthase (allele B_{T0}). The purity of CBGA-predominant plants can vary, depending on the impact of the mutation involved. Genotypes that are homozygous for the alleles B_{D0}^1, B_{D0}^2, and B_{T0}, typically express CBGA proportions of 90%, nearly 100%, and 85% respectively, in the cannabinoid fraction. Regardless of the underlying genotype, all CBGA-rich chemotypes share the morphological feature of white opaque glandular trichome heads (Fig. 5.3B and C). It is remarkable that Gorshkova et al. (1988) characterized this same morphological phenotype as indicative of an absence of cannabinoids. There is no obvious inhibitory feedback in cannabinoid metabolism if the normal end products CBDA and/or THCA are absent or are only poorly formed. After some committed breeding effort the absolute cannabinoid contents of CBGA-predominant plants now reach levels similar to high-content THCA and CBDA plants (Table 5.1). In 2003, Plant Breeders Rights were obtained for the Italian, CBGA-rich fiber hemp cultivar Carma. The average CBGA proportion in the cannabinoid fraction of this cultivar is c.55%, with a residual fraction of mainly CBDA (G. Grassi, personal communication).

5.5.2.4 CBCA-rich and -predominant chemotypes

CBCA is often considered a minor cannabinoid and usually occurs only in proportions of 0–5% in the cannabinoid fraction of most mature *Cannabis* plants of all chemotypes. It is more prominent in juvenile profiles (e.g., Morimoto et al. 1997, 1998; Rowan and Fairbairn 1977; Shoyama et al. 1975). Morphological mutants were found in Afghan hashish and Korean fiber landraces that maintain somewhat higher proportions of CBCA (15–30% of the cannabinoid fraction) throughout the course of the life cycle (de Meijer et al. 2009b). These mutations have in common the suppression of the formation of bracts and bracteoles and thereby, that of stalked glandular trichomes. This leads to a relative abundance of sessile trichomes on the floral tissues (Fig. 5.3E). Besides these inheritable morphological factors we have never found any indication that the variation in CBCA content is attributable to allelism at a "biochemical locus" encoding an active and an inactive CBCA synthase (de Meijer et al. 2009b). The breeding strategy to obtain pure CBCA plants was therefore based on "stacking" the different morphological mutations and obstructing the competitive pathways from CBGA to THCA and/or CBDA. This was realized by establishing a B_{D0}^2/B_{D0}^2 genotype at locus B. In selected clones, CBCA purities at maturity of up to 95% of the cannabinoid fraction were achieved, with CBCA-C_1, CBCA-C_3, cannabicyclol (CBL, a CBCA degradant), THCA (cis and trans isomers), and CBGA as additional trace compounds. In terms of the genetic model, these optimized clones have the genotype: O/O-$A_{pe}^{1\ to\ n}/A_{pe}^{1\ to\ n}$- B_{D0}^2/B_{D0}^2 - PJC_{mono}/PJC_{mono}-PJC_{poly}. As an inherent effect of the absence of bracts and bracteoles that carry the highly productive stalked trichomes, such plants can only attain a relatively low overall cannabinoid content. So far, the maximum content in a dry homogenized BRM appears to be 3–3.5% w/w.

Unlike other chemotypes, the CBCA-rich chemotype shows a certain sensitivity to its environment. At high light intensities, the total cannabinoid content may increase at the expense of the CBCA purity (de Meijer et al. 2009a). This is probably due to the fact that CBCA synthase quickly reaches its catalytic maximum and then leaves a surplus of the CBGA substrate unconverted.

CBCA-rich clones have not been submitted for Plant Breeders Rights but the chemotype is categorically protected by a patent (WO2009/125198).

5.5.2.5 THCVA- and other propyl cannabinoid-rich chemotypes

Generally, propyl cannabinoids occur in low proportions (< 2%) of the total cannabinoid fraction. In situ, THCVA appears the only compound that is occasionally found in more substantial

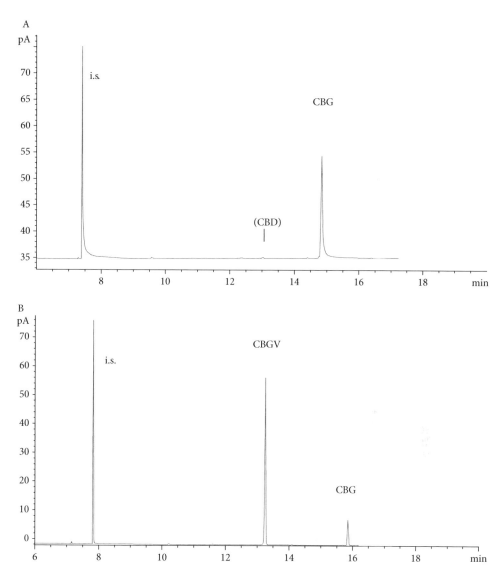

Fig. 5.4 Chromatograms of unusual chemotypes obtained using a gas chromatograph with flame ionization detector (GC-FID). Peaks indicate cannabinoids in decarboxylated form. Data originate from different GC runs and between chromatograms retention times cannot be compared. I.s. = added internal standard. (A) clone M281, CBG purity ≤ 99.9%; (B) clone M350, CBGV purity 87%; (C) clone M408, THCV purity 92%; (D) clone M277, CBDV purity 73%; (E) clone M394, CBC purity 95%; (F) seedling 2012.16.3.26.6, CBCV purity 76%; (G) clone M299, cannabinoid-free.

proportions. It can reach various levels, up to 70% of the cannabinoid fraction, in plants from populations belonging to different crop-use groups. These often originate in China (fiber and seed landraces) and Southern Africa (marijuana landraces). In terms of the genetic model, THCVA-rich plants carry a number of A_{pr} alleles at the multiple locus A and are homozygous B_T/B_T at locus B. Geographical isolation is a possible explanation of why in situ the A_{pr} alleles do

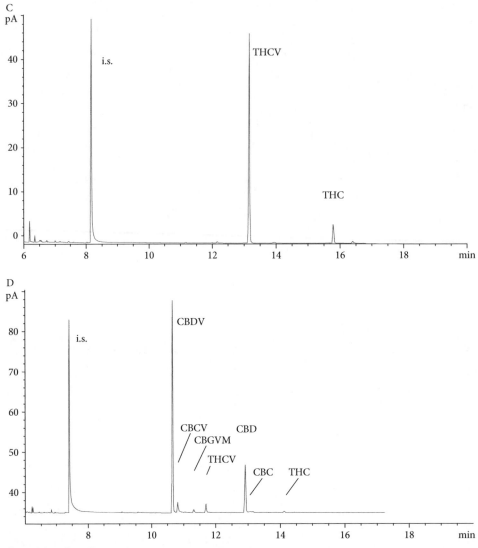

Fig. 5.4 (continued)

not usually occur in combination with a B_D/B_D and B_0/B_0 genotype or with the morphological PJC factors in order to produce CBDVA-, CBGVA-, or CBCVA-rich chemotypes, respectively. In our breeding program we were successful in producing CBDVA- and CBGVA-predominant clones whereas the breeding of CBCVA-predominant plants is still in an early stage. Further improvement of the propyl cannabinoid purity in these chemotypes is ongoing and promising. For THCVA, a level of over 92% of the cannabinoid fraction has already been achieved by stacking A_{pr} alleles from different progenitors in hybrid offspring (Fig. 5.4C). THCA is the main residual cannabinoid in THCVA-predominant plants and its presence is undesirable as it requires chemical purification to avoid the presence of psychoactive, and possibly THCV-counteracting, THC in THCV-based medicines. The purities currently achieved for CBGVA, CBDVA, and CBCVA are

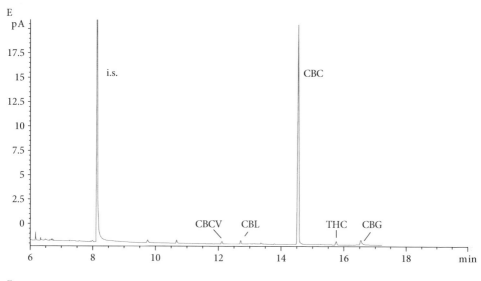

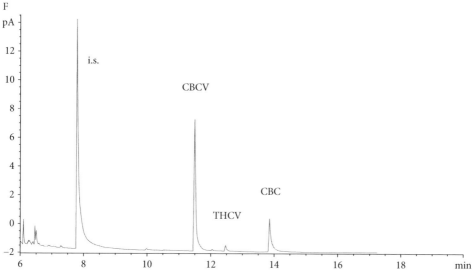

Fig. 5.4 (continued)

87%, 73%, and 76% and in chemotypes with these compounds, the corresponding pentyl homo-logues also form the main residual cannabinoid (Fig. 5.4B, D, and F). The characteristic trichome morphology of CBGA- and CBCA-predominant chemotypes (Fig. 5.3B, C, and E) is also associated to the CBGVA- and CBCVA-predominant chemotypes.

The molecular basis of the C_3/C_5 regulation at the postulated locus A remains to be clarified. We compared flower transcriptomes of C_3-rich- and pure C_5 segregant bulks of segregating, single plant progenies. In the phenolic pathway, meaningful variation in gene sequence or gene expression was not found at the level of the candidate genes AAE1, TKS, and OAC (data unpublished). This suggests that the $C_3:C_5$ ratio is regulated by still unknown genes involved in the production of the short-chain fatty acid precursors: butanoate and hexanoate.

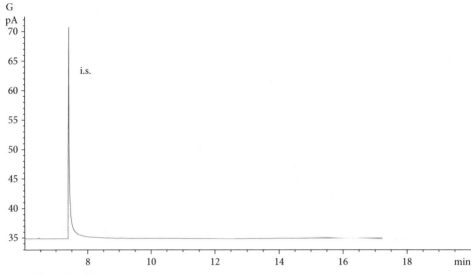

Fig. 5.4 (continued)

Currently, no Plant Breeders Rights or patents are known for THCVA- or other propyl-rich materials.

5.5.2.6 Cannabinoid-free chemotype

Our cannabinoid-free chemotype appears to be the consequence of an obstacle in the phenolic pathway towards the resorcinolic acids (de Meijer et al. 2009b). In terms of our genetic model, these plants carry a mutant allele in the homozygous state at the single locus O. It is conceivable that other mechanisms also induce an absence of cannabinoids. Gorshkova et al. (1988) reported on a cannabinoid-free chemotype attributable to a total absence of glandular trichomes. Nonfunctional trichomes, an obstacle in the terpenoid pathway towards geranylpyrophosphate or a mutation in GOT, thereby disabling the terpeno-phenolic condensation, would also obstruct cannabinoid production, but as yet there are no reports on cannabinoid-free chemotypes induced by such mechanisms.

The cannabinoid knockout gene expressed in our clones was derived from a low-cannabinoid-content fiber cultivar. In certain specimens of this cultivar there were no detectable cannabinoids. When crossed with high-content plants, an F_1 with low cannabinoid levels (ca 1/10 of that of the high-content parent) was produced, whereas F_2 generations obtained from self-fertilized F_1 individuals segregated in three discrete chemotypes: cannabinoid-free, low-content (as F_1), and high-content individuals in a monogenic 1:2:1 ratio. The severe reduction in the cannabinoid content of the heterozygous groups suggests that the knockout factor is not a mutated structural pathway gene. It is more likely to be a regulator, in this case probably a dominant repressor of OLS/TKS (F. Licausi, unpublished data). Repeated backcrossing of the first-generation cannabinoid-free plants with high-content materials has resulted in a range of cannabinoid-free plants with a dense, branched habitus, high trichome density, and a strong fragrance. Knockout homologues with a strong resemblance to the Sativex® THCA and CBDA clones (Fig. 5.5) plus a series of cannabinoid-free clones predominant in each one of the monoterpenes: pinene, myrcene, terpinolene, carene, and limonene, have all been bred through backcrossing. The fact that these clones contain terpenes (mono- and sesqui-) in normal quantities, demonstrates that neither the

A

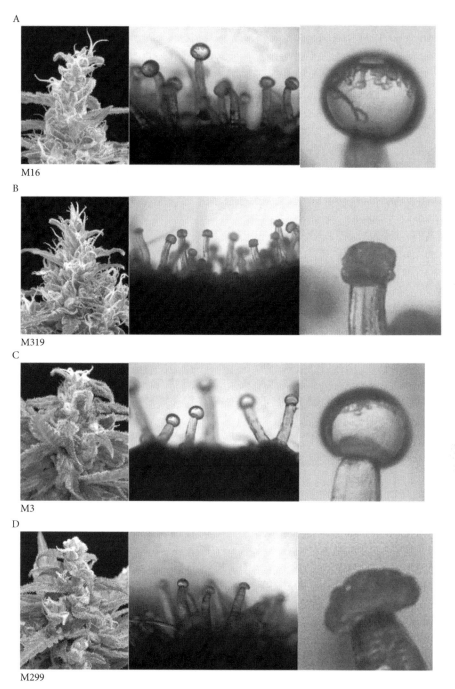

M16

B

M319

C

M3

D

M299

Fig. 5.5 (See also colour plate section.) Macro- and microscopic photos of clones used for Sativex®
raw material production, M16 (CBD) and M3 (THC), and their respective cannabinoid-free
homologues M319 and M299. The homologues were selected from backcross progenies
(e.g., M299 = M3 × (M3 × (M3 × knockout progenitor))) and share 87.5% genetic identity with
the corresponding "original."

© T.J. Wilkinson.

terpenoid pathway nor the functionality of the trichomes is affected by the knockout factor. Such materials could play a role in clarifying cannabinoid-terpenoid interactions ("entourage effects"; Russo 2011). The incorporation of purified cannabinoids (or combinations thereof) into various cannabinoid-free BRMs would enable a systematic study of the possible differential physiological effects of pure cannabinoids versus cannabinoids extracts. Another obvious application of the knockout factor is in breeding cannabinoid-free fiber hemp and seed hemp. The absence of the usual terpenophenolic end products together with the presence of most of the pathway enzymes has made our cannabinoid-free plants useful as chemical-analytical reference material and as crude enzyme sources for in vitro assays.

Patent protection has been obtained for cannabinoid-free clones and their use as a reference plant (WO2008/146006).

5.5.3 Chemotype and evolutionary fitness

Cannabinoids can reach extremely high concentrations in above-ground plant tissues. Various theories, all relating to the defense against biotic and abiotic stress, attribute ecological benefits to the presence of cannabinoids in general, or to the presence of certain cannabinoids in particular (Appendino et al. 2008; Lydon et al. 1987; Morimoto et al. 2007; Pate 1983). Our breeding experiments and the crop production of different chemotypes take place in a protected indoor environment, but they should still reveal some relationship between chemotype and fitness, if it does exist. The chemotype segregating progenies obtained from a single self-fertilized parent, where all individuals are highly related sister plants, are particularly suitable to compare the strengths or susceptibilities of contrasting chemotypes. However, compelling associations between chemotype (including the cannabinoid-free plants) and features such as seed set, plant size, and infestation with insects or fungi have so far not been observed.

5.6 Molecular studies of chemotype regulation

5.6.1 Historic overview

A more molecular approach to the underlying genetics of *Cannabis* chemotype perhaps commenced with the in vitro testing of crude *Cannabis* enzyme extracts (e.g., Shoyama et al. 1984). This was followed by the purification and characterization of the important pathway enzymes THCA synthase, CBDA synthase, and CBCA synthase by Taura et al. (1995b, 1996) and Morimoto et al. (1998), respectively. THCA synthase and CBDA synthase were also the first pathway genes to be sequenced, by Sirikantaramas et al. (2004) and Taura et al. (2007), respectively. THCA synthase is polymorphic and Kojoma et al. (2006) published sequence variants found in plants with a THCA-predominant, CBDA-predominant, and mixed THCA/CBDA chemotype. A number of these sequence variants encodes an active synthase whereas, in the CBDA-predominant plants, only inactive or minimally active THCA sequences occur, with many amino acid substitutions compared to the active ones. Different molecular markers (PCR products) associated with CBDA or THCA synthase sequences have been developed (e.g., de Meijer et al. 2003; Kojoma et al. 2006; Pacifico et al. 2006; Rotherham and Harbison 2010). Very recently, Shoyama et al. (2012) elucidated the structure–function relationship of the active THCA synthase protein.

One step upstream in the pathway, the prenyl transferase GOT, that catalyzes the condensation of the resorcinolic acids with geranylpyrophosphate into CBGA type products, was sequenced by Page and Boubakir (2011).

Further upstream in the phenolic pathway, three crucial genes for the *n*-alkyl-resorcinolic acid synthesis have now been sequenced. Stout et al. (2012) identified the acyl activating enzyme AAE1 that binds coenzyme-A to the short-chain fatty acids hexanoate, butanoate, and malonate. The process of the condensation of the fatty acid-CoA substrates into resorcinolic acids by a polyketide type mechanism has long been unclear, but was recently clarified by Gagne et al. 2012. For this two-step reaction both a TKS and an OAC are required. TKS had already been sequenced by Taura et al. (2009) under the name olivetol synthase (OLS). OAC was sequenced by Gagne et al. (2012). In 2011 the first entire draft genomes for *Cannabis*, based on two different THCA-predominant drug strains, were published by McKernan et al. (see http://www.medicinalgenomics.com). Van Bakel et al. (2011) published the transcriptomes (expressed genes) of various tissues of a high-content THCA drug strain and a low-content CBDA-predominant oil seed cultivar as well as the draft genomes of these accessions and a low-content fiber cultivar.

Although the cannabinoid pathways have now largely been elucidated, there are still some important issues to be resolved: the CBCA synthase sequence, the regulation of the methoxylation of CBGA type structures into monomethyl ethers, and the mechanism of the cannabinoid alkyl side chain regulation. In order to study these topics, F_2 progenies, obtained from self-fertilized parents which segregate the relevant chemotypes, would be more promising plant materials than unrelated drug and fiber strains.

5.6.2 Prospects for novel chemotype breeding

As has been presented here, conventional plant breeding, with the inclusion of the cannabinoid knockout, has resulted in nine fairly pure chemotypes. Additionally, an increase in the proportions of CBGA type monomethyl ethers (CBGAM and CBGVAM) might be possible. Since the conventional approach appears to have reached its limit, it is opportune to explore the prospects of molecular techniques for a further expansion of the chemotype portfolio. With cannabinoid contents up to 25–30% of the floral dry weight already achieved, there is no urgency to improve the quantitative aspects of chemotype, a situation quite different from that with plants producing opiates, artemisin, taxol, etc. Innovations such as (1) chemotypes containing substantial proportions of truly novel terpenophenolic compounds (e.g., with branched alkyl- or aromatic side chains); (2) chemotypes with dramatically increased proportions of known, but currently very minor substances (e.g., rich in methyl- or butyl cannabinoids, rich in farnesyl cannabinoids); (3) chemotypes lacking naturally associated, undesirable compounds (e.g., CBDA-predominant plants devoid of THCA) would be more valuable. Page and Boubakir (2011) mention the possibility of mutating their sequenced prenyltransferase gene (GOT) in order to enhance cannabinoid production or to obtain cannabinoid-free plants by gene inactivation. Van Bakel et al. (2011) speculate that the identification of candidate pathway genes may eventually result in the development of cannabinoid-free hemp cultivars and CBCA-rich materials. McKernan et al. (2011, http://www.medicinalgenomics.com) hope that their draft genome, once further annotated, will help to enhance the expression of some, currently minor, cannabinoids. These ambitions are remarkably modest and largely aimed at existing chemotypes.

Modification of the phenolic pathway achieved by exploiting recent advances in *Cannabis* molecular biology could be an interesting new direction. Currently available homologues with the same aromatic structure but a different alkyl side chain, such as THC and THCV, can show totally different activity. The *Cannabis* gene(s) regulating the C_3:C_5 cannabinoid ratio, once identified, would be an interesting target for site-specific mutagenesis. This may lead to a substantial production of resorcinolic acids with alkyl chains other than propyl or pentyl. Alternatively, there might be a transgenic option to modify this pathway. Some other plant species do produce resorcinols, resorcinolic acids, and even terpenophenolic acids, often in a different form from that of *Cannabis*. It is likely that such plants carry genes homologous to certain cannabinoid pathway genes. Transfer to, and heterologous expression of, such genes in *Cannabis* may result in variant precursors and products. One uncertainty with both site-specific mutagenesis and heterologous expression is that the desired incorporation of alternative precursors into cannabinoid end products requires substrate promiscuity of the enzymes downstream. Shoyama et al. (2012) suggest that their structure–function study of THCA synthase allows the development of mutants with altered substrate preference or catalytic activity. This could lead to novel THCA derivatives. In the plant, suitable substrates other than CBGA and cannabinerolic acid homologues do not occur naturally, but they could result from an artificially modified phenolic pathway. Altered catalytic activity of THCA (and CBDA) synthase would also be of practical interest were it to result in new cyclization products.

References

Anderson, L.C. (1980). Leaf variation among *Cannabis* species from a controlled garden. *Harvard University Botanical Museum Leaflets*, **28**, 61–69.

Appendino, G., Gibbons, S., Giana, A., *et al.* (2008). Antibacterial cannabinoids from *Cannabis sativa*: a structure-activity study. *Journal of Natural Products*, **71**, 1427–1430.

Bakel, H. van, Stout, J.M., Cote, A.G., *et al.* (2011). The draft genome and transcriptome of *Cannabis sativa*. *Genome Biology*, **12**, R102.

Berg, R.G. van den (1999). Cultivar-group classification. In: S. Andrews, A.C. Leslie, and C. Alexander (eds.). *Taxonomy of Cultivated Plants, III*[rd] *International Symposium of Cultivated Plants*. Kew: Royal Botanic Gardens, pp. 135–143.

Berg, R.G. van den (2004). The crop concept in cultonomic classification. In: C.G. Davidson and P. Trehane (eds.). IVth Int. Symp. of Cultivated Plants. *Acta Horticulturae*, **634**, 141–144.

Bohlmann, F. and Hoffmann, E. (1979). Cannabigerol-ähnliche verbindungen aus *Helichrysum umbraculigerum*. *Phytochemistry*, **18**, 1371–1374.

Brickell, C.D., Baum, B.R., Hetterscheid, W.L.A., *et al.* (2004). International Code of Nomenclature for Cultivated Plants. *Acta Horticulturae*, 647.

ElSohly, M.A. and Slade, D. (2005). Chemical constituents of marijuana: the complex mixture of natural cannabinoids. *Life Sciences*, **78**, 539–548.

Fellermeier, M. and Zenk, M.H. (1998). Prenylation of olivetolate by a hemp transferase yields cannabigerolic acid, the precursor of tetrahydrocannabinol. *FEBS Letters*, **427**, 283–285.

Fellermeier, M., Eisenreich, W., Bacher, A., and Zenk, M.H. (2001). Biosynthesis of cannabinoids. Incorporation experiments with ^{13}C-labeled glucoses. *European Journal of Biochemistry*, **268**, 1596–1604.

Fournier, G., Richez-Dumaois, C., Duvezin, J., Mathieu, J.P., and Paris, M. (1987). Identification of a new chemotype in *Cannabis sativa*: cannabigerol-dominant plants, biogenetic and agronomic prospects. *Planta Medica*, **53**, 277–280.

Gagne, S.J., Stout, J.M., Liu, E., Boubakir, Z., Clark, S.M., and Page J. (2012). Identification of olivetolic acid cyclase from *Cannabis sativa* reveals a unique catalytic route to plant polyketides. *Proceedings of the National Academy of Sciences of the United States of America*, **109**, 12811–12816.

Gorshkova, L.M., Senchenko, G.I., and Virovets, V.G. (1988). Method of evaluating hemp plants for content of cannabinoid compounds [Russian]. *Referativnyi Zhurnal*, 12.65.322.

Hillig, K.W. and Mahlberg, P.G. (2004). A chemotaxonomic analysis of cannabinoid variation in *Cannabis* (Cannabaceae). *American Journal of Botany*, **91**, 966–975.

Kojoma, M., Seki, H., Yoshida, S., and Muranaka, T. (2006). DNA polymorphisms in the tetrahydrocannabinolic acid (THCA) synthase gene in "drug type" and "fibre type" *Cannabis sativa* L. *Forensic Science International*, **159**, 132–140.

Lydon, J. and Teramura, A.H. (1987). Photochemical decomposition of cannabidiol in its resin base. *Phytochemistry*, **26**, 1216–1217.

Lydon, J., Teramura, A.H., and Coffman, C.B. (1987). UV-B radiation effects on photosynthesis, growth and cannabinoid production of two *Cannabis sativa* chemotypes. *Photochemistry and Photobiology*, **46**, 201–206.

Meijer, E.P.M. de, Bagatta, M., Carboni, A., *et al.* (2003). The inheritance of chemical phenotype in *Cannabis sativa* L. *Genetics*, **163**, 335–346.

Meijer, E.P.M. de and Hammond, K.M. (2005). The inheritance of chemical phenotype in *Cannabis sativa* L. (II): cannabigerol predominant plants. *Euphytica*, **145**, 189–198.

Meijer, E.P.M. de, Hammond, K.M., and Micheler, M. (2009a). The inheritance of chemical phenotype in *Cannabis sativa* L. (III): variation in cannabichromene proportion. *Euphytica*, **165**, 293–311.

Meijer, E.P.M. de, Hammond, K.M., and Sutton, A. (2009b). The inheritance of chemical phenotype in *Cannabis sativa* L. (IV): cannabinoid-free plants. *Euphytica*, **168**, 95–112.

Meijer, E.P.M. and Keizer, L.C.P. (1996). Patterns of diversity in *Cannabis*. *Genetic Resources and Crop Evolution*, **43**, 41–52.

Morimoto, S., Komatsu, K., Taura, F., and Shoyama, Y. (1997). Enzymological evidence for cannabichromenic acid biosynthesis. *Journal of Natural Products*, **60**, 854–857.

Morimoto, S., Komatsu, K., Taura, F., and Shoyama, Y. (1998). Purification and characterisation of cannabichromenic acid synthase from Cannabis sativa. *Phytochemistry*, **49**, 1525–1529.

Morimoto, S., Tanaka, Y. and Sasaki, K., *et al.* (2007). Identification and characterisation of cannabinoids that induce cell death through mitochondrial permeability transition in *Cannabis* leaf cells. *The Journal of Biological Chemistry*, **282**, 20739–20751.

Pacifico, D., Miselli, F., Micheler, M., Carboni, A., Ranalli, P., and Mandolino, G. (2006). Genetics and marker-assisted selection of the chemotype in *Cannabis sativa* L. *Molecular Breeding*, **17**, 257–268.

Page, J.E. and Boubakir, Z. (2011). Aromatic prenyltransferase from *Cannabis*. Patent WO 2011/017798 A1.

Pate, D.W. (1983). Possible role of ultraviolet radiation in evolution of *Cannabis* chemotypes. *Economic Botany*, **37**, 396–405.

Pollastro, F., Taglialatela-Scafati, O. and Allarà, M., *et al.* (2011). Bioactive prenylogous cannabinoid from fiber hemp (*Cannabis sativa*). *Journal of Natural Products*, **74**, 2019–2022.

Raederstorff, D., Schwager, J., and Schueler, G. (2012). Nutraceutical and pharmaceutical compositions and use thereof for the treatment, co-treatment or prevention of inflammatory disorders. US Patent 8158681.

Raharjo, T.J., Chang, W.T., Choi, Y.H., Peltenburg-Looman, A.M.G., and Verpoorte, R. (2004). Olivetol as product of a polyketide synthase in *Cannabis sativa* L. *Plant Science*, **166**, 381–385.

Rotherham, D. and Harbison, S. (2010). Differentiation of drug and non-drug *Cannabis* using a single nucleotide polymorphism (SNP) assay. *Forensic Science International*, **207**, 193–197.

Rowan, M.G. and Fairbairn, J.W. (1977). Cannabinoid patterns in seedlings of *Cannabis sativa* L. and their use in the determination of chemical race. *Journal of Pharmacy and Pharmacology*, **29**, 491–494.

Russo, E.B. (2011). Taming THC: potential cannabis synergy and phytocannabinoid-terpenoid entourage effects. *British Journal of Pharmacology*, **163**, 1344–1364.

Samuelsson, G. (1999). *Drugs of Natural Origin*. 4th edn. Stockholm: Swedish Pharmaceutical Press.

Schultes, R.E., Klein, W.M., Plowman, T., and Lockwood, T.E. (1974). *Cannabis*: an example of taxonomic neglect. *Harvard University Botanical Museum Leaflets*, **23**, 337–367.

Sirikantaramas, S., Morimoto, S., Shoyama, S., *et al.* (2004). The gene controlling marijuana psychoactivity. Molecular cloning and heterologous expression of Δ^1-tetrahydrocannabinolic acid synthase from *Cannabis sativa* L. *The Journal of Biological Chemistry*, **279**, 39767–39774.

Shoyama, Y., Hirano, H., and Nishioka, I. (1984). Biosynthesis of propyl cannabinoid acid and its biosynthetic relationship with pentyl and methyl cannabinoid acids. *Phytochemistry*, **23**, 1909–1912.

Shoyama, Y., Tamada, T. and Kurihara, K., *et al.* (2012). Structure and function of Δ1-tetrahydrocannabinolic acid (THCA) synthase, the enzyme controlling the psychoactivity of *Cannabis sativa. Journal of Molecular Biology*, **423**, 96–105.

Shoyama, Y., Yagi, M., and Nishioka, I. (1975). Biosynthesis of cannabinoid acids. *Phytochemistry*, **14**, 2189–2192.

Shoyama, Y., Yamauchi, T., and Nishioka, I. (1970) Cannabis. V. Cannabigerolic acid monomethyl ether and cannabinolic acid. *Chemical and Pharmaceutical Bulletin (Tokyo)*, **18**, 1327–1332.

Small, E. and Beckstead, H.D. (1973). Common cannabinoid phenotypes in 350 stocks of *Cannabis. Lloydia*, **36**, 144–165.

Small, E. and Cronquist, A. (1976). A practical and natural taxonomy for *Cannabis. Taxon*, **25**, 405–435.

Stout, J.M., Boubakir, Z., Ambrose, S.J., Purves, R.W., and Page, J.E. (2012). The hexanoyl-CoA precursor for cannabinoid biosynthesis is formed by an acyl-activating enzyme in *Cannabis sativa* trichomes. *The Plant Journal*, **71**, 353–365.

Taura, F., Morimoto, S., and Shoyama, Y. (1995). Cannabinerolis acid, a cannabinoid from *Cannabis sativa. Phytochemistry*, **39**, 457–458.

Taura, F., Morimoto, S., and Shoyama, Y. (1995). First direct evidence for the mechanism of delta-1-tetrahydrocannabinolic acid biosynthesis. *Journal of the American Chemical Society*, **38**, 9766–9767.

Taura, F., Morimoto, S., and Shoyama, Y. (1996). Purification and characterization of cannabidiolic-acid synthase from Cannabis sativa L. *The Journal of Biological Chemistry*, **271**, 17411–17416.

Taura, F., Sirikantaramas, S., Shoyama, Y., Yoshikai, K., Shoyama, Y., and Morimoto, S. (2007). Cannabidiolic-acid synthase, the chemotype-determining enzyme in the fiber-type *Cannabis sativa. FEBS Letters*, **581**, 2929–2934.

Taura, F., Tanaka, S., Taguchi, C., *et al.* (2009). Characterization of olivetol synthase, a polyketide synthase putatively involved in cannabinoid biosynthetic pathway. *FEBS Letters*, **583**, 2061–2066.

Toyota, M., Kinugawa, T., Asakawa, Y. (1994). Bibenzyl cannabinoid and bisbibenzyl derivative from the liverwort *Radula perrottetii. Phytochemistry*, **37**, 859–862.

Toyota, M., Shimamura, T., Ishii, H., Renner, M., Braggins, J. and Asakawa, Y. (2002). New bibenzyl cannabinoid from the New Zealand liverwort *Radula marginata. Chemical and Pharmaceutical Bulletin (Tokyo)*, **50**, 1390–1392.

Part 2

Pharmacology, Pharmacokinetics, Metabolism, and Forensics

Roger G. Pertwee

Part 2 Overview

Part 2 contains 11 chapters (Chapters 6–16). The first of these chapters, by Pertwee and Cascio, summarizes the known pharmacological actions of four phytocannabinoid constituents of cannabis that have been shown to activate cannabinoid CB_1 and/or CB_2 receptors with significant potency: Δ^8- and Δ^9-tetrahydrocannabinol, Δ^9-tetrahydrocannabivarin, and cannabinol. This chapter also presents evidence that cannabinoid CB_2 receptors can be activated by the nonphytocannabinoid constituent of cannabis, (E)-β-caryophyllene. Chapter 7 by Cascio and Pertwee extends this theme by describing the known pharmacological actions of nine other phytocannabinoid constituents of cannabis: (1) cannabichromene; (2) cannabidiol, cannabigerol, and their propyl analogues, cannabidivarin and cannabigerovarin; (3) cannabidiolic acid and cannabigerolic acid; and (4) Δ^9-tetrahydrocannabidiolic acid and its propyl analogue, Δ^9-tetrahydrocannabivarinic acid.

In Chapter 8, Szabo summarizes current knowledge of how neurotransmission is affected by Δ^9-tetrahydrocannabinol and other phytocannabinoids both within and outside the brain through their known actions on cannabinoid and/or noncannabinoid receptors, and identifies some important neuropharmacological questions about these compounds that still need to be addressed.

In Chapter 9, Gardner discusses cannabis dependence, and presents evidence indicating first, that its incidence in humans who take cannabis is low, second that it is attributable primarily to the main psychoactive constituent of cannabis, Δ^9-tetrahydrocannabinol, and third, that two other phytocannabinoid constituents of cannabis could well possess anti-addictive efficacy.

In Chapter 10, Patel, Hill, and Hillard present current knowledge about the adverse and/or potentially beneficial effects that cannabis, tetrahydrocannabinol, and other cannabinoids have both on anxiety and mood, and on anxiety and mood disorders such as panic attacks, posttraumatic stress disorder, and depression. The chapter also mentions what has already been discovered about how cannabis and certain individual phytocannabinoids interact with the endocrine system, for example, to alter levels of glucocorticoid, thyroid and growth hormones, and of melatonin.

In Chapter 11, O'Sullivan reviews the known effects on the cardiovascular system, mainly of cannabis and Δ^9-tetrahydrocannabinol, but also of cannabinol, cannabidiol, tetrahydrocannabivarin, and cannabigerol, the cardiovascular effects of which have been much less investigated than those of Δ^9-tetrahydrocannabinol. Both in vivo and in vitro data obtained from human or animal experiments are presented.

In Chapter 12, Duncan and Izzo describe both how cannabis and individual phytocannabinoids can affect the functioning of the gastrointestinal tract, and preclinical and clinical evidence that some of these substances might be effective against gastrointestinal disorders such as irritable bowel syndrome, inflammatory bowel disease, and colon cancer.

In Chapter 13, Stuart, Leishman, and Bradshaw consider the effects of cannabis and tetrahydrocannabinol on human and nonhuman reproductive function and sexual behavior in males and females, and on pregnancy and birth outcomes. The mechanisms underlying some of these effects are also discussed, as is the involvement in these effects of the endocrine system, and the part played by cannabinoid receptors in reproductive function.

In Chapter 14, Cabral, Raborn, and Ferreira outline how the phytocannabinoids, tetrahydrocannabinol, cannabinol, and cannabidiol, affect the immune system. As well as discussing their immunomodulatory effects, this chapter also considers the anti-inflammatory effects these three compounds produce both in vitro and in vivo, effects of tetrahydrocannabinol on host resistance to viral, bacterial, and fungal infections, and the part played by cannabinoid receptors, particularly CB_2 receptors, in immunomodulation.

Chapter 15 by McPartland and Russo includes descriptions of the known pharmacological effects of some of the flavonoid and terpenoid constituents of cannabis, and on pharmacological interactions that have been found to occur between phytocannabinoid and terpenoid constituents of cannabis, and indeed, between certain phytocannabinoids.

Finally, Chapter 16 by Huestis and Smith presents what is currently known about the absorption, distribution, metabolism, and elimination of phytocannabinoids following their administration to humans in cannabis, in cannabis extracts, or as pure compounds (e.g., tetrahydrocannabinol) by one or other of a wide range of different routes, as indicated by the levels of these compounds or their metabolites measured in plasma, urine, feces, oral fluid, sweat, or hair. Possible answers to the questions both of how best to detect cannabinoids for forensic purposes, and of how best to assess the length of time before such testing that the most recent exposure to cannabis/cannabinoids occurred, are also considered.

Chapter 6

Known Pharmacological Actions of Delta-9-Tetrahydrocannabinol and of Four Other Chemical Constituents of Cannabis that Activate Cannabinoid Receptors

Roger G. Pertwee and Maria Grazia Cascio

6.1 Introduction

Cannabis is the unique natural source of a set of chemicals known as phytocannabinoids (ElSohly et al. 2005), and it is one of these phytocannabinoids, (−)-*trans*-delta-9-tetrahydrocannabinol (Δ^9-THC; Fig. 6.1), that is primarily responsible for producing the well-documented effects on perception, mood, emotion, and cognition that together constitute the psychotropic effects of cannabis (Pertwee 1988). The finding that Δ^9-THC is the main psychoactive constituent of cannabis prompted a search for the pharmacological basis for its psychotropic effects, and this led to three further important discoveries: first, of two new G protein-coupled receptors that were named cannabinoid receptor type 1 (CB_1) and type 2 (CB_2); second, that these receptors can both be activated by Δ^9-THC; and third, that this phytocannabinoid produces many of its effects on brain function by activating the CB_1 receptor (Howlett et al. 2002; Pertwee 1997, 2005).

As discussed in greater detail elsewhere (Howlett et al. 2002; Pertwee 2005), cannabinoid CB_1 receptors are found mainly at the terminals of central and peripheral neurons, where they usually mediate inhibition of ongoing release of a number of different excitatory and inhibitory neurotransmitters. The distribution of these receptors within the central nervous system is such that their activation can affect processes such as cognition and memory, alter the control of motor function, and induce signs of analgesia. CB_1 receptors are also expressed by certain non-neuronal cells, including immune cells. As to cannabinoid CB_2 receptors, these are located predominantly in immune cells and, when activated, they can modulate immune cell migration and cytokine release both outside and within the brain (Cabral and Staab 2005; Howlett et al. 2002; Pertwee et al. 2010). There is also evidence that CB_2 receptors are expressed by some neurons in the brain and elsewhere (Pertwee et al. 2010). However, the role of neuronal CB_2 receptors remains to be established. There is evidence too, first, that CB_1 receptors can signal through both $G_{i/o}$ and G_s proteins, second, that CB_1 receptor agonism can cause $G_{i/o}$ protein-mediated activation of A-type and inwardly rectifying potassium currents, and inhibition of N-type and P/Q-type calcium currents, and third, that either CB_1 or CB_2 receptor agonism can lead to $G_{i/o}$ protein-mediated inhibition of adenylyl cyclase and activation of mitogen-activated protein kinase (Howlett 2005; Howlett et al. 2002; Pertwee 2005). Cannabinoid receptors can be activated not only by exogenously administered compounds, but also by endogenous cannabinoids such as

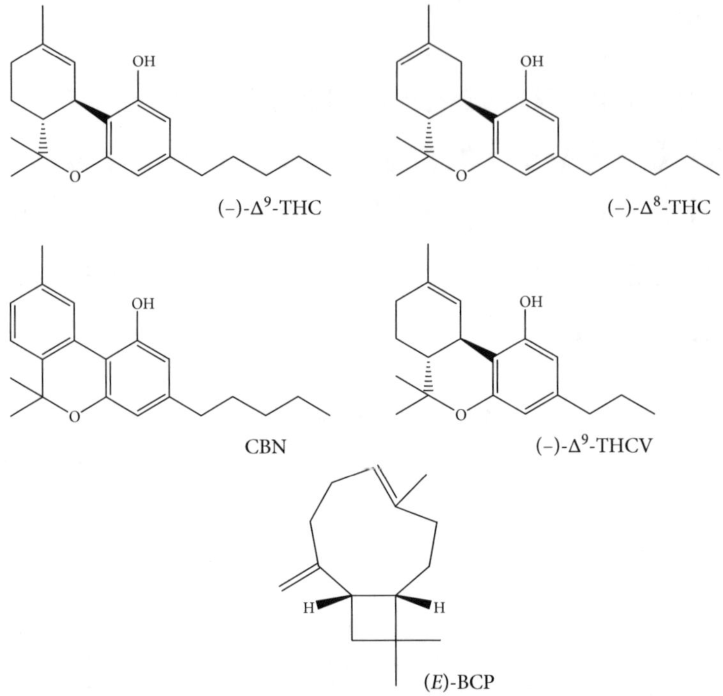

Fig. 6.1 Structures of (–)-*trans*-Δ^9- and (–)-*trans*-Δ^8-tetrahydrocannabinol ((–)-Δ^9-THC and (–)-Δ^8-THC), cannabinol (CBN), (–)-*trans*-Δ^9-tetrahydrocannabivarin ((–)-Δ^9-THCV), and (*E*)-β-caryophyllene ((*E*)-BCP).

N-arachidonoylethanolamine (anandamide) and 2-arachidonoyl glycerol that are synthesized by neurons and other cells and are known as endocannabinoids (Howlett et al. 2002; Pertwee 2005).

This review focuses on Δ^9-THC, and on four other constituents of growing and/or harvested cannabis that have been discovered to activate CB_1 and/or CB_2 receptors: the phytocannabinoids, cannabinol (CBN), (–)-*trans*-delta-8-tetrahydrocannabinol (Δ^8-THC) and (–)-*trans*-delta-9-tetrahydrocannabivarin (Δ^9-THCV), and the sesquiterpene, (*E*)-β-caryophyllene ((*E*)-BCP) (Fig. 6.1). It begins with a brief description of the in vivo and in vitro bioassays that have been used to investigate the ability of these compounds to activate cannabinoid receptors.

6.2 Bioassays for measuring drug-induced activation of cannabinoid receptors in vitro or in vivo

Two in vitro bioassays that are particularly widely used to provide a measure of cannabinoid receptor activation, exploit the ability of CB_1 and CB_2 receptors to signal through $G_{i/o}$ proteins by monitoring the ability of a compound either to increase [^{35}S]GTPγS binding to cell membranes or to inhibit forskolin-induced stimulation of cyclic adenosine monophosphate (AMP) production by whole cells (Howlett et al. 2002; Pertwee 1999; 2005). The strength (efficacy) with which an active compound (agonist) induces receptor activation (agonism) in these assays is usually determined by measuring the size of the maximal response that it can induce (E_{max}), whereas an indication of its potency is usually obtained by establishing the concentration (EC_{50}) at which it produces a half- maximal response.

A third frequently used in vitro bioassay measures the ability of putative cannabinoid receptor agonists to produce complete displacement, from specific binding sites in cannabinoid receptor-expressing membranes, of an established cannabinoid CB_1 and/or CB_2 receptor ligand that has been radiolabeled with tritium (Howlett et al. 2002; Pertwee 1999, 2005). Tritiated cannabinoids often used in such experiments are $[^3H]CP55940$ and $[^3H]R(+)$-WIN55212, which bind to both CB_1 and CB_2 receptors, the CB_1-selective ligand, $[^3H]SR141716A$, and the CB_2-selective ligand,

Table 6.1 Examples of K_i values of Δ^9-THC, Δ^8-THC, CBN, Δ^9-THCV, and (E)-BCP for the in vitro displacement of $[^3H]CP55940$, $[^3H]HU$-243, or $[^3H]SR141716A$ from CB_1- and CB_2-specific binding sites

Displacing compound	CB_1 K_i (nM)	CB_2 K_i (nM)	Reference
Δ^9-THC	5.05	3.13	Iwamura et al. 2001
	8.33[a]	1.73[b]	Iwamura et al. 2001
	13.5[c]	6.8[c]	Iwamura et al. 2001
	21; 40.7[c]	36.4	Showalter et al. 1996
	35.3[c]	3.9[c]	Rinaldi-Carmona et al. 1994
	39.5[d, e]	40[e]	Bayewitch et al. 1996
	47.7[c]	ND	Booker et al. 2009
	53.3	75.3	Felder et al. 1995
	66.5[c,e]; 80.3[d,e]	32.2[e]	Rhee et al. 1997
Δ^8-THC	44[c]	44	Huffman et al. 1999
	47.6[c]	39.3[a]	Busch-Petersen et al. 1996
CBN	120.2	100	MacLennan et al. 1998
	129.3[c]	ND	Booker et al. 2009
	392.2[c,e]; 211.2[d,e]	126.4[e]	Rhee et al. 1997
	326	96.3	Showalter et al. 1996
	1130	301	Felder et al. 1995
Δ^9-THCV	46.6[a]	ND	Pertwee et al. 2007
	75.4[a]	62.8	Thomas et al. 2005
	286[c,f]	ND	Hill et al. 2010
	ND	145	Bolognini et al. 2012
	ND	225	Bolognini et al. 2010
(E)-BCP	>10,000	155	Gertsch et al. 2008

Abbreviations: CBN, cannabinol; Δ^9-THC, (–)-trans-Δ^9-tetrahydrocannabinol; Δ^8-THC, (–)-trans-Δ^8-tetrahydrocannabinol; Δ^9-THCV, (–)-trans-Δ^9-tetrahydrocannabivarin; (E)-BCP, (E)-β-caryophyllene; ND, not determined.

Experiments performed with: [a] mouse brain (CB_1) or mouse spleen (CB_2) membranes; [b] membranes from cultured cells transfected with mouse cannabinoid receptors; [c] rat brain (CB_1) or rat spleen (CB_2) membranes; [d] membranes from cultured cells transfected with rat cannabinoid receptors; [e] $[^3H]HU$-243; [f] $[^3H]SR141716A$. All other data are from experiments performed with $[^3H]CP55940$ and/or with membranes from cultured cells transfected with human cannabinoid receptors. See Fig. 6.1 for the structures of the compounds listed in this table.

[^{3}H]SR144528. The potency of an active compound in these binding assays is expressed either as the concentration (IC_{50}) at which it produces 50% displacement of one of these tritiated cannabinoids or as its K_i value (Table 6.1), which can be calculated from its IC_{50} value. K_i values are directly related to the affinities of ligands for their receptors, whereas IC_{50} values are, of course, inversely related to these affinity values.

Moving on to quantitative in vivo bioassays for cannabinoid receptor agonists, these are usually performed with mice or rats, although sometimes with other species, including dogs, pigeons, and nonhuman primates (Howlett et al. 2002). Apparent CB_1 receptor-mediated effects that most often serve as measured responses to drugs in such bioassays are:

- hypolocomotion, hypothermia, antinociception, and catalepsy which, when measured in parallel using mice, constitute the widely used "mouse tetrad" test
- subjective effects which can be distinguished by animals in "drug discrimination" assays from effects produced by substances that do not activate cannabinoid receptors
- impairment of learning and memory as measured, for example, in radial mazes or in the Morris water maze.

Antinociception in the mouse tetrad is most often monitored using tail-flick or hot-plate tests, which provide measures of relief from acute pain induced by heat, whereas catalepsy is often monitored by noting the length of time that mice remain immobile when subjected to a "ring test" that was originally developed in 1972 (Pertwee 1972), or to a "bar test."

As to in vivo indications of CB_2 receptor activation that are exploited in bioassays, these include the reduction of signs of inflammatory paw pain induced in rats or mice by an intraplantar injection of carrageenan or formalin, and the reduction of rat or mouse paw edema induced by intraplantar carrageenan (Bolognini et al. 2010; Guindon and Hohmann 2008).

Importantly, confirmatory evidence that apparent signs of cannabinoid receptor binding or activation observed in CB_1 or CB_2 receptor-transfected cells, or in membranes obtained from these cells, are indeed cannabinoid receptor-mediated can be obtained by establishing whether these signs are, or are not, detectable in untransfected cells. Activation of CB_1 or CB_2 receptors should also be undetectable when an in vitro or in vivo bioassay is performed with animals or tissues from which these receptors have been genetically deleted (Howlett et al. 2002). In addition, a compound that can truly activate CB_1 or CB_2 receptor in an in vivo or in vitro bioassay is expected to be antagonized with appropriate potency by a CB_1-selective antagonist such as SR141716A, AM251, or AM281 and/or by a CB_2-selective antagonist such as SR144528 or AM630 (Howlett et al. 2002; Pertwee 2005).

6.3 Δ^9-tetrahydrocannabinol

6.3.1 Δ^9-THC can activate CB_1 and CB_2 receptors

That Δ^9-THC can activate CB_1 receptors in vivo is strongly supported by the findings, first, that it can, in mice, suppress locomotor activity and induce hypothermia, immobility (catalepsy) in the ring test, and antinociception in the tail-flick test, all at similar doses (Martin et al. 1991), and, second, that its ability to produce each of these tetrad test effects is readily blocked by the selective CB_1 receptor antagonist, SR141716A (Varvel et al. 2005; Wiley et al. 2001). In addition, Δ^9-THC has been found not to affect locomotor activity or to induce hypothermia or ring immobility in mice bred on a C57BL/6J background from which the CB_1 receptor has been genetically deleted (Di Marzo et al. 2000; Zimmer et al. 1999). This genetic deletion also abolished Δ^9-THC-induced antinociception in the hot-plate test, although unexpectedly, not in the tail-flick test.

There is evidence as well that Δ^9-THC can activate CB_2 receptors. Thus, for example, experiments with female mice have shown that Δ^9-THC shares the ability of the CB_2-selective agonist, JWH-133, to decrease the growth rate of xenografts derived from cells that had been isolated from a CB_1- and CB_2-expressing breast cancer tumor, and also, that this effect of Δ^9-THC, and of JWH-133, can be reduced by the CB_2-selective antagonist SR144528 but not by SR141716A (Caffarel et al. 2010). In addition, there has been a report that Δ^9-THC can reduce signs of paw pain in a rat model of arthritis and that this reduction can be attenuated by SR144528 (Cox et al. 2007). This antinociceptive effect of Δ^9-THC was also decreased by SR141716A, suggesting that it was produced through the activation of both CB_1 and CB_2 receptors. It is noteworthy too that, as expected for a CB_2 receptor agonist, Δ^9-THC can decrease carrageenan-induced mouse paw edema (Wise et al. 2008). However, the likely involvement of CB_2 receptors in this effect was not investigated.

Δ^9-THC also behaves as both a CB_1 and a CB_2 receptor agonist in vitro. This is indicated, for example, by its ability to stimulate [^{35}S]GTPγS binding or to inhibit forskolin-induced production of cyclic AMP with significant potency in tissues that express CB_1 receptors, either naturally or after CB_1 receptor transfection (Pertwee 1997; 1999). These effects can be produced by concentrations of Δ^9-THC in the low nanomolar range, although even so, with a potency that is usually less than that displayed by certain other established CB_1/CB_2 receptor agonists such as CP55940 and HU-210 (Pertwee 1997, 1999). Confirmatory evidence that some of these in vitro effects of Δ^9-THC are CB_1 receptor-mediated comes from the finding that they can be prevented by genetic deletion of the CB_1 receptor in the [^{35}S]GTPγS binding assay performed with mouse cerebellar homogenates (Monory et al. 2002), and that cell lines that do not express CB_1 receptors naturally, only exhibit signs of Δ^9-THC-induced CB_1 receptor activation in the cyclic AMP assay if they have first been transfected with this receptor (Matsuda et al. 1990; Slipetz et al. 1995). As expected from the results obtained in these functional in vitro bioassays, it has also been found that Δ^9-THC can fully displace cannabinoid receptor ligands such as [^{3}H]CP55940 from specific binding sites on cannabinoid CB_1 and CB_2 receptors with K_i values in the low nanomolar range (Table 6.1). These K_i values are similar for each of these receptors, but significantly higher than those of the synthetic cannabinoid receptor agonists, CP55940 and HU-210 (Howlett et al. 2002; Pertwee 1997), an indication that Δ^9-THC has less affinity than these other compounds for both CB_1 and CB_2 receptors.

6.3.2 Δ^9-THC is a cannabinoid receptor partial agonist

In several cannabinoid receptor-containing tissue preparations, the maximal sizes (E_{max} values) of apparent CB_1 or CB_2 receptor-mediated effects produced by Δ^9-THC are well below those of certain other established CB_1/CB_2 receptor agonists. This is an indication that Δ^9-THC possesses less CB_1 and CB_2 efficacy than these other agonists and should, therefore, be classified as a partial agonist for these receptors (Pertwee 1997; 1999). Cannabinoids that have been found to display greater CB_1 receptor efficacy than Δ^9-THC, in some in vitro bioassays, include the 11-hydroxy primary metabolite of Δ^9-THC (Matsuda et al. 1990), and the synthetic cannabinoid receptor agonists, CP55940 and HU-210 (Pertwee 1997; 1999). They also include the synthetic cannabinoid, nabilone (Matsuda et al. 1990), which like Δ^9-THC, has been a licensed medicine for many years (Pertwee and Thomas 2009).

Importantly, cannabis is increasingly being taken recreationally together with synthetic "designer drugs" that can activate CB_1 receptors much more strongly than Δ^9-THC (Seely et al. 2012). Just two notable examples of these compounds are JWH-018 and JWH-073, both of which have been reported to stimulate [^{35}S]GTPγS binding to mouse brain membranes with markedly greater efficacy than Δ^9-THC (Brents et al. 2011; 2012). Pharmacological and toxicological consequences of the recreational use of CB$_1$ receptor agonists that possess significantly higher efficacy than Δ^9-THC have still to be fully explored.

6.3.3 Δ^9-THC can both activate and block CB$_1$ and CB$_2$ receptors

Since Δ^9-THC displays relatively low efficacy as an agonist at CB$_1$ and CB$_2$ receptors, it is to be expected that the maximum size of the effect that it can produce when it activates these receptors will be greatly influenced by the proportion of them that are in an "active state" (Bolognini et al. 2012), as well as by their expression level and coupling efficiency, and hence will not be the same in all cannabinoid receptor-expressing tissues. Thus, for example, the size of the maximal effect that Δ^9-THC can produce in tissues in which cannabinoid receptors are particularly highly expressed, or in which they signal with particularly high efficiency, is likely to be quite large. However, in tissues in which cannabinoid receptors are poorly expressed or signal with low efficiency, Δ^9-THC could well fail to produce any detectable sign of cannabinoid receptor activation at all. Indeed, since it would still be expected to possess unchanged affinity for these receptors, Δ^9-THC might possibly antagonize the effects of higher efficacy cannabinoid receptor agonists in such tissues.

It is noteworthy, therefore, that in some in vitro investigations, the maximal sizes of apparent cannabinoid CB$_1$ receptor-mediated effects of Δ^9-THC have been found to match those of higher efficacy agonists such as CP55940 (Pertwee 1997, 1999), whereas in other investigations, Δ^9-THC has been found to produce signs of antagonism, or even of inverse agonism, at CB$_1$ or CB$_2$ receptors either in vitro or in vivo. More specifically, Paronis et al. (2012) have found that in mice, a maximal hypothermic dose of Δ^9-THC (30 mg kg^{-1} s.c.) produced a significant rightward shift in the log dose–response curve of the cannabinoid receptor agonist, AM2389, for its production of hypothermia. By itself, Δ^9-THC behaved as a partial agonist, displaying less hypothermic efficacy than AM2389. There has also been a report that in a mouse model in which CP55940 and R-(+)-WIN55212 each produced an apparent anxiolytic effect, Δ^9-THC shared the ability of the CB$_1$-selective antagonists, SR141716A and AM251, to induce signs of increased anxiety (Patel and Hillard 2006). In addition, in other experiments, Δ^9-THC was found to reduce stimulation of [^{35}S]GTPγS binding to rat cerebellar membranes produced by R-(+)-WIN55212 (Sim et al. 1996), to attenuate R-(+)-WIN55212- and 2-arachidonoyl glycerol-induced inhibition of glutamatergic synaptic transmission induced in rat or mouse cultured hippocampal neurons (Kelley and Thayer 2004; Shen and Thayer 1999; Straiker and Mackie 2005), or to antagonize CB$_2$ receptor-mediated inhibition of cyclic AMP production in CB$_2$-transfected cells (Bayewitch et al. 1996). Moreover, in another investigation, it was found that although Δ^9-THC did, as expected, stimulate [^{35}S]GTPγS binding to membranes obtained from CB$_1$-transfected cells, it inhibited such binding to membranes obtained from CB$_2$-transfected cells (Govaerts et al. 2004), an indication that Δ^9-THC can behave as a CB$_2$ receptor *inverse* agonist. There have also been in vitro investigations in which Δ^9-THC has been found to produce no detectable CB$_2$ receptor-mediated inhibition of cyclic AMP production (Pertwee 1997, 1999).

6.3.4 CB$_1$ and CB$_2$ receptor-independent actions of Δ^9-THC

Among the known CB$_1$ and CB$_2$ receptor-independent actions of Δ^9-THC (Table 6.2 and 6.3), are several that it can display at submicromolar concentrations in at least some bioassays and that are, therefore, likely to reduce its CB$_1$ and CB$_2$ receptor selectivity. Thus, Δ^9-THC has been reported:

Table 6.2 A selection of receptors and ion channels that Δ^9-THC has been reported to target in vitro

Concentration of Δ^9-THC§	Pharmacological target and effect	Reference
	Receptors and channels	
<1 µM	CB$_1$ receptor (A or B)	¶
	CB$_2$ receptor (A or B)	¶
	GPR18 (A)	McHugh et al. 2012
	GPR55 (A)*	Pertwee 2010†
	5-HT$_{3A}$ ligand-gated ion channel (B)	Pertwee 2010†
	Glycine ligand-gated ion channels, including α1 and α1 β1 (P)	Pertwee 2010†
	TRPA1 cation channel (A)*; TRPV2 cation channel (A)*; TRPM8 cation channel (B)	De Petrocellis and Di Marzo 2010†; De Petrocellis et al. 2008, 2011
	PPARγ nuclear receptor (A)	O'Sullivan et al. 2005
	Putative non-CB$_1$, non-CB$_2$, non-TRPV1 receptors on capsaicin-sensitive perivascular sensory neurons mediating CGRP release (+)	Zygmunt et al. 2002
1–10 µM	β-adrenoceptor (P)	Pertwee 2010†
	µ-opioid receptors (D)	Pertwee 2010†
	Allosteric modulation of µ- and δ-opioid receptors (–)	Pertwee 2010†
	GPR55 (A or B)	Anavi-Goffer et al. 2012
	PPARγ nuclear receptor (A)	O'Sullivan et al. 2005
	TRPV3 cation channel (A)	De Petrocellis et al. 2012†
	TRPV4 cation channel (A)	De Petrocellis et al. 2012†
	T-type calcium (Ca$_v$3) voltage gated ion channels (–)	Pertwee 2010†
	Potassium K$_v$1.2 voltage gated ion channels (–)	Pertwee 2010†
	Conductance in Na$^+$ voltage gated ion channels (–)	Oz 2006†
	Conductance in gap junctions between cells (–)	Oz 2006†
>10 µM	TRPA1 cation channel (A)	De Petrocellis and Di Marzo 2010†
	TRPV2 cation channel (A)	De Petrocellis and Di Marzo 2010†

Abbreviations: 5-HT, 5-hydroxytryptamine; A, activation; B, blockade; CGRP, calcitonin gene-related peptide; D, displacement from binding sites; P, potentiation; PPAR, peroxisome proliferator-activated receptor; TRP transient receptor potential; see also footnote to Table 6.1.

(+), enhancement; (–), inhibition; § EC$_{50}$ or IC$_{50}$ when this has been determined; † review article; * see also effect of 1–10 µM or of >10 µM; ¶ see this review for further details.

Table 6.3 A selection of enzymes and cellular uptake or other processes that Δ^9-THC has been reported to target in vitro

Concentration of Δ^9-THC§	Pharmacological target and effect	Reference
	Enzymes	
<1 µM	Phospholipase(s) (+)*	Pertwee 1988†
	Lysophosphatidylcholine acyl transferase (–)	Greenberg et al. 1978
1–10 µM	Phospholipase(s) (+)	Pertwee 1988†
	Lipoxygenase (–)	Evans 1991
	Na^+-K^+-ATPase activity (–)	Pertwee 1988†
	Mg^{2+}-ATPase activity (±)	Pertwee 1988†
	CYP1A1 (–); CYP1A2 (–); CYP1B1 (–)	Yamaori et al. 2010
	CYP2B6 (–)	Yamaori et al. 2011b
	CYP2C9 (–)	Yamaori et al. 2012
	Norepinephrine-induced melatonin biosynthesis (–)	Koch et al. 2006
	Monoamine oxidase activity (–)	Pertwee 1988†
	Synaptic conversion of tyrosine to noradrenaline and dopamine (+)	Pertwee 1988†
>10 µM	Cyclooxygenase (–)	Evans 1991
	CYP2A6 (–)	Yamaori et al. 2011b
	CYP2D6 (–)	Yamaori et al. 2011c
	CYP3A4 (–); CYP3A5 (–); CYP3A7 (–)	Yamaori et al. 2011a
	Transporters and cellular uptake	
<1 µM	Adenosine uptake by cultured microglia and macrophages (–)	Carrier et al. 2006
	Synaptosomal uptake of dopamine (±)*	Pertwee 1988†
	Synaptosomal uptake of noradrenaline (+)*	Pertwee 1988†
	Synaptosomal uptake of 5-hydroxytryptamine (–)*	Pertwee 1988†
1–10 µM	Cellular uptake of anandamide (–)	Rakhshan et al. 2000
	Synaptosomal uptake of dopamine (–)	Pertwee 1988†
	Synaptosomal uptake of noradrenaline (–)	Pertwee 1988†
	Synaptosomal uptake of 5-hydroxytryptamine (±)	Pertwee 1988†
	Synaptosomal uptake of γ-aminobutyric acid (–)	Pertwee 1988†
	Synaptosomal uptake of choline (–)	Pertwee 1988†
	Other actions or effects	
1–10 µM	Oxidative stress (–)	Marsicano et al. 2002
	Human keratinocyte proliferation (–)	Wilkinson and Williamson 2007
>10 µM	Fluidity of synaptic plasma membranes (+); (–)	Hillard et al. 1985

Abbreviations: (+),enhancement; (–), inhibition; see also footnote to Table 6.1. § EC_{50} or IC_{50} when this has been determined; * see also effect of 1–10 µM or of >10 µM; †review article.

- to inhibit 5-HT_{3A}-mediated currents induced by 5-HT in human embryonic kidney 293 (HEK293) cells stably transfected with the functional 3A subunit of the human 5-HT_3 receptor (IC_{50} = 38 nM), possibly by acting through an allosteric mechanism (Barann et al. 2002)

- to enhance the activation of glycine receptors naturally expressed in rat isolated ventral teg-mental area neurons (EC_{50} = 115 nM), and of both homomeric α1 and heteromeric α1β1 subunits of human glycine receptors transfected into *Xenopus laevis* oocytes (EC_{50} = 86 nM and 73 nM, respectively), again possibly in an allosteric manner (Hejazi et al. 2006)

- to elevate calcium levels in HEK293 cells stably overexpressing high levels of the transient receptor potential (TRP) cation channels, TRPA1 or TRPV2 (EC_{50} = 230 nM and 650 nM, respectively), and to desensitize TRPV2 cation channels to activation by lysophosphatidylcho-line (IC_{50} = 800 nM) (De Petrocellis et al. 2008, 2011)

- to reduce elevations of intracellular calcium levels induced by the TRPM8 agonists, icilin or menthol, in HEK293 cells stably overexpressing recombinant rat TRPM8 cation channels (IC_{50} = 160 nM and 150 nM, respectively (De Petrocellis et al. 2008; 2011)

- to activate the nuclear receptor, peroxisome proliferator-activated receptor gamma (PPARγ), at concentrations of 100 nM and above in a luciferase reporter gene assay performed with HEK293 cells transiently expressing this receptor (O'Sullivan et al. 2005)

- to activate the G protein-coupled receptor, GPR18 in HEK293 cells transfected with this recep-tor (EC_{50} = 960 nM; McHugh et al. 2012).

In some in vitro investigations, submicromolar concentrations of Δ^9-THC have also been found to activate GPR55 in HEK293 cells transfected with this deorphanized receptor, both in a β-arrestin assay, albeit with rather low efficacy (Yin et al. 2009), and in a $[^{35}S]GTPγS$ binding assay (EC_{50} = 8 nM; Ryberg et al. 2007). In other in vitro investigations, however, Δ^9-THC induced signs of GPR55 activation only at concentrations in the micromolar range (Anavi-Goffer et al. 2012; Lauckner et al. 2008), or lacked detectable activity as a GPR55 agonist altogether (Pertwee 2010; Pertwee et al. 2010). It is also noteworthy that in one of these investigations (Anavi-Goffer et al. 2012), a concentration of Δ^9-THC (1 μM) that did not seem to activate GPR55, induced a signifi-cant downward shift in the log concentration–response curve of an endogenous agonist for this receptor (L-α-lysophosphatidylinositol), when the measured response was stimulation of extra-cellular receptor kinases 1/2 (ERK1/2) phosphorylation by human GPR55-transfected HEK293 cells.

6.4 Δ^8-tetrahydrocannabinol

Although the pharmacological profile of Δ^8-THC (Fig. 6.1) has been little investigated, there is evidence that it does share the ability of Δ^9-THC to target cannabinoid CB_1 receptors as a par-tial agonist. Thus, it has been reported to inhibit forskolin-induced production of cyclic AMP in Chinese hamster ovary (CHO) cells transfected with CB_1 receptors with a potency slightly less than that of Δ^9-THC, but an efficacy similar to that of Δ^9-THC and hence less than that of CP55940 (Gérard et al. 1991; Matsuda et al. 1990). This effect of Δ^8-THC was presumably CB_1 receptor-mediated as it was not observed in untransfected CHO cells. In addition, it has been reported first, that Δ^8-THC can fully displace $[^3H]CP55940$ from specific binding sites on can-nabinoid CB_1 receptors with a similar potency to Δ^9-THC (Table 6.1), and second, that it also displays similar potency to Δ^9-THC in vivo in the mouse tetrad test (Martin et al. 1993). It has also been found that 11-hydroxy-Δ^8-THC, which is a primary metabolite of Δ^8-THC (Yamamoto et al. 2003), can bind to rat CB_1 and human CB_2 (hCB_2) receptors present in membranes obtained from

African green monkey kidney (COS-7) cells transfected with these receptors, with K_i values in the low nanomolar range (Rhee et al. 1997). Other results obtained in this investigation showed that 11-hydroxy-Δ^8-THC could also inhibit forskolin-induced cyclic AMP production by these cells. Interestingly, however, it displayed much lower CB_2 than CB_1 efficacy as an agonist in the cyclic AMP assay, and yet higher CB_2 than CB_1 affinity in the binding assays.

There is evidence too that Δ^8-THC can induce ataxia in dogs and cannabis-like psychopharmacological effects in human subjects and rhesus monkeys, albeit with less potency than Δ^9-THC (Pertwee 1988). However, whether or not any of these in vivo effects of Δ^8-THC can be opposed by a selective CB_1 receptor antagonist has yet to be investigated. It is noteworthy, therefore, that there have been reports first, that intraperitoneal (i.p.) administration of a low dose of Δ^8-THC can increase food intake by mice, and that this effect can be prevented by the CB_1-selective antagonist, SR141716A (Avraham et al. 2004), and second, that antinociceptive effects induced in a mouse model of acute pain by intracerebroventricular or intrathecal injections of Δ^8-THC, or indeed of Δ^9-THC, can be blocked by this antagonist when it is administered intracerebroventricularly or intraperitoneally (Welch et al. 1998). Finally, again like Δ^9-THC, Δ^8-THC has been found to displace [^{3}H]CP55940 from CB_2 receptors no less potently than it displaces this tritiated ligand from CB_1 receptors (Table 6.1). The likely possibility that Δ^8-THC also activates CB_2 receptors still needs to be investigated, as indeed does the extent to which Δ^8-THC has Δ^9-THC-like CB_1 and CB_2 receptor-independent modes of action.

6.5 **Cannabinol**

CBN (Fig. 6.1) has been found to bind less potently than Δ^8- or Δ^9-THC to CB_1 and CB_2 receptors, and to possess slightly higher CB_2 than CB_1 affinity (Table 6.1). In addition, it has been found to display lower efficacy than Δ^9-THC as a CB_1 receptor agonist in vitro in both [^{35}S]GTPγS and cyclic AMP assays performed with CB_1-transfected CHO cells, mouse N18TG2 cells, or rat or mouse brain tissue (Pertwee 1999). There has also been one report that CBN activates CB_2 receptors with greater efficacy than Δ^9-THC in the cyclic AMP assay (Rhee et al. 1997), although another report that it behaves as a CB_2 receptor inverse agonist in the [^{35}S]GTPγS binding assay (MacLennan et al. 1998). There is evidence as well that CBN can activate CB_1 receptors in vivo. Thus, it has been found that CBN shares the ability of Δ^9-THC to suppress acetic acid-induced abdominal stretching behavior in mice and that this effect of CBN, like that of Δ^9-THC, can be blocked by SR141716A, but not by SR144528 (Booker et al. 2009). SR141716A has also been reported to prevent increases in food consumption induced in rats by CBN (Farrimond et al. 2012).

Interestingly, 11-hydroxy-CBN seems to target both CB_1 and CB_2 receptors with greater potency than CBN (Table 6.1), since it has been reported to bind to rat CB_1 and hCB_2 receptors with K_i values of 38.0 and 26.6 nM, respectively (Rhee et al. 1997). This 11-hydroxy metabolite of CBN (Yamamoto et al. 2003), has also been found: (1) to activate CB_1 receptors with significant potency (EC_{50} = 58.1 nM), in the cyclic AMP assay performed with rat CB_1-transfected COS-7 cells, but (2) to display little activity as an agonist in this assay (EC_{50} > 10 μM) when it was performed with hCB_2-transfected COS-7 cells, behaving instead as an antagonist of the potent synthetic CB_1/CB_2 receptor agonist, HU-210 (Rhee et al. 1997). Δ^9-THC behaved similarly to 11-hydroxy-CBN in this investigation, displaying significant potency as a CB_1 receptor agonist (EC_{50} = 11 nM) but not as a CB_2 receptor agonist (EC_{50} > 1 μM).

Finally, submicromolar concentrations of CBN have also been found to inhibit CYPA1, CYP1A2, and CYP1B1 enzymes (IC_{50} = 740 nM, 188 nM and 278 nM, respectively), to desensitize

Table 6.4 A selection of receptors, ion channels, enzymes and cellular uptake or other processes that CBN or Δ^9-THCV has been reported to target in vitro

Compound and its concentration§		Pharmacological target and effect	Reference
		Receptors and channels	
CBN	<1 µM	CB$_1$ receptor (A)	Pertwee 1999†; Rhee et al. 1997
		CB$_2$ receptor (A)	Pertwee 1999†; Rhee et al. 1997;
		TRPA1 cation channel (A)*	De Petrocellis et al. 2011
		TRPM8 cation channel (B)	De Petrocellis et al. 2011
	1–10 µM	TRPV1 cation channel (A) (low efficacy)	De Petrocellis et al. 2011
		TRPV3 cation channel (A)	De Petrocellis et al. 2012†
		Conductance in gap junctions between cells (−)	Oz 2006†
		Putative non-CB$_1$, non-CB$_2$, non-TRPV1 receptors on capsaicin-sensitive perivascular sensory neurons mediating CGRP release (+)	Zygmunt et al. 2002
	>10 µM	TRPA1 cation channel (A)	De Petrocellis and Di Marzo 2010†
		TRPV2 cation channel (A)	De Petrocellis and Di Marzo 2010†
		TRPV4 cation channel (A)	De Petrocellis et al. 2012
Δ^9-THCV	<1 µM	CB$_1$ receptor (B)	¶
		CB$_2$ receptor (A)	¶
		TRPM8 cation channel (B)	De Petrocellis et al. 2011
	1–10 µM	GPR55 (A or B)	Anavi-Goffer et al. 2012
		TRPA1 cation channel (A)	De Petrocellis et al. 2011
		TRPV1 cation channel (A)	De Petrocellis et al. 2011
		TRPV2 cation channel (A)	De Petrocellis et al. 2011
		TRPV3 cation channel (A)	De Petrocellis et al. 2012†
		TRPV4 cation channel (A)	De Petrocellis et al. 2012†
		Enzymes	
CBN	<1 µM	CYP1A1 (−); CYP1A2 (−); CYP1B1 (−)	Yamaori et al. 2010
	1–10 µM	Phospholipase(s) (+)	Burstein et al. 1982
		Lipoxygenase (−)	Evans 1991
		CYP2B6 (−)	Yamaori et al. 2011b
		CYP2C9 (−)	Yamaori et al. 2012
	>10 µM	Cyclooxygenase (−)	Evans 1991
		CYP3A4 (−); CYP3A5 (−); CYP3A7 (−)	Yamaori et al. 2011a
		CYP2A6 (−)	Yamaori et al. 2011b
		CYP2D6 (−)	Yamaori et al. 2011c

Table 6.4 (continued) A selection of receptors, ion channels, enzymes and cellular uptake or other processes that CBN or Δ^9-THCV has been reported to target in vitro

Compound and its concentration§		Pharmacological target and effect	Reference
		Norepinephrine-induced melatonin biosynthesis (−)	Koch et al. 2006
		Transporters and cellular uptake	
CBN	1–10 μM	Synaptosomal uptake of dopamine (−)	Poddar and Dewey 1980
		Synaptosomal uptake of noradrenaline (−)*	Poddar and Dewey 1980
	>10 μM	Synaptosomal uptake of noradrenaline (−)	Banerjee et al. 1975
		Synaptosomal uptake of 5-hydroxytryptamine (−)	Banerjee et al. 1975
		Synaptosomal uptake of γ-aminobutyric acid (−)	Banerjee et al. 1975
		Other actions or effects	
CBN	1–10 μM	Oxidative stress (−)	Marsicano et al. 2002
		Human keratinocyte proliferation (−)	Wilkinson and Williamson 2007
	>10 μM	Fluidity of synaptic plasma membranes (+); (−)	Hillard et al. 1985

Abbreviations: A, activation; B, blockade; TRP transient receptor potential; see also footnote to Table 6.1.

(+), enhancement; (−), inhibition; § EC_{50} or IC_{50} when this has been determined; † review article; * see also effect of 1–10 μM or of >10 μM; ¶ see this review for further details.

TRPA1 cation channels to activation by allyl isothiocyanate (IC_{50} = 400 nM) and, like Δ^9-THC, to activate TRPA1 (EC_{50} = 180 nM), and block TRPM8 cation channels (IC_{50} = 210 nM) (De Petrocellis et al. 2011; Yamaori et al. 2010; see also Table 6.4). At higher concentrations, CBN can target additional CYP enzymes and TRP cation channels, as well as other receptors or enzymes, and transmitter uptake processes (Table 6.4).

6.6 Δ^9-tetrahydrocannabivarin

6.6.1 Δ^9-tetrahydrocannabivarin is a CB_2 receptor partial agonist

Δ^9-THCV (Fig. 6.1) can fully displace [^{3}H]CP55940 from specific binding sites in CB_2 receptors located in membranes obtained from hCB_2-transfected CHO cells with a potency similar to that of Δ^9-THC (Table 6.1). There is also evidence that Δ^9-THCV shares the ability of Δ^9-THC both to inhibit forskolin-induced stimulation of cyclic AMP production by hCB_2-transfected CHO cells and to stimulate [^{35}S]GTPγS binding to membranes obtained from these cells (Bolognini et al. 2010). The mean E_{max} value of Δ^9-THCV was significantly less than that of CP55940 in both these assays, evidence that it activates CB_2 receptors with less efficacy than CP55940 and is, therefore, a CB_2 receptor partial agonist. Neither compound inhibited forskolin-induced stimulation of cyclic AMP production in CHO cells that had not been transfected with CB_2 receptors.

As is to be expected for a partial agonist, the ability of Δ^9-THCV to activate CB_2 receptors seems to be influenced by the expression level of these receptors. Thus, it produced a significant stimulation of $[^{35}S]GTP\gamma S$ binding to hCB_2 CHO cell membranes in which CB_2 receptors were expressed at a level of 215 pmol mg^{-1}, but no detectable stimulation of such binding to cell membranes in which these receptors were expressed at the lower level of 72.57 pmol mg^{-1} (Bolognini et al. 2010). Indeed, Δ^9-THCV antagonized CP55940-induced stimulation of $[^{35}S]GTP\gamma S$ binding to these lower CB_2-expressing membranes (Thomas et al. 2005), an indication that Δ^9-THCV possesses the typical mixed agonist-antagonist properties of a partial agonist, inducing signs of agonism when its receptors are highly expressed, but signs of antagonism when they are less highly expressed.

It has also been found that Δ^9-THCV can stimulate $[^{35}S]GTP\gamma S$ binding to membranes obtained from mouse spleen, and that such stimulation is not produced by Δ^9-THCV in membranes obtained from mice from which the CB_2 receptor has been genetically deleted (Bolognini et al. 2010). Hence Δ^9-THCV can activate CB_2 receptors not only in cells that have been transfected with CB_2 receptors but also in a tissue that expresses these receptors naturally. Additionally, it has been found: (1) that like the CB_2-selective agonist, JWH-015, Δ^9-THCV can stimulate fibroblastic colony formation by bone marrow cells, and (2) that this stimulation by Δ^9-THCV is reduced by the CB_2-selective antagonist, AM630 (Scutt and Williamson 2007).

There is evidence as well that CB_2 receptors can be activated by Δ^9-THCV in vivo. This has come from experiments with mice showing: (1) that this compound resembles established CB_2 receptor agonists by displaying an ability to decrease both carrageenan-induced paw edema and signs of inflammatory pain exhibited in the formalin paw test, and (2) that both these effects of Δ^9-THCV can be attenuated by the CB_2-selective antagonist SR144528 (Bolognini et al. 2010). However, the effect of Δ^9-THCV in the second of these bioassays was opposed by the CB_1 selective antagonist, SR141716A too, and although Δ^9-THCV also suppressed carrageenan-induced hind paw hyperalgesia, this effect was attenuated by neither SR144528 nor SR141716A. In addition, Δ^9-THCV attenuated the first and second phases of formalin-induced pain behavior at a dose of 5 mg kg^{-1} i.p., but only the second of these phases at the lower dose of 1 mg kg^{-1} i.p. (Bolognini et al. 2010). This is of interest since several established CB_2-selective agonists have been found to suppress only phase 2 of the formalin test (Guindon and Hohmann 2008).

Further evidence that Δ^9-THCV can activate CB_2 receptors in vivo comes from the finding that in mice that had received intrastriatal injections of lipopolysaccharide (LPS), it can produce signs of neuroprotection similar to those produced by the CB_2-selective agonist, HU-308 (García et al. 2011). It has been found too that signs of hepatic ischemia/reperfusion injury in mice can be attenuated by Δ^8-THCV in a manner that can be opposed by the CB_2-selective antagonist, SR144528 (Bátkai et al. 2012). This investigation also showed that Δ^8-THCV and 11-hydroxy-Δ^8-THCV display similar potency to Δ^9-THCV in vitro, both as CB_2 agonists in cyclic AMP assays performed with hCB_2-transfected CHO cells, and as displacers of $[^3H]CP55940$ from specific binding sites in membranes obtained from these cells.

6.6.2 Δ^9-tetrahydrocannabivarin also targets CB_1 receptors

Δ^9-THCV can induce a complete displacement of $[^3H]CP55940$ as potently from CB_1 receptors as from CB_2 receptors (Table 6.1), and has also been found to displace $[^3H]R$-$(+)$-WIN55212 and $[^3H]SR141716A$ from specific binding sites on mouse brain membranes with about the same potency as that with which it displaces $[^3H]CP55940$ from these sites (Thomas et al. 2005). Importantly, however, evidence has also emerged from both in vitro and in vivo experiments that, at doses at which it activates CB_2 receptors, Δ^9-THCV behaves as a CB_1 receptor antagonist.

Turning first to the in vitro evidence, Δ^9-THCV has been found:

- to produce significant parallel dextral shifts in the log concentration–response curves of CP55940 and R-(+)-WIN55212 for their stimulation of [^{35}S]GTPγS binding to mouse whole brain membranes at 1 μM (Pertwee et al. 2007; Thomas et al. 2005)

- to produce such antagonism of R-(+)-WIN55212 at concentrations of 100 nM to 5 μM, when this assay is performed with membranes obtained from mouse cerebellum or piriform cortex (Dennis et al. 2008)

- to share the ability of one established CB_1-selective antagonist, SR141716A, to oppose inhibition of electrically evoked contractions of mouse isolated vasa deferentia induced by cannabinoid receptor agonists such as CP55940, R-(+)-WIN55212, and Δ^9-THC (Pertwee et al. 1995, 2007; Thomas et al. 2005)

- to share the ability of another such antagonist, AM251, to reverse R-(+)-WIN55212-induced decreases of miniature inhibitory postsynaptic current frequency at mouse cerebellar interneuron–Purkinje cell synapses (Ma et al. 2008).

Interestingly, Δ^9-THCV appeared to act solely as a competitive CB_1 antagonist in the first of these investigations, but not in the second one, a difference that merits further investigation. So, too, does the finding that although the potency that Δ^9-THCV displayed as an antagonist of Δ^9-THC in mouse isolated vasa deferentia was very similar to the potency it displayed as an antagonist of R-(+)-WIN55212 or CP55940 in [^{35}S]GTPγS binding assays performed with mouse whole brain membranes, the potency with which it antagonized R-(+)-WIN55212 or CP55940 was significantly higher in vasa deferentia than in brain membranes.

When administered by itself, at concentrations of up to 10 μM, Δ^9-THCV has been found neither to stimulate nor to inhibit [^{35}S]GTPγS binding to mouse whole brain membranes (Pertwee et al. 2007). Similar results have been obtained in experiments with membranes obtained from mouse cerebellum or piriform cortex or from rat cerebral cortex (Dennis et al. 2008; Hill et al. 2010), although in those investigations Δ^9-THCV was found to exert an inhibitory effect on [^{35}S]GTPγS binding at concentrations above 10 μM. However, in contrast to these findings, Δ^9-THCV has been found to induce signs of CB_1 receptor inverse agonism at 10, 100, and 1000 nM in experiments with human CB_1 (hCB_1) CHO cells, as indicated by its ability to enhance forskolin-induced stimulation of cyclic AMP production (Bolognini et al. 2010). This effect was most likely CB_1 receptor-mediated since it was not observed in cells that had been pre-incubated with pertussis toxin, a pretreatment expected to abolish $G_{i/o}$ protein-linked receptor signaling.

Turning now to evidence that Δ^9-THCV can also block CB_1 receptors in vivo, this came initially from experiments with mice showing that, at intravenous (i.v.) doses of 0.3 and/or 3 mg kg^{-1}, both Δ^9-THCV and Δ^8-THCV opposed the ability of Δ^9-THC to induce antinociception in a mouse model of acute pain (tail-flick test), and hypothermia (Pertwee et al. 2007). When injected at a dose of 2 mg kg^{-1} i.p., Δ^9-THCV has also been found to display significant potency as an antagonist both of CP55940-induced antinociception in a rat model of acute pain (hot-plate test), and of CP55940-induced inhibition of rat locomotor activity (García et al. 2011). In addition, Δ^8-THCV, but not Δ^9-THCV, has been reported to antagonize (1) Δ^9-THC-induced immobility in the mouse ring test at 0.3 and 3 mg kg^{-1} i.v. (Pertwee et al. 2007) and (2) Δ^9-THC induced antinociception in a mouse model of visceral pain at a subcutaneously administered dose of 50 mg kg^{-1} (Booker et al. 2009). It is also noteworthy that when injected intraperitoneally at doses of 2, 3, 10, or 30 mg kg^{-1}, Δ^9-THCV shares the ability both of AM251 to suppress food consumption and body weight in nonfasted mice (Riedel et al. 2009), and of SR141716A to reduce signs of motor inhibition displayed by 6-hydroxydopamine-lesioned "parkinsonian" rats (García et al. 2011).

Although there is no doubt that Δ^9-THCV can block CB_1 receptors, there is also evidence that its in vivo administration at high doses can lead to an activation of these receptors. Thus, Gill et al. (1970) discovered that Δ^9-THCV could induce catalepsy in the mouse ring test with an intraperitoneal potency 4.8 times less than that of Δ^9-THC, and it was also found in more recent experiments that when administered to mice intravenously at doses of 3, 10, 30, and/or 56 mg kg^{-1}: (1) Δ^8-THCV could produce both antinociception in the tail-flick test and hypothermia, (2) Δ^9-THCV could produce the first but not the second of these effects, and (3) Δ^8- and Δ^9-THCV could both produce immobility in the ring test (Pertwee et al. 2007). SR141716A was found to block Δ^8- and Δ^9-THCV-induced antinociception in the tail-flick test, although not Δ^8- or Δ^9-THCV-induced immobility in the ring test or Δ^8-THCV-induced hypothermia, findings that require further investigation (Pertwee et al. 2007). Further research is also still needed to investigate why Δ^8- and Δ^9-THCV block CB_1 receptors at low doses both in vivo and in vitro, but can produce signs of CB_1 receptor activation at high doses, in vivo but not in vitro.

6.6.3 CB_1 and CB_2 receptor-independent actions of Δ^9-tetrahydrocannabivarin

At concentrations above those at which it interacts with CB_1 and CB_2 receptors as an agonist or antagonist, Δ^9-THCV has been reported to activate or block certain TRP cation channels that are also targeted by Δ^9-THC (Table 6.4). There is also evidence that Δ^9-THCV can activate GPR55 with similar potency to but greater efficacy than Δ^9-THC. This has come from experiments with human GPR55-expressing HEK293 cells in which both these phytocannabinoids were found to stimulate ERK1/2 phosphorylation at concentrations above 1 µM (Anavi-Goffer et al. 2012). It was also found in the same investigation that when administered at a concentration of 1 µM, Δ^9-THCV produced a downward shift in the log concentration–response curve of L-α-lysophosphatidylinositol for its apparent activation of GPR55 that was greater in magnitude than the downward shift produced by 1 µM Δ^9-THC.

The extent to which Δ^9-THCV interacts with other pharmacological targets remains to be established. Further research is also needed to identify the mechanisms by which this phytocannabinoid inhibits firstly, electrically-evoked contractions of the mouse isolated vas deferens, at concentrations of 10 µM or more, in an apparent CB_1 receptor-independent manner (Thomas et al. 2005), and secondly, [^{35}S]GTPγS binding to the membranes of CHO cells expressing dopamine D_2, but most probably not cannabinoid CB_1 or CB_2 receptors (Dennis et al. 2008).

6.7 Caryophyllene activates CB_2 receptors

Convincing evidence has been obtained that there is at least one non-phytocannabinoid constituent of cannabis that can activate cannabinoid receptors. This is the sesquiterpene, (E)-BCP (Fig. 6.1), which appears to have the ability to activate CB_2 receptors. Thus, Gertsch et al. (2008) have found that this compound can:

- displace [^{3}H]CP55940 from specific binding sites on membranes obtained from hCB_2 receptor-expressing HEK293 cells with significant potency (Table 6.1)
- inhibit forskolin-induced stimulation of cyclic AMP production by hCB_2-transfected CHO cells (EC_{50} = 1.9 µM)
- stimulate calcium release within CB_2-expressing human promyelocytic leukemia (HL60) cells (EC_{50} = 11.5 µM), but not within HL60 cells devoid of CB_2 receptor surface expression, in a manner that could be blocked by 1 µM SR144528

- induce a rapid phosphorylation of ERK1/2 in both human monocytes and CB_2-expressing HL60 cells, at a concentration of 1 μM, and in a manner that could be blocked by 1 μM SR144528

- inhibit LPS-induced-stimulation of expression of the cytokines, TNF-α and IL-1β, in human whole blood at 500 nM in a manner that could be opposed by the CB_2 receptor antagonist, AM630, at 5 μM.

At this 5 μM concentration, AM630 has also been found to oppose the ability of 10 μM (*E*)-BCP to decrease LPS-induced proinflammatory cytokine expression in a rat intestinal epithelium-derived cell line (Bento et al. 2011).

As to in vivo evidence that (*E*)-BCP can activate CB_2 receptors, this has come from experiments showing that:

- oral administration of (*E*)-BCP at doses of 5 and 10 mg kg^{-1} could induce an apparent CB_2 receptor-mediated anti-inflammatory effect in mice, as indicated by its ability to attenuate intraplantar carrageenan-induced paw edema (Gertsch et al. 2008)

- an intraperitoneal (*E*)-BCP dose of 10 mg kg^{-1} could lessen the dysfunction and ameliorate the histological injury caused by cisplatin in mouse kidneys (Horváth et al. 2012)

- an orally administered (*E*)-BCP dose of 50 mg kg^{-1} could reduce signs of colitis induced in mice by dextran sulfate sodium (Bento et al. 2011).

These in vivo effects all appear to have been CB_2 receptor-mediated since the first two of them could be detected in wild-type mice, but not in mice from which the CB_2 receptor had been genetically deleted, and since the third effect was no longer produced by (*E*)-BCP if it was coadministered with a dose of AM630, 10 mg kg^{-1} i.p. or orally, that by itself did not affect dextran sulfate sodium-induced signs of colitis. It is noteworthy, however, that the PPARγ antagonist, GW9662, was also found to oppose the ability of (*E*)-BCP to inhibit these signs of colitis (Bento et al. 2011), suggesting that activation of CB_2 receptors may trigger PPARγ activation, or even that these nuclear receptors can be directly targeted by (*E*)-BCP. There is now a need for further research aimed at characterizing the pharmacology of (*E*)-BCP more fully, especially since there is already evidence that this compound is not only anti-inflammatory, but also possesses anticarcinogenic, antibiotic, antioxidant, and local anesthetic activity, as well as an ability to increase membrane permeability (Ghelardini et al. 2001; Legault and Pichette 2007).

Although (*E*)-BCP displays significant potency at displacing [^{3}H]CP554940 from specific binding sites on hCB_2 receptors, it has been found to induce only a slight displacement of this tritiated ligand from hCB_1 receptors in HEK293 cell membranes, even at the rather high concentration of 10 μM (Gertsch et al. 2008). It differs, therefore, from all other constituents of cannabis that are currently known to activate CB_2 receptors (Δ^9-THC, Δ^8-THC, CBN and Δ^9-THCV), since they all possess significant affinity for CB_1 receptors as well (Table 6.1).

6.8 Conclusions and future directions

Constituents of cannabis that have so far been found to activate cannabinoid receptors fall essentially into three pharmacological categories. These are first, the phytocannabinoids, Δ^8-THC, Δ^9-THC, and CBN, which activate both CB_1 and CB_2 receptors, second, the phytocannabinoid, Δ^9-THCV, which behaves as a CB_1 receptor antagonist at doses at which it activates CB_2 receptors, and third, the sesquiterpene, (*E*)-BCP, which can activate CB_2 receptors but lacks significant potency as a CB_1 agonist or antagonist. Further research is now required to establish whether any of the many other constituents of cannabis can activate CB_1 and/or CB_2 receptors with significant potency.

It is important to note that Δ^9-THC and Δ^9-THCV are both cannabinoid receptor *partial* agonists, since this is most probably the reason why they activate CB_2 receptors in some bioassays but block these receptors in other bioassays, and indeed, why Δ^9-THC can also behave as both an agonist and antagonist at the CB_1 receptor. Still to be investigated, however, is first, whether Δ^8-THC or CBN, which are also partial cannabinoid receptor agonists, share the ability of Δ^9-THC to both activate and block cannabinoid receptors, and second, both why Δ^9-THCV appears to activate the CB_1 receptor at doses above those at which it blocks this receptor, and why such activation is detectable in vivo but not in vitro.

At doses at or above those at which it activates CB_1 and CB_2 receptors, Δ^9-THC also interacts with a number of other pharmacological targets (Table 6.2 and 6.3). Further research is now required to identify any additional actions of Δ^9-THC, and to investigate the impact of the many cannabinoid receptor-independent actions of this phytocannabinoid on its in vivo pharmacology, for example, by seeking out any toxic or potentially beneficial effects that these other actions cause. It will also be important to characterize the non-CB_1, non-CB_2 receptor pharmacology of Δ^8-THC, CBN, Δ^9-THCV and (*E*)-BCP more fully, and to establish the extent to which the complex pharmacological "fingerprint" of Δ^9-THC overlaps with the pharmacological fingerprints of these other constituents of cannabis and indeed, of synthetic and endogenous compounds that are known to activate CB_1 or CB_2 receptors.

References

Anavi-Goffer, S., Baillie, G., Irving, A.J., *et al.* (2012). Modulation of L-α-lysophosphatidylinositol/GPR55 mitogen-activated protein kinase (MAPK) signaling by cannabinoids. *Journal of Biological Chemistry*, **287**, 91–104.

Avraham, Y., Ben-Shushan, D., Breuer, A., *et al.* (2004). Very low doses of Δ^8-THC increase food consumption and alter neurotransmitter levels following weight loss. *Pharmacology Biochemistry and Behavior*, **77**, 675–684.

Banerjee, S.P., Snyder, S.H., and Mechoulam, R. (1975). Cannabinoids: influence on neurotransmitter uptake in rat brain synaptosomes. *Journal of Pharmacology and Experimental Therapeutics*, **194**, 74–81.

Barann, M., Molderings, G., Brüss, M., Bönisch, H., Urban, B.W., and Göthert, M. (2002). Direct inhibition by cannabinoids of human 5-HT_{3A} receptors: probable involvement of an allosteric modulatory site. *British Journal of Pharmacology*, **137**, 589–596.

Bátkai, S., Mukhopadhyay, P., Horváth, B., *et al.* (2012). Δ^8-tetrahydrocannabivarin prevents hepatic ischaemia/reperfusion injury by decreasing oxidative stress and inflammatory responses through cannabinoid CB_2 receptors. *British Journal of Pharmacology*, **165**, 2450–2461.

Bayewitch, M., Rhee, M-H., Avidor-Reiss, T., Breuer, A., Mechoulam, R., and Vogel, Z. (1996). (−)-Δ^9-tetrahydrocannabinol antagonizes the peripheral cannabinoid receptor-mediated inhibition of adenylyl cyclase. *Journal of Biological Chemistry*, **271**, 9902–9905.

Bento, A.F., Marcon, R., Dutra, R.C., *et al.* (2011). β-caryophyllene inhibits dextran sulfate sodium-induced colitis in mice through CB_2 receptor activation and PPARγ pathway. *American Journal of Pathology*, **178**, 1153–1166.

Bolognini, D., Cascio, M.G., Parolaro, D., and Pertwee, R.G. (2012). AM630 behaves as a protean ligand at the human cannabinoid CB_2 receptor. *British Journal of Pharmacology*, **165**, 2561–2574.

Bolognini, D., Costa, B., Maione, S., *et al.* (2010). The plant cannabinoid Δ^9-tetrahydrocannabivarin can decrease signs of inflammation and inflammatory pain in mice. *British Journal of Pharmacology*, **160**, 677–687.

Booker, L., Naidu, P.S., Razdan, R.K., Mahadevan, A., and Lichtman, A.H. (2009). Evaluation of prevalent phytocannabinoids in the acetic acid model of visceral nociception. *Drug and Alcohol Dependence*, **105**, 42–47.

Brents, L.K., Gallus-Zawada, A., Radominska-Pandya, A., *et al.* (2012). Monohydroxylated metabolites of the K2 synthetic cannabinoid JWH-073 retain intermediate to high cannabinoid 1 receptor (CB1R) affinity and exhibit neutral antagonist to partial agonist activity. *Biochemical Pharmacology*, **83**, 952–961.

Brents, L.K., Reichard, E.E., Zimmerman, S.M., Moran, J.H., Fantegrossi, W.E., and Prather, P.L. (2011). Phase I hydroxylated metabolites of the K2 synthetic cannabinoid JWH-018 retain in vitro and in vivo cannabinoid 1 receptor affinity and activity. *PLoS ONE*, **6**.

Burstein, S., Hunter, S.A., Sedor, C., and Shulman, S. (1982). Prostaglandins and cannabis - IX. Stimulation of prostaglandin E_2 synthesis in human lung fibroblasts by Δ^1-tetrahydrocannabinol. *Biochemical Pharmacology*, **31**, 2361–2365.

Busch-Petersen, J., Hill, W.A., Fan, P., *et al.* (1996). Unsaturated side chain β-11-hydroxyhexahydrocannabinol analogs. *Journal of Medicinal Chemistry*, **39**, 3790–3796.

Cabral, G.A. and Staab, A. (2005) Effects on the immune system. In: R.G. Pertwee (ed.). *Cannabinoids. Handbook of Experimental Pharmacology*. Vol. **168**. Heidelberg: Springer-Verlag, pp. 385–423.

Caffarel, M.M., Andradas, C., Mira, E., *et al.* (2010). Cannabinoids reduce ErbB2-driven breast cancer progression through Akt inhibition. *Molecular Cancer*, **9**, 196.

Carrier, E.J., Auchampach, J.A., and Hillard, C.J. (2006). Inhibition of an equilibrative nucleoside transporter by cannabidiol: a mechanism of cannabinoid immunosuppression. *Proceedings of the National Academy of Sciences of the United States of America*, **103**, 7895–7900.

Cox, M.L., Haller, V.L., and Welch, S.P. (2007). The antinociceptive effect of Δ9-tetrahydrocannabinol in the arthritic rat involves the CB_2 cannabinoid receptor. *European Journal of Pharmacology*, **570**, 50–56.

De Petrocellis, L. and Di Marzo, V. (2010). Non-CB_1, non-CB_2 receptors for endocannabinoids, plant cannabinoids, and synthetic cannabimimetics: focus on G-protein-coupled receptors and transient receptor potential channels. *Journal of Neuroimmune Pharmacology*, **5**, 103–121.

De Petrocellis, L., Ligresti, A., Moriello, A.S., *et al.* (2011). Effects of cannabinoids and cannabinoid-enriched *Cannabis* extracts on TRP channels and endocannabinoid metabolic enzymes. *British Journal of Pharmacology*, **163**, 1479–1494.

De Petrocellis, L., Orlando, P., Moriello, A.S., *et al.* (2012). Cannabinoid actions at TRPV channels: effects on TRPV3 and TRPV4 and their potential relevance to gastrointestinal inflammation. *Acta Physiologica*, **204**, 255–266.

De Petrocellis, L., Vellani, V., Schiano-Moriello, A., *et al.* (2008). Plant-derived cannabinoids modulate the activity of transient receptor potential channels of ankyrin type-1 and melastatin type-8. *Journal of Pharmacology and Experimental Therapeutics*, **325**, 1007–1015.

Dennis, I., Whalley, B.J., and Stephens, G.J. (2008). Effects of Δ^9-tetrahydrocannabivarin on [^{35}S]GTPγS binding in mouse brain cerebellum and piriform cortex membranes. *British Journal of Pharmacology*, **154**, 1349–1358.

Di Marzo, V., Breivogel, C.S., Tao, Q., *et al.* (2000). Levels, metabolism, and pharmacological activity of anandamide in CB1 cannabinoid receptor knockout mice: evidence for non-CB_1, non-CB_2 receptor-mediated actions of anandamide in mouse brain. *Journal of Neurochemistry*, **75**, 2434–2444.

ElSohly, M.A. and Slade, D. (2005). Chemical constituents of marijuana: the complex mixture of natural cannabinoids. *Life Sciences*, **78**, 539–548.

Evans, F.J. (1991). Cannabinoids: the separation of central from peripheral effects on a structural basis. *Planta Medica*, **57**, S60–S67.

Farrimond, J.A., Whalley, B.J., and Williams, C.M. (2012). Cannabinol and cannabidiol exert opposing effects on rat feeding patterns. *Psychopharmacology*, **223**, 117–129.

Felder, C.C., Joyce, K.E., Briley, E.M., *et al.* (1995). Comparison of the pharmacology and signal transduction of the human cannabinoid CB_1 and CB_2 receptors. *Molecular Pharmacology*, **48**, 443–450.

García, C., Palomo-Garo, C., García-Arencibia, M., Ramos, J.A., Pertwee, R.G., and Fernández-Ruiz, J. (2011). Symptom-relieving and neuroprotective effects of the phytocannabinoid Δ^9-THCV in animal models of Parkinson's disease. *British Journal of Pharmacology*, **163**, 1495–1506.

Gérard, C.M., Mollereau, C., Vassart, G., and Parmentier, M. (1991). Molecular cloning of a human cannabinoid receptor which is also expressed in testis. *Biochemical Journal*, **279**, 129–134.

Gertsch, J., Leonti, M., Raduner, S., *et al.* (2008). Beta-caryophyllene is a dietary cannabinoid. *Proceedings of the National Academy of Sciences of the United States of America*, **105**, 9099–9104.

Ghelardini, C., Galeotti, N., Di Cesare Mannelli, L., Mazzanti, G., and Bartolini, A. (2001). Local anaesthetic activity of β-caryophyllene. *Il Farmaco*, **56**, 387–389.

Gill, E.W., Paton, W.D.M., and Pertwee, R.G. (1970). Preliminary experiments on the chemistry and pharmacology of cannabis. *Nature*, **228**, 134–136.

Govaerts, S.J., Hermans, E., and Lambert, D.M. (2004). Comparison of cannabinoid ligands affinities and efficacies in murine tissues and in transfected cells expressing human recombinant cannabinoid receptors. *European Journal of Pharmaceutical Sciences*, **23**, 233–243.

Greenberg, J.H., Mellors, A., and McGowan, J.C. (1978). Molar volume relationships and specific inhibition of a synaptosomal enzyme by psychoactive cannabinoids. *Journal of Medicinal Chemistry*, **21**, 1208–1212.

Guindon, J. and Hohmann, A.G. (2008). Cannabinoid CB$_2$ receptors: a therapeutic target for the treatment of inflammatory and neuropathic pain. *British Journal of Pharmacology*, **153**, 319–334.

Hejazi, N., Zhou, C., Oz, M., Sun, H., Ye, J.H., and Zhang, L. (2006). Δ^9-tetrahydrocannabinol and endogenous cannabinoid anandamide directly potentiate the function of glycine receptors. *Molecular Pharmacology*, **69**, 991–997.

Hill, A.J., Weston, S.E., Jones, N.A., *et al.* (2010). Δ^9-tetrahydrocannabivarin suppresses in vitro epileptiform and in vivo seizure activity in adult rats. *Epilepsia*, **51**, 1522–1532.

Hillard, C.J., Harris, R.A., and Bloom, A.S. (1985). Effects of the cannabinoids on physical properties of brain membranes and phospholipid vesicles: fluorescence studies. *Journal of Pharmacology and Experimental Therapeutics*, **232**, 579–588.

Horváth, B., Mukhopadhyay, P., Kechrid, M., *et al.* (2012). β-Caryophyllene ameliorates cisplatin-induced nephrotoxicity in a cannabinoid 2 receptor-dependent manner. *Free Radical Biology and Medicine*, **52**, 1325–1333.

Howlett, A.C. (2005). Cannabinoid receptor signaling. In: R.G. Pertwee (ed.). *Cannabinoids. Handbook of Experimental Pharmacology*. Vol. **168**. Heidelberg: Springer-Verlag, pp. 53–79.

Howlett, A.C., Barth, F., Bonner, T.I., *et al.* (2002). International Union of Pharmacology. XXVII. Classification of cannabinoid receptors. *Pharmacological Reviews*, **54**, 161–202.

Huffman, J.W., Liddle, J., Yu, S., *et al.* (1999). 3-(1′,1′-dimethylbutyl)-1-deoxy-Δ^8-THC and related compounds: synthesis of selective ligands for the CB$_2$ receptor. *Bioorganic and Medicinal Chemistry*, **7**, 2905–2914.

Iwamura, H., Suzuki, H., Ueda, Y., Kaya, T., and Inaba, T. (2001). In vitro and in vivo pharmacological characterization of JTE-907, a novel selective ligand for cannabinoid CB$_2$ receptor. *Journal of Pharmacology and Experimental Therapeutics*, **296**, 420–425.

Kelley, B.G. and Thayer, S.A. (2004). Δ^9-tetrahydrocannabinol antagonizes endocannabinoid modulation of synaptic transmission between hippocampal neurons in culture. *Neuropharmacology*, **46**, 709–715.

Koch, M., Dehghani, F., Habazettl, I., Schomerus, C., and Korf, H-W. (2006). Cannabinoids attenuate norepinephrine-induced melatonin biosynthesis in the rat pineal gland by reducing arylalkylamine N-acetyltransferase activity without involvement of cannabinoid receptors. *Journal of Neurochemistry*, **98**, 267–278.

Lauckner, J.E., Jensen, J.B., Chen, H-Y., Lu, H-C., Hille, B., and Mackie, K. (2008). GPR55 is a cannabinoid receptor that increases intracellular calcium and inhibits M current. *Proceedings of the National Academy of Sciences of the United States of America*, **105**, 2699–2704.

Legault, J. and Pichette, A. (2007). Potentiating effect of β-caryophyllene on anticancer activity of α-humulene, isocaryophyllene and paclitaxel. *Journal of Pharmacy and Pharmacology*, **59**, 1643–1647.

Ma, Y-L., Weston, S.E., Whalley, B.J., and Stephens, G.J. (2008). The phytocannabinoid Δ^9-tetrahydrocannabivarin modulates inhibitory neurotransmission in the cerebellum. *British Journal of Pharmacology*, **154**, 204–215.

MacLennan, S.J., Reynen, P.H., Kwan, J., and Bonhaus, D.W. (1998). Evidence for inverse agonism of SR141716A at human recombinant cannabinoid CB_1 and CB_2 receptors. *British Journal of Pharmacology*, **124**, 619–622.

Marsicano, G., Moosmann, B., Hermann, H., Lutz, B., and Behl, C. (2002). Neuroprotective properties of cannabinoids against oxidative stress: role of the cannabinoid receptor CB_1. *Journal of Neurochemistry*, **80**, 448–456.

Martin, B.R., Compton, D.R., Semus, S.F., *et al.* (1993). Pharmacological evaluation of iodo and nitro analogs of Δ^8-THC and Δ^9-THC. *Pharmacology Biochemistry and Behavior*, **46**, 295–301.

Martin, B.R., Compton, D.R., Thomas, B.F., *et al.* (1991). Behavioral, biochemical, and molecular modeling evaluations of cannabinoid analogs. *Pharmacology Biochemistry and Behavior*, **40**, 471–478.

Matsuda, L.A., Lolait, S.J., Brownstein, M.J., Young, A.C., and Bonner, T.I. (1990). Structure of a cannabinoid receptor and functional expression of the cloned cDNA. *Nature*, **346**, 561–564.

McHugh, D., Page, J., Dunn, E., and Bradshaw, H.B. (2012). Δ^9-tetrahydrocannabinol and *N*-arachidonyl glycine are full agonists at GPR18 receptors and induce migration in human endometrial HEC-1B cells. *British Journal of Pharmacology*, **165**, 2414–2424.

Mechoulam, R. (1973). Cannabinoid chemistry. In: R. Mechoulam (ed.). *Marijuana*. New York: Academic Press, pp. 1–99.

Monory, K., Tzavara, E.T., Lexime, J., *et al.* (2002). Novel, not adenylyl cyclase-coupled cannabinoid binding site in cerebellum of mice. *Biochemical and Biophysical Research Communications*, **292**, 231–235.

O'Sullivan, S.E., Tarling, E.J., Bennett, A.J., Kendall, D.A., and Randall, M.D. (2005). Novel time-dependent vascular actions of Δ^9-tetrahydrocannabinol mediated by peroxisome proliferator-activated receptor gamma. *Biochemical and Biophysical Research Communications*, **337**, 824–831.

Oz, M. (2006). Receptor-independent actions of cannabinoids on cell membranes: focus on endocannabinoids. *Pharmacology & Therapeutics*, **111**, 114–144.

Paronis, C.A., Nikas, S.P., Shukla, V.G., and Makriyannis, A. (2012). Δ^9-tetrahydrocannabinol acts as a partial agonist/antagonist in mice. *Behavioural Pharmacology*, **23**, 802–805.

Patel, S. and Hillard, C.J. (2006). Pharmacological evaluation of cannabinoid receptor ligands in a mouse model of anxiety: further evidence for an anxiolytic role for endogenous cannabinoid signaling. *Journal of Pharmacology and Experimental Therapeutics*, **318**, 304–311.

Pertwee, R.G. (1972). The ring test: a quantitative method for assessing the 'cataleptic' effect of cannabis in mice. *British Journal of Pharmacology*, **46**, 753–763.

Pertwee, R.G. (1988). The central neuropharmacology of psychotropic cannabinoids. *Pharmacology and Therapeutics*, **36**, 189–261.

Pertwee, R.G. (1997). Pharmacology of cannabinoid CB_1 and CB_2 receptors. *Pharmacology and Therapeutics*, **74**, 129–180.

Pertwee, R.G. (1999). Pharmacology of cannabinoid receptor ligands. *Current Medicinal Chemistry*, **6**, 635–664.

Pertwee, R.G. (2005). Pharmacological actions of cannabinoids. In: R.G. Pertwee (ed.). *Cannabinoids. Handbook of Experimental Pharmacology*. Vol. **168**. Heidelberg: Springer-Verlag, pp. 1–51.

Pertwee, R.G. (2010). Receptors and channels targeted by synthetic cannabinoid receptor agonists and antagonists. *Current Medicinal Chemistry*, **17**, 1360–1381.

Pertwee, R.G., Griffin, G., Lainton, J.A.H., and Huffman, J.W. (1995). Pharmacological characterization of three novel cannabinoid receptor agonists in the mouse isolated vas deferens. *European Journal of Pharmacology*, **284**, 241–247.

Pertwee, R.G., Howlett, A.C., Abood, M.E., *et al.* (2010). International Union of Basic and Clinical Pharmacology. LXXIX. Cannabinoid receptors and their ligands: beyond CB_1 and CB_2. *Pharmacological Reviews*, **62**, 588–631.

Pertwee, R.G. and Thomas, A. (2009). Therapeutic applications for agents that act at CB_1 and CB_2 receptors. In: P. Reggio (ed.). *The Cannabinoid Receptors*. New York: Humana Press, pp. 361–392.

Pertwee, R.G., Thomas, A., Stevenson, L.A., *et al.* (2007). The psychoactive plant cannabinoid, Δ^9-tetrahydrocannabinol, is antagonized by Δ^8- and Δ^9-tetrahydrocannabivarin in mice in vivo. *British Journal of Pharmacology*, **150**, 586–594.

Poddar, M.K. and Dewey, W.L. (1980). Effects of cannabinoids on catecholamine uptake and release in hypothalamic and striatal synaptosomes. *Journal of Pharmacology and Experimental Therapeutics*, **214**, 63–67.

Rakhshan, F., Day, T.A., Blakely, R.D., and Barker, E.L. (2000). Carrier-mediated uptake of the endogenous cannabinoid anandamide in RBL-2H3 cells. *Journal of Pharmacology and Experimental Therapeutics*, **292**, 960–967.

Rhee, M-H., Vogel, Z., Barg, J., *et al.* (1997). Cannabinol derivatives: binding to cannabinoid receptors and inhibition of adenylylcyclase. *Journal of Medicinal Chemistry*, **40**, 3228–3233.

Riedel, G., Fadda, P., McKillop-Smith, S., Pertwee, R.G., Platt, B., and Robinson, L. (2009). Synthetic and plant-derived cannabinoid receptor antagonists show hypophagic properties in fasted and non-fasted mice. *British Journal of Pharmacology*, **156**, 1154–1166.

Rinaldi-Carmona, M., Barth, F., Héaulme, M., *et al.* (1994). SR141716A, a potent and selective antagonist of the brain cannabinoid receptor. *FEBS Letters*, **350**, 240–244.

Ryberg, E., Larsson, N., Sjögren, S., *et al.* (2007). The orphan receptor GPR55 is a novel cannabinoid receptor. *British Journal of Pharmacology*, **152**, 1092–1101.

Scutt, A. and Williamson, E.M. (2007). Cannabinoids stimulate fibroblastic colony formation by bone marrow cells indirectly via CB_2 receptors. *Calcified Tissue International*, **80**, 50–59.

Seely, K.A., Lapoint, J., Moran, J.H., and Fattore, L. (2012). Spice drugs are more than harmless herbal blends: a review of the pharmacology and toxicology of synthetic cannabinoids. *Progress in Neuro-Psychopharmacology & Biological Psychiatry*, **39**, 234–243.

Shen, M. and Thayer, S.A. (1999). Δ^9-tetrahydrocannabinol acts as a partial agonist to modulate glutamatergic synaptic transmission between rat hippocampal neurons in culture. *Molecular Pharmacology*, **55**, 8–13.

Showalter, V.M., Compton, D.R., Martin, B.R., and Abood, M.E. (1996). Evaluation of binding in a transfected cell line expressing a peripheral cannabinoid receptor (CB_2): identification of cannabinoid receptor subtype selective ligands. *Journal of Pharmacology and Experimental Therapeutics*, **278**, 989–999.

Sim, L.J., Hampson, R.E., Deadwyler, S.A., and Childers, S.R. (1996). Effects of chronic treatment with Δ^9-tetrahydrocannabinol on cannabinoid-stimulated $[^{35}S]GTP\gamma S$ autoradiography in rat brain. *Journal of Neuroscience*, **16**, 8057–8066.

Slipetz, D.M., O'Neill, G.P., Favreau, L., *et al.* (1995). Activation of the human peripheral cannabinoid receptor results in inhibition of adenylyl cyclase. *Molecular Pharmacology*, **48**, 352–361.

Straiker, A. and Mackie, K. (2005). Depolarization-induced suppression of excitation in murine autaptic hippocampal neurones. *Journal of Physiology*, **569**, 501–517.

Thomas, A., Stevenson, L.A., Wease, K.N., *et al.* (2005). Evidence that the plant cannabinoid Δ^9-tetrahydrocannabivarin is a cannabinoid CB_1 and CB_2 receptor antagonist. *British Journal of Pharmacology*, **146**, 917–926.

Varvel, S.A., Bridgen, D.T., Tao, Q., Thomas, B.F., Martin, B.R., and Lichtman, A.H. (2005). Δ^9-tetrahydrocannabinol accounts for the antinociceptive, hypothermic, and cataleptic effects of marijuana in mice. *Journal of Pharmacology and Experimental Therapeutics*, **314**, 329–337.

Welch, S.P., Huffman, J.W., and Lowe, J. (1998). Differential blockade of the antinociceptive effects of centrally administered cannabinoids by SR141716A. *Journal of Pharmacology and Experimental Therapeutics*, **286**, 1301–1308.

Wiley, J.L., Jefferson, R.G., Grier, M.C., Mahadevan, A., Razdan, R.K., and Martin, B.R. (2001). Novel pyrazole cannabinoids: insights into CB_1 receptor recognition and activation. *Journal of Pharmacology and Experimental Therapeutics*, **296**, 1013–1022.

Wilkinson, J.D. and Williamson, E.M. (2007). Cannabinoids inhibit human keratinocyte proliferation through a non-CB_1/CB_2 mechanism and have a potential therapeutic value in the treatment of psoriasis. *Journal of Dermatological Science*, **45**, 87–92.

Wise, L.E., Cannavacciulo, R., Cravatt, B.F., Martin, B.F., and Lichtman, A.H. (2008). Evaluation of fatty acid amides in the carrageenan-induced paw edema model. *Neuropharmacology*, **54**, 181–188.

Yamamoto, I., Watanabe, K., Matsunaga, T., Kimura, T., Funahashi, T., and Yoshimura, H. (2003). Pharmacology and toxicology of major constituents of marijuana - on the metabolic activation of cannabinoids and its mechanism. *Journal of Toxicology - Toxin Reviews*, **22**, 577–589.

Yamaori, S., Ebisawa, J., Okushima, Y., Yamamoto, I., and Watanabe, K. (2011a). Potent inhibition of human cytochrome P450 3A isoforms by cannabidiol: role of phenolic hydroxyl groups in the resorcinol moiety. *Life Sciences*, **88**, 730–736.

Yamaori, S., Koeda, K., Kushihara, M., Hada, Y., Yamamoto, I., and Watanabe, K. (2012). Comparison in the in vitro inhibitory effects of major phytocannabinoids and polycyclic aromatic hydrocarbons contained in marijuana smoke on cytochrome P450 2C9 activity. *Drug Metabolism and Pharmacokinetics*, **27**, 294–300.

Yamaori, S., Kushihara, M., Yamamoto, I., and Watanabe, K. (2010). Characterization of major phytocannabinoids, cannabidiol and cannabinol, as isoform-selective and potent inhibitors of human CYP1 enzymes. *Biochemical Pharmacology*, **79**, 1691–1698.

Yamaori, S., Maeda, C., Yamamoto, I., and Watanabe, K. (2011b). Differential inhibition of human cytochrome P450 2A6 and 2B6 by major phytocannabinoids. *Forensic Toxicology*, **29**, 117–124.

Yamaori, S., Okamoto, Y., Yamamoto, I., and Watanabe, K. (2011c). Cannabidiol, a major phytocannabinoid, as a potent atypical inhibitor for CYP2D6. *Drug Metabolism and Disposition*, **39**, 2049–2056.

Yin, H., Chu, A., Li, W., *et al.* (2009). Lipid G protein-coupled receptor ligand identification using β-arrestin PathHunter™ assay. *Journal of Biological Chemistry*, **284**, 12328–12338.

Zimmer, A., Zimmer, A.M., Hohmann, A.G., Herkenham, M., and Bonner, T.I. (1999). Increased mortality, hypoactivity, and hypoalgesia in cannabinoid CB_1 receptor knockout mice. *Proceedings of the National Academy of Sciences of the United States of America*, **96**, 5780–5785.

Zygmunt, P.M., Andersson, D.A., and Högestätt, E.D. (2002). Δ^9-tetrahydrocannabinol and cannabinol activate capsaicin-sensitive sensory nerves via a CB_1 and CB_2 cannabinoid receptor-independent mechanism. *Journal of Neuroscience*, **22**, 4720–4727.

Chapter 7

Known Pharmacological Actions of Nine Nonpsychotropic Phytocannabinoids

Maria Grazia Cascio and Roger G. Pertwee

7.1 Introduction

The plant *Cannabis sativa* contains more than 100 chemical compounds, known collectively as phytocannabinoids. Four of these compounds, Δ^9- and Δ^8-tetrahydrocannabinol (Δ^9- and Δ^8-THC), Δ^9-tetrahydrocannabivarin (Δ^9-THCV), and cannabinol (CBN), can activate cannabinoid receptor type 1 (CB_1) and/or type 2 (CB_2) receptors, both in vitro at submicromolar concentrations and in vivo, and we have recently presented current information about their pharmacological actions elsewhere (Pertwee and Cascio, Chapter 6, this volume). No other phytocannabinoid investigated to date has been reported to activate CB_1 or CB_2 receptors with significant potency. These other phytocannabinoids are cannabichromene (CBC), cannabidiol (CBD), cannabidivarin (CBDV), cannabidiolic acid (CBDA), cannabigerol (CBG), cannabigerovarin (CBGV), cannabigerolic acid (CBGA), Δ^9-tetrahydrocannabinolic acid (THCA), and Δ^9-tetrahydrocannabivarinic acid (THCVA). In this chapter we provide an overview of what is currently known about the pharmacological actions of each of these nine phytocannabinoids.

7.2 Cannabichromene (CBC)

CBC (Fig. 7.1) is, together with THC, CBD, and CBN, one of the most abundant naturally occurring cannabinoids (Brown and Harvey 1990). Even so, relatively few studies have yet been directed at identifying the pharmacological actions of this phytocannabinoid. What has been found so far is that CBC shows significant potency at targeting certain transient receptor potential (TRP) cation channels. Thus, for example, De Petrocellis et al. (2011, 2012) have reported that at concentrations below 10 μM, CBC can activate TRP ankyrin-type 1 (TRPA1) cation channels ($EC_{50} = 90$ nM), desensitize these channels to activation by allyl isothiocyanate ($IC_{50} = 370$ nM), activate TRPV4 and TRPV3 cation channels ($EC_{50} = 600$ nM and 1.9 μM, respectively), and desensitize TRPV2 and TRPV4 channels to their activation by an agonist ($IC_{50} = 6.5$ and 9.9 μM, respectively) (Table 7.1). It was also found in one or other of these investigations (Table 7.1) that CBC can, albeit with somewhat lower potency, activate TRPV1 channels ($EC_{50} = 24.2$ μM), desensitize TRPV3 channels to their activation by an agonist ($IC_{50} = 200.8$ μM), and block the activation of TRPM8 cation channels ($IC_{50} = 40.7$ μM). In addition, it has been reported that CBC displays an ability to inhibit both the cellular uptake of one endocannabinoid, anandamide ($IC_{50} = 12.3$ μM) and the metabolism by monoacylglycerol lipase of another endocannabinoid, 2-arachidonoyl glycerol ($IC_{50} = 50.1$ μM) (De Petrocellis et al. 2011; Tables 7.1–7.3). CBC has also been found to: (1) induce antinociception by itself and to potentiate the antinociceptive effect of THC in the mouse tail-flick assay (Davis and Hatoum 1983), and (2) stimulate the

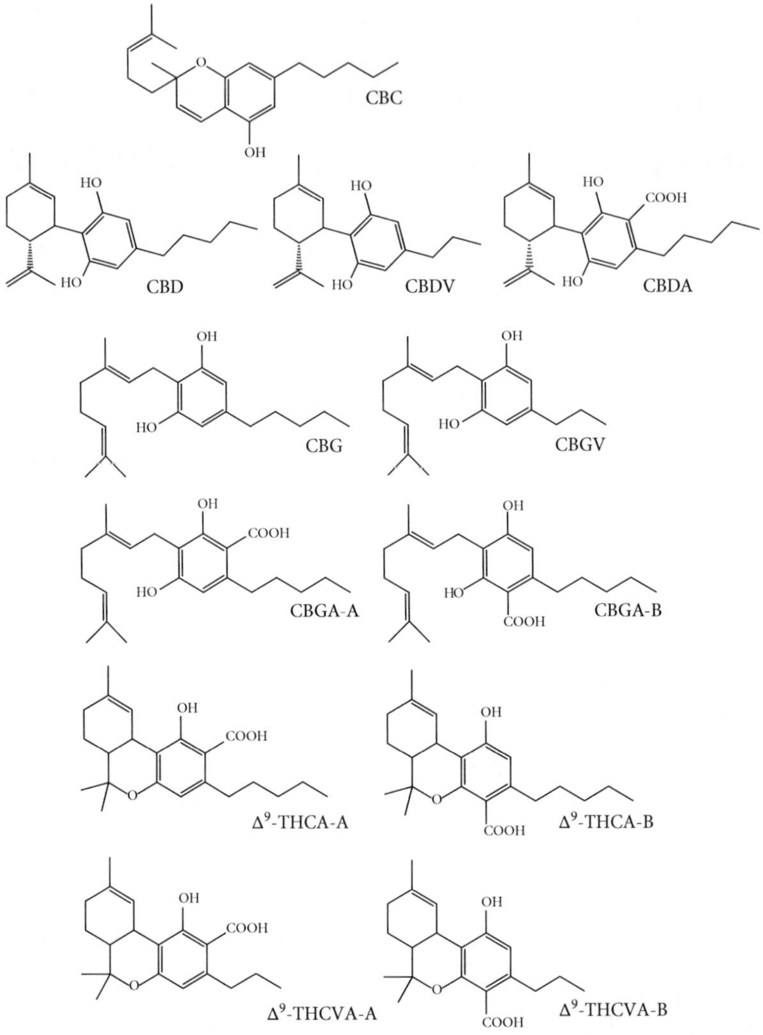

Fig. 7.1 The chemical structures of cannabichromene (CBC), cannabidiol (CBD), cannabidivarin (CBDV), cannabidiolic acid (CBDA), cannabigerol (CBG), cannabigerovarin (CBGV), cannabigerolic acid A (CBGA-A), cannabigerolic acid B (CBGA-B), Δ^9-tetrahydrocannabinolic acid A (THCA-A), Δ^9-tetrahydrocannabinolic acid B (Δ^9-THCA-B), Δ^9-tetrahydrocannabivarinic acid A (Δ^9-THCVA-A), and Δ^9-tetrahydrocannabivarinic acid B (Δ^9-THCVA-B).

descending pathway of antinociception in rat ventrolateral periaqueductal gray (Maione et al. 2011). It was also found by Maione et al. (2011) that intracerebrally injected CBC reduced tail flick-related nociception in anesthetized rats in a manner that could be blocked by intracerebral administration of the CB_1-selective antagonist, AM251, the adenosine A_1-selective antagonist, DPCPX, and the TRPA1-selective antagonist, AP18, although not by the TRPV1-selective antagonist, 5′-iodo-resiniferatoxin. The extent to which CBC induces antinociception by activating/desensitizing TRP channels, by somehow increasing the activation of adenosine A_1 receptors

Table 7.1 A selection of receptors and ion channels that CBC, CBD, CBDV, or CBDA has been reported to target in vitro

Compound and its concentration§		Pharmacological target and effect	Reference
		Receptors and channels	
CBC	< 1 µM	TRPA1 cation channel (A)	De Petrocellis et al. 2008, 2011
		TRPV4 cation channel (A)	De Petrocellis et al. 2012
	1–10 µM	TRPV3 cation channel (A)	De Petrocellis et al. 2012
	>10 µM	TRPV1 cation channel (A)	De Petrocellis et al. 2011
		TRPM8 cation channel (B)	De Petrocellis et al. 2011
CBD	< 1 µM	CB_1 receptor (B)	Thomas et al. 2007
		CB_2 receptor (B)	Thomas et al. 2007
		GPR55 (B)	Pertwee et al. 2010†
		$5\text{-}HT_{1A}$ receptor (P)	Rock et al. 2012
		$5\text{-}HT_{3A}$ ligand-gated ion channel (B)‡	Yang et al. 2010
		TRPM8 cation channel (B)	De Petrocellis et al. 2008, 2011
		TRPA1 cation channel (A)	De Petrocellis et al. 2008, 2011
		TRPV4 cation channel (A)	De Petrocellis et al. 2012
	1–10 µM	CB_1 receptor (D)	Pertwee 2008†
		CB_2 receptor (D)	Pertwee et al. 2010†
		PPARγ nuclear receptor (A)	Pertwee et al. 2010†
		Ca_V3 T-type Ca^{2+} voltage gated ion channels (−)	Ross et al. 2008
		TRPV1 cation channel (A)	De Petrocellis et al. 2011
		TRPV2 cation channel (A)	De Petrocellis et al. 2011
		TRPV3 cation channel (A)	De Petrocellis et al. 2012
		α3 glycine ligand-gated ion channel (P)	Xiong et al. 2012
	>10 µM	GPR18 (A or B)	McHugh et al. 2012
		$5\text{-}HT_{1A}$ receptor (A)	Pertwee 2008†; Russo et al. 2005
		µ and δ opioid receptors (B)‡	Pertwee 2008†
		α1 and α1β glycine ligand-gated ion channels (P)‡	Ahrens et al. 2009
CBDV	< 1 µM	TRPA1 cation channel (A)	De Petrocellis et al. 2011
		TRPM8 cation channel (B)	De Petrocellis et al. 2011
		TRPV4 cation channel (A)	De Petrocellis et al. 2012
	1–10 µM	TRPV1 cation channel (A)	De Petrocellis et al. 2011
		TRPV2 cation channel (A)	De Petrocellis et al. 2011
		TRPV3 cation channel (A)	De Petrocellis et al. 2012

Table 7.1 (continued) A selection of receptors and ion channels that CBC, CBD, CBDV, or CBDA has been reported to target in vitro

Compound and its concentration§		Pharmacological target and effect	Reference
CBDA	< 1 µM	5-HT$_{1A}$ receptor (P)	Bolognini et al. 2013
	1–10 µM	GPR55 (B)	Anavi-Goffer et al. 2012
		TRPM8 cation channel (B)	De Petrocellis et al. 2008, 2011
		TRPA1 cation channel (A)	De Petrocellis et al. 2011
		TRPV4 cation channel (A)	De Petrocellis et al. 2012
	>10 µM	TRPA1 cation channel (A)	De Petrocellis et al. 2008
		TRPV1 cation channel (A)	De Petrocellis et al. 2011; Ligresti et al. 2006

Abbreviations: 5-HT, 5-hydroxytryptamine; A, activation; B, blockade; CBC, cannabichromene; CBD, cannabidiol; CBDV, cannabidivarin; CBDA, cannabidiolic acid; D, displacement of [^{3}H]CP55940 or [^{3}H]HU243 from specific binding sites; P, potentiation; PPAR, peroxisome proliferator-activated receptor; TRP, transient receptor potential; (–), inhibition or antagonism. † review article; § EC$_{50}$ or IC$_{50}$ when this has been determined; ‡ apparent allosteric modulation.

Table 7.2 A selection of enzymes that CBC, CBD, CBDV, CBDA, CBG, CBGA, or THCA has been reported to target in vitro

Compound and its concentration§		Pharmacological target and effect	Reference
		Enzymes	
CBC	>10 µM	Monoacylglycerol lipase (–)	De Petrocellis et al. 2011; Ligresti et al. 2006
CBD	< 1 µM	CYP1A1(–)	Yamaori et al. 2010
	1–10 µM	CYP1A2 and CYP1B1 (–)	Yamaori et al. 2010
		CYP2B6 (–)	Yamaori et al. 2011b
		CYP2C9 (–)	Yamaori et al. 2012
		CYP2D6 (–)	Yamaori et al. 2011c
		CYP3A5 (–)	Yamaori et al. 2011a
		Mg^{2+}-ATPase (–)	Pertwee 2008†
		Arylalkylamine N-acetyltransferase (–)	Koch et al. 2006
		Indoleamine-2,3-dioxygenase (–)	Jenny et al. 2009
		15-lipoxygenase (–)	Takeda et al. 2009
		Phospholipase A$_2$ (+)	Pertwee 2008†
		Glutathione peroxidase (+)	Massi et al. 2006; Usami et al. 2008
		Glutathione reductase (+)	Massi et al. 2006; Usami et al. 2008

Table 7.2 (continued) A selection of enzymes that CBC, CBD, CBDV, CBDA, CBG, CBGA, or THCA has been reported to target in vitro

Compound and its concentration§		Pharmacological target and effect	Reference
	>10 µM	CYP2A6 (–)	Yamaori et al. 2011b
		CYP3A4 and CYP3A7 (–)	Yamaori et al. 2011a
		Fatty acid amide hydrolase (–)	De Petrocellis et al. 2011
		Cyclooxygenase (–)	Evans 1991
		5-lipoxygenase (–)	Takeda et al. 2009
		Superoxide dismutase (–)	Usami et al. 2008
		Catalase (–)	Usami et al. 2008
		NAD(P)H-quinone reductase (–)	Usami et al. 2008
		Progesterone 17α-hydroxylase (–)	Funahashi et al. 2005; Watanabe et al. 2005
		Testosterone 6β-hydroxylase (–)	Watanabe et al. 2005
		Testosterone 16α -hydroxylase (–)	Watanabe et al. 2005
		Phosphatases (induction)	Sreevalsan et al. 2011
CBDV	>10 µM	Diacylglycerol lipase α (–)	De Petrocellis et al. 2011
		NAAA (–)	De Petrocellis et al. 2011
CBDA	1–10 µM	Cyclooxygenase-2 (–)	Takeda et al. 2008
	>10 µM	NAAA (–)	De Petrocellis et al. 2011
		Diacylglycerol lipase α (–)	De Petrocellis et al. 2011
		Cyclooxygenase-1 (–)	Ruhaak et al. 2011; Takeda et al. 2008
CBG	1–10 µM	Lipoxygenase (–)	Evans 1991
	>10 µM	Monoacylglycerol lipase (–)	De Petrocellis et al. 2011
		Phospholipase A_2 (+)	Evans 1991
		Cyclooxygenase-2 (–)	Ruhaak et al. 2011
CBGA	>10 µM	Diacylglycerol lipase α (–)	De Petrocellis et al. 2011
		Cyclooxygenase-1 (–)	Ruhaak et al. 2011
		Cyclooxygenase-2 (–)	Ruhaak et al. 2011
THCA	>10 µM	Monoacylglycerol lipase (–)	De Petrocellis et al. 2011
		Diacylglycerol lipase α (–)	De Petrocellis et al. 2011
		Cyclooxygenase-1 (–)	Ruhaak et al. 2011
		Cyclooxygenase-2 (–)	Ruhaak et al. 2011

Abbreviations: CBC, cannabichromene; CBD, cannabidiol; CBDV, cannabidivarin;, CBDA, cannabidiolic acid; CBG, cannabigerol; CBGA cannabigerolic acid; NAAA, N-acylethanolamine-hydrolyzing acid amidase; THCA, Δ^9-tetrahydrocannabinolic acid. (+) activation; (–) inhibition; † review article. § EC_{50} or IC_{50} when this has been determined.

Table 7.3 A selection of cellular uptake or other processes that CBC, CBD, CBDV, CBDA, CBG, CBGA, or THCA has been reported to target in vitro

Compound and its concentration§		Pharmacological target and effect	Reference
		Transporters and cellular uptake	
CBC	>10 μM	Cellular uptake of anandamide (–)	De Petrocellis et al. 2011; Ligresti et al. 2006
CBD	< 1 μM	Adenosine uptake by cultured microglia and macrophages (–)	Pertwee 2008†
		Synaptosomal uptake of calcium (–)	Pertwee 2008†
	1–10 μM	Synaptosomal uptake of dopamine (–)	Pertwee 2008†
		Synaptosomal uptake of norepinephrine(–)	Pertwee 2008†
		Synaptosomal uptake of 5-hydroxytryptamine (–)	Pertwee 2008†
		Synaptosomal uptake of γ-aminobutyric acid (–)	Pertwee 2008†
		Cellular uptake of anandamide (–)	De Petrocellis et al. 2011; Ligresti et al. 2006; Rakhshan et al. 2000
		P-glycoprotein (drug efflux transporter) (–)	Zhu et al. 2006
	>10 μM	Choline uptake by rat hippocampal homogenates (–)	Pertwee 2008†
CBDV	>10 μM	Cellular uptake of anandamide (–)	De Petrocellis et al. 2011
CBG	>10 μM	Cellular uptake of anandamide (–)	De Petrocellis et al. 2011; Ligresti et al. 2006
		Synaptosomal uptake of norepinephrine (–)	Banerjee et al. 1975
		Synaptosomal uptake of 5-hydroxytryptamine (–)	Banerjee et al. 1975
		Synaptosomal uptake of γ-aminobutyric acid (–)	Banerjee et al. 1975
		Other actions or effects	
CBD	< 1 μM	Membrane fluidity (↑)	Pertwee 2004a†
	1–10 μM	Signs of neuroprotection	Fernández-Ruiz et al. 2012; Pertwee 2004a
		Oxidative stress (↓)	Pertwee 2004a†
		Release of certain cytokines (↑ or ↓)	Pertwee 2004a†
		Membrane stability (↑)	Pertwee 2004a†
	>10 μM	Release of certain cytokines (↑ or ↓)	Pertwee 2004a†

Abbreviations: CBC, cannabichromene; CBD, cannabidiol; CBDV, cannabidivarin; CBG, cannabigerol. (–), inhibition; ↑, increase; ↓, decrease; † review article; § EC_{50} or IC_{50} when this has been determined.

and by activating CB_1 receptors indirectly, by elevating extracellular levels of endocannabinoids through inhibition of their cellular uptake or metabolism, remains to be established.

7.3 **Cannabidiol (CBD)**

CBD (Fig. 7.1; Tables 7.1–7.3), was first isolated from the cannabis plant in the late 1930s and early 1940s, and its structure was elucidated in 1963 by Mechoulam and Shvo (Mechoulam and Hanus 2002). Unlike the main psychotropic component of cannabis, Δ^9-THC, CBD lacks psychotropic activity but does have therapeutic potential, both for the management of disorders such as inflammation, anxiety, emesis, and nausea, and as a neuroprotective agent and antioxidant (Pertwee 2004a, 2004b). Indeed, together with Δ^9-THC, CBD is a major constituent of Sativex®, a medicine developed by GW Pharmaceuticals that is used to ameliorate cancer pain and for the relief of neuropathic pain and spasticity due to multiple sclerosis.

7.3.1 **CBD interacts with cannabinoid CB_1 and CB_2 receptors**

The ability of CBD to target cannabinoid receptors has been explored in several investigations, and a brief summary of some of the assays used in that research can be found elsewhere (Pertwee and Cascio, Chapter 6, this volume). It has been found in some of these investigations that CBD displaces [^{3}H]CP55940 from cannabinoid CB_1 and CB_2 receptors at concentrations in the micromolar range (Table 7.1). In addition, in some functional in vitro assays, CBD has been found to behave as a low-potency CB_1 receptor inverse agonist as indicated by its ability at 10 μM to inhibit [^{35}S]GTPγS binding to membranes obtained either from C57BL/6 mouse brains or human CB_1-Chinese hamster ovary (hCB_1-CHO) cells (Thomas et al. 2007), or from rat cerebellum (Petitet et al. 1998). This inverse effect may or may not have been CB_1 receptor-mediated since, although CBD was found to inhibit [^{35}S]GTPγS binding to brain membranes obtained from mice from which the CB_1 receptor had been genetically deleted ($CB_1^{-/-}$ mice), it did not inhibit such binding to membranes obtained from untransfected CHO cells (Thomas et al. 2007).

Interestingly, CBD displays significant potency as an antagonist of cannabinoid receptor agonists such as CP55940 and R-(+)-WIN55212. Thus, there have been reports that CBD antagonizes:

- CP55940-induced stimulation of [^{35}S]GTPγS binding to rat cerebellar membranes at 10 μM (Petitet et al. 1998)
- CP55940 and R-(+)-WIN55212 in the mouse isolated vas deferens with apparent K_B values in the low nanomolar range (Pertwee et al. 2002)
- CP55940- and R-(+)-WIN55212-induced stimulation of [^{35}S]GTPγS binding to mouse brain membranes with apparent K_B values (79 and 138 nM, respectively) well below the K_i value of CBD (4.9 μM) for its displacement of [^{3}H]CP55940 from specific binding sites on these membranes (Thomas et al. 2007).

These in vitro findings are consistent with previous reports that CBD can block various in vivo responses to Δ^9-THC in rabbits, rats, mice, and human subjects (Pertwee 2004a, 2004b).

It has also been found that CBD can oppose CP55940-induced stimulation of [^{35}S]GTPγS binding to hCB_2-Chinese hamster ovary (hCB_2-CHO) cell membranes (Thomas et al. 2007). Its apparent K_B value for this antagonism was 65 nM, which is far less than its K_i value for the displacement of [^{3}H]CP55940 from such membranes (4.2 μM). CBD was also found in this investigation to inhibit [^{35}S]GTPγS binding to hCB_2-CHO cell membranes, an indication that it is a CB_2 receptor inverse agonist. Since there is convincing evidence that CB_2 receptor inverse agonists reduce immune cell migration and have anti-inflammatory effects (Lunn et al. 2006), the ability of CBD to behave as a CB_2 receptor inverse agonist could account, at least in part, for its well-documented anti-inflammatory properties (Izzo et al. 2009; Pertwee 2004a, 2004b), and for its capacity to inhibit immune cell migration as demonstrated, for example, in Boyden chamber experiments performed with murine microglial cells or macrophages (Sacerdote et al. 2005; Walter et al. 2003), or with human neutrophils (McHugh and Ross 2005).

CBD is not generally regarded as being a cannabinoid receptor agonist. It is noteworthy, therefore, that there has been one report that submicromolar concentrations of this phytocannabinoid can produce a small but significant stimulation of $[^{35}S]GTP\gamma S$ binding to membranes obtained from CHO cells in which the hCB_1 receptor is highly expressed, but not to membranes obtained from CHO cells that do not express this receptor (Thomas et al. 2007). It may be, therefore, that CBD is a very low-efficacy CB_1 receptor partial agonist that can induce signs of CB_1 receptor agonism in tissues in which these receptors are highly expressed. Whether CBD can also behave in this way in vivo remains to be established. It is noteworthy, however, that there is already evidence that microsomal enzymes catalyze the metabolism of CBD to Δ^9-THC-like compounds such as 6β-hydroxymethyl-Δ^9-THC, which may well be psychotropic since it has been found to produce catalepsy, antinociception, and hypothermia in mice, albeit with less potency than Δ^9-THC (Nagai et al. 1993; Yamamoto et al. 2003). There have also been reports first, that CBD can reduce signs of compulsive behavior in mice and tail flick-related nociception in anesthetized rats in a manner that can be antagonized by the CB_1-selective antagonist AM251, and second, that CBD can elevate brain levels of the endogenous CB_1 receptor agonist, 2-arachidonoyl glycerol, in rats (Casarotto et al. 2010; Maione et al. 2011).

7.3.2 CB_1 and CB_2 receptor-independent actions of CBD

CBD has the ability to produce a large number of cannabinoid receptor-independent effects in vitro (Tables 7.1–7.3). Among these are several that it can produce at concentrations in the sub-micromolar range (see Tables 7.1–7.3 for references): (1) antagonism of the G protein-coupled receptor, GPR55, and of the TRP cation channel, TRPM8 (IC_{50} = 60 or 80 nM); (2) activation of TRPA1 (EC_{50} = 96 or 110 nM) and TRPV4 cation channels (EC_{50} = 800 nM), and desensitization of the TRPA1 cation channel to activation by allyl isothiocyanate (IC_{50} = 80, 140, or 160 nM); (3) desensitization of TRPV1 and TRPV3 cation channels to activation by an agonist (IC_{50} = 600 and 900 nM, respectively); (4) potentiation of the activation of the G protein-coupled $5-HT_{1A}$ receptor and of the ligand-gated ion channel, $5-HT_{3A}$; (5) inhibition of the human cytochrome P450 enzyme, CYP1A1; (6) inhibition of the cellular uptake of adenosine and of the synaptosomal uptake of calcium. Importantly, as indicated in sections 7.3.2.1–7.3.2.4, there is evidence that several of the in vitro effects of CBD listed earlier or in Tables 7.1, 7.2, or 7.3 can also be produced by this phytocannabinoid in vivo. There is also evidence that when administered repeatedly to mice or rats, CBD can induce hepatic CYP3A, CYP2B10, and CYP2C enzymes (Pertwee 2004a).

7.3.2.1 Evidence that CBD can increase $5-HT_{1A}$ receptor activation in vitro

In vitro evidence that CBD can potentiate the activation of $5-HT_{1A}$ receptors came from the finding that it can enhance stimulation of $[^{35}S]GTP\gamma S$ binding to rat brainstem membranes induced by the $5-HT_{1A}$ receptor agonist, 8-hydroxy-2-(di-*n*-propylamino)tetralin (8-OH-DPAT) (Rock et al. 2012). This enhancement was found to be produced by CBD at a concentration of 100 nM, but not at concentrations of 1, 10, 31.62, or 1000 nM, indicating its concentration–response curve to be bell-shaped. This is a noteworthy finding since the dose–response curves of CBD for its production in vivo of several effects that seem to be $5-HT_{1A}$ receptor-mediated have been found to be biphasic or bell-shaped (section 7.3.2.2). It is also noteworthy that CBD did not displace [^{3}H]8-OH-DPAT from specific binding sites on rat brainstem membranes at 100 nM, or indeed, at other concentrations between 0.1 nM and 10 µM, suggesting that it did not enhance the activation of 5-HT$_{1A}$ receptors by interacting directly with sites on these receptors that are targeted by 8-OH-DPAT. Whether CBD produces this enhancement by interacting allosterically with the 5-HT$_{1A}$ receptor or by acting on a different target which then somehow augments 5-HT- or 8-OH-DPAT-induced 5-HT$_{1A}$ receptor activation through an indirect mechanism remains to be established.

7.3.2.2 Evidence that CBD can increase 5-HT$_{1A}$ receptor activation *in vivo*

7.3.2.2.1 **CBD induces an apparent 5-HT$_{1A}$ receptor-mediated attenuation of nausea and vomiting** CBD (5 mg kg^{-1} i.p.) has been found to attenuate cisplatin-induced (Kwiatkowska et al. 2004) and lithium chloride-induced (Parker et al. 2004) vomiting and anticipatory retching (Parker et al. 2006) in shrews (*Suncus murinus*), as well as conditioned gaping (nausea-like behavior) induced by lithium chloride in rats (Rock et al. 2012). These effects of CBD all appear to be mediated by 5-HT$_{1A}$ receptors. Thus, WAY100135, a well-established 5-HT$_{1A}$ antagonist, and/or WAY100635, a more selective 5-HT$_{1A}$ antagonist, have been found to oppose the ability of CBD to reduce nicotine, cisplatin, and lithium chloride-induced vomiting in shrews, and to interfere with the establishment of lithium chloride-induced conditioned gaping in rats (Rock et al. 2011b). Moreover, when injected directly into the rat dorsal raphe nucleus: (1) WAY100635 reversed the antinausea-like effects of systemic CBD, and (2) CBD suppressed nausea-like behavior in a manner that could be opposed by systemic WAY100635 (Rock et al. 2012). It has also been found that CBD and the 5-HT$_{1A}$ receptor agonist, 8-OH-DPAT, interact synergistically to suppress nausea-like behavior in rats (Rock et al. 2012). It is noteworthy too that CBD was found to affect toxin-induced vomiting in shrews in a biphasic manner, potentiating this vomiting at doses above those at which it had a suppressant effect (Kwiatkowska et al. 2004; Parker et al. 2004). These in vivo findings are all in line with the in vitro evidence that CBD can potentiate the activation of 5-HT$_{1A}$ receptors, and that its concentration–response curve for the production of this potentiation is bell-shaped (section 7.3.2.1). When considered together, these in vivo and in vitro findings strongly support the hypothesis that CBD suppresses vomiting in shrews and nausea-like behavior in rats by somehow augmenting the activation of 5-HT$_{1A}$ receptors in the brainstem by endogenously released 5-HT (Rock et al. 2012).

7.3.2.2.2 **CBD induces an apparent 5-HT$_{1A}$ receptor-mediated attenuation of cerebral infarction** CBD has been found to produce a significant reduction in infarct volume in a mouse middle cerebral artery occlusion model of cerebral infarction with a bell-shaped dose–response curve (Mishima et al. 2005). This neuroprotective effect of CBD was opposed by WAY100135, but not by the CB$_1$ receptor antagonist, rimonabant, or the TRPV1 antagonist, capsazepine. CBD (3 mg kg^{-1} i.p.) also increased cerebral blood flow to the cortex, and this effect too was opposed by WAY100135. These findings suggest that these effects of CBD on cerebral blood flow and infarct volume were both 5-HT$_{1A}$ receptor-mediated.

7.3.2.2.3 **CBD induces apparent 5-HT$_{1A}$ receptor-mediated anxiolytic effects** When injected directly into the dorsolateral periaqueductal gray of rats, CBD has been found to produce signs of anxiolysis in both the elevated plus maze and the Vogel conflict test (Campos and Guimarães 2008). These effects were opposed by WAY100635, but not by AM251, supporting the hypothesis that CBD produced these apparent anxiolytic effects by targeting 5-HT$_{1A}$ receptors in the dorsolateral periaqueductal gray. The elevated plus maze experiments were performed with several doses of CBD and the shape of the resultant dose–response curve was bell-shaped. More recently, it has also been found that when CBD is injected directly into the bed nucleus of the stria termi-nalis of rats, it reduces both signs of anxiety in these two bioassays, and the expression of con-textual fear conditioning, in a manner that can be prevented by WAY100635 (Gomes et al. 2011, 2012). Intraperitoneally administered CBD has also been found to produce signs of anxiolysis in rats, and this effect was also blocked by WAY100635 (Resstel et al. 2009). In addition, there have been reports that CBD can block panic-like responses in rats when administered intracerebrally, that its repeated intraperitoneal administration can reduce signs of anxiety in rats in a predator exposure model of posttraumatic stress disorder, and that WAY100635 antagonizes the produc-tion by CBD of both these effects (Campos et al. 2012; de Paula Soares et al. 2010).

7.3.2.2.4 **Other apparent 5-HT$_{1A}$ receptor-mediated effects produced by CBD** In experiments performed with mice, CBD has been found to share the ability of the well-established antidepres-sant, imipramine, to reduce immobility time in the forced swim test, without affecting explora-tory behavior in an open field arena (Zanelati et al. 2010). This effect of CBD was blocked by WAY100635, suggesting that it was 5-HT$_{1A}$ receptor-mediated. It was produced by CBD at a dose of 30 mg kg^{-1} but not by lower or higher intraperitoneal doses of this phytocannabinoid. It has also been found that repeated administration of CBD (i.p.) can induce apparent improvements in mouse locomotion and cognition following their impairment by bile duct ligation, and that these improvements can be prevented by WAY100635 (Magen et al. 2010). Finally, WAY100635 has been reported to oppose the ability of CBD to reduce tail flick-related nociception in anesthetized rats when both these compounds were injected directly into the ventrolateral periaqueductal gray (Maione et al. 2011). The dose–response curve of CBD for its production of this antinociceptive effect was bell-shaped.

7.3.2.3 Evidence that CBD can inhibit adenosine uptake both in vitro and in vivo

Release of adenosine is evoked during cellular stress and inflammation and constitutes an endog-enous mechanism of immunosuppression, an effect of adenosine that is terminated by its cel-lular uptake and can therefore be enhanced by inhibitors of this uptake (Carrier et al. 2006). It is noteworthy, therefore, that CBD has been found to: (1) decrease the uptake of [^{3}H]adeno-sine into murine microglia and RAW264.7 macrophages; (2) bind to an adenosine transporter, the equilibrative nucleoside transporter 1, at submicromolar concentrations; and (3) decrease lipopolysaccharide-induced tumor necrosis factor-α production in mice in vivo in a manner that could be prevented both by an antagonist of the adenosine A$_{2A}$ receptor and by genetic dele-tion of this receptor (Carrier et al. 2006). Similarly, Liou et al. (2008) have found that CBD can inhibit adenosine uptake into rat retinal microglial cells, that it can also oppose increases in tumor necrosis factor-α production in rat retina in vivo that had been triggered by lipopolysaccharide, and that this in vivo effect of CBD could be prevented by the adenosine A$_{2A}$ receptor antagonist, ZM241385. More recently, this antagonist was also found to oppose anti-inflammatory effects induced by CBD in vivo in a mouse model of acute lung injury (Ribeiro et al. 2012). There has been a report too that the ability of intracerebrally injected CBD to reduce tail flick-related noci-ception in anesthetized rats can be prevented by intracerebral administration of the selective adenosine A$_1$ receptor antagonist, DPCPX (Maione et al. 2011).

7.3.2.4 Other actions that CBD seems to display in vivo

There is also some evidence that CBD can interact with TRPA1 and TRPV1 cation channels, α3 glycine ligand-gated ion channels, and the peroxisome proliferator-activated receptor-γ (PPARγ) not only in vitro (Tables 7.1 and 7.2) but also in vivo.

7.3.2.4.1 **TRP cation channels** Long et al. (2006) have found that the ability of CBD to reverse disruption of prepulse inhibition induced by MK-801 in mice in vivo could be prevented by the TRPV1 antagonist, capsazepine. It is also possible that TRPV1 activation could be at least partly responsible for the bell shape of some dose–response curves produced by CBD in vivo (e.g., see section 7.3.2.2) (Campos et al. 2012). There has also been a report that the ability of CBD injected into the ventrolateral periaqueductal gray to reduce tail flick-related nociception in anesthetized rats could be prevented by the TRPA1-selective antagonist, AP18, and, albeit less strongly, by the TRPV1 selective antagonist, 5′-iodo-resiniferatoxin, when they were injected into this brain area (Maione et al. 2011). It is noteworthy, however, that this effect of CBD was also blocked by the CB_1-selective antagonist, AM251 (section 7.3.1), the 5-HT_{1A}-selective antagonist, WAY100635 (section 7.3.2.2), and the adenosine A_1-selective antagonist, DPCPX (section 7.3.2.3).

7.3.2.4.2 **Glycine ligand-gated ion channels** It has been found by Xiong et al. (2012) that genetic deletion of the α3 glycine channel, although not of the cannabinoid CB_1 or CB_2 receptor, can abolish suppression by CBD (50 mg kg^{-1} i.p.) of signs of inflammatory pain produced in mice by injecting complete Freund's adjuvant into a hind paw.

7.3.2.4.3 **Peroxisome proliferator-activated receptor-γ (PPARγ)** Esposito et al. (2011) have found that the ability of CBD (10 mg kg^{-1} i.p.) to produce neuroprotective effects in an in vivo model of Alzheimer's disease when it was administered repeatedly could be completely prevented by the selective PPARγ antagonist, GW9662, although not by the selective PPARα antagonist, MK886. This was a model in which neuroinflammation was induced in rats by intrahippocampal injection of fibrillar Aβ peptide.

7.4 **Cannabidiolic acid (CBDA)**

The pharmacology of CBDA, the natural precursor of CBD in cannabis, has as yet been little investigated. What has been found so far, from in vitro experiments, is that this phytocannabinoid can target the receptor GPR55 and the cation channels TRPA1, TRPV1, and TRPM8, albeit only at concentrations between 1 and 10 μM (Table 7.1). At even higher concentrations, CBDA has also been reported to activate the cation channel, TRPV1, and to inhibit the enzymes, N-acylethanolamine-hydrolyzing acid amidase (NAAH) and diacylglycerol lipase α (DAGLα) (Tables 7.1 and 7.2). Consistent with the presence of a salicylic acid moiety in its structure, CBDA has, in addition, been reported be a cyclooxygenase inhibitor (Table 7.2). Thus, Takeda et al. (2008) have found that CBDA can inhibit both cycooxygenase-1 (IC_{50} = 20 μM) and cyclooxygenase-2 (IC_{50} = 2.2 μM). In contrast, CBD, which does not have a salicyclic acid moiety in its structure, did not inhibit either of these enzymes significantly even at a concentration of 100 μM. More recently, however, Ruhaak et al. (2011) reported that CBDA inhibited cyclooxygenase-1 with much lower potency (IC_{50} = 470 μM), and cyclooxygenase-2 by less than 30%, even at a concentration of 27.8 μM. Like Takeda et al. (2008), they also found CBD, and indeed $Δ^9$-THC, to lack significant activity for the inhibition of either of these enzymes.

In contrast, CBDA does appear to share the ability of CBD (sections 7.3.2.1 and 7.3.2.2) to display marked potency, both in vitro and in vivo, as an enhancer of 5-HT_{1A} receptor activation (Bolognini et al. 2013). Thus, in vitro experiments have shown that, at concentrations ranging from 0.1 to 100 nM, CBDA can significantly increase the maximal stimulatory effect of 8-OH-DPAT on [^{35}S]GTPγS binding to rat brainstem membranes. The dose–response curve of CBDA for the production of this effect was bell-shaped, as no such enhancement was produced by CBDA at concentrations of either 0.01 nM or 1 μM. It is also noteworthy that CBDA produced this effect over a wider concentration range and with greater potency than CBD, as indicated by data obtained with CBD in a previous investigation (section 7.3.2.1). Turning now to the in vivo experiments, these showed first, that CBDA (0.01 and 0.1 mg kg^{-1} i.p.) suppressed nausea-like behavior in rats, and second, that this effect could be blocked by the selective 5-HT$_{1A}$ receptor antagonist, WAY100635, but not by the selective CB$_1$ receptor antagonist/inverse agonist, SR141716A (rimonabant). Again, the dose–response curve of CBDA was bell-shaped: no anti-nausea effect was produced by this phytocannabinoid at doses of 0.5 or 5 mg kg^{-1} i.p. The manner in which CBDA interacted with 5-HT$_{1A}$ receptors in these experiments remains to be established, since (like CBD) it did not displace [^{3}H]8-OH-DPAT from specific binding sites in rat brainstem membranes at concentrations ranging from 0.1 to 1000 nM. Bolognini et al. (2013) also found that, in contrast to CBD (section 7.3.1), CBDA did not display significant activity as either an agonist or an inverse agonist at cannabinoid CB$_1$ receptors in mouse whole brain membranes, even at a concentration 100,000-fold higher than a concentration (0.1 nM) at which it potentiated 8-OH-DPAT in rat brainstem membranes.

7.5 Cannabigerol (CBG)

CBG (Fig 7.1, Tables 7.2–7.4), is a little-investigated phytocannabinoid that has been found not to induce Δ^9-THC-like psychotropic effects in vivo (Grunfeld and Edery 1969). The structure of CBG was first established by Gaoni and Mechoulam who also performed the first synthesis of this compound (Gaoni and Mechoulam 1971). Effects that CBG has been found to produce in vitro at concentrations in the submicromolar range (Table 7.4) include:

- displacement of [^{3}H]CP55940 from specific binding sites on mouse brain membranes with a K$_i$ value of 381 nM (Cascio et al. 2010)
- α_2-adrenoceptor agonism in both mouse brain (EC$_{50}$ = 0.2 nM) and mouse vas deferens (EC$_{50}$ = 72.8 nM)
- antagonism of the cation channel, TRPM8 (IC$_{50}$ = 160 nM)
- activation of the cation channel, TRPA1 (EC$_{50}$ = 700 nM) (De Petrocellis et al. 2011).

Evidence has also been obtained from in vitro experiments that CBG can oppose the activation of both CB$_1$ and 5-HT$_{1A}$ receptors with significant potency. Thus, it has been found to antagonize the stimulation of [^{35}S]GTPγS binding to mouse whole brain membranes by the 5-HT$_{1A}$ receptor agonist, 8-OH-DPAT, at 1 µM, and by the CB$_1$/CB$_2$ receptor agonists, anandamide and CP55040, at 10 µM (Cascio et al. 2010). The apparent K$_B$ values of CBG for this antagonism, which appeared to be competitive in nature, were in the submicromolar range: 19.6 nM, 483 nM and 936 nM, for the antagonism of 8-OH-DPAT, anandamide and CP55040, respectively. There is evidence as well that CBG can activate α_2-adrenoceptors and block 5-HT$_{1A}$ receptors when administered in vivo.

7.5.1 Evidence that CBG can activate α_2-adrenoceptors in vivo

Evidence has recently emerged that CBG can act through α_2-adrenoceptors in mice to induce signs of antinociception. Thus, Comelli et al. (2012) have reported that CBG (10 mg kg^{-1} i.p.) shares the ability of the established α_2-adrenoceptor agonist, clonidine (0.2 mg kg^{-1} i.p.), to reduce signs of persistent inflammatory pain that were induced by injecting formalin or λ-carrageenan into the hind paws of mice. The pain behavior induced by formalin usually occurs in two phases: a short, transient early phase that is followed a few minutes later by a slightly longer late phase (Guindon and Hohmann, 2008). CBG and clonidine displayed antinociceptive activity in both these phases. Importantly, at a dose of 1 mg kg^{-1} i.p., the α_2-adrenoceptor antagonist, yohimbine, significantly attenuated antinociception induced by CBG and clonidine both in the λ-carrageenan

Table 7.4 A selection of receptors and ion channels that CBG, CBGV, CBGA, THCA, or THCVA has been reported to target in vitro

Compound and its concentration§		Pharmacological target and effect	Reference
		Receptors and channels	
CBG	< 1 μM	CB_1 receptor (D)	Cascio et al. 2010
		TRPA1 cation channel (A)	De Petrocellis et al. 2011
		TRPM8 cation channel (B)	De Petrocellis et al. 2008, 2011
		α_2-adrenoceptor (A)	Cascio et al. 2010
	1–10 μM	CB_1 receptor (B)	Cascio et al. 2010
		CB_2 receptor (D)	Cascio et al. 2010
		$5\text{-}HT_{1A}$ receptor (B)	Cascio et al. 2010
		TRPA1 cation channel (A)	De Petrocellis et al. 2008
		TRPV1 cation channel (A)	De Petrocellis et al. 2011
		TRPV2 cation channel (A)	De Petrocellis et al. 2011
		TRPV3 cation channel (A)	De Petrocellis et al. 2012
		TRPV4 cation channel (A)	De Petrocellis et al. 2012
CBGV	1–10 μM	TRPA1 cation channel (A)	De Petrocellis et al. 2011
		TRPV1 cation channel (A)	De Petrocellis et al. 2011
		TRPV2 cation channel (A)	De Petrocellis et al. 2011
		TRPV3 cation channel (A)	De Petrocellis et al. 2012
		TRPM8 cation channel (B)	De Petrocellis et al. 2011
	>10 μM	TRPV4 cation channel (A)	De Petrocellis et al. 2012
CBGA	1–10 μM	TRPA1 cation channel (A)	De Petrocellis et al. 2011
		TRPM8 cation channel (B)	De Petrocellis et al. 2011
	>10 μM	TRPV1 cation channel (A)	De Petrocellis et al. 2011
		TRPV3 cation channel (A)	De Petrocellis et al. 2012
		TRPV4 cation channel (A)	De Petrocellis et al. 2012
THCA	< 1 μM	TRPM8 cation channel (B)	De Petrocellis et al. 2008, 2011
		TRPA1 cation channel (A)	De Petrocellis et al. 2008
	1–10 μM	TRPA1 cation channel (A)	De Petrocellis et al. 2011
		TRPV4 cation channel (A)	De Petrocellis et al. 2012
	>10 μM	TRPV2 cation channel (A)	De Petrocellis et al. 2011
THCVA	1–10 μM	TRPV4 cation channel (A)	De Petrocellis et al. 2012
		TRPM8 cation channel (B)	De Petrocellis et al. 2011
	>10 μM	TRPA1 cation channel (A)	De Petrocellis et al. 2011
		TRPV1 cation channel (A)	De Petrocellis et al. 2011
		TRPV3 cation channel (A)	De Petrocellis et al. 2012

Abbreviations: A, activation; B, blockade; CBG, cannabigerol; CBGV, cannabigevarin; CBGA cannabigerolic acid; D, displacement of [^{3}H]CP55940 from specific binding sites; THCA, Δ^9-tetrahydrocannabinolic acid; THCVA, Δ^9-tetrahydrocannabivarinic acid; TRP, transient receptor potential. † review article; § EC_{50} or IC_{50} when this has been determined.

test and in the late phase, but not the early phase, of the formalin test. That CBG is able to interact with the α_2-adrenoceptor and shares the ability of clonidine to modulate pain in animals is very interesting, since the chemical structure of CBG differs greatly from that of well-established α_2-adrenoceptors ligands. Hence, CBG may constitute a lead compound for the development of a new class of α_2-adrenoceptor agonists/analgesic drugs.

7.5.2 Evidence that CBG can block 5HT$_{1A}$ receptors in vivo

In vivo evidence that CBG is a 5-HT$_{1A}$ receptor antagonist has come from the finding that it can prevent the 5-HT$_{1A}$ receptor agonist, 8-OH-DPAT, from inducing antinausea effects in rats with significant potency (5 mg kg^{-1} i.p.) (Rock et al. 2011a). Since there is evidence that CBD can induce a 5-HT$_{1A}$ receptor-mediated attenuation of both nausea in rats and vomiting in shrews (section 7.3.2.1), it is also noteworthy that CBG (5 mg kg^{-1} i.p.) has been found to prevent CBD-induced suppression of both lithium chloride-induced nausea in rats and lithium chloride-induced vomiting in shrews (Rock et al. 2011a).

7.6 Other phytocannabinoids

7.6.1 Δ^9-tetrahydrocannabinolic acid (THCA), Δ^9-tetrahydrocannabivarinic acid (THCVA), and cannabigerolic acid (CBGA)

THCA, THCVA, and CBGA (Fig 7.1, Tables 7.1 and 7.2) are the immediate natural precursors in cannabis of THC, THCV, and CBG, respectively. As indicated in Table 7.4, in vitro experiments already performed with these compounds have provided evidence that they can block the activation of TRPM8 cation channels, activate certain other TRP cation channels, or desensitize some of these channels to activation by an agonist. More specifically, there have been reports (De Petrocellis et al. 2011, 2012) that at concentrations of 10 µM or less:

- THCA blocks TRPM8 (IC$_{50}$ = 150 nM), activates TRPA1 and TRPV4 (EC$_{50}$ = 2.7 and 3.4 µM, respectively), and desensitizes TRPV2 and TRPV4 cation channels (IC$_{50}$ = 9.8 and 8.8 µM, respectively)
- THCVA blocks TRPM8 (IC$_{50}$ = 1.33 µM) and activates TRPV4 cation channels (EC$_{50}$ = 4.4 µM)
- CBGA blocks TRPM8 (IC$_{50}$ = 1.31 µM), activates TRPA1 (EC$_{50}$ = 8.4 µM), and desensitizes TRPA1, TRPV3, and TRPV4 cation channels (IC$_{50}$ = 7.14, 7.4, and 3.6 µM, respectively).

Reported effects of higher concentrations of these three phytocannabinoids on TRP cation channels are also listed in Table 7.4. In addition, THCA and CBGA, but not THCVA, have been found to inhibit DAGLα, monoacylglycerol lipase, cyclooxygenase-1, and/or cyclooxygenase-2, again at concentrations above 10 µM (Table 7.2). Finally, as indicated in Fig 7.1, there are both A and B forms of THCA, THCVA, and CBGA, and it is not always clear whether it was the A or the B form that was used in the investigations mentioned in this section or in Tables 7.2 and 7.4.

7.6.2 Cannabidivarin (CBDV) and cannabigerovarin (CBGV)

Relatively few in vitro experiments have so far been performed with CBDV and CBGV (Fig. 7.1). These have provided evidence that both compounds can block the activation of TRPM8 cation channels, activate certain other TRP channels, and desensitize some of these channels to activation by an agonist (Table 7.4). More specifically, it has been reported by De Petrocellis et al. (2011, 2012) that:

◆ CBDV and CBGV can block the activation of TRPM8 (IC_{50} = 0.9 and 1.71 µM, respectively)

◆ CBDV can both activate TRPA1, TRPV1, TRPV2, TRPV3, and TRPV4 (EC_{50} = 0.42, 3.6, 7.3, 1.7, and 0.9 µM, respectively), and desensitize these cation channels (IC_{50} = 1.29, 10.0, 31.1, 25.2, and 2.9 µM, respectively)

◆ CBGV can also activate all these TRPA and TRPV cation channels (EC_{50} = 1.6, 2.0, 1.41, 2.4, and 22.2 µM, respectively), and desensitize them (IC_{50} = 2.02, 2.3, 0.7, 0.8, and 1.8 µM, respectively).

It has been reported too by De Petrocellis et al. (2011) that CBDV, but not CBGV, can inhibit: (1) NAAA, which catalyzes the metabolic degradation of palmitoylethanolamide; (2) a second enzyme, DAGLα; and (3) the cellular uptake of anandamide, albeit in each case only at rather high concentrations (Tables 7.2 and 7.3).

7.7 Conclusions and future directions

In conclusion it is now generally accepted that three of the nine phytocannabinoids featured in this review each displays significant potency at producing at least one action that has been detected both in vitro and in vivo. These actions are:

◆ the potentiation of $5-HT_{1A}$ receptor activation by CBDA and CBD

◆ the inhibition of the cellular uptake of adenosine by CBD

◆ the activation of $α_2$-adrenoceptors by CBG

◆ the antagonism of $5-HT_{1A}$ receptors by CBG

◆ the targeting of certain TRP cation channels by CBD and CBG.

Further research is now needed to investigate the extent to which these actions could be exploited therapeutically. It could well be, for example, that in the clinic: (1) CBDA would induce a $5-HT_{1A}$-mediated suppression of chemotherapy-induced nausea and vomiting, (2) CBG would induce $α_2$-adrenoceptor-mediated analgesia and perhaps also reduce negative signs of schizophrenia through the blockade of $5-HT_{1A}$ receptors, and (3) CBD might induce PPARγ-mediated neu-roprotective effects in neurodegenerative disorders such as Alzheimer's disease. It will also be important to complete the pharmacological characterization, not only of the phytocannabinoids mentioned in this review, and of their metabolites, but also of the many other as yet uninvesti-gated phytocannabinoids that are known to be present in cannabis. Such research would advance our understanding not only of the therapeutic potential of individual phytocannabinoids, admin-istered alone or together with one or more other phytocannabinoid or with nonphytocannabi-noid, but also of the likely myriad of pharmacological effects produced by cannabis when it is self-administered either as a recreational drug or for self-medication.

References

Ahrens, J., Demir, R., Leuwer, M., *et al.* (2009). The nonpsychotropic cannabinoid cannabidiol modulates and directly activates alpha-1 and alpha-1-beta glycine receptor function. *Pharmacology*, **83**, 217–222.

Anavi-Goffer, S., Baillie, G., Irving, A.J., *et al.* (2012). Modulation of L-alpha-lysophosphatidylinositol/ GPR55 mitogen-activated protein kinase (MAPK) signaling by cannabinoids. *Journal of Biological Chemistry*, **287**, 91–104.

Banerjee, S.P., Snyder, S.H., and Mechoulam, R. (1975). Cannabinoids: influence on neurotransmitter uptake in rat brain synaptosomes. *Journal of Pharmacology and Experimental Therapeutics*, **194**, 74–81.

Bolognini, D., Rock, E., Cascio, M.G., *et al.* (2013). Cannabidiolic acid prevents vomiting in *Suncus murinus* and nausea-induced behaviour in rats by enhancing 5-HT$_{1A}$ receptor activation. *British Journal of Pharmacology*, **168**, 1456–1470.

Brown, N.K. and Harvey, D.J. (1990). In vitro metabolism of cannabichromene in 7 common laboratory animals. *Drug Metabolism and Disposition*, **18**, 1065–1070.

Campos, A.C., Ferreira, F.R., and Guimarães, F.S. (2012). Cannabidiol blocks long-lasting behavioral consequences of predator threat stress: possible involvement of 5HT1A receptors. *Journal of Psychiatric Research*, **46**, 1501–1510.

Campos, A.C. and Guimarães, F.S. (2008). Involvement of 5HT1A receptors in the anxiolytic-like effects of cannabidiol injected into the dorsolateral periaqueductal gray of rats. *Psychopharmacology*, **199**, 223–230.

Campos, A.C., Moreira, F.A., Gomes, F.V., Del Bel, E.A., and Guimarães, F.S. (2012). Multiple mechanisms involved in the large-spectrum therapeutic potential of cannabidiol in psychiatric disorders. *Philosophical Transactions of the Royal Society of London. Series B, Biological Sciences*, **367**, 3364–3378.

Carrier, E.J., Auchampach, J.A., and Hillard, C.J. (2006). Inhibition of an equilibrative nucleoside transporter by cannabidiol: a mechanism of cannabinoid immunosuppression. *Proceedings of the National Academy of Sciences of the United States of America*, **103**, 7895–7900.

Casarotto, P.C., Gomes, F.V., Resstel, L.B.M., and Guimara, F.S. (2010). Cannabidiol inhibitory effect on marble-burying behaviour: involvement of CB1 receptors. *Behavioural Pharmacology*, **21**, 353–358.

Cascio, M.G., Gauson, L.A., Stevenson, L.A., Ross, R.A., and Pertwee, R.G. (2010). Evidence that the plant cannabinoid cannabigerol is a highly potent alpha(2)-adrenoceptor agonist and moderately potent 5HT(1A) receptor antagonist. *British Journal of Pharmacology*, **159**, 129–141.

Comelli, F., Filippi, G., Papaleo, E., De Gioaia, L., Pertwee, R.G., and Costa, B. (2012). Evidence that the phytocannabinoid cannabigerol can induce antinociception by activating α_2-adrenoceptors: a computational and pharmacological study. In: *Symposium on the Cannabinoids*. Freiburg: International Cannabinoid Research Society, p. 44.

Davis, W.M. and Hatoum, N.S. (1983). Neurobehavioral actions of cannabichromene and interactions with Δ^9-tetrahydrocannabinol. *General Pharmacology*, **14**, 247–252.

de Paula Soares, V., Campos, A.C., de Bortoli, V.C., Zangrossi, H., Guimarães, F.S., and Zuardi, A.W. (2010). Intra-dorsal periaqueductal gray administration of cannabidiol blocks panic-like response by activating 5-HT1A receptors. *Behavioural Brain Research*, **213**, 225–229.

De Petrocellis, L., Ligresti, A., Moriello, A.S., *et al.* (2011). Effects of cannabinoids and cannabinoid-enriched *Cannabis* extracts on TRP channels and endocannabinoid metabolic enzymes. *British Journal of Pharmacology*, **163**, 1479–1494.

De Petrocellis, L., Orlando, P., Moriello, A.S., *et al.* (2012). Cannabinoid actions at TRPV channels: effects on TRPV3 and TRPV4 and their potential relevance to gastrointestinal inflammation. *Acta Physiologica*, **204**, 255–266.

De Petrocellis, L., Vellani, V., Schiano-Moriello, A., *et al.* (2008). Plant-derived cannabinoids modulate the activity of transient receptor potential channels of ankyrin type-1 and melastatin type-8. *Journal of Pharmacology and Experimental Therapeutics*, **325**, 1007–1015.

Esposito, G., Scuderi, C., Valenza, M., *et al.* (2011). Cannabidiol reduces Aβ-induced neuroinflammation and promotes hippocampal neurogenesis through PPARγ involvement. *PLoS ONE*, **6**, e28668.

Evans, F.J. (1991). Cannabinoids – the separation of central from peripheral effects on a structural basis. *Planta Medica*, **57**, S60–S67.

Fernández-Ruiz, J., Sagredo, O., Pazos, M.R., *et al.* (2012). Cannabidiol for neurodegenerative disorders: important new clinical applications for this phytocannabinoid? *British Journal of Clinical Pharmacology*, **75**, 323–333.

Funahashi, T., Ikeuchi, H., Yamaori, S., Kimura, T., Yamamoto, I., and Watanabe, K. (2005). In vitro inhibitory effects of cannabinoids on progesterone 17 alpha-hydroxylase activity in rat testis microsomes. *Journal of Health Science*, **51**, 369–375.

Gaoni, Y. and Mechoulam, R. (1971). The isolation and structure of Δ^1-tetrahydrocannabinol and other neutral cannabinoids from hashish. *Journal of the American Chemical Society*, **93**, 217–224.

Gomes, F.V., Reis, D.G., Alves, F.H.F., Correa, F.M.A., Guimaraes, F.S., and Resstel, L.B.M. (2012). Cannabidiol injected into the bed nucleus of the stria terminalis reduces the expression of contextual fear conditioning via 5-HT$_{1A}$ receptors. *Journal of Psychopharmacology*, **26**, 104–113.

Gomes, F.V., Resstel, L.B.M., and Guimarães, F.S. (2011). The anxiolytic-like effects of cannabidiol injected into the bed nucleus of the stria terminalis are mediated by 5-HT1A receptors. *Psychopharmacology*, **213**, 465–473.

Grunfeld, Y. and Edery, H. (1969). Psychopharmacological activity of the active constituents of hashish and some related cannabinoids. *Psychopharmacologia*, **14**, 200–210.

Guindon, J. and Hohmann, A.G. (2008). Cannabinoid CB$_2$ receptors: a therapeutic target for the treatment of inflammatory and neuropathic pain. *British Journal of Pharmacology*, **153**, 319–334.

Izzo, A.A., Borrelli, F., Capasso, R., Di Marzo, V., and Mechoulam, R. (2009). Non-psychotropic plant cannabinoids: new therapeutic opportunities from an ancient herb: Trends Pharmacol. Sci. 30 (2009) 515–527. *Trends in Pharmacological Sciences*, **30**, 609.

Jenny, M., Santer, E., Pirich, E., Schennach, H., and Fuchs, D. (2009). Delta 9-tetrahydrocannabinol and cannabidiol modulate mitogen-induced tryptophan degradation and neopterin formation in peripheral blood mononuclear cells in vitro. *Journal of Neuroimmunology*, **207**, 75–82.

Koch, M., Dehghani, F., Habazettl, I., Schomerus, C., and Korf, H.W. (2006). Cannabinoids attenuate norepinephrine-induced melatonin biosynthesis in the rat pineal gland by reducing arylalkylamine N-acetyltransferase activity without involvement of cannabinoid receptors. *Journal of Neurochemistry*, **98**, 267–278.

Kwiatkowska, M., Parker, L.A., Burton, P., and Mechoulam, R. (2004). A comparative analysis of the potential of cannabinoids and ondansetron to suppress cisplatin-induced emesis in the *Suncus murinus* (house musk shrew). *Psychopharmacology*, **174**, 254–259.

Ligresti, A., Moriello, A.S., Starowicz, K., *et al.* (2006). Antitumor activity of plant cannabinoids with emphasis on the effect of cannabidiol on human breast carcinoma. *Journal of Pharmacology and Experimental Therapeutics*, **318**, 1375–1387.

Liou, G.I., Auchampach, J.A., Hillard, C.J., *et al.* (2008). Mediation of cannabidiol anti-inflammation in the retina by equilibrative nucleoside transporter and A$_{2A}$ adenosine receptor. *Investigative Ophthalmology & Visual Science*, **49**, 5526–5531.

Long, L.E., Malone, D.T., and Taylor, D.A. (2006). Cannabidiol reverses MK-801-induced disruption of prepulse inhibition in mice. *Neuropsychopharmacology*, **31**, 795–803.

Lunn, C.A., Fine, J.S., Rojas-Triana, A., *et al.* (2006). A novel cannabinoid peripheral cannabinoid receptor-selective inverse agonist blocks leukocyte recruitment in vivo. *Journal of Pharmacology and Experimental Therapeutics*, **316**, 780–788.

Magen, I., Avraham, Y., Ackerman, Z., Vorobiev, L., Mechoulam, R., and Berry, E.M. (2010). Cannabidiol ameliorates cognitive and motor impairments in bile-duct ligated mice via 5-HT$_{1A}$ receptor activation. *British Journal of Pharmacology*, **159**, 950–957.

Maione, S., Piscitelli, F., Gatta, L., *et al.* (2011). Non-psychoactive cannabinoids modulate the descending pathway of antinociception in anaesthetized rats through several mechanisms of action. *British Journal of Pharmacology*, **162**, 584–596.

Massi, P., Vaccani, A., Bianchessi, S., Costa, B., Macchi, P., and Parolaro, D. (2006). The non-psychoactive cannabidiol triggers caspase activation and oxidative stress in human glioma cells. *Cellular and Molecular Life Sciences*, **63**, 2057–2066.

McHugh, D. and Ross, R.A. (2005). Endocannabinoids and phytocannabinoids inhibit human neutrophil migration. In: *Symposium on the Cannabinoids.* Burlington, VT: International Cannabinoid Research Society, p. 38.

McHugh, D., Page, J., Dunn, E., and Bradshaw, H.B. (2012). Δ^9-Tetrahydrocannabinol and *N*-arachidonyl glycine are full agonists at GPR18 receptors and induce migration in human endometrial HEC-1B cells. *British Journal of Pharmacology*, **165**, 2414–2424.

Mechoulam, R. and Hanus, L. (2002). Cannabidiol: an overview of some chemical and pharmacological aspects. Part I: chemical aspects. *Chemistry and Physics of Lipids*, **121**, 35–43.

Mishima, K., Hayakawa, K., Abe, K., *et al.* (2005). Cannabidiol prevents cerebral infarction via a serotonergic 5-hydroxytryptamine$_{1A}$ receptor-dependent mechanism. *Stroke*, **36**, 1071–1076.

Nagai, K., Watanabe, K., Narimatsu, S., *et al.* (1993). *In vitro* metabolic formation of a new metabolite, 6β-hydroxymethyl-Δ^9-tetrahydrocannabinol from cannabidiol through an epoxide intermediate and its pharmacological effects on mice. *Biological & Pharmaceutical Bulletin*, **16**, 1008–1013.

Parker, L.A., Kwiatkowska, M., Burton, P., and Mechoulam, R. (2004). Effect of cannabinoids on lithium-induced vomiting in the *Suncus murinus* (house musk shrew). *Psychopharmacology*, **171**, 156–161.

Parker, L.A., Kwiatkowska, M., and Mechoulam, R. (2006). Delta-9-tetrahydrocannabinol and cannabidiol, but not ondansetron, interfere with conditioned retching reactions elicited by a lithium-paired context in *Suncus murinus*: an animal model of anticipatory nausea and vomiting. *Physiology & Behavior*, **87**, 66–71.

Pertwee, R.G. (2004a). The pharmacology and therapeutic potential of cannabidiol. In: V. Di Marzo (ed.). *Cannabinoids.* New York: Kluwer Academic/Plenum Publishers, pp. 32–83.

Pertwee, R.G. (2004b). Pharmacological and therapeutic targets for Δ^9-tetrahydrocannabinol and cannabidiol. *Euphytica*, **140**, 73–82.

Pertwee, R.G. (2008). The diverse CB$_1$ and CB$_2$ receptor pharmacology of three plant cannabinoids: Δ^9-tetrahydrocannabinol, cannabidiol and Δ^9-tetrahydrocannabivarin. *British Journal of Pharmacology*, **153**, 199–215.

Pertwee, R.G., Howlett, A.C., Abood, M.E., *et al.* (2010). International Union of Basic and Clinical Pharmacology. LXXIX. Cannabinoid receptors and their ligands: beyond CB$_1$ and CB$_2$. *Pharmacological Reviews*, **62**, 588–631.

Pertwee, R.G., Ross, R.A., Craib, S.J., and Thomas, A. (2002). (–)-Cannabidiol antagonizes cannabinoid receptor agonists and noradrenaline in the mouse vas deferens. *European Journal of Pharmacology*, **456**, 99–106.

Petitet, F., Jeantaud, B., Reibaud, M., Imperato, A., and Dubroeucq, M.-C. (1998). Complex pharmacology of natural cannabinoids: evidence for partial agonist activity of Δ^9-tetrahydrocannabinol and antagonist activity of cannabidiol on rat brain cannabinoid receptors. *Life Sciences*, **63**, PL1–PL6.

Rakhshan, F., Day, T.A., Blakely, R.D., and Barker, E.L. (2000). Carrier-mediated uptake of the endogenous cannabinoid anandamide in RBL-2H3 cells. *Journal of Pharmacology and Experimental Therapeutics*, **292**, 960–967.

Resstel, L.B.M., Tavares, R.F., Lisboa, S.F.S., Joca, S.R.L., Corrêa, F.M.A., and Guimarães, F.S. (2009). 5-HT$_{1A}$ receptors are involved in the cannabidiol-induced attenuation of behavioural and cardiovascular responses to acute restraint stress in rats. *British Journal of Pharmacology*, **156**, 181–188.

Ribeiro, A., Ferraz-de-Paula, V., Pinheiro, M.L., *et al.* (2012). Cannabidiol, a non-psychotropic plant-derived cannabinoid, decreases inflammation in a murine model of acute lung injury: role for the adenosine A$_{2A}$ receptor. *European Journal of Pharmacology*, **678**, 78–85.

Rock, E.M., Bolognini, D., Limebeer, C.L., *et al.* (2012). Cannabidiol, a non-psychotropic component of cannabis, attenuates vomiting and nausea-like behaviour via indirect agonism of 5-HT$_{1A}$ somatodendritic autoreceptors in the dorsal raphe nucleus. *British Journal of Pharmacology*, **165**, 2620–2634.

Rock, E.M., Goodwin, J.M., Limebeer, C.L., *et al.* (2011a). Interaction between non-psychotropic cannabinoids in marihuana: effect of cannabigerol (CBG) on the anti-nausea or anti-emetic effects of cannabidiol (CBD) in rats and shrews. *Psychopharmacology*, **215**, 505–512.

Rock, E.M., Limebeer, C.L., Mechoulam, R., Piomelli, D., and Parker, L.A. (2011b). The effect of cannabidiol and URB597 on conditioned gaping (a model of nausea) elicited by a lithium-paired context in the rat. *Psychopharmacology*, **196**, 389–395.

Ross, H.R., Napier, I., and Connor, M. (2008). Inhibition of recombinant human T-type calcium channels by Δ^9-tetrahydrocannabinol and cannabidiol. *Journal of Biological Chemistry*, **283**, 16124–16134.

Ruhaak, L.R., Felth, J., Karlsson, P.C., Rafter, J.J., Verpoorte, R., and Bohlin, L. (2011). Evaluation of the cyclooxygenase inhibiting effects of six major cannabinoids isolated from *Cannabis sativa*. *Biological & Pharmaceutical Bulletin*, **34**, 774–778.

Russo, E.B., Burnett, A., Hall, B., and Parker, K.K. (2005). Agonistic properties of cannabidiol at 5-HT1a receptors. *Neurochemical Research*, **30**, 1037–1043.

Sacerdote, P., Martucci, C., Vaccani, A., *et al.* (2005). The nonpsychoactive component of marijuana cannabidiol modulates chemotaxis and IL-10 and IL-12 production of murine macrophages both in vivo and in vitro. *Journal of Neuroimmunology*, **159**, 97–105.

Sreevalsan, S., Joseph, S., Jutooru, I., Chadalapaka, G., and Safe, S.H. (2011). Induction of apoptosis by cannabinoids in prostate and colon cancer cells is phosphatase dependent. *Anticancer Research*, **31**, 3799–3807.

Takeda, S., Misawa, K., Yamamoto, I., and Watanabe, K. (2008). Cannabidiolic acid as a selective cyclooxygenase-2 inhibitory component in cannabis. *Drug Metabolism and Disposition*, **36**, 1917–1921.

Takeda, S., Usami, N., Yamamoto, I., and Watanabe, K. (2009). Cannabidiol-2',6'-dimethyl ether, a cannabidiol derivative, is a highly potent and selective 15-lipoxygenase inhibitor. *Drug Metabolism and Disposition*, **37**, 1733–1737.

Thomas, A., Baillie, G.L., Phillips, A.M., Razdan, R.K., Ross, R.A., and Pertwee, R.G. (2007). Cannabidiol displays unexpectedly high potency as an antagonist of CB_1 and CB_2 receptor agonists in vitro. *British Journal of Pharmacology*, **150**, 613–623.

Usami, N., Yamamoto, I., and Watanabe, K. (2008). Generation of reactive oxygen species during mouse hepatic microsomal metabolism of cannabidiol and cannabidiol hydroxy-quinone. *Life Sciences*, **83**, 717–724.

Walter, L., Franklin, A., Witting, A., *et al.* (2003). Nonpsychotropic cannabinoid receptors regulate microglial cell migration. *Journal of Neuroscience*, **23**, 1398–1405.

Watanabe, K., Motoya, E., and Matsuzawa, N., *et al.* (2005). Marijuana extracts possess the effects like the endocrine disrupting chemicals. *Toxicology*, **206**, 471–478.

Xiong, W., Cui, T.X., Cheng, K.J., *et al.* (2012). Cannabinoids suppress inflammatory and neuropathic pain by targeting α3 glycine receptors. *Journal of Experimental Medicine*, **209**, 1121–1134.

Yamamoto, I., Watanabe, K., Matsunaga, T., Kimura, T., Funahashi, T., and Yoshimura, H. (2003). Pharmacology and toxicology of major constituents of marijuana – on the metabolic activation of cannabinoids and its mechanism. *Journal of Toxicology – Toxin Reviews*, **22**, 577–589.

Yamaori, S., Ebisawa, J., Okushima, Y., Yamamoto, I., and Watanabe, K. (2011a). Potent inhibition of human cytochrome P450 3A isoforms by cannabidiol: role of phenolic hydroxyl groups in the resorcinol moiety. *Life Sciences*, **88**, 730–736.

Yamaori, S., Koeda, K., Kushihara, M., Hada, Y., Yamamoto, I., and Watanabe, K. (2012). Comparison in the in vitro inhibitory effects of major phytocannabinoids and polycyclic aromatic hydrocarbons contained in marijuana smoke on cytochrome P450 2C9 activity. *Drug Metabolism and Pharmacokinetics*, **27**, 294–300.

Yamaori, S., Kushihara, M., Yamamoto, I., and Watanabe, K. (2010). Characterization of major phytocannabinoids, cannabidiol and cannabinol, as isoform-selective and potent inhibitors of human CYP1 enzymes. *Biochemical Pharmacology*, **79**, 1691–1698.

Yamaori, S., Maeda, C., Yamamoto, I., and Watanabe, K. (2011b). Differential inhibition of human cytochrome P450 2A6 and 2B6 by major phytocannabinoids. *Forensic Toxicology*, **29**, 117–124.

Yamaori, S., Okamoto, Y., Yamamoto, I., and Watanabe, K. (2011c). Cannabidiol, a major phytocannabinoid, as a potent atypical inhibitor for CYP2D6. *Drug Metabolism and Disposition*, **39**, 2049–2056.

Yang, K.H., Galadari, S., Isaev, D., Petroianu, G., Shippenberg, T.S., and Oz, M. (2010). The nonpsycho-active cannabinoid cannabidiol inhibits 5-hydroxytryptamine$_{3A}$ receptor-mediated currents in *Xenopus laevis* oocytes. *Journal of Pharmacology and Experimental Therapeutics*, **333**, 547–554.

Zanelati, T.V., Biojone, C., Moreira, F.A., Guimaraes, F.S., and Joca, S.R.L. (2010). Antidepressant-like effects of cannabidiol in mice: possible involvement of 5-HT$_{1A}$ receptors. *British Journal of Pharmacology*, **159**, 122–128.

Zhu, H.J., Wang, J.S., Markowitz, J.S., *et al*. (2006). Characterization of P-glycoprotein inhibition by major cannabinoids from marijuana. *Journal of Pharmacology and Experimental Therapeutics*, **317**, 850–857.

Chapter 8

Effects of Phytocannabinoids on Neurotransmission in the Central and Peripheral Nervous Systems

Bela Szabo

8.1 Introduction

This chapter focuses on the neuronal effects of phytocannabinoids. Phytocannabinoids are constituents of *Cannabis sativa*. Fig. 8.1 shows the chemical structures of some important phytocannabinoids. Only a few phytocannabinoids have known effects on synaptic transmission, and the effects of these compounds will be discussed: delta-9-tetrahydrocannabinol (Δ^9-THC), delta-9-tetrahydrocannabivarin (Δ^9-THCV), cannabinol, cannabidiol, and cannabigerol. It is important to note that far more information is available on the effects on neuronal systems of Δ^9-THC than of these other phytocannabinoids.

8.2 Interaction of phytocannabinoids with cannabinoid receptors

Here the basic interactions of neuronally active phytocannabinoids with the G protein-coupled cannabinoid receptors type 1 (CB_1) and type 2 (CB_2), are described. Δ^9- and Δ^8-THC are partial agonists of both receptors (Bayewitch et al. 1996; Breivogel et al. 2004; Kelley and Thayer 2004; Shen and Thayer 1998; Sim et al. 1996). Cannabinol is a low-potency partial agonist at CB_1 and CB_2 receptors (Bayewitch et al. 1996; Munro et al. 1993; Rhee et al. 1997; Showalter et al. 1996; Thomas et al. 1998). In some studies, Δ^9-THCV behaves as a CB_2 agonist and CB_1 inverse agonist (Bolognini et al. 2010), in other studies as a CB_1 and CB_2 receptor antagonist (Ma et al. 2008; Pertwee et al. 2007; Thomas et al. 2005). Cannabidiol possesses only low affinity for CB_1 and CB_2 receptors in radioligand binding studies (Showalter et al. 1996; Thomas et al. 1998). In more recent functional studies, cannabidiol appeared to be a rather potent antagonist of CB_1 receptors and an antagonist/inverse agonist at CB_2 receptors (Thomas et al. 2004, 2007). Remarkably, cannabidiol is also an antagonist at the G protein-coupled receptor 55 (GPR55), a recently "deorphanized" receptor for which several phytocannabinoids, endocannabinoids, and synthetic cannabinoids possess affinity (Ryberg et al. 2007).

8.3 Distribution of cannabinoid receptors in the nervous system

Knowledge of the localization of cannabinoid receptors in the nervous system is important for understanding the effects of cannabinoids on neurons.

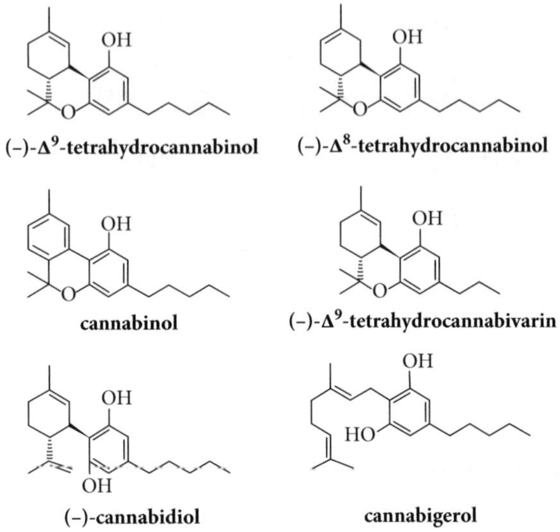

Fig. 8.1 Chemical structures of important phytocannabinoids.

8.3.1 **CB$_1$ receptor**

The CB$_1$ receptor can be found at low concentration in some peripheral non-neuronal tissues, for example, the heart, liver, fat tissue, stomach, and testis (Cota et al. 2003; Gerard et al. 1991; Mukhopadhyay et al. 2007; Pazos et al. 2008; Shire et al. 1995; Staender et al. 2005; Teixeira-Clerc et al. 2006). However, its main localization is in the nervous system. In situ hybridization studies, autoradiographic studies with radiolabeled cannabinoids, and immunohistochemical studies identified CB$_1$ receptors in most brain regions (Cristino et al. 2006; Dove Pettit et al. 1998; Egertova et al. 2003; Herkenham et al. 1991b; Matsuda et al. 1993; Tsou et al. 1998; Van Laere et al. 2008; Westlake et al. 1994; for review see Mackie 2005). The high density of CB$_1$ receptors in the brain is remarkable: it is thought that compared with other G protein-coupled receptors CB$_1$ receptors have the highest density in the brain. The concentration of CB$_1$ receptors in the brainstem and in the spinal cord is relatively low.

CB$_1$ receptors were also identified in the peripheral nervous system. Thus, CB$_1$ receptors are found in some sensory neurons (e.g., Hohmann and Herkenham 1999; Ständer et al. 2005), in many postganglionic sympathetic neurons (e.g., Calignano et al. 2000; Ishac et al. 1996), and in neurons of the parasympathetic nervous system. The gut nervous system is also rich in CB$_1$ receptors (e.g., Sibaev et al. 2009).

A characteristic feature of neuronal CB$_1$ receptors is that after their synthesis in the somatodendritic region, they are transported to the axon terminals. The concentration of CB$_1$ receptors in the axonal membrane is usually much higher than in the membrane of the somatodendritic region of neurons (Herkenham et al. 1991a; Katona et al. 1999; Leterrier et al. 2006; Nyiri et al. 2005; Yoshida et al. 2006).

8.3.2 **CB$_2$ receptor**

Originally, the CB$_2$ receptor was thought to be restricted to peripheral immune-related organs like the tonsils, spleen, thymus, and bone marrow and to cells involved in immune responses like B lymphocytes, monocytes, macrophages, mast cells, and microglial cells (Galiègue et al. 1995;

Munro et al. 1993). However, more recent observations point to the presence of CB_2 receptors also in neurons. Thus, CB_2 receptor mRNA or protein was shown to be present in a series of regions: cerebral cortex, hippocampal pyramidal cells, globus pallidus, cerebellar Purkinje cells, cerebellar granule cells, cerebellar nuclei, vestibular nuclei, dorsal motor nucleus of the vagus, nucleus ambiguous, spinal trigeminal nucleus, and spinal sensory neurons (Brusco et al. 2008; Gong et al. 2006; Lanciego et al. 2011; Skaper et al. 1996; Suarez et al. 2008; Van Sickle et al. 2005; Wotherspoon et al. 2005). Compared with the CB_1 receptors, the distribution of CB_2 receptors in the nervous system is more restricted, and the density of CB_2 receptors is much lower.

8.4 Cannabinoids inhibit synaptic transmission

This chapter provides an overview of the main effects of cannabinoids on synaptic transmission. Most of the knowledge in this field has been obtained by using certain synthetic cannabinoids that behave consistently as full agonists of cannabinoid receptors, and whose use for research purposes is not legally restricted.

8.4.1 Involvement of CB_1 receptors

The most frequently reported neuronal effect of CB_1 receptor agonists is inhibition of synaptic transmission (for review, see Freund et al. 2003; Szabo and Schlicker 2005). Fig. 8.2 shows CB_1 receptor-mediated inhibition of synaptic transmission schematically, and Fig. 8.3 shows an example of synaptic inhibition by the synthetic cannabinoid receptor agonist, WIN 55,212-2. It has been shown that glutamatergic, gamma-aminobutyric acid (GABA)-ergic, cholinergic, and noradrenergic neurotransmission all are inhibited after activation of CB_1 receptors, and inhibition has been shown in many regions of the central nervous system and in the peripheral nervous system of several species. Inhibition of synaptic transmission after activation of CB_1 receptors has also been shown to occur in the human brain (Kovacs et al. 2011; Nakatsuka et al. 2003). Corresponding to the presence of CB_1 receptors in the presynaptic axon terminals, the basis of the inhibition of synaptic transmission is inhibition of transmitter release from the axon terminals. Several mechanisms have been implicated in this presynaptic inhibition. Most frequently, inhibition of axon terminal voltage-gated calcium channels has been shown to contribute to the decrease in transmitter release resulting from CB_1 receptor activation (see Fig. 8.2) (Brown et al. 2004; Engler et al. 2006; Kushmerick et al. 2004). In many cases, direct inhibition of the vesicular release machinery after CB_1 receptor activation has also been found to contribute to the decrease in transmitter release (e.g., Freiman et al. 2006; Szabo et al. 2004). It is thought that voltage-gated calcium channels and the vesicle release machinery are inhibited by the $\beta\gamma$-subunits released from the heterotrimeric G protein complex (Blackmer et al. 2005) (Fig. 8.2). Some evidence exists also for the involvement of axon terminal potassium channels in the presynaptic inhibition of transmitter release by cannabinoids (e.g., Daniel et al. 2004).

Compared with the ubiquitous presynaptic inhibition seen after the activation of CB_1 receptors, somatodendritic effects of CB_1 agonists are usually not observed. Thus, for example, there have been reports that in neurons which synthesize CB_1 receptors, a CB_1 receptor-mediated inhibition is seen at their axon terminals, whereas no CB_1-mediated effects are detectable in the somatodendritic region of the same neurons (Freiman and Szabo 2005; Freiman et al. 2006). Although somatodendritic effects are usually not observed, signs of such effects have sometimes been detected. For example, Bacci et al. (2004) have shown that low-threshold-spiking neocortical interneurons respond with hyperpolarization to an endocannabinoid released by the neuron itself, and that this process was mediated by CB_1 receptors.

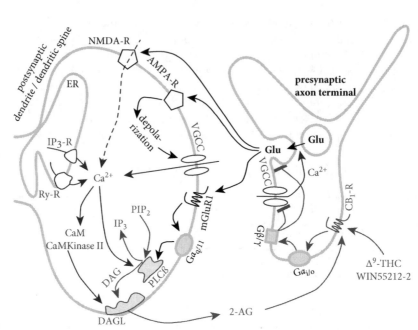

Fig. 8.2 Inhibition of synaptic transmission by exogenous cannabinoids and the endocannabinoid 2-arachidonoylglycerol (2-AG) (retrograde signaling). Glutamate (Glu) released from the presynaptic axon terminal activates postsynaptic (α-amino-3-hydroxy-5-methyl-4-isoxazolepropionic acid (AMPA), N-methyl-D-aspartate receptor (NMDA), and mGluR1 receptors. The CB_1 receptor (CB_1-R) is localized at the presynaptic axon terminal. Its activation leads via $G\alpha_{i/o}$- and $G\beta/\gamma$ proteins to inhibition of voltage-gated calcium channels (VGCCs), direct inhibition of the synaptic vesicle release machinery and finally to inhibition of glutamate release. The CB_1-R can be activated by exogenous cannabinoids (e.g., Δ^9-tetrahydrocannabinol (Δ^9-THC) and WIN 55,212-2) or by the endocannabinoid 2-AG. 2-AG is released from the dendritic spine of the postsynaptic neuron. 2-AG is produced from phosphatidylinositol diphosphate (PIP_2) via diacylglycerol (DAG) by the enzymes phospholipase C-β (PLC-β) and diacylglycerol lipase (DAGL). The production of 2-AG can be stimulated by calcium, which flows into the neuron through VGCCs or the NMDA receptor/ion channel. Activation of the $G\alpha_{q/11}$ protein-coupled mGluR1 glutamate receptor can also trigger 2-AG production. After retrograde diffusion through the synaptic cleft 2-AG activates the CB_1 receptor at the presynaptic axon terminal. The action of 2-AG is terminated by monoacylglycerol lipase (MAGL) localized at the presynaptic site (not shown).

The presynaptic CB_1 receptor can also be activated by endocannabinoids. Usually, an endocannabinoid is produced in the postsynaptic neuron, diffuses through the synaptic cleft to the presynaptic axon terminal, and activates the CB_1 receptor there (see Fig. 8.2). This endocannabinoid-mediated retrograde signaling operates in many brain regions (for reviews, see Castillo et al. 2012; Heifets and Castillo 2009; Kano et al. 2009; Lovinger 2008). The trigger for endocannabinoid production in the postsynaptic neuron is an increase in the intracellular calcium concentration or the activation of a $G\alpha_{q/11}$ protein-coupled receptor on the surface of the postsynaptic neuron (see Fig. 8.2). The endocannabinoid released from the postsynaptic neuron has been repeatedly identified as 2-arachidonoylglycerol (2-AG) (e.g., Szabo et al. 2006; Tanimura et al. 2010).

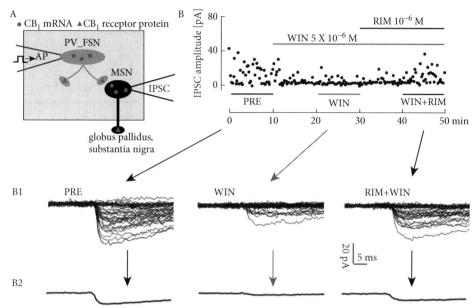

Fig. 8.3 Inhibition of synaptic transmission by the synthetic cannabinoid agonist WIN 55,212-2. The experiments that generated these data were performed on mouse brain slices containing the caudate-putamen (see Freiman et al. 2006). (A) CB_1 receptor mRNA and protein are localized in fast spiking neurons (FSNs) and medium spiny neurons (MSNs) of the caudate-putamen. The presynaptic FSN was depolarized via a patch-clamp pipette to elicit action potentials (APs). The resulting GABAergic inhibitory postsynaptic currents (IPSCs) were registered with a patch-clamp pipette in the postsynaptic MSN. (B) Course of the experiment: after the initial reference period (PRE) the synthetic CB_1/CB_2 agonist WIN 55,212-2 (WIN) was superfused, followed later by the CB_1 antagonist rimonabant (RIM). The points represent the amplitudes of the individual IPSCs. (B1) Individual synaptic events (IPSCs) during the three phases of the experiment. (B2) Averages of synaptic events during the three experimental phases. This experiment demonstrates a strong inhibition of FSN → MSN synaptic transmission by the synthetic cannabinoid receptor agonist. The antagonism by RIM verifies the involvement of CB_1 receptors.

8.4.2 Involvement of CB_2 receptors

Neuronal effects have been repeatedly observed in vivo which can be best explained by involvement of neuronal CB_2 receptors. For example, 2-AG inhibited emesis induced by morphine-6-glucuronide in a CB_2 receptor-dependent fashion (Van Sickle et al. 2005). Another example is that activation of CB_2 receptors leads to profound inhibition of mesolimbic dopaminergic neurons and interferes with the behavioral effects of cocaine (Xi et al. 2011). However, observations of CB_2 receptor-mediated effects on identified neurons are rare. It has been shown recently that activation of CB_2 receptors on pyramidal neurons of the prefrontal cortex leads to activation of calcium-dependent chloride channels (den Boon et al. 2012).

A role for natural CB_2 receptors in synaptic inhibition has not yet been demonstrated. In a recent study it was shown, however, that activation of CB_2 receptors artificially expressed in cultured mouse hippocampal neurons can lead to presynaptic inhibition of synaptic transmission which is very similar to the inhibition observed after activation of CB_1 receptors (Atwood et al. 2012).

8.5 **Effects of phytocannabinoids on synaptic transmission**

8.5.1 **Effects of Δ^9-THC**

8.5.1.1 Effects of Δ^9-THC in the central nervous system

Most observations were made in patch-clamp electrophysiological experiments (Table 8.1). In some studies, conclusions on synaptic transmission were drawn from observations of intracellular calcium changes. Data exist only on glutamatergic and GABAergic neurotransmission, probably because only neurotransmission by these two transmitters can be (easily) studied with electrophysiological techniques. When Δ^9-THC inhibited synaptic transmission, the involvement of CB_1 receptors was usually verified. When Δ^9-THC inhibited synaptic transmission, the basis for this was inhibition of transmitter release from the presynaptic axon terminal.

Surprisingly, the effects of Δ^9-THC have been studied only in hippocampal slices and in hippocampal neuronal cultures. Δ^9-THC inhibited glutamatergic synaptic transmission in some studies (Hoffman et al. 2010; Roloff and Thayer 2009; Shen and Thayer 1999). Remarkably, Δ^9-THC was found to be only a partial agonist, capable of antagonizing the effects of full agonists, like WIN 55,212-2 or 2-AG (Kelley and Thayer 2004; Roloff and Thayer 2009). 2-AG-mediated retrograde synaptic transmission was also antagonized by Δ^9-THC (Roloff and Thayer 2009). In cultured mouse hippocampal neurons, Δ^9-THC itself did not affect glutamatergic synaptic transmission at all but did prevent inhibition by the synthetic agonist WIN 55,212-2 (Straiker and Mackie 2005). In this latter study, Δ^9-THC also prevented endocannabinoid-mediated retrograde synaptic transmission. In an important study, the effects of Δ^9-THC were analyzed on cultured mouse hippocampal neurons transfected with the human CB_1 receptor (hCB_1) and its splice variants (hCB_{1a}, hCB_{1b}; Straiker et al. 2012). Δ^9-THC did not affect glutamatergic synaptic transmission in neurons transfected with hCB_1, hCB_{1a}, or hCB_{1b}.

The summary of these observations is that Δ^9-THC can inhibit glutamatergic synaptic transmission. However, Δ^9-THC is only a partial agonist, and so sometimes fails to activate the CB_1 receptor (especially the human CB_1 receptor). Due to its low intrinsic activity, Δ^9-THC can act as an antagonist. It is interesting in this respect that endocannabinoid-mediated synaptic plasticity processes can be antagonized by this phytocannabinoid, also in humans.

GABAergic synaptic transmission was inhibited by Δ^9-THC in mouse hippocampal slices (Laaris et al. 2010). The inhibition was presynaptic in nature, and Δ^9-THC behaved as a full agonist, producing an inhibition as strong as that produced by the synthetic agonist WIN 55,212-2.

As already indicated, Δ^9-THC appears to behave as a full CB_1 receptor agonist at GABAergic synapses but only as a partial CB_1 agonist at glutamatergic synapses. A similar difference between the efficacy or potency of Δ^9-THC was also observed in the case of synthetic CB_1 receptor agonists (Ohno-Shosaku et al. 2002). This difference is most probably due to the difference in the number of CB_1 receptors in the axon terminals: their density is high in the GABAergic terminals and much lower in the glutamatergic axon terminals.

8.5.1.2 Effects of Δ^9-THC in the peripheral nervous system

Neurotransmission between sympathetic or parasympathetic axons and innervated tissues has been most often studied by measuring electrically evoked contractions of the target tissues (Table 8.2). When Δ^9-THC inhibited neurotransmission, it was always shown that this inhibition was due to presynaptic inhibition. In a few cases, electrically evoked release of [^{3}H]norepinephrine was determined. When inhibition of neurotransmission by Δ^9-THC was observed, the involvement of CB_1 receptors was verified in most cases.

Table 8.1 Effects of phytocannabinoids on synaptic transmission in the central nervous system

Neurotransmitter	Species	Region	Method	Phytocannabinoid	Effect	Reference
Glutamate	Rat	Hippocampus (cell culture)	Electrophysiology (patch clamp); microfluorometry (Ca^{2+} spikes analyzed)	Δ^9-THC	Δ^9-THC inhibits transmission; Δ^9-THC is a partial agonist	Shen and Thayer 1999
Glutamate	Rat	Hippocampus (cell culture)	Microfluorometry (Ca^{2+} spikes analyzed)	Δ^9-THC	Δ^9-THC blocks the inhibition of transmission by 2-AG	Kelley and Thayer 2004
Glutamate	Rat	Hippocampus (cell culture)	Electrophysiology (patch clamp)	Δ^9-THC	Δ^9-THC inhibits EPSCs; Δ^9-THC blocks the inhibition of EPSCs by WIN 55,212-2; Δ^9-THC occludes DSE	Roloff and Thayer 2009
Glutamate	Rat/mouse	Hippocampus (brain slice)	Electrophysiology (patch clamp)	Δ^9-THC	Δ^9-THC inhibits fEPSPs/EPSCs (the degree of inhibition depends on the level of activation of A_1 adenosine receptors)	Hoffman et al. 2010
Glutamate	Mouse	Hippocampus (cell culture)	Electrophysiology (patch clamp); autaptic EPSCs	Δ^9-THC	Δ^9-THC does *not* inhibit EPSCs; Δ^9-THC blocks the inhibition of EPSCs by WIN 55,212-2; Δ^9-THC blocks DSE	Straiker and Mackie 2005
Glutamate	Mouse; expression of human cb_1 receptors (hcb_1, cb_{1a}, hcb_{1b})	Hippocampus (cell culture)	Electrophysiology (patch clamp); autaptic EPSCs	Δ^9-THC	Δ^9-THC does *not* affect EPSCs	Straiker et al. 2012

Table 8.1 (continued) Effects of phytocannabinoids on synaptic transmission in the central nervous system

Neurotransmitter	Species	Region	Method	Phytocannabinoid	Effect	Reference
Glutamate	Rat	Hippocampus (cell culture, brain slice)	Electrophysiology (patch clamp, fEPSPs)	Cannabidiol	Cannabidiol lowers the frequency of synaptically driven action potentials.Cannabidiol inhibits fEPSPs; CB_1 receptors and $5-HT_{1A}$ receptors are involved in these effects	Ledgerwood et al. 2011
Glutamate	Rat/mouse	Hippocampus (brain slice)	Electrophysiology (patch-clamp); microfluorometry	Cannabidiol	Cannabidiol antagonizes the GPR55-mediated effects of LPI and O-1602 (increase in mEPSC frequency and presynaptic axon terminal calcium concentration)	Sylantyev et al. 2013
GABA	Mouse	Hippocampus (brain slice)	Electrophysiology (patch clamp)	Δ^9-THC	Δ^9-THC inhibits IPSCs; Δ^9-THC is a full agonist	Laaris et al. 2010
GABA	Mouse	Cerebellum (brain slice)	Electrophysiology (patch clamp)	Δ^9-THCV	Δ^9-THCV increases mIPSC frequency	Ma et al. 2008

Abbreviations: 2-AG, 2-arachidonoylglycerol; Δ^9-THC, delta-9-tetrahydrocannabinol; Δ^9-THCV, delta-9-tetrahydrocannabivarin; EPSCs, excitatory postsynaptic currents; DSE, depolarization-induced suppression of excitation; fEPSPs, extracellular field excitatory postsynaptic potentials; GABA, gamma-aminobutyric acid; IPSCs, inhibitory postsynaptic currents; mIPSCs, miniature inhibitory postsynaptic currents.

Table 8.2 Effects of phytocannabinoids on neuroeffector transmission in the peripheral nervous system

Neurotransmitter	Species	Tissue	Phytocannabinoid	Measured parameter	Effect	Reference
Norepinephrine	Rat	Vas deferens, heart atrium	Δ^9-THC	Electrically evoked [^{3}H] norepinephrine release	Inhibition of transmission	Ishac et al. 1996
Norepinephrine, ATP	Rat	Vas deferens	Δ^9-THC	Electrically evoked [^{3}H] norepinephrine release	Inhibition of transmission	Graham et al. 1974
Norepinephrine, ATP	Mouse	Vas deferens	Δ^9-THC	Electrically evoked contraction	Inhibition of transmission	Pertwee et al. 1992a, 1993, 1995
Norepinephrine, ATP	Mouse	Vas deferens	Δ^9-THC	Electrically evoked contraction	Inhibition of transmission	Lay et al. 2000
Acetylcholine, ATP	Mouse	Urinary bladder	Δ^9-THC	Electrically evoked contraction	Inhibition of transmission	Pertwee and Fernando 1996
Acetylcholine	Rat	Ileum	Δ^9-THC	Electrically evoked contraction	Inhibition of transmission	Makwana et al. 2010
Acetylcholine	Guinea pig	Ileum	Δ^9-THC	Electrically evoked contraction	Inhibition of transmission	Pertwee et al. 1992a, 1996
CGRP	Rat	Mesenteric artery	Δ^9-THC	Electrically evoked relaxation	Inhibition of transmission (not CB_1/CB_2-mediated)	Duncan et al. 2004
Norepinephrine, ATP	Mouse	Vas deferens	Cannabidiol	Electrically evoked contraction	Antagonism of the effects of WIN 55,212-2 and CP55940 (not CB_1/CB_2-mediated)	Pertwee et al. 1992b
Norepinephrine, ATP	Mouse	Vas deferens	Δ^9-THCV	Electrically evoked contraction	Antagonism of CB_1-mediated inhibition of transmission	Thomas et al. 2005; Pertwee et al. 2007
Norepinephrine, ATP	Mouse	Vas deferens	Cannabigerol	Electrically evoked contraction	Inhibition of transmission (mediated by α_2-adrenoceptors)	Cascio et al. 2010

Abbreviations: CGRP, calcitonin gene-related peptide; Δ^9-THC, delta-9-tetrahydrocannabinol; Δ^9-THCV, delta-9-tetrahydrocannabivarin.

Δ^9-THC inhibited sympathetic neuroeffector transmission in the rat heart and vas deferens (Ishac et al. 1996). It was shown in many studies that Δ^9-THC inhibits contractions of the mouse vas deferens elicited by electrical stimulation of sympathetic axons (e.g., Pertwee et al. 1992a; 1995). Remarkably, in one study, Δ^9-THC did not affect responses elicited by sympathetic stimulation of the mouse heart atrium, rat heart atrium, rat mesenteric artery, or rat vas deferens (Lay et al. 2000).

Cholinergic neuroeffector transmission was inhibited by Δ^9-THC in the mouse urinary bladder and in the rat and guinea pig ileum (Makwana et al. 2010; Pertwee and Fernando 1996; Pertwee et al. 1992a, 1996).

Δ^9-THC suppressed the calcitonin gene-related peptide (CGRP)-mediated relaxation of mesenteric arteries elicited by electrical stimulation of sensory mesenteric axons (Duncan et al. 2004). However, this suppression was not prevented by CB_1 or CB_2 antagonists.

8.5.2 Effects of cannabidiol, Δ^9-THCV, and cannabigerol

8.5.2.1 Cannabidiol

In a recent study, Ledgerwood et al. (2011) showed that cannabidiol inhibits synaptic transmission between cultured hippocampal neurons and glutamatergic synaptic transmission in hippocampal slices. The inhibition was attenuated by CB_1 antagonists and was presynaptic in nature. These findings are remarkable in the light of observations that cannabidiol has only low affinity for CB_1 receptors in some studies (Thomas et al. 1998; Showalter et al. 1996) or behaves as a CB_1 antagonist in other studies (Thomas et al. 2004, 2007).

In the mouse vas deferens, cannabidiol antagonized suppression of the electrically evoked twitch response by the synthetic cannabinoids WIN 55,212-2 and CP-55940 (Pertwee et al. 1992b). CB_1 and CB_2 receptors were, however, not involved in this antagonism.

In 2007, Ryberg et al. reported that many cannabinoids possess affinity for GPR55. In that study it was also shown that cannabidiol is an antagonist at GPR55: it prevented G protein activation elicited by GPR55 agonists. In a more recent study it was shown that exogenous GPR55 agonists (O-1602 and lysophosphatidyl inositol) and an unidentified endogenous GPR55 agonist each enhance transmitter release from glutamatergic axons in rat hippocampal slices (Sylantyev et al. 2013). Cannabidiol acted as an antagonist of the synaptic stimulation elicited by the exogenous and the endogenous agonists.

8.5.2.2 Δ^9-THCV

In mouse cerebellar cortical brain slices Δ^9-THCV antagonized the inhibition of GABAergic synaptic transmission between interneurons and Purkinje cells elicited by the synthetic cannabinoid receptor agonist WIN 55,212-2 (Ma et al. 2008). Interestingly, Δ^9-THCV alone enhanced synaptic transmission between the interneurons and Purkinje cells (Ma et al. 2008): this may have been due either to antagonism of the effect of an endogenous cannabinoid or to inverse agonistic action at constitutively active CB_1 receptors. Although not yet shown, it is expected that Δ^9-THCV will share the ability of synthetic CB_1 receptor antagonists to prevent endocannabinoid-mediated retrograde signaling in the brain (see Fig. 8.2).

In the mouse vas deferens, synthetic cannabinoids and endocannabinoids inhibited the twitch response elicited by stimulation of sympathetic axons (Pertwee et al. 2007; Thomas et al. 2005). Δ^9-THCV prevented this inhibition by acting as a competitive CB_1 antagonist.

8.5.2.3 Cannabigerol

The phytocannabinoid cannabigerol inhibited electrically evoked twitch responses in the mouse vas deferens (Cascio et al. 2010). Surprisingly, this inhibition was antagonized by yohimbine, pointing to an involvement of α_2-adrenoceptors.

8.6 **Conclusions and future directions**

By acting on CB_1 receptors, the main psychoactive phytocannabinoid, Δ^9-THC, inhibits gluta-matergic and GABAergic synaptic transmission in the hippocampus and neuroeffector transmission mediated by norepinephrine, acetylcholine, and ATP in a series of peripheral tissues. The basis of this inhibition is inhibition of transmitter release from the presynaptic axon terminals. In some of the studies Δ^9-THC appeared to be a partial agonist.

Remarkably, the effects of Δ^9-THC have been studied only in the hippocampus and in peripheral tissues of animals: no observations on human tissues exist. Future research should demonstrate the effect of Δ^9-THC in additional central nervous system regions and, more importantly, in human central nervous and peripheral tissues.

Interference of Δ^9-THC with endocannabinoid-mediated retrograde signaling should be systemically studied: it is hypothesized that due to its low intrinsic activity, Δ^9-THC will attenuate retrograde signaling in many tissues and brain regions.

In future studies it should be clarified how Δ^9-THCV interferes with the function of CB_1 receptors in situ in tissues: Does it inhibit endocannabinoid-mediated retrograde signaling? Does it suppress constitutively active presynaptic receptors?

Phytocannabinoids possess affinity not only for CB_1 and CB_2 receptors, but also for many other receptors, ion channels, transporters, and enzymes. For example, at submicromolar concentrations, Δ^9-THC has affinity for GPR55, 5- hydroxytryptamine (5-HT)-$_{3A}$ receptors, transient receptor potential (TRP)-A1 receptors, TRPV2 receptors, adenosine transporters, monoamine transporters, and phospholipases (Pertwee and Cascio, Chapter 6, this volume). Likewise, Δ^9-THCV possesses affinity in the submicromolar range also for TRPM8 receptors (Pertwee and Cascio, Chapter 6, this volume). In this same concentration range, cannabidiol can target, in addition to CB_1 and CB_2 receptors, GPR55, 5-HT_{1A}-receptors, 5-HT_{3A}-receptors, TRPA1 receptors, TRPM8 receptors, TRPV4 receptors, and the CYP1A1 microsomal enzyme (Cascio and Pertwee, Chapter 7, this volume). No information is available on how these non-CB_1- and non-CB_2-mediated effects of the phytocannabinoids contribute to their effects on synaptic transmission. Research in the future should eliminate this deficit in knowledge.

References

Atwood, B.K., Straiker, A., and Mackie, K. (2012). CB_2 cannabinoid receptors inhibit synaptic transmission when expressed in cultured autaptic neurons. *Neuropharmacology*, **63**, 514–523.

Bacci, A., Huguenard, J.R., and Prince D.A. (2004). Long-lasting self-inhibition of neocortical interneurons mediated by endocannabinoids. *Nature*, **431**, 312–316.

Bayewitch, M., Rhee, M.-H., Avidor-Reiss, T., Breuer, A., Mechoulam, R., and Vogel, Z. (1996). (-)-Δ^9-Tetrahydrocannabinol antagonizes the peripheral cannabinoid receptor-mediated inhibition of adenylyl cyclase. *Journal of Biological Chemistry*, **271**, 9902–9905.

Blackmer, T., Larsen, E.C., Bartleson, C., *et al.* (2005). G protein βγ directly regulates SNARE protein fusion machinery for secretory granule exocytosis. *Nature Neuroscience*, **8**, 412–425.

Bolognini, D., Costa, B., Maione, S., *et al.* (2010). The plant cannabinoid Δ^9-tetrahydrocannabivarin can decrease signs of inflammation and inflammatory pain in mice. *British Journal of Pharmacology*, **160**, 677–687.

Breivogel, C.S., Walker, M.J., Huang, S.M., Roy, M.B., and Childers, S.R. (2004). Cannabinoid signaling in rat cerebellar granule cells: G-protein activation, inhibition of glutamate release and endogenous cannabinoids. *Neuropharmacology*, **47**, 81–91.

Brown, S.P., Safo, P.K., and Regehr, W.G. (2004). Endocannabinoids inhibit transmission at granule cell to Purkinje cell synapses by modulating three types of presynaptic calcium channels. *Journal of Neuroscience*, **24**, 5623–5631.

Brusco, A., Tagliaferro, P., Saez, T., and Onaivi, E.S. (2008). Postsynaptic localization of CB2 cannabinoid receptors in the rat hippocampus. *Synapse*, **62**, 944–949.

Calignano, A., Katona, I., Desarnaud, F., *et al.* (2000). Bidirectional control of airway responsiveness by endogenous cannabinoids. *Nature*, **408**, 96–101.

Cascio, M.G., Gauson, L.A., Stevenson, L.A., Ross, R.A., and Pertwee, R.G. (2010). Evidence that the plant cannabinoid cannabigerol is a highly potent α_2-adrenoceptor agonist and moderately potent 5HT1A receptor antagonist. *British Journal of Pharmacology*, **159**, 129–141.

Castillo, P.E., Younts, T.J., Chavez, A.E., and Hashimotodani, Y. (2012). Endocannabinoid signaling and synaptic function. *Neuron*, **76**, 70–81.

Cota, D., Marsicano, G., Tschop, M., *et al.* (2003). The endogenous cannabinoid system affects energy balance via central orexigenic drive and peripheral lipogenesis. *Journal of Clinical Investigation*, **112**, 423–431.

Cristino, L., De Petrocellis, L., Pryce, G., Baker, D., Guglielmotti, V., and Di Marzo, V. (2006). Immunohistochemical localization of cannabinoid type 1 and vanilloid transient receptor potential vanilloid type 1 receptors in the mouse brain. *Neuroscience*, **139**, 1405–1415.

Daniel, H., Rancillac, A., and Crepel, F. (2004). Mechanisms underlying cannabinoid inhibition of presynaptic Ca^{2+} influx at parallel fibre synapses of the rat cerebellum. *Journal of Physiology (London)*, **557**, 159–174.

Den Boon, F.S., Chameau, P., Schaafsma-Zhao, Q., *et al.* (2012). Excitability of prefrontal cortical pyramidal neurons is modulated by activation of intracellular type-2 cannabinoid receptors. *Proceedings of the National Academy of Sciences of the United States of America*, **109**, 3534–3539.

Dove Pettit, D.A., Harrison, M.P., Olson, J.M., Spencer, R.F., and Cabral, G.A. (1998). Immunohistochemical localization of the neural cannabinoid receptor in rat brain. *Journal of Neuroscience Research*, **51**, 391–402.

Duncan, M., Kendall, D.A., and Ralevic, V. (2004). Characterization of cannabinoid modulation of sensory neurotransmission in the rat isolated mesenteric arterial bed. *Journal of Pharmacology and Experimental Therapeutics*, **311**, 411–419.

Egertova, M., Cravatt, B.F., and Elphick, M.R. (2003). Comparative analysis of fatty acid amide hydrolase and CB1 cannabinoid receptor expression in the mouse brain: evidence of a widespread role for fatty acid amide hydrolase in regulation of endocannabinoid signaling. *Neuroscience*, **119**, 481–496.

Engler, B., Freiman, I., Urbanski, M., and Szabo, B. (2006). Effects of exogenous and endogenous cannabinoids on GABAergic neurotransmission between the caudate-putamen and the globus pallidus in the mouse. *Journal of Pharmacology and Experimental Therapeutics*, **316**, 608–617.

Freiman, I., Anton, A., Monyer, H., Urbanski, M.J. and Szabo, B. (2006). Analysis of the effects of cannabinoids on identified synaptic connections in the caudate-putamen by paired recordings in transgenic mice. *Journal of Physiology (London)*, **575**, 789–806.

Freiman, I. and Szabo, B. (2005). Cannabinoids depress excitatory neurotransmission between the subthalamic nucleus and the globus pallidus. *Neuroscience*, **133**, 305–313.

Freund, T.F., Katona, I., and Piomelli, D. (2003). Role of endogenous cannabinoids in synaptic signaling. *Physiological Reviews*, **83**, 1017–1066.

Galiègue, S., Mary, S., Marchand, J., *et al.* (1995). Expression of central and peripheral cannabinoid receptors in human immune tissues and leukocyte subpopulations. *European Journal of Biochemistry*, **232**, 54–61.

Gerard, C.M., Mollereau, C., Vassart, G., and Parmentier, M. (1991). Molecular cloning of a human cannabinoid receptor which is also expressed in testis. *Biochemical Journal*, **279**, 129–134.

Gong, J.-P., Onaivi, E.S., Ishiguro, H., *et al.* (2006). Cannabinoid CB_2 receptors: immunohistochemical localization in rat brain. *Brain Research* **1071**, 10–23.

Graham, J.D.P., Lewis, M.J., and Li, D.M.F. (1974). The effect of delta-1-tetrahydrocannabinol on the release of [3H]-(-)-noradrenaline from the isolated vas deferens of the rat. *British Journal of Pharmacology*, **52**, 223–236.

Heifets, B.D. and Castillo, P.E. (2009). Endocannabinoid signaling and long-term synaptic plasticity. *Annual Review of Physiology*, **71**, 283–306.

Herkenham, M., Lynn, A.B., De Costa, B.R., and Richfield, E.K. (1991a). Neuronal localization of cannabinoid receptors in the basal ganglia of the rat. *Brain Research*, **547**, 267–274.

Herkenham, M., Lynn, A.B., Johnson, R.M., Melvin, L.S., de Costa, B.R. and Rice, K.C. (1991b). Characterization and localization of cannabinoid receptors in rat brain: a quantitative in vitro autoradiographic study. *Journal of Neuroscience*, **11**, 563–583.

Hoffman, A.F., Laaris, N., Kawamura, M., Masino, S.A. and Lupica, C.R. (2010). Control of cannabinoid CB_1 receptor function on glutamate axon terminals by endogenous adenosine acting at A_1 receptors. *Journal of Neuroscience*, **30**, 545–555.

Hohmann, A.G. and Herkenham, M. (1999). Cannabinoid receptors undergo axonal flow in sensory nerves. *Neuroscience*, **92**, 1171–1175.

Ishac, E.J.N., Jiang, L., Lake, K.D., Varga, K., Abood, M.E., and Kunos, G. (1996). Inhibition of exocytotic noradrenaline release by presynaptic cannabinoid CB1 receptors on peripheral sympathetic nerves. *British Journal of Pharmacology*, **118**, 2023–2028.

Kano, M., Ohno-Shosaku, T., Hashimotodani, Y., Uchigashima, M., and Watanabe, M. (2009). Endocannabinoid-mediated control of synaptic transmission. *Physiological Reviews*, **89**, 309–380.

Katona, I., Sperlagh, B., Sik, A., *et al.* (1999). Presynaptically located CB_1 cannabinoid receptors regulate GABA release from axon terminals of specific hippocampal interneurons. *Journal of Neuroscience*, **19**, 4544–4558.

Kelley, B.G. and Thayer, S.A. (2004). Δ^9-Tetrahydrocannabinol antagonizes endocannabinoid modulation of synaptic transmission between hippocampal neurons in culture. *Neuropharmacology*, **46**, 709–715.

Kovacs, F.E., Illes, P., and Szabo, B. (2011). Purinergic receptor-mediated endocannabinoid production and retrograde synaptic signaling in the cerebellar cortex. *British Journal of Pharmacology*, **162**, 974–988.

Kushmerick, C., Price, G.D., Taschenberger, H., *et al.* (2004). Retroinhibition of presynaptic Ca^{2+} currents by endocannabinoids released via postsynaptic mGluR activation at a calyx synapse. *Journal of Neuroscience*, **24**, 5955–5965.

Laaris, N., Good, C.H., and Lupica, C.R. (2010). Δ^9-tetrahydrocannabinol is a full agonist at CB_1 receptors on GABA neuron axon terminals in the hippocampus. *Neuropharmacology*, **59**, 121–127.

Lanciego, J.L., Barroso-Chinea, P., Rico, A.J., *et al.* (2011). Expression of the mRNA coding the cannabinoid receptor 2 in the pallidal complex of *Macaca fascicularis*. *Journal of Psychopharmacology*, **25**, 97–104.

Lay, L., Angus, J.A., and Wright, C.E. (2000). Pharmacological characterization of cannabinoid CB_1 receptors in the rat and mouse. *European Journal of Pharmacology*, **391**, 151–161.

Ledgerwood, C.J., Greenwood, S.M., Brett, R.R., Pratt, J.A., and Bushell, T.J. (2011). Cannabidiol inhibits synaptic transmission in rat hippocampal cultures and slices via multiple receptor pathways. *British Journal of Pharmacology*, **162**, 286–294.

Leterrier, C., Laine, J., Darmon, M., Boudin, H., Rossier, J., and Lenkei, Z. (2006). Constitutive activation drives compartment-selective endocytosis and axonal targeting of type 1 cannabinoid receptors. *Journal of Neuroscience*, **26**, 3141–3153.

Lovinger, D.M. (2008). Presynaptic modulation by endocannabinoids. *Handbook of Experimental Pharmacology*, **184**, 435–477.

Ma, Y.-L., Weston, S., Whalley, B., and Stephens, G. (2008). The phytocannabinoid Δ^9-tetrahydrocannabivarin modulates inhibitory neurotransmission in the cerebellum. *British Journal of Pharmacology*, **154**, 204–215.

Mackie, K. (2005). Distribution of cannabinoid receptors in the central and peripheral nervous system. *Handbook of Experimental Pharmacology*, **168**, 299–325.

Makwana, R., Molleman, A., and Parsons, M.E. (2010). Evidence for both inverse agonism at the cannabinoid CB_1 receptor and the lack of an endogenous cannabinoid tone in the rat and guinea-pig isolated ileum myenteric plexus-longitudinal muscle preparation. *British Journal of Pharmacology*, **160**, 615–626.

Matsuda, L.A., Bonner, T.I., and Lolait, S.J. (1993). Localization of cannabinoid receptor mRNA in rat brain. *Journal of Comparative Neurology*, **327**, 535–550.

Mukhopadhyay, P., Batkai, S., Rajesh, M., *et al.* (2007). Pharmacological inhibition of CB_1 cannabinoid receptor protects against doxorubicin-induced cardiotoxicity. *Journal of the American College of Cardiologists*, **50**, 528–536.

Munro, S., Thomas, K.L., and Abu-Shaar, M. (1993). Molecular characterization of a peripheral receptor for cannabinoids. *Nature*, **365**, 61–65.

Nakatsuka, T., Chen, H.-X., Roper, S.N., and Gu, J.G. (2003). Cannabinoid receptor-1 activation suppresses inhibitory synaptic activity in human dentate gyrus. *Neuropharmacology*, **45**, 116–121.

Nyiri, G., Cserep, C., Szabadits, E., Mackie, K., and Freund, T.F. (2005). CB_1 cannabinoid receptors are enriched in the perisynaptic annulus and on preterminal segments of hippocampal GABAergic axons. *Neuroscience*, **136**, 811–822.

Ohno-Shosaku, T., Tsubokawa, H., Mizushima, I., Yoneda, N., Zimmer, A., and Kano, M. (2002). Presynaptic cannabinoid sensitivity is a major determinant of depolarization-induced retrograde suppression at hippocampal synapses. *Journal of Neuroscience*, **22**, 3864–3872.

Pazos, M.R., Tolon, R.M., Benito, C., *et al.* (2008). Cannabinoid CB_1 receptors are expressed by parietal cells of the human gastric mucosa. *Journal of Histochemistry and Cytochemistry*, **56**, 511–516.

Pertwee, R.G. and Fernando, S.R. (1996). Evidence for the presence of cannabinoid CB_1 receptors in mouse urinary bladder. *British Journal of Pharmacology*, **118**, 2053–2058.

Pertwee, R.G., Fernando, S.R., Nash, J.E., and Coutts, A.A. (1996). Further evidence for the presence of cannabinoid CB_1 receptors in guinea-pig small intestine. *British Journal of Pharmacology*, **118**, 2199–2205.

Pertwee, R., Griffin, G., Fernando, S., Li, X., Hill, A., and Makriyannis, A. (1995). AM630, a competitive cannabinoid receptor antagonist. *Life Sciences*, **56**, 1949–1955.

Pertwee, R.G., Ross, R.A., Craib, S.J., and Thomas, A. (2002). (-)-Cannabidiol antagonizes cannabinoid receptor agonists and noradrenaline in the mouse vas deferens. *European Journal of Pharmacology*, **456**, 99–106.

Pertwee, R.G., Stevenson, L.A., Elrick, D.B., Mechoulam, R., and Corbett, A.D. (1992a). Inhibitory effects of certain enantiomeric cannabinoids in the mouse vas deferens and the myenteric plexus preparation of guinea-pig small intestine. *British Journal of Pharmacology*, **105**, 980–984.

Pertwee, R.G., Stevenson, L.A., and Griffin, G. (1993). Cross-tolerance between delta-9-tetrahydrocannabinol and the cannabimimetic agents, CP 55,940, WIN 55,212-2 and anandamide. *British Journal of Pharmacology*, **110**, 1483–1490.

Pertwee, R.G., Thomas, A., Stevenson, L.A., *et al.* (2007). The psychoactive plant cannabinoid, Δ^9-tetrahydrocannabinol, is antagonized by Δ^8- and Δ^9-tetrahydrocannabivarin in mice in vivo. *British Journal of Pharmacology*, **150**, 586–594.

Rhee, M.-H., Vogel, Z., Barg, J., *et al.* (1997). Cannabinol derivatives: binding to cannabinoid receptors and inhibition of adenylylcyclase. *Journal of Medicinal Chemistry*, **40**, 3228–3233.

Roloff, A.M. and Thayer, S.A. (2009). Modulation of excitatory synaptic transmission by Δ^9-tetrahydrocannabinol switches from agonist to antagonist depending on firing rate. *Molecular Pharmacology*, **75**, 892–900.

Ryberg, E., Larsson, N., Sjögren, S., *et al.* (2007). The orphan receptor GPR55 is a novel cannabinoid receptor. *British Journal of Pharmacology*, **152**, 1092–1101.

Shen, M. and Thayer, S.A. (1998). Cannabinoid receptor agonists protect cultured rat hippocampal neurons from excitotoxicity. *Molecular Pharmacology*, **54**, 459–462.

Shen, M. and Thayer, S.A. (1999). Delta9-Tetrahydrocannabinol acts as a partial agonist to modulate gluta-matergic synaptic transmission between rat hippocampal neurons in culture. *Molecular Pharmacology*, **55**, 8–13.

Shire, D., Carillon, C., Kaghad, M., *et al.* (1995). An amino-terminal variant of the central cannabinoid receptor resulting from alternative splicing. *Journal of Biological Chemistry*, **270**, 3726–3731.

Showalter, V.M., Compton, D.R., Martin, B.R., and Abood, M.E. (1996). Evaluation of binding in a trans-fected cell line expressing a peripheral cannabinoid receptor (CB_2): Identification of cannabinoid recep-tor subtype selective ligands. *Journal of Pharmacology and Experimental Therapeutics*, **278**, 989–999.

Sibaev, A., Yüce, B., Kemmer, M., *et al.* (2009). Cannabinoid-1 (CB_1) receptors regulate colonic propulsion by acting at motor neurons within the ascending motor pathways in mouse colon. *American Journal of Physiology, Gastrointestinal and Liver Physiology*, **296**, G119–G128.

Sim, L.J., Hampson, R.E., Deadwyler, S.A., and Childers, S.R. (1996). Effects of chronic treatment with delta-9-tetrahydrocannabinol on cannabinoid-stimulated [35S]GTP-gamma-S autoradiography in rat brain. *Journal of Neuroscience*, **16**, 8057–8066.

Skaper, S.D., Buriani, A., Dal Toso, R., *et al.* (1996). The ALIAmide palmitoylethanolamide and cannabi-noids, but not anandamide, are protective in a delayed postglutamate paradigm of excitotoxic death of cerebellar granule neurons. *Proceedings of the National Academy of Sciences of the United States of America*, **93**, 3984–3989.

Ständer, S., Schmelz, M., Metze, D., Luger, T., and Rukwied, R. (2005). Distribution of cannabinoid receptor 1 (CB_1) and 2 (CB_2) on sensory nerve fibers and adnexal structures in human skin. *Journal of Dermatological Sciences*, **38**, 177–188.

Straiker A. and Mackie K. (2005). Depolarization-induced suppression of excitation in murine autaptic hippocampal neurones. *Journal of Physiology (London)*, **569**, 501–517.

Straiker, A., Wager-Miller, J., Hutchens, J., and Mackie, K. (2012). Differential signalling in human can-nabinoid CB_1 receptors and their splice variants in autaptic hippocampal neurones. *British Journal of Pharmacology*, **165**, 2660–2671.

Suarez, J., Bermudez-Silva, F., Mackie, K., *et al.* (2008). Immunohistochemical description of the endog-enous cannabinoid system in the rat cerebellum and functionally related nuclei. *Journal of Comparative Neurology*, **509**, 400–421.

Szabo, B. and Schlicker, E. (2005). Effects of cannabinoids on neurotransmission. *Handbook of Experimental Pharmacology*, **168**, 327–365.

Szabo, B., Than, M., Thorn, D., and Wallmichrath, I. (2004). Analysis of the effects of cannabinoids on synaptic transmission between basket and Purkinje cells in the cerebellar cortex of the rat. *Journal of Pharmacology and Experimental Therapeutics* **310**, 915–925.

Szabo, B., Urbanski, M.J., Bisogno, T., *et al.* (2006). Depolarization-induced retrograde synaptic inhibi-tion in the cerebellar cortex is mediated by 2-arachidonoylglycerol. *Journal of Physiology (London)*, **577**, 263–280.

Sylantyev, S., Jensena, T.P., Ross, R.A., and Rusakova, D.A. (2013). Cannabinoid- and lysophosphatidylinositol-sensitive receptor GPR55 boosts neurotransmitter release at central synapses. *Proceedings of the National Academy of Sciences of the United States of America*, **110**, 5193–5198.

Tanimura, A., Yamazaki, M., Hashimotodani, Y., *et al.* (2010). The endocannabinoid 2-arachidonoylglycerol produced by diacylglycerol lipase α mediates retrograde suppression of synaptic transmission. *Neuron*, **65**, 320–327.

Teixeira-Clerc, F., Julien, B., Grenard, P., *et al.* (2006). CB_1 cannabinoid receptor antagonism: a new strat-egy for the treatment of liver fibrosis. *Nature Medicine*, **12**, 671–675.

Thomas, A., Baillie, G.L., Phillips, A.M., Razdan, R.K., Ross, R.A., and Pertwee, R.G. (2007). Cannabidiol displays unexpectedly high potency as an antagonist of CB_1 and CB_2 receptor agonists in vitro. *British Journal of Pharmacology*, **150**, 613–623.

Thomas, A., Ross, R.A., Saha, B., Mahadevan, A., Razdan, R.K. and Pertwee, R.G. (2004). 6"-Azidohex-2"-yne-cannabidiol: a potential neutral, competitive cannabinoid CB_1 receptor antagonist. *European Journal of Pharmacology*, **487**, 213–221.

Thomas, A., Stevenson, L.A. and Wease, K.N., *et al.* (2005). Evidence that the plant cannabinoid Δ^9-tetrahydrocannabivarin is a cannabinoid CB_1 and CB_2 receptor antagonist. *British Journal of Pharmacology*, **146**, 917–926.

Thomas, B.F., Gilliam, A.F., Burch, D.F., Roch, e M.J., and Seltzman, H.H. (1998). Comparative receptor binding analyses of cannabinoid agonists and antagonists. *Journal of Pharmacology and Experimental Therapeutics*, **285**, 285–292.

Tsou, K., Brown, S., Sanudo-Pena, M.C., Mackie, K., and Walker, J.M. (1998). Immunohistochemical distribution of cannabinoid CB_1 receptors in the rat central nervous system. *Neuroscience*, **83**, 393–411.

Van Laere, K., Goffin, K., Casteels, C., *et al.* (2008). Gender-dependent increases with healthy aging of the human cerebral cannabinoid-type 1 receptor binding using [18F]MK-9470 PET. *Neuroimage*, **39**, 1533–1541.

Van Sickle, M.D., Duncan, M., and Kingsley, P.J., *et al.* (2005). Identification and functional characterization of brainstem cannabinoid CB_2 receptors. *Science*, **310**, 329–332.

Westlake, T.M., Howlett, A.C., Bonner, T.I., Matsuda, L.A., and Herkenham, M. (1994). Cannabinoid receptor binding and messenger RNA expression in human brain: an in vitro receptor autoradiography and in situ hybridization histochemistry study of normal aged and Alzheimer's brains. *Neuroscience*, **63**, 637–652.

Wotherspoon, G., Fox, A., McIntyre, P., Colley, S., Bevan, S., and Winter J. (2005). Peripheral nerve injury induces cannabinoid receptor 2 protein expression in rat sensory neurons. *Neuroscience*, **135**, 235–245.

Xi, Z.-X., Peng, X.-Q., Li, X., *et al.* (2011). Brain cannabinoid CB_2 receptors modulate cocaine´s actions in mice. *Nature Neuroscience*, **14**, 1160–1166.

Yoshida, T., Fukaya, M., Uchigashima, M., *et al.* (2006). Localization of diacylglycerol lipase-a around post-synaptic spine suggests close proximity between production site of an endocannabinoid, 2-arachidonoyl-glycerol, and presynaptic cannabinoid CB_1 receptor. *Journal of Neuroscience*, **26**, 4740–4751.

Chapter 9

Cannabinoids and Addiction

Eliot L. Gardner

9.1 Brain mechanisms and substrates of addiction

Over the past 60 years, many of the brain substrates, circuits, and mechanisms underlying addiction have been elucidated (Gardner 1999, 2000, 2005, 2011; Gardner and David 1999; Gardner and Wise 2009; O'Brien and Gardner 2005).

It is now well accepted that abusable drugs derive their addictive potential from activating the core pleasure/reward circuitry of the brain (Gardner 2005, 2011). That circuitry originates in the anterior bed nuclei of the medial forebrain bundle (MFB), descends caudally in a myelinated moderately fast-conducting pathway (of unknown neurotransmitter type) within the MFB to synapse on dopamine (DA) neurons within the ventral tegmental area (VTA) of the limbic midbrain. Axons from those VTA DA cell bodies ascend rostrally within the medial forebrain bundle to synapse within the nucleus accumbens (NAc) of the limbic forebrain. Collateral reward-encoding DA axons also ascend rostrally to innervate the olfactory tubercle and frontal cortex. From the NAc, additional reward-encoding neurons—using gamma-aminobutyric acid and endogenous opiate peptides as their neurotransmitter—project to the ventral pallidum (VP). Although this MFB–VTA–MFB–NAc–VP system is commonly spoken of as encoding reward, it is in truth very much more functionally complex and heterogeneous. This system also encodes degree of reward, reward anticipation, disconfirmation of reward expectancy, reward prediction error (e.g., Chang et al. 1994; Lee 1999; Peoples and Cavanaugh 2003; Peoples et al. 1999; Schulz 1994; Schulz et al. 1992, 1993) and very likely additional reward-related neural computations.

Given the centrality of drug-induced reward enhancement to the disease of addiction, a number of workers have postulated that—to a degree—addiction results from a basal reward-deficiency state which addictive drugs counteract, giving them much of their powerful motivational properties (e.g., Blum et al. 1996; Comings and Blum 2000; Gardner 1999; Koob 2013).

As the disease of addiction develops, drug-seeking and drug-taking become progressively less driven by drug-induced reward and drug-induced positive hedonic states, and progressively more driven by negative reinforcement. Such negative reinforcement can be based upon concurrent "opponent process" hedonic and motivational mechanisms (Gardner 2011; Koob and Wee 2010; Nazzaro et al. 1981) or upon rebound withdrawal dysphoria (Der-Avakian and Markou 2012; Epping-Jordan et al. 1998; Kenny et al. 2003; Kokkinidis and McCarter 1990; Koob 2009a, 2009b; Koob and Le Moal 2008) or both. The drug user then comes to use addictive drugs not to get "high" but rather to get "straight" (i.e., to push his/her chronically depressed subjective hedonic state back toward normal). Another neurobiological change occurs during the progression of the addictive process—drug-seeking and drug-taking behavior become less reward driven and more habit driven (Robbins and Everitt 2002), although "chasing the remembered 'high'" remains a powerful motivation (O'Brien and Gardner 2005). This progression from reward-driven drug-taking to habit-driven drug-taking corresponds to a progressive change in locus of control over behavior from the reward-encoding ventral striatal domains of the NAc to the habit-mediating neural circuitry of the dorsal neostriatum (Haber et al. 2000; Robbins and Everitt 2002).

Even in drug addicts or alcoholics who have succeeded in achieving long-term sobriety and abstinence, the control over such sobriety and abstinence often remains extremely fragile (Hubbard et al. 2003; Milkman et al. 1983–84; Milton and Everitt 2012). This fragility can last for decades, is associated with significant relapse to drug-seeking and drug-taking behavior, and is associated with increased mortality (Woody et al. 2007). It has been long understood, since the pioneering work done by Alcoholics Anonymous in the 1930s, that there are three principal triggers to relapse—re-exposure to addictive drug (and it needn't be the drug that the addict was formerly addicted to; so-called "cross-triggering" from one addictive drug to another is well-described), stress, and re-exposure to the environmental cues (sights, sounds, smells) that were previously associated with drinking or drugging. Using animals models of relapse to drug-seeking and drug-taking behavior (e.g., Cooper et al. 2007; Crombag et al. 2008; Epstein et al. 2006; Shaham et al. 2002), a great deal has been learned recently about the neural circuits, substrates, and mechanisms underlying relapse to drug-seeking and drug-taking behaviors (e.g., Bossert et al. 2005; Lê and Shaham 2002; Shalev et al. 2002; Vorel et al. 2001). Drug-triggered relapse appears to be mediated by the rostrally projecting mesolimbic DA fiber bundle within the MFB—which sends axonal projections not only to the NAc but also to the olfactory tubercle, amygdala, and frontal cortex. Stress-triggered relapse appears to involve two distinctly separate brain substrates. One is a neural circuit that arises in the central nucleus of the amygdala and projects axonal terminals into the bed nucleus of the stria terminalis; this system uses corticotrophin-releasing factor as its neurotransmitter. The other is a neural circuit that arises in lateral tegmental nucleus A2 in the brain stem and projects axonal terminals into the hypothalamus, bed nucleus of stria terminalis, NAc, and amygdala; this system uses norepinephrine as its neurotransmitter. Relapse triggered by environmental cues appears to involve two brain systems. One is a neural circuit that arises in the ventral subiculum of the hippocampus and projects axonal terminals into the VTA and thence secondarily to the NAc (Vorel et al. 2001). The other is a neural circuit that arises in the basolateral complex of the amygdala and projects to the NAc (Hayes et al. 2003). Both systems appear to use glutamate as their primary neurotransmitter.

9.2 **Common features of addictive drugs**

By reference to the *Chemical Abstracts* compound count of all known chemicals and all known chemical congeners, it appears that approximately 30 million chemicals are known to the human species. Approximately 100 of these have addictive potential (Gardner 2000, 2005, 2011). The question arises—what do these 100 compounds have in common that distinguishes them from the other 30 million? The answers are straightforward and instructive (Gardner 2000, 2005, 2011). First, addictive drugs activate the VTA–NAc DA neural axis that encodes reward and pleasure. Second, addictive drugs elevate NAc DA. Third, addictive drugs enhance electrical brain-stimulation reward (BSR) within the core VTA–NAc reward-encoding neural axis. Fourth, addictive drugs inhibit BSR upon drug withdrawal (this is considered to be an electrophysiological measure of withdrawal dysphoria; see, e.g., Kokkinidis and McCarter 1990). Fifth, addictive drugs produce conditioned place preferences (CPP). Sixth, addictive drugs are voluntarily (often avidly) systemically self-administered. Seventh, addictive drugs are voluntarily self-administered into the core VTA–NAc reward-encoding neural axis. Eighth, addictive drugs trigger relapse to previously-extinguished drug-seeking behavior.

9.3 **Cannabis and psychoactive phytocannabinoids**

The *Cannabis sativa* plant has been used by humans for thousands of years, for both recreational and medicinal use (Maldonado et al. 2011). There appear to be over 100 compounds—termed phytocannabinoids—in *C. sativa*, at least some of which are known to be pharmacologically active. Among these are Δ^9-tetrahydrocannabinol (THC), Δ^8-tetrahydrocannabinol, cannabidiol (CBD), and cannabinol (Pertwee 2005). Other phytocannabinoid derivatives of the cannabis plant include cannabichromene, cannabigerol, cannabicyclol, cannabitriol, cannabivarin, cannabidivarin, cannabinolic acid, and Δ^9-tetrahydrocannabivarin (Δ^9-THCV) (Elsohly and Slade 2005; Mechoulam et al. 1970; Turner et al. 1980). It is generally agreed that the principal psychoactive phytocannabinoid—having agonist actions—is THC (Gaoni and Mechoulam 1964).

9.4 **Addictive actions of Δ^9-tetrahydrocannabinol**

9.4.1 **Phytocannabinoid agonists activate the VTA–NAc core reward neural axis**

THC, the principal psychoactive constituent of marijuana and hashish, neurophysiologically activates the VTA–NAc core reward neural axis by enhancing VTA–NAc DA neuronal firing (e.g., French 1997; French et al. 1997). Cannabinoid activation of VTA–NAc DA neuronal firing appears to be mediated by action within the VTA. Single-neuron electrophysiological recording studies have shown that THC enhances neuronal firing rates in the VTA, both in intact animals (e.g., French et al. 1997; Gessa et al. 1998; Wu and French 2000) and in VTA-containing brain slices (e.g., Cheer et al. 2000). Crucially, cannabinoid agonist-induced enhancement of VTA–NAc DA neuronal firing is accompanied by increased DA neuronal burst-firing (e.g., Diana et al. 1998; French et al. 1997). This is important because DA neuronal burst-firing dramatically augments terminal axonal DA release (e.g., Gonon 1988). Equally important is the fact that cannabinoid agonist-enhanced DA neuronal firing is attenuated by cannabinoid receptor type 1 (CB_1) antagonism—implicating an endocannabinoid underlying mechanism. The straightforward interpretation of such findings is that cannabinoid agonist-induced enhancement of the VTA–NAc DA core reward- and addiction-related neural axis (which then produces enhanced extracellular NAc DA—see section 9.4.2) results from cannabinoid agonist-induced enhancement of DA neuronal firing and burst firing of VTA DA neurons. This action appears on the basis of best present evidence to be indirect (although see section 9.4.7).

9.4.2 **Phytocannabinoid agonists elevate NAc DA**

THC elevates NAc DA (Chen et al. 1990; Tanda et al. 1997). This NAc DA elevation is calcium dependent and naloxone blockable (Chen et al. 1990; Tanda et al. 1997). Importantly, this THC-induced NAc DA elevation is qualitatively indistinguishable from the NAc DA elevations produced by opioids (e.g., DiChiara and Imperato 1988), amphetamine (e.g., Carboni et al. 1989), cocaine (e.g., Carboni et al. 1989), ethanol (e.g., DiChiara and Imperato 1988), nicotine (DiChiara and Imperato 1988), barbiturates (e.g., DiChara and Imperato 1986), or addictive dissociative anesthetics such as phencyclidine (e.g., Carboni et al. 1989). These effects are tetrodotoxin sensitive (indicating that the DA is neuronal) and blocked by endocannabinoid CB_1 receptor antagonism (indicating mediation of these effects via a CB_1 receptor-linked neuronal cascade). Importantly, local intracerebral microinjections or microperfusions of THC elevate extracellular DA in the VTA–NAc reward-encoding neural axis, whether the THC is microinjected into the VTA or NAc (Chen et al. 1993).

9.4.3 **Phytocannabinoid agonists enhance electrical brain-stimulation reward in the VTA–MFB–NAc reward-encoding neural axis**

THC augments electrical BSR in the VTA–MFB–NAc reward-encoding neural axis (Lepore et al. 1996). It must be noted that this cannabinoid-enhancing effect on BSR is a left-shift in electrophysiological brain-reward functions, i.e., a reward-enhancing or euphorigenic effect. It should also be noted that the BSR-enhancing effect of THC is qualitatively indistinguishable from the BSR-enhancing effects of such addictive compounds as morphine (e.g., Tzschentke and Schmidt 2000), methamphetamine (Spiller et al. 2008), and cocaine (e.g., Tzschentke and Schmidt 2000).

9.4.4 **Phytocannabinoid agonist withdrawal inhibits electrical brain-stimulation reward in the VTA–MFB–NAc reward-encoding neural axis**

Withdrawal from THC administration inhibits (depresses) BSR in the VTA–MFB–NAc reward-encoding neural axis (Gardner and Vorel 1998). This inhibiting effect on BSR produced by THC withdrawal is a right-shift in electrophysiological brain-reward functions, i.e., a reward-inhibiting or dysphorigenic effect. It should also be noted that the inhibiting effect on BSR produced by THC withdrawal is qualitatively indistinguishable from the BSR-inhibiting effects produced by withdrawal from virtually all addictive compounds—including cocaine (e.g., Kokkinidis and McCarter 1990).

9.4.5 **Phytocannabinoid agonists induce conditioned place preference**

Conditioned place preference (CPP) is an animal behavioral paradigm that measures the ability of environmental contexts paired with addictive drug administration to evoke drug-seeking behavior in the absence of drug (see Tzschentke 1998, 2007). Thus, it is an animal model of both drug-induced reward and of incentive motivation to seek drug. It has therefore been commonly used as an animal model in addiction research (Gardner and Wise 2009). THC induces CPP (Lepore et al. 1995; Valjent and Maldonado 2000), which is qualitatively indistinguishable from the CPP produced by opioid agonists (e.g., Ashby et al. 2003), cocaine (e.g., Ashby et al. 2002), or nicotine (e.g., Horan et al. 2001; Pak et al. 2006). Importantly, THC microinfusions directly into the VTA–MFB–NAc reward-encoding neural axis also produce CPP (Zangen et al. 2006), and the CPP produced by such cannabinoid agonist microinfusions into the VTA–MFB–NAc neural axis is qualitatively indistinguishable from the CPP produced by VTA–MFB–NAc microinfusions of such addictive psychostimulants as amphetamine or cocaine (e.g., Liao et al. 2000).

9.4.6 **Phytocannabinoid agonists are self-administered in animal models of drug-taking behavior**

For many, the *sine qua non* of an addictive substance is whether or not it will sustain voluntary self-administration in animal models (see, e.g., Gardner and Wise 2009). For many years, voluntary self-administration of THC in animal models was elusive. However, this elusiveness has been definitively put to rest by the pioneering work of Goldberg and colleagues (e.g., Justinova et al. 2003) who have successively achieved, and replicated under exacting experimental conditions, voluntary THC self-administration in laboratory animals. Importantly, such THC self-administration is qualitatively indistinguishable from the intravenous self-administration that is supported by other addictive substances, such as cocaine (e.g., Xi et al. 2004). Importantly and compellingly too, THC is voluntarily micro-infused by laboratory animals into both the VTA and NAc loci of the VTA–MFB–NAc reward-encoding neural axis of the mesolimbic midbrain and forebrain (Zangen et al. 2006). Equally importantly and compellingly, such voluntary cannabinoid agonist self-administration directly into the VTA–MFB–NAc neural axis is qualitatively indistinguishable from the voluntary self-administration directly into the VTA–MFB–NAc neural axis supported by other addictive substances such as cocaine (e.g., Carlezon et al. 1995).

Thus, THC does not qualitatively differ to any significant degree from other addictive compounds in its ability to meet the earlier-noted cardinal characteristics of drugs possessing addictive potential.

9.4.7 Brain sites of pro-addiction phytocannabinoid action

The pro-addictive actions of phytocannabinoid CB_1 agonists have conventionally been viewed as being mediated within the VTA (see sections 9.4.5 and 9.4.6). However, as long ago as 1993, Chen and colleagues demonstrated (Chen et al. 1993) that THC activates brain substrates of addictive drug action at both the level of the VTA (nucleus of origin of the VTA–MFB–NAc DA addiction-related neural axis) and the level of the NAc (major terminal locus of the VTA–MFB–NAc DA addiction-related neural axis). Specifically, local microinjections of THC directly into the VTA enhance local VTA extracellular DA overflow while local microinjections of THC directly into the NAc enhance local NAc extracellular DA overflow, as measured by in vivo brain microdialysis (Chen et al. 1993). This suggestion of dual sites of action for cannabinoid-enhanced brain reward and reward-related behaviors has been more recently confirmed. Cannabinoid agonist-induced reward is activated by THC microinjections into either the VTA or NAc (Zangen et al. 2006).

9.5 Cannabis addiction at the human level

9.5.1 Cannabis self-administration at the human laboratory level

One of the major advances in addiction research in recent decades has been the emulation of animal models of addiction (see section 9.4) in human beings under controlled laboratory situations. There is a high degree of consistency between the drugs that are abused by humans and the drugs that nonhuman animals will self-administer, demonstrating that the mechanisms mediating drug reinforcement are largely conserved across species (Balster 1991; Brady et al. 1987; Lile and Nader 2003). However, many have argued that the leap from animal models to the human clinical situation—while obviously having face validity—is too broad to have adequate construct or predictive validity (e.g., Haney 2009). Therefore, cannabis self-administration has been carried out with humans in controlled laboratory settings starting several decades ago (e.g., Mendelson et al. 1976). Such studies have shown that marijuana is reinforcing. Active marijuana is self-administered significantly more than placebo marijuana (Chait and Zacny 1992; Haney et al. 1997; Mendelson and Mello 1984; Ward et al. 1997). Such cannabis self-administration is dose-dependent, i.e., marijuana smokers choose to smoke high-potency cigarettes over low-potency cigarettes (Chait and Burke 1994; Kelly et al. 1997). Furthermore, a distinct cannabis withdrawal syndrome—characterized by irritability, craving, and disrupted sleep and food intake—is observed upon cessation of marijuana or THC intake (Budney et al. 2004; Haney 2005; Kouri and Pope 2000). This withdrawal syndrome manifests itself after approximately 24 h of abstinence (Budney et al. 2004; Haney 2005) and lasts for several weeks (Kouri and Pope 2000). In the human laboratory setting, this withdrawal syndrome is rapidly alleviated by re-administration of marijuana or THC in double-blind fashion (Haney et al. 1999, 2004; Hart et al. 2002).

9.5.2 **Cannabis addiction at the human clinical level**

Cannabis is the most widely used illicit drug in the world (Anthony et al. 1994). Approximately 100 million Americans have used illicit marijuana, with approximately 8–10% developing cannabis dependence (Crean et al. 2011). In the US, approximately 25% of all high school seniors state that they have smoked marijuana within the last 30 days, with approximately 2–3 million new marijuana users every year, two-thirds of them being between the ages of 12 and 17 (Compton et al. 2004; ONDCP 2008; SAMHSA 2008). Furthermore, 16% of all substance abuse treatment admissions to hospital in the US are for cannabis-related disorders; second only to alcohol-related hospital admissions (Crean et al. 2011). In Canada, the prevalence of past-year cannabis use by youth was approximately 25% in 2010 (Health Canada 2012). In the UK, approximately one-third of all adults have tried marijuana, and 2.5 million (mostly 16–29-year-olds) have used it in the past year (Hoare 2009). In Australia, cannabis is the most widely used illicit substance (AIHW 2005).

The *Diagnostic and Statistical Manual of Mental Disorders*, Fourth Edition, Text Revision and the International Classification of Diseases, Tenth Revision both include a diagnostic category for cannabis addiction and dependence (Anthony et al. 1994; Cottler et al. 1995), and the Fifth Edition of the *Diagnostic and Statistical Manual of Mental Disorders* includes cannabis dependence as a medically recognized drug addiction syndrome.

The essential feature of addiction to a chemical substance is a cluster of cognitive, behavioral, and physiological symptoms—all centering around the fact that the addicted individual continues use of the substance despite significant harm to his/her health, lifestyle, work, and significant others (such as family members). Thus, a diagnosis of drug addiction is made if three or more of the following criteria occur at any time during the same 1-year period (American Psychiatric Association 1994): (1) tolerance, as defined by either a need for increased amounts of the substance to achieve intoxication or the desired effect, or a markedly diminished effect on the user with continued use of the substance; (2) withdrawal, as manifested by either characteristic withdrawal symptoms—"drug-opposite" to the effects produced by the dependence-producing drug (O'Brien 2001)—such as insomnia, drug craving, restlessness, loss of appetite, difficulty in concentration, sweating, mood swings, depression, irritability, anger, or hyperthermia; or the fact that the same or a chemically closely-related substance is taken to avoid or relieve withdrawal symptoms; (3) the substance is often taken in larger amounts or over a longer period of time than was originally intended; (4) there is persistent desire to reduce substance use, or unsuccessful attempts to do so; (5) considerable time and effort is spent obtaining the substance; (6) social, occupational, or recreational activities are given up or reduced because of use of the substance; (7) the substance is used despite knowledge of persistent or recurrent physical or psychological problems caused by the substance.

Clinically, drug addiction manifests as a syndrome of compulsive drug-seeking behavior characterized by: (1) impaired control over drug self-administration, (2) compulsive drug self-administration, (3) continued self-administration despite obvious harm to self and significant others, and (4) drug craving. Clinicians in addiction medicine often characterize drug addiction as "the disease with the 5 Cs": Chronic disease with impaired Control, Compulsive use, Continued use despite harm, and Craving for the drug(s) to which the individual has become addicted.

It is sometimes assumed that addictive drug-seeking and drug-taking are driven solely by the negative consequences of drug dependence, that is, by a desire to mitigate or avoid the unpleasant physical consequences of drug withdrawal (for review, see Gardner 2005). Indeed, avoidance of withdrawal symptoms can serve as a motivation for drug-taking in human addicts, and some addicts do worry about the onset of withdrawal symptoms. But the pursuit of the drug-induced "high" remains the goal. Congruently, addictive drug-seeking and drug-taking are now viewed as being closely linked to the appetitive properties of addictive drugs (for reviews, see Gardner 2000, 2005; O'Brien 2001). This view has been driven in large measure by the facts that: (1) drugs that are addictive at the human level are voluntarily self-administered by laboratory animals (Gardner 2000); (2) such self-administration can take place in the absence of tolerance, physical dependence, withdrawal, or previous drug-taking behavior (e.g., Ternes et al. 1984); (3) the reward produced by addictive drugs summates with the reward produced by electrical BSR, thus presumably activating the same neural substrates (Wise 1989, 1996); and (4) addictive drugs are voluntarily self-administered intracerebrally only into brain loci known to be associated with the brain's reward substrates (for reviews, see Gardner 2000, 2005; Wise and Gardner 2002). Thus, brain-reward mechanisms are currently considered to constitute the fundamental substrate upon which addictive drugs act to produce their reinforcing and incentive motivational effects (Wise 1996; Wise and Gardner 2002; Gardner 2005).

9.5.3 Can cannabis be considered to be an addictive substance at the human level?

It seems irrefutable that cannabis can be considered to be addictive at the human level. Winstock and colleagues have delineated some useful criteria for assessing cannabis addiction upon initial clinical interview (Winstock et al. 2010). First, does the patient use cannabis on a regular (daily, weekly) basis? Second, does the patient seek to reduce his/her cannabis use, but fail to achieve reduction in use? Third, is there evidence of physical dependence upon cannabis? Fourth, does the patient experience withdrawal symptoms upon cessation of cannabis use? Fifth, does the patient's cannabis use produce harm to himself/herself or others? Along somewhat similar lines, Budney has proffered a distinction between cannabis dependence and cannabis abuse (Budney 2006). Under the category of "dependence" come the following: (1) tolerance; (2) withdrawal; (3) using for a longer period of time or more than intended; (4) persistent desire or unsuccessful efforts to quit or cut down; (5) considerable time spent buying, using, or recovering from the effects; (6) important activities are given up because of use; (7) continued use despite persistent or recurrent psychological or physical problems related to use. Under the category of "abuse" come the following: (1) recurrent use resulting in failure to fulfill major role obligations; (2) recurrent use in situations that are physically hazardous; (3) recurrent legal problems related to use; (4) continued use despite persistent social or interpersonal problems related to use.

It seems fairly clear that most cannabis users do so for its euphoriant and relaxant effects (Bromberg 1934; Costa 2007; Grinspoon et al. 2005; Grotenhermen 2007; Winstock et al. 2010), as well as for additional effects such as enhanced sensory perception, distorted sense of time, and increased appetite (Winstock et al. 2010). It seems equally clear that tolerance develops to such effects with repeated cannabis use (Swift et al. 1998). A cannabis withdrawal syndrome has been well described (Budney and Hughes 2006; Budney et al. 2001, 2003), and is reported by up to one-third of heavy cannabis users and more than one-half of those seeking treatment for cannabis dependence (Budney and Hughes 2006). Compellingly, this withdrawal syndrome is rapidly alleviated by readministration of cannabis or THC in both human laboratory (Haney et al. 1999, 2004; Hart et al. 2002) and clinical (Budney et al. 1999, 2007; Stephens et al. 1993; 2000) settings. Understandably, the cannabis withdrawal syndrome can serve as a negative reinforcer for relapse to cannabis use among cannabis users attempting to maintain abstinence (Budney and Hughes 2006; Copersino et al. 2006).

Under the category of continued use despite harm to self and/or others, it now seems clear that dependent cannabis use fits this criterion of addiction also. Impaired attention and memory have been reported to be hallmarks of cannabis use (Ranganathan and D'Souza 2006), as has severe motor incoordination (Li et al. 2012; Papafotiou et al. 2005). Additional probable harmful effects associated with chronic cannabis use include cognitive deficits (decision-making, planning, concept formation, organization and processing of complex information), pulmonary disease, oropharyngeal and lung cancers, and decreased female fertility (Crean et al. 2011; Lundqvist 2005; Winstock et al. 2010). Cannabis dependence in adolescence appears to be especially harmful, being associated with codependence upon alcohol and other addictive substances, poor academic and educational achievement, truancy, delinquency, criminal behavior, unemployment, poor interpersonal relationships, and exacerbation of anxiety, depression, and schizophrenia (Sofuoglu et al. 2010; Winstock et al. 2010). Chronic cannabis use is associated with twice the normal risk of schizophrenia, with evidence that starting cannabis use before age 16 substantially increases the risk (Moore et al. 2007).

9.6 Two additional interesting phytocannabinoids with possible relevance for addiction

9.6.1 Cannabidiol

CBD is abundantly present in cannabis (Mechoulam et al. 2007; Pertwee 2004; Russo 2011) and displays the interesting property of antagonizing CB_1 receptors at low nanomolar concentrations in the presence of THC, despite having little binding affinity at that site (Pertwee 2008; Russo 2011; Thomas et al. 2007). A number of laboratories have reported that pharmacological blockade or genetic deletion of the CB_1 receptor in laboratory rodents markedly attenuates the actions of addictive drugs (e.g., heroin, cocaine) in several animal models of drug addiction—including electrical brain-stimulation reward, enhanced nucleus accumbens dopamine, intravenous drug self-administration, and reinstatement of drug-seeking behavior after behavioral extinction of the drug self-administration habit (e.g., De Vries et al. 2001; Fattore et al. 2005; Li et al. 2009; Xi et al. 2006, 2008). This raises the question—might CBD show anti-addiction properties? Two preliminary pieces of evidence suggest that this might be so. Ren et al. (2009) found that, in laboratory rats, CBD significantly attenuates heroin-seeking behavior reinstated by exposure to a conditioned environmental cue previously uniquely associated with heroin-taking behavior. This effect was exceedingly prolonged—still present 2 weeks after acute CBD administration. In addition, CBD normalized the abnormal CB_1 receptor expression observed in the NAc associated with stimulus cue-induced relapse to heroin-seeking behavior. On the other hand, CBD did not alter stable heroin self-administration, extinction responding after replacement of heroin by saline, or heroin-primed reinstatement of heroin-seeking behavior. In humans, Morgan et al. (2010) found that CBD attenuates the appetitive effects of THC in smoked cannabis.

9.6.2 THCV

While CB_1 receptor *antagonists* may possess anti-addiction efficacy (see earlier sections), CB_2 receptor *agonists* may possess similar properties (Xi et al. 2011). Both Δ^9- and Δ^8-THCV appear to have antagonist action at the CB_1 receptor and agonist action at the CB_2 receptor (Bátkai et al. 2012; Pertwee et al. 2007). Given these effects of Δ^9- and Δ^8-THCV at CB_1 and at CB_2 receptors, the possibility arises that these cannabinoids could show anti-addiction effects in standard models of addiction. Future experiments may yield an answer.

9.7 **Concluding remarks**

On the basis of evidence at the animal laboratory, human laboratory, and human clinical levels, it appears that cannabis use carries with it the risk of cannabis addiction. At all three levels, cannabis addiction appears to fit the criteria for addiction established for such other addictive substances as alcohol, nicotine, opioids, and psychostimulants. The rate of cannabis addiction appears to be low—in the range of 8–10% of users (Wagner and Anthony 2002; Winstock et al. 2010). Two interesting phytocannabinoids—CBD and THCV—may possess anti-addiction efficacy.

Disclosure statement

Author's contribution to the Work was done as part of the Author's official duties as an NIH employee and is a Work of the United States Government. Therefore, copyright may not be established in the United States. Apart from his salary from the National Institute on Drug Abuse, the author receives no funding from any source that could be construed as constituting a conflict of interest.

References

AIHW (Australian Institute of Health and Welfare). (2005). *2004 National Drug Strategy Household Survey: First Results* (AIHW Cat. No. PHE 57; Drug Statistics Series No. 13). Canberra: Australian Institute of Health and Welfare.

American Psychiatric Association. (1994). *Diagnostic and Statistical Manual of Mental Disorders.* 4th ed. Washington, DC: American Psychiatric Association.

Anthony, J., Warner, L. and Kessler, R. (1994). Comparative epidemiology of dependence on tobacco, alcohol, controlled substances, and inhalants: basic findings from the National Comorbity Survey. *Experimental and Clinical Psychopharmacology*, **2**, 244–268.

Ashby, C.R. Jr., Paul, M., Gardner, E.L., *et al.* (2002). Systemic administration of 1R,4S-4-amino-cyclopent-2-ene-carboxylic acid, a reversible inhibitor of GABA transaminase, blocks expression of conditioned place preference to cocaine and nicotine in rats. *Synapse*, **44**, 61–63.

Ashby, C.R. Jr., Paul, M., Gardner, E.L., Heidbreder, C.A., and Hagan, J.J. (2003). Acute administration of the selective D3 receptor antagonist SB-277011A blocks the acquisition and expression of the conditioned place preference response to heroin in male rats. *Synapse*, **48**, 154–156.

Balster, R.L. (1991). Drug abuse potential evaluation in animals. *British Journal on Addictions*, **86**, 1549–1558.

Bátkai, S., Mukhopadhyay, P., Horváth, B., *et al.* (2012). Δ^8-Tetrahydrocannabivarin prevents hepatic ischaemia/reperfusion injury by decreasing oxidative stress and inflammatory responses through cannabinoid CB_2 receptors. *British Journal of Pharmacology*, **165**, 2450–2461.

Blum, K., Sheridan, P.J., Wood, R.C., *et al.* (1996). The D2 dopamine receptor gene as a determinant of reward deficiency syndrome. *Journal of the Royal Society of Medicine*, **89**, 396–400.

Bossert, J.M., Ghitza, U.E., Lu, L., Epstein, D.H., and Shaham, Y. (2005). Neurobiology of relapse to heroin and cocaine seeking: an update and clinical implications. *European Journal of Pharmacology*, **526**, 36–50.

Brady, J.V., Griffiths, R.R., Hienz, R.D., Ator, N.A., Lukas, S.E., and Lamb, R.J. (1987). Assessing drugs for abuse liability and dependence potential in laboratory primates. In: M.A. Bozarth (ed.). *Methods of Assessing the Reinforcing Properties of Abused Drugs*. New York: Springer Verlag, pp. 45–86.

Bromberg, W. (1934). Marihuana intoxication: a clinical study of *Cannabis sativa* intoxication. *American Journal of Psychiatry*, **91**, 303–330.

Budney, A.J. (2006). Are specific dependence criteria necessary for different substances: how can research on cannabis inform this issue? *Addiction*, **101**(Suppl. 1), 125–133.

Budney, A.J. and Hughes, J.R. (2006). The cannabis withdrawal syndrome. *Current Opinion in Psychiatry*, **19**, 233–238.

Budney, A.J., Hughes, J.R., Moore, B.A., and Novy, P.L. (2001). Marijuana abstinence effects in marijuana smokers maintained in their home environment. *Archives of General Psychiatry*, **58**, 917–924.

Budney, A.J., Hughes, J.R., Moore, B.A., and Vandrey, R. (2004). Review of the validity and significance of cannabis withdrawal syndrome. *American Journal of Psychiatry*, **161**, 1967–1977.

Budney, A.J., Moore, B.A., Vandrey, R.G., and Hughes, J.R. (2003). The time course and significance of cannabis withdrawal. *Journal of Abnormal Psychology*, **112**, 393–402.

Budney, A.J., Novy, P.L., and Hughes, J.R. (1999). Marijuana withdrawal among adults seeking treatment for marijuana dependence. *Addiction*, **94**, 1311–1321.

Budney, A.J., Vandrey, R.G., Hughes, J.R., Moore, B.A., and Bahrenburg, B. (2007). Oral delta-9-tetrahydrocannabinol suppresses cannabis withdrawal symptoms. *Drug and Alcohol Dependence*, **86**, 22–29.

Carboni, E., Imperato, A., Perezzani, L., and Di Chiara, G. (1989). Amphetamine, cocaine, phencyclidine and nomifensine increase extracellular dopamine concentrations preferentially in the nucleus accumbens of freely moving rats. *Neuroscience*, **28**, 653–661.

Carlezon, W.A. Jr., Devine, D.P., and Wise, R.A. (1995). Habit-forming actions of nomifensine in nucleus accumbens. *Psychopharmacology*, **122**, 194–197.

Chait, L.D. and Burke, K.A. (1994). Preference for high- versus low-potency marijuana. *Pharmacology Biochemistry and Behavior*, **49**, 643–647.

Chait, L.D. and Zacny, J.P. (1992). Reinforcing and subjective effects of oral Δ^9-THC and smoked marijuana in humans. *Psychopharmacology*, **107**, 255–262.

Chang, J.-Y., Sawyer, S.F., Lee, R.-S., and Woodward, D.J. (1994). Electrophysiological and pharmacological evidence for the role of the nucleus accumbens in cocaine self-administration in freely moving rats. *Journal of Neuroscience*, **14**, 1224–1244.

Cheer, J.F., Marsden, C.A., Kendall, D.A., and Mason, R. (2000). Lack of response suppression follows repeated ventral tegmental cannabinoid administration: an *in vitro* electrophysiological study. *Neuroscience*, **99**, 661–667.

Chen, J., Paredes, W., Li, J., Smith, D., Lowinson, J., and Gardner, E.L. (1990). Δ^9-tetrahydrocannabinol produces naloxone-blockable enhancement of presynaptic basal dopamine efflux in nucleus accumbens of conscious, freely-moving rats as measured by intracerebral microdialysis. *Psychopharmacology*, **102**, 156–162.

Chen, J., Marmur, R., Pulles, A., Paredes, W., and Gardner, E.L. (1993). Ventral tegmental microinjection of Δ^9-tetrahydrocannabinol enhances ventral tegmental somatodendritic dopamine levels but not forebrain dopamine levels: evidence for local neural action by marijuana's psychoactive ingredient. *Brain Research*, **621**, 65–70.

Comings, D.E. and Blum, K. (2000). Reward deficiency syndrome: genetic aspects of behavioral disorders. *Progress in Brain Research*, **126**, 325–341.

Compton, W.M., Grant, B.F., Colliver, J.D., Glantz, M.D., and Stinson, F.S. (2004). Prevalence of marijuana use disorders in the United States: 1991-1992 and 2001-2002. *JAMA*, **291**, 2114–2121.

Cooper, A., Barnea-Ygael, N., Levy, D., Shaham, Y., and Zangen, A. (2007). A conflict rat model of cue-induced relapse to cocaine seeking. *Psychopharmacology*, **194**, 117–125.

Copersino, M.L., Boyd, S.J., Tashkin, D.P., *et al.* (2006). Cannabis withdrawal among non-treatment-seeking adult cannabis users. *American Journal on Addictions*, **15**, 8–14.

Costa, B. (2007). On the pharmacological properties of Δ^9-tetrahydrocannabinol (THC). *Chemistry and Biodiversity*, **4**, 1664–1677.

Cottler, L.B., Schuckit, M.A., Helzer, J.E., *et al.* (1995). The DSM-IV field trial for substance use disorders: major results. *Drug and Alcohol Dependence*, **38**, 59–69.

Crean, R.D., Crane, N.A., and Mason, B.J. (2011). An evidence-based review of acute and long-term effects of cannabis use on executive cognitive functions. *Journal of Addiction Medicine*, **5**, 1–8.

Crombag, H.S., Bossert, J.M., Koya, E., and Shaham, Y. (2008). Context-induced relapse to drug seeking: a review. *Philosophical Transactions of the Royal Society. Series B, Biological Sciences*, **363**, 3233–3243.

Der-Avakian, A. and Markou, A. (2012). The neurobiology of anhedonia and other reward-related deficits. *Trends in Neurosciences*, **35**, 68–77.

De Vries, T.J., Shaham, Y., Homberg, J.R., *et al.* (2001). A cannabinoid mechanism in relapse to cocaine seeking. *Nature Medicine*, **7**, 1151–1154.

Diana, M., Melis, M., and Gessa, G.L. (1998). Increase in meso-prefrontal dopaminergic activity after stimulation of CB1 receptors by cannabinoids. *European Journal of Neuroscience*, **10**, 2825–2830.

Di Chiara, G. and Imperato, A. (1986). Preferential stimulation of dopamine release in the nucleus accumbens by opiates, alcohol, and barbiturates: studies with transcerebral dialysis in freely moving rats. *Annals of the New York Academy of Sciences*, **473**, 367–381.

Di Chiara, G. and Imperato, A. (1988). Drugs abused by humans preferentially increase synaptic dopamine concentrations in the mesolimbic system of freely moving rats. *Proceedings of the National Academy of Sciences of the United States of America*, **85**, 5274–5278.

Elsohly, M.A. and Slade, D. (2005). Chemical constituents of marijuana: the complex mixture of natural cannabinoids. *Life Sciences*, **78**, 539–548.

Epping-Jordan, M.P., Watkins, S.S., Koob, G.F., and Markou, A. (1998). Dramatic decreases in brain reward function during nicotine withdrawal. *Nature*, **393**, 76–79.

Epstein, D.H., Preston, K.L., Stewart, J., and Shaham, Y. (2006). Toward a model of drug relapse: an assessment of the validity of the reinstatement procedure. *Psychopharmacology*, **189**, 1–16.

Fattore, L., Spano, S., Cossu, G., Deiana, S., Fadda, P., and Fratta, W. (2005). Cannabinoid CB_1 antagonist SR 141716A attenuates reinstatement of heroin self-administration in heroin-abstinent rats. *Neuropharmacology*, **48**, 1097–1104.

French, E.D. (1997). Δ^9-Tetrahydrocannabinol excites rat VTA dopamine neurons through activation of cannabinoid CB_1 but not opioid receptors. *Neuroscience Letters*, **226**, 159–162.

French, E.D., Dillon, K., and Wu, X. (1997). Cannabinoids excite dopamine neurons in the ventral tegmentum and substantia nigra. *Neuroreport*, **8**, 649–652.

Gaoni, Y. and Mechoulam, R. (1964). Isolation, structure and partial synthesis of an active constituent of hashish. *Journal of the American Chemical Society*, **86**, 1646–1647.

Gardner, E.L. (1999). Neurobiology and genetics of addiction: implications of "reward deficiency syndrome" for therapeutic strategies in chemical dependency. In: J. Elster (ed.), *Addiction: Entries and Exits*. New York: Russell Sage Foundation, pp. 57–119.

Gardner, E.L. (2000). What we have learned about addiction from animal models of drug self-administration. *American Journal on Addictions*, **9**, 285–313.

Gardner, E.L. (2005). Brain reward mechanisms. In: J.H. Lowinson, P. Ruiz, R.B. Millman, and J.G. Langrod (eds.). *Substance Abuse: A Comprehensive Textbook*. 4th ed. Philadelphia, PA: Lippincott Williams & Wilkins, pp. 48–97.

Gardner, E.L. (2011). Addiction and brain reward and anti-reward pathways. *Advances in Psychosomatic Medicine*, **30**, 22–60.

Gardner, E.L. and David, J. (1999). The neurobiology of chemical addiction. In: J. Elster, and O.-J. Skog (eds.). *Getting Hooked: Rationality and Addiction*. Cambridge: Cambridge University Press, pp. 93–136.

Gardner, E.L. and Vorel, S.R. (1998). Cannabinoid transmission and reward-related events. *Neurobiology of Disease*, **5**, 502–533.

Gardner, E.L. and Wise, R.A. (2009). Animal models of addiction. In: D.S. Charney, and E.J. Nestler (eds.). *Neurobiology of Mental Illness*. 3rd ed. Oxford: Oxford University Press, pp. 757–774.

Gonon, F.G. (1988). Nonlinear relationship between impulse flow and dopamine released by rat midbrain dopaminergic neurons as studied by in vivo electrochemistry. *Neuroscience*, **24**, 19–28.

Grinspoon, L., Bakalar, J.B. and Russo, E. (2005). Marijuana: clinical aspects. In: J.H. Lowinson, P. Ruiz, R.B. Millman, and J.G. Langrod (eds.). *Substance Abuse: A Comprehensive Textbook*. 4th ed. Philadelphia, PA: Lippincott Williams & Wilkins, pp. 263–276.

Grotenhermen, F. (2007). The toxicology of cannabis and cannabis prohibition. *Chemistry and Biodiversity*, **4**, 1744–1769.

Haber, S.N., Fudge, J.L., and McFarland, N.R. (2000). Striatonigrostriatal pathways in primates form an ascending spiral from the shell to the dorsolateral striatum. *Journal of Neuroscience*, **20**, 2369–2382.

Haney, M. (2005). The marijuana withdrawal syndrome: diagnosis and treatment. *Current Psychiatry Reports*, **7**, 360–366.

Haney, M. (2009). Self-administration of cocaine, cannabis and heroin in the human laboratory: benefits and pitfalls. *Addiction Biology*, **14**, 9–21.

Haney, M., Comer, S.D., Ward, A.S., Foltin, R.W., and Fischman, M.W. (1997). Factors influencing marijuana self-administration by humans. *Behavioural Pharmacology*, **8**, 101–112.

Haney, M., Ward, A.S., Comer, S.D., Foltin, R.W., and Fischman, M.W. (1999). Abstinence symptoms following smoked marijuana in humans. *Psychopharmacology*, **4**, 395–404.

Haney, M., Hart, C.L., Vosburg, S.K., *et al.* (2004). Marijuana withdrawal in humans: effects of oral THC or divalproex. *Neuropsychopharmacology*, **29**, 158–170.

Hart, C., Ward, A.S., Haney, M., Comer, S.C., Foltin, R.W., and Fischman, M.W. (2002). Comparison of smoked marijuana and oral Δ^9-tetrahydrocannabinol in humans. *Psychopharmacology*, **154**, 407–415.

Hayes, R.J., Vorel, S.R., Spector, J., Liu, X., and Gardner, E.L. (2003). Electrical and chemical stimulation of the basolateral complex of the amygdala reinstates cocaine-seeking behavior in the rat. *Psychopharmacology*, **168**, 75–83.

Health Canada (2012). *Canadian Alcohol and Drug Use Monitoring Survey, Summary of Results For 2010.* Ottawa, Ontario: Office of Drugs and Alcohol Research and Surveillance, Controlled Substances and Tobacco Directorate, Health Canada.

Hoare, J. (2009). *Drug Misuse Declared: Findings from the 2008/09 British Crime Survey.* London: Home Office.

Horan, B., Gardner, E.L., Dewey, S.L., Brodie, J.D., and Ashby, C.R. Jr. (2001). The selective σ1 receptor agonist, 1-(3,4-dimethoxyphenethyl)-4-(phenylpropyl)piperazine (SA4503), blocks the acquisition of the conditioned place preference response to (-)-nicotine in rats. *European Journal of Pharmacology*, **426**, R1–R2.

Hubbard, R.L., Craddock, S.G., and Anderson, J. (2003). Overview of 5-year follow-up outcomes in the Drug Abuse Treatment Outcome Study (DATOS). *Journal of Substance Abuse Treatment*, **25**, 125–134.

Justinova, Z., Tanda, G., Redhi, G.H., and Goldberg, S.R. (2003). Self-administration of Δ^9-tetrahydrocannabinol (THC) by drug naive squirrel monkeys. *Psychopharmacology*, **169**, 135–140.

Kelly, T.H., Foltin, R.W., Emurian, C.S., and Fischman, M.W. (1997). Are choice and self-administration of marijuana related to Δ^9-THC content? *Experimental and Clinical Psychopharmacology*, **5**, 74–82.

Kenny, P.J., Polis, I., Koob, G.F., and Markou, A. (2003). Low dose cocaine self-administration transiently increases but high dose cocaine persistently decreases brain reward function in rats. *European Journal of Neuroscience*, **17**, 191–195.

Kokkinidis, L. and McCarter, B.D. (1990). Postcocaine depression and sensitization of brain-stimulation reward: analysis of reinforcement and performance effects. *Pharmacology Biochemistry and Behavior*, **36**, 463–471.

Koob, G.F. (2009a). Dynamics of neuronal circuits in addiction: reward, antireward, and emotional memory. *Pharmacopsychiatry*, **42**(Suppl. 1), S32–S41.

Koob, G.F. (2009b). Neurobiological substrates for the dark side of compulsivity in addiction. *Neuropharmacology*, **56**(Suppl. 1), 18–31.

Koob, G.F. (2013). Theoretical frameworks and mechanistic aspects of alcohol addiction: alcohol addiction as a reward deficit disorder. *Current Topics in Behavioral Neuroscience*, **13**, 3–30.

Koob, G.F. and Le Moal, M. (2008). Neurobiological mechanisms for opponent motivational processes in addiction. *Philosophical Transactions of the Royal Society. Series B, Biological Sciences*, **363**, 3113–3123.

Koob, G.F. and Wee, S. (2010). The role of the dynorphin-kappa opioid system in the reinforcing effects of drugs of abuse. *Psychopharmacology*, **210**, 121–135.

Kouri, E.M. and Pope, H.G. Jr. (2000). Abstinence symptoms during withdrawal from chronic marijuana use. *Experimental and Clinical Psychopharmacology*, **8**, 483–492.

Lê, A. and Shaham, Y. (2002). Neurobiology of relapse to alcohol in rats. *Pharmacology and Therapeutics*, **94**, 137–156.

Lee, R.-S., Criado, J.R., Koob, G.F., and Henriksen, S.J. (1999). Cellular responses of nucleus accumbens neurons to opiate-seeking behavior: I. sustained responding during heroin self-administration. *Synapse*, **33**, 49–58.

Lepore, M., Vorel, S.R., Lowinson, J., and Gardner, E.L. (1995). Conditioned place preference induced by Δ^9-tetrahydrocannabinol: comparison with cocaine, morphine, and food reward. *Life Sciences*, **56**, 2073–2080.

Lepore, M., Liu, X., Savage, V., Matalon, D., and Gardner, E.L. (1996). Genetic differences in Δ^9-tetrahydrocannabinol-induced facilitation of brain stimulation reward as measured by a rate-frequency curve-shift electrical brain stimulation paradigm in three different rat strains. *Life Sciences [Pharmacology Letters]*, **58**, PL365–PL372.

Li, M.-C., Brady, J.E., DiMaggio, C.J., Lusardi, A.R., Tzong, K.Y., and Li, G. (2012). Marijuana use and motor vehicle crashes. *Epidemiologic Reviews*, **34**, 65–72.

Li, X., Hoffman, A.F., Peng, X.-Q., Lupica, C.R., Gardner, E.L., and Xi, Z.-X. (2009). Attenuation of basal and cocaine-enhanced locomotion and nucleus accumbens dopamine in cannabinoid CB1-receptor-knockout mice. *Psychopharmacology*, **204**, 1–11.

Liao, R.-M., Chang, Y.-H., Wang, S.-H., and Lan, C.-H. (2000). Distinct accumbal subareas are involved in place conditioning of amphetamine and cocaine. *Life Sciences*, **67**, 2033–2043.

Lile, J.A. and Nader, M.A. (2003). The abuse liability and therapeutic potential of drugs evaluated for cocaine addiction as predicted by animal models. *Current Neuropharmacology*, **1**, 21–46.

Lundqvist, T. (2005). Cognitive consequences of cannabis use: comparison with abuse of stimulants and heroin with regard to attention, memory and executive functions. *Pharmacology Biochemistry and Behavior*, **81**, 319–330.

Maldonado, R., Berrendero, F., Ozaita, A., and Robledo, P. (2011). Neurochemical basis of cannabis addiction. *Neuroscience*, **181**, 1–17.

Mechoulam, R., Shani, A., Edery, H., and Grunfeld, Y. (1970). Chemical basis of hashish activity. *Science*, **169**, 611–612.

Mechoulam, R., Peters, M., Murillo-Rodriguez, E., and Hanuš, L.O. (2007). Cannabidiol – recent advances. *Chemistry and Biodiversity*, **4**, 1678–1692.

Mendelson, J.H. and Mello, N.K. (1984). Reinforcing properties of oral Δ^9-tetrahydrocannabinol, smoked marijuana, and nabilone: influence of previous marijuana use. *Psychopharmacology*, **83**, 351–356.

Mendelson, J.H., Kuehnle, J.C., Greenberg, I., and Mello, N.K. (1976). Operant acquisition of marijuana in man. *Journal of Pharmacology and Experimental Therapeutics*, **198**, 42–53.

Milkman, H., Weiner, S.E., and Sunderwirth, S. (1983-84). Addiction relapse. *Advances in Alcohol and Substance Abuse*, **3**, 119–134.

Milton, A.L. and Everitt, B.J. (2012). The persistence of maladaptive memory: addiction, drug memories and anti-relapse treatments. *Neuroscience and Biobehavioral Reviews*, **36**, 1119–1139.

Moore, T.H.M., Zammit, S., Lingford-Hughes, A., *et al.* (2007). Cannabis use and risk of psychotic or affective mental health outcomes: a systematic review. *Lancet*, **370**, 319–328.

Morgan, C.J., Freeman, T.P., Schafer, G.L., and Curran, H.V. (2010). Cannabidiol attenuates the appetitive effects of Δ^9-tetrahydrocannabinol in humans smoking their chosen cannabis. *Neuropsychopharmacology*, **35**, 1879–1885.

Nazzaro, J.M., Seeger, T.F., and Gardner, E.L. (1981). Morphine differentially affects ventral tegmental and substantia nigra brain reward thresholds. *Pharmacology Biochemistry and Behavior*, **14**, 325–331.

O'Brien, C.P. (2001). Drug addiction and drug abuse. In: J.G. Hardman, L.E. Limbird, and A.G. Gilman (eds.). *Goodman and Gilman's The Pharmacological Basis of Therapeutics*. 10th ed. New York: McGraw-Hill, pp. 621–642.

O'Brien, C.P. and Gardner, E.L. (2005). Critical assessment of how to study addiction and its treatment: human and non-human animal models. *Pharmacology and Therapeutics*, **108**, 18–58.

ONDCP (Office of National Drug Control Policy). (2008). *Marijuana: the Greatest Cause of Illegal Drug Abuse (2008 Marijuana Sourcebook)*. Washington, DC: Office of National Drug Control Policy, Executive Office of the President.

Pak, A.C., Ashby, C.R. Jr., Heidbreder, C.A., *et al.* (2006). The selective dopamine D_3 receptor antagonist SB-277011A reduces nicotine-enhanced brain reward and nicotine-paired environmental cue functions. *International Journal of Neuropsychopharmacology*, **9**, 585–602.

Papafotiou, K., Carter, J.D., and Stough, C. (2005). The relationship between performance on the standardised field sobriety tests, driving performance and the level of Δ9-tetrahydrocannabinol (THC) in blood. *Forensic Science International*, **155**, 172–178.

Peoples, L.L. and Cavanaugh, D. (2003). Differential changes in signal and background firing of accumbal neurons during cocaine self-administration. *Journal of Neurophysiology*, **90**, 993–1010.

Peoples, L.L., Uzwiak, A.J., Gee, F., *et al.* (1999). Phasic accumbal firing may contribute to the regulation of drug taking during intravenous cocaine self-administration sessions. *Annals of the New York Academy of Sciences*, **877**, 781–787.

Pertwee, R.G. (2004). The pharmacology and therapeutic potential of cannabidiol. In: V. DiMarzo (ed.). *Cannabinoids*. Dordrecht: Kluwer Academic Publishers, pp. 32–83.

Pertwee, R.G. (2005). Pharmacological actions of cannabinoids. *Handbook of Experimental Pharmacology*, **168**, 1–51.

Pertwee, R.G., Thomas, A., Stevenson, L.A., *et al.* (2007). The psychoactive plant cannabinoid, Δ^9-tetrahydrocannabinol, is antagonized by Δ^8- and Δ^9-tetrahydrocannabivarin in mice *in vivo*. *British Journal of Pharmacology*, **150**, 586–594.

Pertwee, R.G. (2008). The diverse CB_1 and CB_2 receptor pharmacology of three plant cannabinoids: Δ^9-tetrahydrocannabinol, cannabidiol and Δ^9-tetrahydrocannabivarin. *British Journal of Pharmacology*, **153**, 199–215.

Ranganathan, M. and D'Souza, D.C. (2006). The acute effects of cannabinoids on memory in humans: a review. *Psychopharmacology*, **188**, 425–444.

Robbins, T.W. and Everitt, B.J. (2002). Limbic-striatal memory systems and drug addiction. *Neurobiology of Learning and Memory*, **78**, 625–636.

Russo, E.B. (2011). Taming THC: potential cannabis synergy and phytocannabinoid-terpenoid entourage effects. *British Journal of Pharmacology*, **163**, 1344–1364.

SAMHSA (Substance Abuse and Mental Health Services Administration; Office of Applied Studies, U.S. Department of Health and Human Services). (2008). *Results From the 2008 National Survey on Drug Use and Health: National Findings* (NSDUH Series H-36, HHS Publication No. SMA 09-4434). Rockville, Maryland: Substance Abuse and Mental Health Services Administration.

Schultz, W., Apicella, P., Scarnati, E., and Ljungberg, T. (1992). Neuronal activity in monkey ventral striatum related to the expectation of reward. *Journal of Neuroscience*, **12**, 4595–4610.

Schultz, W., Apicella, P., and Ljungberg, T. (1993). Responses of monkey dopamine neurons to reward and conditioned stimuli during successive steps of learning a delayed response task. *Journal of Neuroscience*, **13**, 900–913.

Schultz, W. (1994). Behavior-related activity of primate dopamine neurons. *Revue Neurologique*, **150**, 634–639.

Shaham, Y., Shalev, U., Lu, L., De Wit, H., and Stewart, J. (2002). The reinstatement model of drug relapse: history, methodology and major findings. *Psychopharmacology*, **168**, 3–20.

Shalev, U., Grimm, J.W., and Shaham, Y. (2002). Neurobiology of relapse to heroin and cocaine seeking: a review. *Pharmacological Reviews*, **54**, 1–42.

Sofuoglu, M., Sugarman, D.E., and Carroll, K.M. (2010). Cognitive function as an emerging treatment target for marijuana addiction. *Experimental and Clinical Psychopharmacology*, **18**, 109–119.

Spiller, K., Xi, Z.-X. and Peng, X.-Q., *et al.* (2008). The selective dopamine D_3 receptor antagonists SB-277011A and NGB 2904 and the putative partial D_3 receptor agonist BP-897 attenuate methamphetamine-enhanced brain-stimulation reward in rats. *Psychopharmacology*, **196**, 533–542.

Stephens, R.S., Roffman, R.A., and Simpson, E.E. (1993). Adult marijuana users seeking treatment. *Journal of Consulting and Clinical Psychology*, **61**, 1100–1114.

Stephens, R.S., Roffman, R.A., and Curtin, L. (2000). Comparison of extended versus brief treatments for marijuana use. *Journal of Consulting and Clinical Psychology*, **68**, 898–908.

Swift, W., Hall, W., and Copeland, J. (1998). Characteristics of long term cannabis users in Sydney, Australia. *European Addiction Research*, **4**, 190–197.

Tanda, G., Pontieri, F.E., and Di Chiara, G. (1997). Cannabinoid and heroin activation of mesolimbic dopamine transmission by a common μ_1 opioid receptor mechanism. *Science*, **276**, 2048–2050.

Ternes, J.W., Ehrman, R., and O'Brien, C.P. (1984). Nondependent monkeys self-administer hydromorphone. *Behavioral Neuroscience*, **99**, 583–588.

Thomas, A., Baillie, G.L., Phillips, A.M., Razdan, R.K., Ross, R.A., and Pertwee, R.G. (2007). Cannabidiol displays unexpectedly high potency as an antagonist of CB_1 and CB_2 receptor agonists *in vitro*. *British Journal of Pharmacology*, **150**, 613–623.

Turner, C.E., Elsohly, M.A., and Boeren, E.G. (1980). Constituents of *Cannabis sativa* L. XVII. A review of the natural constituents. *Journal of Natural Products*, **43**, 169–234.

Tzschentke, T.M. (1998). Measuring reward with the conditioned place preference paradigm: a comprehensive review of drug effects, recent progress and new issues. *Progress in Neurobiology*, **56**, 613–672.

Tzschentke, T.M. (2007). Measuring reward with the conditioned place preference (CPP) paradigm: update of the last decade. *Addiction Biology*, **12**, 227–462.

Tzschentke, T.M. and Schmidt, W.J. (2000). Effects of the non-competitive NMDA-receptor antagonist memantine on morphine- and cocaine-induced potentiation of lateral hypothalamic brain stimulation reward. *Psychopharmacology*, **149**, 225–234.

Valjent, E. and Maldonado, R. (2000). A behavioural model to reveal place preference to Δ^9-tetrahydrocannabinol in mice. *Psychopharmacology*, **147**, 436–438.

Vorel, S.R., Liu, X., Hayes, R.J., Spector, J.A., and Gardner, E.L. (2001). Relapse to cocaine-seeking after hippocampal theta burst stimulation. *Science*, **292**, 1175–1178.

Wagner, F.A. and Anthony, J.C. (2002). From first drug use to drug dependence; developmental periods of risk for dependence upon marijuana, cocaine, and alcohol. *Neuropsychopharmacology*, **26**, 479–488.

Ward, A.S., Comer, S.D., Haney, M., Foltin, R.W., and Fischman, M.W. (1997). The effects of a monetary alternative on marijuana self-administration. *Behavioural Pharmacology*, **8**, 275–286.

Winstock, A.R., Ford, C., and Witton, J. (2010). Assessment and management of cannabis use disorders in primary care. *British Medical Journal*, **340**, 800–804.

Wise, R.A. (1989). The brain and reward. In: J.M. Liebman and S.J. Cooper (eds.). *The Neuropharmacological Basis of Reward*. Oxford: Oxford University Press, pp. 377–424.

Wise, R.A. (1996). Addictive drugs and brain stimulation reward. *Annual Review of Neuroscience*, **19**, 319–340.

Wise, R.A. and Gardner, E.L. (2002). Functional anatomy of substance-related disorders. In: H. D'haenen, J.A. den Boer, and P. Willner (eds.) *Biological Psychiatry*. New York: Wiley, pp. 509–522.

Woody, G.E., Kane, V., Lewis, K., and Thompson, R. (2007). Premature deaths after discharge from methadone maintenance: a replication. *Journal of Addiction Medicine*, **1**, 180–185.

Wu, X. and French, E.D. (2000). Effects of chronic Δ^9-tetrahydrocannabinol on rat midbrain neurons: an electrophysiological assessment. *Neuropharmacology*, **39**, 391–398.

Xi, Z.-X., Gilbert, J., Campos, A.C., *et al.* (2004). Blockade of mesolimbic dopamine D_3 receptors inhibits stress-induced reinstatement of cocaine-seeking in rats. *Psychopharmacology*, **176**, 57–65.

Xi, Z.-X., Gilbert, J.G., Peng, X.-Q., Pak, A.C., Li, X., and Gardner, E.L. (2006). Cannabinoid CB_1 receptor antagonist AM251 inhibits cocaine-primed relapse in rats: role of glutamate in the nucleus accumbens. *Journal of Neuroscience*, **26**, 8531–8536.

Xi, Z.-X., Spiller, K., Pak, A.C., *et al.* (2008). Cannabinoid CB1 receptor antagonists attenuate cocaine's rewarding effects: experiments with self-administration and brain-stimulation reward in rats. *Neuropsychopharmacology*, **33**, 1735–1745.

Xi, Z.-X., Peng, X.-Q., Li, X., *et al.* (2011). Brain cannabinoid CB_2 receptors modulate cocaine's actions in mice. *Nature Neuroscience*, **14**, 1160–1166.

Zangen, A., Solinas, M., Ikemoto, S., Goldberg, S.R., and Wise, R.A. (2006). Two brain sites for cannabinoid reward. *Journal of Neuroscience*, **26**, 4901–4907.

Chapter 10

Effects of Phytocannabinoids on Anxiety, Mood, and the Endocrine System

Sachin Patel, Matthew N. Hill, and Cecilia J. Hillard

10.1 Introduction

The earliest systematic studies of cannabis and the phytocannabinoids focused on their effects on mood, anxiety, and the endocrine system. The reasons for this include the prominent effects of the phytocannabinoids on these important aspects of human psychological and physiological function. Our understanding of the mechanisms by which delta-9-tetrahydrocannabinol (THC) and other cannabinoid receptor type $1(CB_1)$ agonists affect neural processes involved in mood and anxiety regulation is very advanced; however, very little is known about the other phytocannabinoids, despite hints that cannabidiol (CBD) in particular has effects on both mood and anxiety. Finally, our understanding of the effects of THC and other phytocannabinoids on endocrine signaling has lagged behind that of other aspects of these compounds, with the exception of their effects on the hypothalamic–pituitary–adrenal (HPA) axis. It is possible that some of the effects of the phytocannabinoids on mood in particular are mediated by endocrine changes. The purpose of this chapter is to review our current knowledge of the interactions of the phytocannabinoids with the processing of anxiety, setting of mood, and regulation of the HPA axis, thyroid and growth hormone, and melatonin.

10.2 Phytocannabinoids and anxiety

Among the diverse psychophysiological consequences of cannabis intoxication and use, effects on anxiety-related emotional processes are perhaps the best documented (Moreira and Wotjak 2010). Here we will review the scientific literature examining the relationship between underlying trait anxiety and anxiety disorders, and cannabis use disorders; the adverse effects of acute cannabis intoxication on anxiety-related symptoms; and the therapeutic potential of cannabinoid/endocannabinoid-based treatment approaches for anxiety disorders.

10.2.1 Why people use cannabis, and what's anxiety got to do with it?

Anxiety disorders are the most common psychiatric disorders in the general population, and there is a particularly high incidence of cannabis use in patients with symptoms of anxiety and anxiety disorders (Crippa et al. 2009). Several hypotheses have been proposed to account for this unusually high comorbidity. The "tension-reduction hypothesis" posits that cannabis is used to self-medicate anxiety symptoms, whereas an alternate hypothesis contends that chronic use of cannabis increases anxiety symptoms and results in increased vulnerability to anxiety disorders (Hyman and Sinha 2009). As we describe in the following paragraphs, it is likely that both of these hypotheses are correct and that cannabis users, like the users of other drugs with dependence liability, exhibit a trajectory from casual use to dependence and problematic use.

According to the "tension-reduction hypothesis" of cannabis use, negative affect (i.e., feelings or mood) associated with anxiety disorders could promote cannabis use in an attempt to reduce symptom severity (Buckner et al. 2007). There is evidence to support this hypothesis. For example, the most common reason chronic users give for their continued cannabis use is to reduce anxiety and relieve tension (Hyman and Sinha 2009; Reilly et al. 1998). In addition, cannabis users increase consumption during times of stress (Kaplan et al. 1986), and very often report that coping with stress is an important reason that they use cannabis (Bujarski et al. 2012b; Chabrol et al. 2005; Fox et al. 2011; Hyman and Sinha 2009).

Recent studies indicate that individuals who utilize cannabis for stress coping report higher rates of arousal, worry and agoraphobic cognition, and higher frequency of cannabis use than subjects who use cannabis for other reasons (Bonn-Miller et al. 2008). Additionally, heavy cannabis users who meet criteria for being clinically anxious exhibit greater severity and numbers of marijuana-related problems and nonanxiety psychopathology than nonanxious cannabis users (Van Dam et al. 2012). Social anxiety is associated with higher cannabis use, cannabis-related problems, and avoidance/coping motives for cannabis use, especially in males (Buckner et al. 2012). Most convincingly, a 14-year, longitudinal prospective study found that social anxiety disorder at study entry was associated with a 6.5 greater odds for cannabis dependence at follow-up (Buckner et al. 2008). Overall, it appears that coping motives for cannabis use are widespread and the presence of anxiety symptoms and anxiety disorders (especially social anxiety disorder) are associated with increased risk for cannabis use, supporting the tension-reduction hypothesis of cannabis use disorders.

Bonn-Miller and colleagues have hypothesized that although initial use of cannabis can reduce anxiety symptoms, long-term use could contribute to worsening of anxiety, increased cannabis use, and cannabis-related problems (Bonn-Miller et al. 2008). Furthermore, these authors suggest that some individuals use cannabis to avoid social contact and develop avoidant coping strategies to stress, which are risk factors for the development of future anxiety disorders. Such a process may explain the relationship between frequency of cannabis use and risk of developing anxiety symptoms and disorders (Hayatbakhsh et al. 2007; Patton et al. 2002; Zvolensky et al. 2006, 2008). Taken together, these data suggest that chronic heavy cannabis use could have deleterious effects on anxiety symptoms. Indeed, cannabis use can be associated with the emergence of acute adverse effects including anxiety symptoms and panic as described in later sections; however, a definitive causal link between chronic cannabis use and the development of anxiety disorders per se remains speculative.

Laboratory studies in animals provide support for the tension-reduction hypothesis, as well as cannabis-induced anxiety states. In support of the tension-reduction hypothesis, numerous studies have demonstrated that acute administration of low doses of CB_1 receptor agonists can reduce anxiety behaviors in a variety of animal models (Moreira and Wotjak 2010; Ruehle et al. 2012), likely through activation of CB_1 receptors on glutamatergic nerve terminals (Rey et al. 2012). On the other hand, 12 days of high-dose cannabinoid treatment increases anxiety behaviors and neuroendocrine responses to acute stress in rats (Hill and Gorzalka 2006). Thus, preclinical studies support the hypothesis that low doses and infrequent exposure to cannabis constituents can reduce feelings of anxiety and stress but that chronic use of large amounts has the opposite effect and could contribute to the development of anxiety and other psychiatric disorders.

10.2.2 Phytocannabinoids and panic disorder

Panic attacks and panic disorder are a subclass of anxiety-related disorders that have been particularly linked to cannabis use. Epidemiological studies have demonstrated a significant correlation between cannabis dependence and lifetime presence of panic attacks (Zvolensky et al. 2006). Interestingly, subjects with comorbid cannabis use and panic attacks reported age of onset of panic attacks 8.6 years earlier than noncannabis users. Evidence supporting a causal relationship between cannabis use and panic disorders comes from a prospective study examining the effects of cannabis use, abuse, or dependence at age 16 on the presence of panic attacks or panic disorder at age 24 (Zvolensky et al. 2008). The results of this study indicate an odds ratio between 3.7 and 4.9 for the presence of panic attacks and panic disorder, respectively, in cannabis-dependent subjects. However, in a further analysis of these data, the effects of cannabis on the development of panic attacks and panic disorder were not independent from cigarette smoking, so it is difficult to parse out the contributions of each substance (Zvolensky et al. 2008). Patients with comorbid cannabis dependence and panic disorder do not differ in their responses rates to standard antidepressant treatment for panic disorder (Dannon et al. 2004).

Several case reports and clinical studies have described subjects who experience acute anxiety and panic-like reactions to cannabis intoxication, and subsequently developed recurrent panic attacks in the absence of cannabis use (Dannon et al. 2004; Deas et al. 2000; Langs et al. 1997). Thus, a subgroup of individuals are particularly susceptible to the anxiogenic effects of cannabis and these individuals experience recurrent panic attacks and develop panic disorder even if they never use cannabis again.

Although further studies are clearly needed, emerging evidence suggests that cannabis use and dependence could represent risk factors for the development of panic attacks and panic disorder, at least in a subset of susceptible individuals.

10.2.3 Phytocannabinoids and posttraumatic stress disorder

Experiencing or witnessing severe traumatic events can cause posttraumatic stress disorder (PTSD), which is characterized by re-experiencing the event, avoidance, and hypervigilance. A PTSD diagnosis is associated with greater risk for cannabis use than stimulant use (Calhoun et al. 2000; Cougle et al. 2011), and rates of PTSD are higher among patients with a cannabis use disorder diagnosis compared with other substance use disorder groups (Bonn-Miller et al. 2012). These data suggest that patients with PTSD could be more susceptible to tension-reduction motivated cannabis use (Potter et al. 2011), and that individuals with PTSD could have increased susceptibility to the development of cannabis use disorders (Cornelius et al. 2010). In support of these hypotheses, past 2-week PTSD symptoms significantly predicted coping motives but not social, enhancement, or conformity motives for cannabis use (Bujarski et al. 2012a). In addition, lack of improvement in PTSD symptoms during residential treatment of veterans predicted greater frequency of cannabis use 4 months after treatment (Bonn-Miller et al. 2011). Also consistent with this hypothesis, use of the synthetic cannabinoid, nabilone, reduced nightmare frequency and reduced daytime flashbacks in a subset of patients (Fraser 2009), and case-report-level evidence has suggested cannabis could reduce the severity of PTSD symptoms (Passie et al. 2012). Overall, these data suggest a strong association between PTSD and cannabis use, and that subjects with PTSD use cannabis to reduce PTSD symptom severity. However, whether long-term outcomes are improved or worsened by cannabis use in PTSD patients remains to be determined.

Studies in laboratory animals support a prominent role for cannabinoids in the regulation of fear responses to traumatic experiences (de Bitencourt et al. 2013; Neumeister 2013; Ruehle et al. 2012).

For example, many studies find that reduced CB_1 receptor function impairs the ability of animals to extinguish conditioned fear behaviors (Lutz 2007; Marsicano et al. 2002) while activating CB_1 receptors with direct or indirect CB_1 agonists can facilitate extinction of fear memories (Chhatwal et al. 2009; Gunduz-Cinar et al. 2013; Lin et al. 2009; Pamplona et al. 2008). Together these data indicate that activation of CB_1 receptors reduces the expression of fear in response to reminders of traumatic experiences, which is consistent with the symptom relief reported by PTSD sufferers when they use cannabis. Overall, these animal data are consistent with the clinical studies reviewed earlier, in that they provide experimental support for the tension-reduction motive for cannabis use in patients with PTSD.

10.2.4 Adverse anxiety reactions to cannabis intoxication

The most commonly provided reasons for continued use by chronic cannabis users are to promote relaxation and reduce tension (Reilly et al. 1998). Paradoxically, the most consistently documented adverse effect of cannabis intoxication is the appearance of anxiety and panic-like reactions (Thomas 1996). Bialos documented a case series of subjects experiencing several distinct anxiety states he classified into "free-floating" anxiety and anxiety following psychotomimetic symptoms (Bialos 1970). In general, higher doses of cannabis consumption were associated with higher incidence of adverse reactions, while "hysterical" or "histrionic" individuals who utilize primitive defenses, including repression and denial, could be more susceptible to anxious reactions as conflicted materials emerge during the intoxication experience (Bialos 1970). Lastly, Bialos noted that stressful or anxiety-provoking environmental situations were often associated with worse anxiety-related adverse reactions to cannabis intoxication.

These insights are supported by larger studies. Halikas noted that 5% of subjects described anxious or fearful feelings greater than 50% of the time, while 54% of subjects reported experiencing these effects occasionally (Halikas et al. 1971). Similarly, 22% of cannabis users reported anxiety or panic attacks after cannabis use (Thomas 1996). Interestingly, the rates of panic attacks were significantly higher in females (30%) than males (14%). Based on these high rates, Thomas has suggested that anxiety-related symptoms are the most common adverse reactions to cannabis use (Thomas 1996, 1993).

Consistent with these human studies suggesting anxiety reactions are common adverse reactions of cannabis use, laboratory studies using rodents also clearly demonstrate a biphasic effect of cannabinoids on anxiety-related behaviors (Patel and Hillard 2006; Rey et al. 2012). Low doses of THC and synthetic cannabinoids can reduce anxiety in some models. In contrast, higher doses, or administration of cannabinoids under stressful environmental conditions, uniformly produce anxiogenic effects in animal studies (Hill and Gorzalka 2004). There is evidence that increased neuronal activity in the amygdala underlies the interaction between environmental stress and anxiety responses induced by cannabis (Patel et al. 2005). In general, there exists a complex biphasic dose–response for the effects of cannabinoids on anxiety-like behaviors. Importantly, this curve appears to undergo a leftward shift under stressful environmental conditions, but may also undergo a rightward shift under socially permissive situations. This dynamic dose–response relationship could also be shifted by personality factors and the existence of comorbid mood or anxiety disorders as discussed earlier.

10.2.5 The therapeutic potential of cannabinoid/endocannabinoid-based treatment approaches for anxiety disorders

There is great interest in advancing cannabinoid and endocannabinoid-based treatment approaches for anxiety disorders. Overall, three primary approaches have been advocated: (1) the use of cannabis-based products, i.e., medicinal marijuana; (2) the use of synthetic cannabinoids; and (3) the use of pharmaceutical agents that modulate concentrations of endogenously produced cannabinoids. The use of cannabis products in the form of oral THC or sublingual THC:CBD (Sativex®) combinations for the treatment of anxiety disorders is not likely to be beneficial due to their narrow therapeutic window. For example, oral THC and Sativex® both increased anxiety in a group of healthy cannabis-using subjects (Karschner et al. 2011; Martin-Santos et al. 2012). Although this effect was not clinically significant, one could reasonably presume that this response would be more pronounced in patients with anxiety disorders. Additionally, the effects of both formulations on anxiety were dose-dependent, increasing the chance of potentially worsening symptoms in patients with anxiety disorders (Karschner et al. 2011). Interestingly, several recent human and animal studies have suggested that CBD, a phytocannabinoid that does not activate CB_1 or CB_2 receptors (Mechoulam et al. 2002), can reduce anxiety in humans (Bergamaschi et al. 2011; Crippa et al. 2011; Das et al. 2013) and in laboratory animals (Campos et al. 2013; Uribe-Marino et al. 2012). Some authors have suggested these effects could be, in part, mediated via activation of serotonin 1A receptor subtypes in the brain (Gomes et al. 2011). Further studies into the efficacy and mechanisms by which CBD modulates anxiety are needed, but initial results suggest this could be a promising new approach for the treatment of anxiety disorders.

The third approach, which is currently focused on pharmacological blockade of endocannabinoid degradation, has many advantages (Hill and Gorzalka 2009a; Ruehle et al. 2012). Specifically, inhibition of fatty acid amide hydrolase (FAAH), the enzyme that degrades the endocannabinoid N-arachidonoylethanolamine, reduces anxiety and facilitates extinction of conditioned fear via activation of CB_1 receptors in preclinical studies (Gunduz-Cinar et al. 2013; Kathuria et al. 2003; Patel and Hillard 2006). Importantly, inhibition of FAAH does not synergize with stress to activate the amygdala (Patel et al. 2005) and does not exhibit a biphasic dose response common to direct acting CB_1 receptor agonists (Patel and Hillard 2006). More recently, inhibition of monoacylglycerol lipase, the enzyme that degrades the endocannabinoid, 2-arachidonoylglycerol, has also been shown to exhibit anxiolytic effects (Kinsey et al. 2011; Sciolino et al. 2011; Sumislawski et al. 2011). Given the prominent role for cannabinoid systems in the modulation of anxiety-related behaviors, the development of novel therapeutic approaches for the treatment of anxiety disorders based on this system is well supported by clinical and preclinical findings. However, a caveat is that chronic activation of CB_1 receptor signaling could exacerbate current anxiety disorders and/or predispose development of more severe disorders in susceptible individuals.

10.3 **Phytocannabinoids, mood, and depression**

In addition to its ability to reduce anxiety and produce relaxation, cannabis use is commonly reported to elevate mood and cause euphoria (Halikas et al. 1971). The mood-enhancing effect of cannabis likely contributes to the association between mood disorders, particularly depression, and cannabis use. Similar to the "tension reduction" hypothesis relating cannabis use to anxiety disorders, a "mood elevating" hypothesis can be proposed to explain the relationship between cannabis use and depression. In this section, we will review the scientific evidence regarding the mood effects of cannabinoids, including the evidence that cannabinoids have antidepressant and pro-depressant properties.

10.3.1 **Cannabinoids as antidepressants**

Studies examining the ability of cannabis and cannabinoids to reduce depression have yielded contradictory findings. One study that examined depressive symptoms in a survey of nearly 4500 individuals found that cannabis users had fewer depressive symptoms than nonusers (Denson and Earleywine 2006). Similarly, case report studies of five individuals suffering from depression who used cannabis indicated that depression preceded cannabis use in most of the individuals studied and found evidence of antidepressant effects (Gruber et al. 1996). Self-report question-naires examining the reasons for cannabis use found that 22% engaged in cannabis use to con-trol symptoms of depression (Ware et al. 2005). While no systematic studies have been carried out, anecdotal reports of bipolar patients indicate that cannabis use helps regulate symptoms of depression (Ashton et al. 2005). Multiple studies examining cannabis use in populations suffer-ing from chronic diseases also report reductions in depression and elevation in mood following cannabis use (Amtmann et al. 2004; Lahat et al. 2012; Page et al. 2003; Williamson and Evans 2000; Woolridge et al. 2005). Taken together, these data are consistent with the hypothesis that cannabis use has mood elevating and antidepressant properties, particularly in patients with chronic disease.

In contrast to these reports, two studies that examined the effect of THC administration to depressed individuals did not find evidence for any clinical antidepressant effect; in fact, consid-erable dysphoria was observed in some patients (Ablon and Goodwin 1974; Kotin et al. 1973). There are several factors that could contribute to the differing results of these studies compared to those discussed previously. First, the subjects to which the THC was administered were primar-ily naïve to cannabis and thus the psychoactive effects could have been viewed as undesirable. Self-medication with cannabis by an experienced user likely represents a fundamentally different process than administration of THC alone to a noncannabis user given the range of positive and negative reactions to cannabis that individuals report (Halikas et al. 1971; Williamson and Evans 2000). Second, these studies looked exclusively at THC administration, while cannabis itself contains a wide array of other phytocannabinoids which can synergize, moderate, or oppose the effects of THC (Russo 2011). For example, pure THC administration has been found to increase anxiety while co-administration of CBD can counter this effect (Zuardi et al. 1982). Thus, the presence of CBD could contribute to some of the reported antidepressant effects of cannabis, which would be absent in studies administering THC alone.

10.3.2 Cannabis use can predispose to depression

Multiple studies have demonstrated that individuals who engaged in excessive cannabis use dur-ing adolescence exhibit increased rates of depression later in life (Bovasso 2001; Chen et al. 2002; Degenhardt et al. 2003; Fairman and Anthony 2012; Green and Ritter 2000; Lynskey et al. 2004). Light to moderate use of cannabis, even during adolescence, did not correlate with the occurrence of later depression, indicating that heavy use patterns are key determinants in this relationship. Harder and colleagues found that the relationship between cannabis and depression was not sig-nificant when other variables were included in the analysis (Harder et al. 2006). These investiga-tors suggested an alternative hypothesis that other factor(s) could be at play that both increase risk for depression and the choice to engage in cannabis use (Harder et al. 2006). For example, individ-uals who have experienced early life adversity exhibit an increased risk of developing depression in adulthood (Heim and Nemeroff 2001) and increased propensity to use cannabis (Hayatbakhsh et al. 2013). Alternately, a study examining twin-pairs in which one exhibits cannabis dependency and the other does not reported that the cannabis-dependent twin exhibits a 2.5–2.9-fold greater risk of suicidal ideation and suicide attempts than the nondependent twin, which was even greater if cannabis use initiated before the age of 17 (Lynskey et al. 2004). Taken together, these data suggest that excessive cannabis use during adolescence is associated with increased likelihood of developing depression in adulthood; however, the causative relationship is not understood.

10.3.3 Animal studies examining the relationship between cannabinoids and depressive symptoms

The phytocannabinoids THC (Bambico et al. 2012; El-Alfy et al. 2010; Elbatsh et al. 2012; Haring et al. 2013) and CBD (Campos et al. 2013; El-Alfy et al. 2010; Zanelati et al. 2010) have been reported to produce antidepressant effects in animal models. The antidepressant effects of THC are mediated by activation of CB_1 receptors and can be mimicked by direct and indirect CB_1 receptor agonists (Hill et al. 2009a). On the other hand, CBD appears to exert its antidepressant action through a direct action on serotonergic 5-HT_{1A} receptors (Zanelati et al. 2010). In contradiction to these data, a few reports have shown that acute administration of THC, or direct CB_1 receptor agonists, can produce depressive-like behavioral responses (Egashira et al. 2008; Sano et al. 2009; Shearman et al. 2003). These effects, however, are likely due to the motor suppressant effects of higher doses of cannabinoid ligands which can confound interpretation of behaviors in the forced swim test. In summary, there is a substantial body of preclinical evidence supporting the hypothesis that the phytocannabinoids THC and CBD possess antidepressant actions, and these effects appear to be primarily mediated by serotonin and catecholaminergic systems (Bambico et al. 2007; Banerjee et al. 1975; Fisar 2010; McLaughlin et al. 2012).

Preclinical studies support a relationship between cannabinoid exposure during adolescence and the development of depression in adulthood. In particular, administration of escalating doses of THC during adolescence results in increased rates of depressive-like behavior in adulthood (Bambico et al. 2010; Realini et al. 2011; Rubino et al. 2008, 2009). The mechanism for this effect is likely compromised function of the endocannabinoid system in adulthood. For example, escalating doses of THC during adolescence results in a downregulation of CB_1 receptors throughout limbic regions in the brain known to mediate the effects of cannabinoids on emotionality (Rubino et al. 2008). In addition, administration to adults of drugs that increase endocannabinoid activation of CB_1 receptors is sufficient to reverse the depressive-like phenotype induced by adolescent exposure to THC (Realini et al. 2011).

10.4 Phytocannabinoids and regulation of endocrine systems

Considerable data demonstrate that processes involved in the regulation of homeostasis, including the autonomic nervous system and endocrine systems, are dysregulated in individuals with anxiety and mood disorders. In this section, we will examine the effects of the phytocannabinoids on several endocrine systems that are known to be stress responsive or otherwise contribute to mood disorders.

10.4.1 Cannabinoids and the HPA axis

HPA axis dysfunction is present in many individuals with major depression and has been hypothesized to contribute to its etiology and symptomatology (Holsboer 2000). Basal cortisol concentrations are elevated in approximately 66% of depressed individuals, particularly those with the most severe depressive symptoms (Holsboer 2000). Inability of patients to suppress cortisol release following dexamethasone challenge is considered diagnostic of depressive mood disorders (Rush et al. 1996). Long-term treatment with all of the effective antidepressant drugs and electroconvulsive shock therapy result in reductions in basal and stress-induced activation of the HPA axis (Gorzalka and Hill 2011). Thus, hyperactivity of the HPA axis accompanies depression in many individuals, and attenuation of hyperactive HPA axis activity is a common feature of effective antidepressant therapies.

Despite the mood elevating properties of cannabis consumption, studies seem to reliably demonstrate that acute consumption of cannabis (Cone et al. 1986) or THC (D'Souza et al. 2004, 2008; Kleinloog et al. 2012; Klumpers et al. 2012; Ranganathan et al. 2009) increases the secretion of cortisol in individuals who were either naïve to cannabis or infrequent users. When examined in chronic cannabis users, the ability of THC administration to increase cortisol levels was blunted indicating that tolerance develops with regular cannabis use (D'Souza et al. 2008; Ranganathan et al. 2009).

Some (King et al. 2011; Somaini et al. 2012), but not all (Block et al. 1991), studies have also reported that chronic cannabis users exhibit elevated basal cortisol levels, suggesting that there may be dysregulation in both the basal and stimulated responses of the HPA axis. Consistent with this hypothesis, it has been reported that stress-induced activation of the HPA axis is blunted in chronic adult and adolescent cannabis users (Somaini et al. 2012; van Leeuwen et al. 2011). In adolescents with an early onset of use, chronic cannabis use is associated with altered diurnal cortisol rhythms such that cortisol concentrations are higher than normal at night and blunted in the morning (Huizink and Mulder 2006).

The only study that has examined the effect of CBD on the HPA axis in humans found that this phytocannabinoid attenuated the diurnal decline in cortisol levels, consistent with an HPA stimulatory effect (Zuardi et al. 1993).

Preclinical studies of the effects of cannabinoids on HPA axis function have demonstrated effects of the phytocannabinoids that parallel their effects in humans. Administration of THC to rodents increases circulating concentrations of corticosterone (the rodent analog of cortisol) (Steiner and Wotjak 2008) as does CBD (Zuardi et al. 1984). While THC administration increases HPA axis activity, low doses of other CB_1 receptor agonists reduce basal and stress-induced HPA axis responses in rodents (Patel et al. 2004; Saber-Tehrani et al. 2010). These differential responses are likely due to distinct neuroanatomical circuits. For example, CB_1 receptors within the paraventricular nucleus (PVN) of the hypothalamus or the basolateral amygdala have been found to constrain activation of the HPA axis and decrease corticosterone secretion (Di et al. 2003; Evanson et al. 2010; Ganon-Elazar and Akirav 2009; Hill et al. 2010; Hill et al. 2009b), while pharmacological blockade of noradrenergic or serotonergic receptors, but not glutamatergic receptors, attenuates cannabinoid-induced corticosterone secretion (McLaughlin et al. 2009). These data suggest that the ability of cannabinoids to increase HPA axis activity is secondary to activation of monoaminergic hindbrain nuclei, while the inhibitory effects of cannabinoids on corticosterone secretion is due to direct actions on limbic and hypothalamic circuitry.

10.4.2 Cannabinoids and the hypothalamic–pituitary–thyroid (HPT) axis

The thyroid hormones, L-thyroxin (T_4) and 3,5,3'-triiodothyrionine (T_3) are vital for proper development and metabolic regulation in many mammalian tissues. The thyroid hormones exert the majority of their effects through binding to nuclear receptors that function as transcription factors acting through thyroid hormone response elements (Flamant et al. 2007). The brain is an important target of thyroid hormones and hypothyroidism during the perinatal period in particular results in irreversible, severe cognitive deficits (Bernal 2007). Disorders of the HPT axis are associated with depressed mood in adults (Joffe 2011). Thyroid hormones and endocannabinoids both participate in the regulation of energy homeostasis; thyroid hormones increase basal metabolic rate and energy expenditure while endocannabinoids, acting through CB_1 receptors, increase food consumption and energy conservation. Although untested as yet, these data suggest the hypothesis that CB_1 receptor regulation of the release of thyrotropin-releasing hormone (TRH) could be the mechanism by which starvation suppresses thyroid hormone release.

In a study of chronic cannabis users, Bonnett found that thyrotropin (TSH), T_3 and T_4 concentrations were all within normal limits and did not correlate with concentrations of THC or its major metabolites (Bonnet 2013). These findings suggest that chronic exposure of adults to THC does not produce a long-lasting impact on HPT axis function. However, in light of the importance of thyroid hormones during development, it is quite possible that cannabis use during pregnancy could have adverse effects on fetal development through dysregulation of the HPT axis. There is evidence that THC could reduce thyroid hormone efficacy during development. In particular, treatment of a trophoblast cell line with micromolar concentrations of THC results in inhibition of proliferation and a nearly threefold reduction in the expression of thyroid receptor β1 (TRβ1) (Khare et al. 2006). This effect on TRβ1 expression is similar to what occurs in fetal growth restriction (FGR) (Ohara et al. 2004). As marijuana use has been associated with FGR (Zuckerman et al. 1989), these data suggest that THC exposure during pregnancy could interfere with growth as a result of downregulation of TRβ1.

Treatment of adult rats with THC reduces concentrations of T_3 and T_4 in the circulation (Hillard et al. 1984; Nazar et al. 1977; Rosenkrantz and Esber 1980). High doses of a synthetic CB receptor agonist inhibit T_3 release without affecting TSH release, suggesting a site of action in the thyroid gland (Porcella et al. 2002). On the other hand, studies in anterior pituitary explants support an inhibitory effect of CB_1 receptor activation on pituitary TSH release (Veiga et al. 2008). However, the majority of available evidence indicates a primary role for THC to inhibit TRH release through effects in the hypothalamus or higher CNS regions (Deli et al. 2009; Hillard et al. 1984). Glucocorticoid-induced mobilization of endocannabinoid signaling has been shown to inhibit glutamate release onto TRH positive neurons in the PVN (Di et al. 2003), suggesting that endocannabinoids could link stress and activation of the HPT axis.

10.4.3 Phytocannabinoids and regulation of growth hormone

Growth hormone (GH), also known as somatotropin, is a polypeptide that is synthesized and released from somatotrophic cells in the anterior pituitary. GH is an anabolic hormone that stimulates growth and regulates energy homeostasis. GH secretion is regulated by the coordinated effects of two hypothalamic peptides: somatostatin (inhibitory) and growth hormone-releasing hormone (GHRH; stimulatory). The release of somatostatin and GHRH are regulated by biogenic amines, metabolic status, sex hormones, and sleep. GH is released in a pulsatile manner, with the largest GH peak occurring about an hour after the onset of sleep (Takahashi et al. 1968). Surges in GH release occur during waking as well, with a frequency of approximately 3–5 h (Natelson et al. 1975).

There is only one study of the effects of phytocannabinoids in humans. Prolonged administration to human males of THC (more than 200 mg per day) decreased serum GH concentrations evoked by insulin, which is the gold-standard test of GH axis integrity (Benowitz et al. 1976). The effects of more moderate THC doses are unknown.

Preclinical studies have demonstrated that acute and chronic THC treatment of adult and adolescent rodents decreases basal circulating GH concentrations (Dalterio et al. 1981, 1983; Kokka and Garcia 1974). THC also suppresses episodic release of GH in unrestrained male rats (Falkenstein and Holley 1992). The effect of THC is not affected by dexamethasone (Kokka and Garcia 1974) or by castration (Dalterio et al. 1983), suggesting that it is not secondary to either increased HPA axis activation or suppression of sex hormone release.

The effect of THC is mimicked by acute administration of very low doses of the synthetic CB_1 receptor agonist, HU-210 (Martin-Calderon et al. 1998), suggesting a CB_1 receptor role in the effects of THC. The suppressive effect of THC on GH occurs when THC is injected into the third ventricle (Rettori et al. 1988) and incubation of median eminence fragments or the mediobasal hypothalamus with THC at concentrations as low as 1 nM increases somatostatin release (Rettori et al. 1990), leading to the hypothesis that the mechanism of THC is to increase somatostatin. However, CB_1 receptors are present on human GH secreting cells in the pituitary and CB_1 receptor agonist treatment inhibits GH secretion from acromegaly-associated pituitary adenomas in culture (Pagotto et al. 2001), although another study found no effect of THC on GH release from isolated pituitary cells (Rettori et al. 1988).

Acute exposure of mice to 50 mg/kg of the nonpsychoactive phytocannabinoid, cannabinol increased plasma GH concentrations in unstressed male mice (Dalterio et al. 1981). The mechanism for this effect is not known.

10.4.4 Phytocannabinoids and melatonin

Melatonin is synthesized in the pineal gland during the night and plays an important role in the sleep wake cycle in mammals. Melatonin biosynthesis is controlled by norepinephrine (NE) released from sympathetic fibers that innervate the gland. NE acts through both alpha and beta receptors to increase cAMP and calcium concentrations, which regulate transcriptional and post-translational activation of the penultimate enzyme of melatonin biosynthesis, arylalkylamine N-acetyltransferase (AANAT).

A study of the effects of THC on melatonin secretion in man found that 10 mg of THC administered by smoking in mid-afternoon (when melatonin concentrations are low) produced a 30-fold increase in melatonin concentrations 1 and 2 h later in eight of nine subjects (Lissoni et al. 1986). Interestingly, the remaining subject had very high basal melatonin concentrations and THC treatment reduced melatonin concentrations in this individual. Although untested, the increase in melatonin concentrations several hours after cannabis use could contribute to the well-known crash, or sleepiness, experienced after a bout of cannabis use.

This observation has not been well studied in preclinical models. There are multiple mechanisms by which CB_1 receptor activity could regulate NE release in the pineal. Systemic administration of CB_1 receptor agonists increase the firing rate (Muntoni et al. 2006) and c fos expression (Oropeza et al. 2005; Patel and Hillard 2003) in midbrain noradrenergic neurons; and increase NE synthesis (Moranta et al. 2009) and release (Oropeza et al. 2005) in terminal regions. Thus, THC could increase melatonin release as a result of increased NE drive onto the pineal. On the other hand, immunohistochemical evidence indicates that the CB_1 receptor is expressed by NE terminals in the pineal gland (Koch et al. 2008). If the presynaptic CB_1 receptor inhibits NE release in the pineal as it does in other brain regions (Tzavara et al. 2003), then endocannabinoid-CB_1 receptor signaling could also regulate melatonin release as a result of inhibition of the release of NE in the pineal. It is tempting to speculate that the first mechanism is operative when NE drive onto the pineal is low while the second becomes more important when NE drive is high. This could explain the divergent effects of THC in the human study outlined earlier.

Incubation of primary cultures of rat pineal glands with micromolar concentrations of THC, CBD, and CBN inhibits melatonin synthesis through direct inhibition of AANAT activity (Koch et al. 2006). This effect of the phytocannabinoids is not CB receptor mediated; in fact the phytocannabinoids inhibit AANAT activity in cell free systems, suggesting a direct inhibition of the enzyme (Koch et al. 2006).

10.5 Summary

The phytocannabinoid THC can exert bidirectional effects on anxiety and mood. Considerable human and animal data support the hypothesis that THC-mediated activation of the CB_1 receptor likely contributes to the reported antianxiety and antidepressant effects of cannabis. However, excessive cannabis use during adolescence can downregulate endocannabinoid/CB_1 receptor function, which could predispose an individual to either anxiety disorders or depression. In support of this hypothesis, treatment of humans with a CB_1 receptor antagonist resulted in a significant increase in indices of anxiety, depression, and suicidal ideation in otherwise mentally healthy individuals (Hill and Gorzalka 2009b; Nissen et al. 2008). In addition, individuals with major depression exhibit reduced levels of endocannabinoids in their circulation (Hill et al. 2008, 2009c) and circulating endocannabinoid concentrations are inversely related to anxiety measures (Hill et al., 2008). Together, these findings suggest that compromised endocannabinoid signaling is sufficient to increase risk for anxiety and depression in humans, and as such, the downregulation of endocannabinoid function following excessive cannabis use could be the bridge linking excessive cannabis use with risk for these psychiatric disorders in humans.

While the effects of the phytocannabinoids on the HPA axis and reproductive hormones are well described in human and preclinical studies, we know far less about the interactions of THC and other phytocannabinoids with other endocrine systems. This is particularly striking for GH and melatonin in light of earlier findings that these hormones are significantly altered by cannabis. Since GH and melatonin are both implicated in regulation of mood and altered by stress, an untested hypothesis is that the endocannabinoids contribute to the link between these hormones and mood.

Acknowledgments

The authors wish to acknowledge the following for support during the writing of this chapter: NIH grants R01 DA026996 (CJH), K08 MH090412 (SP) and the Canadian Institutes of Health-Research Canada Research Chairs Program (MNH).

References

Ablon, S.L. and Goodwin, F.K. (1974). High frequency of dysphoric reactions to tetrahydrocannabinol among depressed patients. *American Journal of Psychiatry*, **131**, 448–453.

Amtmann, D., Weydt, P., Johnson, K.L., Jensen, M.P., and Carter, G.T. (2004). Survey of cannabis use in patients with amyotrophic lateral sclerosis. *American Journal of Hospice Palliative Care*, **21**, 95–104.

Ashton, C.H., Moore, P.B., Gallagher, P., and Young, A.H. (2005). Cannabinoids in bipolar affective disorder: a review and discussion of their therapeutic potential. *Journal of Psychopharmacology*, **19**, 293–300.

Bambico, F.R., Hattan, P.R., Garant, J.P., and Gobbi, G. (2012). Effect of delta-9-tetrahydrocannabinol on behavioral despair and on pre- and postsynaptic serotonergic transmission. *Progress in Neuro-Psychopharmacology & Biological Psychiatry*, **38**, 88–96.

Bambico, F.R., Katz, N., Debonnel, G., and Gobbi, G. (2007). Cannabinoids elicit antidepressant-like behavior and activate serotonergic neurons through the medial prefrontal cortex. *Journal of Neuroscience*, **27**, 11700–11711.

Bambico, F.R., Nguyen, N.T., Katz, N., and Gobbi, G. (2010). Chronic exposure to cannabinoids during adolescence but not during adulthood impairs emotional behaviour and monoaminergic neurotransmission. *Neurobiology of Disease*, **37**, 641–655.

Banerjee, A., Poddar, M.K., Saha, S., and Ghosh, J.J. (1975). Effect of delta9-tetrahydrocannabinol on monoamine oxidase activity of rat tissues in vivo. *Biochemical Pharmacology*, **24**, 1435–1436.

Benowitz, N.L., Jones, R.T., and Lerner, C.B. (1976). Depression of growth hormone and cortisol response to insulin-induced hypoglycemia after prolonged oral delta-9-tetrahydrocannabinol administration in man. *Journal of Clinical Endocrinology and Metabolism*, **42**, 938–941.

Bergamaschi, M.M., Queiroz, R.H., Chagas, M.H., *et al.* (2011). Cannabidiol reduces the anxiety induced by simulated public speaking in treatment-naive social phobia patients. *Neuropsychopharmacology*, **36**, 1219–1226.

Bernal, J. (2007). Thyroid hormone receptors in brain development and function. *Nature Clinical Practice Endocrinology & Metabolism*, **3**, 249–259.

Bialos, D.S. (1970). Adverse marijuana reactions: a critical examination of the literature with selected case material. *American Journal of Psychiatry*, **127**, 819–823.

Block, R.I., Farinpour, R., and Schlechte, J.A. (1991). Effects of chronic marijuana use on testosterone, luteinizing hormone, follicle stimulating hormone, prolactin and cortisol in men and women. *Drug and Alcohol Dependence*, **28**, 121–128.

Bonn-Miller, M.O., Harris, A.H., and Trafton, J.A. (2012). Prevalence of cannabis use disorder diagnoses among veterans in 2002, 2008, and 2009. *Psychological Services*, **9**, 404–416.

Bonn-Miller, M.O., Vujanovic, A.A., and Drescher, K.D. (2011). Cannabis use among military veterans after residential treatment for posttraumatic stress disorder. *Psychology of Addictive Behaviors*, **25**, 485–491.

Bonn-Miller, M.O., Zvolensky, M.J., Bernstein, A., and Stickle, T.R. (2008). Marijuana coping motives interact with marijuana use frequency to predict anxious arousal, panic related catastrophic thinking, and worry among current marijuana users. *Depression and Anxiety*, **25**, 862–873.

Bonnet, U. (2013). Chronic cannabis abuse, delta-9-tetrahydrocannabinol and thyroid function. *Pharmacopsychiatry*, **46**, 35–36.

Bovasso, G.B. (2001). Cannabis abuse as a risk factor for depressive symptoms. *American Journal of Psychiatry*, **158**, 2033–2037.

Buckner, J.D., Bonn-Miller, M.O., Zvolensky, M.J., and Schmidt, N.B. (2007). Marijuana use motives and social anxiety among marijuana-using young adults. *Addictive Behaviors*, **32**, 2238–2252.

Buckner, J.D., Schmidt, N.B., Lang, A.R., Small, J.W., Schlauch, R.C., and Lewinsohn, P.M. (2008). Specificity of social anxiety disorder as a risk factor for alcohol and cannabis dependence. *Journal of Psychiatric Research*, **42**, 230–239.

Buckner, J.D., Zvolensky, M.J., and Schmidt, N.B. (2012). Cannabis-related impairment and social anxiety: the roles of gender and cannabis use motives. *Addictive Behaviors*, **37**, 1294–1297.

Bujarski, S.J., Feldner, M.T., Lewis, S.F., *et al.* (2012a). Marijuana use among traumatic event-exposed adolescents: posttraumatic stress symptom frequency predicts coping motivations for use. *Addictive Behaviors*, **37**, 53–59.

Bujarski, S.J., Norberg, M.M., and Copeland, J. (2012b). The association between distress tolerance and cannabis use-related problems: the mediating and moderating roles of coping motives and gender. *Addictive Behaviors*, **37**, 1181–1184.

Calhoun, P.S., Sampson, W.S., Bosworth, H.B., *et al.* (2000). Drug use and validity of substance use self-reports in veterans seeking help for posttraumatic stress disorder. *Journal of Consulting and Clinical Psychology*, **68**, 923–927.

Campos, A.C., Ortega, Z., Palazuelos, J., *et al.* (2013). The anxiolytic effect of cannabidiol on chronically stressed mice depends on hippocampal neurogenesis: involvement of the endocannabinoid system. *International Journal of Neuropsychopharmacology*, **16**, 1407–1419.

Chabrol, H., Duconge, E., Casas, C., Roura, C., and Carey, K.B. (2005). Relations between cannabis use and dependence, motives for cannabis use and anxious, depressive and borderline symptomatology. *Addictive Behaviors*, **30**, 829–840.

Chen, C.Y., Wagner, F.A., and Anthony, J.C. (2002). Marijuana use and the risk of major depressive episode. Epidemiological evidence from the United States National Comorbidity Survey. *Social Psychiatry and Psychiatric Epidemiology*, **37**, 199–206.

Chhatwal, J.P., Gutman, A.R., Maguschak, K.A., *et al.* (2009). Functional interactions between endocannabinoid and CCK neurotransmitter systems may be critical for extinction learning. *Neuropsychopharmacology*, **34**, 509–521.

Cone, E.J., Johnson, R.E., Moore, J.D., and Roache, J.D. (1986). Acute effects of smoking marijuana on hormones, subjective effects and performance in male human subjects. *Pharmacology Biochemistry and Behavior*, **24**, 1749–1754.

Cornelius, J.R., Kirisci, L., Reynolds, M., Clark, D.B., Hayes, J., and Tarter, R. (2010). PTSD contributes to teen and young adult cannabis use disorders. *Addictive Behaviors*, **35**, 91–94.

Cougle, J.R., Bonn-Miller, M.O., Vujanovic, A.A., Zvolensky, M.J., and Hawkins, K.A. (2011). Posttraumatic stress disorder and cannabis use in a nationally representative sample. *Psychology of Addictive Behaviors*, **25**, 554–558.

Crippa, J.A., Derenusson, G.N., Ferrari, T.B., *et al.* (2011). Neural basis of anxiolytic effects of cannabidiol (CBD) in generalized social anxiety disorder: a preliminary report. *Journal of Psychopharmacology*, **25**, 121–130.

Crippa, J.A., Zuardi, A.W., Martin-Santos, R., *et al.* (2009). Cannabis and anxiety: a critical review of the evidence. *Human Psychopharmacology*, **24**, 515–523.

D'Souza, D.C., Perry, E., MacDougall, L., *et al.* (2004). The psychotomimetic effects of intravenous delta-9-tetrahydrocannabinol in healthy individuals: implications for psychosis. *Neuropsychopharmacology*, **29**, 1558–1572.

D'Souza, D.C., Ranganathan, M., Braley, G., *et al.* (2008). Blunted psychotomimetic and amnestic effects of delta-9-tetrahydrocannabinol in frequent users of cannabis. *Neuropsychopharmacology*, **33**, 2505–2516.

Dalterio, S.L., Mayfield, D.L., Michael, S.D., Macmillan, B.T., and Bartke, A. (1983). Effects of delta 9-THC and castration on behavior and plasma hormone levels in male mice. *Pharmacology Biochemistry and Behavior*, **18**, 81–86.

Dalterio, S.L., Michael, S.D., Macmillan, B.T., and Bartke, A. (1981). Differential effects of cannabinoid exposure and stress on plasma prolactin, growth hormone and corticosterone levels in male mice. *Life Sciences*, **28**, 761–766.

Dannon, P.N., Lowengrub, K., Amiaz, R., Grunhaus, L., and Kotler, M. (2004). Comorbid cannabis use and panic disorder: short term and long term follow-up study. *Human Psychopharmacology*, **19**, 97–101.

Das, R.K., Kamboj, S.K., Ramadas, M., *et al.* (2013). Cannabidiol enhances consolidation of explicit fear extinction in humans. *Psychopharmacology*, **226**, 781–792.

de Bitencourt, R.M., Pamplona, F.A., and Takahashi, R.N. (2013). A current overview of cannabinoids and glucocorticoids in facilitating extinction of aversive memories: potential extinction enhancers. *Neuropharmacology*, **64**, 389–395.

Deas, D., Gerding, L., and Hazy, J. (2000). Marijuana and panic disorder. *Journal of the American Academy of Child and Adolescent Psychiatry*, **39**, 1467.

Degenhardt, L., Hall, W., and Lynskey, M. (2003). Exploring the association between cannabis use and depression. *Addiction*, **98**, 1493–1504.

Deli, L., Wittmann, G., Kallo, I., *et al.* (2009). Type 1 cannabinoid receptor-containing axons innervate hypophysiotropic thyrotropin-releasing hormone-synthesizing neurons. *Endocrinology*, **150**, 98–103.

Denson, T.F. and Earleywine, M. (2006). Decreased depression in marijuana users. *Addictive Behaviors*, **31**, 738–742.

Di, S., Malcher-Lopes, R., Halmos, K.C., and Tasker, J.G. (2003). Nongenomic glucocorticoid inhibition via endocannabinoid release in the hypothalamus: a fast feedback mechanism. *Journal of Neuroscience*, **23**, 4850–4857.

Egashira, N., Matsuda, T., Koushi, E., *et al.* (2008). Delta(9)-tetrahydrocannabinol prolongs the immobility time in the mouse forced swim test: Involvement of cannabinoid CB(1) receptor and serotonergic system. *European Journal of Pharmacology*, **589**, 117–121.

El-Alfy, A.T., Ivey, K., Robinson, K., *et al.* (2010). Antidepressant-like effect of delta9-tetrahydrocannabinol and other cannabinoids isolated from *Cannabis sativa* L. *Pharmacology Biochemistry and Behavior*, **95**, 434–442.

Elbatsh, M.M., Moklas, M.A., Marsden, C.A., and Kendall, D.A. (2012). Antidepressant-like effects of Delta(9)-tetrahydrocannabinol and rimonabant in the olfactory bulbectomised rat model of depression. *Pharmacology Biochemistry and Behavior*, **102**, 357–365.

Evanson, N.K., Tasker, J.G., Hill, M.N., Hillard, C.J., and Herman, J.P. (2010). Fast feedback inhibition of the HPA axis by glucocorticoids is mediated by endocannabinoid signaling. *Endocrinology*, **151**, 4811–4819.

Fairman, B.J. and Anthony, J.C. (2012). Are early-onset cannabis smokers at an increased risk of depression spells? *Journal of Affective Disorders*, **138**, 54–62.

Falkenstein, B.A. and Holley, D.C. (1992). Effect of acute intravenous administration of delta-9-tetrahydrocannabinol on the episodic secretion of immunoassayable growth hormone in the rat. *Life Sciences*, **50**, 1109–1116.

Fisar, Z. (2010). Inhibition of monoamine oxidase activity by cannabinoids. *Naunyn-Schmiedeberg's Archives of Pharmacology*, **381**, 563–572.

Flamant, F., Gauthier, K., and Samarut, J. (2007). Thyroid hormones signaling is getting more complex: STORMs are coming. *Molecular Endocrinology*, **21**, 321–333.

Fox, C.L., Towe, S.L., Stephens, R.S., Walker, D.D., and Roffman, R.A. (2011). Motives for cannabis use in high-risk adolescent users. *Psychology of Addictive Behaviors*, **25**, 492–500.

Fraser, G.A. (2009). The use of a synthetic cannabinoid in the management of treatment-resistant nightmares in posttraumatic stress disorder (PTSD). *CNS Neuroscience & Therapeutics*, **15**, 84–88.

Ganon-Elazar, E. and Akirav, I. (2009). Cannabinoid receptor activation in the basolateral amygdala blocks the effects of stress on the conditioning and extinction of inhibitory avoidance. *Journal of Neuroscience*, **29**, 11078–10788.

Gomes, F.V., Resstel, L.B., and Guimaraes, F.S. (2011). The anxiolytic-like effects of cannabidiol injected into the bed nucleus of the stria terminalis are mediated by 5-HT1A receptors. *Psychopharmacology (Berlin)*, **213**, 465–473.

Gorzalka, B.B. and Hill, M.N. (2011). Putative role of endocannabinoid signaling in the etiology of depression and actions of antidepressants. *Progress in Neuro-Psychopharmacology and Biological Psychiatry*, **35**, 1575–1585.

Green, B.E. and Ritter, C. (2000). Marijuana use and depression. *Journal of Health and Social Behavior*, **41**, 40–49.

Gruber, A.J., Pope, H.G., Jr., and Brown, M.E. (1996). Do patients use marijuana as an antidepressant? *Depression*, **4**, 77–80.

Gunduz-Cinar, O., Macpherson, K.P., Cinar, R., et al. (2013). Convergent translational evidence of a role for anandamide in amygdala-mediated fear extinction, threat processing and stress-reactivity. *Molecular Psychiatry*, **18**, 813–823.

Halikas, J.A., Goodwin, D.W., and Guze, S.B. (1971). Marihuana effects. A survey of regular users. *JAMA*, **217**, 692–694.

Harder, V.S., Morral, A.R., and Arkes, J. (2006). Marijuana use and depression among adults: Testing for causal associations. *Addiction*, **101**, 1463–1472.

Haring, M., Grieb, M., Monory, K., Lutz, B., and Moreira, F.A. (2013). Cannabinoid CB(1) receptor in the modulation of stress coping behavior in mice: the role of serotonin and different forebrain neuronal subpopulations. *Neuropharmacology*, **65**, 83–89.

Hayatbakhsh, M.R., Najman, J.M., Jamrozik, K., Mamun, A.A., Alati, R., and Bor, W. (2007). Cannabis and anxiety and depression in young adults: a large prospective study. *Journal of the American Academy of Child and Adolescent Psychiatry*, **46**, 408–417.

Hayatbakhsh, R., Williams, G.M., Bor, W., and Najman, J.M. (2013). Early childhood predictors of age of initiation to use of cannabis: a birth prospective study. *Drug and Alcohol Review*, **32**, 232–240.

Heim, C. and Nemeroff, C.B. (2001). The role of childhood trauma in the neurobiology of mood and anxiety disorders: preclinical and clinical studies. *Biological Psychiatry*, **49**, 1023–1039.

Hill, M.N. and Gorzalka, B.B. (2004). Enhancement of anxiety-like responsiveness to the cannabinoid CB(1) receptor agonist HU-210 following chronic stress. *European Journal of Pharmacology*, **499**, 291–295.

Hill, M.N. and Gorzalka, B.B. (2006). Increased sensitivity to restraint stress and novelty-induced emotionality following long-term, high dose cannabinoid exposure. *Psychoneuroendocrinology*, **31**, 526–536.

Hill, M.N. and Gorzalka, B.B. (2009a). The endocannabinoid system and the treatment of mood and anxiety disorders. *CNS & Neurological Disorders Drug Targets*, **8**, 451–458.

Hill, M.N. and Gorzalka, B.B. (2009b). Impairments in endocannabinoid signaling and depressive illness. *JAMA*, **301**, 1165–1166.

Hill, M.N., Hillard, C.J., Bambico, F.R., Patel, S., Gorzalka, B.B., and Gobbi, G. (2009a). The therapeutic potential of the endocannabinoid system for the development of a novel class of antidepressants. *Trends in Pharmacological Sciences*, **30**, 484–493.

Hill, M.N., Karatsoreos, I.N., Hillard, C.J., and McEwen, B.S. (2010). Rapid elevations in limbic endocannabinoid content by glucocorticoid hormones in vivo. *Psychoneuroendocrinology*, **35**, 1333–1338.

Hill, M.N., McLaughlin, R.J., Morrish, A.C., *et al.* (2009b). Suppression of amygdalar endocannabinoid signaling by stress contributes to activation of the hypothalamic-pituitary-adrenal axis. *Neuropsychopharmacology*, **34**, 2733–2745.

Hill, M.N., Miller, G.E., Carrier, E.J., Gorzalka, B.B., and Hillard, C.J. (2009c). Circulating endocannabinoids and N-acyl ethanolamines are differentially regulated in major depression and following exposure to social stress. *Psychoneuroendocrinology*, **34**, 1257–1262.

Hill, M.N., Miller, G.E., Ho, W.S., Gorzalka, B.B., and Hillard, C.J. (2008). Serum endocannabinoid content is altered in females with depressive disorders: a preliminary report. *Pharmacopsychiatry*, **41**, 48–53.

Hillard, C.J., Farber, N.E., Hagen, T.C., and Bloom, A.S. (1984). The effects of delta 9-tetrahydrocannabinol on serum thyrotropin levels in the rat. *Pharmacology Biochemistry and Behavior*, **20**, 547–550.

Holsboer, F. (2000). The corticosteroid receptor hypothesis of depression. *Neuropsychopharmacology*, **23**, 477–501.

Huizink, A.C. and Mulder, E.J. (2006). Maternal smoking, drinking or cannabis use during pregnancy and neurobehavioral and cognitive functioning in human offspring. *Neuroscience & Biobehavioral Reviews*, **30**, 24–41.

Hyman, S.M. and Sinha, R. (2009). Stress-related factors in cannabis use and misuse: implications for prevention and treatment. *Journal of Substance Abuse Treatment*, **36**, 400–413.

Joffe, R.T. (2011). Hormone treatment of depression. *Dialogues in Clinical Neuroscience*, **13**, 127–138.

Kaplan, H.B., Martin, S.S., Johnson, R.J., and Robbins, C.A. (1986). Escalation of marijuana use: application of a general theory of deviant behavior. *Journal of Health and Social Behavior*, **27**, 44–61.

Karschner, E.L., Darwin, W.D., McMahon, R.P., *et al.* (2011). Subjective and physiological effects after controlled Sativex and oral THC administration. *Clinical Pharmacology & Therapeutics*, **89**, 400–407.

Kathuria, S., Gaetani, S., Fegley, D., *et al.* (2003). Modulation of anxiety through blockade of anandamide hydrolysis. *Nature Medicine*, **9**, 76–81.

Khare, M., Taylor, A.H., Konje, J.C., and Bell, S.C. (2006). Delta9-tetrahydrocannabinol inhibits cytotrophoblast cell proliferation and modulates gene transcription. *Molecular Human Reproduction*, **12**, 321–333.

King, G.R., Ernst, T., Deng, W., *et al.* (2011). Altered brain activation during visuomotor integration in chronic active cannabis users: relationship to cortisol levels. *Journal of Neuroscience*, **31**, 17923–17931.

Kinsey, S.G., O'Neal, S.T., Long, J.Z., Cravatt, B.F., and Lichtman, A.H. (2011). Inhibition of endocannabinoid catabolic enzymes elicits anxiolytic-like effects in the marble burying assay. *Pharmacology Biochemistry and Behavior*, **98**, 21–27.

Kleinloog, D., Liem-Moolenaar, M., Jacobs, G., *et al.* (2012). Does olanzapine inhibit the psychomimetic effects of Delta(9)-tetrahydrocannabinol? *Journal of Psychopharmacology*, **26**, 1307–1316.

Klumpers, L.E., Cole, D.M., Khalili-Mahani, N., *et al.* (2012). Manipulating brain connectivity with delta(9)-tetrahydrocannabinol: a pharmacological resting state FMRI study. *Neuroimage*, **63**, 1701–1711.

Koch, M., Dehghani, F., Habazettl, I., Schomerus, C., and Korf, H.W. (2006). Cannabinoids attenuate norepinephrine-induced melatonin biosynthesis in the rat pineal gland by reducing arylalkylamine N-acetyltransferase activity without involvement of cannabinoid receptors. *Journal of Neurochemistry*, **98**, 267–278.

Koch, M., Habazettl, I., Dehghani, F., and Korf, H.W. (2008). The rat pineal gland comprises an endocannabinoid system. *Journal of Pineal Research*, **45**, 351–360.

Kokka, N. and Garcia, J.F. (1974). Effects of delta 9-THC on growth hormone and ACTH secretion in rats. *Life Sciences*, **15**, 329–338.

Kotin, J., Post, R.M., and Goodwin, F.K. (1973). Delta9-tetrahydrocannabinol in depressed patients. *Archives of General Psychiatry*, **28**, 345–348.

Lahat, A., Lang, A., and Ben-Horin, S. (2012). Impact of cannabis treatment on the quality of life, weight and clinical disease activity in inflammatory bowel disease patients: a pilot prospective study. *Digestion*, **85**, 1–8.

Langs, G., Fabisch, H., Fabisch, K., and Zapotoczky, H. (1997). Can cannabis trigger recurrent panic attacks in susceptible patients? *European Psychiatry*, **12**, 415–419.

Lin, H.C., Mao, S.C., Su, C.L., and Gean, P.W. (2009). The role of prefrontal cortex CB_1 receptors in the modulation of fear memory. *Cerebral Cortex*, **19**, 165–175.

Lissoni, P., Resentini, M., Mauri, R., *et al.* (1986). Effects of tetrahydrocannabinol on melatonin secretion in man. *Hormone and Metabolic Research*, **18**, 77–78.

Lutz, B. (2007). The endocannabinoid system and extinction learning. *Molecular Neurobiology*, **36**, 92–101.

Lynskey, M.T., Glowinski, A.L., Todorov, A.A., *et al.* (2004). Major depressive disorder, suicidal ideation, and suicide attempt in twins discordant for cannabis dependence and early-onset cannabis use. *Archives of General Psychiatry*, **61**, 1026–1032.

Marsicano, G., Wotjak, C.T., Azad, S.C., *et al.* (2002). The endogenous cannabinoid system controls extinction of aversive memories. *Nature*, **418**, 530–534.

Martin-Calderon, J.L., Munoz, R.M., Villanua, M.A., *et al.* (1998). Characterization of the acute endocrine actions of (-)-11-hydroxy-delta8-tetrahydrocannabinol-dimethylheptyl (HU-210), a potent synthetic cannabinoid in rats. *European Journal of Pharmacology*, **344**, 77–86.

Martin-Santos, R., Crippa, J.A., Batalla, A., *et al.* (2012). Acute effects of a single, oral dose of Δ^9-tetrahydrocannabinol (THC) and cannabidiol (CBD) administration in healthy volunteers. *Current Pharmaceutical Design*, **18**, 4966–4979.

McLaughlin, R.J., Hill, M.N., Bambico, F.R., *et al.* (2012). Prefrontal cortical anandamide signaling coordinates coping responses to stress through a serotonergic pathway. *European Neuropsychopharmacology*, **22**, 664–671.

McLaughlin, R.J., Hill, M.N., and Gorzalka, B.B. (2009). Monoaminergic neurotransmission contributes to cannabinoid-induced activation of the hypothalamic-pituitary-adrenal axis. *European Journal of Pharmacology*, **624**, 71–76.

Mechoulam, R., Parker, L.A., and Gallily, R. (2002). Cannabidiol: an overview of some pharmacological aspects. *Journal of Clinical Pharmacology*, **42**, 11S–19S.

Moranta, D., Esteban, S., and Garcia-Sevilla, J.A. (2009). Chronic treatment and withdrawal of the cannabinoid agonist WIN 55,212-2 modulate the sensitivity of presynaptic receptors involved in the regulation of monoamine syntheses in rat brain. *Naunyn Schmiedebergs Arch Pharmacol*, **379**, 61–72.

Moreira, F.A. and Wotjak, C.T. (2010). Cannabinoids and anxiety. *Current Topics in Behavioral Neurosciences*, **2**, 429–450.

Muntoni, A.L., Pillolla, G., Melis, M., Perra, S., Gessa, G.L., and Pistis, M. (2006). Cannabinoids modulate spontaneous neuronal activity and evoked inhibition of locus coeruleus noradrenergic neurons. *European Journal of Neuroscience*, **23**, 2385–2394.

Natelson, B.H., Holaday, J., Meyerhoff, J., and Stokes, P.E. (1975). Temporal changes in growth hormone, cortisol, and glucose: relation to light onset and behavior. *American Journal of Physiology*, **229**, 409–415.

Nazar, B., Kairys, D.J., Fowler, R., and Harclerode, J. (1977). Effects of delta9-tetrahydrocannabinol on serum thyroxine concentrations in the rat. *Journal of Pharmacology and Pharmacotherapeutics*, **29**, 778–779.

Neumeister, A. (2013). The endocannabinoid system provides an avenue for evidence-based treatment development for PTSD. *Depression and Anxiety*, **30**, 93–96.

Nissen, S.E., Nicholls, S.J., Wolski, K., *et al.* (2008). Effect of rimonabant on progression of atherosclerosis in patients with abdominal obesity and coronary artery disease: the STRADIVARIUS randomized controlled trial. *JAMA*, **299**, 1547–1560.

Ohara, N., Tsujino, T., and Maruo, T. (2004). The role of thyroid hormone in trophoblast function, early pregnancy maintenance, and fetal neurodevelopment. *Journal of Obstetrics and Gynaecology Canada*, **26**, 982–990.

Oropeza, V.C., Page, M.E., and Van Bockstaele, E.J. (2005). Systemic administration of WIN 55,212-2 increases norepinephrine release in the rat frontal cortex. *Brain Research*, **1046**, 45–54.

Page, S.A., Verhoef, M.J., Stebbins, R.A., Metz, L.M., and Levy, J.C. (2003). Cannabis use as described by people with multiple sclerosis. *Canadian Journal of Neurological Sciences*, **30**, 201–205.

Pagotto, U., Marsicano, G., Fezza, F., *et al.* (2001). Normal human pituitary gland and pituitary adenomas express cannabinoid receptor type 1 and synthesize endogenous cannabinoids: first evidence for a direct role of cannabinoids on hormone modulation at the human pituitary level. *Journal of Clinical Endocrinology and Metabolism*, **86**, 2687–2696.

Pamplona, F.A., Bitencourt, R.M., and Takahashi, R.N. (2008). Short- and long-term effects of cannabinoids on the extinction of contextual fear memory in rats. *Neurobiology of Learning and Memory*, **90**, 290–293.

Passie, T., Emrich, H.M., Karst, M., Brandt, S.D., and Halpern, J.H. (2012). Mitigation of post-traumatic stress symptoms by *Cannabis* resin: a review of the clinical and neurobiological evidence. *Drug Testing and Analysis*, **4**, 649–659.

Patel, S., Cravatt, B.F., and Hillard, C.J. (2005). Synergistic interactions between cannabinoids and environmental stress in the activation of the central amygdala. *Neuropsychopharmacology*, **30**, 497–507.

Patel, S. and Hillard, C.J. (2003). Cannabinoid-induced Fos expression within A10 dopaminergic neurons. *Brain Research*, **963**, 15–25.

Patel, S. and Hillard, C.J. (2006). Pharmacological evaluation of cannabinoid receptor ligands in a mouse model of anxiety: further evidence for an anxiolytic role for endogenous cannabinoid signaling. *Journal of Pharmacology and Experimental Therapeutics*, **318**, 304–311.

Patel, S., Roelke, C.T., Rademacher, D.J., Cullinan, W.E., and Hillard, C.J. (2004). Endocannabinoid signaling negatively modulates stress-induced activation of the hypothalamic-pituitary-adrenal axis. *Endocrinology*, **145**, 5431–5438.

Patton, G.C., Coffey, C., Carlin, J.B., Degenhardt, L., Lynskey, M., and Hall, W. (2002). Cannabis use and mental health in young people: cohort study. *BMJ*, **325**, 1195–1198.

Porcella, A., Marchese, G., Casu, M.A., *et al.* (2002). Evidence for functional CB1 cannabinoid receptor expressed in the rat thyroid. *European Journal of Endocrinology*, **147**, 255–261.

Potter, C.M., Vujanovic, A.A., Marshall-Berenz, E.C., Bernstein, A., and Bonn-Miller, M.O. (2011). Posttraumatic stress and marijuana use coping motives: the mediating role of distress tolerance. *Journal of Anxiety Disorders*, **25**, 437–443.

Ranganathan, M., Braley, G., Pittman, B., *et al.* (2009). The effects of cannabinoids on serum cortisol and prolactin in humans. *Psychopharmacology (Berlin)*, **203**, 737–744.

Realini, N., Vigano, D., Guidali, C., Zamberletti, E., Rubino, T., and Parolaro, D. (2011). Chronic URB597 treatment at adulthood reverted most depressive-like symptoms induced by adolescent exposure to THC in female rats. *Neuropharmacology*, **60**, 235–243.

Reilly, D., Didcott, P., Swift, W., and Hall, W. (1998). Long-term cannabis use: characteristics of users in an Australian rural area. *Addiction*, **93**, 837–846.

Rettori, V., Aguila, M.C., Gimeno, M.F., Franchi, A.M., and McCann, S.M. (1990). In vitro effect of delta 9-tetrahydrocannabinol to stimulate somatostatin release and block that of luteinizing hormone-releasing hormone by suppression of the release of prostaglandin E2. *Proceedings of the National Academy of Sciences of the United States of America*, **87**, 10063–10066.

Rettori, V., Wenger, T., Snyder, G., Dalterio, S., and McCann, S.M. (1988). Hypothalamic action of delta-9-tetrahydrocannabinol to inhibit the release of prolactin and growth hormone in the rat. *Neuroendocrinology*, **47**, 498–503.

Rey, A.A., Purrio, M., Viveros, M.P., and Lutz, B. (2012). Biphasic effects of cannabinoids in anxiety responses: CB_1 and GABA(B) receptors in the balance of GABAergic and glutamatergic neurotransmission. *Neuropsychopharmacology*, **37**, 2624–2634.

Rosenkrantz, H. and Esber, H.J. (1980). Cannabinoid-induced hormone changes in monkeys and rats. *Journal of Toxicology and Environmental Health*, **6**, 297–313.

Rubino, T., Guidali, C., Vigano, D., *et al.* (2008). CB_1 receptor stimulation in specific brain areas differently modulate anxiety-related behaviour. *Neuropharmacology*, **54**, 151–160.

Rubino, T., Realini, N., Braida, D., *et al.* (2009). The depressive phenotype induced in adult female rats by adolescent exposure to THC is associated with cognitive impairment and altered neuroplasticity in the prefrontal cortex. *Neurotoxicity Research*, **15**, 291–302.

Ruehle, S., Rey, A.A., Remmers, F., and Lutz, B. (2012). The endocannabinoid system in anxiety, fear memory and habituation. *Journal of Psychopharmacology*, **26**, 23–39.

Rush, A.J., Giles, D.E., Schlesser, M.A., *et al.* (1996). The dexamethasone suppression test in patients with mood disorders. *Journal of Clinical Psychiatry*, **57**, 470–484.

Russo, E.B. (2011). Taming THC: potential cannabis synergy and phytocannabinoid-terpenoid entourage effects. *British Journal of Pharmacology*, **163**, 1344–1364.

Saber-Tehrani, A., Naderi, N., Hosseini Najarkolaei, A., Haghparast, A., and Motamedi, F. (2010). Cannabinoids and their interactions with diazepam on modulation of serum corticosterone concentration in male mice. *Neurochemical Research*, **35**, 60–66.

Sano, K., Koushi, E., Irie, K., *et al.* (2009). Delta(9)-tetrahydrocannabinol enhances an increase of plasma corticosterone levels induced by forced swim-stress. *Biological & Pharmaceutical Bulletin*, **32**, 2065–2067.

Sciolino, N.R., Zhou, W., and Hohmann, A.G. (2011). Enhancement of endocannabinoid signaling with JZL184, an inhibitor of the 2-arachidonoylglycerol hydrolyzing enzyme monoacylglycerol lipase, produces anxiolytic effects under conditions of high environmental aversiveness in rats. *Pharmacology Research*, **64**, 226–234.

Shearman, L.P., Rosko, K.M., Fleischer, R., *et al.* (2003). Antidepressant-like and anorectic effects of the cannabinoid CB_1 receptor inverse agonist AM251 in mice. *Behavioural Pharmacology*, **14**, 573–582.

Somaini, L., Manfredini, M., Amore, M., *et al.* (2012). Psychobiological responses to unpleasant emotions in cannabis users. *European Archives of Psychiatry and Clinical Neurosciences*, **262**, 47–57.

Steiner, M.A. and Wotjak, C.T. (2008). Role of the endocannabinoid system in regulation of the hypothalamic-pituitary-adrenocortical axis. *Progress in Brain Research*, **170**, 397–432.

Sumislawski, J.J., Ramikie, T.S., and Patel, S. (2011). Reversible gating of endocannabinoid plasticity in the amygdala by chronic stress: a potential role for monoacylglycerol lipase inhibition in the prevention of stress-induced behavioral adaptation. *Neuropsychopharmacology*, **36**, 2750–2761.

Takahashi, Y., Kipnis, D.M., and Daughaday, W.H. (1968). Growth hormone secretion during sleep. *Journal of Clinical Investigation*, **47**, 2079–20790.

Thomas, H. (1993). Psychiatric symptoms in cannabis users. *British Journal of Psychiatry*, **163**, 141–149.

Thomas, H. (1996). A community survey of adverse effects of cannabis use. *Drug and Alcohol Dependence*, **42**, 201–207.

Tzavara, E.T., Davis, R.J., Perry, K.W., *et al.* (2003). The CB_1 receptor antagonist SR141716A selectively increases monoaminergic neurotransmission in the medial prefrontal cortex: implications for therapeutic actions. *British Journal of Pharmacology*, **138**, 544–553.

Uribe-Marino, A., Francisco, A., Castiblanco-Urbina, M.A., *et al.* (2012). Anti-aversive effects of cannabidiol on innate fear-induced behaviors evoked by an ethological model of panic attacks based on a prey vs the wild snake *Epicrates cenchria crassus* confrontation paradigm. *Neuropsychopharmacology*, **37**, 412–421.

Van Dam, N.T., Bedi, G., and Earleywine, M. (2012). Characteristics of clinically anxious versus non-anxious regular, heavy marijuana users. *Addictive Behaviors*, **37**, 1217–1223.

van Leeuwen, A.P., Verhulst, F.C., Reijneveld, S.A., Vollebergh, W.A., Ormel, J., and Huizink, A.C. (2011). Can the gateway hypothesis, the common liability model and/or, the route of administration model predict initiation of cannabis use during adolescence? A survival analysis – the TRAILS study. *Journal of Adolescent Health*, **48**, 73–78.

Veiga, M., Bloise, F., Costa, E.S.R., *et al.* (2008). Acute effects of endocannabinoid anandamide and CB_1 receptor antagonist, AM251 in the regulation of thyrotropin secretion. *Journal of Endocrinology*, **199**, 235–242.

Ware, M.A., Adams, H., and Guy, G.W. (2005). The medicinal use of cannabis in the UK: results of a nationwide survey. *International Journal of Clinical Practice*, **59**, 291–295.

Williamson, E.M. and Evans, F.J. (2000). Cannabinoids in clinical practice. *Drugs*, **60**, 1303–1314.

Woolridge, E., Barton, S., Samuel, J., Osorio, J., Dougherty, A., and Holdcroft, A. (2005). Cannabis use in HIV for pain and other medical symptoms. *Journal of Pain and Symptom Management*, **29**, 358–367.

Zanelati, T.V., Biojone, C., Moreira, F.A., Guimaraes, F.S., and Joca, S.R. (2010). Antidepressant-like effects of cannabidiol in mice: possible involvement of 5-HT1A receptors. *British Journal of Pharmacology*, **159**, 122–128.

Zuardi, A.W., Guimaraes, F.S., and Moreira, A.C. (1993). Effect of cannabidiol on plasma prolactin, growth hormone and cortisol in human volunteers. *Brazilian Journal of Medical and Biological Research*, **26**, 213–217.

Zuardi, A.W., Shirakawa, I., Finkelfarb, E., and Karniol, I.G. (1982). Action of cannabidiol on the anxiety and other effects produced by delta 9-THC in normal subjects. *Psychopharmacology (Berlin)*, **76**, 245–250.

Zuardi, A.W., Teixeira, N.A., and Karniol, I.C. (1984). Pharmacological interaction of the effects of delta 9-trans-tetrahydrocannabinol and cannabidiol on serum corticosterone levels in rats. *Archives internationales de pharmacodynamie et de thérapie*, **269**, 12–19.

Zuckerman, B., Frank, D.A., Hingson, R., *et al.* (1989). Effects of maternal marijuana and cocaine use on fetal growth. *New England Journal of Medicine*, **320**, 762–768.

Zvolensky, M.J., Bernstein, A., Sachs-Ericsson, N., Schmidt, N.B., Buckner, J.D., and Bonn-Miller, M.O. (2006). Lifetime associations between cannabis, use, abuse, and dependence and panic attacks in a representative sample. *Journal of Psychiatric Research*, **40**, 477–486.

Zvolensky, M.J., Lewinsohn, P., Bernstein, A., *et al.* (2008). Prospective associations between cannabis use, abuse, and dependence and panic attacks and disorder. *Journal of Psychiatric Research*, **42**, 1017–1023.

Chapter 11

Phytocannabinoids and the Cardiovascular System

Saoirse E. O'Sullivan

11.1 Introduction

The plethora of ailments for which cannabis was taken historically included atherosclerosis, cardiac palpitations, and hypertension (see Lambert 2001; Zuardi 2006), implying actions on the cardiovascular system, which have been investigated scientifically since the 1970s. Most studies have investigated the effects of delta-9-tetrahydrocannabinol (THC) or cannabis/marijuana smoking, and few studies have documented the cardiovascular effects of some of the lesser known phytocannabinoids. In vivo studies revealed a complex response to THC/cannabis, dependent on whether the studies were carried out under anesthesia, and in what species. Later studies looked at the direct effects of phytocannabinoids, primarily THC, on isolated preparations of the heart, whole vascular beds, and individual arteries, again revealing complex actions of phytocannabinoids in the vasculature. In Chapter 11, the effects of phytocannabinoids under these various experimental conditions will be discussed and summarized. This chapter will conclude with an overall summary and identification of gaps in our current knowledge in this area.

11.2 Acute in vivo cardiovascular responses to phytocannabinoids

11.2.1 In vivo responses to THC in anesthetized animals

Early studies examined the hemodynamic response (the forces involved in the circulation of blood) to THC in anesthetized animals. In anesthetized dogs, THC (2.5 mg/kg, intravenously (i.v.)) causes a decrease in heart rate (bradycardia), blood pressure, and peripheral vascular resistance 15–30 min post administration (Jandhyala et al. 1976). A similar response was seen in anesthetized rats, where administration of THC (up to 30 mg/kg, i.v.) caused an initial pressor (increase in blood pressure) effect (<1 min) followed by a depressor (decrease in blood pressure) effect accompanied by bradycardia (Adams et al. 1976). Estrada et al. (1987) also reported a bradycardic and depressor response to THC (up to 5 mg/kg, i.v.) in anesthetized rats. Siqueira et al. (1979) found a more complex triphasic response to THC (2–10 mg/kg, i.v.) with an immediate and short-lived decrease in blood pressure, a brief hypertensive response, and then a longer-lasting hypotensive response. Bradycardic and depressor responses to i.v. administration of THC have also been observed in anesthetized cats (1 mg/kg, i.v.) (Innemee et al. 1979) and anesthetized pregnant sheep (1 mg/kg, pulmonary artery infusion) (Cotterill et al. 1984).

11.2.1.1 Mechanism of action

The bradycardic response to THC is reported to be due to changes in the autonomic nervous system. Cavero et al. (1973) showed that blockade of either parasympathetic or sympathetic activity to the heart partially prevented the bradycardia induced by THC in anesthetized dogs (up to 5 mg/kg, i.v), and that blockade of both pathways completely abolished the bradycardic effects of THC. When the hearts of anesthetized dogs were paced to eliminate the effects of bradycardia, the reduction in blood pressure and total peripheral resistance were not altered (Jandhyala et al. 1976). This suggests that the effect of THC on blood pressure is not solely due to changes in heart rate. However, Siqueira et al. (1979) found the immediate fall in blood pressure was due to bradycardia and was vagally mediated, while the long-lasting hypotensive response to THC was due to inhibition of the sympathetic nervous system, as evidenced by its inhibition by pithing, sympathetic ganglion blockade, and alpha adrenergic inhibition. Under anesthesia, other cannabinoids have been shown to inhibit norepinephrine release from postganglionic sympathetic axons (Niederhoffer and Szabo 1999; Varga et al. 1996). Together, this suggests that the blood pressure response to THC in anesthetized animals has an early vagal component related to the fall in heart rate, and a longer-lasting component related to inhibition of the sympathetic nervous system.

Other mechanisms of action may also contribute to the hemodynamic responses to THC. Burstein and colleagues (1982) showed that aspirin, a cyclooxygenase (COX) inhibitor, significantly reduced the hypotensive effect of THC (0.45 mg/kg, i.v.), and also to a lesser extent the reduction in heart rate. More recently, it was shown that the bradycardic and depressor effect of THC (0.2 mg/kg, i.v.) in anesthetized rats is inhibited by systemic or hindbrain administration of a COX inhibitor (Krowicki 2012). These studies suggest that vasoactive prostaglandins produced by THC may play a role in in vivo responses. The production of vasoactive prostaglandins is a mechanism of action also proposed for some of the direct actions of THC in isolated vascular preparations (see section 11.5.1).

In 1997, Lake et al. showed that THC (4 mg/kg, i.v.) in anesthetized rats causes a brief pressor response followed by hypotension and bradycardia. These hemodynamic responses to THC, except the brief pressor response, were all inhibited by a CB_1 receptor antagonist. Although earlier studies didn't have the pharmacological tools to assess a potential role for cannabinoid receptors, it might be assumed that the universally observed bradycardic and depressor response to THC in anesthetized animals might also be CB_1 mediated.

11.2.1.2 The effects of THC on regional blood flow in anesthetized animals

Observations that cannabis smoking might have beneficial effects in glaucoma led several investigators to look at the effects of THC on intraocular blood pressure. In anesthetized rabbits, i.v. THC increased total eye blood flow by about 12% (Green et al. 1978). THC (up to 1 mg/kg, i.v.) also decreased intraocular pressure in anesthetized cats (Innemee et al. 1979). Other vascular beds/arteries that have increased blood flow after THC administration in anesthetized animals include the pulmonary artery (Jandhyala et al. 1976) and umbilical artery (Cotterill et al. 1984). However, interarterial administration of THC also causes increased perfusion pressure of the hindquarters in an anesthetized rat (Adams et al. 1976; see also section 11.5.3).

11.2.2 In vivo responses to THC in conscious animals and man

In anesthetized animals, a depressor and bradycardic response to THC is consistently seen across species. However, in the conscious animal, a different response is observed. Jandhyala and Buckley (1977) showed various anesthetic agents have a significant effect on the cardiovascular response to THC. In conscious dogs, THC (1 mg/kg, i.v.) caused a slight decrease in heart rate, which was potentiated by pentobarbital or urethane anesthesia. Under morphine and chloralose anesthesia, THC caused tachycardia (increase in heart rate), which could be inhibited by vagotomy, methylatropine (inhibits muscarinic acetylcholine receptors), or propranolol (nonselective beta adrenergic receptor blocker), suggesting sympathetic and parasympathetic nervous system involvement. In conscious dogs, THC did not affect blood pressure, but caused a depressor effect in those animals anesthetized with either pentobarbital, urethane, or chloralose. Jandhyala and Hamed (1978) also showed the hypotensive effect of THC was detectable in anesthetized but not conscious dogs.

In conscious, freely moving Spague Dawley rats, i.v. administration of THC (1 mg/kg) causes an acute (over 60 min) decrease in heart rate and an increase in blood pressure. This was accompanied by vasoconstriction in the renal and mesenteric vascular beds, and vasodilation of the hindquarters (O'Sullivan et al. 2007). Both the pressor and regional vascular (but not heart rate) responses to THC were inhibited by a CB_1 receptor antagonist. A similar hemodynamic response has been observed to other cannabinoids in conscious rats, which could be blocked by CB_1 antagonism and neurohumoral blockade and is likely to be due to sympathoexcitation (Gardiner et al. 2001). To this end, Niederhoffer and Szabo (2000) showed in conscious rabbits that centrally administered CB_1 agonists increase blood pressure, sympathetic nerve activity, and plasma norepinephrine. Since the depressor effects of THC in anesthetized animals appears to be due to CB_1-mediated sympathetic inhibition, the sympathoexcitatory versus inhibitory effects of THC (resulting in a pressor versus depressor response) may be due to the basal level of sympathetic activity at the time of administration, which is known to be reduced in anesthesia. Alternatively, the central effects of THC on the cardiovascular system may be susceptible to general anesthesia.

11.2.2.1 In vivo responses to THC/cannabis in man

In contrast to the findings in conscious animals where no effect (dogs) or bradycardia (rats) was observed, investigations in humans have consistently shown that administration of THC, Sativex® (THC and CBD in an approximately 1:1 ratio), THC analogues such as nabilone or dronabinol, or smoking marijuana, causes tachycardia (Bedi et al. 2013; Crawford and Merritt 1979; Karschner et al. 2011; Mathew et al. 1992a, 1992b; Schwope et al. 2012). The tachycardic response to THC in man can be inhibited by a CB_1 receptor antagonist (Huestis et al. 2001; Klumpers et al. 2013) and is also subject to the development of tolerance, the effect being smaller in chronic cannabis users (Benowitz et al. 1975; Boles Ponto et al. 2004; O'Leary et al. 2002).

The effect of THC or cannabis smoking on blood pressure in humans is more variable. Some studies have reported no change in mean arterial blood pressure (Gorelick et al. 2005; Mathew et al. 1992a, 1992b), a decrease in blood pressure (Crawford and Merritt 1979), or an increase in blood pressure (Boles Ponto et al. 2004). Other studies found that diastolic, but not systolic blood pressure, is affected by THC (Karschner et al. 2011; Schwope et al. 2012). Conversely, nabilone and dronabinol selectively decrease systolic blood pressure (Bedi et al. 2013).

Some people who take THC/cannabis experience dizziness on standing, known as postural or orthostatic hypotension. This may be related to the reduction in diastolic blood pressure sometimes observed with THC and/or an inability to compensate for the fall in blood pressure (the baroreflex), which is normally brought about by sympathetically mediated vasoconstriction to increase peripheral resistance. Mathew et al. (1992c) observed that after marijuana smoking, some volunteers had increased orthostatic hypotension, related to a fall in cerebral blood flow velocity (Mathew et al. 1992c, 2003). Subjects who experienced the most severe symptoms of dizziness had the greatest fall in blood pressure and a larger reduction in cerebral blood velocity.

Gorelick et al. (2005) showed that a CB_1 antagonist administered before marijuana smoking decreased the incidence of symptomatic orthostatic hypotension. Also, Benowitz and Jones (1976, 1981) reported that the orthostatic hypotensive response to THC diminishes with repeated THC administration. Together, this suggests a role for CB_1-mediated inhibition of sympathetic activity involved in orthostatic hypotension, which is subject to the development of tolerance.

11.2.2.2 Changes in regional blood flow with THC/cannabis smoking

Smoking marijuana increases regional cerebral blood flow (Mathew et al. 1992a) and middle cerebral artery velocity (Mathew et al. 1992b). Cerebral blood flow is also increased after dronabinol (Mathew et al. 2002). More specifically, Mathew and colleagues (2002) showed that cerebral blood flow was increased for up to 2 h post-THC (0.25 mg/kg i.v.), and the areas of the brain that were most affected included the frontal, insular, and anterior cingulate regions. Smoking marijuana (Hepler and Frank 1971) and orally administered dronabinol (7.5 mg) (Plange et al. 2006) reduces intraocular pressure in humans. Forearm blood flow is increased by i.v. administration of THC in healthy volunteers (Benowitz and Jones 1981).

11.2.2.3 Summary

To summarize the complex hemodynamic effects of THC in vivo, in anesthetized animals, THC causes a CB_1-mediated reduction in heart rate and blood pressure. In conscious animals, THC causes bradycardia and a pressor response in some animals, also mediated by CB_1. However, in conscious humans, THC causes tachycardia and variable changes in blood pressure, again mediated by CB_1 and subject to the development of tolerance. It is clear that there are species differences in the cardiovascular response to THC. For example, in the conscious state, THC causes little change in heart rate in dogs, bradycardia in rats, and tachycardia in humans. Similarly, in the conscious state, THC causes little change in blood pressure in dogs, a pressor response in rats, and a variable response in humans. However, the route of administration in animal studies is generally i.v., while in humans it is oral or by inhalation, which should be taken into consideration. Additionally, although studies that have probed a mechanism of action for THC have revealed an important role for CB_1, it should be noted that other possible receptor target sites of action have not been tested to date.

11.2.3 In vivo responses to cannabidiol in animals and man

In anesthetized rats, CBD (50 micrograms/kg but not 10 micrograms/kg, i.v.) causes a significant but transient 16 mmHg fall in mean arterial blood pressure without affecting heart rate (Walsh et al. 2010). A single dose of CBD (10 or 20 mg/kg i.p.) also reduces the heart rate and blood pressure response to conditioned fear (Resstel et al. 2006) or to acute restraint stress (Resstel et al. 2009) without affecting baseline blood pressure or heart rate. The inhibitory effect of CBD on the cardiovascular response to stress was shown to be inhibited by a serotonin receptor ($5HT_{1A}$) antagonist. This effect appears to be mediated centrally, as the response to CBD was observed when CBD was injected into the bed nucleus of the stria terminalis (Gomes et al. 2013).

11.3 Cardiac effects of phytocannabinoids

The most consistently observed cardiovascular responses to THC or cannabis smoking are on heart rate, and some investigators have employed a Langendorff preparation (a perfused isolated heart) to investigate the direct effects of phytocannabinoids on the heart. In the 1970s, Smiley and colleagues (1976) found that THC and cannabinol (CBN) increased heart rate and decreased the force of contraction, while CBD decreased both heart rate and contraction, and produced arrhythmias. Nahas and Trouve (1985) also found THC increased heart rate which was associated with a decrease in coronary blood flow and a decrease in pulse pressure (the pressure difference between the systolic and diastolic pressures). CBD had little effect on heart rate, but significantly increased coronary blood flow and pulse pressure. Interestingly, when THC and CBD were co-administered (as would occur in the medication Sativex®), the effects of CBD predominated. CBN decreased heart rate and pulse pressure with a relatively stable blood flow. A more recent study confirmed that THC decreases coronary blood flow and left ventricular pressure in isolated rat hearts (Wagner et al. 2005). These effects were not inhibited by CB_1 antagonism, and were in fact slightly enhanced by CB_1 antagonism. Interestingly, the bradycardic response to THC was also enhanced in the presence of a CB_1 antagonist, suggesting that CB_1 receptors may be coupled to positive chronotropy (O'Sullivan et al. 2007). Wagner et al. (2005) found that abnormal CBD (abn-CBD) caused an increase in coronary blood flow and left ventricular pressure, as observed previously for CBD.

In anesthetized dogs, THC (2.5 mg/kg, i.v.) reduces cardiac output, stroke volume, left ventricular pressure, and left ventricular end diastolic pressure, even in paced hearts (i.e. unrelated to the reduction in heart rate) (Cavero et al. 1973, 1974). Rather than an effect on cardiac contractility, the reduced cardiac output and stroke volume was related to decreased venous return. This could be inhibited by ligating the splanchnic artery, suggesting vasodilatation of the splanchnic vasculature.

Tashkin et al. (1977) showed that the tachycardia observed with THC in humans was associated with an increase in cardiac output and a small decrease in stroke volume. Echocardiographic studies did not find any effects of chronic THC treatment on indices of left ventricular function. Benowitz and Jones (1981) showed the tachycardic response to THC (30–50 micrograms/kg, i.v.) was partly blocked by pretreatment with either atropine or propranolol, and abolished by the combination of both, suggesting THC stimulates the sympathetic and inhibits parasympathetic activity at the heart.

11.4 Cardiovascular responses to chronic phytocannabinoid administration

11.4.1 Cardiovascular response to chronic THC/cannabis administration

Jandhyala et al. (1976) showed that 7 days of administration with 1 mg/kg THC in dogs did not affect basal heart rate, except when they were under anesthesia, when a reduced heart rate was observed in the THC-treated dogs. THC-treated dogs also had a reduced bradycardic response to vagal stimulation, while the tachycardic response to sympathetic stimulation was unaffected (both under anesthesia). More prolonged treatment with THC for 35 days led to changes in reflex bradycardia mediated by enhanced withdrawal of sympathetic tone (Jandhyala 1978). The same study found reductions in the resistance of the mesenteric and femoral vascular beds, and no adverse effect on myocardial function of chronic THC administration.

In young male volunteers, 5–15 days of treatment with THC (210 mg once daily) results in a decrease in resting blood pressure and heart rate, which returned to pretreatment values within a day of stopping THC (Benowitz et al. 1975). In contrast, Tashkin et al. (1977) did not find any effect of chronic THC administration (64 days of unlimited marijuana smoking) on heart rate, stroke volume, cardiac output, or indices of left ventricular function. However, another study has shown that cessation of cannabis use is associated with a significant increase in blood pressure and heart rate (Vandrey et al. 2011), suggesting these are affected by chronic use. Chronic cannabis users are reported to have decreased cerebral blood flow (Jacobus et al. 2012; Tunvig et al. 1985), which also increases on the cessation of cannabis use.

In humans, the cardiovascular responses to THC or cannabis/marijuana smoking diminish with repeated use such that the tachycardic (Benowitz and Jones 1981; Benowitz et al. 1975; Boles Ponto et al. 2004; O'Leary et al. 2002), blood pressure (Benowitz and Jones 1981) and orthostatic intolerance (Benowitz and Jones 1981; Benowitz et al. 1975) responses are smaller after chronic use or in chronic compared to occasional users. Benowitz et al. 1975) also found that THC treatment caused an increased fall in blood pressure in response to standing (associated with dizziness), a decreased blood pressure response to exercise and an increased heart rate response to exercise. THC treatment was associated with an increase in plasma volume. The authors suggest that together this profile is suggestive of decreased sympathetic activity with THC treatment. The same group also showed that THC treatment (14 days, up to 210 mg daily) increased the blood pressure response to atropine, but had no effect on the response to either alpha or beta adrenoceptor stimulation, suggesting increased parasympathetic activity (Benowitz and Jones 1976).

11.4.2 Cardiovascular response to chronic CBD administration

In humans, 5–12 days of treatment with CBD (up to 600 mg per day) did not result in any changes in heart rate or blood pressure (Benowitz and Jones 1981). Similarly, in a recent review, Bergamaschi et al. (2011) report that CBD treatment in humans does not result in changes in blood pressure or heart rate.

11.5 Direct vascular actions of phytocannabinoids in isolated vascular preparations

11.5.1 Acute vasorelaxation response to THC

A number of studies have shown that application of THC causes acute relaxation (within minutes) of isolated preconstricted vascular preparations including rabbit kidney arterioles, rabbit cerebral arterioles, rat mesenteric arteries, rat hepatic arteries, and the rat aorta (Ellis et al. 1995; Fleming et al. 1999; O'Sullivan et al. 2005a, 2005b, 2005c; Zygmunt et al. 2002). We have also shown that THC relaxes human mesenteric arteries, although the magnitude of this response was blunted compared to that seen in animals (Stanley et al. 2011). The vasorelaxant effect of THC, unlike that of other cannabinoids like anandamide, is not universal. No effect of THC has been observed in rabbit carotid arteries or porcine coronary arteries, and some studies have reported a contractile effect of THC, which will be discussed in section 11.5.3.

A variety of mechanisms have been proposed to underlie the vasorelaxant response to THC in various vascular preparations. These include a role for the production of vasoactive prostaglandins, activation of sensory nerves and the release of vasoactive neuropeptides. There is, however, little evidence for a role for the endothelium (except perhaps in the rat aorta), no evidence for a role for the CB_1 receptor and only one study showing a role for CB_2 in the rat aorta. There is also evidence to suggest that THC causes vasorelaxation through modulation of ion channels. The evidence for each of these mechanisms will be discussed in the following sections.

11.5.1.1 A role for metabolism

The first paper showing the vasorelaxant properties of THC in an isolated organ preparation came from Kaymakcalan and Türker (1975), who showed that THC causes a concentration-dependent decrease in the perfusion pressure of approximately 25 mmHg of an isolated kidney. This effect was inhibited by aspirin, a COX inhibitor, suggesting that the involvement of vasodilator prostaglandins. Ellis et al. (1995) later showed that topical application of THC causes concentration-dependent vasodilatation of cerebral arteries (maximal effect was about 25% relaxation) measured using a cranial window technique in an anesthetized rabbit. This effect was also inhibited by a COX inhibitor.

In 1999, Fleming and colleagues showed that THC causes acute, maximal vasorelaxation of isolated rabbit mesenteric arteries, but not rabbit carotid arteries, or porcine coronary arteries. The effect of THC in the mesenteric arteries was inhibited by diclofenac, another COX inhibitor. However, in rat mesenteric arteries, indomethacin has no effect on THC-induced relaxation (O'Sullivan et al. 2005a). The relaxation produced by THC in the work by Zygmunt and colleagues (2002) was produced in the presence of indomethacin, also suggesting COX is not involved in relaxation to THC in rat mesenteric arteries. This may reflect a species difference (rabbit versus rat), or could be due to differences in the mechanisms underpinning THC's effects in different vascular beds (renal or cerebral arteries versus mesenteric arteries). Interestingly, a role for prostanoids has also been implicated in mediating the vasoconstrictor effects of THC in the rabbit lung, rat superior mesenteric artery and the rat aorta (see section 11.5.3). Therefore, THC may have the potential to cause both vasoconstriction and vasorelaxation depending on the prostanoid produced (a vasorelaxant versus a vasoconstrictor prostanoid), the balance of both vasorelaxant or vasoconstrictor prostanoids produced, or the prostanoid receptors expressed on that particular artery.

11.5.1.2 A role for sensory nerves

Zygmunt et al. (2002) showed that THC caused concentration-dependent vasorelaxation of rat hepatic and mesenteric arteries, which could be abolished by pretreatment with the TRPV1 agonist capsaicin, which depletes the sensory neurotransmitters in the artery. However, in similar arteries (rat mesenteric resistance) we have shown that vasorelaxation to THC was unaffected by incubation with the TRPV1 receptor agonist capsaicin, except in the presence of L-NAME and indomethacin, which were the experimental conditions of Zygmunt and colleagues (O'Sullivan et al. 2005a). This might suggest that this pathway becomes more prevalent when other vasodilator pathways are suppressed. In the rat aorta, vasorelaxation to THC was inhibited by capsaicin pretreatment (O'Sullivan et al. 2005b), which may reflect differences between small versus large arteries.

Interestingly, Zygmunt and colleagues showed that the vasorelaxant response to THC in mesenteric arteries persists in TRPV1 knockout mice, and that vasorelaxation to THC was sensitive to ruthenium red, which inhibits several other members of the TRPV family. This suggests that another member of the TRPV family must be responsible, perhaps TRPV4, -5, or -6 (Zygmunt et al. 2002). Vasorelaxation to THC in rat mesenteric arteries is not sensitive to the TRPV1 receptor antagonist, capsazepine, further evidence that TRPV1 is not involved (O'Sullivan et al. 2005a; Zygmunt et al. 2002).

The vasorelaxant response to THC was inhibited by a calcitonin gene-related peptide (CGRP) antagonist, suggesting that this is the vasoactive neurotransmitter responsible for mediating the effects of THC (Zygmunt et al. 2002). This was confirmed by the detection of CGRP release from mesenteric arteries in response to THC (10 µM), that could be inhibited by ruthenium red (Zygmunt et al. 2002). Wilkinson et al. (2007) later confirmed that THC (1 and 10 µM) causes the release of CGRP from perfused rat mesenteric beds. The release of CGRP by THC in the first 30 min was inhibited by ruthenium red but not capsazepine, but the sustained release of CGRP

(30 min to 2 h) was inhibited by capsazepine, although the authors suggest this might be due to capsazepine inhibiting other ion channels.

In addition to the evidence that THC stimulates sensory nerves to cause vasorelaxation, there is evidence that THC can also inhibit sensory nerves. In the whole perfused rat mesenteric bed, Duncan et al. (2004) showed that THC concentration-dependently reduces the vasorelaxant response to electrical field stimulation (EFS), which normally causes the release of CGRP and vasorelaxation. THC did not directly affect the vasorelaxant response to CGRP or capsaicin administration, suggesting this effect is prejunctional. This was confirmed by Wilkinson et al. (2007) who also showed that THC significantly reduced the amount of CGRP released and vasorelaxation by the whole mesenteric bed caused by EFS. This response to THC was insensitive to capsazepine, but was sensitive to ruthenium red, as in the studies of Zygmunt and colleagues (2002). In rat isolated resistance mesenteric arteries, THC (1 μM) did not affect nerve-mediated contractions induced by EFS (Lay et al. 2000).

In summary, in the vasculature, THC can activate sensory nerves to release vasoactive neuro-transmitters causing relaxation of the artery or vascular bed. However, THC can also inhibit the release of vasoactive neurotransmitters, and the vasorelaxation that would accompany this through a prejunctional site. Both of these responses to THC appear to be mediated by members of the TRPV receptor family, but not TRPV1.

11.5.1.3 A role for the endothelium

The effects of THC are not inhibited by removal of the endothelium in rabbit mesenteric arteries (Fleming et al. 1999), rat hepatic or mesenteric arteries (O'Sullivan et al. 2005a; Zygmunt et al. 2002). However, in the rat aorta, vasorelaxation to THC was inhibited by removal of the endothe-lium (O'Sullivan et al. 2005b). We have also found that a time-dependent vasorelaxant effect of THC can be observed in the rat aorta that was sensitive to removal of the endothelium (O'Sullivan et al. 2005c, see section 11.5.2). Together, this might suggest that a role for the endothelium in vas-orelaxation to THC is only observed in the aorta, or perhaps other large conduit arteries, but this is yet to be tested. As THC is not sensitive to removal of the endothelium, this suggests that THC does not act via the cannabinoid receptor that is proposed to exist on the endothelium, sometimes termed CB_e (Begg et al. 2005; Jarai et al. 1999).

11.5.1.4 A role for cannabinoid receptors

The vasorelaxant effects of many cannabinoids such as anandamide are at least partly mediated by activation of the CB_1 receptor in the vasculature in a number of different arteries (see Randall et al. 2004). Although THC has similar affinity and efficacy as anandamide at CB_1, CB_1 receptor antagonism does not affect the vasorelaxant effect of THC in rat mesenteric or hepatic arteries (O'Sullivan et al. 2005a; Zygmunt et al. 2002) or rat aorta (O'Sullivan et al. 2005b). The reduction in the vasorelaxant response to EFS by THC in the whole mesenteric bed is also not sensitive to CB_1 (Duncan et al. 2004; Wilkinson et al. 2007).

Many of the studies investigating the direct vascular effects of THC have not probed activation of CB_2 as a mechanism of action, possibly because previous studies have shown there is little role for CB_2 in the vascular responses to cannabinoids. However, one study showed that vasorelaxa-tion to THC in the rat aorta was inhibited by in vivo pretreatment with pertussis toxin (inhibits $G_{i/o}$ protein coupled receptors) and also by CB_2 receptor antagonism (O'Sullivan et al. 2005b). In pathological situations such as atherosclerosis, activation of CB_2 by THC may play a more impor-tant role (see Fernández-Ruiz et al. Chapter 27, this volume).

We have observed that THC-induced vasorelaxation in resistance arteries of the mesenteric bed is inhibited by pertussis toxin (PTX), but not CB_1, suggesting THC might act through an as yet unidentified G protein coupled receptor (O'Sullivan et al. 2004). As THC is not sensitive to removal of the endothelium in these arteries, it is unlikely to be the proposed endothelial cannabinoid receptor (Begg et al. 2005; Jarai et al. 1999). We have therefore suggested that perhaps there is another as yet uncloned cannabinoid receptor in the vasculature that is expressed on the vascular smooth muscle and that is activated by THC.

11.5.1.5 A role for ion channel modulation

There is evidence to show that THC can modulate ion channel activity, which might be coupled to receptor activation, or might be a direct effect of THC. In rat mesenteric resistance arteries, vasorelaxation to THC was inhibited when arteries were contracted with a high potassium solution, implicating the activation of potassium channels as a mechanism by which THC causes relaxation (O'Sullivan et al. 2005a). The use of specific inhibitors indicated that THC activates large and small calcium-activated potassium channels and the voltage-dependent inward rectifier potassium channel, but not the K_{ATP} or K_v channels (O'Sullivan et al. 2005a).

In rat mesenteric resistance arteries, THC (10 and 100 µM) inhibits the contractile response to the addition of calcium (Ca^{2+}) to a Ca^{2+}-free, high potassium buffer, suggesting that THC blocks Ca^{2+} influx (O'Sullivan et al. 2005a). This was not altered by CB_1 receptor antagonism. In the rat aorta and superior mesenteric artery, THC (10 µM) also inhibits the contractile response to calcium in the same experimental protocol (O'Sullivan et al. 2006), indicating this response to THC is observed in arteries of different sizes.

11.5.2 Time-dependent responses to THC in isolated arteries

In section 11.5.1, evidence was reviewed on the acute effects of THC in isolated vascular preparations. In these experiments, the vasorelaxant response to THC in preconstricted arteries was generally observed within minutes. THC (10 µM) also causes a time-dependent (over 2 h) vasorelaxation of rat aortae (approximately 50%) and the superior mesenteric artery (approximately 25%) compared with vehicle treated vessels (O'Sullivan et al. 2005c). A time-dependent effect of THC was not observed in resistance arteries of the mesenteric bed (O'Sullivan et al. 2006). This suggests that the time-dependent effects of THC are only observed in larger conduit arteries, and also that the acute vasorelaxant effects of THC in small resistance arteries is transient.

On probing the mechanisms underpinning the time-dependent effects of THC, it was found that the effect of THC was inhibited by an antagonist of the peroxisome proliferator-activated receptor gamma (PPARγ) nuclear receptor, in a similar manner to other PPARγ ligands like rosiglitazone (O'Sullivan et al. 2005c). The time-dependent response to THC was not inhibited by CB_1 antagonism, but was inhibited by inhibition of protein synthesis, removal of the endothelium, nitric oxide synthase (NOS) inhibition and superoxide dismutase (SOD) inhibition. These findings are similar to those observed with PPARγ ligands in the vasculature.

In a subsequent study, when either the aorta or superior mesenteric arteries were incubated with THC (10 µM) for 2 h (but not 10 min), subsequent vasoconstrictor responses to methoxamine were blunted (O'Sullivan et al. 2006). Vasorelaxant responses to acetylcholine were also enhanced, but only in the superior mesenteric artery. The blunting of methoxamine responses was not inhibited by PPARγ antagonism or NOS inhibition, but was reduced by catalase, suggesting a role for hydrogen peroxide production. It was also partly reduced by a SOD inhibitor. The enhanced vasorelaxant response to acetylcholine by THC was reduced by PPARγ antagonism, catalase and SOD inhibition. Together, these data suggest that PPARγ agonism by THC in conduit arteries reduces contractile responses and enhances vasorelaxation through increased SOD activity producing hydrogen peroxide.

11.5.3 Vasoconstrictor responses to THC

While many studies have shown vasorelaxant effects of THC in various vascular preparations, others have shown that THC causes vasoconstriction. Kaymakcalan and Türker (1975) showed that THC injected into the pulmonary artery causes a concentration-dependent increase in the perfusion pressure of an isolated lung (but relaxation of the isolated kidney), which could be inhibited by aspirin and by SC19220, a selective antagonist of the prostanoid EP_1 receptor. Interarterial administration of THC also causes a dose-dependent increase in perfusion pressure (of about 30 mmHg) of the hindquarters (Adams et al. 1976). This could be inhibited by alpha adrenergic blockade with phentolamine, or reserpine, which depletes catecholamines, both suggesting an action on the release of norepinephrine from sympathetic nerve terminals. Barbosa et al. (1981) found that THC caused a concentration-dependent increase in the perfusion pressure of the rabbit ear artery, which could be inhibited by artery denervation or reserpine.

Some investigators have found that THC causes vasoconstriction of the whole perfused mesenteric bed (Duncan et al. 2004; Wagner et al. 1999). This is clearly in contrast to the numerous studies showing THC can relax isolated mesenteric arteries. These opposing vascular responses to THC may be dependent on the artery being examined based on the findings that THC causes relaxation of third- and second-order (to a lesser extent) branches of the mesenteric bed, but has little effect in the first order branches of the mesenteric bed, and causes a contractile response in the isolated superior mesenteric artery (O'Sullivan et al. 2005a; see Fig. 11.1).

In the superior mesenteric artery, the vasoconstriction caused by THC was inhibited by removal of the endothelium and a CB_1 receptor antagonist, but not by an endothelin (ET_A) receptor antagonist (O'Sullivan et al. 2005a). Interestingly, COX inhibition revealed a relaxant response to THC in lower concentration ranges, suggesting the production of a vasoconstrictor prostanoid which is masking any vasorelaxant effect of THC in the superior mesenteric artery. Similarly, the vasorelaxant response to THC in the rat aorta was enhanced after COX inhibition (O'Sullivan et al. 2005c). In an unconstricted rat aorta, THC causes concentration-dependent vasoconstriction that can be inhibited by PTX, CB_1 antagonism and COX inhibition (O'Sullivan et al. 2005b).

Together, these studies suggest that when THC causes vasoconstriction, it is through a CB_1-dependent, endothelium-dependent mechanism involving the production of vasoconstrictor

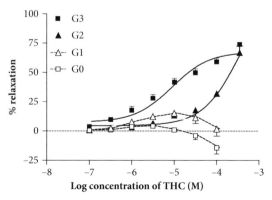

Fig. 11.1 THC causes vasorelaxant and vasoconstrictor responses in descending branches of the mesenteric bed (O'Sullivan et al. 2005a). G0, superior mesenteric artery (SMA); G1, first-order branch of the SMA; G2, second-order branch of the SMA; G3, third-order branch of the SMA.

prostaglandins. In some vascular beds, the vasoconstrictor effect of THC is brought about by sympathetic stimulation. The vasoconstrictor response to THC appears to be dependent on the artery size, being more prevalent in larger conduit arteries. It also seems more likely that a constrictor effect would be seen in a whole perfused vascular bed where the balance of the contribution of larger and smaller arteries to perfusion pressure may favor the effects of THC in larger arteries. The vasoconstrictor response to THC also may depend on the vascular bed being studied, for example, a contractile effect of THC has been observed in the mesenteric bed and lung, but not in the kidney.

11.5.4 Other actions of THC in isolated vascular preparations

In addition to the direct vasorelaxant and vasoconstrictor responses to THC seen in isolated arteries, THC can inhibit the responses to other agonists that cause vasorelaxation such as acetylcholine, bradykinin, carbachol, and anandamide. Fleming et al. (1999) first showed that THC (30 μM) inhibits the vasorelaxant response to acetylcholine in rabbit carotid and mesenteric arteries in the presence of NO and COX inhibition, and these authors suggested that THC inhibits endothelium-derived hyperpolarizing factor (EDHF) release. This was partly inhibited by the CB_1 antagonist SR141716A, although at a very high concentration (30 μM) that is probably having many off target effects. The same group went on to show that THC also inhibits bradykinin relaxation in porcine coronary arteries, which was inhibited by an ERK inhibitor (Brandes et al. 2002). THC also inhibits the vasorelaxant effect of the endogenous cannabinoid anandamide, but not through the CB_1 or TRPV1 receptor (O'Sullivan et al. 2005a). In rat mesenteric arteries, THC (10 μM) inhibits the vasorelaxant response to acetylcholine in the presence of a NOS inhibitor (i.e. not by inhibiting nitric oxide) (O'Sullivan et al. 2006), However, when EDHF was blocked, there was no longer any effect of THC, giving further evidence that THC is capable of inhibiting agonist-stimulated production of EDHF in resistance arteries.

11.5.5 Summary of the direct vascular effects of THC in the vasculature

In summary, THC has complex actions in isolated vascular preparations. The acute vasorelaxant effects of THC involves the production of vasodilator prostaglandins, activation of TRPV channels on sensory nerves and the release of the vasoactive neuropeptide CGRP, activation of potassium channels and inhibition of calcium channels. No major role for the endothelium or cannabinoid receptors has been identified. The acute response to THC is also transient.

In contrast, THC inhibits the vasorelaxant response of the whole mesenteric bed via sensory nerve stimulation and TRPV activation, and also inhibits the vasorelaxant response to a number of vasorelaxant agonists through inhibition of EDHF or its communication through gap junctions. A vasoconstrictor response to THC is observed in some preparations through sympathetic stimulation, CB_1 activation and the production of vasoconstrictor prostanoids.

THC also causes a time-dependent vasorelaxation that is only observed in larger conduit arteries and is dependent on PPARγ activation, the endothelium, NO, and SOD. Incubation of arteries with THC for 2 h blunts subsequent methoxamine responses and enhances acetylcholine responses in conduit arteries. This is mediated by PPARγ, SOD, and the production of hydrogen peroxide.

11.5.6 Acute vascular responses to CBD and abnormal CBD

Despite the wealth of literature on the vascular effects of THC, only a limited number of studies to date have investigated the direct vascular responses to CBD in isolated arteries. Jarai and colleagues (1999) found no effect of CBD (10 μM) on vascular tone in phenylephrine-constricted rat whole mesenteric beds. However, in isolated mesenteric arterial segments, CBD caused a concentration-dependent near-maximal vasorelaxation (Offertaler et al. 2003). Unfortunately, this study did not probe the mechanisms underlying this response. Topical administration of CBD decreases intraocular pressure in the cat (Colasanti et al. 1984). In rat aortae, 10 min of incubation with CBD causes a concentration-dependent (in the micromolar range) inhibition of the contractile response to calcium, suggesting that CBD inhibits calcium channels (O'Sullivan et al. 2009).

In human mesenteric arteries, CBD causes vasorelaxation of preconstricted arterial segments with a pEC_{50} in the mid-micromolar range similar to that observed in rat mesenteric arteries (Stanley and O'Sullivan 2012). However, CBD-induced vasorelaxation in human arteries has a lower maximal response (~45% reduction of preimposed tone). Investigations into the mechanisms underpinning the CBD-induced vasorelaxation in human mesenteric arteries showed an involvement of CB_1 and TRPV1 activation, nitric oxide release and potassium channel activation. Vasorelaxation to CBD in human mesenteric arteries is also endothelium-dependent, but was not affected by antagonism of CB_e.

The vascular effects of the CBD analogue, abn-CBD, have been better characterized in the vasculature, as this compound is suggested to be an agonist of CB_e. Jarai et al. (1999) showed that abn-CBD causes hypotension in both $CB_1^{+/+}/CB_2^{+/+}$ and $CB_1^{-/-}/CB_2^{-/-}$ mice, and the acute vasorelaxant effects of abn-CBD were inhibited by high concentrations of SR141716A, endothelium denudation and CBD. In this study, CBD antagonized the vasorelaxant effects of abn-CBD and anandamide. Begg et al. (2003) showed that abn-CBD causes hyperpolarization through PTX-sensitive activation of large conductance calcium activated potassium channels (BK_{Ca}) in human umbilical vein endothelial cells. In isolated rat mesenteric arteries, abn-CBD causes vasorelaxation that is dependent on the endothelium, SR141716A sensitive pathways and potassium channel hyperpolarization through calcium activated potassium channels (Ho and Hiley 2003). More recently it has been shown that abn-CBD causes vasorelaxation in the human isolated pulmonary artery through similar mechanisms (Kozlowska et al. 2007).

11.5.7 Time-dependent responses to CBD

CBD is a weak/partial agonist at the PPARγ receptor which increases PPARγ transcriptional activity, and binds to the PPARγ ligand binding domain with an $IC_{50} \approx 5$ μM (O'Sullivan et al. 2009). CBD (at concentrations above 100 nM) also causes a time-dependent vasorelaxation of rat aortae. This time-dependent vasorelaxation was inhibited by PPARγ antagonism or SOD inhibition, but was not inhibited by PTX treatment, CB_1 or CB_2 antagonism, capsaicin pretreatment, removal of the endothelium, or NOS inhibition. In human mesenteric arteries, CBD causes a time-dependent response, but this effect is not inhibited by a PPARγ antagonist.

11.5.8 Summary of the direct vascular effects of CBD

In summary, CBD causes acute relaxation of animal arteries through unknown mechanisms that might partly involve inhibition of calcium channels, and causes a time-dependent vasorelaxant effect in rat aortae through PPARγ and SOD. In human mesenteric arteries, CBD causes vasorelaxation through activation of CB_1, TRPV1, the endothelium, NO release, and potassium channel activation. Abn-CBD causes acute vasorelaxation of animal and human arteries through the proposed endothelial cannabinoid receptor and potassium channel activation. CBD is suggested to antagonize this endothelial cannabinoid receptor, although data obtained from human arteries do not support this.

11.6 **Vascular effects of other phytocannabinoids**

Few studies have investigated the direct vascular effects of lesser known phytocannabinoids. Cannabinol (CBN) relaxes isolated rat hepatic arteries, which is antagonized by ruthenium red, but not capsazepine, indicating actions at a TRPV channel other than TRPV1 (Zygmunt et al. 2002). Topical application of both CBN and cannabigerol (CBG) decrease intraocular pressure in the cat (Colasanti et al. 1984). Tetrahydrocannabivarin (THCV) causes a modest vasorelaxant effect in small resistance arteries of the rat mesenteric bed, which reverses at higher concentrations (S.E. O'Sullivan, unpublished observations). In unconstricted vessels, THCV has no effect on vascular tone until 10 μM, and then causes contraction. The contractile effects of THCV in rat mesenteric arteries were not affected by removal of the endothelium, CB_1 antagonism or COX inhibition. THCV (100 nM) does not antagonize the vasorelaxant effect of anandamide and, at 1 μM, does not affect the contractile response to methoxamine in mesenteric resistance arteries (S.E. O'Sullivan, unpublished observations).

11.7 **Action of phytocannabinoids in vascular cell lines**

Some studies have employed vascular cell lines as a means of further exploring the mechanisms that might underlie the vascular responses to phytocannabinoids.

In porcine endothelial cells, gap junction communication was reversibly reduced by 15 min of incubation with THC (30 μM) to a level observed with a gap junction inhibitor (Brandes et al. 2002). This was partially inhibited by a CB_1 receptor antagonist. In human vein endothelial cells, the same study showed that THC increases connexin 43 phosphorylation (a gap junction protein) via ERK signaling. These findings tie in with the in vitro experiments in isolated arteries discussed in section 11.5.4 showing that THC can inhibit the vasorelaxant response to a number of vasorelaxant agents through inhibition of EDHF or its communication through gap junctions. In confluent endothelial cells, THC decreased cytochrome P450 enzyme activity and isoprenaline-induced cAMP levels (Fleming et al. 1999). Cytochrome P450 is suggested to be involved in the production of EDHF in some vascular beds, and so this might be a mechanism by which THC inhibits EDHF production.

In human vein endothelial cells, CBD inhibited cell proliferation at concentrations above 9 μM and cell migration above 1 μM (Solinas et al. 2012). CBD also inhibited angiogenesis and down-regulated some of the key proteins involved in angiogenesis. This is suggested to be a mechanism by which CBD might be beneficial as an antitumor agent (see Velasco et al. Chapter 35, this volume).

In rat brain microvascular endothelial cells, CBD inhibits the basal to apical transport of a fluorescent probe (Zhu et al. 2006). Although not tested in that cell line, it was suggested by the authors to be due to inhibition of the P-glycoprotein transporter, a drug efflux transporter, which could potentially influence the absorption and disposition of drugs at the blood–brain barrier.

In cultured smooth muscle cells, THC, CBD, and CBN decrease low-density lipoprotein-induced cholesteryl ester formation in the low micromolar range (Cornicelli et al. 1981). Phospholipids and triglycerides were not affected, so this is unlikely to be due to a general effect on lipid metabolism, and THC, CBD, and CBN were not found to bind to the low-density lipoprotein receptor. The authors suggest that these phytocannabinoids compartmentalize cholesterol, making it unavailable for metabolism, and that this might represent an antiatherosclerotic mechanism of these drugs (see Fernández-Ruiz et al. Chapter 27, this volume).

11.8 **Chapter summary**

It is clear that phytocannabinoids have interesting and complex effects throughout the cardiovascular system. However, most studies to date have focused on the effects of THC, and we know little about other phytocannabinoids, even CBD. In vivo, THC causes a fall in blood pressure and heart rate in anesthetized animals, and increase in blood pressure and decrease in heart rate in conscious animals, but an increase in heart rate and variable effects on blood pressure in humans. CBD does not appear to elicit hemodynamic responses in vivo. The effects of THC involve changes in the activity of the autonomic nervous system and appear to be mediated by CB_1, which is potentially why we don't see similar hemodynamic responses to CBD, which is not thought to activate CB_1. In vitro, both vasorelaxation (THC, CBD, CBN, THCV) and vasoconstriction (THC, THCV) to phytocannabinoids have been observed. Vasorelaxation to THC is mediated by prostaglandins, activation of sensory nerves, modulation of ion channels, and activation of PPARγ. Vasoconstriction to THC is mediated by prostanoids, CB_1 and sympathetic stimulation. One study in human arteries suggests CBD causes vasorelaxation by activation of CB_1, TRPV1, and nitric oxide. THC also inhibits the vasorelaxation caused by sensory nerve activation, or by agonists such as acetylcholine, bradykinin and anandamide, which is suggested to be through inhibition of EDHF.

11.9 **Directions for future research**

◆ Further investigation into the acute and chronic in vivo hemodynamic effects of phytocannabinoids are warranted, especially for CBD, THCV, CBN, and CBG which haven't been fully investigated in animals or humans. The mechanisms of how phytocannabinoids act in vivo have only been probed in studies from the 1990s onward with the advent of antagonists and deeper knowledge of the cannabinoid system, therefore further studies are required to establish any potential role of receptors other than CB_1.

◆ Many of the human studies were carried out in volunteers who were not drug naïve (although sometimes drug free at the time of experimentation). Since the in vivo responses to cannabis and THC seem to be CB_1 mediated and subject to tolerance, the hemodynamic responses might be underestimated. Most studies in humans have been in healthy volunteers and therefore the cardiovascular effects of phytocannabinoids in people who might have cardiovascular disorders, for example, hypertension, remain unknown.

◆ In in vitro studies, research has focused on the effects of THC, and CBD to a lesser extent. Further investigations into these and other phytocannabinoids are required to understand their pharmacology in the vasculature, particularly in vascular beds other than the mesentery such as the coronary and cerebral vasculature.

◆ Only one study to date has investigated the direct effects of phytocannabinoids in human arteries. It is difficult to tell at this stage whether the mechanisms underpinning the effects of CBD, or indeed other phytocannabinoids, are different between animals and humans, because they have never been fully probed in animals.

◆ It is unlikely that all the target sites of action for phytocannabinoids in the vasculature have been identified. For example, which are the other members of the TRP family that phytocannabinoids act at? Is there a role for CB_2? Is there a vascular smooth muscle site that has yet to be identified? Is there a role for GPR55?

◆ There are surprisingly few studies in vascular cell lines examining the cellular effects, and underpinning mechanisms of action of phytocannabinoids in the vasculature.

♦ No studies have looked at the effects of chronic phytocannabinoid treatment on the direct vascular responses to phytocannabinoids in isolated arterial preparations to establish if there are any changes in these responses with repeated use.

References

Adams, M.D., Earnhardt, J.T., Dewey, W.L., and Harris, L.S. (1976). Vasoconstrictor actions of delta8- and delta9-tetrahydrocannabinol in the rat. *Journal Pharmacology and Experimental Therapeutics*, **196**, 649–656.

Barbosa, P.P., Lapa, A.J., Lima-Landman, M.T., and Valle, J.R. (1981). Vasoconstriction induced by delta 9-tetrahydrocannabinol on the perfused rabbit ear artery. *Archives Internationales de Pharmacodynamie et de Thérapie*, **252**, 253–2561.

Bedi, G., Cooper, Z.D., and Haney, M. (2013). Subjective, cognitive and cardiovascular dose-effect profile of nabilone and dronabinol in marijuana smokers. *Addiction Biology*, **18**, 872–881.

Begg, M., Mo, F.-M., Offertaler, L., *et al.* (2003). G protein-coupled endothelial receptor for atypical cannabinoid ligands modulates a Ca^{2+}-dependent K^+ current. *Journal of Biological Chemistry*, **278**, 46188–46194.

Benowitz, N.L. and Jones, R.T. (1975). Cardiovascular effects of prolonged delta-9-tetrahydrocannabinol ingestion. *Clinical Pharmacology & Therapeutics*, **18**, 287–297.

Benowitz, N.L. and Jones, R.T. (1977). Prolonged delta-9-tetrahydrocannabinol ingestion. Effects of sympathomimetic amines and autonomic blockades. *Clinical Pharmacology & Therapeutics*, **21**, 336–342.

Benowitz, N.L. and Jones, R.T. (1981). Cardiovascular and metabolic considerations in prolonged cannabinoid administration in man. *Clinical Pharmacology & Therapeutics*, **21**, 214S–223S.

Bergamaschi, M.M., Queiroz, R.H., Zuardi, A.W., and Crippa, J.A. (2011). Safety and side effects of cannabidiol, a *Cannabis sativa* constituent. *Current Drug Safety*, **6**, 237–249.

Brandes, R.P., Popp, R., Ott, G., *et al.* (2002). The extracellular regulated kinases (ERK) 1/2 mediate cannabinoid-induced inhibition of gap junctional communication in endothelial cells. *British Journal Pharmacology*, **136**, 709–716.

Burstein, S., Ozman, K., Burstein, E., Palermo, N., and Smith, E. (1982). Prostaglandins and cannabis – XI. Inhibition of delta 1-tetrahydrocannabinol-induced hypotension by aspirin. *Biochemical Pharmacology*, **31**, 591–592.

Cavero, I., Lokhandwala, M.F., Buckley, J.P., and Jandhyala, B.S. (1974). The effect of (minus)-delta 9-trans-tetrahydrocannibinol on myocardial contractility and venous return in anesthetized dogs. *European Journal of Pharmacology*, **29**, 74–82.

Cavero, I., Solomon, T., Buckley, J.P., and Jandhyala, B.S. (1973). Studies on the bradycardia induced by (-)- -trans-tetrahydrocannabinol in anesthetized dogs. *European Journal of Pharmacology*, **22**, 263–269.

Colasanti, B.K., Craig, C.R., and Allara, R.D. (1984). Intraocular pressure, ocular toxicity and neurotoxicity after administration of cannabinol or cannabigerol. *Experimental Eye Research*, **39**, 251–259.

Cornicelli, J.A., Gilman, S.R., Krom, B.A., and Kottke, B.A. (1981). Cannabinoids impair the formation of cholesteryl ester in cultured human cells. *Arteriosclerosis*, **1**, 449–454.

Cotterill, R.W., Penney, L.L., Vaughn, D.L., Reimann, B.E. and Rauls, D.O. (1984). Acute cardiovascular effects of delta-9-tetrahydrocannabinol in pregnant anesthetized sheep. *Biological Research in Pregnancy and Perinatology*, **5**, 1–5.

Crawford, W.J. and Merritt, J.C. (1979). Effects of tetrahydrocannabinol on arterial and intraocular hypertension. *International Journal of Clinical Pharmacology and Biopharmacy*, **17**, 191–196.

Duncan, M., Kendall, D.A., and Ralevic, V. (2004). Characterization of cannabinoid modulation of sensory neurotransmission in the rat isolated mesenteric arterial bed. *Journal of Pharmacology and Experimental Therapeutics*, **311**, 411–419.

Ellis, E.F., Moore, S.F., and Willoughby, K.A. (1995). Anandamide and delta 9-THC dilation of cerebral arterioles is blocked by indomethacin. *American Journal of Physiology*, **269**, H1859–1864.

Estrada, U., Brase, D.A., Martin, B.R., and Dewey, W.L. (1987). Cardiovascular effects of delta 9- and delta 9(11)-tetrahydrocannabinol and their interaction with epinephrine. *Life Science*, **41**, 79–87.

Fleming, I., Schermer, B., Popp, R., and Busse, R. (1999). Inhibition of the production of endothelium-derived hyperpolarizing factor by cannabinoid receptor agonists. *British Journal of Pharmacology*, **126**, 949–960.

Gardiner, S.M., March, J.E., Kemp, P.A., and Bennett, T. (2001). Regional haemodynamic responses to the cannabinoid agonist, WIN 55212-2, in conscious, normotensive rats, and in hypertensive, transgenic rats. *British Journal of Pharmacology*, **133**, 445–453.

Gomes, F.V., Alves, F.H., Guimaraes, F.S., Correa, F.M., Resstel, L.B., and Crestani, C.C. (2013). Cannabidiol administration into the bed nucleus of the stria terminalis alters cardiovascular responses induced by acute restraint stress through 5-HT(1A) receptor. *European Neuropsychopharmacology*, **23**, 1096–1104.

Gorelick, D.A., Heishman, S.J., Preston, K.L., Nelson, R.A., Moolchan, E.T., and Huestis, M.A. (2006). The cannabinoid CB_1 receptor antagonist rimonabant attenuates the hypotensive effect of smoked marijuana in male smokers. *American Heart Journal*, **151**, 754.e1–754.e5.

Green, K., Wynn, H., and Padgett, D. (1978). Effects of delta9-tetrahydrocannabinol on ocular blood flow and aqueous humor formation. *Experimental Eye Research*, **26**, 65–69.

Hepler, R.S. and Frank, I.R. (1971). Marihuana smoking and intraocular pressure. *JAMA*, **217**, 1392.

Ho, W.S. and Hiley, C.R. (2003). Vasodilator actions of abnormal-cannabidiol in rat isolated small mesenteric artery. *British Journal of Pharmacology*, **138**, 1320–1332.

Huestis, M.A., Gorelick, D.A., Heishman, S.J., *et al.* (2001). Blockade of effects of smoked marijuana by the CB_1-selective cannabinoid receptor antagonist SR141716. *Archives of General Psychiatry*, **58**, 322–328.

Innemee, H.C., Hermans, A.J., and van Zwieten, P.A. (1979). The influence of delta 9-tetrahydrocannabinol on intraocular pressure in the anaesthetized cat. *Advances in Ophthalmology*, **48**, 235–241.

Jacobus, J., Goldenberg, D., Wierenga, C.E., Tolentino, N.J., Liu, T.T., and Tapert, S.F. (2012). Altered cerebral blood flow and neurocognitive correlates in adolescent cannabis users. *Psychopharmacology (Berlin)*, **222**, 675–684.

Jandhyala, B.S. (1978). Effects of prolonged administration of delta 9-tetrahydrocannabinol on the autonomic and cardiovascular function and regional hemodynamics in mongrel dogs. *Research Communications in Chemical Pathology and Pharmacology*, **20**, 489–508.

Jandhyala, B.S. and Buckley, J.P. (1977). Influence of several anesthetic agents on the effect of delta9-tetrahydrocannabinol on the heart rate and blood pressure of the mongrel dog. *European Journal of Pharmacology*, **44**, 9–16.

Jandhyala, B.S. and Hamed, A.T. (1978). Pulmonary and systemic hemodynamic effects of delta9-tetrahydrocannabinol in conscious and morphine-chloralose-anesthetized dogs: anesthetic influence on drug action. *European Journal of Pharmacology*, **53**, 63–68.

Jandhyala, B.S., Malloy, K.P., and Buckley, J.P. (1976a). Effects of acute administration of delta9-tetrahydrocannabinol on pulmonary hemodynamics of anesthetized dogs. *European Journal of Pharmacology*, **38**, 183–187.

Jandhyala, B.S., Malloy, K.P., and Buckley, J.P. (1976b). Effects of chronic administration of delta9-tetrahydrocannabinol on the heart rate of mongrel dogs. *Research Communications in Chemical Pathology and Pharmacology*, **14**, 201–204.

Jarai, Z., Wagner, J.A., Varga, K.R., *et al.* (1999). Cannabinoid-induced mesenteric vasodilation through an endothelial site distinct from CB_1 or CB_2 receptors. *Proceedings of the National Academy of Sciences of the United States of America*, **96**, 14136–14141.

Karschner, E.L., Darwin, W.D., McMahon, R.P., *et al.* (2011). Subjective and physiological effects after controlled Sativex and oral THC administration. *Clinical Pharmacology & Therapeutics*, **89**, 400–407.

Kaymakcalan, S. and Türker, R.K. (1975). The evidence of the release of prostaglandin-like material from rabbit kidney and guinea-pig lung by (minus)-trans-delta9-tetrahydrocannabinol. *Journal of Pharmacy and Pharmacology*, **27**, 564–568.

Klumpers, L.E., Roy, C., Ferron, G., *et al.* (2013). Surinabant, a selective CB$_1$ antagonist, inhibits THC-induced central nervous system and heart rate effects in humans. *British Journal of Clinical Pharmacology*, **76**, 65–77.

Kozlowska, H., Baranowska, M., Schlicker, E., Kozlowski, M., Laudanski, J., and Malinowska, B. (2007). Identification of the vasodilatory endothelial cannabinoid receptor in the human pulmonary artery. *Journal of Hypertension*, **25**, 2240–2248.

Krowicki, Z.K. (2012). Involvement of hindbrain and peripheral prostanoids in gastric motor and cardio-vascular responses to delta-9-tetrahydrocannabinol in the rat. *Journal of Physiology and Pharmacology*, **63**, 581–588.

Lake, K.D., Compton, D.R., Varga, K., Martin, B.R., and Kunos, G. (1997). Cannabinoid-induced hypo-tension and bradycardia in rats mediated by CB$_1$-like cannabinoid receptors. *Journal Pharmacology and Experimental Therapeutics*, **281**, 1030–1107.

Lambert, D.M. (2001). Medical use of cannabis through history. *Journal of Pharmacy Belgium*, **56**, 111–118.

Lay, L., Angus, J.A. and Wright, C.E. (2000). Pharmacological characterisation of cannabinoid CB$_1$ recep-tors in the rat and mouse. *European Journal of Pharmacology*, **391**, 151–161.

Mathew, R.J., Wilson, W.H. and Davis, R. (2003). Postural syncope after marijuana: a transcranial Doppler study of the hemodynamics. *Pharmacology Biochemistry & Behavior*, **75**, 309–318.

Mathew, R.J., Wilson, W.H., Humphreys, D., Lowe, J.V., and Wiethe, K.E. (1992a). Middle cerebral artery velocity during upright posture after marijuana smoking. *Acta Psychiatrica Scandinavica*, **86**, 173–178.

Mathew, R.J., Wilson, W.H., Humphreys, D.F., Lowe, J.V., and Wiethe, K.E. (1992b). Changes in middle cerebral artery velocity after marijuana. *Biological Psychiatry*, **32**, 164–169.

Mathew, R.J., Wilson, W.H., Humphreys, D.F., Lowe, J.V., and Wiethe, K.E. (1992c). Regional cerebral blood flow after marijuana smoking. *Journal of Cerebral Blood Flow & Metabolism*, **12**, 750–758.

Nahas, G. and Trouve, R. (1985). Effects and interactions of natural cannabinoids on the isolated heart. *Proceedings of the Society for Experimental Biology and Medicine*, **180**, 312–316.

Niederhoffer, N. and Szabo, B. (1999). Effect of the cannabinoid receptor agonist WIN55212-2 on sympa-thetic cardiovascular regulation. *British Journal of Pharmacology*, **126**, 457–466.

Niederhoffer, N. and Szabo, B. (2000). Cannabinoids cause central sympathoexcitation and bradycardia in rabbits. *Journal Pharmacology and Experimental Therapeutics*, **294**, 707–713.

O'Leary, D.S., Block, R.I., Koeppel, J.A., *et al.* (2002). Effects of smoking marijuana on brain perfusion and cognition. *Neuropsychopharmacology*, **26**, 802–816.

O'Sullivan, S.E., Kendall, D.A. and Randall, M.D. (2005a). The effects of Delta9-tetrahydrocannabinol in rat mesenteric vasculature, and its interactions with the endocannabinoid anandamide. *British Journal of Pharmacology*, **145**, 514–526.

O'Sullivan, S.E., Kendall, D.A. and Randall, M.D. (2005b). Vascular effects of delta 9-tetrahydrocannabinol (THC), anandamide and N-arachidonoyldopamine (NADA) in the rat isolated aorta. *European Journal of Pharmacology*, **507**, 211–221

O'Sullivan, S.E., Kendall, D.A. and Randall, M.D. (2006). Further characterization of the time-dependent vascular effects of delta9-tetrahydrocannabinol. *Journal Pharmacology and Experimental Therapeutics*, **317**, 428–438.

O'Sullivan, S.E., Randall, M.D., and Gardiner, S.M. (2007). The in vitro and in vivo cardiovascular effects of Delta9-tetrahydrocannabinol in rats made hypertensive by chronic inhibition of nitric-oxide syn-thase. *Journal Pharmacology and Experimental Therapeutics*, **321**, 663–672.

O'Sullivan, S.E., Sun, Y., Bennett, A.J., Randall, M.D., and Kendall, D.A. (2009). Time-dependent vascu-lar actions of cannabidiol in the rat aorta. *European Journal of Pharmacology*, **612**, 61–68.

O'Sullivan, S.E., Tarling, E.J., Bennett, A.J., Kendall, D.A., and Randall, M.D. (2005c). Novel time-dependent vascular actions of Delta9-tetrahydrocannabinol mediated by peroxisome proliferator-activated receptor gamma. *Biochemical and Biophysical Research Communications*, **337**, 824–831.

Offertaler, L., Mo, F.-M., Bátka, S., *et al.* (2003). Selective ligands and cellular effectors of a G protein-coupled endothelial cannabinoid receptor. *Molecular Pharmacology*, **63**, 699–705.

Plange, N., Arend, K.O., Kaup, M., *et al.* (2007). Dronabinol and retinal hemodynamics in humans. *American Journal of Ophthalmology*, **143**, 173–174.

Ponto, L.L., O'Leary, D.S., Koeppel, J., *et al.* (2004). Effect of acute marijuana on cardiovascular function and central nervous system pharmacokinetics of [(15)O]water: effect in occasional and chronic users. *Journal of Clinical Pharmacology*, **44**, 751–66.

Randall, M.D., Kendall, D.A., and O'Sullivan, S. (2004). The complexities of the cardiovascular actions of cannabinoids. *British Journal of Pharmacology*, **142**, 20–26.

Resstel, L.B., Joca, S.R., Moreira, F.A., Correa, F.M. and Guimaraes, F.S. (2006). Effects of cannabidiol and diazepam on behavioral and cardiovascular responses induced by contextual conditioned fear in rats. *Behavioural Brain Research*, **172**, 294–298.

Resstel, L.B., Tavares, R.F., Lisboa, S.F., Joca, S.R., Correa, F.M. and Guimaraes, F.S. (2009). 5-HT1A receptors are involved in the cannabidiol-induced attenuation of behavioural and cardiovascular responses to acute restraint stress in rats. *British Journal of Pharmacology*, **156**, 181–188.

Schwope, D.M., Bosker, W.M., Ramaekers, J.G., Gorelick, D.A. and Huestis, M.A. (2012). Psychomotor performance, subjective and physiological effects and whole blood Δ^9-tetrahydrocannabinol concentrations in heavy, chronic cannabis smokers following acute smoked cannabis. *Journal of Analytical Toxicology*, **36**, 405–412.

Siqueira, S.W., Lapa, A.J., and Ribeiro do Valle, J. (1979). The triple effect induced by delta 9-tetrahydrocannabinol on the rat blood pressure. *European Journal of Pharmacology*, **58**, 351–357.

Smiley, K.A., Karler, R., and Turkanis, S.A. (1976). Effects of cannabinoids on the perfused rat heart. *Research Communications in Chemical Pathology and Pharmacology*, **14**, 659–675.

Solinas, M., Massi, P., Cantelmo, A.R., *et al.* (2012). Cannabidiol inhibits angiogenesis by multiple mechanisms. *British Journal of Pharmacology*, **167**, 1218–1231.

Stanley, C., Manning, G., and O'Sullivan, S. (2011). Cannabinoid induced vasorelaxation of human mesenteric arteries. *Proceedings of the International Cannabinoid Research Society*. Available at: http://bps.conference-services.net/resources/344/2336/pdf/BPSWINTER10_0158.pdf.

Stanley, C.P. and O'Sullivan, S.E. (2012). Cannabidiol induced vasorelaxation of human mesenteric arteries is mediated by the endothelium, CB_1 and TRPV1. *Proceedings of the International Cannabinoid Research Society*, P1-25. Available at: http://www.icrs.co/SYMPOSIUM.2012/ICRS2012.Final.Programme.and.Abstracts.pdf.

Tashkin, D.P., Levisman, J.A., Abbasi, A.S., Shapiro, B.J., and Ellis, N.M. (1977). Short-term effects of smoked marihuana on left ventricular function in man. *Chest*, **72**, 20–26.

Tunving, K., Thulin, S.O., Risberg, J., and Warkentin, S. (1986). Regional cerebral blood flow in long-term heavy cannabis use. *Psychiatry Research*, **17**, 15–21.

Vandrey, R., Umbricht, A., and Strain, E.C. (2011). Increased blood pressure after abrupt cessation of daily cannabis use. *Journal of Addiction Medicine*, **5**, 16–20.

Varga, K., Lake, K.D., Huangfu, D., Guyenet, P.G., and Kunos, G. (1996). Mechanism of the hypotensive action of anandamide in anesthetized rats. *Hypertension*, **28**, 682–686.

Wagner, J.A., Abesser, M., Karcher, J., Laser, M., and Kunos, G. (2005). Coronary vasodilator effects of endogenous cannabinoids in vasopressin-preconstricted unpaced rat isolated hearts. *Journal of Cardiovascular Pharmacology*, **46**, 348–355.

Wagner, J.A., Varga, K., Jarai, Z., and Kunos, G. (1999). Mesenteric vasodilation mediated by endothelial anandamide receptors. *Hypertension*, **33**, 429–434.

Walsh, S.K., Hepburn, C.Y., Kane, K.A., and Wainwright, C.L. (2010). Acute administration of cannabidiol in vivo suppresses ischaemia-induced cardiac arrhythmias and reduces infarct size when given at reperfusion. *British Journal of Pharmacology*, **160**, 1234–1242.

Wilkinson, J.D., Kendall, D.A., and Ralevic, V. (2007). Delta 9-tetrahydrocannabinol inhibits electrically-evoked CGRP release and capsaicin-sensitive sensory neurogenic vasodilatation in the rat mesenteric arterial bed. *British Journal of Pharmacology*, **152**, 709–716.

Zhu, H.J., Wang, J.S., Markowitz, J.S., *et al.* (2006). Characterization of P-glycoprotein inhibition by major cannabinoids from marijuana. *Journal of Pharmacology and Experimental Therapeutics*, **317**, 850–857.

Zuardi, A.W. (2006). History of cannabis as a medicine: a review. *Revista Brasileira de Psiquiatria*, **28**, 153–157.

Zygmunt, P.M., Andersson, D.A., and Hogestatt, E.D. (2002). Delta 9-tetrahydrocannabinol and cannabinol activate capsaicin-sensitive sensory nerves via a CB_1 and CB_2 cannabinoid receptor-independent mechanism. *Journal of Neuroscience*, **22**, 4720–4727.

Chapter 12

Phytocannabinoids and the Gastrointestinal System

Marnie Duncan and Angelo A. Izzo

12.1 Introduction

Phytocannabinoids include about 100 meroterpenoids (prenylated polyketides), accumulated in tiny epidermal resinous glands of the cannabis plant and characterized, in most instances, by specific and potent pharmacological activities (Appendino et al. 2011). For obvious reasons, most attention has been paid to Δ^9-tetrahydrocannabinol (THC), which is the most important psychotropic component. The THC content in cannabis extracts is extremely variable, reaching 15% in some varieties currently available in the illegal market (Appendino et al. 2011). In addition to THC, the plant cannabis also contains nonpsychotropic cannabinoids of potential therapeutic interest. These include cannabigerol (CBG), cannabichromene (CBC), THC, and their corresponding acids (Izzo et al. 2009).

The benefits of cannabis extracts for gastrointestinal (GI) disorders have been well documented for centuries. Cannabis has been used to treat conditions such as emesis, gastric ulcer, abdominal pain, gastroenteritis, diarrhea, and intestinal inflammation. Scientific evidence for empirical traditional uses of cannabis for GI disorders emerged about 35 years ago, when it was demonstrated that a crude cannabis extract exerted protective effects in an experimental model of gastric ulceration (De Souza et al. 1978).

This chapter focuses on the pharmacological effects and the modes of action of phytocannabinoids in the digestive tract both under normal and pathophysiological conditions.

12.2 Main phytocannabinoid targets and their localization in the gut

Phytocannabinoid may activate—or modulate the activity of—the classical targets of the endogenous cannabinoids. These include cannabinoid receptors types 1 and 2 (CB_1 and CB_2), enzymes involved in the degradation of endocannabinoids, i.e., monoacylglycerol lipase (MAGL, mostly involved in 2-arachidonoylglycerol (2-AG) catabolism) and fatty acid amide hydrolase (FAAH, mostly involved in anandamide enzymatic degradation), as well as transient receptor potential (TRP) channels, G protein-coupled receptor 55 (GPR55), and peroxisome proliferator-activated receptors (PPARs). A brief discussion on the localization and role of these targets in the gut is reported in sections 12.2.1 to 12.2.5.

12.2.1 Cannabinoid receptors

THC, the main psychotropic cannabis ingredient, is a CB_1 and CB_2 receptor partial agonist and, in line with classical pharmacology, it evokes pharmacological responses which are clearly influenced both by the expression level and signaling efficiency of cannabinoid receptors (Pertwee 2008). Cannabinol (CBN), another phytocannabinoid, is a weak CB_1 partial agonist, with approximately 10% of the activity of THC (Izzo et al. 2009). By contrast, nonpsychotropic phytocannabinoids generally do not activate cannabinoid receptors efficiently. An exception is THCV, which has been shown to behave as a CB_2 receptor agonist and CB_1 receptor antagonist in vitro and to attenuate inflammation in vivo (Bolognini et al. 2010; Pertwee 2008). THCV also shares the ability of synthetic CB_1 antagonists to reduce food intake in mice (Riedel et al. 2009). Finally, CBD has been shown to display unexpectedly high potency as an antagonist of CB1 and CB2 receptor agonists in vitro (Thomas et al. 2007).

In the digestive tract, CB_1 receptors are located predominantly in the excitatory motor neurons of the myenteric plexus, which regulate gut motility. In vitro activation of these receptors inhibits contraction mainly by the inhibition of acetylcholine release from prejunctional neurons, and these findings have also been confirmed in vivo (Izzo and Coutts 2005). The inhibitory actions of CB_1 receptors on GI motility are thought to be predominantly via enteric receptors, and this has been confirmed using a peripherally restricted cannabinoid receptor agonist SAB378 (Cluny et al. 2010). In the submucosal plexus, CB_1 receptors are localized on secretomotor and vaso-motor neurons. Cannabinoids are thought to inhibit secretion via activation of CB_1 receptors on these neurons (Duncan et al. 2005). In addition to being localized within the gut, CB_1 receptors are also present on peripheral nerve fibers within the brain-gut axis. CB_1 receptors may influence motility and secretion via these receptors as well as modulate food intake and emesis (Duncan et al. 2005). CB_1 receptors may play a role in intestinal inflammation as they are upregulated in response to an inflammatory insult such as mustard oil, croton oil, or dinitrobenzene sulfonic acid (DNBS) (Izzo et al. 2001; Kimball et al. 2010; Massa et al. 2004). CB_1 receptors are also expressed in GI epithelia, human parietal cells, and macrophages within the gut wall (Izzo and Sharkey 2010; Wright et al. 2005).

CB_2 receptors have been reported to be expressed on excitatory motor neurons, but not on inhibitory motor neurons or enteric glia. CB_2 receptors are not thought to modulate motility in the gut under normal conditions, but do normalize deregulated motility in inflammatory conditions by reducing neuronal activation (Duncan et al. 2008a; Mathison et al. 2004). CB_2 receptors are also expressed in GI epithelia, and can be upregulated by probiotic treatment or IBS (Izzo and Sharkey 2010; Wright et al. 2005, 2008).

12.2.2 Enzymes involved in endocannabinoid degradation

Both fatty acid amide hydrolase (FAAH, an enzyme mostly involved in the anandamide degradation) and MAGL (monoacylglycerol lipase, an enzyme mostly involved in 2-AG degradation) have been shown to be targets for some phytocannabinoids. For example, CBD has been shown to inhibit FAAH activity in biochemical assays (Bisogno et al. 2001) as well as FAAH protein expression in the inflamed gut (De Filippis et al. 2008). In addition, CBC has been shown to be a weak inhibitor of MAGL (De Petrocellis et al. 2011).

FAAH is a membrane-bound enzyme which hydrolyzes and therefore terminates the actions of anandamide and 2-AG. FAAH is expressed throughout the GI tract in myenteric neurons (Duncan et al. 2005). Inhibition of FAAH delays GI motility by increasing local levels of endocannabinoids in a manner that increases CB_1 receptor activation. FAAH is thought to be protective under pathophysiological conditions as FAAH$^{-/-}$ mice show less inflammation in models of colitis (Massa et al. 2004). In addition, the FAAH inhibitor URB597 and the anandamide membrane transport inhibitor VDM11 significantly reduced inflammation in such models. These effects were abolished in CB_1 and CB_2 receptor gene-deficient mice (Storr et al. 2008). Moreover, FAAH inhibition can reverse the actions of lipopolysaccharide (LPS) on GI transit via CB_1 and CB_2 receptors (Bashashati et al. 2012).

MAGL is the principal 2-AG-hydrolyzing enzyme, and is expressed throughout the rodent gut. MAGL is expressed in neurons in the myenteric and submucosal plexuses (Duncan et al. 2008b). MAGL is also expressed in the epithelium. The protein levels of MAGL progressively increase from the duodenum through to the colon. Conversely, the highest activity is observed in the duodenum and progressively decreases toward the colon. Inhibition of MAGL can reduce whole-gut transit in a dose-dependent manner. This is thought to be due to an increase in local endocannabinoid levels which then activate CB_1 receptors in the enteric nervous system as it was not observed in CB_1 knockout mice (Duncan et al. 2008b). In human samples, MAGL was detected in fibers of the enteric nervous system and in epithelial cells, but not in human smooth muscle and mucosal layers (Marquez et al. 2009). In samples from patients with ulcerative colitis, an increase of MAGL expression in the colonic epithelium was observed, suggesting an increase of 2-AG turnover during the inflammation (Marquez et al. 2009). 2-AG may also be protective in the stomach, since the MAGL inhibitor JZL184 prevented diclofenac-induced gastric hemorrhage. This protective effect is thought to result from increased stomach levels of 2-AG that possibly induce a CB_1 receptor-mediated inhibition of increased release of gastric interleukin (IL)-1β, IL-10, IL-6, tumor necrosis factor (TNF)-α and granulocyte colony-stimulating factor (Kinsey et al. 2011).

12.2.3 **G protein-coupled receptor 55**

There have been several reports that the GPR55 gene is present within the GI tract, although to date, there have been no localization studies to determine if this expression is neuronal, muscular, or mucosal (Ross et al. 2012). The atypical cannabinoid O-1602 inhibits neurogenic contractions in the mouse colon via GPR555; these finding were confirmed using CB_1 and CB_2 knockout tissues as controls (Ross et al. 2012). Although the effects were predominantly prejunctional, some were postjunctional at high concentrations and effects on calcium influx have been ruled out. GPR55 appears to be upregulated (at gene and protein level) by inflammation in the duodenum, ileum, and colon in a LPS model of sepsis (Lin et al. 2011); the upregulation of GPR55 was reversed by CBD and O-1602. CBD is thought to be an antagonist at GPR55, whereas O-1602 is an agonist. The authors speculate that GPR55 could be pro-inflammatory in the gut, and that CBD exerted its anti-inflammatory effect by acting as a GPR55 antagonist (Lin et al. 2011).

12.2.4 **Transient receptor potential channels**

TRP channels play an important role in GI motility, GI sensation, and GI disorders. In addition, CB_1 receptors and TRPV1 channels are colocalized in primary afferent nerves in the gut (Izzo and Sharkey 2010), and the endocannabinoid, anandamide, can activate both these pharmacological targets. Certain phytocannabinoids can also activate TRP channels. De Petrocellis and coworkers have reported that CBD, CBG, CBGV, and THCV stimulate and desensitize human TRPV1, and also that the majority of phytocannabinoids activate and desensitize TRPV2 (De Petrocellis et al. 2011). These channels are expressed on visceral afferents and epithelial cells: TRPV1 is thought to have a role in visceral chemoception, mechanoception, and nociception. However, the role of TRPV2 in gut is still unknown (Boesmans et al. 2011).

Both experimentally and in the clinic, phytocannabinoids can be administered as standardized cannabis extracts enriched with particular phytocannabinoids. Such an extract is commonly termed "botanic drug substance" (BDS). CBG BDS (i.e., cannabis standardized extract enriched in CBG) and THCV BDS (i.e., cannabis standardized extract enriched in THCV) are potent rat TRPM8 antagonists (De Petrocellis et al. 2011). The implications of this are unclear as this channel, located on visceral afferents, is activated by cooling or menthol. However, menthol actions in gut are reported to be TRPM8 independent and so the physiological function of this channel in the GI tract is unknown (Boesmans et al. 2011).

CBC, CBD, THCV, and CBN are TRPA1 agonists and desensitizers (De Petrocellis et al. 2011). The TRPA1 channel is activated by pungent compounds such as mustard oil and is expressed in visceral afferents. This channel contributes to mechanosensation, and is thought to play a role in mast cell activation and in the regulation of 5-hydroxytryptamine release in enterochromaffin cells (Boesmans et al. 2011). The TRPA1 channel may represent an important pharmacological target for cannabinoids in the gut.

A recent paper reported that the plant cannabinoid CBC affects TRPV1, TRPV3, and TRPV4 expression in the GI tract that had been increased by an inflammatory insult (De Petrocellis et al. 2012). A further study found that CBC normalized croton oil-induced hypermotility in vivo, and reduced electrically and acetylcholine-induced contractions. These actions were not mediated by cannabinoid receptors or TRPA1 channels (Izzo et al. 2012). These data indicate that CBC can modify TRP channel expression under inflammatory conditions but does not appear to interact directly with such channels (at least in motility/contractility studies).

12.2.5 Peroxisome proliferator-activated receptors

Endogenous, synthetic, and plant-derived cannabinoids are known to activate PPARs, a family of nuclear receptors comprising three isoforms—α, β, and γ—which regulate cell differentiation, metabolism, and immune function. Anandamide and oleoylethanolamide (a structural analogue of anandamide) may activate PPARα (Borrelli and Izzo 2009; Capasso and Izzo 2008), which is expressed by neurons in the myenteric and submucosal plexuses throughout the GI tract. Furthermore, anandamide and 2-AG, and ajulemic acid, a structural analogue of THC, elicit anti-inflammatory effects via PPARγ activation (O'Sullivan and Kendall 2010). Among the phytocannabinoids, THC and CBD are known to activate PPARγ (O'Sullivan and Kendall 2010). CBD has been shown to exert antiproliferative effects in colorectal carcinoma cells with a mechanism involving, at least in part, PPARγ activation (Aviello et al. 2012). Similarly, CBD has been found to reduce the expression of S100β and inducible nitric oxide synthase (iNOS) proteins in intestinal biopsies of ulcerative colitis patients in a PPARγ-antagonist sensitive manner (De Filippis et al. 2011).

12.3 Pharmacological actions

12.3.1 Gastric acid secretion and gastroprotection

Cannabinoids decrease acid production in rodents via CB_1 receptor activation (Adami et al. 2002, Coruzzi et al. 2006). The site of action is on vagal efferent pathways to the gastric mucosa and not on parietal cells because CB_1 receptor activation results in a reduction in acid secretion induced by 2-deoxy-D-glucose and pentagastrin (which increases acid secretion through the release of acetylcholine), but not by histamine, which directly activates H_2 receptors on parietal cells (Adami et al. 2002). In agreement with a gastric antisecretory action, CB_1 receptor activation by cannabinoids is protective in animal models in which gastric ulcers have been induced by: (1) aspirin (Rutkowska and Fereniec-Gołebiewska 2009), (2) water immersion and restraint stress

(Dembiński et al. 2006; Warzecha et al. 2011), or (3) cold/restraint stress (Germanò et al. 2011). Similarly, FAAH inhibitors also show gastroprotective effects (Naidu et al. 2009; Sasso et al. 2012), while CB_1 receptor antagonists both increase acid production in vitro and aggravate experimentally induced gastric lesions (Borrelli 2007; Dembiński et al., 2006).

Studies on plant-derived cannabinoids were first performed before the discovery of cannabinoid receptors. An acute treatment with a *Cannabis sativa* extract affected the lesion pattern and incidence of ulcerations associated with restraint-induced gastric ulcerations in rats (De Souza et al. 1978). THC produced a marked reduction in gastric ulcer formation in the pylorus-ligated rat test (Sofia et al. 1978). This reduction was more pronounced after subcutaneous than oral administration. THC reduced gastric juice volume, while free and total gastric acid content was not modified (Sofia et al. 1978). In an in vitro study, THC did not modify resting acid production in rats, but did inhibit gastric acid secretion induced by histamine (Rivas and Josè 1980), which is suggestive of a direct action of THC on parietal cells that is most likely not mediated by CB_1 receptors (see earlier in this section). Nevertheless, the quite recent discovery of CB_1 receptors on human parietal cells (Pazos et al. 2008) points to species differences and suggests that further studies are needed to fully establish the mode of action of THC in the control of GI acid secretion.

12.3.2 **Lower esophageal sphincter**

The lower esophageal sphincter (LES) is a specialized, involuntary, ring-shaped, smooth muscle located at the base of the esophagus that allows the passage of a swallowed bolus and prevents the reflux of gastric contents into the esophagus. Defects in LES relaxation can lead to gastroesophageal reflux disease (GERD). CB_1 receptor activation has been shown to inhibit transient LES relaxations in dogs and ferrets (Beaumont et al. 2009; Lehmann et al. 2002; Partosoedarso et al. 2003), the effect being associated, at least in the dog, with the inhibition of gastroesophageal reflux (Beaumont et al. 2009; Lehmann et al. 2002). Central and peripheral vagal mechanisms are involved in these functional changes (Beaumont et al. 2009). Similarly, in healthy volunteers, THC (10 mg and 20 mg) both inhibited the increase in transient LES relaxations evoked by meal ingestion, and reduced spontaneous swallowing as well as basal LES pressure (Beaumont et al. 2009). After intake of 20 mg THC, half of the subjects experienced nausea and vomiting leading to premature termination of the study. Other side effects were hypotension, tachycardia, and central effects (Beaumont et al. 2009). Intriguingly, a placebo-controlled, double-blind, randomized, crossover study demonstrated that the CB_1 receptor antagonist, rimonabant, inhibited the meal-induced increase in transient LES relaxation, increased postprandial LES pressure leading to a lower number of acid reflux events, and increased the duration of distal esophageal peristaltic waves (Scarpellini et al. 2011).

12.3.3 **Gastrointestinal motility**

Cannabinoid receptor agonists have been shown to reduce gastric, small intestinal, and colonic motility both in isolated segments and in in vivo studies in rodents (Pinto et al. 2002a). The effect is largely due to CB_1 receptor activation, although CB_2 receptors may be involved in some pathophysiological states (see sections 12.3.5–12.3.8). In vitro, cannabinoids act on prejunctional CB_1 receptors to reduce smooth muscle contractility and peristalsis in different regions of the rodent GI tract (Aviello et al. 2008; Izzo and Sharkey 2010). A number of cannabinoid receptor agonists have shown high potency as inhibitors of electrically induced contractions in several intestinal isolated preparations, including human ones. Notably, the plant cannabinoids THC and CBN have been shown to reduce electrically evoked contractions in the guinea pig (Pertwee et al. 1992, 1996; R.A. Ross et al. 1998) and rat (Makwana et al. 2010) ileum. The mechanism by which cannabinoid receptor activation reduces contractility is mainly related to reduction of acetylcholine release from myenteric nerves. Conversely, cannabinoid receptor antagonists/inverse agonists have been shown to increase electrically evoked contractions in isolated rodent intestinal segments and to accelerate gastric emptying and intestinal motility in vivo (Di Marzo et al. 2008; Pertwee et al. 1996; Pinto et al. 2002b; Storr et al. 2010).

The ability of plant cannabinoids to reduce intestinal motility was already known before the discovery of cannabinoid receptors. In 1972, Dewey and colleagues were the first to report that THC reduced the rate of passage of a charcoal meal along the mouse small intestine (Dewey et al. 1972). These findings were confirmed in other studies (Anderson et al. 1974; Chesher et al. 1973; Jackson et al. 1976; Shook et al. 1986). In each of these early experiments THC was administered intraperitoneally or subcutaneously and it was found to be six to ten times less potent than morphine in slowing the transit. However, when administered intravenously, THC was equipotent with morphine (Shook and Burks 1989). Interestingly, THC antagonized (at low doses, i.e., 0.25 mg/kg) or potentiated (at a higher dose, i.e., 1 mg/kg) the decreased motility induced by prostaglandin E_2 in mice (Jackson et al. 1976).

In a more complete study, Shook and Bruks showed that THC and CBN slowed the rate of gastric emptying and small intestinal transit when injected intravenously in mice and rats. Whereas THC equally inhibited gastric emptying and small intestinal transit, CBN had only minimal effects on gastric emptying. THC produced greater inhibition of gastric emptying and small intestinal transit than of large bowel transit, indicating a relative selectivity for the more proximal section of the gut. When THC was injected intracerebroventricularly, it inhibited transit, but only at doses which were also active when injected intravenously, implying that it was acting at a peripheral site (Shook and Burks 1989). In more recent years, with the availability of selective receptor antagonists, other investigators have shown that the inhibitory effects of THC and CBN on GI motility are mediated by cannabinoid receptor activation (Izzo et al. 2000; Krowicki et al. 1999; Pinto et al. 2002b). Specifically, intraperitoneally administered CBN reduces the passage of charcoal in the mouse small intestine and increases the time of expulsion of a bead inserted in the mouse colon in a CB_1 antagonist-sensitive way (Izzo et al. 2000; Pinto et al. 2002b). Similarly, the CB_1 receptor antagonist rimonabant counteracted the long-lasting decrease in rat intragastric pressure and pyloric contractility evoked by intravenously administered THC (Krowicki et al. 1999). The effect of THC on gastric motility was abolished by bilateral vagotomy at the mid cervical level and by hexamethonium, but not by transection of the cervical spinal cord suggesting that this phytocannabinoid produces its inhibitory effects on the stomach partly by acting on the dorsal vagal complex of the hindbrain to modulate vagal (parasympathetic) outflow to gastric smooth muscle (Krowicki et al. 1999).

Recently, the nonpsychotropic phytocannabinoids CBD and CBC have been evaluated as modulators of intestinal motility, both in isolated intestinal segments and in in vivo studies on transit. Neither compound modified intestinal motility in control mice in vivo, but both of them did normalize motility following the administration of an inflammatory insult (Capasso et al. 2008a; Izzo et al. 2012; Lin et al. 2009; see also later sections). In the isolated mouse intestine, CBD reduced acetylcholine- and KCl-induced contractions, suggesting a nonspecific antispasmodic effect (Capasso et al. 2008a). In the same tissue, CBC preferentially reduced electrically induced contractions—rather than acetylcholine-induced contractions—by a mechanism involving neuronal N-type Ca^{2+} channels (Izzo et al. 2012).

12.3.4 **Intestinal fluid secretion**

An adequate fluid secretion is required for the normal passage of gut contents along the bowel. In the colon, fluid is absorbed, limiting water content; a failure to absorb water or any situation of excessive secretion leads to diarrhea. Studies on isolated intestinal segments have shown that activation of CB_1 receptors may produce an antisecretory effect through a neuronal mechanism involving the inhibition of neurotransmitter(s) release from submucosal plexus neurons and extrinsic primary afferents (MacNaughton et al. 2004; Tyler et al. 2000). In vivo, cannabinoid receptor agonists reduce intestinal hypersecretion induced by cholera toxin in mice (Izzo et al. 2003).

The effect of plant-derived cannabinoids on intestinal water and electrolyte transport has not been thoroughly evaluated. Early studies showed that THC enhanced net water absorption in the rat ileum, and this effect was not associated with a reduced content of prostaglandin E_2-like material (Coupar and Taylor 1983).

12.3.5 **Visceral sensation**

Experimental evidence suggests that CB_1 or CB_2 receptor activation inhibits visceral sensitivity and pain in rodents. The CB_1 receptor-mediated analgesic effect is associated with downregulation of TRPV1, whilst CB_2 receptor agonist inhibition of visceral pain responses appears to be due to inhibition of the algesic responses to bradykinin (Izzo and Sharkey 2010). Booker and colleagues assessed the antinociceptive effect of a number of plant-derived cannabinoids in the acetic acid stretching test, a rodent visceral pain model. It was found that THC and CBN exerted a CB_1 antagonist-sensitive, but not a CB_2 antagonist-sensitive antinociceptive effect at doses lower than those necessary to produce locomotor suppression. Also, consistent with its CB_1 receptor antagonistic properties, THCV had no effect when administered alone, but did counteract the antinociceptive effect of THC (Booker et al. 2010). A previous report showed that both a crude marijuana extract, and THC, CBN, but not CBD, displayed a significant analgesic effect in the acetic acid stretching test, with THC being as active as morphine (Sofia et al. 1975).

12.3.6 **Intestinal inflammation**

Animal studies have shown that cannabinoids, via CB_1 or CB_2 receptor activation, as well as via elevation of endocannabinoid levels, effectively attenuate inflammation in well-established models of inflammatory bowel disease (IBD) (Alhouayek et al. 2011, 2012; Bento et al. 2011; D'Argenio et al. 2006; Engel et al. 2006, 2010; Kimball et al. 2006; Massa et al. 2004; Singh et al. 2012; Storr et al. 2008, 2009). Conversely, experimental inflammation is exacerbated in CB_1 or CB_2 receptor knockout mice or in mice treated with CB_1 or CB_2 receptor antagonists (Engel et al. 2010; Massa et al. 2004). In the gut of patients with IBD, adaptive changes of the endogenous cannabinoid system (e.g., changes in cannabinoids receptors and/or in endocannabinoid levels resulting from modifications of one or more of the enzymes involved in endocannabinoid biosynthesis or degradation) have been observed (D'Argenio et al. 2006; Di Sabatino et al. 2011; Wright et al. 2005).

Concerning plant-derived cannabinoids, THC, CBD, CBC, and CBG have proved to be beneficial in experimental models of IBD. Jamontt and colleagues showed that THC reduced signs of damage, inflammation, and functional disturbance in the trinitrobenzene sulfonic acid (TNBS) rat model of IBD. THC also improved the function of cholinergic motoneurons, while sulfasalazine (a standard treatment for IBD) did not show any protective effect on TNBS-induced changes in motility (Jamontt et al., 2010). THC also restored the increased permeability induced by ethylenediaminetetraacetic acid (EDTA) in intestinal epithelial cells (Alhamoruni et al. 2010).

The first demonstration of a beneficial action of CBD in intestinal inflammation was provided by Borrelli and colleagues, who demonstrated that this phytocannabinoid, given intraperitoneally, reduced the degree of intestinal inflammation caused by intracolonic administration of dinitrobenzene sulfonic acid (DNBS) in mice. The protective effect of CBD was associated with downregulation of iNOS (but not cyclooxygenase-2) expression and modulation of cytokine (IL-1β and IL-10) levels, whereas it did not involve interference with endocannabinoid inactivation mechanisms such as FAAH inhibition (Borrelli et al. 2009). The beneficial effect of CBD in mice has recently been confirmed by Schicho and Storr, who, by demonstrating that not only intraperitoneal administration but also intrarectal treatment with CBD led to a significant improvement of disease parameters, have provided evidence that intrarectal delivery of cannabidiol may represent a useful therapeutic administration route for the treatment of colonic inflammation (Schicho and Storr, 2012). Finally, CBD proved beneficial in the TNBS model of colitis in rats with its dose–response relationship showing a bell-shaped pattern for the majority of parameters investigated (Jamontt et al. 2010). CBD not only reduced inflammation, but also lowered the occurrence of functional disorders; in addition, CBD acted additively or synergistically with THC to reduce inflammation and to protect cholinergic nerves (Jamontt et al. 2010).

Experiments on isolated intestinal cells have confirmed the beneficial effect of CBD against inflammatory insults. In colorectal carcinoma (Caco-2) cells, CBD prevented oxidative stress, which may be one of the underlying factors leading to mucosal protection in vivo (Borrelli et al., 2009). Also, CBD was able to restore the increased permeability induced by EDTA or cytokine in the Caco-2 cell culture model of intestinal permeability (Alhamoruni et al. 2010, 2012). The effect was sensitive to a cannabinoid CB_1 receptor antagonist, but not to CB_2 receptor, TRPV1, PPARγ, or PPARα antagonists. Finally, in intestinal segments obtained from mice with LPS-induced intestinal inflammation, CBD was found to counteract reactive enteric gliosis, an effect associated with a massive reduction in the astroglial signaling neurotrophin S100β (De Filippis et al. 2011). Similarly, CBD reduced the expression of S100β and iNOS proteins in human biopsy samples obtained from patients with ulcerative colitis (De Filippis et al. 2011).

Recently, CBG and CBC have been shown to exert preventive and therapeutic effect in the DNBS murine model of colitis (Borrelli et al. 2013; Romano et al. 2013). Both CBC and CBG reduced the colon weight/colon length ratio (a simple and reliable marker of intestinal inflammation), myeloperoxidase activity, and intestinal permeability in DNBS-treated mice. More in-depth studies showed that the beneficial effect of CBG was associated with modulation of cytokine (IL-1β, IL-10, and interferon-γ) levels and downregulation of iNOS (but not cyclooxygenase-2) expression. In intestinal epithelial cells, CBG prevented reactive oxygen species production, which may help to explain the protective effect of this phytocannabinoid that has been observed in vivo (Borrelli et al. 2013).

12.3.7 **Motility dysfunctions in the inflamed gut**

Changes in the endogenous cannabinoid system during inflammation may alter and/or contribute to motility changes that occur in IBD patients. Experimental evidence suggests that, depending on the inflammatory insult, both CB_1 and CB_2 receptor activation may reduce hypermotility associated with gut inflammation (Duncan et al. 2008a; Izzo 2004; Mathison et al. 2004; Wright et al. 2008). Thus, intestinal inflammation induced by croton oil is characterized by disruption of the mucosa and an infiltration of lymphocytes into the sub mucosa (Pol and Puig 1997), and such changes are associated with decreased anandamide and palmitoylethanolamide levels, as well as with upregulation of cannabinoid CB_1 receptors and TRPA1 channels (Capasso et al. 2001;

Izzo et al. 2001, 2012). Motility in the croton oil model of ileitis can be attenuated by a number of drugs including CB_1 and CB_2 receptor agonists (Capasso et al. 2008b; Izzo et al. 2001). CBN, CBD, and CBC have been evaluated for their ability to alter the motility changes associated with the intestinal inflammation induced by oral croton oil administration, as detailed in section 3.7.

Like other cannabinoid receptor agonists, CBN (a partial cannabinoid CB_1 receptor agonist) reduced intestinal motility both in control and in croton oil-treated animals, displaying greater inhibitory activity in pathological states. Interestingly, this inhibitory effect was accompanied not only by a leftward shift in the in vivo log dose–response curve of CBN, but also by an increase in the size of its maximal effect (Izzo et al. 2001). The synthetic agonist CP55940, which has higher CB_1 efficacy than CBN, exhibited a potency increase but no change in its maximal effect (Izzo et al. 2001). The low doses of CBN that are needed to reduce motility during intestinal inflammation are of interest in the light of possible therapeutic applications of such a compound in IBD.

More recently, the nonpsychotropic phytocannabinoids CBD and CBC have been evaluated in the croton oil model of intestinal hypermotility. Although neither CBD nor CBC modify intestinal motility in control mice, both of them do normalize intestinal motility in inflamed mice (Capasso et al. 2008a; Izzo et al. 2012). The inhibitory effect of CBD could involve CB_1 receptors via elevation of endocannabinoid levels at these receptors induced by FAAH inhibition, which is consistent with the ability of this phytocannabinoid to reduce FAAH expression in the inflamed—but not in the normal—mouse gut (De Filippis et al. 2008). On the other hand, the inhibitory effect of CBC did not involve cannabinoid receptors or TRPA1 channels. In vitro, both CBC and CBD exerted spasmolytic actions in ilea from control and croton oil-treated animals. More in depth studies on CBC showed that this phytocannabinoid altered the ex vivo expression of a number of TRP channels, such as TRPA1, TRPV1, TRPV3, and TRPV4, in the gut of croton oil-treated mice (De Petrocellis et al. 2012; Izzo et al. 2012). Overall, the in vivo ability of both CBC and CBD to normalize motility in the inflamed gut, without slowing the rate of transit in healthy animals, is of potential clinical interest since currently used antidiarrheal agents are often associated with constipating effects.

Finally, Lin and colleagues found that CBD normalized hypomotility and inflammatory responses in the LPS mouse model of septic ileus (Lin et al. 2011). The possibility that CBD acts as a systemic anti-inflammatory agent in this model of intestinal dysfunction cannot be ruled out (Lin et al. 2011).

12.3.8 Colon cancer

Cannabinoids exert antiproliferative, antimetastatic, and proapoptotic actions in colorectal carcinoma epithelial cells (Izzo and Camilleri 2009). In experimental in vivo models of colon cancer, cannabinoid agonists might be protective in different stages of colon cancer progression either directly, through activation of CB_1 or CB_2 receptors, or indirectly, through elevation of endocannabinoid levels via FAAH inhibition (Cianchi et al. 2008; Izzo et al. 2008; Wang et al. 2008). Their antitumor actions may be mediated by either CB_1 or CB_2 receptor activation (Izzo and Camilleri 2009). The mechanism of CB_1-mediated apoptosis involves inhibition of both the RAS–MAPK/ERK and PI3K–Akt survival signaling cascades and downregulation of the antiapoptotic factor survivin. The proapoptotic lipid ceramide could be involved in both CB_1- and CB_2-mediated antitumor effects (Izzo and Camilleri 2009).

Recently, the phytocannabinoid CBD has been evaluated for its possible chemopreventive effect in a murine model of colon cancer induced by the carcinogenic agent azoxymethane (AOM). CBD effectively reduced AOM-induced preneoplastic lesions, polyps and tumors in the colon, an effect that was associated with downregulation of phospho-Akt and upregulation of caspase-3. Studies on colorectal carcinoma cells suggested that CBD protected DNA damage caused by an oxidative insult and exerted antiproliferative effects through multiple mechanisms, including involvement of CB_1 receptors, TRPV1 and PPARγ (Aviello et al. 2012).

The oxidation of cannabis constituents leads to the formation of the corresponding quinones, which have been demonstrated to be cytotoxic agents. The quinone of CBD, named HU-331, exerts antiangiogenic and proapoptotic properties and also inhibits topoisomerase II (Peters and Kogan 2007). Unlike other quinones, it is not cardiotoxic and does not induce the formation of free radicals. A comparative in vivo study in mice has shown HU-331 to be less toxic and more effective than doxorubicin in a nude mouse HT-29 colon carcinoma model (Kogan et al. 2007).

12.4 **Clinical studies**

12.4.1 **Gastrointestinal motility, visceral sensation, and IBS**

Visceral hypersensitivity to distension and altered GI motility are thought to play an important role in the pathophysiology of the irritable bowel syndrome (IBS). Both visceral sensation and GI motility have been evaluated in human volunteers after THC administration. Thus, nine male and four female experienced cannabis users underwent gastric emptying studies that used radiolabeled solid food as a marker, after they had received THC (at a dose of 10 mg/m^2 of body surface area) or placebo. Gastric emptying after THC was slower than after placebo in all subjects. However, no correlation was found between plasma THC levels and the delay in gastric emptying. The authors concluded that THC, at a dose that can prevent chemotherapy-induced nausea and vomiting, significantly delayed gastric emptying of solid food in humans (McCallum et al. 1999). The inhibitory effect of THC on gastric emptying has been confirmed more recently by Esfandyari and colleagues, in a randomized, double-blind study performed with 30 healthy volunteers who received THC (5 mg twice a day) or placebo. Gastric emptying was measured noninvasively. An overall retardation of gastric emptying with THC compared to placebo was observed, the effect being more pronounced in females than in males (Esfandyari et al. 2006).

In a further randomized, double-blind trial, Esfandyari and colleagues assessed colonic compliance, motility, tone, and sensation in 52 volunteers who had received a single dose of 7.5 mg THC. An overall significant increase in colonic compliance, a borderline effect on relaxation in fasting colonic tone, inhibition of postprandial colonic tone, and inhibition of fasting and postprandial phasic pressure was observed. Collectively, the results suggest that THC relaxes the colon and reduces postprandial colonic motility and tone in humans (Esfandyari et al. 2007).

More recently, Wong and colleagues compared the effects of THC (5 mg) with those of placebo on colonic motility and sensation in patients with IBS, and also conducted a pharmacogenetic analysis that explored the influence of genetic variation in the CB_1 receptor, FAAH and MAGL on the ability of THC to alter diarrhea and colonic transit in IBS with diarrhea patients (Wong et al. 2011). In all patients (35 with IBS with constipation, 35 with IBS with diarrhea, and 5 with alternating IBS) THC did not alter sensation or tone but decreased the fasting proximal left colonic motility index compared with placebo, and increased colonic compliance. The effects of THC were greatest in patients with IBS with diarrhea or with alternating IBS. FAAH and CNR1 variants influenced the effect of THC on colonic motility (Wong et al. 2011). In a subsequent study, the same authors found that THC (2.5 and 5 mg) had no effect on gut transit in IBS patients with diarrhea, although a treatment-by-genotype effect was observed, whereby THC preferentially delayed colonic transit in patients with the CNR1 rs806378 CT/TT genotypes (Wong et al. 2012).

Finally, Klooker and colleagues evaluated the effect of THC on rectal sensitivity in ten IBS patients and 12 healthy volunteers. THC did not alter baseline rectal perception to distension compared to placebo either in volunteers or in IBS patients. Similarly, after sigmoid stimulation there were no significant differences between placebo and THC in sensory thresholds of discomfort (Klooker et al. 2011).

In conclusion, studies in humans suggest that THC may affect gastric emptying and colonic motility in healthy and/or IBS patients, particularly in a subset of IBS with diarrhea patients, based on a specific genetic variation in the CB_1 receptor. Further studies of cannabinoid pharmacogenetics could identify a subset of IBS with diarrhea patients in which cannabinoid therapy may be effective. Conversely, THC does not seem to affect visceral perception in humans, a result which illustrates the importance of doing translational studies when investigating a possible clinical use of a cannabinoid.

12.4.2 Inflammatory bowel disease

Some IBD patients anecdotally report that they can obtain relief by smoking marijuana. Recently, three studies, by showing beneficial effects of cannabis use in humans, seem to confirm such reports.

Naftali and colleagues performed a retrospective observational study examining disease activity, use of medication, need for surgery before and after cannabis use in 30 Crohn's disease (CD) patients (26 males). Of the 30 patients, 21 improved significantly after treatment with cannabis. The need for other medication was significantly reduced and the number of patients requiring surgery decreased during cannabis use (Naftali et al. 2011).

Lal and colleagues evaluated cannabis use in 291 IBD patients, who completed a questionnaire regarding current and previous cannabis use. About 50% of these IBD patients, particularly those with a history of abdominal surgery, chronic abdominal pain and/or a low quality of life, reported lifetime or current cannabis use. Patients who had used cannabis were more likely than nonusers to express an interest in participating in a hypothetical therapeutic trial of cannabis for IBD. Collectively such results suggest that cannabis use for symptom relief is common in patients with IBD (Lal et al. 2011).

Finally, a pilot prospective study involving 13 patients with long-standing IBD assessed whether treatment with inhaled cannabis (cigarettes) improved quality of life, reduced disease activity, and promoted weight gain in IBD patients. After 3 months' treatment, patients reported improvement in general health perception, social functioning, ability to work, pain, and depression. cannabis also promoted weight gain and induced a rise in body mass index (Lahat et al. 2012).

12.6 Conclusions

There is anecdotal evidence, spanning many centuries, that cannabis is therapeutically beneficial for a variety of human GI disease conditions. Recently, however, in-depth research efforts have begun to document the detailed pharmacological actions of specific plant-derived cannabinoids, which have been shown to modulate several critically important functions in the GI tract (e.g., motility, sensation, inflammation, tissue proliferation, and carcinogenesis). The resurgence of interest in the study of plant-based cannabinoids has probably been encouraged by the approval of Sativex® for the treatment of multiple sclerosis spasticity and pain. Concerning the GI tract, areas of major interest are those related to widespread diseases such as IBS, IBD, and colon cancer and, at least for IBD and IBS, promising, albeit preliminary, clinical data are already available.

The challenge now is to achieve a favorable balance between the beneficial effects of cannabinoids on GI disorders and the unwanted effects that can result from CB_1 receptor activation, for example, by focusing on the particularly promising potential approach of exploiting the apparent ability of nonpsychoactive plant cannabinoids to ameliorate GI disorders.

References

Adami, M., Frati, P., Bertini, S., *et al.* (2002). Gastric antisecretory role and immunohistochemical localization of cannabinoid receptors in the rat stomach. *British Journal of Pharmacology*, **135**, 598–606.

Adami, M., Zamfirova, R., Sotirov, E., *et al.* (2004). Gastric antisecretory effects of synthetic cannabinoids after central or peripheral administration in the rat. *Brain Research Bulletin*, **64**, 357–361.

Alhouayek, M., Lambert, D.M., Delzenne, N.M., *et al.* (2011). Increasing endogenous 2-arachidonoylglycerol levels counteracts colitis and related systemic inflammation. *FASEB Journal*, **25**, 2711–2721.

Alhouayek, M. and Muccioli, G.G. (2012). The endocannabinoid system in inflammatory bowel diseases: from pathophysiology to therapeutic opportunity. *Trends in Molecular Medicine*, **18**, 615–625.

Alhamoruni, A., Lee, A.C., Wright, K.L., *et al.* (2010). Pharmacological effects of cannabinoids on the Caco-2 cell culture model of intestinal permeability. *Journal of Pharmacology and Experimental Therapeutics*, **335**, 92–102.

Alhamoruni, A., Wright, K.L., Larvin, M., and O'Sullivan, S.E. (2012). Cannabinoids mediate opposing effects on inflammation-induced intestinal permeability. *British Journal of Pharmacology*, **165**, 2598–2610.

Anderson, P.F., Jackson, D.M., and Chesher, G.B. (1974). Interaction of delta9-tetrahydrocannabinol and cannabidiol on intestinal motility in mice. *Journal of Pharmacy and Pharmacology*, **26**, 136–137.

Appendino, G., Chianese, G., and Taglialatela-Scafati O. (2011). Cannabinoids: occurrence and medicinal chemistry. *Current Medicinal Chemistry*, **18**, 1085–1099.

Aviello, G., Romano, B., and Borrelli, F., *et al.* (2012). Chemopreventive effect of the non-psychotropic phytocannabinoid cannabidiol on experimental colon cancer. *Journal of Molecular Medicine*, **90**, 925–934.

Aviello, G., Romano, B., and Izzo, A.A. (2008). Cannabinoids and gastrointestinal motility: animal and human studies. *European Review for Medical and Pharmacological Sciences*, **12**(Suppl. 1), 81–93.

Bashashati, M., Storr, M.A., and Nikas, S.P. (2012). Inhibiting fatty acid amide hydrolase normalizes endotoxin-induced enhanced gastrointestinal motility in mice. *British Journal of Pharmacology*, **165**, 1556–1571.

Beaumont, H., Jensen, J., Carlsson, A., Ruth, M., Lehmann, A., and Boeckxstaens, G. (2009). Effect of delta9-tetrahydrocannabinol, a cannabinoid receptor agonist, on the triggering of transient lower oesophageal sphincter relaxations in dogs and humans. *British Journal of Pharmacology*, **156**, 153–162.

Bento, A.F., Marcon, R., Dutra, R.C., *et al.* (2011). β-Caryophyllene inhibits dextran sulfate sodium-induced colitis in mice through CB2 receptor activation and PPARγ pathway. *American Journal of Pathology*, **178**, 1153–1166.

Bisogno, T., Hanus, L., De Petrocellis, L., *et al.* (2001). Molecular targets for cannabidiol and its synthetic analogues: effect on vanilloid VR1 receptors and on the cellular uptake and enzymatic hydrolysis of anandamide. *British Journal of Pharmacology*, **134**, 845–852.

Boesmans, W., Owsianik, G., Tack, J., Voets, T., and Vanden Berghe, P. (2011). TRP channels in neurogastroenterology: opportunities for therapeutic intervention. *British Journal of Pharmacology*, **162**, 18–37.

Bolognini, D., Costa, B., Maione, S., *et al.* (2010). The plant cannabinoid Delta9- tetrahydrocannabivarin can decrease signs of inflammation and inflammatory pain in mice. *British Journal of Pharmacology*, **160**, 677–87.

Booker, L., Naidu, P.S., Razdan, R.K., Mahadevan, A., and Lichtman, A.H. (2009). Evaluation of prevalent phytocannabinoids in the acetic acid model of visceral nociception. *Drug and Alcohol Dependence*, **105**, 42–47.

Borrelli, F. (2007). Cannabinoid CB_1 receptor and gastric acid secretion. *Digestive Disease and Sciences*, **52**, 3102–3103.

Borrelli, F., Aviello, G., Romano, B., *et al.* (2009). Cannabidiol, a safe and non-psychotropic ingredient of the marijuana plant *Cannabis sativa*, is protective in a murine model of colitis. *Journal of Molecular Medicine*, **87**, 1111–1121.

Borrelli, F. and Izzo, A.A. (2009). Role of acylethanolamides in the gastrointestinal tract with special reference to food intake and energy balance. *Best Practice and Research Clinical Endocrinology and Metabolism*, **23**, 33–49.

Borrelli, F., Fasolino, I., Romano, B., *et al.* (2013). Beneficial effect of the non-psychotropic plant cannabinoid cannabigerol on experimental inflammatory bowel disease. *Biochemical Pharmacology*, **85**, 1306–1316.

Capasso, R., Borrelli, F., Aviello, G., *et al.* (2008a). Cannabidiol, extracted from *Cannabis sativa*, selectively inhibits inflammatory hypermotility in mice. *British Journal of Pharmacology*, **154**, 1001–1008.

Capasso, R., Borrelli, F., Cascio, M.G., *et al.* (2008b). Inhibitory effect of salvinorin A, from Salvia divinorum, on ileitis-induced hypermotility: cross-talk between kappa-opioid and cannabinoid CB_1 receptors. *British Journal of Pharmacology*, **155**, 681–689.

Capasso, R. and Izzo, A.A. (2008). Gastrointestinal regulation of food intake: general aspects and focus on anandamide and oleoylethanolamide. *Journal of Neuroendocrinology*, **20**(Suppl. 1), 39–46.

Capasso, R., Izzo, A.A., Fezza, F., *et al.* (2001). Inhibitory effect of palmitoylethanolamide on gastrointestinal motility in mice. *British Journal of Pharmacology*, **134**, 945–950.

Chesher, G.B., Dahl, C.J., Everingham, M., *et al.* (1973). The effect of cannabinoids on intestinal motility and their antinociceptive effect in mice. *British Journal of Pharmacology*, **49**, 588–594.

Cianchi, F., Papucci, L., Schiavone, N., *et al.* (2008). Cannabinoid receptor activation induces apoptosis through tumor necrosis factor alpha-mediated ceramide de novo synthesis in colon cancer cells. *Clinical Cancer Research*, **14**, 7691–7700.

Cluny, N.L., Keenan, C.M., Duncan, M., Fox, A., Lutz, B., and Sharkey, K.A. (2010). Naphthalen-1-yl-(4-pentyloxynaphthalen-1-yl)methanone (SAB378), a peripherally restricted cannabinoid CB1/CB2 receptor agonist, inhibits gastrointestinal motility but has no effect on experimental colitis in mice. *Journal of Pharmacology and Experimental Therapeutics*, **334**, 973–980.

Coruzzi, G., Adami, M., Guaita, E., *et al.* (2006). Effects of cannabinoid receptor agonists on rat gastric acid secretion: discrepancy between *in vitro* and *in vivo* data. *Digestive Disease and Sciences*, **51**, 310–317.

Coupar, I.M. and Taylor, D.A. (1983). Effect of delta-9-tetrahydrocannabinol on prostaglandin concentrations and fluid absorption rates in the rat small intestine. *Journal of Pharmacy and Pharmacology*, **35**, 392–394.

D'Argenio, G., Valenti, M., Scaglione, G., Cosenza, V., Sorrentini, I., and Di Marzo, V. (2006). Up-regulation of anandamide levels as an endogenous mechanism and a pharmacological strategy to limit colon inflammation. *FASEB Journal*, **20**, 568–570.

De Filippis, D., Esposito, G., Cirillo, C., *et al.* (2011). Cannabidiol reduces intestinal inflammation through the control of neuroimmune axis. *PLoS One*, **6**, e28159.

De Filippis, D., Iuvone, T., D'amico, A., *et al.* (2008). Effect of cannabidiol on sepsis-induced motility disturbances in mice: involvement of CB receptors and fatty acid amide hydrolase. *Neurogastroenterology and Motility*, **20**, 919–927.

De Petrocellis, L., Ligresti, A., and Moriello, A.S. (2011). Effects of cannabinoids and cannabinoid-enriched *Cannabis* extracts on TRP channels and endocannabinoid metabolic enzymes. *British Journal of Pharmacology*, **163**, 1479–1494.

De Petrocellis, L., Orlando, P., Moriello, A.S., *et al.* (2012). Cannabinoid actions at TRPV channels: effects on TRPV3 and TRPV4 and their potential relevance to gastrointestinal inflammation. *Acta Physiologica*, **204**, 255–266.

De Souza, H., Trajano, E., de Carvalho, F.V., and Palermo Neto, J. (1978). Effects of acute and long-term cannabis treatment of restraint-induced gastric ulceration in rats. *Japanese Journal of Pharmacology*, **28**, 507–510.

Dembiński, A., Warzecha, Z., Ceranowicz, P., *et al.* (2006). Cannabinoids in acute gastric damage and pancreatitis. *Journal of Physiology Pharmacology*, **57**(Suppl. 5), 137–154.

Dewey, W.L., Harris, L.S., and Kennedy, J.S. (1972). Some pharmacological and toxicological effects of 1-trans-8 and 1-trans-9-tetrahydrocannabinol in laboratory rodents. *Archives Internationales de Pharmacodynamie et de Thérapie*, **196**, 133–145.

Di Marzo, V., Capasso, R., Matias, I., *et al.* (2008). The role of endocannabinoids in the regulation of gastric emptying: alterations in mice fed a high-fat diet. *British Journal of Pharmacology*, **153**, 1272–1280.

Di Sabatino, A., Battista, N., Biancheri, P., *et al.* (2011). The endogenous cannabinoid system in the gut of patients with inflammatory bowel disease. *Mucosal Immunology*, **4**, 574–583.

Duncan, M., Davison, J.S., and Sharkey, K.A. (2005). Review article: endocannabinoids and their receptors in the enteric nervous system. *Alimentary Pharmacology and Therapeutics*, **22**, 667–683.

Duncan, M., Mouihate, A., Mackie, K., *et al.* (2008a). Cannabinoid CB_2 receptors in the enteric nervous system modulate gastrointestinal contractility in lipopolysaccharide-treated rats. *American Journal of Physiology – Gastrointestinal and Liver Physiology*, **295**, G78–G87.

Duncan, M. Thomas, A.D., Cluny, N.L., *et al.* (2008b). Distribution and function of monoacylglyc-erol lipase in the gastrointestinal tract. *American Journal of Physiology – Gastrointestinal and Liver Physiology*, **295**, G1255–G1265.

Engel, M.A., Kellermann, C.A., Burnat, G., *et al.* (2010). Mice lacking cannabinoid CB1-, CB2-receptors or both receptors show increased susceptibility to trinitrobenzene sulfonic acid (TNBS)-induced colitis. *Journal of Physiology and Pharmacology*, **61**, 89–97.

Engel, M.A., Kellermann, C.A., Rau, T., Burnat, G., Hahn, E.G., and Konturek, P.C. (2008). Ulcerative colitis in AKR mice is attenuated by intraperitoneally administered anandamide. *Journal of Physiology and Pharmacology*, **59**, 673–689.

Esfandyari, T., Camilleri, M., Busciglio, I., Burton, D., Baxter, K. and Zinsmeister, A.R. (2007). Effects of a cannabinoid receptor agonist on colonic motor and sensory functions in humans: a randomized, placebo-controlled study. *American Journal of Physiology – Gastrointestinal and Liver Physiology*, **293**, G137–G145.

Esfandyari, T., Camilleri, M., Ferber, I., Burton, D., Baxter, K. and Zinsmeister, A.R. (2006). Effect of a cannabinoid agonist on gastrointestinal transit and postprandial satiation in healthy human subjects: a randomized, placebo-controlled study. *Neurogastroenterology and Motility*, **18**, 831–838.

Germanò, M.P., D'Angelo, V., Mondello, M.R., *et al.* (2001). Cannabinoid CB_1-mediated inhibition of stress-induced gastric ulcers in rats. *Naunyn-Schmiedeberg's Archives of Pharmacology*, **363**, 241–244.

Izzo, A.A. (2004). Cannabinoids and intestinal motility: welcome to CB_2 receptors. *British Journal of Pharmacology*, **142**, 1201–1202.

Izzo, A.A., Aviello, G., Petrosino, S., *et al.* (2008). Increased endocannabinoid levels reduce the development of precancerous lesions in the mouse colon. *Journal of Molecular Medicine*, **86**, 89–98.

Izzo, A.A., Borrelli, F. Capasso, R., Di Marzo, V., and Mechoulam, R .(2009). Non-psychotropic plant cannabinoids: new therapeutic opportunities from an ancient herb. *Trends in Pharmacological Sciences*, **30**, 515–527.

Izzo, A.A. and Camilleri, M. (2009). Cannabinoids in intestinal inflammation and cancer. *Pharmacological Research*, **60**, 117–125.

Izzo, A.A, Capasso, R., Aviello, G., *et al.* (2012). Inhibitory effect of cannabichromene, a major non-psychotropic cannabinoid extracted from Cannabis sativa, on inflammation-induced hypermotility in mice. *British Journal of Pharmacology*, **166**, 1444–1460.

Izzo, A.A., Capasso, F., Costagliola, A., *et al.* (2003). An endogenous cannabinoid tone attenuates cholera toxin-induced fluid accumulation in mice. *Gastroenterology*, **125**, 765–774.

Izzo, A.A. and Coutts, A.A. (2005). Cannabinoids and the digestive tract. *Handbook of Experimental Pharmacology*, **168**, 573–598.

Izzo, A.A., Fezza, F., Capasso, R., *et al.* (2001). Cannabinoid CB_1-receptor mediated regulation of gastro-intestinal motility in mice in a model of intestinal inflammation. *British Journal of Pharmacology*, **134**, 563–570.

Izzo, A.A., Pinto, L., Borrelli, F., Capasso, R., Mascolo, N. and Capasso, F. (2000). Central and periph-eral cannabinoid modulation of gastrointestinal transit in physiological states or during the diarrhoea induced by croton oil. *British Journal of Pharmacology*, **129**, 1627–1632.

Izzo, A.A. and Sharkey, K.A. (2010). Cannabinoids and the gut: new developments and emerging concepts. *Pharmacology and Therapeutics*, **126**, 21–38.

Jackson, D.M., Malor, R., Chesher, G.B., Starmer, G.A., Welburn, P.J., and Bailey, R. (1976). The inter-action between prostaglandin E1 and delta 9-tetrahydrocannabinol on intestinal motility and on the abdominal constriction response in the mouse. *Psychopharmacologia*, **47**, 187–193.

Jamontt, J.M., Molleman, A., Pertwee, R.G., and Parsons, M.E. (2010). The effects of Delta-tetrahydrocannabinol and cannabidiol alone and in combination on damage, inflammation and *in vitro* motility disturbances in rat colitis. *British Journal of Pharmacology*, **160**, 712–723.

Kimball, E.S., Schneider, C.R. Wallace, N.H., and Hornby, P.J. (2006). Agonists of cannabinoid receptor 1 and 2 inhibit experimental colitis induced by oil of mustard and by dextran sulfate sodium. *American Journal of Physiology – Gastrointestinal and Liver Physiology*, **291**, G364–G371.

Kimball, E.S., Wallace, N.H., Schneider, C.R, D'Andrea, M.R., and Hornby, P.J. (2010). Small intestinal cannabinoid receptor changes following a single colonic insult with oil of mustard in mice. *Frontiers in Pharmacology*, **1**, 132.

Kinsey, S.G., Nomura, D.K. and O'Neal, S.T., *et al.* (2011). Inhibition of monoacylglycerol lipase attenuates nonsteroidal anti-inflammatory drug-induced gastric hemorrhages in mice. *Journal of Pharmacology and Experimental Therapeutics*, **338**, 795–802.

Klooker, T.K., Leliefeld, K.E., Van Den Wijngaard, R.M., and Boeckxstaens, G.E. (2011). The cannabi-noid receptor agonist delta-9-tetrahydrocannabinol does not affect visceral sensitivity to rectal disten-sion in healthy volunteers and IBS patients. *Neurogastroenterology and Motility*, **23**, 30–5e2.

Kogan, N.M., Schlesinger, M., Peters, M., Marincheva, G., Beeri, R., and Mechoulam, R. (2007). A can-nabinoid anticancer quinone, HU-331, is more potent and less cardiotoxic than doxorubicin: a com-parative *in vivo* study. *Journal of Pharmacology and Experimental Therapeutics*, **322**, 646–653.

Krowicki, Z.K., Moerschbaecher, J.M., Winsauer, P.J., Digavalli, S.V., and Hornby, P.J. (1999). Delta9-tetrahydrocannabinol inhibits gastric motility in the rat through cannabinoid CB_1 receptors. *European Journal of Pharmacology*, **371**, 187–196.

Lahat, A., Lang, A., and Ben-Horin, S. (2012). Impact of cannabis treatment on the quality of life, weight and clinical disease activity in inflammatory bowel disease patients: a pilot prospective study. *Digestion*, **85**, 1–8.

Lal, S., Prasad, N., Ryan, M., *et al.* (2011). Cannabis use amongst patients with inflammatory bowel dis-ease. *European Journal of Gastroenterology and Hepatology*, **23**, 891–896.

Lehmann, A., Blackshaw, L.A., and Brändén, L. (2002). Cannabinoid receptor agonism inhibits transient lower esophageal sphincter relaxations and reflux in dogs. *Gastroenterology*, **123**, 1129–1134.

Lin, X.H., Yuece, B., Li, Y.Y., *et al.* (2011). A novel CB receptor GPR55 and its ligands are involved in regu-lation of gut movement in rodents. *Neurogastroenterology and Motility*, **23**, 862–e342.

MacNaughton, W.K., Van Sickle, M.D., Keenan, C.M., Cushing, K., Mackie, K., and Sharkey, K.A. (2004). Distribution and function of the cannabinoid-1 receptor in the modulation of ion transport in the guinea pig ileum: relationship to capsaicin-sensitive nerves. *American Journal of Physiology – Gastrointestinal and Liver Physiology*, **286**, G863–G871.

Makwana, R., Molleman, A., and Parsons, M.E. (2010). Pharmacological characterization of cannabinoid receptor activity in the rat-isolated ileum myenteric plexus-longitudinal muscle preparation. *British Journal of Pharmacology*, **159**, 1608–1622.

Marquéz, L., Suárez, J., Iglesias, M., Bermudez-Silva, F.J., Rodríguez de Fonseca, F., and Andreu, M. (2009). Ulcerative colitis induces changes on the expression of the endocannabinoid system in the human colonic tissue. *PLoS One*, **4**, e6893.

Massa, F., Marsicano, G., Hermann, H., *et al.* (2004). The endogenous cannabinoid system protects against colonic inflammation. *Journal of Clinical Investigation*, **113**, 1202–1209.

Mathison, R., Ho, W., Pittman, Q.J., Davison, J.S., and Sharkey, K.A. (2004). Effects of cannabinoid receptor-2 activation on accelerated gastrointestinal transit in lipopolysaccharide-treated rats. *British Journal of Pharmacology*, **142**, 1247–1254.

McCallum, R.W., Soykan, I., Sridhar, K.R., Ricci, D.A., Lange, R.C., and Plankey, M.W. (1999). Delta-9-tetrahydrocannabinol delays the gastric emptying of solid food in humans: a double-blind, randomized study. *Alimentary Pharmacology and Therapeutics*, **13**, 77–80.

Naftali, T., Lev, L.B., Yablecovitch, D., Half, E., and Konikoff, F.M. (2011). Treatment of Crohn's disease with cannabis: an observational study. *Israel Medical Association Journal*, **13**, 455–458.

Naidu, P.S., Booker, L., Cravatt, B.F., and Lichtman, A.H. (2009). Synergy between enzyme inhibitors of fatty acid amide hydrolase and cyclooxygenase in visceral nociception. *Journal of Pharmacology and Experimental Therapeutics*, **329**, 48–56.

Partosoedarso, E.R., Abrahams, T.P., Scullion, R.T., Moerschbaecher, J.M., and Hornby, P.J. (2003). Cannabinoid1 receptor in the dorsal vagal complex modulates lower oesophageal sphincter relaxation in ferrets. *Journal of Physiology*, **550**, 149–158.

Pazos, M.R., Tolón, R.M., Benito, C., *et al.* (2008). Cannabinoid CB1 receptors are expressed by parietal cells of the human gastric mucosa. *Journal of Histochemistry and Cytochemistry*, **56**, 511–516.

Pertwee, R.G. (2008). The diverse CB1 and CB2 receptor pharmacology of three plant cannabinoids: delta9-tetrahydrocannabinol, cannabidiol and delta9-tetrahydrocannabivarin. *British Journal of Pharmacology*, **153**, 199–215.

Pertwee, R.G., Fernando, S.R., Nash, J.E. and Coutts, A.A. (1996). Further evidence for the presence of cannabinoid CB1 receptors in guinea-pig small intestine. *British Journal of Pharmacology*, **118**, 2199–2205.

Pertwee, R.G., Stevenson, L.A., Elrick, D.B., Mechoulam, R., and Corbett, A.D. (1992). Inhibitory effects of certain enantiomeric cannabinoids in the mouse vas deferens and the myenteric plexus preparation of guinea-pig small intestine. *British Journal of Pharmacology*, **105**, 980–984.

Peters, M. and Kogan, N.M. (2007). HU-331: a cannabinoid quinone, with uncommon cytotoxic properties and low toxicity. *Expert Opinion on Investigational Drugs*, **16**, 1405–1413.

Pinto, L, Capasso, R., Di Carlo, G., and Izzo, A.A. (2002a). Endocannabinoids and the gut. *Prostaglandins, Leukotrienes and Essential Fatty Acids*, **66**, 333–341.

Pinto, L., Izzo, A.A., Cascio, M.G., *et al.* (2002b). Endocannabinoids as physiological regulators of colonic propulsion in mice. *Gastroenterology*, **123**, 227–234.

Pol, O. and Puig, M.M. (1997). Reversal of tolerance to the antitransit effects of morphine during acute intestinal inflammation in mice. *British Journal of Pharmacology*, **122**, 1216–1222.

Riedel, G., Fadda, P., McKillop-Smith, S., Pertwee, R.G., Platt, B., and Robinson, L. (2009). Synthetic and plant-derived cannabinoid receptor antagonists show hypophagic properties in fasted and non-fasted mice. *British Journal of Pharmacology*, **156**, 1154–1166.

Rivas, V. and Josè, F. (1980). Inhibition of histamine-stimulated gastric acid secretion by delta9-tetrahydrocannabinol in rat isolated stomach. *European Journal of Pharmacology*, **65**, 317–318.

Romano, B., Borrelli, F., Fasolino, I., *et al.* (2013). The cannabinoid TRPA1 agonist cannabichromene inhibits nitric oxide production in macrophages and ameliorates murine colitis. *British Journal of Pharmacology*, **169**, 213–229.

Ross, G.R., Lichtman, A., Dewey, W.L., and Akbarali, H.I. (2012). Evidence for the putative cannabinoid receptor (GPR55)-mediated inhibitory effects on intestinal contractility in mice. *Pharmacology*, **90**, 55–65.

Ross, R.A., Brockie, H.C., Fernando, S.R., Saha, B., Razdan, R.K., and Pertwee, R.G. (1998). Comparison of cannabinoid binding sites in guinea-pig forebrain and small intestine. *British Journal of Pharmacology*, **125**, 1345–1351.

Rutkowska, M. and Fereniec-Gołebiewska, L. (2009). Involvement of nitric oxide in the gastroprotective effect of ACEA, a selective cannabinoid CB_1 receptor agonist, on aspirin-induced gastric ulceration. *Pharmazie*, **64**, 595–597.

Sasso, O., Bertorelli, R., and Bandiera, T. (2012). Peripheral FAAH inhibition causes profound antinociception and protects against indomethacin-induced gastric lesions. *Pharmacological Research*, **65**, 553–563.

Scarpellini, E., Blondeau, K., and Boecxstaens, V. (2011). Effect of rimonabant on oesophageal motor function in man. *Alimentary Pharmacology and Therapeutics*, **33**, 730–737.

Schicho, R. and Storr, M. (2012). Topical and systemic cannabidiol improves trinitrobenzene sulfonic acid colitis in mice. *Pharmacology*, **89**, 149–155.

Shook, J.E. and Burks, T.F. (1989). Psychoactive cannabinoids reduce gastrointestinal propulsion and motility in rodents. *Journal of Pharmacology and Experimental Therapeutics*, **249**, 444–449.

Shook, J.E., Dewey, W.L., and Burks, T.F. (1986). The central and peripheral effects of delta-9-tetrahydrocannabinol on gastrointestinal transit in mice. *NIDA Research Monograph*, **67**, 222–227.

Singh, U.P., Singh, N.P., Singh, B., Price, R.L., Nagarkatti, M., and Nagarkatti, P.S. (2012). Cannabinoid receptor-2 (CB_2) agonist ameliorates colitis in IL-10$^{-/-}$ mice by attenuating the activation of T cells and promoting their apoptosis. *Toxicology and Applied Pharmacology*, **258**, 256–267.

Sofia, R.D., Diamantis, W., and Edelson, J. (1978). Effect of delta9-tetrahydrocannabinol on the gastrointestinal tract of the rat. *Pharmacology*, **17**, 79–82.

Sofia, R.D., Vassar, H.B., and Knobloch, L.C. (1975). Comparative analgesic activity of various naturally occurring cannabinoids in mice and rats. *Psychopharmacologia*, **40**, 285–295.

Storr, M.A., Keenan, C.M., and Emmerdinger, D. (2008). Targeting endocannabinoid degradation protects against experimental colitis in mice: involvement of CB_1 and CB_2 receptors. *Journal of Molecular Medicine*, **86**, 925–936.

Storr, M.A., Keenan, C.M., Zhang, H., Patel, K.D., Makriyannis, A., and Sharkey, K.A. (2009). Activation of the cannabinoid 2 receptor (CB_2) protects against experimental colitis. *Inflammatory Bowel Disease*, **15**, 1678–1685.

Storr, M.A., Bashashati, M. and Hirota, C., *et al.* (2010). Differential effects of CB_1 neutral antagonists and inverse agonists on gastrointestinal motility in mice. *Neurogastroenterology and Motility*, **22**, 787–796, e223.

Thomas, A., Baillie, G.L., Phillips, A.M., Razdan, R.K., Ross, R.A., and Pertwee, R.G. (2007). Cannabidiol displays unexpectedly high potency as an antagonist of CB_1 and CB_2 receptor agonists *in vitro*. *British Journal of Pharmacology*, **150**, 613–623.

Tyler, K., Hillard, C.J., and Greenwood-Van Meerveld B. (2000). Inhibition of small intestinal secretion by cannabinoids is CB1 receptor-mediated in rats. *European Journal of Pharmacology*, **409**, 207–211.

Wang, D., Wang, H., Ning, W., *et al.* (2008). Loss of cannabinoid receptor 1 accelerates intestinal tumor growth. *Cancer Research*, **68**, 6468–6476.

Warzecha, Z., Dembinski, A., and Ceranowicz, P. (2011). Role of sensory nerves in gastroprotective effect of anandamide in rats. *Journal of Physiology and Pharmacology*, **62**, 207–217.

Wong, B.S., Camilleri, M., Busciglio, I., *et al.* (2011). Pharmacogenetic trial of a cannabinoid agonist shows reduced fasting colonic motility in patients with nonconstipated irritable bowel syndrome. *Gastroenterology*, **141**, 1638–1647.

Wong, B.S., Camilleri, M., Eckert, D., *et al.* (2012). Randomized pharmacodynamic and pharmacogenetic trial of dronabinol effects on colon transit in irritable bowel syndrome-diarrhea. *Neurogastroenterology and Motility*, **24**, 358–e169.

Wright, K., Rooney, N., Feeney, M., *et al.* (2005). Differential expression of cannabinoid receptors in the human colon: cannabinoids promote epithelial wound healing. *Gastroenterology*, **129**, 437–453.

Wright, K.L., Duncan, M. and Sharkey, K.A. (2008). Cannabinoid CB_2 receptors in the gastrointestinal tract: a regulatory system in states of inflammation. *British Journal of Pharmacology*, **153**, 263–270.

Chapter 13

Reproduction and Cannabinoids: Ups and Downs, Ins and Outs

Jordyn M. Stuart, Emma Leishman, and Heather B. Bradshaw

13.1 Introduction

According to Wikipedia, reproduction is "the biological process by which new 'offspring' individual organisms are produced from their 'parents.' Reproduction is a fundamental feature of all known life; each individual organism exists as the result of reproduction." This seems simple enough; however, the suite of biological, psychological, and social influences of this simple process within the human species has arguably been the basis for many of life's greatest triumphs and defeats. Reproduction sciences span from conception to development (including in utero through puberty and adulthood) to andropause and menopause. From the purely basic science standpoint, it is often argued that there are "reproductive" and "nonreproductive" areas of the brain and body; however, it can also be argued that the myriad of processes that drive reproduction require (or hijack) all of the body and mind. Indeed circuitry that drives sexual motivation is the same that provides the rewarding effects of psychoactive drugs. Therefore, when approaching the topic of cannabinoids and reproduction one could take the view of how basic biology is affected, such as focusing on cannabinoids and the hypothalamic–pituitary–gonadal (HPG) axis and the reproductive tracts. However, the focus on the sensual aspects of reproduction cannot truly be discussed outside of the social/cultural view of reproduction and the range of freedoms and constraints that are imposed among different societies and how that plays a role in or is mirrored in cannabinoid use. In working on the integration of these points of view we draw on an ideology of our field (neuroscience) that posits that *everything psychological is simultaneously biological*. This phrase defines the understanding that there can be no behavior, thought, or feeling that is not a result of the biological activity of the body and brain. Here, we will review what is known about the biological role of the cannabinoid system in the context of sexuality, how that likely drives the outcomes of cannabinoid use in both the functional and sensual aspects of sexuality, and how this may differ in the context of gender and culture.

13.2 Cannabis as an aphrodisiac?

Folklore of cannabis use as an aphrodisiac has been passed down for thousands of years. One of the earliest stories is told within Hindu mythology. The story states that what we know now as psychoactive hemp, the plant most associated with the deity Shiva, was linked with his persona characterized with eroticism, asceticism, and healing. It was thought, "the gods gave humans hemp out of compassion so that they could attain enlightenment, lose their fear, and maintain their sexual excitement" (Rätsch 2001). In other cultures, such as Ukraine, young girls were said to use hemp seeds as an aphrodisiac. They referred to hemp as "love magic," and thought that the wetting of the seeds with water in their mouths "would result in the pursuit of a bed partner and disrobed frolicking" (Rätsch 2001). In Tibet, it was believed that hemp's aphrodisiac properties could be exploited to treat mental illness; the idea being that the increase in sexual activity would help heal the mind (Rätsch 2001). Still, as with many myths and folklore, it is impossible to determine which came first: the story of the gods' involvement in the use of cannabis or the use of cannabis, which was then attributed and "legitimized" by the story of the gods. Either way, multiple societies have been documented in their associations with cannabis use for socialization rites and rituals, including sexuality, which in itself provides reliability if not validity.

Inherent in the discussion of sex and drugs is the belief that there is a direct relationship between the risky uses of both. Indeed, there is some correlation between the two. A survey of 8656 people found that frequent users of cannabis were more likely to report two or more sexual partners within the year before the interview was conducted. It also found that female cannabis users were more likely to have contracted a sexually transmitted disease than noncannabis-smoking women (Smith et al. 2010). Another survey, done on a population of HIV-positive German men who had sex with other men, showed a significant correlation between cannabis use and risky sexual behavior, including unprotected anal intercourse (Dirks et al. 2012). While it is very possible that those who are phenotypically more prone to generalized risk would be more likely to engage in all risky behaviors, it is also possible that the motivational aspects of sex could be acting synergistically to increase the likelihood of those risks involved with sex and drugs.

Although it has been suggested that cannabis was used as a libido enhancer since ancient times, it was not until the 1970s that more data on how cannabis use actually affected sexual function became more widely available through published papers. Surveys of men and women, using self-reported recall, were used to examine correlations between sexual experiences and cannabis use (Gorzalka et al. 2010). In these early studies, women typically reported increased sexual responsiveness, specifically heightened sensitivity to touch and relaxation. Yet, they did not report a simultaneous effect on vaginal lubrication, orgasm frequency, or orgasm strength (Gorzalka et al. 2010). Koff has proposed a dose-dependent effect of cannabis on female sexual desire. When participants reported only smoking one cannabis joint, 71% of females reported an increase in sexual motivation, yet the same females indicated a decrease in sexual desire after smoking more than one joint (Koff 1974). Another study in 1982 found a positive correlation between female cannabis use and sexual pleasure. After smoking cannabis, 90% of women reported their sexual experience was more satisfying and 40% reported having improved orgasm quality. The population of the respondents self-identified as regular marijuana users, meaning that they had used marijuana on more than 50 separate occasions during a time period lasting more than 6 months. In fact, the average duration of marijuana use at that time was more than 2 years, with an average frequency of two to three times per week (Halikas et al. 1982). Therefore, there may be a phenotype of this population that makes these comparisons suspect. For example, could the increase in pleasure be an effect of a decrease in potential withdrawal symptoms from lack of use? Could their HPG axis be altered by chronic cannabis use such that there is a maladaptation of this circuitry that then requires the use of cannabis to re-engage this access? Or, did these individuals adapt to the chronic use of cannabis for another reason all together (e.g., relief of pain, posttraumatic stress disorder) and the side effect of the perception of heightened sexual pleasure added to the therapeutic effects?

Perceptions of heightened sexual experiences were likewise noted in men. Three different surveys of cannabis users showed that over 70% of males claimed an increase in sexual pleasure.

Similarly, most men noted an increase in the quality of orgasm in two of these surveys. Over a quarter of males in these surveys stated that the cannabis enabled them to have sexual intercourse for longer (Halikas et al. 1982; Kolodny et al. 1979; Tart 1970). These positive attributes were found to be dose dependent: one joint smoked was concluded to ameliorate sexual desire, whereas two or more joints smoked potentially dampened sexual motivation (Abel 1981; Koff 1974). Chronic cannabis use has also been shown to have detrimental effects on sexual functioning. Vallejo-Medina and Sierra found in males that consumed on average 2.7 g/day (roughly two to three joints) and had been in withdrawal for at least 2 weeks had significantly poorer sexual functioning than a nondrug use group in four areas of sexual functioning: pleasure, desire, arousal, and orgasm (Vallejo-Medina and Sierra 2013a, 2013b). Here, again one could hypothesize that increases in perceptions of sexual pleasure with chronic cannabis use may be a function of the suppression of withdrawal symptoms.

The complexity of human sexual response that combines biological, psychological, environmental/cultural, and interpersonal factors makes it difficult to understand what is causing the positive *aphrodisiac* effects reported in these studies (i.e., mechanism of action). One hypothesis states that the smoking of marijuana may slow temporal perception, which could in turn increase concentration and therefore enhance focus on the sexual act itself while also changing the perception of the length of the sexual act (Gorzalka et al. 2010; Melges 1971; Shamloul and Bella 2011). This hypothesis was taken further through the suggestion that this proposed increase in focus would develop into a heightened sensory focus that would cause an erotic experience to occur not just in specific erogenous zones, but throughout the entire body, in a manner that would boost sexual pleasure (Gorzalka et al. 2010). Another hypothesis is that the perceived positive effects of cannabis on sexual function are due purely to the placebo effect. Thus, since cannabis has a reputation for being an aphrodisiac, users' sexual experiences may be influenced by their sexual expectations of the substance (Crenshaw and Goldberg 1996; Rosen 1991). Therefore, the relationship between cannabis and sexual outcomes, such as sexual motivation, orgasm intensity, and pleasure indices may be a coincidental change in perception and not a change in physiological functions of the genitals. It is possible that sexual function may be enhanced indirectly through cannabis' anxiolytic effects. A person under the influence of cannabis may be more relaxed; which in turn could enhance sexual functioning by reducing the pressures of performance anxiety, a trait unique to humans. This brings us back to the biopsychosocial aspect of how cannabinoids affect all facets of reproduction and where to begin if we want to get a clearer understanding of their relationships.

13.3 Biological basis for cannabinoid activity in reproduction

Additional chapters in this book discuss the myriad of endogenous cannabinoid receptors both established and putative, biosynthetic and metabolic enzymes, as well as endogenous and exogenous ligands that interact with each of these; therefore, we will not revisit this information. Within the realm of the biological basis of reproduction the cannabinoid (CB) system has been linked to regulation of the following systems: (1) HPG axis, (2) sperm and ova mobility, (3) implantation, (4) reproductive tract physiology, and (5) sexual/mating behavior (Bradshaw and Allard 2011; Bradshaw et al. 2006; Maccarone et al. 2000, 2004; Sun and Dey 2012; Wang et al. 2004). Here, we will attempt to focus on the biological bases for effects of phytocannabinoids on reproduction. For a more detailed review of the endogenous cannabinoid system's role in sexual motivation, please refer to Leishman et al. (2013).

13.3.1 Cannabinoids and the hypothalamic–pituitary–gonadal axis

First coined by Phoenix and colleagues in 1959, the "organizational/activational" hypothesis asserts that there are two key time points in sexual differentiation in the brain (Phoenix et al. 1959). The first is the critical period of early development, which is primarily organizational, when exposure to steroid hormones causes sexual differentiation of neural circuitry and sex-specific reproductive tract physiology. The second begins in adolescence and is labeled the "activational" phase, when gonadal steroids bind to their respective receptors in the previously organized neuronal circuits and reproductive tissues driving divergence in reproductive neurophysiology. Sex steroid hormones alone do not organize these circuits; rather, it is the cellular cascades and signaling pathways they initiate that organize the brain (McCarthy 2010). CBs have multiple roles in driving these cascades and shaping this organization (Krebs-Kraft et al. 2010; Leishman et al. 2013). Three main lines of evidence suggest that the CB and gonadal hormone signaling systems interact. Firstly, endogenous CBs and their receptors are present throughout the HPG axis and changes to the CB system cause changes in the HPG axis. Second, changes in HPG axis can affect the expression of multiple components of the CB system. Finally, the CB system mediates mating behaviors, which are also mediated by gonadal hormones (Gorzalka and Dang 2012). As an example, chronic use of delta-9-tetrahydrocannabinol (Δ^9-THC) has been implicated in negative reproductive outcomes, including the inhibition of ovulation in women (Brown and Dobs 2002) and lower serum luteinizing hormone (LH) and testosterone (T) in men (Lopez 2010). How this occurs at the molecular level is perhaps more telling in terms of long-range implications of CB influence on reproductive neurophysiology and behavior.

CB regulation of gonadal (sex steroid) hormones is primarily through the regulation of gonadotropin-releasing hormone (GnRH) release. GnRH is the central peptide that regulates pituitary levels of LH and follicle-stimulating hormone (FSH), which are the stimulating hormones for gonads in both sexes that drive production of sex steroids. Sex steroids, in turn, regulate and are regulated by GnRH neurons in the brain, which are necessary for both the development and control of reproduction and sexual behaviors (Bakker and Brock 2010). GnRH-producing neurons are under regulation by gamma-aminobutyric acid (GABA)-ergic and glutamatergic neuronal and astrocytic control. These neurons and astrocytes express hormone as well as CB receptors. Blocking CB signaling disrupts GABAergic postsynaptic currents that alter GnRH-dependent depolarization (Glanowska and Moenter 2011). Likewise, CBs can reduce basal GABAergic transmission to GnRH neurons via a metabotropic glutamate receptor-dependent mechanism, by activating presynaptic CB_1 receptors to inhibit GABA release, and/or by altering glial transmission (Farkas et al. 2010).

A growing body of data points to the involvement of the CB system within the organizational effects of puberty and adolescence, including how CBs play a role in the onset of puberty. This involvement may depend at least in part on the ability of CBs to inhibit peripubertal GnRH neurons. Lopez hypothesizes that estradiol (E2) release from the ovaries at the time of puberty helps remove the CB "brake" on reproductive functioning (Lopez 2010). The overall relationship between E2 and CBs can be described as "bidirectional." In one direction, CB activity downregulates HPG axis activity, leading to reduced E2 levels. In contrast, by decreasing fatty acid amide hydrolase (FAAH) activity and modulating CB_1 expression, E2 upregulates anandamide (AEA) production (Gorzalka and Dang 2012).

Neuronal circuitry of sexual motivation likely involves the CB system in multiple regions of the brain (Gorzalka et al. 2010: Shamloul and Bella 2011). In rodents, striatal and cerebral CB_1 receptor stimulation may produce reduced motor activity and increased coordination (Egashira et al.

2002). CB_1 receptors may be able to regulate stress responses and emotional behavior due to their presence in the corticolimbic structures (mainly prefrontal cortex, amygdala, and hippocampus), thereby indirectly affecting sexual behavior (McLaughlin et al. 2007). Activation of CB_1 receptors within the dorsal raphe (cell bodies for serotonergic input to forebrain) and the ventral tegmental area (VTA) (cell bodies for dopaminergic input to forebrain) modulate the synaptic release of both serotonin and dopamine (DA), each of which is intricately involved in the regulation of genital reflexes, sexual motivation, and inhibition (Giraldi et al. 2004; Matyas et al. 2008). Finally, CB_1 receptors within the hypothalamus regulate the release of several peptides important for sexual activity, physiology, and reproductive neuroendocrinology, such as oxytocin (Sabatier and Leng 2006) and gonadotropin-releasing hormone (Gammon et al. 2005).

Growing evidence suggests that Δ^9-THC affects males and females differently. This is not to say that there is not a large variation in response within the sexes, but there have been enough intersex differences shown to suggest gonadal steroid modulation of exogenous cannabinoid effects, including reward. After showing that CB_1 receptor agonists induce stronger analgesic and motor suppressing effects in female rats than in male rats, Craft and colleagues investigated whether activational effects of gonadal hormones were responsible for these differences. In males, T attenuated the motor effects of Δ^9-THC. In females, E2 was linked to increased antinociception. Ovariectomized (OVX) females showed less analgesia in response to Δ^9-THC than OVX females given E2. In addition, intact estrous females showed more antinociception than diestrous females (Craft and Leitl 2008). Fattore and colleagues determined that female rats found the CB_1 agonist WIN55,212-2 (WIN) more rewarding than male rats. Compared to male rats and OVX females, female rats showed faster acquisition of WIN self-administration and higher overall drug intake. However, gonad-intact female rats showed faster extinction from WIN self-administration. One explanation is that there is a higher hedonistic value on cannabinoids for females (Fattore et al. 2007). On the other hand, E2 may attenuate the disruptive effects of Δ^9-THC on learning, leaving female rats less affected by the drug's negative side effects (Daniel et al. 2002). It is possible that the greater response to Δ^9-THC seen in female rats is due to E2 modulation of DA signaling in the VTA and nucleus accumbens (NAc). However, the precise interactions between CBs and E2 in these regions are not well understood (Lopez 2010). It may be, however, that hormones are not the only answer and that the sex differences in development (both organizational and activational effects) also cause some effects of cannabis to be different in men and women.

13.4 Cannabinoids and male reproduction and sexuality: the ups and downs

In male rodents, the effect of cannabis on sexual behavior was examined after intraperitoneal injections of Δ^9-THC followed by exposure of the male to a receptive female. Data showed that at doses as low as 0.5 mg/kg inhibited sexual behavior by reducing the number of mounts and the ejaculation frequency (Gorzalka et al. 2010; Merari et al. 1973). Higher doses increased latency before the first mount, latency to ejaculate, and latency to mount following ejaculation. Doses as high as 10 mg/kg of Δ^9-THC impair sexual motivation across all species exhibiting this effect (mice, humans); the underlying mechanism has yet to be determined, one possibility being that this impairment arises from motor deficits resulting from catalepsy. This dose dependence was also tested with intraperitoneal injections of AEA. At lower doses ejaculation frequency was increased slightly, whereas with higher doses mount, intromission, and ejaculation latencies were all increased (Martinez-Gonzalez et al. 2004). This suggests the CB system may have an inhibitory function as well as a facilitatory function in regulating sexual behavior (Gorzalka et al. 2010).

To test this duality, the CB_1 receptor agonist HU-210 was examined for effects on copulation rates. HU-210 reduced male rat copulation in a dose-dependent manner even at doses that did not affect motor function, whereas the CB_1 receptor antagonist/inverse agonist AM251 led to dose-dependent facilitation of ejaculation in male rats (Ferrari et al. 2000; Gorzalka et al. 2008). Recent evidence has shown that AM251 is not specific to CB_1 in that it also blocks the NAGly responsive receptor, GPR18, a finding that may explain some of this duality (McHugh et al. 2012).

Cannabis as an aphrodisiac may seem at the least less linked to "medical treatments" than many conditions. However, pathophysiological conditions associated with sex may have a closer link to justified medicinal use. Sexual headaches have a close resemblance to migraines as they both respond to a common mechanism of vascular hyperactivity (Álvaro et al. 2002). Men who develop these headaches are more prone to develop ischemic symptoms and stroke. Since cannabis use can induce swings in blood pressure, it is thought that in one case study, the alterations of blood pressure from cannabis use along with the alterations in blood pressure of orgasm caused a man to have a stroke (Álvaro et al. 2002). Interestingly, this link with changes in vascular tone may be related to the relationship of cannabis use and impotence. Cohen found that 19% of daily cannabis users had a prevalence of erectile dysfunction when compared to 8% in the control group (Cohen 1982). One study highlighted a correlation between cannabis use in young males (mean age 30) and erectile dysfunction exhibited by endothelial dysfunction and vascular damage (Aversa et al. 2008). It is thought that chronic cannabis smoking may alter both the endothelial dependent and independent vasodilatatory pathways (Aversa et al. 2008). In a related case study of two male subjects with erectile dysfunction, the discontinuing of use of the drug allowed one male to regain erectile functioning (Gorzalka et al. 2010).

Alternatively, animal and in vitro studies provide evidence to connect the CB system with the inhibition of erectile dysfunction. Oxytocin-producing neurons located in the paraventricular nucleus (PVN) of the hypothalamus are responsible for regulating male copulatory behavior including male erection. These neurons contain CB_1 receptors whose blockade has been found to increase penile erection. This is thought to be through the decrease in the release of the neurotransmitter GABA and an increase in glutamate, which signals the production of nitric oxide (NO) via NO synthase (NOS) in the oxytocinergic neurons. Oxytocin release, which is responsible for penile erections, is triggered by the increase in NO. Administering SR141716A, a CB_1 antagonist, into the PVN of male rats induced erections (Shamloul and Bella 2011).

To induce and maintain a penile erection, the cavernous smooth muscle in the corpus cavernosum must relax. Both CB_1 and CB_2 receptors are expressed on NOS-containing nerves in the corpus cavernosum of rhesus monkeys and humans (Gratzke et al. 2010). AEA administration antagonized the relaxation of the corpus cavernosum in the rhesus monkeys (Gratzke et al. 2010). CB_1 has also been found in the corpus cavernosum of rats and rabbits. The effect of AEA in rats is different from that of the rhesus monkey, as it increases relaxation in this species. This highlights that although CB signaling may have a peripheral role in sexual behavior, it may be species dependent (Shamloul and Bella 2011).

Cannabis use in males has also been associated with adverse effects on male fertility at both a hormonal and spermatogenesis level (Kumar et al. 2009). In males, it is believed that Δ^9-THC blocks release of GnRH, ultimately decreasing testosterone production (Kumar et al. 2009). THC consumption also has a negative effect on sperm mobility. It is believed that marijuana smoke causes a cannabinoid dependent increase in reactive oxidative species (ROS). An imbalance between the amount of ROS and antioxidants in a cell can lead to oxidative stress. Oxidative stress, the major cause of DNA damage in the male germ line, is associated with poor sperm quality, low fertilization rates, impaired preimplantation development, increased abortion rates, and elevated incidence of disease in offspring. It also alters another essential sperm function, that of the acrosome reaction, the reaction occurring when the sperm fuses to the plasma membrane of the egg, impairing the acrosome reactions of the poorer sperm at recreational concentrations of THC. Finally, the expression/activity of CB_1 controls the physiological alterations of DNA packaging during spermatogenesis and epididymal transit. Therefore, smoking cannabis may impair fertility outcomes as well (Pasqualotto and Pasqualotto 2012).

13.5 Cannabinoids and female reproduction and sexuality: the ins and outs

One of the first documented uses of cannabis in relation to the female reproductive system was by the Egyptian civilization in 2350 BC. An ancient passage reads, "Another (to cool the uterus and eliminate its heat): shemshemet (cannabis); ground in honey; introduced into her vagina . . . causing a contraction" (Russo 2007). These writings generated the conclusion that cannabis was used as an obstetric aid. An archeological dig of a tomb in Israel during the early 1990s revealed a skeleton of a young woman and the skeleton of her partially born fetus (still within her pelvis). Traces of Δ^8-THC, a trace component of cannabis, was found in her abdominal area denoting that cannabis had been used during the attempted childbirth (Zias et al. 1993). It has since been determined that cannabis was also used in the treatment of: menstrual irregularity, menorrhagia, dysmenorrhea, threatened abortion, hyperemesis gravidarum, childbirth, postpartum hemorrhage, toxemic seizures, dysuria, urinary frequency, urinary retention, gonorrhea, menopausal symptoms, decreased libido, and as a possible abortifacient (Russo 2002).

The dual effect of cannabis on sexual behavior in female rats also appears to be dose dependent, with high doses impairing lordosis but having a facilitatory effect at low doses (Gorzalka et al. 2010). In a study performed on female hamsters, the administration of Δ^9-THC stimulated lordosis and ultrasound production, a form of communication used to assess sexual proceptivity (Turley and Floody 1981). Lordosis, or in general sexual receptivity, was also stimulated by the addition of low doses of THC in E2-treated female rats (Mani et al. 2001b). This effect was diminished when SR141716A was administered (Mani et al. 2001b). An adrenalectomy was also done on these females to test the hypothesis that Δ^9-THC was acting like an ovarian steroid or by enhancing adrenal secretions that would facilitate lordosis. Even with the adrenals removed the facilitory effect remained, suggesting that Δ^9-THC was probably acting on the central nervous system (Gordon et al. 1978). Additionally, they showed that Δ^9-THC did not induce sexual receptivity when ovarian hormones were removed and it did not function like progesterone in E2-treated rats (Gordon et al. 1978). Antagonizing the CB_1 receptor has also been seen to block DA- and progesterone-induced sexual facilitation, whereas blocking the progesterone and DA receptors demonstrated the sexually enhancing effect of THC. Sexual behavior in the female rat therefore depends on the linking of CB_1 with dopaminergic and progesterone pathways, all three of which are found within different regions of the hypothalamus involved in sexual behavior regulation (Gorzalka et al. 2010; Mani et al. 2001a). In two studies, the potent agonists CP55,940 and HU-210, were administered and were found to lessen instead of enhance female receptivity and motivation. CP55,940 produced its effects in a dose-dependent manner, a higher dose (~40 micrograms/kg) inhibiting sexual motivation to a greater extent than a lower dose (~20 micrograms/kg). However, a dosage that high also attenuates a female's social motivation, and so may not be targeting sexual behavior specifically (Gorzalka et al. 2010; Lopez et al. 2009). Another study found that AM251 significantly increased, rather than decreased, sexual motivation, receptivity, and proceptivity in the female rat (Lopez et al. 2009). Interestingly, differences in methodology could be the reason for discrepancies among these studies in that the types of mating strategies used in these studies were varied. Female rats will only show conditioned placed preference (CPP) and upregulation of DA for mating when provided a paced-mating opportunity, whereas, no CPP or DA upregulation occurs during standard mating (Martinez and Paredes 2001). Therefore, when the mating situations did not drive changes in DA circuits, the effects of CBs may not have been as strong.

Unsurprisingly, there is very little focus on the neurophysiology of human female sexual response that would be analogous to the work in men in the context of cannabinoids. There are no published data on cannabinoids and the clitoris that could be found through any literature search engines at our disposal, whereas, there are data on cannabinoids and penis function highlighted previously in this chapter. Somewhat predictably, of the five reports listed when the search was "cannabinoids and the vagina," three of them are aimed at sperm motility studies and the other two were animal studies on disease transmission rates. Perhaps this is simply a reflection of the overwhelming lack of research on the subject of female sexual arousal as a whole and not on cannabinoid research specifically. There is, however, a rapidly growing literature on the aspects of the female reproductive tract that are specifically geared toward pregnancy. Given the logical constraints of human experimentation during pregnancy, all of the experimental data are gathered in animal models, though observational data do exist for humans. How translational the animal findings are, like most basic science using animal models, remains to be determined. Many of these findings do provide strong evidence for important CB roles in cyclic changes in the reproductive tract, fertilization, implantation, and parturition; therefore, each will be summarized here.

Much of the female reproductive tract physiology produces each of the major constituents of the CB system: CB_1, CB_2, AEA, 2-arachidonoyl glycerol, and FAAH have been discovered in the uterus, ovaries, and fallopian tubes of both humans and rats (Bradshaw and Allard 2011; Habayeb et al. 2002; Sun and Dey 2012; Taylor et al. 2010b). Specifically in humans, CB_1 was localized in the ovary, while CB_1 and CB_2 were localized in oocytes, and the myometrium and endometrium of the uterus (Taylor et al. 2010b). Immunohistochemistry was used to localize the CB_1 protein, which was found in the smooth muscle of the wall, endothelial vessels, and luminal epithelium of the fallopian tube (Horne et al. 2008). Within the epithelial glands and stroma, CB_2 was observed most prominently in the late proliferation phase whereas CB_1 was more intense in the glands than the stroma (not tested across cycle) (Taylor et al. 2010a, 2010c). The localization of both CB_1 and CB_2 expression also changed throughout the different stages of oocyte maturation (Maccarrone 2009). CB_1 expression in the pregnant uterus was seen by the detection of CB_1 mRNA in woman with ectopic pregnancies (Horne et al. 2008). This expression of CB_1 mRNA was also seen in the pregnant and ovariectomized mouse uterus (Das et al. 1995).

In species with estrous cycles, such as rodents, females are only sexually active during estrus, referred to as behavioral estrus, which coincides with the time of ovulation. In contrast, many primate species with menstrual cycles are sexually active at any time in their cycle, though some data suggest a stronger drive for mating around the time of ovulation in these species as well. The onset of ovulation is dependent on the release of LH via HPG axis regulation. Exogenous cannabinoids such as Δ^9-THC have been shown to suppress plasma FSH and the preovulatory surge of LH, which inhibits ovulation (Taylor et al. 2007). AEA has a similar effect, decreasing levels of serum prolactin and LH (Wenger et al. 1999). This seems contradictory to the finding that the success of pregnancy (a result of mating) correlates with higher levels of AEA in plasma during the time of ovulation (Maccarrone 2009). However, it is supported by an observation by Lazzarin et al. (2004) that both a significant increase in AEA and a significant decrease in FAAH activity occurred during ovulation. The variation in FAAH activity during the ovulation/hormonal cycle also seems to be influenced by the concentration of progesterone, illustrating another example of signaling synergy between sex hormones and the CB system (Lazzarin et al. 2004).

Successful mating not only involves access and a drive to copulate, timed events for ovulation, and availability of viable mates; it also relies heavily on the next initiation event in the cascade, which is implantation of a developed blastocyst. For implantation to occur and the blastocyst to attach to the luminal epithelium of the uterus in a mammalian species, the uterus must first enter a receptive phase and the blastocyst must be implantation competent (Maccarrone 2009). Blastocysts actually release a FAAH activator, which helps to dispose of anandamide at the implantation site (Karasu et al. 2011). Therefore, an upregulation in AEA is correlated with uterine refractoriness, inversely related to uterine receptivity (Park et al. 2004). Interestingly, levels of AEA are lowest at the actual site of implantation and highest at the interimplantation sites (Park et al. 2004). AEA is hypothesized to act on a CB_1-mediated pathway influencing implantation. This notion was solidified by the addition of CP55,940, a synthetic cannabinoid, during the preimplantation phase, as this was found successfully to prevent implantation (Park et al. 2004). Finally, the human fallopian tube has a varied expression of CB_1 mRNA in the endometrium of women with ectopic pregnancy. It has been hypothesized that malfunctioned endocannabinoid signaling is responsible for the incorrect positioning of implantation (Helliwell et al. 2004).

13.5.1 Cannabis use during pregnancy: short-term and long-term consequences

In a descriptive study of almost 25,000 women referred to a hospital in Brisbane, Australia for antenatal care, 2.6% of women surveyed used cannabis during pregnancy (Hayatbakhsh et al. 2012). This is similar to estimates of the prevalence of cannabis use during pregnancy in the US, which is around 2.9% (Huizink and Mulder 2006). However, 9.5% of the women surveyed in the Australian study reported regular cannabis use before becoming pregnant, showing that even regular cannabis users often abstain during pregnancy. Even after controlling for use of alcohol, tobacco, and other drugs, cannabis use in pregnancy was associated with low birth weight, preterm labor, babies who were small for gestational age, and admission to the neonatal intensive care unit (Hayatbakhsh et al. 2012).

Although cannabis use during pregnancy has been associated with preterm delivery and low birth weight (Hayatbakhsh et al. 2012), the demographic characteristics of women who use cannabis during pregnancy are often different from those of women who do not use drugs during pregnancy. Van Gelder and colleagues gathered structured interviews regarding illicit drug use during pregnancy from 5871 women in the US. Women who reported use of cannabis, cocaine, or stimulants during pregnancy were more likely to be young, be unemployed, have a low education level, and to have a low income level than women who abstained from illicit drug use during pregnancy. Although women who used illicit drugs during pregnancy were more likely to be underweight, the cannabis-using women were actually more likely to have excessive weight gain during pregnancy. Illicit drug use during pregnancy was also associated with low folic acid intake. Interestingly, the women who reported cannabis use were less likely to have already had children but were more likely to have had an abortion in the past. Illicit drug use during pregnancy was also significantly associated with alcohol and tobacco use during pregnancy (van Gelder et al. 2010). Hayatbakhsh's study of Australian women also reported similar demographic differences: cannabis-using women were more likely to be younger and less educated than women who did not use cannabis during pregnancy (Hayatbakhsh et al. 2012). Despite differences in demographics between the cannabis using and noncannabis using mothers, van Gelder and colleagues reported no significant association between cannabis use and mean birth weight or gestational age (van Gelder et al. 2010).

The frequency of cannabis use during pregnancy may have an effect on birth outcomes. For example, Fergusson's group surveyed 12,000 British pregnant women between 18 and 20 weeks of gestation about frequency of drug use before and during pregnancy (Fergusson et al. 2002). The surveys were then correlated with birth outcomes that included: late fetal and perinatal death, admission to the infant intensive care unit, birth weight, birth length, and head circumference. Use of cannabis during pregnancy was associated with lower maternal income and age, and was also associated with the use of alcohol, tobacco, caffeine, and other hard drugs during pregnancy. With cannabis use during pregnancy as the only factor, there was no link between cannabis use and fetal death or infant intensive care. However, the babies born to cannabis using mothers were more likely to be smaller, with a lower birth weight, length, and head circumference. After adjusting for use of other drugs, the association between cannabis use and small infants was no longer significant, except for women who used cannabis at least once per week before and throughout pregnancy (Fergusson et al. 2002). In a meta-analysis of studies that examined the effect of marijuana use during pregnancy on birth weight controlling for cigarette smoking, English and colleagues found that there was substantial heterogeneity among studies (English et al. 1997). They found that a frequency of marijuana use of once per week or less was actually correlated with an increase in mean birth weight. It was not until women frequently consumed marijuana multiple times a week during pregnancy that there was a reduction in birth weight, and most women who use cannabis during pregnancy do not smoke nearly that much. Therefore, the authors concluded that cannabis is unlikely to contribute to low birth weight when used in the amount typically taken by pregnant women (English et al. 1997).

Longitudinal studies tracking the development of children who were prenatally exposed to marijuana have shown that there are potentially lasting effects of marijuana use during pregnancy. Several studies have been based on the Maternal Health Practices and Child Development Study (MHPCD), which followed a "high-risk" cohort of American women with low socioeconomic status (Huizink and Mulder 2006). In this cohort, 19% of subjects reported using marijuana during pregnancy and 5% smoked one or more joints every day during their pregnancy (Goldschmidt et al. 2000). The first follow-up study examined babies born to the women in the MHPCD at age 3 years. The children's intelligence levels were measured with the Stanford–Binet intelligence scale, which is a composite of verbal reasoning, visual reasoning, quantitative reasoning, and short-term memory. Overall, maternal marijuana use during pregnancy had no effect on the Stanford–Binet scores. However, there was a trending effect of marijuana use during the second trimester of pregnancy on the short-term memory subscale of the testing. Interestingly, for the white children in the study, daycare attendance moderated effects of prenatal marijuana exposure to offset negative consequences, but no such moderation was seen in African American children (Day et al. 1994). Using the same subjects as the Day group, Leech and colleagues found that 6-year-old children exposed to cannabis in the second trimester were more impulsive in a continuous performance task (Leech et al. 1999). Surveys filled out by the children's teachers indicated that the children prenatally exposed to marijuana exhibited more delinquent behavior (Leech et al. 1999). At age 10, these same children were assessed for hyperactivity, impulsivity, and inattention by self-reported surveys filled out by their mothers and for the presence of externalizing psychopathology by another survey filled out by the mothers. Prenatal marijuana exposure during the first and third trimesters significantly predicted increased hyperactivity, inattention, and impulsivity symptoms. Additionally, the children exposed to marijuana were more likely to score higher on ratings of delinquency and externalizing disorders, although this was a result of marijuana-induced inattentive symptoms (Goldschmidt et al. 2000).

A similar longitudinal study is the Ottawa Prenatal Prospective Study (OPPS), which began in 1978 and focused on a group of mostly white, middle-class women. At 1 year of age, children born to mothers who used cannabis prenatally were not significantly different than nonexposed infants in measurements of motor and mental development. At age 2, the prenatally exposed children scored lower on a test of language comprehension, but this was not significant after controlling for the children's home environments. Furthermore, at age 3 there was no effect of prenatal marijuana exposure on language expression and comprehension or on cognition. It was not until age 4 that significant effects of prenatal marijuana exposure became more profound; however, the association between prenatal exposure and lower memory and verbal scores was only significant for children of mothers who smoked marijuana heavily (five or more joints per week) during pregnancy. When cognitive tests were performed on the same children at ages 9–12, there was no link between prenatal marijuana exposure and full-scale IQ, however exposed children performed more poorly on tests of visual–spatial organization and impulse control. Although exposed children did score higher in reports of delinquent behavior filled out by their mothers, the correlation was not significant once extraneous variables were controlled for (Fried and Smith 2001). Interestingly, neither of the longitudinal studies found an effect of maternal marijuana use on miscarriage rates, duration of gestation, or frequency of labor complications. Contrary to other studies, prenatal marijuana use was actually linked with higher birth weight in both the MHPCD and OPPS cohorts (Fried and Smith 2001).

Many of the published studies on cannabis use during pregnancy rely on self-report surveys. Given that discovery of illicit drug use during pregnancy can have negative legal and social consequences for pregnant women, there may be reluctance to report use (Hayatbakhsh et al. 2012). In a study of Dutch women, El Marroun's group found substantial agreement between self-reports of cannabis use during pregnancy and positive urinalysis for cannabis exposure (El Marroun et al. 2011). However, although 92 women (2.3%) reported using cannabis in pregnancy, only 33 of them had positive urine screens. 7.6% of women who used cannabis before pregnancy but quit during pregnancy had a positive urine screen, which could perhaps be a result of the long half-life of the THC metabolite, $11\text{-nor-}\Delta^9\text{-THC-9-COOH}$. Only 0.4% of women who had never used cannabis had a positive urine screen, suggesting that false positives for cannabis use during pregnancy are rare (El Marroun et al. 2011).

Although prenatal exposure to marijuana has been correlated with future vulnerability to addiction (Huizink and Mulder 2006), the potential biochemical mechanisms that increase the risk of addiction have not been well characterized in humans. Aiming to identify a mechanism, DiNieri's group examined human fetal brain tissue from fetuses terminated between 18 and 22 weeks of gestation (DiNieri et al. 2011). Some of the fetal brains had been exposed to THC, as determined by maternal self-report and urinalysis, and these were compared to brains that had not been exposed to cannabis. Maternal alcohol and tobacco use was assessed by self-report, and there was no significant difference in maternal alcohol or tobacco use between groups. The authors hypothesized that differences would be found in the dopaminergic system of cannabis-exposed brains because this circuit is involved in addiction. Using in situ hybridization histochemistry, DiNieri's group found decreased DA D2 receptor mRNA levels in the NAc of fetuses exposed to THC, but did not find any significant differences in DA D1 receptor mRNA. In contrast, brains from fetuses exposed to alcohol but not cannabis had lower expression of both DA receptors in the dorsal striatum. Interestingly, the alcohol exposed fetuses had normal levels of D2 expression in the NAc (DiNieri et al. 2011).

In an animal model of prenatal THC exposure, male rats born to mothers who were injected with 0.15 mg/kg THC daily from gestation day five (GD5) to postnatal day two (PND2) had lower D2 receptor mRNA levels and fewer DA D2 receptor binding sites in the NAc than control rats. These changes persisted into adulthood. Interestingly, there were also behavioral effects of prenatal THC exposure: rats prenatally exposed to THC exhibited a higher sensitivity to heroin self-administration and showed higher conditioned place preference for morphine compared to vehicle-exposed rats (DiNieri et al. 2011).

Cannabis use during human pregnancy has been correlated with poor birth outcomes and may have some lasting effects on cognition. However, all of the studies are epidemiological in nature and do not allow for any conclusions to be made regarding causality. Given the differences in income and education levels between mothers who use cannabis in pregnancy and mothers who abstain from drugs in pregnancy, it is not surprising that there could also be differences in their offspring. Although it is not certain that smoking cannabis when pregnant harms the fetus, it is probably unwise to subject a developing nervous system to exogenous cannabinoids because it could potentially disrupt the endogenous cannabinoid system, a system that ensures proper neural development.

13.6 Conclusions

"It's hugely difficult to forecast the business cycle. Understanding an organism as complex as the economy is very hard": Jan Hatzius, Chief economist for Goldman Sachs as quoted in Nate Silver's book, *The Signal and the Noise: Why So Many Predictions Fail-but Some Don't* (Silver 2012). To borrow from this quotation of Jan Hatzius: "understanding an organism as complex as the *human* is very hard." Humans do not have sex simply for procreation, on this point we can (mostly) agree. Likewise, humans do not use cannabis simply for recreation, also on this point we can (mostly) agree. That these recreational, procreative, and social outlets for human behavior have the opportunity to be positively and negatively synergistic is both fascinating and predictable. Much of our evolutionary processes are geared toward maintaining balance. Pharmacology has long been one of our answers to restoring balance. We need a deeper understanding of the mechanisms of action by which cannabinoids induce changes in neuroendocrine circuits that drive reproductive and sexual phenotypes as well as how cannabis use affects functional physiology of the reproductive tract. Animal studies have greatly advanced our knowledge; however, there is a great need for human studies. Those working in the cannabinoid field are acutely aware of the difficulties of conducting cannabis experiments with humans. We applaud those brave few who also combine studies in sexuality. Thank you for your many efforts.

References

Abel, E.L. (1981). Marihuana and sex: a critical survey. *Drug and Alcohol Dependence*, **8**, 1–22.

Álvaro, L.C., Iriondo, I., and Villaverde, F.J. (2002). Sexual headache and stroke in a heavy cannabis smoker. *Headache: The Journal of Head and Face Pain*, **42**, 224–226.

Aversa, A., Rossi, F., Francomano, D., *et al.* (2008). Early endothelial dysfunction as a marker of vasculogenic erectile dysfunction in young habitual cannabis users. *International Journal of Impotence Research*, **20**, 566–573.

Bakker, J. and Brock, O. (2010). Early oestrogens in shaping reproductive networks: evidence for a potential organisational role of oestradiol in female brain development. *Journal of Neuroendocrinology*, **22**, 728–735.

Bradshaw, H. and Allard, C. (2011). Endogenous cannabinoid production in the rat female reproductive tract is regulated by changes in the hormonal milieu. *Pharmaceuticals*, **4**, 933–949.

Bradshaw, H.B., Rimmerman, N., Krey, J.F., and Walker, J.M. (2006). Sex and hormonal cycle differences in rat brain levels of pain-related cannabimimetic lipid mediators. *American Journal of Physiology – Regulatory, Integrative and Comparative Physiology*, **291**, R349–358.

Brown, T.T. and Dobs, A.S. (2002). Endocrine effects of marijuana. *Journal of Clinical Pharmacology*, **42**, 90S–96S.

Cohen, S. (1982). Cannabis and sex: multifaceted paradoxes. *Journal of Psychoactive Drugs*, **14**, 55–58.

Craft, R.M. and Leitl, M.D. (2008). Gonadal hormone modulation of the behavioral effects of Delta9-tetrahydrocannabinol in male and female rats. *European Journal of Pharmacology*, **578**, 37–42.

Crenshaw, T.L. and Goldberg, J.P. (1996). Marijuana and other illegal drugs. In: *Sexual Pharmacology: Drugs That Affect Sexual Functioning*. New York: W.W. Norton & Company, pp. 189–193.

Daniel, J.M., Winsauer, P.J., Brauner, I.N., and Moerschbaecher, J.M. (2002). Estrogen improves response accuracy and attenuates the disruptive effects of delta9-THC in ovariectomized rats responding under a multiple schedule of repeated acquisition and performance. *Behavioral Neuroscience*, **116**, 989–998.

Das, S.K., Paria, B.C., Chakraborty, I., and Dey, S.K. (1995). Cannabinoid ligand-receptor signaling in the mouse uterus. *Proceedings of the National Academy of Sciences of the United States of America*, **92**, 4332–4336.

Day, N.L., Richardson, G.A., Goldschmidt, L. *et al.* (1994). Effect of prenatal marijuana exposure on the cognitive development of offspring at age three. *Neurotoxicology and Teratology*, **16**, 169–175.

DiNieri, J.A., Wang, X., Szutorisz, H., *et al.* (2011). Maternal cannabis use alters ventral striatal dopamine D2 gene regulation in the offspring. *Biological Psychiatry*, **70**, 763–769.

Dirks, H., Esser, S., Borgmann, R., *et al.* (2012). Substance use and sexual risk behaviour among HIV-positive men who have sex with men in specialized out-patient clinics. *HIV Medicine*, **13**, 533–540.

Egashira, N., Mishima, K., Iwasaki, K., and Fujiwara, M. (2002). Intracerebral microinjections of Delta9-tetrahydrocannabinol: search for the impairment of spatial memory in the eight-arm radial maze in rats. *Brain Research*, **952**, 239–245.

El Marroun, H., Tiemeier, H., Jaddoe, V.W., *et al.* (2011). Agreement between maternal cannabis use during pregnancy according to self-report and urinalysis in a population-based cohort: the Generation R Study. *European Journal of Addiction Research*, **17**, 37–43.

English, D.R., Hulse, G.K., Milne, E., Holman, C.D., and Bower, C.I. (1997). Maternal cannabis use and birth weight: a meta-analysis. *Addiction*, **92**, 1553–1560.

Farkas, I., Kallo, I., Deli, L. *et al.* (2010). Retrograde endocannabinoid signaling reduces GABAergic synaptic transmission to gonadotropin-releasing hormone neurons. *Endocrinology*, **151**, 5818–5829.

Fattore, L., Spano, M.S., Altea, S., Angius, F., Fadda, P., and Fratta, W. (2007). Cannabinoid self-administration in rats: sex differences and the influence of ovarian function. *British Journal of Pharmacology*, **152**, 795–804.

Fergusson, D.M., Horwood, L.J., and Northstone, K. (2002). Maternal use of cannabis and pregnancy outcome. *British Journal of Gynaecology*, **109**, 21–27.

Ferrari, F., Ottani, A., and Giuliani, D. (2000). Inhibitory effects of the cannabinoid agonist HU 210 on rat sexual behaviour. *Physiology & Behavior*, **69**, 547–554.

Fried, P.A. and Smith, A.M. (2001). A literature review of the consequences of prenatal marihuana exposure. An emerging theme of a deficiency in aspects of executive function. *Neurotoxicology and Teratology*, **23**, 1–11.

Gammon, C.M., Freeman, G.M., Xie, W., Petersen, S.L., and Wetsel, W.C. (2005). Regulation of gonadotropin-releasing hormone secretion by cannabinoids. *Endocrinology*, **146**, 4491–4499.

Giraldi, A., Marson, L., Nappi, R., *et al.* (2004). Physiology of female sexual function: animal models. *The Journal of Sexual Medicine*, **1**, 237–253.

Glanowska, K.M. and Moenter, S.M. (2011). Endocannabinoids and prostaglandins both contribute to GnRH neuron-GABAergic afferent local feedback circuits. *Journal of Neurophysiology*, **106**, 3073–3081.

Goldschmidt, L., Day, N.L., and Richardson, G.A. (2000). Effects of prenatal marijuana exposure on child behavior problems at age 10. *Neurotoxicology and Teratology*, **22**, 325–336.

Gordon, J.H., Bromley, B.L., Gorski, R.A., and Zimmermann, E. (1978). Delta9-tetrahydrocannabinol enhancement of lordosis behavior in estrogen treated female rats. *Pharmacology, Biochemistry and Behavior*, **8**, 593–596.

Gorzalka, B., Morrish, A., and Hill, M. (2008). Endocannabinoid modulation of male rat sexual behavior. *Psychopharmacology*, **198**, 479–486.

Gorzalka, B.B. and Dang, S.S. (2012). Minireview: endocannabinoids and gonadal hormones: bidirectional interactions in physiology and behavior. *Endocrinology*, **153**, 1016–1024.

Gorzalka, B.B., Hill, M.N., and Chang, S.C. (2010). Male-female differences in the effects of cannabinoids on sexual behavior and gonadal hormone function. *Hormones and Behavior*, **58**, 91–99.

Gratzke, C., Christ, G.J., Stief, C.G., Andersson, K.-E., and Hedlund, P. (2010). Localization and function of cannabinoid receptors in the corpus cavernosum: basis for modulation of nitric oxide synthase nerve activity. *European Urology*, **57**, 342–349.

Habayeb, O.M., Bell, S.C., and Konje, J.C. (2002). Endogenous cannabinoids: metabolism and their role in reproduction. *Life Sciences*, **70**, 1963–1977.

Halikas, J., Weller, R., and Morse, C. (1982). Effects of regular marijuana use on sexual performance. *Journal of Psychoactive Drugs*, **14**, 59–70.

Hayatbakhsh, M.R., Flenady, V.J., Gibbons, K.S., et al. (2012). Birth outcomes associated with cannabis use before and during pregnancy. *Pediatric Research*, **71**, 215–219.

Helliwell, R.J.A., Chamley, L.W., Blake-Palmer, K., et al. (2004). Characterization of the endocannabinoid system in early human pregnancy. *Journal of Clinical Endocrinology & Metabolism*, **89**, 5168–5174.

Horne, A.W., Phillips, J.A., III, Kane, N., et al. (2008). CB1 expression is attenuated in fallopian tube and decidua of women with ectopic pregnancy. *PLoS ONE*, **3**, e3969.

Huizink, A.C. and Mulder, E.J. (2006). Maternal smoking, drinking or cannabis use during pregnancy and neurobehavioral and cognitive functioning in human offspring. *Neuroscience and Biobehavioral Reviews*, **30**, 24–41.

Karasu, T., Marczylo, T.H., Maccarrone, M., and Konje, J.C. (2011). The role of sex steroid hormones, cytokines and the endocannabinoid system in female fertility. *Human Reproduction Update*, **17**, 347–361.

Koff, W.C. (1974). Marijuana and sexual activity. *Journal of Sex Research*, **10**, 194–204.

Kolodny, R.C., Masters, W.H., and Johnson, V.E. (1979). *Textbook of Sexual Medicine*. Boston, MA: Little, Brown.

Krebs-Kraft, D.L., Hill, M.N., Hillard, C.J., and McCarthy, M.M. (2010). Sex difference in cell proliferation in developing rat amygdala mediated by endocannabinoids has implications for social behavior. *Proceedings of the National Academy of Sciences of the United States of America*, **107**, 20535–20540.

Kumar, S., Kumari, A., and Murarka, S. (2009). Lifestyle factors in deteriorating male reproductive health. *Indian Journal of Experimental Biology*, **47**, 615–624.

Lazzarin, N., Valensise, H., Bari, M., et al. (2004). Fluctuations of fatty acid amide hydrolase and anandamide levels during the human ovulatory cycle. *Gynecological Endocrinology*, **18**, 212–218.

Leech, S.L., Richardson, G.A., Goldschmidt, L., and Day, N.L. (1999). Prenatal substance exposure: effects on attention and impulsivity of 6-year-olds. *Neurotoxicology and Teratology*, **21**, 109–118.

Leishman, E., Kokesh, K.J., and Bradshaw, H.B. (2013). Lipids and addiction: how sex steroids, prostaglandins, and cannabinoids interact with drugs of abuse. *Annals of the New York Academy of Sciences*, **1282**, 25–38.

Lopez, H.H. (2010). Cannabinoid-hormone interactions in the regulation of motivational processes. *Hormones and Behavior*, **58**, 100–110.

Lopez, H.H., Webb, S.A., and Nash, S. (2009). Cannabinoid receptor antagonism increases female sexual motivation. *Pharmacology, Biochemistry and Behavior*, **92**, 17–24.

Maccarrone, M. (2009). Endocannabinoids: friends and foes of reproduction. *Progress in Lipid Research*, **48**, 344–354.

Maccarrone, M., Gasperi, V., Fezza, F., Finazzi-Agro, A., and Rossi, A. (2004). Differential regulation of fatty acid amide hydrolase promoter in human immune cells and neuronal cells by leptin and progesterone. *European Journal of Biochemistry*, **271**, 4666–4676.

Maccarrone, M., Salvati, S., Bari, M., and Finazzi, A. (2000). Anandamide and 2-arachidonoylglycerol inhibit fatty acid amide hydrolase by activating the lipoxygenase pathway of the arachidonate cascade. *Biochemical and Biophysical Research Communications*, **278**, 576–583.

Mani, S.K., Mitchell, A., and O'Malley, B.W. (2001a). Progesterone receptor and dopamine receptors are required in Delta 9-tetrahydrocannabinol modulation of sexual receptivity in female rats. *Proceedings of the National Academy of Sciences of the United States of America*, **98**, 1249–1254.

Mani, S.K., Mitchell, A., and O'Malley, B.W. (2001b). Progesterone receptor and dopamine receptors are required in Delta 9-tetrahydrocannabinol modulation of sexual receptivity in female rats. *Proceedings of the National Academy of Sciences of the United States of America*, **98**, 1249–1254.

Martinez-Gonzalez, D., Bonilla-Jaime, H., Morales-Otal, A., Henriksen, S.J., Velazquez-Moctezuma, J., and Prospero-Garcia, O. (2004). Oleamide and anandamide effects on food intake and sexual behavior of rats. *Neuroscience Letters*, **364**, 1–6.

Martinez, I. and Paredes, R.G. (2001). Only self-paced mating is rewarding in rats of both sexes. *Hormones and Behavior*, **40**, 510–517.

Matyas, F., Urban, G.M., Watanabe, M., *et al.* (2008). Identification of the sites of 2-arachidonoylglycerol synthesis and action imply retrograde endocannabinoid signaling at both GABAergic and glutamatergic synapses in the ventral tegmental area. *Neuropharmacology*, **54**, 95–107.

McCarthy, M.M. (2010). How it's made: organisational effects of hormones on the developing brain. *Journal of Neuroendocrinology*, **22**, 736–742.

McHugh, D., Page, J., Dunn, E., and Bradshaw, H.B. (2012). Delta(9)-tetrahydrocannabinol and N-arachidonyl glycine are full agonists at GPR18 receptors and induce migration in human endometrial HEC-1B cells. *British Journal of Pharmacology*, **165**, 2414–2424.

McLaughlin, R.J., Hill, M.N., Morrish, A.C., and Gorzalka, B.B. (2007). Local enhancement of cannabinoid CB1 receptor signalling in the dorsal hippocampus elicits an antidepressant-like effect. *Behavioural Pharmacology*, **18**, 431–438.

Melges, F.T., Tinklenberg, J.R., Hollister, L.E., and Gillespie, H.K. (1971). Marihuana and the temporal span of awareness. *Archives of General Psychiatry*, **24**, 564–567.

Merari, A., Barak, A., and Plaves, M. (1973). Effects of 1(2) -tetrahydrocannabinol on copulation in the male rat. *Psychopharmacologia*, **28**, 243–246.

Park, B., McPartland, J.M., and Glass, M. (2004). Cannabis, cannabinoids and reproduction. *Prostaglandins, Leukotrienes and Essential Fatty Acids*, **70**, 189–197.

Pasqualotto, F.F. and Pasqualotto, E.B. (2012). Recreational drugs and ROS production in mammalian spermatozoa. In: A. Agarwal, R.J. Aitken, and J.G. Alvarez (eds.). *Studies on Men's Health and Fertility*. New York: Humana Press, pp. 417–431.

Phoenix, C.H., Goy, R.W., Gerall, A.A., and Young, W.C. (1959). Organizing action of prenatally administered testosterone propionate on the tissues mediating mating behavior in the female guinea pig. *Endocrinology*, **65**, 369–382.

Rätsch, C. (2001). *Marijuana Medicine: A World Tour of the Healing and Visionary Powers of Cannabis*. Rochester, VT: Inner Traditions/Bear.

Rosen, R.C. (1991). Alcohol and drug effects on sexual response: human experimental and clinical studies. *Annual Review of Sex Research*, **2**, 119–179.

Russo, E. (2002). Cannabis treatments in obstetrics and gynecology: a historical review. *Journal of Cannabis Therapeutics*, **2**, 5–35.

Russo, E.B. (2007). History of cannabis and its preparations in saga, science, and sobriquet. *Chemistry and Biodiversity*, **4**, 1614–1648.

Sabatier, N. and Leng, G. (2006). Presynaptic actions of endocannabinoids mediate MSH-induced inhibition of oxytocin cells. *American Journal of Physiology – Regulatory, Integrative and Comparative Physiology*, **290**, R577–R584.

Shamloul, R. and Bella, A.J. (2011). Impact of cannabis use on male sexual health. *Journal of Sexual Medicine*, **8**, 971–975.

Silver, N. (2012). *The Signal and the Noise: Why So Many Predictions Fail – But Some Don't*. New York: Penguin.

Smith, A., Ferris, J.A., Simpson, J.M., Shelley, J., Pitts, M.K., and Richters, J. (2010). Cannabis use and sexual health. *The Journal of Sexual Medicine*, **7**, 787–793.

Sun, X. and Dey, S.K. (2012). Endocannabinoid signaling in female reproduction. *American Chemical Society Chemical Neuroscience*, **3**, 349–355.

Tart, C.T. (1970). Marijuana intoxication: common experiences. *Nature*, **226**, 701–704.

Taylor, A., Abbas, M., Habiba, M., and Konje, J. (2010a). Histomorphometric evaluation of cannabinoid receptor and anandamide modulating enzyme expression in the human endometrium through the menstrual cycle. *Histochemistry and Cell Biology*, **133**, 557–565.

Taylor, A.H., Abbas, M.S., Habiba, M.A., and Konje, J.C. (2010b). Histomorphometric evaluation of cannabinoid receptor and anandamide modulating enzyme expression in the human endometrium through the menstrual cycle. *Histochemistry and Cell Biology*, **133**, 557–565.

Taylor, A.H., Amoako, A.A., Bambang, K., *et al.* (2010c). Endocannabinoids and pregnancy. *Clinica Chimica Acta*, **411**, 921–930.

Taylor, A.H., Ang, C., Bell, S.C., and Konje, J.C. (2007). The role of the endocannabinoid system in gametogenesis, implantation and early pregnancy. *Human Reproduction Update*, **13**, 501–513.

Turley Jr, W.A. and Floody, O.R. (1981). Delta-9-tetrahydrocannabinol stimulates receptive and proceptive sexual behaviors in female hamsters. *Pharmacology Biochemistry and Behavior*, **14**, 745–747.

Vallejo-Medina, P. and Sierra, J.C. (2013a). Adaptation, equivalence, and validation of the Changes in Sexual Functioning Questionnaire-Drugs (CSFQ-D) in a sample of drug-dependent males. *Journal of Sex & Marital Therapy*, 368–384.

Vallejo-Medina, P. and Sierra, J.C. (2013b). Effect of drug use and influence of abstinence on sexual functioning in a Spanish male drug-dependent sample: a multisite study. *The Journal of Sexual Medicine*, 333–341.

van Gelder, M.M., Reefhuis, J., Caton, A.R., Werler, M.M., Druschel, C.M., and Roeleveld, N. (2010). Characteristics of pregnant illicit drug users and associations between cannabis use and perinatal outcome in a population-based study. *Drug and Alcohol Dependence*, **109**, 243–247.

Wang, H., Guo, Y., Wang, D., *et al.* (2004). Aberrant cannabinoid signaling impairs oviductal transport of embryos. *Nature Medicine*, **10**, 1074–1080.

Wenger, T., Tóth, B.E., Juanéda, C., Leonardelli, J., and Tramu, G. (1999). The effects of cannabinoids on the regulation of reproduction. *Life Sciences*, **65**, 695–701.

Zias, J., Stark, H., Sellgman, J., *et al.* (1993). Early medical use of cannabis. *Nature*, **363**, 215.

Chapter 14

Phytocannabinoids and the Immune System

Guy A. Cabral, Erinn S. Raborn,
and Gabriela A. Ferreira

14.1 Phytocannabinoids

Phytocannabinoids are a class of compounds from the marijuana plant, *Cannabis sativa*. These include the major nonpsychoactive components cannabidiol (CBD), cannabinol (CBN), cannabigerol (CBG), and the major psychoactive component delta-9-tetrahydrocannabinol (THC). The purification and structural analysis of THC have led to the synthesis of analogs that have been used in structure–activity studies to characterize cannabinoid-mediated effects and define their mechanism of action. Such studies led to the recognition that THC exhibits specificity of action at the physiological and pharmacological levels and can act through the G inhibitory (G_i) protein-coupled receptors, cannabinoid receptor type 1 (CB_1R), and cannabinoid receptor type 2 (CB_2R). The CB_1R accounts for most, if not all, of the centrally mediated effects of cannabinoids and is concentrated in areas of the brain that control movement, coordination, sensory perception, learning, memory, reward, emotions, hormonal function, and body temperature. The CB_2R has been implicated as relevant in immune modulation. Since the discovery of the CB_1R and CB_2R, major advances in cannabinoid pharmacology and physiology have taken place, including the recognition that phytocannabinoids such as CBD, CBN, and THC have immune modulatory properties. However, while immune modulatory effects of THC have been linked to the CB_2R, those of CBD and CBN have been attributed generally to noncannabinoid receptor-mediated actions.

14.2 Effects of phytocannabinoids on the immune system

14.2.1 In vivo models

Experimental animals have offered unique insights into the effects of phytocannabinoids on immune function. Due to their well-defined immune systems, statistically significant data with minimal confounding variables have been obtained. Rosenkrantz et al. (1975) administered THC to rats before, during, and after intraperitoneal (i.p.) injection of sheep red blood cells (sRBCs) and found a reduction in the induction and production of anti-sRBC antibodies. Zimmerman et al. (1977) compared the effects of CBD, CBN, and THC on the antibody response and found that THC elicited a dose-dependent depression of immune responsiveness while CBD and CBN did not, suggesting a specificity of action. Baczynsky et al. (1983a, 1983b) examined the effects of CBD, CBN, and THC on the primary and secondary antibody immune responses to sRBCs in mice. While CBD and CBN elicited no effect, THC administered during the primary immunization period suppressed the primary (i.e., immunoglobulin M (IgM)) antibody response but when administered during the secondary immunization period had no effect. Jan et al. (2007) reported that CBD attenuated the serum level of IgM and IgG anti-ovalbumin (OVA) antibodies in OVA-sensitized mice.

Phytocannabinoids have also been reported to dampen cytokine responses. Malfait et al. (2000) reported that CBD blocked the production of inflammatory cytokines associated with disease progression in a collagen-induced rheumatoid arthritis DBA/1 mouse model. Draining lymph node cells from CBD-treated mice exhibited decreased levels of interferon (IFN)-γ while knee synovial cells yielded decreased release of tumor necrosis factor (TNF)-α. CBD was shown also to block bacterial lipopolysaccharide (LPS)-induced increase in serum TNF-α in C57/BL mice. Weiss et al. (2006, 2008) reported that CBD lowered the incidence of diabetes in nonobese diabetes-prone mice. This decrease was accompanied by reduced plasma levels of IFN-γ and TNF-α, lowered pro-inflammatory cytokine production in vitro, and augmented production of the anti-inflammatory cytokines interleukin (IL)-4 and IL-10. El-Remessy et al. (2006) reported that CBD reduced oxidative stress, retinal neuronal cell death, and vascular permeability in streptozotocin (STZ)-induced diabetic rats, effects that are associated with increased levels of TNF-α, vascular endothelial growth factor (VEGF), and the intercellular adhesion molecule (ICAM)-1. Esposito et al. (2007) indicated that CBD inhibited inducible nitric oxide synthase (iNOs) and IL-1β expression in an amyloid-beta injected mouse model of Alzheimer disease-related neuroinflammation. Borrelli et al. (2009) examined the effect of intracolonic administration of CBD in a mouse model of dinitrobenzene sulfonic acid (DNBS)-induced colitis and noted that disease improvement was accompanied by a decrease in the level of IL-1β. Recently, Liu et al. (2010) reported that CBD attenuated delayed-type hypersensitivity (DTH) by suppressing T-lymphocyte and macrophage reactivity to subcutaneous OVA challenge to the footpads of mice sensitized previously with OVA. CBD suppressed the infiltration of T lymphocytes and macrophages in the footpad and inhibited the expression of the proinflammatory cytokines IFN-γ and TNF-α while augmenting the level of the anti-inflammatory cytokine IL-10. Thus, CBD promotes a switch in cytokine profile from that of a proinflammatory (Th1) type to that of an anti-inflammatory (Th2) type in a number of animal models.

The effects of phytocannabinoids on immune function appear to differ with age. Pross et al. (1990) examined THC-mediated suppression of mouse lymphoid cell proliferative responses to the mitogens concanavalin A (ConA) and phytohemagglutinin (PHA) in adult versus juvenile mice. Thymus cells were suppressed more readily than spleen cells in adults while spleen cells from mice under 2 weeks of age were suppressed more readily than those from older mice. Snella et al. (1995) found that lymphoid cells from 2- and 18-month-old mice, as compared with adult mice, were resistant to THC-mediated proliferation when stimulated by their CD3 receptor. Ramarathinam et al. (1997) demonstrated that lymphoid cells from young and old mice exhibited different immunological responses to THC in terms of their ability to produce cytokines following stimulation with either ConA or anti-CD3 antibody. Levels of IL-4 and IL-10 were upregulated in spleen cell cultures from the older animals. In vivo administration of THC resulted in an upregulation of the proliferative response of lymphoid cells from young adult mice.

14.2.2 In vitro/ex vivo models

14.2.2.1 Effects on mixed cell populations

In order to garner insight regarding the immunocyte population targeted by phytocannabinoids, mixed cell and purified immunocyte subpopulations (Table 14.1) have been examined. Lefkowitz and Klager (1978) assessed the effect of in vivo THC administration on in vitro sRBC sensitization

Table 14.1 Major immune cell types in humans

Immune cell types	Function	% of leukocyte population†	Cannabinoid receptor expression
B lymphocytes	Antibody production; antigen presentation (MHCII)	1–7%	$CB_2R >> CB_1R$
CD4+ T lymphocytes	Cell-mediated immunity	4–20%	CB_2R
Th1	inflammation (TGF-β, IFN-γ)		
Th2	Antibody-mediated immunity (IL-4, IL-5, IL-13)		
Treg	Immune homeostasis (IL-10, TGF-β)		
CD8+ T lymphocytes	Kill virally infected cell and tumor cells	2–11%	$CB_2R > CB_1R$
Macrophages/monocytes	Phagocytosis; process/present antigen (MHCII); chemokine/cytokine secretion	2–12%	$CB_2R > CB_1R$
Microglia	Resident macrophage of CNS		$CB_2R > CB_1R$
Natural killer cells	Rapid innate immune response, release cytolytic factors to induce apoptosis/lysis of infected cells	1–6%	$CB_2R > CB_1R$

† leukocytes account for 0.1–0.2% of blood cells.

Data from Galiegue, S., Mary, S., and Marchand, J., et al., Expression of central and peripheral cannabinoid receptors in human immune tissues and leukocyte subpopulations. *European Journal of Biochemistry*, 232, pp. 54–61 © 1995, John Wiley and Sons, Inc and Graham, E.S., Angel, C.E., Schwarcz, L.E., Dunbar, P.R., and Glass, M., Detailed characterisation of CB2 receptor protein expression in peripheral blood immune cells from healthy human volunteers using flow cytometry, *International Journal of Immunopathology and Pharmacology*, 23, pp.25–34 © 2010, BIOLIFE, s.a.s.

of mouse splenic lymphocytes. THC depressed the anti-sRBC antibody response, an outcome that was obtained when THC was added directly in vitro. Baczynsky et al. (1983b) reported that CBD, CBN, and THC acted differentially on mouse spleen cells in vitro since CBN did not depress the primary immune response. Pross et al. (1992) found that, when ConA or PHA was used to stimulate THC-treated splenocytes, a downregulation of lymphocyte proliferation occurred. In contrast, when splenocytes were stimulated directly with anti-CD3 antibody that ligates to CD3 on T lymphocytes and activates their proliferation, THC at low concentrations enhanced proliferation. It was indicated also that THC suppressed the expression of IL-2 and the IL-2 receptor. The T-cell mitogen anti-CD3 produced an opposite effect when combined with THC since it increased T-lymphocyte proliferation and the response of IL-2. Nakano et al. (1992) demonstrated that THC-related modulation of IL-2 activity corresponded with changes in blastogenic activity and with variation in numbers of Tac antigen-positive cells, T lymphocytes that are activated in the autologous mixed lymphocyte reaction that regulate the generation of killer T cells. Jan et al. (2007) found that i.p. injection of CBD resulted in suppression of antigen-specific antibody production and inhibition of splenocyte production of IL-2 and IFN-γ in OVA-sensitized mice upon ex vivo stimulation.

14.2.2.2 Effects on mononuclear cells, macrophages, and macrophage-like cells

Phytocannabinoids have been reported to suppress macrophage phagocytosis, bactericidal activity, and cell spreading (Friedman et al. 1991; Klein and Friedman 1990) and to alter cytokine expression. Zheng et al. (1992) indicated that THC caused a decrease in TNF-α production by mouse peritoneal macrophages in response to LPS and IFN-γ. Fisher-Stenger et al. (1993) examined the effects of THC on TNF-α production by mouse RAW264.7 macrophage-like cells and reported that it altered its conversion from a 26-kDa presecretory form to the 17 kDa secretory product. Klein and Friedman (1990) indicated that the activity of IL-1 increased in supernatants of mouse macrophage cultures treated with LPS and THC. The higher activity was attributed to increase in release of the premature IL-1α and mature IL-1β forms. A subsequent report suggested that Bcl-2 and caspase-1 (i.e., IL-1 converting enzyme that proteolytically cleaves the precursor form of IL-1β) played a role in this process (Zhu et al. 1998). Steffens et al. (2005), using a mouse model of atherosclerosis, showed that oral administration of THC resulted in inhibition of disease progression associated with lymphoid cell diminished proliferation and IFN-γ secretion.

THC also has been reported to alter cytokine expression by microglia, macrophage-like cells resident in the central nervous system (CNS) and eye. Puffenbarger et al. (2000) reported that THC caused a reduction in levels of LPS-induced rat microglial mRNAs for IL-1α, IL-1β, IL-6, and TNF-α. This reduction was linked to neither the CB_1R nor the CB_2R. Chang et al. (2001) using mouse J774 macrophage-like cells compared the effects of THC with those of the endocannabinoids, anandamide (AEA), and 2-arachidonoylglycerol (2-AG), and of indomethacin morpholinylamide (IMMA). A differential effect was exerted since THC, IMMA, and AEA diminished LPS-induced nitric oxide (NO) and IL-6 production, while 2-AG inhibited the production of IL-6.

CBD also alters the expression of cytokines by macrophage-like cells. Weiss et al. (2006) indicated that the production of Th1 (i.e., proinflammatory) cytokines by ex vivo activated peritoneal macrophages was reduced in CBD-treated mice, whereas that of Th2-associated (i.e., anti-inflammatory) cytokines such as IL-4 and IL-10 was increased. El-Remessy et al. (2008) using a rat model of diabetes and glaucoma, reported that CBD inhibited LPS-induced production of TNF-α and NO in rat microglia. Kozela et al. (2010) demonstrated that CBD and THC decreased the production and release of IL-1β, IL-6, and IFN-β from LPS-activated mouse BV-2 microglial-like cells. The anti-inflammatory action appeared not to involve the CB_1R, the CB_2R, or the abnormal (abn)-CBD-sensitive receptor. De Filippis et al. (2011) reported that CBD reduced intestinal inflammation through a process that involved control at the level of the neuro-immune axis. CBD counteracted reactive enteric gliosis in LPS-treated mice through the reduction of astroglial signaling by neurotrophin S100B. The S100B decrease was associated with fewer mast cells and macrophages in the intestine. Moreover, treatment of LPS-mice with CBD reduced TNF-α expression. Similar results were obtained with cultures of colonic biopsies from ulcerative colitis patients. The activity of CBD was attributed, at least in part, to activation of the peroxisome proliferator-activated receptor (PPAR)-γ pathway. Juknat et al. (2012b) found that CBD affected the expression of mouse BV-2 cell genes involved in zinc homeostasis, suggesting that regulation of zinc levels could be a means through which CBD exerted its antioxidant and anti-inflammatory effects. Juknat et al. (2012a) also reported that CBD and THC elicited a differential transcriptional profile in BV-2 cells since CBD altered the expression of many more genes. The CBD-stimulated genes were implicated as under the control of nuclear factors known to be involved in the regulation of stress responses and inflammation.

Phytocannabinoids also have been reported to alter a variety of other macrophage-like cell functions. Burnette-Curley and Cabral (1995) reported that THC inhibition of cell contact-dependent tumor cell cytolysis was linked to targeting of a TNF-dependent pathway. Coffey et al. (1996) implied that an early step in NO production by mouse peritoneal macrophages, such as NO synthase (NOS) gene transcription or NOS synthesis, was affected by THC. A structure–activity order of effectiveness in inhibition was noted for THC analogs used with potency being highest for Δ^8-tetrahydrocannabinol and decreasing in order for THC >CBD ≥11-OH-THC >CBN. The investigators concluded that inhibition of NO was mediated partly by a stereoselective cannabinoid receptor/cAMP pathway and partly by a nonselective molecular process. Jeon et al. (1996), using the mouse RAW264.7 macrophage cell line, demonstrated that THC inhibited NOS transcription factors such as nuclear factor (NF)-κB/RelA, suggesting a mode by which this cannabinoid altered NO production. THC has also been reported to alter macrophage processing of antigens that is necessary for the activation of CD4+ T lymphocytes (McCoy et al. 1995). The THC-mediated processing defect was shown to involve the CB_2R (McCoy et al. 1999). This observation was confirmed by Buckley et al. (2000) using knockout mice with a targeted deletion for the CB_2R. Matveyeva et al. (2000) suggested that THC caused an antigen-dependent defect in the ability of macrophages to activate T-helper cells in a CB_2R-linked fashion by selectively increasing aspartyl cathepsin D proteolytic activity. Chuchawankul et al. (2004) reported that the CB_2R also played a role in THC-mediated inhibition of macrophage function by targeting costimulatory activity. Carrier et al. (2006) found that THC and CBD inhibited mouse EOC-20 microglial cell proliferation through inhibition of adenosine uptake, consistent with a cannabinoid receptor-independent mode of action for CBD-induced decreased inflammation.

In addition, phytocannabinoids have been shown to alter the migratory activities of macrophage-like cells. Sacerdote et al. (2005) reported that CBD decreased chemotaxis of mouse macrophages in vivo and in vitro in response to the peptide fMet-Leu-Phe. Walter et al. (2003) reported that CBN and CBD inhibited microglial cell migration in response to the endocannabinoid 2-AG. The migration enhancing effect of 2-AG was reported to occur through the CB_2R and the abn-CBD-sensitive receptor, with subsequent activation of the extracellular signal-regulated kinase 1/2 signal transduction pathway. CBN and CBD prevented the 2-AG-induced cell migration by antagonizing the two receptors. Rajesh et al. (2010) indicated that CBD attenuated high glucose-induced monocyte adhesion to endothelial cells and reduced transendothelial monocyte migration.

14.2.2.3 Effects on B lymphocytes

B lymphocytes express relatively high levels of the CB_2R (Carayon et al. 1998; Galiègue et al. 1995; Lynn and Herkenham 1994). Thus, it is not surprising that functional activities of these immune cells are affected by phytocannabinoids acting through this receptor. Klein et al. (1985) noted that the addition of THC to mouse splenocyte cultures suppressed B lymphocytes in response to LPS. Derocq et al. (1995) reported that THC at low nanomolar concentrations had an enhancing effect on human tonsillar B-cell growth. It was proposed that the growth-enhancing activity observed on B cells at very low concentrations of THC was mediated through the CB_2R.

14.2.2.4 Effects on T lymphocytes

Nahas and colleagues reported as early as 1977 that THC altered human T-lymphocyte functions (Nahas et al. 1977). Numerous investigators since have expanded on this observation. Klein et al. (1991) found that THC altered the activity of mouse cytotoxic T lymphocytes (CTLs) through a step beyond the binding of the CTL to its target cell. THC appeared to suppress the development of CTLs from precursors to mature cells. Fischer-Stenger et al. (1992) found that THC inhibited CTL cytoplasmic polarization toward herpes simplex virus (HSV)-infected target cells. CTL granule reorientation toward the target cell that followed cell–cell conjugation occurred at a lower frequency in co-cultures containing CTLs from THC-treated mice. Yebra et al. (1992) examined the effect of THC on mobilization of cytosolic free calcium [Ca²⁺], one of the earliest events in

T-cell activation, and suggested that the proliferation defect in THC-treated lymphocytes was related to inhibition of $[Ca^{2+}]$ mobilization. Karmaus et al. (2012) reported that THC suppression of CTL function occurred independently of the CB_1R and CB_2R. An allogeneic model of major histocompatibility complex (MHC) I mismatch was used to elicit CTLs in CB_1R/CB_2R double knockout mice to determine the requirement for these receptors. THC suppressed CTL function independently of the CB_1R and CB_2R.

Schatz et al. (1993) proposed that THC selectively inhibited T-cell-dependent humoral (i.e., antibody) immune responses. Oral administration of THC to mice produced a selective inhibition of primary antibody (i.e., IgM) responses to the T-cell-dependent antigen sRBC. In contrast, no inhibitory effect on antibody responses to the T-cell-independent antigen DNP-Ficoll was obtained. Phytocannabinoid-mediated defects in cytokine expression also have been reported. Condie et al. (1996) found that treatment of murine thymoma-derived EL4T cells with CBN or THC disrupted the adenylate cyclase signaling cascade by inhibiting forskolin-stimulated cAMP accumulation. It was suggested that inhibition of the adenylate cyclase/cAMP signal transduction pathway led to T-cell dysfunction by decreasing the level of IL-2 gene transcription. Jan et al. (2002) reported that CBN enhanced IL-2 expression by T cells that was associated with an increase in IL-2 distal nuclear factor of activated T cell (NFAT) activity. Enhancement of IL-2 was demonstrated also with THC and CBD, suggesting that the enhanced effect was not unique to CBN. It was indicated that increased IL-2 secretion by CBN was mediated through the enhancement of IL-2 gene transcription through activation of NF-AT in a CB_1R/CB_2R-independent manner. Yuan et al. (2002) stimulated human T cells with allogeneic dendritic cells and reported that THC suppressed T-cell proliferation, inhibited the production of IFN-γ and shifted the balance of Th1/Th2 cytokines. It was indicated that THC decreased the steady-state levels of mRNA encoding for Th1 cytokines, while increasing those for Th2 cytokines by a CB_2R-dependent pathway.

In order to gain insight into the mechanisms involved in phytocannabinoid-mediated T-cell dysfunction, Rao and Kaminski (2006) investigated the ability of various cannabinoid compounds to elevate intracellular calcium concentration $[Ca^{2+}]_i$ in CB_2R-expressing human peripheral blood acute lymphoid leukemia (HPB-ALL) T cells. It was found that the $[Ca^{2+}]_i$ elevation elicited by CBN and compounds structurally similar to THC was independent of the CB_1R and CB_2R. Lee et al. (2008) demonstrated that thymocytes and EL-4 thymoma cells were susceptible to CBD-induced apoptosis and suggested a role for reactive oxygen species in the induction of apoptosis. Lu et al. (2009) reported that THC suppressed the expression of an inducible co-stimulatory (ICOS) receptor related to CD28 that is essential for T-lymphocyte activation and function. Inhibition of this receptor appeared to occur at the transcriptional level through THC-mediated modulation of NFAT signaling. Rao et al. (2004) suggested that cannabinoid receptors were linked to T-lymphocyte dysfunction by inducing an influx of extracellular calcium in resting cells. THC elevated $[Ca^{2+}]_i$ in purified murine splenic T cells and the HPB-ALL but had a minimal effect on human Jurkat E6-1 cells that exhibit dysfunctional expression of the CB_2R. Rao and Kaminski (2006) reported that the induction of $[Ca^{2+}]_i$ elevation by THC in T lymphocytes involved transient receptor potential channel (TRPC)1 channels, ion channels that are located on the plasma membrane. It was concluded that the THC-induced elevation in $[Ca^{2+}]_i$ was attributable to extracellular calcium influx, which is independent of $[Ca^{2+}]_i$ store depletion and was mediated, at least partially, through diacylglycerol-sensitive TRPC1 channels.

On the other hand, Borner et al. (2007) implicated a role for the CB_1R in T-lymphocyte dysfunction. It was reported that transcription of the CB_1R gene was induced in response to THC, whereas the CB_2R gene was not. However, the induction of CB_1R gene expression was found to be mediated by the CB_2R, the consequent upregulation facilitating or enhancing T-lymphocyte immunomodulatory effects related to phytocannabinoids. The release of IL-4 protein from these cells was proposed as necessary for the induction of the CB_1R gene. Recently, Lombard et al. (2011) reported that perinatal exposure of mice to THC triggers defects in T-cell differentiation and function in fetal and postnatal stages of life. These THC-mediated outcomes were attributed to activation of cannabinoid receptors. Thymic atrophy induced in the fetus correlated with caspase-dependent apoptosis in thymocytes. Perinatal exposure to THC also had a profound effect on the immune response during postnatal life.

14.2.2.5 Effects on natural killer cells

Kawakami et al. (1988) reported that THC suppressed IL-2-induced killing activity and proliferation using the NKB61A2 natural killer (NK) cell line (Warner and Dennert 1982). Similarly, THC was reported to suppress proliferation of murine spleen cells stimulated with recombinant human IL-2. In addition, spleen cells previously stimulated in culture with IL-2, and then incubated with THC prior to addition to target cells, displayed suppressed cytolytic activity. The results indicated that THC could suppress IL-2-linked functions, including clonal expansion of lymphocytes, expansion of killer cell populations, and stimulation of killer cell cytotoxic activity. Studies have shown also that THC suppresses the killing activity of mouse and human NK cells (Klein et al. 1998a, 1998b). This THC-mediated inhibition has been attributed partly to a decrease in the number of high-affinity and intermediate-affinity IL-2 binding sites, suggesting suppression in the expression of IL-2 receptor (IL-2R) proteins (Zhu et al. 1993). Indeed, THC has since been shown to increase cellular levels of IL-2Rα and β proteins, to decrease levels of the γ-protein, and to decrease the function of the IL-2R (Zhu et al. 1995). It was concluded that THC disturbed the relative expression of various IL-2R chains, resulting in overall receptor dysfunction and responsiveness to IL-2. Daaka et al. (1997), using NKB61A2 cells, suggested a functional link of the CB_1R to these THC-mediated effects and implicated involvement of the universal transcription factor NF-κB and the IL-2Rα gene. Massi et al. (2000) reported that THC administered to mice resulted in inhibition of NK cytolytic activity and a reduction in production of IFN-γ. It was suggested that the CB_1R and CB_2R were both involved in the THC-affected network that mediated NK cytolytic activity.

14.2.2.6 Effects on cytokines

The collective data suggest that select phytocannabinoids such as THC and CBD alter the expression of cytokines (Table 14.2). They converge to inhibit the production of the Th1-type (i.e., pro-inflammatory) cytokines while promoting that of the Th2-type (anti-inflammatory) cytokines, although the respective mechanisms may differ. Blanchard et al. (1986) and Cabral et al. (1986a) reported that the induction of IFN-α/β was suppressed by THC treatment of mice. Watzl et al. (1991) reported that cytokine activity in cultured human peripheral blood mononuclear cells was modulated by THC. CBD also modulated cytokine production and/or secretion, leading to the suggestion that a noncannabinoid receptor-mediated mode of action was involved. Berdyshev et al. (1997) examined the effects of THC on the production of TNF-α, IL-4, IL-6, IL-8, IL-10, IFN-γ, p55, and, p75 TNF-α soluble receptors by stimulated human peripheral blood mononuclear cells. THC exerted a biphasic effect on Th1 cytokine production in that TNF-α, IL-6, IL-8, and INF-γ synthesis was inhibited by a low concentration of THC (i.e., 3 nM) but stimulated by a high concentration of THC (i.e., 3 μM). Srivastava et al. (1998) examined the effect of THC and CBD on cytokine production by human leukemic T, B, eosinophilic, and CD8+ NK lines in vitro. THC decreased the constitutive production of IL-8, macrophage inflammatory protein (MIP)-1α, MIP-1β, and RANTES (regulated upon activation normal T-cell expressed and secreted) protein.

Table 14.2 Select cytokines produced by immune cells

Cytokine	Producing immune cell	Action
IL-1α/β	Monocytes/macrophages, microglia, B lymphocytes, dendritic cells, endothelial cells	Proinflammatory, acute inflammation, fever, acute phase protein production
IL-4	T lymphocytes, mast cells	Anti-inflammatory, B- and T-lymphocyte differentiation factor
IL-6	T lymphocytes, monocytes/macrophages, microglia, endothelial cells	Proinflammatory, acute inflammation, fever, acute phase protein productionAnti-inflammatory, inhibits TNF-α and IL-1, activates IL-10, B- and T-lymphocyte differentiation factor
IL-8	Macrophages, microglia, endothelial cells, epithelial cells	Proinflammatory, chemotactic factor for neutrophils and T lymphocytes; activates neutrophils
IL-10	Monocytes/macrophages, microglia, Th2 and Treg lymphocytes, B lymphocytes	Anti-inflammatory, inhibits proinflammatory cytokine production, suppresses antigen presentation capacity of APCs
IL-12	Macrophages, microglia, dendritic cells, B lymphocytes	Proinflammatory, stimulates differentiation of CD4 T cells to Th1, stimulates production of TNF-α and IFN-γ
IFN-γ	T lymphocytes (Th1, CD8+), natural killer cells	Proinflammatory, activates macrophages, stimulates differentiation of CD4 T cells to Th1 while suppressing Th2
TNF-α	Macrophages, microglia, CD4+ T lymphocytes, natural killer cells	Proinflammatory, localized inflammation, fever

Phorbol ester-stimulated production of TNF-α, granulocyte-macrophage colony-stimulating factor (GM-CSF), and IFN-γ by NK cells also was affected. These results indicated that THC and CBD could alter production of cytokines across a diverse array of immune cell lineages.

It is highly relevant that phytocannabinoids have been reported to alter the expression of chemokines and cytokines in various disease paradigms. Zhu et al. (2000) reported that THC promoted tumor growth by inhibiting antitumor immunity by a CB_2R-mediated, cytokine-dependent pathway. Levels of the immune inhibitory Th2 cytokines IL-10 and transforming growth factor (TGF) were augmented while those of the immune stimulatory Th1 cytokine IFN-γ were downregulated at both the tumor site and in the spleens of THC-treated mice. McKallip et al. (2005) reported that exposure of mice to THC led to elevated tumor growth and metastasis of the mouse mammary carcinoma 4T1 due to inhibition of the specific antitumor immune response in vivo. Exposure to THC led to increased production of IL-4 and IL-10 and suppression of the antitumor immune response was mediated primarily through the CB_2R. Li et al. (2001) reported that THC had an immunosuppressive effect in STZ-induced autoimmune diabetes. In addition to ablating the elevation in serum glucose and loss of pancreatic insulin, it reduced STZ-induced levels of IFN-γ, TNF-α, and IL-12 mRNA. El-Remessy et al. (2006) found that CBD treatment of STZ-induced diabetic rats reduced oxidative stress, decreased levels of TNF-α, VEGF, and ICAM-1, and prevented retinal cell death and vascular hyperpermeability in the retina. Napimoga et al. (2009) reported that CBD decreased bone resorption by inhibiting RANK/RANKL expression and proinflammatory cytokines during experimental periodontitis in rats. Gingival tissues from the CBD-treated rats showed decreased neutrophil migration associated with lower production of IL-1β and TNF-α. Ribeiro et al. (2012) demonstrated that administration of CBD prior to the induction of LPS-induced acute lung injury decreased neutrophil migration into the lungs, albumin concentration in the bronchoalveolar lavage fluid, myeloperoxidase activity in the lung tissue, and the production of the cytokines TNF and IL-6 and the chemokines monocyte chemoattractant protein (MCP)-1 and macrophage inflammatory protein (MIP)-2. Li et al. (2012) suggested that CBD played an anti-inflammatory role in i.p. cerulein-induced acute pancreatitis in C57BL mice. CBD treatment improved the pathological changes of mice with acute pancreatitis and decreased levels of IL-6 and TNF-α. De Filippis et al. (2011) investigated the effect of CBD using intestinal biopsies from patients with ulcerative colitis and from intestinal segments of mice with LPS-induced intestinal inflammation. Treatment of LPS-mice with CBD reduced the level of TNF-α. Similar results were obtained in ex vivo cultured human-derived colonic biopsies.

14.3 Effects of phytocannabinoids on host resistance to viral, bacterial, and fungal infections

14.3.1 In vitro infections

In view of the multiplicity of effects on immunity in vivo and in vitro, it is not surprising that phytocannabinoids have been implicated in modulating resistance to a variety of infectious agents. Blevins and Dumic (1980) indicated that THC exerted a protective effect against HSV infection in vitro. On the other hand, THC has been reported to inhibit macrophage extrinsic anti-HSV activity (Cabral and Vásquez 1991, 1992), a process whereby macrophages normally suppress virus replication in the virus-infected cells to which they attach (Morahan et al. 1980; Stohlman et al. 1982). Noe et al. (1998) reported that THC enhanced syncytia formation in MT-2 cells infected with the human immunodeficiency virus (HIV), a process that has been reported to serve as an indicator of HIV infection and cytopathicity. Raborn and Cabral (2010) reported that THC inhibited human U937 macrophage-like cell migration to the trans-activating (Tat) protein of HIV-1 and that this effect was linked to the CB_2R. Fraga and Raborn et al. (2011) showed that THC also inhibited migration of BV-2 microglial-like cells to the HIV protein Tat. Recently, Chen et al. (2012), using a surrogate mouse model to induce polyclonal T cell responses against gp120, the major envelope glycoprotein of HIV, reported that THC altered mouse CD8[+] T cell proliferation and the gp120-specific CTL response dependent on the magnitude of the IFN-γ response.

Phytocannabinoids have also been reported to alter resistance to microbial agents other than viruses. Arata et al. (1991, 1992) reported that THC could overcome the restriction of the growth of *Legionella pneumophila*, a facultative intracellular pathogen that replicates in macrophages. While pretreatment of macrophages with THC did not affect ingestion or replication of *Legionella*, treatment following infection resulted in increased numbers of intracellular bacteria. Stimulation of macrophages with LPS resulted in a reduction in *Legionella* growth. Furthermore, treatment of these LPS-activated macrophages with THC resulted in greater growth of *Legionella*, indicating that THC abolished the LPS-induced enhanced resistance. Gross et al. (2000) reported that THC ablated infection of macrophages by the intracellular gram-negative bacterium *Brucella suis*. THC also has been reported to alter the capacity of macrophages to kill *Naegleria fowleri* (Burnette-Curley et al. 1993), the causative agent of primary amoebic meningoencephalitis (PAME) (Marciano-Cabral 1988), and to decrease neonatal rat microglial levels of mRNA for IL-1α, IL-1β, and TNF-α elicited in response to *Acanthamoeba* (Cabral and Marciano-Cabral, 2004).

14.3.2 **In vivo infections**

Bradley et al. (1977) demonstrated that THC enhanced the susceptibility of mice to live or killed gram-negative bacteria. Subsequently, Morahan et al. (1979) demonstrated that mice exposed to THC were compromised in their ability to resist infection to *Listeria monocytogenes* or to HSV-2. Mishkin and Cabral (1985) and Cabral et al. (1986a, b) demonstrated that THC increased the susceptibility to HSV-2 genital infection in guinea pigs and mice based on greater severity of herpes genitalis, higher mortalities, and higher mean titers of virus shed from the vagina. Cabral et al. (1986b) also noted that THC caused a reduction of the splenocyte proliferative response to HSV-2. Buchweitz et al. (2007) reported that THC increased influenza A viral load and decreased macrophage and lymphocyte recruitment into the lungs. It was indicated that effects on the immune and airway epithelial cell responses to challenge with influenza A virus in THC-treated mice involved both CB_1R/CB_2R-dependent and -independent mechanisms (Buchweitz et al. 2008). In addition, THC (dronabinol) treatment has been reported to lead to severity of disease in mice infected with vaccinia virus (Huemer et al. 2011). Paradise and Friedman (1993), using a hamster model of syphilis, indicated that THC enhanced infection with *Treponema pallidum*. A greater degree of enhancement was exhibited also in rabbits in that treponemes proliferated more readily during treatment with THC. Also, Marciano-Cabral et al. (2001) reported that THC exacerbated brain infection in mice by *Acanthamoeba* spp.

There is also evidence that phytocannabinoids have the ability to alter resistance to retroviruses. Specter et al. (1991) reported that THC augmented murine retroviral-induced immunosuppression and infection. THC administered in vitro to spleen cells from mice infected with Friend leukemia virus (FLV) resulted in a decrease, beyond that seen with virus or THC alone, in lymphocyte blastogenesis and NK cell activity. When both FLV and THC were administered to mice concurrently infected with HSV, mortality attributed to FLV infection occurred significantly more rapidly than in the absence of HSV or THC. Roth et al. (2005) reported that THC suppressed immune function and enhanced HIV replication in the huPBL-SCID mouse. In this hybrid model, human peripheral blood leukocytes (huPBLs) were implanted into severe combined immunodeficient mice (huPBL-SCID) followed by infection with an HIV reporter construct in the presence or absence of THC exposure. The results suggested that exposure to THC in vivo suppressed immune function, increased the expression of CCR5 and CXCR4 chemokine receptors that serve as HIV co-receptors, and acted as a cofactor to significantly enhance HIV replication. On the other hand, Winsauer et al. (2011) using the simian immune deficiency virus (SIV)-infected rhesus macaque model of HIV infection, demonstrated that chronic administration of THC resulted in a decrease in neuroinflammation and lower viral load in the CNS. Similarly, Molina et al. (2011) reported that chronic THC administration decreased early mortality from SIV infection in macaques, and that this outcome was associated with attenuation of plasma and cerebral spinal fluid viral load and retention of body mass. It was speculated that reduced levels of SIV, retention of body mass, and attenuation of inflammation were likely modalities for THC-mediated moderation of disease progression. LeCapitaine et al. (2011) investigated whether prolonged THC administration affected lymphocyte counts, lymphocyte phenotype, and lymphocyte proliferation induced in young adult rhesus macaques infected with SIV over a 12-month period. Chronic THC administration did not alter lymphocyte subtypes, naive and memory subsets, and proliferation or apoptosis of T lymphocytes. However, an increase in CXCR4 expression in both $CD4^+$ and $CD8^+$ T lymphocytes was observed. It was suggested that chronic THC administration produced changes in T-cell phenotype, a condition that, it has been suggested, could contribute to host immunomodulation to infectious challenge.

14.4 **Summary and conclusions**

The mode through which phytocannabinoids such as THC and CBD converge to inhibit immune functional activities has not been fully elucidated. These two phytocannabinoids exert a commonality of action by altering the production of chemokines and cytokines, usually causing a switch from promoting elicitation of Th1 cytokines such as IFN-γ, TNF-α, IL-1β, and IL-2 to that of Th2 cytokines such as IL-10 and IL-4 (Cabral and Marciano-Cabral, 2004; Klein et al. 2000; Lu et al. 2006; Newton et al. 1994). However, phytocannabinoids such as THC have been reported to induce cytokine-mediated mortality of mice infected with *L. pneumophila* by augmenting proinflammatory responses, thereby exacerbating infection and disease (Klein et al. 1993). Smith et al. (1997) examined the effects of CBD and CBN on sublethal infection of inbred BALB/c mice, animals that are relatively resistant to infection with *L. pneumophila*. Mice receiving THC before and after infection exhibited higher levels of bacteria in their lungs compared to sublethally infected mice not receiving phytocannabinoid. In addition, lung levels of mRNA for IL-6 were increased markedly following treatment of infected animals with THC.

The mechanisms that come into play for CBD versus THC in mediating anti-inflammatory events have not been resolved. THC inhibitory effects on immune cell migration appear to be linked to the CB_2R. However, CBD and THC converge to alter cytokine/chemokines expression but may do so by disparate modes of action. Newton et al. (2009) demonstrated that IFN-γ production was dependent upon signaling through IL-12Rβ2, that THC treatment suppressed splenic β2 message, and that these effects were cannabinoid receptor dependent. Using IL-4 deficient mice, it was observed that increases in IL-4 induced by THC were not involved in the phytocannabinoid effect on β2. It was suggested that both the CB_1R and the CB_2R mediated the THC-induced shift in T-helper activity in *L. pneumophila*-infected mice, with the CB_1R involved in suppressing IL-12Rβ2 and the CB_2R involved in enhancing the trans-activating T-cell specific transcription factor GATA-3.

The recognition that CBD is nonpsychoactive and has immune modulatory properties suggests a potential for its therapeutic application. Several modes of action have been proposed for its therapeutic potential. For example, El Remessy et al. (2006) indicated that CBD reduced neurotoxicity, inflammation, and blood–retinal barrier breakdown in STZ-induced diabetic rats. It also has been reported that CBD blocks *N*-methyl-D-aspartate-, LPS-, or diabetes-induced retinal damage (El Remessy et al. 2003, 2006, 2008). Carrier et al. (2006) reported that CBD inhibited adenosine uptake by acting as a competitive inhibitor at the equilibrative adenosine nucleoside transporter. Hedge et al. (2011) proposed that CBD acted through TRPV1 vanilloid receptors on myeloid-derived suppressor cells that are induced at sites of inflammation and that suppress T-cell functions. CBD has also been reported to induce apoptosis in immortalized lymphocytes, primary lymphocytes, and monocytes. Gallily et al. (2003) reported that γ-irradiation of cultured human HL-60 myeloblastic leukemia cells enhanced apoptosis that was induced by CBD, while monocytes from normal individuals were resistant to either CBD or γ-irradiation. Wu et al. (2010) demonstrated that CBD enhanced apoptosis of freshly isolated monocytes, whereas precultured monocytes were insensitive to CBD. Wu et al. (2012) reported that CBD-induced apoptosis in BV-2 microglial-like cells was mediated through lipid rafts. It was suggested that a proapoptotic effect in microglia occurred through lipid raft coalescence and elevated expression of GM1 ganglioside and caveolin-1.

Although phytocannabinoids such as CBD and THC have been documented to alter immune function in vitro and in experimental animals, a definitive role in susceptibility to infection and/or disease progression in humans remains elusive (Abrams et al. 2003; Bredt et al. 2002; Chao et al.

2008; Struwe et al. 1993). Nevertheless, elucidation of the mechanisms of action through which phytocannabinoids alter immune activities has provided novel insights as to the functional relevance of cannabinoid receptors within the human. Studies on the action of phytocannabinoids on immune cells using experimental animals have led to the identification of an endogenous or endocannabinoid system that is characterized by specific ligands, cognate receptors, and linked metabolizing enzymes. The recognition that CBD has immunomodulatory properties while exhibiting minimal psychotropic effects offers the possibility of its consideration for adjunct therapeutic application, particularly since it has low toxicity, is highly lipophilic, and is bioavailable in the CNS. Investigation of other phytocannabinoids present in cannabis that are not psychoactive, such as cannabigerol, cannabichromene, cannabidivarin, and tetrahydrocannabivarin should reveal whether these also have immunomodulatory properties that have therapeutic potential. Finally, an understanding of the mode through which phytocannabinoids alter immune function and target specified signal transductional cascades has yielded novel insights into the engineering of molecules that have potential for dampening inflammatory responses that are associated with a variety of human pathological processes.

Acknowledgments

Supported by National Institutes of Health awards 1R01 DA005832 and 1R01 DA029532.

References

Abrams, D.I., Hilton, J.F., Leiser, R.J., *et al.* (2003). Short-term effects of cannabinoids in patients with HIV-1 infection: a randomized, placebo-controlled clinical trial. *Annals of Internal Medicine*, **139**, 258–266.

Arata, S., Klein, T.W., Newton, C., and Friedman, H. (1991). Tetrahydrocannabinol treatment suppresses growth restriction of *Legionella pneumophila* in murine macrophage cultures. *Life Sciences*, **49**, 473–479.

Arata, S., Newton, C., Klein, T., and Friedman, H. (1992). Enhanced growth of *Legionella pneumophila* in tetrahydrocannabinol-treated macrophages. *Proceedings of the Society for Experimental Biology and Medicine*, **199**, 65–67.

Baczynsky, W.O. and Zimmerman, A.M. (1983a). Effects of delta 9-tetrahydrocannabinol, cannabinol and cannabidiol on the immune system in mice. I. *In vivo* investigation of the primary and secondary immune response. *Pharmacology*, **26**, 1–11.

Baczynsky, W.O. and Zimmerman, A.M. (1983b). Effects of delta 9-tetrahydrocannabinol, cannabinol and cannabidiol on the immune system in mice. II. *In vitro* investigation using cultured mouse splenocytes. *Pharmacology*, **26**, 12–19.

Berdyshev, E.V., Boichot, E., Germain, N., Allain, N., Anger, J.P., and Lagente, V. (1997). Influence of fatty acid ethanolamides and delta9-tetrahydrocannabinol on cytokine and arachidonate release by mononuclear cells. *European Journal of Pharmacology*, **330**, 231–240.

Blanchard, D.K., Newton, C., Klein, T.W., Stewart, W.E., and Friedman, H. (1986). *In vitro* and *in vivo* suppressive effects of delta-9-tetrahydrocannabinol on interferon production by murine spleen cells. *International Journal of Immunopharmacology*, **8**, 819–824.

Blevins, R.D. and Dumic, M.P. (1980). The effect of delta-9-tetrahydrocannabinol on herpes simplex virus replication. *Journal of General Virology*, **49**, 427–431.

Borner, C., Hollt, V., Sebald, W., and Kraus, J. (2007). Transcriptional regulation of the cannabinoid receptor type 1 gene in T cells by cannabinoids. *Journal of Leukocyte Biology*, **81**, 336–343.

Borrelli, F., Aviello, G., Romano, B., *et al.* (2009). Cannabidiol, a safe and non-psychotropic ingredient of the marijuana plant *Cannabis sativa*, is protective in a murine model of colitis. *Journal of Molecular Medicine*, **87**, 1111–1121.

Bradley, S.G., Munson, A.E., Dewey, W.L., and Harris, L.S. (1977). Enhanced susceptibility of mice to combinations of delta-9-tetrahydrocannabinol and live or killed gram-negative bacteria. *Infection and Immunity*, **17**, 325–329.

Bredt, B.M., Higuera-Alhino, D., Shade, S.B., Hebert, S.J., McCune, J.M., and Abrams, D.I. (2002). Short-term effects of cannabinoids on immune phenotype and function in HIV-1-infected patients. *Journal of Clinical Pharmacology*, **42**, 82S–89S.

Buchweitz, J., Karmaus, P., Harkema, J., Williams, K., and Kaminski, N. (2007). Modulation of airway responses to influenza A/PR/8/34 by Δ^9-tetrahydrocannabinol in C57Bl/6 mice. *Journal of Pharmacology and Experimental Therapeutics*, **323**, 675–683.

Buchweitz, J.P., Karmaus, P.W., Williams, K.J., Harkema, J.R., and Kaminski, N.E. (2008). Targeted deletion of cannabinoid receptors CB1 and CB2 produced enhanced inflammatory responses to influenza A/PR/8/34 in the absence and presence of Delta9-tetrahydrocannabinol. *Journal of Leukocyte Biology*, **83**, 785–796.

Buckley, N.E., McCoy, K.L., Mezey, E., *et al.* (2000). Immunomodulation by cannabinoids is absent in mice deficient for the cannabinoid CB_2 receptor. *European Journal of Pharmacology*, **396**, 141–149.

Burnette-Curley, D. and Cabral, G.A. (1995). Differential inhibition of RAW264.7 macrophage tumoricidal activity by delta 9tetrahydrocannabinol. *Proceedings of the Society for Experimental Biology and Medicine*, **210**, 64–76.

Burnette-Curley, D., Marciano-Cabral, F., Fischer-Stenger, K., and Cabral, G.A. (1993). Delta- 9-Tetrahydrocannabinol inhibits cell contact-dependent cytotoxicity of *Bacillus* Calmette-Guerin-activated macrophages. *International Journal of Immunopharmacology*, **15**, 371–382.

Cabral, G.A., Lockmuller, J.C., and Mishkin, E.M. (1986b). Delta 9-tetrahydrocannabinol decreases alpha/beta interferon response to herpes simplex virus type 2 in the B6C3F1 mouse. *Proceedings of the Society for Experimental Biology and Medicine*, **181**, 305–311.

Cabral, G.A. and Marciano-Cabral, F. (2004). Cannabinoid-mediated exacerbation of brain infection by opportunistic amebae. *Journal of Neuroimmunology*, **147**, 127–30.

Cabral, G.A., Mishkin, E.M., Marciano-Cabral, F., Coleman, P., Harris, L., and Munson, A.E. (1986a). Effect of delta 9-tetrahydrocannabinol on herpes simplex virus type 2 vaginal infection in the guinea pig. *Proceedings of the Society for Experimental Biology and Medicine*, **182**, 181–186.

Cabral, G.A. and Vasquez, R. (1991). Effects of marijuana on macrophage function. *Advances in Experimental Medicine and Biology*, **288**, 93–105.

Cabral, G.A. and Vasquez, R. (1992). Delta 9-Tetrahydrocannabinol suppresses macrophage extrinsic antiherpesvirus activity. *Proceedings of the Society for Experimental Biology and Medicine*, **199**, 255–263.

Carrier, E.J., Auchampach, J.A., and Hillard, C.J. (2006). Inhibition of an equilibrative nucleoside transporter by cannabidiol: a mechanism of cannabinoid immunosuppression. *Proceedings of the National Academy of Sciences of the United States of America*, **103**, 7895–7900.

Carayon, P., Marchand, J., Dussossoy, D., *et al.* (1998). Modulation and functional involvement of CB_2 peripheral cannabinoid receptors during B-cell differentiation. *Blood*, **92**, 3605–3615.

Chang, Y.H., Lee, S.T., and Lin, W.W. (2001). Effects of cannabinoids on LPS-stimulated inflammatory mediator release from macrophages: involvement of eicosanoids. *Journal of Cellular Biochemistry*, **81**, 715–723.

Chao, C., Jacobson, L.P., Tashkin, D., *et al.* (2008). Recreational drug use and T lymphocyte subpopulations in HIV uninfected and HIV-infected men. *Drug and Alcohol Dependence*, **94**, 165–171.

Chen, W., Kaplan, B.L., Pike, S.T., *et al.* (2012). Magnitude of stimulation dictates the cannabinoid-mediated differential T cell response to HIVgp120. *Journal of Leukocyte Biology*, **92**, 1093–1102.

Chuchawankul, S., Shima, M., Buckley, N.E., Hartmann, C.B., and McCoy, K.L. (2004). Role of cannabinoid receptors in inhibiting macrophage costimulatory activity. *International Immunopharmacology*, **4**, 265–278.

Coffey, R.G., Snella, E., Johnson, K., and Pross, S. (1996). Inhibition of macrophage nitric oxide production by tetrahydrocannabinol *in vivo* and *in vitro*. *International Journal of Immunopharmacology*, **18**, 749–752.

Condie, R., Herring, A., Koh, W.S., Lee, M., and Kaminski, N.E. (1996). Cannabinoid inhibition of adenylate cyclase-mediated signal transduction and interleukin 2 (IL-2) expression in the murine T-cell line, EL4.IL-2. *The Journal of Biological Chemistry*, **271**, 13175–13183.

Daaka, Y., Zhu, W., Friedman, H., and Klein, T.W. (1997). Induction of interleukin-2 receptor alpha gene by delta9-tetrahydrocannabinol is mediated by nuclear factor kappaB and CB1 cannabinoid receptor. *DNA and Cell Biology*, **16**, 301–309.

De Filippis, D., Esposito, G., Cirillo, C., *et al.* (2011). Cannabidiol reduces intestinal inflammation through the control of neuroimmune axis. *PLoS One*, **6**, e28159.

Derocq, J.M., Segui, M., Marchand, J., Le Fur, G., and Casellas, P. (1995). Cannabinoids enhance human B-cell growth at low nanomolar concentrations. *FEBS Letters*, **369**, 177–182.

El-Remessy, A., Al-Shabrawey, M., Khalifa, Y., Tsai, N., Caldwell, R.B., and Liou, G. (2006). Neuroprotective and blood-retinal barrier-preserving effects of cannabidiol in experimental diabetes. *American Journal of Pathology*, **168**, 235–244.

El-Remessy, A., Khalil, I., Matragoon, S., *et al.* (2003). Neuroprotective effect of (-) Δ^9-tetrahydrocannabinol and cannabidiol in N-methyl-D-aspartate-induced retinal neurotoxocity: involvement of peroxynitrite. *American Journal of Pathology*, **163**, 1997–2008.

El-Remessy, A., Tang, Y., Zhu, G., *et al.* (2008). Neuroprotective effects of cannabidiol in endotoxin-induced uveitis: critical role of p38 MAPK activation. *Molecular Vision*, **14**, 2190–2203.

Esposito, G., Scuderi, C., Savani, C., *et al.* (2007). Cannabidiol *in vivo* blunts β-amyloid induced neuroinflammation by suppressing IL-1β and iNOS expression. *British Journal of Pharmacology*, **151**, 1272–1279.

Fischer-Stenger, K., Dove Pettit, D.A., and Cabral, G.A. (1993). Delta 9-tetrahydrocannabinol inhibition of tumor necrosis factor-alpha: suppression of post-translational events. *Journal of Pharmacology and Experimental Therapeutics*, **267**, 1558–1565.

Fischer-Stenger, K., Updegrove, A.W., and Cabral, G.A. (1992). Delta 9-tetrahydrocannabinol decreases cytotoxic T lymphocyte activity to herpes simplex virus type 1-infected cells. *Proceedings of the Society for Experimental Biology and Medicine*, **200**, 422–430.

Fraga, D., Raborn, E.S., Ferreira, G.A., and Cabral, G.A. (2011). Cannabinoids inhibit migration of microglial-like cells to the HIV protein Tat. *Journal of Neuroimmune Pharmacology*, **6**, 566–577.

Friedman, H., Klein, T., and Specter, S. (1991). Immunosuppression by marijuana components. In: R. Ader, D.L. Felten, and N. Cohen (eds.). *Psychoneuroimmunology*. San Diego, CA: Academic Press, pp. 931–953.

Gallily, R., Even-Chena, T., Katzavian, G., Lehmann, D., Dagan, A., and Mechoulam, R. (2003). Gamma-irradiation enhances apoptosis induced by cannabidiol, a non-psychotropic cannabinoid, in cultured HL-60 myeloblastic leukemia cells. *Leukemia and Lymphoma*, **44**, 1767–1773.

Galiegue, S., Mary, S., Marchand, J., *et al.* (1995). Expression of central and peripheral cannabinoid receptors in human immune tissues and leukocyte subpopulations. *European Journal of Biochemistry*, **232**, 54–61.

Graham, E.S., Angel, C.E., Schwarcz, L.E., Dunbar, P.R., and Glass, M. (2010). Detailed characterisation of CB2 receptor protein expression in peripheral blood immune cells from healthy human volunteers using flow cytometry. *International Journal of Immunopathology and Pharmacology*, **23**, 25–34.

Gross, A., Terraza, A., Marchant, J., *et al.* (2000). A beneficial aspect of a CB1 cannabinoid receptor antagonist: SR141716A is a potent inhibitor of macrophage infection by the intracellular pathogen *Brucella suis*. *Journal of Leukocyte Biology*, **67**, 335–344.

Hegde, V.L., Nagarkatti, P.S., and Nagarkatti, M. (2011). Role of myeloid-derived suppressor cells in amelioration of experimental autoimmune hepatitis following activation of TRPV1 receptors by cannabidiol. *PLoS One*, **6**, e18281.

Huemer, H.P., Lassnig, C., Bernhard, D., *et al.* (2011). Cannabinoids lead to enhanced virulence of the smallpox vaccine (vaccinia) virus. *Immunobiology*, **216**, 670–677.

Jan, T.R., Rao, G.K., and Kaminski, N.E. (2002). Cannabinol enhancement of IL-2 expression by T cells is associated with an increase in IL-2 distal nuclear factor of activated T cell activity. *Molecular Pharmacology*, **61**, 446–454.

Jan, T.R., Su, S.T., Wu, H.Y., and Liao, M.H. (2007). Suppressive effects of cannabidiol on antigen-specific antibody production and functional activity of splenocytes in ovalbumin-sensitized BALB/c mice. *International Immunopharmacology*, **7**, 773–780.

Jeon, Y.J., Yang, K.H., Pulaski, J.T., and Kaminski, N.E. (1996). Attenuation of inducible nitric oxide synthase gene expression by delta 9-tetrahydrocannabinol is mediated through the inhibition of nuclear factor- kappa B/Rel activation. *Molecular Pharmacology*, **50**, 334–341.

Juknat, A., Pietr, M., Kozela, E., *et al.* (2012a). Differential transcriptional profiles mediated by exposure to the cannabinoids cannabidiol and Delta9-tetrahydrocannabinol in BV-2 microglial cells. *British Journal of Pharmacology*, **165**, 2512–2528.

Juknat, A., Rimmerman, N., Levy, R., Vogel, Z., and Kozela, E. (2012b). Cannabidiol affects the expression of genes involved in zinc homeostasis in BV-2 microglial cells. *Neurochemistry International*, **61**, 923–930.

Karmaus, P.W., Chen, W., Kaplan, B.L., and Kaminski, N.E. (2012). Delta(9)-Tetrahydrocannabinol suppresses cytotoxic T lymphocyte function independent of CB_1 and CB_2, disrupting early activation events. *Journal of Neuroimmune Pharmacology*, **7**, 843–855.

Kawakami, Y., Klein, T.W., Newton, C., Djeu, J.Y., Specter, S., and Friedman, H. (1988). Suppression by delta-9-tetrahydrocannabinol of interleukin 2-induced lymphocyte proliferation and lymphokine-activated killer cell activity. *International Journal of Immunopharmacology*, **10**, 485–488.

Klein, T.W. and Friedman, H. (1990). Modulation of murine immune cell function by marijuana components. In: R. Watson (ed.). *Drugs of Abuse and Immune Function*. Boca Raton, FL: CRC Press, pp. 87–111.

Klein, T.W., Friedman, H., and Specter, S. (1998a). Marijuana, immunity and infection. *Journal of Neuroimmunology*, **83**, 102–115.

Klein, T.W., Kawakami, Y., Newton, C., and Friedman, H. (1991). Marijuana components suppress induction and cytolytic function of murine cytotoxic T cells *in vitro* and *in vivo*. *Journal of Toxicology and Environmental Health*, **32**, 465–477.

Klein, T.W., Newton, C., and Friedman, H. (1998b). Cannabinoid receptors and immunity. *Immunology Today*, **19**, 373–381.

Klein, T.W., Newton, C.A., Nakachi, N., and Friedman, H. (2000). Delta 9-tetrahydrocannabinol treatment suppresses immunity and early IFN-gamma, IL-12, and IL-12 receptor beta 2 responses to *Legionella pneumophila* infection. *Journal of Immunology*, **164**, 6461–6466.

Klein, T.W., Newton, C.A., Widen, R., and Friedman, H. (1985). The effect of delta-9-tetrahydrocannabinol and 11-hydroxy-delta-9-tetrahydrocannabinol on T-lymphocyte and B-lymphocyte mitogen responses. *Journal of Immunopharmacology*, **7**, 451–466.

Klein, T.W., Newton, C., Widen, R., and Friedman, H. (1993). Delta 9-tetrahydrocannabinol injection induces cytokine-mediated mortality of mice infected with *Legionella pneumophila*. *Journal of Pharmacology and Experimental Therapeutics*, **267**, 635–640.

Kozela, E., Pietr, M., Juknat, A., Rimmerman, N., Levy, R., and Vogel, Z. (2010). Cannabinoids Delta(9)-tetrahydrocannabinol and cannabidiol differentially inhibit the lipopolysaccharide-activated NF-kappaB and interferon-beta/STAT proinflammatory pathways in BV-2 microglial cells. *The Journal of Biological Chemistry*, **285**, 1616–1626.

LeCapitaine, N.J., Zhang, P., Winsauer, P., *et al.* (2011). Chronic Delta-9-tetrahydrocannabinol administration increases lymphocyte CXCR4 expression in rhesus macaques. *Journal of Neuroimmune Pharmacology*, **6**, 540–545.

Lee, C.Y., Wey, S.P., Liao, M.H., Hsu, W.L., Wu, H.Y., and Jan, T.R. (2008). A comparative study on cannabidiol-induced apoptosis in murine thymocytes and EL-4 thymoma cells. *International Immunopharmacology*, **8**, 732–740.

Lefkowitz, S.S., and Klager, K. (1978). Effect of delta9-tetrahydrocannabinol on *in vitro* sensitization of mouse splenic lymphocytes. *Immunological Communications*, 7, 557–566.

Li, K., Feng, J.Y., Li, Y.Y., *et al.* (2012). Anti-inflammatory role of cannabidiol and O-1602 in cerulein-induced acute pancreatitis in mice. *Pancreas*, 42, 123–129.

Li, X., Kaminski, N.E., and Fischer, L.J. (2001). Examination of the immunosuppressive effect of delta9-tetrahydrocannabinol in streptozotocin-induced autoimmune diabetes. *International Immunopharmacology*, 4, 699–712.

Liu, D.Z., Hu, C.M., Huang, C.H., Wey, S.P., and Jan, T.R. (2010). Cannabidiol attenuates delayed-type hypersensitivity reactions via suppressing T-cell and macrophage reactivity. *Acta Pharmacologica Sinica*, 31, 1611–1617.

Lombard, C., Hegde, V.L., Nagarkatti, M., and Nagarkatti, P.S. (2011). Perinatal exposure to Delta9-tetrahydrocannabinol triggers profound defects in T cell differentiation and function in fetal and post-natal stages of life, including decreased responsiveness to HIV antigens. *Journal of Pharmacology and Experimental Therapeutics*, 339, 607–617.

Lu, H., Kaplan, B.L., Ngaotepprutaram, T., and Kaminski, N.E. (2009). Suppression of T cell costimulator ICOS by Delta9-tetrahydrocannabinol. *Journal of Leukocyte Biology*, 85, 322–329.

Lu, T., Newton, C., Perkins, I., Friedman, H, and Klein, T. (2006). Role of cannabinoid receptors in delta-9-tetrahydrocannabinol suppression of IL-12p40 in mouse bone marrow-derived dendritic cells infected with *Legionella pneumophila*. *European Journal of Pharmacology*, 532, 170–177.

Lynn, A.B. and Herkenham, M. (1994). Localization of cannabinoid receptors and nonsaturable high-density cannabinoid binding sites in peripheral tissues of the rat: implications for receptor-mediated immune modulation by cannabinoids. *Journal of Pharmacology and Experimental Therapeutics*, 268, 1612–1623.

Malfait, A.M., Gallily, R., Sumariwalla, P.F., *et al.* (2000). The nonpsychoactive cannabis constituent cannabidiol is an oral anti-arthritic therapeutic in murine collagen-induced arthritis. *Proceedings of the National Academy of Sciences of the United States of America*, 97, 9561–9566.

Marciano-Cabral, F.M. (1988). Biology of *Naegleria* spp. *Microbiological Reviews*, 52, 114–133.

Marciano-Cabral, F.M., Ferguson, T., Bradley, S.G., and Cabral, G.A. (2001). Delta-9-tetrahydrocannabinol (THC), the major psychoactive component of marijuana, exacerbates brain infection by *Acanthamoeba*. *Journal of Eukaryotic Microbiology*, Suppl, 4S–5S.

Massi, P., Fuzio, D., Vigano, D., Sacerdote, P., and Parolaro, D. (2000). Relative involvement of cannabinoid CB_1 and CB_2 receptors in the Delta(9)-tetrahydrocannabinol-induced inhibition of natural killer activity. *European Journal of Pharmacology*, 387, 343–347.

Matveyeva, M., Hartmann, C.B., Harrison, M.T., Cabral, G.A., and McCoy, K.L. (2000). Delta(9)-tetrahydrocannabinol selectively increases aspartyl cathepsin D proteolytic activity and impairs lysozyme processing by macrophages. *International Journal of Immunopharmacology*, 22, 373–381.

McCoy, K.L., Gainey, D., and Cabral, G.A. (1995). Delta-9-tetrahydrocannabinol modulates antigen processing by macrophages. *Journal of Pharmacology and Experimental Therapeutics*, 273, 1216–1223.

McCoy, K.L., Matveyeva, M., Carlisle, S.J., and Cabral, G.A. (1999). Cannabinoid inhibition of the processing of intact lysozyme by macrophages: evidence for CB_2 receptor participation. *Journal of Pharmacology and Experimental Therapeutics*, 289, 1620–1625.

McKallip, R.J., Nagarkatti, M., and Nagarkatti, P.S. (2005). Delta-9-tetrahydrocannabinol enhances breast cancer growth and metastasis by suppression of the antitumor immune response. *Journal of Immunology*, 174, 3281–3289.

Mishkin, E.M. and Cabral, G.A. (1985). Delta-9-tetrahydrocannabinol decreases host resistance to herpes simplex virus type 2 vaginal infection in the B6C3F1 mouse. *Journal of General Virology*, 66, 2539–2549.

Molina, P., Winsauer, P., Zhang, P., *et al.* (2011). Cannabinoid administration attenuates the progression of simian immunodeficiency virus. *AIDS Research and Human Retroviruses*, 27, 585–592.

Morahan, P.S., Klykken, P.C., Smith, S.H., Harris, L.S., and Munson, A.E. (1979). Effects of cannabinoids on host resistance to *Listeria monocytogenes* and herpes simplex virus. *Infection and Immunity*, **23**, 670–674.

Morahan, P.S., Morse S.S., and McGeorge M.G. (1980). Macrophage extrinsic antiviral activity during herpes simplex virus infection. *Journal of General Virology*, **46**, 291–300.

Nahas, G.G., Morishima, A., and Desoize, B. (1977). Effects of cannabinoids on macromolecular synthesis and replication of cultured lymphocytes. *Federation Proceedings*, **36**, 1748–1752.

Nakano, Y., Pross, S.H., and Friedman, H. (1992). Modulation of interleukin 2 activity by delta-9-tetrayhydrocannabinol after stimulation with concanavalin A, phytohemagglutinin, or anti-CD3 antibody. *Proceedings of the Society for Experimental Biology and Medicine*, **201**, 165–168.

Napimoga, M.H., Benatti, B.B., Lima, F.O., *et al.* (2009). Cannabidiol decreases bone resorption by inhibiting RANK/RANKL expression and pro-inflammatory cytokines during experimental periodontitis in rats. *International Immunopharmacology*, **9**, 216–222.

Newton, C.A., Chou, P.J., Perkins, I., and Klein, T.W. (2009). CB_1 and CB_2 cannabinoid receptors mediate different aspects of delta-9-tetrahydrocannabinol (THC)-induced T helper cell shift following immune activation by *Legionella pneumophila* infection. *Journal of Neuroimmune Pharmacology*, **4**, 92–102.

Newton, C.A., Klein, T.W., and Friedman, H. (1994). Secondary immunity to *Legionella pneumophila* and Th1 activity are suppressed by delta-9-tetrahydrocannabinol injection. *Infection and Immunity*, **62**, 4015–4020.

Noe, S.N., Nyland, S.B., Ugen, K., Friedman, H., and Klein, T.W. (1998). Cannabinoid receptor agonists enhance syncytia formation in MT-2 cells infected with cell free HIV-1MN. *Advances in Experimental Medicine and Biology*, **437**, 223–229.

Paradise, L.J. and Friedman, H. (1993). Syphilis and drugs of abuse. *Advances in Experimental Medicine and Biology*, **335**, 81–87.

Pross, S.H., Klein, T.W., Newton, C., Smith, J., Widen, R., and Friedman, H. (1990). Age-related suppression of murine lymphoid cell blastogenesis by marijuana components. *Developmental and Comparative Immunology*, **14**, 131–137.

Pross, S.H., Nakano, Y., Widen, R., *et al.* (1992). Differing effects of delta-9-tetrahydrocannabinol (THC) on murine spleen cell populations dependent upon stimulators. *International Journal of Immunopharmacology*, **14**, 1019–1027.

Puffenbarger, R.A., Boothe, A.C., and Cabral, G.A. (2000). Cannabinoids inhibit LPS-inducible cytokine mRNA expression in rat microglial cells. *Glia*, **29**, 58–69.

Raborn, E.S. and Cabral, G.A. (2010). Cannabinoid inhibition of macrophage migration to the trans-activating (Tat) protein of HIV-1 is linked to the CB_2 cannabinoid receptor. *Journal of Pharmacology and Experimental Therapeutics*, **333**, 319–327.

Rajesh, M., Mukhopadhyay, P., Bátkai, S., *et al.* (2010). Cannabidiol attenuates high glucose-induced endothelial cell inflammatory response and barrier disruption. *American Journal of Physiology*, **293**, H610–H619.

Ramarathinam, L., Pross, S., Plescia, O., Newton, C., Widen, R., and Friedman, H. (1997). Differential immunologic modulatory effects of tetrahydrocannabinol as a function of age. *Mechanisms of Ageing and Development*, **96**, 117–126.

Rao, G.K. and Kaminski, N.E. (2006). Induction of intracellular calcium elevation by Delta9-tetrahydrocannabinol in T cells involves TRPC1 channels. *Journal of Leukocyte Biology*, **79**, 202–213.

Rao, G.K., Zhang, W., and Kaminski, N.E. (2004). Cannabinoid receptor-mediated regulation of intracellular calcium by delta(9)-tetrahydrocannabinol in resting T cells. *Journal of Leukocyte Biology*, **75**, 884–892.

Ribeiro, A., Ferraz-de-Paula, V., Pinheiro, M.L., *et al.* (2012). Cannabidiol, a non-psychotropic plant-derived cannabinoid, decreases inflammation in a murine model of acute lung injury: role for the adenosine A(2A) receptor. *European Journal of Pharmacology*, **678**, 78–85.

Rosenkrantz, H., Miller, A.J., and Esber, H.J. (1975). Delta-9-tetrahydrocannabinol suppression of the primary immune response in rats. *Journal of Toxicology and Environmental Health*, **1**, 119–125.

Roth, M.D., Tashkin, D.P., Whittaker, K.M., Choi, R., and Baldwin, G.C. (2005). Tetrahydrocannabinol suppresses immune function and enhances HIV replication in the huPBL-SCID mouse. *Life Sciences*, **77**, 1711–1722.

Sacerdote, P., Martucci, C., Vaccani, A., *et al.* (2005). The nonpsychoactive component of marijuana cannabidiol modulates chemotaxis and IL-10 and IL-12 production of murine macrophages both *in vivo* and *in vitro*. *Journal of Neuroimmunology*, **159**, 97–105.

Schatz, A.R., Koh, W.S., and Kaminski, N.E. (1993). Delta-9-tetrahydrocannabinol selectively inhibits T-cell dependent humoral immune responses through direct inhibition of accessory T-cell function. *Immunopharmacology*, **26**, 129–137.

Smith, M.S., Yamamoto, Y., Newton, C., Friedman, H., and Klein, T. (1997). Psychoactive cannabinoids increase mortality and alter acute phase cytokine responses in mice sublethally infected with *Legionella pneumophila*. *Proceedings of the Society for Experimental Biology and Medicine*, **214**, 69–75.

Snella, E., Pross, S., and Friedman, H. (1995). Relationship of aging and cytokines to the immunomodulation by delta-9-tetrahydrocannabinol on murine lymphoid cells. *International Journal of Immunopharmacology*, **17**, 1045–1054.

Specter, S., Lancz, G., Westrich, G., and Friedman, H. (1991). Delta-9-tetrahydrocannabinol augments murine retroviral induced immunosuppression and infection. *International Journal of Immunopharmacology*, **13**, 411–417.

Srivastava, M.D., Srivastava, B.I., and Brouhard, B. (1998). Delta-9 tetrahydrocannabinol and cannabidiol alter cytokine production by human immune cells. *Immunopharmacology*, **40**, 179–185.

Steffens, S., Veillard, N.R., Arnaud, C., *et al.* (2005). Low dose oral cannabinoid therapy reduces progression of atherosclerosis in mice. *Nature*, **434**, 782–786.

Stohlman, S.A., Woodward, J.G., and Frelinger, J.A. (1982). Macrophage antiviral activity: extrinsic versus intrinsic activity. *Infection and Immunity*, **36**, 672–677.

Struwe, M., Kaempfer, S.H., Geiger, C.J., *et al.* (1993). Effect of dronabinol on nutritional status in HIV infection. *The Annals of Pharmacotherapy*, **27**, 827–831.

Walter, L., Franklin, A., Witting, A., *et al.* (2003). Nonpsychotropic cannabinoid receptors regulate microglial cell migration. *The Journal of Neuroscience* **23**, 1398–1405.

Warner, J.F. and Dennert, G. (1982). Effects of a cloned cell line with NK activity on bone marrow transplants, tumour development and metastasis *in vivo*. *Nature*, **300**, 31–34.

Watzl, B., Scuderi, P., and Watson, R.R. (1991). Marijuana components stimulate human peripheral blood mononuclear cell secretion of interferon-γ and suppress interleukin-1 alpha *in vitro*. *International Journal of Immunopharmacology*, **13**, 1091–1097.

Weiss, L., Zeira, M., Reich, S., *et al.* (2006). Cannabidiol lowers incidence of diabetes in non-obese diabetic mice. *Autoimmunity*, **39**, 143–151.

Weiss, L., Zeira, M., Reich, S., *et al.* (2008). Cannabidiol arrests onset of autoimmune diabetes in NOD mice. *Neuropharmacology*, **54**, 244–249.

Winsauer, P.J., Molina, P.E., Amedee, A.M., *et al.* (2011). Tolerance to chronic delta-9-tetrahydrocannabinol (Delta(9)-THC) in rhesus macaques infected with simian immunodeficiency virus. *Experimental and Clinical Psychopharmacology*, **19**, 154–172.

Wu, H.Y., Chang, A.C., Wang, C.C., *et al.* (2010). Cannabidiol induced a contrasting pro-apoptotic effect between freshly isolated and precultured human monocytes. *Toxicology and Applied Pharmacology*, **246**, 141–147.

Wu, H.Y., Goble, K., Mecha, M., *et al.* (2012). Cannabidiol-induced apoptosis in murine microglial cells through lipid raft. *Glia*, **60**, 1182–1190.

Yebra, M., Klein, T.W., Friedman, H. (1992). Delta 9-tetrahydrocannabinol suppresses concanavalin A induced increase in cytoplasmic free calcium in mouse thymocytes. *Life Sciences*, **51**, 151–160.

Yuan, M., Kiertscher, S.M., Cheng, Q., Zoumalan, R., Tashkin, D.P., and Roth, M.D. (2002). Delta 9-Tetrahydrocannabinol regulates Th1/Th2 cytokine balance in activated human T cells. *Journal of Neuroimmunology*, **133**, 124–131.

Zheng, Z.M., Specter, S., and Friedman, H. (1992). Inhibition by delta-9-tetrahydrocannabinol of tumor necrosis factor alpha production by mouse and human macrophages. *International Journal of Immunopharmacology*, **14**, 1445–1452.

Zhu, L.X., Sharma, S., Stolina, M., *et al.* (2000). Delta-9-tetrahydrocannabinol inhibits antitumor immunity by a CB2 receptor-mediated, cytokine-dependent pathway. *Journal of Immunology*, **165**, 373–380.

Zhu, W., Friedman, H., and Klein, T.W. (1998). Delta9-tetrahydrocannabinol induces apoptosis in macrophages and lymphocytes: involvement of Bcl-2 and caspase-1. *Journal of Pharmacology and Experimental Therapeutics*, **286**, 1103–1109.

Zhu, W., Igarashi, T., Friedman, H., and Klein, T.W. (1995). Delta 9-Tetrahydrocannabinol (THC) causes the variable expression of IL2 receptor subunits. *Journal of Pharmacology and Experimental Therapeutics*, **274**, 1001–1007.

Zhu, W., Igarashi, T., Qi, Z.T., *et al.* (1993). Delta-9-Tetrahydrocannabinol (THC) decreases the number of high and intermediate affinity IL-2 receptors of the IL-2 dependent cell line NKB61A2. *International Journal of Immunopharmacology*, **15**, 401–408.

Zimmerman, S., Zimmerman, A.M., Cameron, I.L., and Laurence, H.L. (1977). Delta 1-tetrahydrocannabinol, cannabidiol and cannabinol effects on the immune response of mice. *Pharmacology*, **15**, 10–23.

Chapter 15

Non-Phytocannabinoid Constituents of Cannabis and Herbal Synergy

John M. McPartland and Ethan B. Russo

15.1 **Introduction**

Therapeutic synergy is gaining respect in the medical world, and describes an interaction between two or more drugs whose combined effect is greater than the sum of their individual effects. Thanks to tractable research methods such as isobolographic analysis, the simultaneous administration of two or more drugs is no longer derided as "black box medicine." Polypharmacy has become the norm in clinical disciplines such as anesthesia, oncology, and infectious disease.

Medicinal plants are inherently polypharmaceutical. Turner et al. (1980) tallied 420 constituents in herbal cannabis. The tally is now over 530, of which 108 are phytocannabinoids (Hanuš 2008). Practitioners of traditional Chinese medicine (TCM) administer several medicinal plants at once, which exponentially increases the polypharmacy. TCM practitioners have used cannabis for centuries (see Russo, Chapter 2, this volume). One herbal remedy known as *má zǐ rén wán* ("hemp seed pill"), was prescribed by Zhāng Zhòngjǐng (*c.*150–219 CE). The exact same formulation is still in use today (Bensky et al. 1993).

Pharmacology as a science began with chemists isolating constituents from medicinal plants and testing them for physiological activity. In 1804, Friedrich Sertürner began analyzing opium extracted from poppy, *Papaver somniferum*. Not until 1817 did he unequivocally report the isolation of pure morphine (Huxtable and Schwarz 2001). Other early discoveries included caffeine from *Coffea arabica* in 1819, quinine from *Cinchona officinalis* in 1820, nicotine from *Nicotiana tabacum* in 1828, atropine from *Atropa belladonna* in 1831, cocaine from *Erythroxylum coca* in 1855, and digitoxin from *Digitalis purpurea* in 1869.

Cannabis drew attention early; Buchholz (1806) conducted the first analytical study, and he extracted a crude resin. The polypharmaceutical resin stymied chemists for over 150 years in their search for the "primary active ingredient." The recalcitrant substance turned out to be a terpenophenol, quite unlike the easy-to-isolate alkaloids listed earlier. Along the way, chemists suspected the primary active ingredient was a component of the resin, an essential oil, or even an alkaloid. Finally Raphael Mechoulam isolated and characterized delta-9-tetrahydrocannabinol (Δ^9-THC) as the primary psychoactive ingredient (Gaoni and Mechoulam 1964). But barely 6 years later Roger Pertwee noted that THC did not act alone in cannabis (Gill et al. 1970).

This chapter begins with an inventory of nonphytocannabinoid constituents of *Cannabis* (the plant) and cannabis (the plant product). We review the concepts of synergy, additivity, and antagonism, and their measurement. This is followed by a historical review of early research that demonstrated the impact of terpenoids upon phytocannabinoids and the endocannabinoid system. Lastly we highlight twenty-first-century research.

15.2 **Non-phytocannabinoid constituents**

Buchholz (1806) extracted 1.6% resin from cannabis with ethyl alcohol. His yield was low, but we wouldn't expect much more, because Bucholz analyzed cannabis *seed*. He extracted much more oil (19.1%) and protein (24.7%). Subsequently, Buchholz (1816) isolated "capsicin" (capsaicin) from Spanish pepper. His decision to work on cannabis and capsaicin was prophetic: nearly 200 years later, the receptor that binds capsaicin, known as TRPV1, would be named "the ionotropic cannabinoid receptor" (Di Marzo et al. 2002).

Tscheppe (1821) described *hanfblätter* (hemp foliage) as "narcotic." Tscheppe isolated a brown extract and a sweetish bitter extract, as well as chlorophyll, wood fiber, lignin, protein, and several salts and minerals. He could not isolate the psychoactive ingredient, possibly because he analyzed low-THC fiber-type German hemp. Schlesinger (1840) analyzed fresh flowering tops and isolated a green resinous ethanolic extract that Mechoulam (1973) characterized as "the first active extract." Schlesinger never described its activity beyond "bitter taste." In retrospect, the odds of finding the psychoactive ingredient were low because he also worked with hemp. O'Shaughnessy (1838–1840) extracted a strongly psychoactive ingredient by boiling Indian *gañjā* in alcohol under pressure. He subsequently utilized the ethanolic extract in many animal studies and clinical trials.

Bohlig (1840) extracted an essential oil from flowering tops of hemp. Essential oil is a volatile, aromatic, hydrophobic liquid derived from plants by steam distillation or solvent extraction. We now recognize the essential oil as a collection of terpenoid compounds. We use the term "terpenoid" broadly, to include terpenes and modified terpenes, where the methyl group has been moved or removed, or oxygen atoms added. The unique smell of *Cannabis* arises from its volatile terpenoids and not its phytocannabinoids. Bohling reasoned that the psychoactive ingredient was volatile, because he experienced somnolence in a field of flowering hemp. The essential oil was soporific, weakly anesthetic, and caused a headache when inhaled or taken internally.

Most terpenoids in cannabis are monoterpenoids ($C_{10}H_{16}$ template) and sesquiterpenoids ($C_{15}H_{24}$ template). Glandular trichomes secrete terpenoids, and they account for up to 10% of gland head contents (Potter 2009). No terpenoids are unique to *Cannabis*, but various types of *Cannabis* produce unique terpenoid profiles (Fischedick et al. 2010a; Hillig 2004; Mediavilla and Steinemann 1997; Nissen et al. 2010). Examples of terpenoids in cannabis are illustrated in (Fig. 15.1).

On an industrial scale, field-cultivated *Cannabis* yields 1.3 L of essential oil per ton of undried plants, or about 10 L ha^{-2} (Mediavilla and Steinemann 1997). Preventing pollination increases the yield. Meier and Mediavilla (1998) obtained 18 L ha^{-2} from *sinsemilla* crops, versus 8 L ha^{-2} from pollinated crops. In a greenhouse setting, Potter (2009) reported a much higher yield of 7.7 mL m^{-2}, equivalent to 77 L ha^{-2}.

Smith and Smith (1847a) analyzed an ethanolic extract of *gañjā*. They isolated the active principle in a resin that tasted "balsamic" and not bitter, like morphine. They determined that the active ingredient was neutral, "altogether destitute of basic properties" (i.e., not an alkaloid). The Smith brothers gave it the name "cannabine" (Smith and Smith 1847b). Its neutral properties were confirmed by de Courtive (1848), who obtained Algerian hashīsh from Jacques-Joseph Moreau. De Courtive named the active ingredient "cannabin."

Personne (in Robiquet 1857) acknowledged the discoveries of the Smith brothers, but reasoned that *another* active principle was volatile, because hashīsh fumes were psychoactive. Personne distilled the essential oil and isolated two fractions that produced psychoactive effects. Valente (1880, 1881) also searched for a volatile principle in hemp, reasoning that workers in Italian hemp fields became gay and giddy. Valente distilled a sesquiterpene (giving the formula as $C_{15}H_{24}$) from the

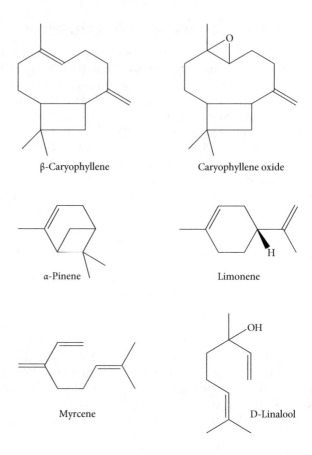

Fig. 15.1 Examples of terpenoids in cannabis: two sesquiterpenoids and four monoterpenoids.

β-Caryophyllene

Caryophyllene oxide

α-Pinene

Limonene

Myrcene

D-Linalool

essential oil. Valieri (1887) tested the essential oil on human subjects. Inhalation of the essential oil provided sedative effects, not unlike the essential oils distilled from other aromatic plants like lemon balm (*Melissa officinalis*) and mint (*Mentha* spp.). Valieri suggested its use immediately prior to treatment with "stronger" preparations made from cannabis resin.

Wood et al. (1896) extracted a monoterpenoid (identified as $C_{10}H_{16}$) and a sesquiterpenoid (identified as $C_{15}H_{24}$) from Punjabi *charas*. They described the physiological action of these substances: "In doses of 0.5 gram they have very little effect and produce none of the characteristic symptoms of cannabis action." Simonsen and Todd (1942) began to name individual terpenoids in *Cannabis*. They extracted *p*-cymene ($C_{10}H_{14}$) and humulene (α-caryophyllene, $C_{15}H_{24}$) from Egyptian hashish.

The list of terpenoids has steadily grown in modern studies that use utilize gas chromatography (GC). Dutt (1957) and Martin et al. (1961) established the presence of myrcene, limonene, α-caryophyllene, and β-caryophyllene in Indian cannabis and Canadian feral hemp, respectively. Nigam et al. (1965) isolated and identified 20 terpenoids from feral Kashmiri cannabis. They also *quantified* individual terpenoid fractions: they measured the areas of individual GC peaks as a percentage of the total area under all GC peaks. The essential oil consisted largely of β-caryophyllene (45.7%), followed by α-humulene (16.0%), with lesser percentages of other terpenoids in the single digits. Hendricks et al. (1975) listed 55 monoterpenoids and 33 sesquiterpenoids, eluted from *Cannabis sativa* strain X obtained from birdseed.

Hood et al. (1973) investigated *Cannabis* "headspace," the *odor* given off by Mexican cannabis, demonstrating a qualitative difference between terpenoids in the headspace and terpenoids in the essential oil. The headspace comprised mostly of monoterpenoids (α-pinene, β-pinene, myrcene, limonene) whereas the processed essential oil consisted of less-volatile oxygenated monoterpenoids (α-terpinenol, linalool, fenchyl alcohol, borneol) and sesquiterpenoids (β-caryophyllene, α-humulene, caryophyllene oxide). Stahl and Kunde (1973) tested seized hashīsh in which primarily the sesquiterpenoids remained. Seemingly, most of the monoterpenoids had out-gassed. They determined that caryophyllene oxide (the oxidation product of β-caryophyllene) was the volatile compound sensed by hashīsh detection dogs.

Ross and ElSohly (1996) measured the retention of essential oil in a "high potency hybrid." Freshly collected cannabis buds, yielded 0.29% v/w essential oil. Week-old buds air-dried at room temperature and stored in a paper bag yielded 0.20%, a loss of 31%. One-month-old buds yielded 0.16%, a loss of 45%. After 3 months the buds yielded 0.13%, a loss of 55%. Freshly-collected buds consisted of 92% monoterpenoids and 7% sesquiterpenoids. In 3-month-old buds the ratio shifted to 62% monoterpenoids and 36% sesquiterpenoids. Their study identified three new monoterpenoids and 14 new sesquiterpenoids not previously reported by Turner et al. (1980)—bringing the total to 60 monoterpenoids and 51 sesquiterpenoids.

Cannabis also produces about 20 flavonoids, which are aromatic, polycyclic phenols. Quercetin, apigenin, and cannaflavin A are anti-inflammatory, antioxidant, analgesic, and possibly prevent cancer (McPartland and Russo 2001). Flavonoids may retain activity in cannabis smoke (Sauer et al. 1983), but they do not vaporize at temperatures below combustion. Products created by combustion show anti-inflammatory activity (Burstein et al. 1976; Spronck et al. 1978), and resulting polycyclic aromatic hydrocarbons (PAHs) may be responsible for antiestrogenic effects (Lee et al. 2005). Other *Cannabis* compounds with pharmacological activity include phytosterols, glycoproteins, alkaloids, and compounds that remain completely unidentified (Gill et al. 1970).

15.3 **Synergy, additivity, and antagonism**

Polypharmacy gives rise to pharmacokinetic and pharmacodynamic drug interactions. *Pharmacokinetic* interactions arise when one drug alters the absorption, distribution, metabolism, or excretion of another drug. For example, the distribution of L-DOPA across the blood–brain barrier is enhanced by adding carbidopa, a combination drug called Sinemet®. Distribution in this case becomes a factor of metabolism, because carbidopa inhibits dopa decarboxylase activity in the periphery, thereby increasing the bioavailability of L-DOPA in the brain. *Pharmacodynamic* interactions arise when one drug potentiates or diminishes the effect of another drug by targeting different receptors or enzymes. For example, dry mouth caused by a sympathomimetic drug is potentiated by an anticholinergic drug.

Fischedick et al. (2010b) tested the binding affinity of compounds at the CB_1 receptor, and found no statistically significant difference between pure Δ^9-THC and cannabis smoke or vapor at equivalent concentrations of THC. Therefore synergy produced by other constituents in smoke or vapor must occur via pharmacokinetic mechanisms or via pharmacodynamic interactions at other targets. One likely target is the endocannabinoid system (ECS). Two well-known ECS ligands are *N*-arachidonylethanolamide (anandamide, AEA) and *sn*-2-arachidonoylglycerol (2-AG). AEA and 2-AG activate several receptors: CB_1, CB_2, GPR55, and several transient receptor potential ion channels (e.g., TRPV1, TRPV2, TRPA1, TRPM8). Other targets include the catabolic enzymes of AEA and 2-AG: fatty acid amide hydrolase (FAAH), monoacylglycerol lipase (MAGL), and cyclooxygenase 2 (COX2, prostaglandin-endoperoxide synthase). We detail these findings in section 15.4.

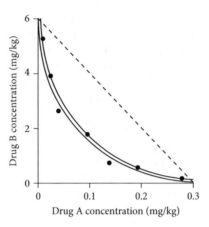

Fig. 15.2 Isobologram analysis: a "line of additivity" (dashed line) is drawn between the ED_{50} values of Drug A and Drug B when given individually. The isobole curve (double line) plots five ED_{50} values when Drug A and Drug B are coadministered at different doses. The isobole bows well below the line of additivity, indicating a synergistic interaction.

Interactions between drugs are usually additive. Departures from additivity are either synergistic ("greater than the sum of the parts") or antagonistic ("less than that expected" or infraadditive). Rector (1922) wrote about synergy, after defining the term, arising in combinations of analgesic drugs. Rector combined *Cannabis indica* with morphine sulfate and magnesium sulfate. Williamson (2001) reviewed the mathematical definitions of synergy. Pharmacologists such as Borisy et al. (2003) cite the pioneering efforts of Walter Siegried Loewe (1884–1963).

Loewe (1928) invented the isobologram to test drug combinations for synergy, additivity, and antagonism. The isobologram uses a two-coordinate graph of drug interactions (Fig. 15.2). The concentrations of single drug A and single drug B that produce x% drug effect (usually EC_{50}) are plotted on the *x*- and *y*-axes. A line that connects two points corresponding to the same x% drug effect becomes "the line of additivity." Then the concentrations of both drugs together that produced the same effect are plotted on the graph. The concentrations of drugs interacting synergistically will be less than the sum of the individual components, and the isobole curve is said to be "concave." The concentrations of drugs interacting antagonistically will be greater than expected, and produce a "convex" isobole (Fig. 15.2).

Loewe emigrated from Germany to the US in 1933, where he added cannabis to his studies of multicomponent medicines and synergy. He demonstrated synergy arising from coadministration of cannabis with butyl-bromallyl-barbituric acid (Loewe 1940). During Congressional hearings regarding the Marihuana Tax Act, Loewe stated to Anslinger, "nobody knows whether there is only one active principle or more than one active principle" (Bureau of Narcotics 1938). Loewe (1945) reported that cannabinol (CBN) exhibited 4% of the potency of "charas tetrahydrocannabinol" in the dog ataxia test. Therefore cannabinol must be included among the compounds having marihuana activity." Loewe served as the pharmacology director of the *LaGuardia Committee on Marihuana* (Loewe 1944), and he conducted the first human clinical trials with individual cannabinoids, including synthetic analogs (Loewe 1946).

15.4 **Combinatorial synergy within cannabis**

Well before synergy was defined, Prain (1893) demonstrated that more than one constituent contributed to cannabis psychoactivity. David Prain (FRS, University of Aberdeen 1857–1944) was a physician-botanist who worked in India. His publication is not well known, and extremely rare (four copies exist in libraries worldwide, according to WorldCat). Prain described "the distinctive gánjá smell, a warm, aromatic, camphoraceous or peppermint-like smell." After 1 year the *gañjā* still smelled aromatic, but the camphoraceous or peppermint odor was gone. After 2 years the aromatic odor diminished. After 3 years the smell was entirely depleted.

Prain weighed fresh *gañjā*, dried it in various ways, and then rehydrated and reweighed it. Predictably, *gañjā* dried at 100°C lost more moisture than *gañjā* dried at room temperature. But rehydration showed that *gañjā* dried at 100°C lost something more: "the volatile constituents were driven off along with the moisture. Exposure to heat must therefore produce a permanent and deleterious change in gánjá."

He then extracted *gañjā* with a series of solvents including water, alcohol, ether, and petroleum-ether. He learned from the alcohol extract that "something is lost by *gánjá* during the first year of storage." Alcohol extracted the essential oil (i.e., terpenoids) that gave *gañjā* its characteristic odor. He calculated that 6.2% of fresh, dried *gañjā* consisted of essential oil. Prain surmised:

> It seems possible that to some extent the *exciting and exhilarating* effect of gánjá resides in an essential oil, which almost disappears by the time the drug has been kept in store for a year. There still, however, remains a considerable *narcotic* effect in gánjá of a year old, though it is much less marked than in fresh ganja. [Italics added for emphasis]

Prain conducted physiological testing of various extracts in cats and isolated the "narcotic fraction" of *gañjā* in a "fixed oil" from the petroleum ether extract. Surprisingly, a resin extracted with pure ether (not petroleum ether) was *not* active. Prain concluded:

> A fixed oil becomes converted into a resin by being oxidised. The quantity of resin increases as the age of the *gánjá* increases, and this increase can only happen at the expense of the substance that constitutes the active principle of the drug.

The petroleum ether contained what we now know as Δ^9-THC, the ether contained CBN, its less potent oxidation product.

Prain's work was continued by David Hooper (1858–1947), appointed as "analyzer" for the Indian Hemp Drugs Commission (IHDC) in 1892. Hooper tested samples of *gañjā* and *charas* obtained from around the subcontinent. Hooper (1908) expanded his earlier analysis of *charas*. He compared 24 samples, 15 from the IHDC report, plus five from Baluchistan, three from Kashgar, and one from Simla. A sample from Kashgar (in modern-day Xinjiang) contained the highest percentage of resin (48.1%). Hooper noted with curiosity that the perceived quality and the cost of three specimens from Kashgar did *not* correlate with resin content: Grade No. 1, 40.2%; Grade No. 2, 40.9%, Grade No. 3, 48.1%.

Hooper added an important analysis not reported in the IHDC report: percentage of essential oil. The Kashgar samples were highest. Intriguingly, the quality and cost of the Kashgar samples correlated with their essential oil content: Grade No. 1 12.7%; Grade No. 2 12.4%; Grade No. 3 12.0%.

Medieval literature indicates that Persian and Arabic physicians prescribed terpenoid-rich citrus fruits to counter the intoxication caused by excessive cannabis (reviewed by Russo 2011): Al-Rāzī (865–925 AD) wrote: "and to avoid these harms, one should drink fresh water and ice or eat any acid fruits." Ibn Sīnā (981–1037) and Ibn-al-Baitār (1197–1248) made similar recommendations. Citrus fruits and especially lemons have been used to treat cannabis overdoses by British physicians (Christison 1850), American homeopaths (Hamilton 1852), Italian physicians (Polli 1865), Āyurvedic practitioners (Shanavaskhan et al. 1997), as well as early American hashīsh littérateurs (Calkins 1871; Ludlow 1857; Taylor 1855) and Afro-Jamaican Rastafarians (Schaeffer 1975). Āyurvedic practitioners espoused calamus root, from *Acorus calamus*, for countering the side effects of cannabis (reviewed by McPartland et al. 2008). The use of pine nuts, pistachio nuts, and terebinth resin, from *Pinus* and *Pistacia* species with their pinene content, also have a rich tradition going back to medieval Arabic physicians and perhaps Pliny that suggest their use as antidotes or modulators of THC intoxication by cannabis (reviewed in Russo 2011).

15.5 **Modern synergy research**

Beginning in the 1970s, a handful of researchers have studied synergy in herbal cannabis. Since then, the pace of research has synergized (see the bottom row in Table 15.1). Gill et al. (1970) proposed that an acetylcholine-like component in whole cannabis extract potentiated the atropinic action of THC ("cotton mouth"). Mechoulam et al. (1972) suggested that THC activity was influenced by other compounds present in herbal cannabis. They proposed that the smell of volatile terpenoids caused a psychological conditioning that potentiated the effects of THC.

Kubena and Barry (1972) reported that rats trained to respond to THC actually showed a greater response to an ethanolic cannabis extract, "a synergistic action of Δ^9-THC with other compounds in the extract." Carlini et al. (1974) determined that cannabis extracts produced effects "two or four times greater than that expected from their THC content." Cannabis extracts were ten times more potent than THC at inhibiting MAO activity in porcine brain (Schurr and Livne 1976). A cannabis ethanol extract plus THC was more potent than an equal amount of THC (Truitt et al. 1976). Fairbairn and Pickens (1981) detected the presence of unidentified "powerful synergists," in cannabis extracts, causing 330% greater activity in mice than THC alone. Cannabis extracts provided greater analgesic activity than individual cannabinoids (Evans et al. 1987; Formukong et al. 1988).

Table 15.1 Interest in *Cannabis*, its constituents, and synergistic effects, estimated by counting the number of studies indexed by PubMed, binned by decade[a]

	1950s	1960s	1970s	1980s	1990s	2000s
Cannabis	40	401	3098	1456	1907	5187
Tetrahydrocannabinol	0	29	1549	1111	1115	1967
Cannabidiol	0	2	169	159	102	353
Cannabinol	0	2	136	103	76	99
Tetrahydrocannabivarin	0	0	2	1	2	16
Cannabichromene	0	5	14	21	8	11
Cannabigerol	0	1	3	12	6	13
Cannabis AND terpenoid[b]	0	0	1	1	0	1
Cannabis AND flavonoid[c]	0	0	2	4	1	14
Cannabis AND synergy[d]	0	0	5	3	2	17

[a] PubMed is a free database accessing life science and biomedical journals, accessible at http://www.ncbi.nlm.nih.gov/pubmed.
[b] Boolean combination of cannabis AND sesquiterpene OR monoterpene OR caryophyllene OR limonene OR linalool OR myrcene OR pinene.
[c] Boolean combination of cannabis AND flavonoid OR flavone OR flavonol OR cannaflavin.
[d] Boolean combination of cannabis AND synergy OR synergism OR synergistic OR isobologram OR isobolographic.

The essential oil of cannabis, devoid of cannabinoids, retained analgesic (Segelman et al. 1974), anti-inflammatory (Burstein et al. 1975), and perhaps even antidepressant effects (Hall 2008; Russo et al. 2000). Terpenoids improve THC pharmacokinetics by increasing vasodilatation of alveolar capillaries (which permits more absorption of THC by the lungs), and by increasing blood–brain barrier permeability (Agrawal et al. 1989).

Individual terpenoids in cannabis essential oil have been assessed for therapeutic properties. Russo (2011) listed some examples:

◆ β-myrcene is analgesic, anti-inflammatory, anti-convulsant, and a skeletal muscle relaxant.

◆ β-caryophyllene is analgesic and anti-inflammatory, eases gut muscle spasms, and is technically a cannabinoid because it binds to CB_2 receptors (but not the CB_1 receptor so it is not psychoactive).

◆ D-limonene is an antioxidant, antidepressant and anticonvulsant, and blocks carcinogenesis induced by benz[a]anthracene, one of the "tars" generated by the combustion of herbal cannabis.

◆ D-linalool is sedative, anxiolytic, analgesic and anti-inflammatory, and induces apoptosis in cancer cells.

◆ α-pinene is anti-inflammatory, aids memory as an acetylcholinesterase inhibitor, and causes bronchodilation.

Russo (2011) reviewed a dozen mechanistic studies that demonstrate the effects of individual terpenoids at clinically relevant dosages. For example, limonene is highly bioavailable with 70% human pulmonary uptake; and 60% of pinene is bioavailable in a similar assay. Inhaling the aroma of terpenoids decreases anxiety, imparts sedation, improves cognitive performance and EEG patterns of alertness in healthy volunteers.

Many studies have specifically identified cannabidiol (CBD) as an "entourage compound" in cannabis that modulates the effects of THC (Russo and Guy 2006). Although Cascio and Pertwee (Chapter 7, this volume) highlight CBD, we add some concepts here. CBD affects the pharmacokinetics of THC:

◆ *Absorption*—CBD is anti-inflammatory, which is one reason why inhaling cannabis smoke caused less airway irritation and inflammation than inhaling pure THC (Tashkin et al. 1977).

◆ *Distribution*—CBD is highly lipophilic, partitions into the lipid bilayer, and fluidizes membrane lipids (Howlett et al. 1989).

◆ *Distribution*—CBD fluidizes cell membranes, increasing the penetration of THC into muscle cells and thereby amplifying THC's muscle-relaxant effects (Wagner 2004).

◆ *Metabolism*—CBD inhibits the hepatic metabolism of drugs, including THC (Loewe 1944; Paton and Pertwee 1972).

◆ *Metabolism*—CBD inhibits two cytochrome P450 enzymes, 3A11 and 2C, that hydroxylate THC to its metabolite 11-hydroxy-Δ^9-THC (Bornheim et al. 1995, 1998).

CBD also alters endocannabinoid pharmacokinetics, by inhibiting FAAH hydrolysis of anandamide. Pharmacodynamically, CBD acts as a "synergistic shotgun," all by itself, by promiscuously targeting many receptors and signaling pathways. CBD enhances many benefits of THC (e.g., analgesic, anticarcinogenic, antiemetic, antiepileptic, anti-inflammatory, antispasmodic, and neuroprotective effects). The importance of CBD led GW Pharmaceuticals to formulate Sativex® as a 50:50 mixture of CBD and THC. 'Sativex can be considered a CBD product with some THC added" (G. Guy, personal communication, 2006).

The ability of CBD to decrease the adverse effects of THC permits the administration of higher doses of the latter, thereby increasing the clinical efficacy and safety of cannabis-based extracts. This "tale of two cannabinoids" (Russo and Guy 2006) is fascinating from an evolutionary perspective: Rottanburg et al. (1982) attributed a high incidence of cannabis-associated psychosis in South Africa to the virtual absence of CBD in plants from that region. Black market *Cannabis* breeders have selected plants for increased THC and decreased CBD, which may pose an increased risk to psychologically susceptible individuals (Potter et al. 2008). Dozens of animal studies and clinical trials have demonstrated CBD's antipsychotic effects, possibly by activating TRPV1 and attenuating dopaminergic effects (reviewed in Russo and Guy 2006) (Leweke et al. 2012; Morgan and Curran 2008).

However, panic reaction and not psychosis is the primary side effect of THC (Weil 1970). Animal studies and clinical trials have demonstrated the anxiolytic benefits of CBD, by suppressing tryptophan degradation, activating 5-HT_{1A} (Russo et al. 2005), and decreasing adenosine uptake (reviewed in Russo and Guy 2006).

15.6 **The twenty-first century**

The twenty-first century began early in the cannabis world: 1998 saw renewed interest in cannabis polypharmacy with a seminal review of therapeutic synergy (McPartland and Pruitt 1998). The same year, Geoffrey Guy and Brian Whittle founded GW Pharmaceuticals on the concept of synergy in whole cannabis extracts. If THC can be characterized as a "silver bullet," then cannabis can be considered a multicomponent "synergistic shotgun" (Izzo et al. 2009; McPartland and Mediavilla 2001; McPartland and Pruitt 1999; McPartland and Russo 2001; Russo 2011; Russo and Guy 2006; Russo and McPartland 2003). Many constituents in cannabis work by multiple mechanisms to modulate the therapeutic effects of THC and mitigate its side effects.

Studies on the combinational effects of THC and CBD have become quite nuanced. The effects of CBD on THC are dose related (Fadda et al. 2004; Vann et al. 2008; Varvel et al. 2006). Timing may be a factor: Zuardi (2008) proposed that preadministration of CBD potentiated the effects of THC via a pharmacokinetic mechanism, whereas coadministration of both compounds caused CBD to antagonize the effects of THC via a pharmacodynamic mechanism.

Williamson (2001) showed that THC reduced muscle spasticity in a mouse model of multiple sclerosis, but was significantly less effective than a cannabis extract containing the same amount of THC. A cannabis extract lacking THC inhibited epileptiform bursting in brain slices, more so than a cannabis extract with THC (Whalley et al. 2004). In an in vitro epilepsy model, the anticonvulsant effects of cannabis extracts were more potent and more rapidly acting than isolated THC (Wilkinson et al. 2003). In some cancer cell lines, a CBD-rich extract inhibited cell growth more potently than pure CBD (Ligresti et al. 2006). Calcium levels in cultured neurons and glia were elevated in a synergistic fashion by adding CBD to THC, but whole cannabis extracts raised calcium levels even more than pure CBD + THC (Ryan et al. 2006). Cannabis extracts provided better antinociceptive efficacy in rats than CBD given alone (Comelli et al. 2008). Cannabis extracts were more potent than pure cannabinoids at the receptors TRPV1, TRPA1, TRPM8 and at inhibiting the enzymes FAAH, DAGLα, and MAGL (De Petrocellis et al. 2011).

As can be seen in Table 15.1, interest in terpenoids still lags. King et al. (2009) demonstrated that pristimerin and euphol inhibit MAGL activity, although these terpenoids do not occur in cannabis. β-caryophyllene has become a focus of attention. It is a component of Sativex® (Guy and Stott 2005), and is the primary sesquiterpenoid in black pepper, *Piper nigrum*. It acts as a full agonist at CB_2 with strong potency (100 nM), the first proven active phytocannabinoid beyond *Cannabis* (Gertsch et al. 2008).

Anonymous (2006) reported interactions between individual terpenoids and THC, apparently based on human bioassays. Drug interactions were assessed with a neuropsychological questionnaire, the Drug Reaction Scale. Limonene added to THC made the drug sensation more "cerebral and euphoric," whereas myrcene made the drug sensation more "physical, mellow, sleepy." Anonymous alleged that THC plus limonene and THC plus myrcene produced stronger cannabimimetic effects than THC alone.

Research in herbal synergy has elicited a predictable reaction—attempts to disprove it. Some scientists have contended that synthetic THC (which is legally available) accounts for all the effects of cannabis. Wachtel et al. (2002) observed no differences in human subjects ingesting or smoking THC versus herbal cannabis. Hart et al. (2002) reported that human subjects experienced "negative" subjective effects after smoking marijuana but not after oral THC consumption. Varvel et al. (2005) reported that THC accounts for all effects in mice subjected to the tetrad test. Ilan et al. (2005) compared the effects of cannabis with high or low CBD and CBC and found no differences in subjective reports and neurophysiological measures. The Wachtel study used cannabis with only 0.05% CBD, likely too low to modulate THC (Russo and McPartland 2003). The other studies share the same problem. Bloor et al. (2008) showed that black market cannabis contains 4.3–8.5 times more terpenoids than cannabis used in NIDA research.

The isobologram has been rediscovered by twenty-first-century cannabinoid researchers: Cichewicz and McCarthy (2003) demonstrated antinociceptive synergy between THC and opioids after oral administration in mice. Cox et al. (2007) showed synergy between THC and morphine in the arthritic rat. DeLong et al. (2010) found an additive effect when combining THC and cannabichromene in mice with LPS-induced inflammation. Four isobolographic studies of endocannabinoids (e.g., anandamide and *N*-arachidonoyl-dopamine) or drugs that block their breakdown (e.g., FAAH inhibitors) also show synergy with analgesics (Farkas et al. 2011; Guindon et al. 2006; Naidu et al., 2009; Sasso et al. 2012). Nearly a dozen isobolographic studies have also demonstrated synergy between synthetic cannabinoids, such as CP55,940 or WIN55,212-2, and a wide range of analgesics, anesthetics, and anticonvulsants, which is beyond the scope of this review on natural constituents.

15.7 **Conclusion**

Evolution (i.e., natural selection) over millions of years creates a phytochemical matrix around key constituents, so they can reach their biochemical targets. Many of our crop plants and medicinal plants exhibit this phenomenon (Spelman 2009). *Cannabis* is no exception. It has likely undergone two rounds of coevolution with animals: perhaps 30 million years of selection to fit mammalian herbivore physiology, followed by thousands of years of accelerated evolution by humans who selected plants for optimal benefit and minimal toxicity (McPartland and Guy 2004). Ehrlich's reductionist "silver bullet" philosophy is being replaced by Loewe's synergistic concepts (Borisy et al. 2003).

The data herein presented strongly support the therapeutic rationale for combining THC with other constituents present in cannabis. The impact of individual terpenoids upon THC requires further animal studies and clinical trials. The formal investigation of the effects of individual flavonoids and other constituents has not yet begun. Should positive outcomes result from such studies, phytopharmaceutical development may follow. Breeding work has already resulted in *Cannabis* chemotypes that produce 97% of monoterpenoid content as myrcene, or 77% as limonene (E. de Meijer, personal communication, 2010). A better future via cannabis phytochemistry may be an achievable goal through further research of the entourage effect in this versatile plant that may help it fulfill its promise as a pharmacological treasure trove.

Conflict of interest statement

JM has been a consultant for GW Pharmaceuticals, and has received travel expenses and research support. ER is Group Senior Medical Advisor to GW Pharmaceuticals and serves as a full-time consultant.

References

Agrawal, A.K., Kumar, P., Gulati, A., and Seth, P.K. (1989). Cannabis-induced neurotoxicity in mice: effects on cholinergic (muscarinic) receptors and blood brain barrier permeability. *Research Communications in Substance Abuse*, **10**, 155–168.

Anonymous. (2006). Studying the effects of terpenes. *O'Shaughnessy's*, Spring, **2**.

Bensky, D., Gamble, A., and Kaptchuk, T. (1993). *Chinese Herbal Medicine: Materia Medica*. Seattle, WA: Eastland Press.

Bloor, R.N., Wang, T.S., Spanel, P., and Smith, D. (2008). Ammonia release from heated 'street' cannabis leaf and its potential toxic effects on cannabis users. *Addiction*, **103**, 1671–1677.

Bohlig, J.F. (1840). *Cannabis sativa* und *Urtica dioica* chemisch analysiert. *Jahrbuch für praktische Pharmacie und verwandte Fächer*, **3**, 1–58.

Borisy, A.A., Elliott, P.J., Hurst, N.W., *et al.* (2003). Systematic discovery of multicomponent therapeutics. *Proceedings of the National Academy of Sciences of the United States of America*, **100**, 7977–7982.

Bornheim, L.M. and Grillo, M.P. (1998). Characterization of cytochrome P450 3A inactivation by cannabidiol: possible involvement of cannabidiol-hydroxyquinone as a P450 inactivator. *Chemical Research in Toxicology*, **11**, 1209–1216.

Bornheim, L.M., Kim, K.Y., Li, J., Perotti, B.Y., and Benet, L.Z. (1995). Effect of cannabidiol pretreatment on the kinetics of tetrahydrocannabinol metabolites in mouse brain. *Drug Metabolism & Disposition*, **23**, 825–831.

Buchholz, C.F. (1806). Beiträge zur pflanzenchemie. Analyse des hanfsamens. *Neues allgemeines Journal der Chemie*, **6**, 615–630.

Buchholz, C.F. (1816). Chemische Untersuchung der trockenen reifen spanischen Pfeffers. *Almanach oder Taschenbuch für Scheidekünstler und Apotheker*, **37**, 1–30.

Bureau of Narcotics. (1938). *Marihuana conference held December 5 1938 in the United States Bureau of Internal Revenue Building (Room 3003)*. Washington, DC: Government Printing Office. Available at: http://www.globalhemp.com/1938/12/marihuana-conference.html.

Burstein, S., Taylor, P., El-Feraly, F.S., and Turner, C. (1976). Prostaglandins and *Cannabis*—V. Identification of p-vinylphenol as a potent inhibitor of prostaglandin synthesis. *Biochemical Pharmacology*, **25**, 2003–2004.

Burstein, S., Varanelli, C., and Slade, L.T. (1975). Prostaglandins and *Cannabis*—III. Inhibition of biosynthesis by essential oil components of marihuana. *Biochemical Pharmacology*, **24**, 1053–1054.

Cichewicz, D.L. and McCarthy, E.A. (2003). Antinociceptive synergy between delta(9)-tetrahydrocannabinol and opioids after oral administration. *Journal of Pharmacology and Experimental Therapeutics*, **304**, 1010–1015.

Calkins, A. (1871). *Opium and the Opium-Appetite: with Notices of Alcoholic Beverages, Cannabis Indica, Tobacco and Coca, and Tea and Coffee, in Their Hygienic Aspects and Pathologic Relationships*. Philadelphia, PA: J.B. Lippincott.

Carlini, E.A., Karniol, I.G., Renault, P.F., and Schuster, C.R. (1974). Effects of marihuana in laboratory animals and man. *British Journal of Pharmacology*, **50**, 299–309.

Christison, A. (1850). On *Cannabis indica*, Indian Hemp. *Transactions and Proceedings of the Botanical Society of Edinburgh*, **4**, 59–69.

Comelli, F., Giagnoni, G., Bettoni, I., Colleoni, M., and Costa, B. (2008). Antihyperalgesic effect of a *Cannabis sativa* extract in a rat model of neuropathic pain: mechanisms involved. *Phytotherapy Research*, **22**(8), 1017–1024.

Cox, M.L., Haller, V.L., and Welch, S.P. (2007). Synergy between delta9-tetrahydrocannabinol and morphine in the arthritic rat. *European Journal of Pharmacology*, **567**, 125–130.

de Courtive, M.E. (1848). *Hashisch. Étude Historique, Chimique et Physiologique*. Paris: Edouard Bautruche.

DeLong, G.T., Wolf, C.E., Poklis, A., and Lichtman, A.H. (2010). Pharmacological evaluation of the natural constituent of *Cannabis sativa*, cannabichromene and its modulation by Δ(9)-tetrahydrocannabinol. *Drug Alcohol Dependence*, **112**(1–2), 126–133.

De Petrocellis, L., Ligresti, A., Moriello, A.S., *et al.* (2011). Effects of cannabinoids and cannabinoid-enriched *Cannabis* extracts on TRP channels and endocannabinoid metabolic enzymes. *British Journal of Pharmacology*, **163**, 1479–1494.

Di Marzo, V., De Petrocellis, L., Fezza, F., Ligresti, A., and Bisogno, T. (2002). Anandamide receptors. *Prostaglandins, Leukotrienes, and Essential Fatty Acids*, **66**, 377–391.

Dutt, S. (1957). Indian *Cannabis sativa* and essential oils derived from the same. *Indian Soap Journal*, **22**, 242–246.

Evans, A.T., Formukong, E.A., and Evans, F.J. (1987). Actions of cannabis constituents on enyzmes of arachidonate: anti-inflammatory potential. *Biochemical Pharmacology*, **36**(12), 2035–2037.

Fairbairn, J.W. and Pickens, J.T. (1981). Activity of *Cannabis* in relation to its Δ-tetrahydrocannabinol content. *British Journal of Pharmacology*, **72**, 401–409.

Fadda, P., Robinson, L., Fratta, W., Pertwee, R.G., and Riedel, G. (2004). Differential effects of THC- or CBD-rich cannabis exacts on working memory in rats. *Neuropharmacology*, **47**, 1170–1179.

Farkas, I., Tuboly, G., Benedek, G., and Horvath, G. (2011). The antinociceptive potency of N-arachidonoyl-dopamine (NADA) and its interaction with endomorphin-1 at the spinal level. *Pharmacology, Biochemistry and Behaviour*, **99**(4), 731–737.

Fischedick, J., Van Der Kooy, F., and Verpoort, R. (2010b). Cannabinoid receptor 1 binding activity and quantitative analysis of *Cannabis sativa* L. smoke and vapor. *Chemical & Pharmaceutical Bulletin*, **58**(2), 201–207.

Fischedick, J.T., Hazekamp. A., Erkelens, T., Choi, Y.H., and Verpoorte, R. (2010a). Metabolic fingerprinting of *Cannabis sativa* L., cannabinoids and terpenoids for chemotaxonomic and drug standardization purposes. *Phytochemistry*, **71**, 2058–2073.

Formukong, E.A., Evans, A.T., and Evans, F.J. (1988). Inhibition of the cataleptic effect of tetrahydrocannabinol by other constituents of *Cannabis sativa* L. *Journal of Pharmacy and Pharmacology*, **40**, 132–134.

Gaoni, Y. and Mechoulam, R. (1964). Isolation, structure, and partial synthesis of an active constituent of hashish. *Journal of the American Chemical Society*, **86**, 1646–1647.

Gertsch, J., Leonti, M., Raduner, S., *et al.* (2008). Beta-caryophyllene is a dietary cannabinoid. *Proceedings of the National Academy of Sciences of the United States of America*, **105**(26), 9099–9104.

Gill, E.W., Paton, W.D.M., and Pertwee, R.G. (1970). Preliminary experiments on the chemistry and pharmacology of *Cannabis*. *Nature*, **228**, 134–136.

Guindon, J., De Léan, A., and Beaulieu, P. (2006). Local interactions between anandamide, an endocannabinoid, and ibuprofen, a nonsteroidal anti-inflammatory drug, in acute and inflammatory pain. *Pain*, **121**, 85–93.

Guy, G.W. and Stott, C.G. The development of Sativex—a natural cannabis-based medicine. In: R. Mechoulam (ed.). *Cannabinoids As Therapeutics*. Basel: Birkhäuser Verlag, pp. 231–263.

Hall, B.P. (2008). *Structure Activity Relationships for Intracellular Loop 2 of the 5HT1a Serotonin Receptor*. Doctoral thesis, Department of Biomedical and Pharmaceutical Sciences, University of Montana, Missoula, MT.

Hamilton, E. (1852). *Flora Homœopathica, Vol. 1*. London: H. Bailliere.

Hanuš, L. (2008). Pharmacological and therapeutic secrets of plant and brain (endo)cannabinoids. *Medicinal Research Reviews*, **29**, 213–271.

Hart, C.L., Ward, A.S., Haney, M., Comer, S.D., Foltin, R.W., and Fischman, M.W. (2002). Comparison of smoked marijuana and oral Delta(9)-tetrahydrocannabinol in humans. *Psychopharmacology*, **164**(4), 407–415.

Hendricks, H., Malingré, T.M., Batterman, S., and Bos, R. (1978). The essential oil of *Cannabis sativa*. *Pharmaceutisch Weekblad*, **113**, 413–424.

Hillig, K.W. (2004). A chemotaxonomic analysis of terpenoid variation in *Cannabis*. *Biochemical Systematics and Ecology*, **32**, 875–891.

Hood, L.V.S., Dames, M.E., and Barry, G.T. (1973). Headspace volatiles of marijuana. *Nature*, **242**, 402–403.

Hooper, D. (1908). Charas of Indian hemp. *Year-Book of Pharmacy*, 1908, 435–444.

Howlett, A.C., Scott, D.K., and Wilken, G.H. (1989). Regulation of adenylate cyclase by cannabinoid drugs. Insights based on thermodynamic studies. *Biochemical Pharmacology*, **38**(19), 3297–3304.

Huxtable, R.J. and Schwarz, S.K.W. (2001). The isolation of morphine—first principles in science and ethics. *Molecular Interventions*, 1(4), 189–191.

Ilan, A.B., Gevins, A., Coleman, M., ElSohly, M.A., and de Wit, H. (2005). Neurophysiological and subjective profile of marijuana with varying concentrations of cannabinoids. *Behavioural Pharmacology*, **16**, 487–496.

Izzo, A.A., Borrell, i F., Capasso, R., Di Marzo, V., and Mechoulam, R. (2009). Non-psychotropic plant cannabinoids: new therapeutic opportunities from an ancient herb. *Trends in Pharmacological Sciences*, **30**(10), 515–527.

King, A.R., Dotsey, E.Y., Lodola, A., *et al.* (2009). Discovery of potent and reversible monoacylglycerol lipase inhibitors. *Chemistry & Biology*, **16**, 1045–1052.

Kubena, R.K. and Barry, H. (1972). Stimulus characteristics of marihuana components. *Nature*, **235**, 397–398.

Lee, S.Y., Oh, S.M., Lee, S.K., and Chung, K.H. (2005). Antiestrogenic effects of marijuana smoke condensate and cannabinoid compounds. *Archives of Pharmacal Research*, **28**(12), 1365–1375.

Leweke, F. M., Piomelli, D., Pahlisch, F. *et al.* (2012). Cannabidiol enhances anandamide signaling and alleviates psychotic symptoms of schizophrenia. *Translational Psychiatry*, **2**, e94.

Ligresti, A., Moriello, A.S., Starowicz, K., *et al.* (2006). Antitumor activity of plant cannabinoids with emphasis on the effect of cannabidiol on human breast carcinoma. *Journal of Pharmacology and Experimental Therapeutics*, **318**(3), 1375–1387.

Loewe, S. (1928). Die quantitative Problem der Pharmakologie. *Ergebnisse der Physiologie*, **27**, 47–187.

Loewe, S. (1940). Synergism of cannabis and butyl-bromallyl-barbituric acid. *Journal of the American Pharmaceutical Association (Scientific edition)*, **29**, 162–163.

Loewe, S. (1944). Studies on the pharmacology of marihuana. In: LaGuardia Committee (eds.). *The Marihuana Problem in the City of New York*. Lancaster, PA: Jaques Cattell Press, pp. 149–212.

Loewe, S. (1945). Marihuana activity of cannabinol. *Science*, **102**, 615–616.

Loewe, S. (1946). Studies on the pharmacology and acute toxicity of compounds with marihuana activity. *Journal of Pharmacology and Experimental Therapeutics*, **88**, 154–164.

Ludlow, F.-H. (1857). *The Hasheesh Eater: Being Passages Form the Life of A Pythagorean*. New York: Harper.

Martin, L., Morison Smith, D., and Farmilo, C.G. (1961). Essential oil from fresh *Cannabis sativa* and its use in identification. *Nature* **191**, 774–776.

McPartland, J.M., Blanchon, D., and Musty, R.E. (2008). Cannabimimetic effects modulated by cholinergic compounds. *Addiction Biology*, **13**, 411–415.

McPartland, J.M. and Mediavilla, V. (2001). Non-cannabinoids in cannabis. In: F. Grotenhermen and E.B. Russo (eds.). *Cannabis and Cannabinoids*. Binghamton, NY: Haworth Press, pp. 401–409.

McPartland, J.M. and Pruitt, P.L. (1998). An herbal "synergistic shotgun" compared to a synthetic "silver bullet": medical marijuana versus tetrahydrocannabinol. *Proceedings 1998 Symposium on the Cannabinoids*. Burlington, VT: International Cannabinoid Research Society, p. 112.

McPartland, J.M. and Pruitt, P.L. (1999). Side effects of pharmaceuticals not elicited by comparable herbal medicines: the case of tetrahydrocannabinol and marijuana. *Alternative Therapies in Health and Medicine* 5, 57–62.

McPartland, J.M. and Russo, E.B. (2001). *Cannabis* and cannabis extracts: greater than the sum of their parts? *Journal of Cannabis Therapeutics* 1(3–4), 103–132.

Mechoulam, R. (1973). Cannabinoid chemisty. In: R. Mechoulam (ed.). *Marijuana*. New York: Academic Press, pp. 1–87.

Mechoulam, R., Ben-Zvi, Z., Shani, A., Zemler, H., and Levy, S. (1972). Cannabinoids and cannabis activity. In: W.D.M. Paton and J. Crown (eds.). *Cannabis and its Derivatives*. London: Oxford University Press, pp. 1–13.

Mediavilla, V. and Steinemann, S. (1997). Essential oil of *Cannabis sativa* L. strains. *Journal of the International Hemp Association*, 4(2), 82–84.

Meier, C. and Mediavilla, V. (1998). Factors influencing the yield and the quality of hemp (*Cannabis sativa* L.) essential oil. *Journal of the International Hemp Association*, 5(1), 16–20.

Morgan, C.J. and Curran, H.V. (2008). Effects of cannabidiol on schizophrenia-like symptoms in people who use cannabis. *British Journal of Psychiatry*, 192, 306–307.

Naidu, P.S., Booker, L., Cravatt, B.F., and Lichtman, A.H. (2009). Synergy between enzyme inhibitors of fatty acid amide hydrolase and cyclooxygenase in visceral nociception. *Journal of Pharmacology and Experimental Therapeutics*, 329, 48–56.

Nigam, M.C., Handa, K.L., Nigam, I.C., and Levi, L. (1965). Essential oils and their constituents. XXIX. The essential oil of marihuana: composition of the genuine Indian *Cannabis sativa* L. *Canadian Journal of Chemistry*, 43, 3372–3376.

Nissen, L., Zatta, A., Stefanini, I., *et al.* (2010). Characterization and antimicrobial activity of essential oils of industrial hemp varieties (*Cannabis sativa* L.). *Fitoterapia*, 81, 413–419.

O'Shaughnessy, W.B. (1838–1840). On the preparations of the Indian hemp, or gunjah *(Cannabis indica)*; Their effects on the animal system in health, and their utility in the treatment of tetanus and other convulsive diseases. *Transactions of the Medical and Physical Society of Bengal*, 71–102, 421–461.

Paton, W.D.M. and Pertwee, R.G. (1972). Effect of cannabis and certain of its constituents on pentobarbitone sleeping time and phenazone metabolism. *British Journal of Pharmacology*, 44(2), 250–261.

Polli, G. (1865). Sull'antidoto dell'haschisch. *Annali di Chimica Applicata alla Medicina*, 40(3), 343–345.

Potter, D. (2009). *The Propagation, Characterisation and Optimisation of Cannabis sativa L. as a Phytopharmaceutical*. Doctoral thesis, London: King's College.

Potter, D.J., Clark, P., and Brown, M.B. (2008). Potency of delta 9-THC and other cannabinoids in cannabis in England in 2005: implications for psychoactivity and pharmacology. *Journal of Forensic Science*, 53, 90–94.

Prain, D. (1893). *Report on the Cultivation and Use of Gánjá*. Calcutta: Bengal Secretariat Press.

Rector, J.M. (1922). Synergistic analgesia: clinical observations. *American Journal of Surgery*, 36(10 Suppl.), 114–119.

Robiquet, E. (1857). *Rapport sur le concours relatif à l'analyse du chanvre présente au nom de la Société de Pharmacie*. Journal de Pharmacie et de Chimie, (Serie 3) 31, 46–51.

Ross, S.A. and ElSohly, M.A. (1996). The volatile oil composition of fresh and air-dried buds of *Cannabis sativa*. *Journal of Natural Products*, 59, 49–51.

Rottanburg, D., Robins, A.H., Ben-Arie, O., Teggin, A., and Elk, R. (1982). Cannabis-associated psychosis with hypomanic features *Lancet*, ii, 1364–1366.

Russo, E.B. (2011). Taming THC: potential cannabis synergy and phytocannabinid-terpeoid entourage effects. *British Journal of Pharmacology*, **163**, 1344–1364.

Russo, E.B. and Guy, G.W. (2006). A tale of two cannabinoids: the therapeutic rationale for combining tetrahydrocannabinol and cannabidiol. *Medical Hypotheses*, **66**, 234–246.

Russo, E., Macarah, C.M., Todd, C.L., Medora, R.S., and Parker, K.K. (2000). Pharmacology of the essential oil of hemp at 5-HT1a and 5-HT2a receptors. Abstract at the 41st Annual Meeting of the American Society of Pharmacognosy, July 22–26, Seattle, WA.

Russo, E.B. and McPartland, J.M. (2003). Cannabis is more than simply delta(9)-tetrahydrocannabinol. *Psychopharmacology*, **165**, 431–432.

Ryan, D., Drysdale, A.J., Pertwee, R.G., and Platt B. (2006). Differential effects of cannabis extracts and pure plant cannabinoids on hippocampal neurones and glia. *Neuroscience Letters*, **408**(3), 236–241.

Sasso, O., Bertorelli, R., Bandiera, T., *et al.* (2012). Peripheral FAAH inhibition causes profound antinociception and protects against indomethacin-induced gastric lesions. *Pharmacological Research*, **65**, 553–563.

Sauer, M.A., Rifka, S.M., Hawks, R.L., Cutler, G.B., and Loriaux, D.L. (1983). Marijuana: interaction with the estrogen receptor. *Journal of Pharmacy and Experimental Therapeutics*, **224**, 404–407.

Schaeffer, J. (1975). The significance of marihuana in a small agricultural community in Jamaica. In V. Rubin (ed.). *Cannabis and Culture*. The Hague: Mouton, pp. 355–388.

Schlesinger, S. (1840). Untersuchung der Cannabis sativa. *Buchner's Repertorium für die Pharmacie*, **21**, 190–208.

Schurr, A. and Livne, A. (1976). Differential inhibition of mitochondrial monoamine oxidase from brain by hashish compounds. *Biochemical Pharmacology*, **25**, 1201–1203.

Segelman, A.B., Sofia, R.D., Segelman, F.P., Harakal, J.J., and Knobloch, L.C. (1974). *Cannabis sativa* L. (marijuana) V: pharmacological evaluation of marijuana aqueous extract and volatile oil. *Journal of Pharmaceutical Sciences*, **63**, 962–964.

Shanavaskhan, A.E., Binu, S., Muraleedharan-Unnithan, C., Santhoshkumar, E.S., and Pushpangadan, P. (1997). Detoxification techniques of traditional physicians of Kerala, India on some toxic herbal drugs. *Fitoterapia*, **68**, 69–74.

Simonsen, J.L. and Todd, A.R. (1942). *Cannabis indica*, Part X. The essential oil from Egyptian hashish. *Journal of the Chemical Society (London)*, **1942**(1), 188–191.

Smith, T. and Smith, H. (1847a). On the resin of Indian hemp. *Pharmaceutical Journal*, **6**, 127–128.

Smith, T. and Smith, H. (1847b). Process for preparing cannabine, or hemp resin. *Pharmaceutical Journal*, **6**, 171–173.

Spelman, K., Wetschler, M.H., and Cech, N.B. (2009). Comparison of alkylamide yield in ethanolic extracts prepared from fresh versus dry *Echinacea purpurea* utilizing HPLC-ESI-MS. *Journal of Pharmaceutical and Biomedical Analysis*, **49**, 1141–1149.

Spronck, H.J., Luteijn, J.M., Salemink, C.A., and Nugteren, D.H. (1978). Inhibition of prostaglandin biosynthesis by derivatives of olivetol formed under pyrolysis of cannabidiol. *Biochemical Pharmacology*, **27**, 607–608.

Stahl, E. and Kunde, R. (1973). Die Leitsubstanzen der Haschisch-Suchhunde. *Kriminalistik*, **9**, 385–388.

Tashkin, D.P., Reiss, S., Shapiro, B.J., Calvarese, B., Olsen, J.L., and Lodge, W. (1977). Bronchial effects of aerosolized Δ^9-tetrahydrocannabinol in healthy and asthmatic subjects. *American Review of Respiratory Disease*, **115**, 57–65.

Taylor, B. (1855). *The Lands of the Saracens*. New York: G.P. Putnam & Sons.

Truitt, E.B., Kinzer, G.W., and Berlow, J.M. (1976). Behavioral activity in various fractions of marijuana smoke condensate in the rat. In: M.C. Braude and S. Szara (eds.). *Pharmacology of Marihuana*. Vol. 2. New York: Raven Press, pp. 463–474.

Tscheppe, F. (Schübler G, *präside*). (1821). *Chemische Untersuchung der Hanfblätter*. Dissertation, Tübingen.

Turner, C.E., ElSohly, M.A., and Boeren, E.G. (1980). Constituents of *Cannabis sativa* L. XVII. A review of the natural constituents. *Journal of Natural Products*, **43**, 169–234.

Valente, L. (1880). Sull' essenza di canapa. *Gazzetta chimica italiana*, **10**, 479–481.

Valente, L. (1881). Sull' idrocarburo estratto dalla canapa. *Gazzetta chimica italiana*, **11**, 196–198.

Valieri, R. (1887). *Sulla canapa nostrana e suoi preparati in sostituzione della Cannabis indica*. Naples: Stabilimento tipografico dell'unione.

Vann, R.E., Gamage, T.F., Warner, J.A., *et al.* (2008). Divergent effects of cannabidiol on the discriminative stimulus and place conditioning effects of delta(9)-tetrahydrocannabinol. *Drug and Alcohol Dependence*, **94**(1–3), 191–198.

Varvel, S.A., Bridgen, D.T., Tao, Q., Thomas, B.F., Martin, B.R., and Lichtman, A.H. (2005). Delta-9-tetrahydrocannbinol accounts for the antinociceptive, hypothermic, and cataleptic effects of marijuana in mice. *Journal of Pharmacology and Experimental Therapeutics*, **314**, 329–337.

Varvel, S.A., Wiley, J.L., Yang, R., *et al.* (2006). Interactions between THC and cannabidiol in mouse models of cannabinoid activity. *Psychopharmacology (Berlin)*, **186**(2), 226–234.

Wachtel, S.R., ElSohly, M.A., Ross, R.A., Ambre, J., and de Wit, H. (2002). Comparison of the subjective effects of delta-9-tetrahydrocannabinol and marijuana in humans. *Psychopharmacology*, **161**, 331–339.

Wagner, H. (2004). Natural products chemistry and phytomedicine research in the new millennium: new developments and challenges. *ARKIVOC Journal of Organic Chemistry*, **7**, 277–284.

Weil, A.T. (1970). Adverse reactions to marihuana, classification and suggested treatment. *New England Journal of Medicine*, **282**, 997–1000.

Whalley, B.J., Wilkinson, J.D., Williamson, E.M., and Constanti, A. (2004). A novel component of cannabis extract potentiates excitatory synaptic transmission in rat olfactory cortex in vitro. *Neuroscience Letters*, **365**(1), 58–63.

Wilkinson, J.D, Whalley, B.J., Baker, D., *et al.* (2003). Medicinal cannabis: is delta9-tetrahydrocannabinol necessary for all its effects? *Journal of Pharmacology and Pharmacotherapeutics*, **55**, 1687–1694.

Williamson, E.M. (2001). Synergy and other interactions in phytomedicines. *Phytomedicine*, **8**, 401–409.

Wood, T.B., Spivey, W.T.N., and Easterfield, T.H. (1896). Charas, the resin of Indian hemp. *Journal of the Chemical Society*, **6**, 539–546.

Zuardi, A.W. (2008). Cannabidiol: from an inactive cannabinoid to a drug with wide spectrum of action. *Revista Brasileira de Psiquiatria*, **30**, 271–280.

Chapter 16

Cannabinoid Pharmacokinetics and Disposition in Alternative Matrices

Marilyn A. Huestis and Michael L. Smith

16.1 Introduction

There is growing interest in the pharmacology and toxicology of natural and synthetic cannabinoids and in cannabinoid pharmacotherapy development. This chapter focuses on human phytocannabinoid pharmacokinetics and interpretation of cannabinoid blood, plasma, oral fluid (OF), sweat, urine, and hair tests. The endogenous cannabinoid system plays a critical role in physiological and behavioral processes. Endogenous cannabinoid neurotransmitters, receptors, and transporters, synthetic cannabinoid agonists and antagonists, and cannabis-based extracts are investigated to identify novel approaches to treat human disorders. Cannabis is one of the oldest and most commonly taken drugs. Knowledge of cannabinoid pharmacokinetics and cannabinoid disposition into biological fluids and tissues is essential to understanding the onset, magnitude and duration of cannabinoid pharmacodynamic effects.

Pharmacokinetics encompasses cannabinoid absorption following diverse routes of administration, distribution throughout the body, metabolism by tissues and organs, elimination in the feces, urine, sweat, OF, and hair, and how these processes change over time. Cannabis plants contain more than 100 cannabinoids including the primary psychoactive component delta-9-tetrahydrocannabinol (THC), and delta-9-tetrahydrocannabinolic acid that decarboxylates with heat producing THC. THC may degrade when exposed to air, heat, or light, and acid exposure can oxidize THC to cannabinol (CBN) that is approximately 10% as potent. THC, containing no nitrogen but with two chiral centers in *trans*-configuration, is described here by the dibenzopyran or delta 9 system.

16.2 THC pharmacokinetics

16.2.1 Absorption

16.2.1.1 Smoked administration

Smoking, the principal cannabis administration route, provides rapid and efficient drug delivery from lungs to brain, contributing to its abuse potential. Intense pleasurable and strongly reinforcing effects are due to immediate central nervous system drug exposure. Early investigations had analytical limitations, but characterized important aspects of smoked cannabis administration. The most important findings from these studies, described in more detail in an earlier review (Huestis 2005), are summarized here.

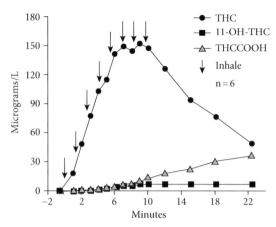

Fig. 16.1 Mean (n = 6) plasma concentrations of Δ^9-tetrahydrocannabinol (THC, ●, 11-hydroxy-Δ^9-tetrahydrocannabinol (11-OH-THC, ■) and 11-nor-9-carboxy-Δ^9-tetrahydrocannabinol (THCCOOH, ▲) during smoking of a single 3.55% THC cigarette. Each arrow represents one inhalation or puff on the cannabis cigarette.

Reproduced from *Handbook of Experimental Pharmacology*, 168, p. 660, Pharmacokinetics and Metabolism of the Plant Cannabinoids, Δ 9-Tetrahydrocannibinol, Cannabidiol and Cannabinol,M. A. Huestis, fig. 1 (c) 2005, Springer Science and Business Media. With kind permission from Springer Science and Business Media.

- Bioavailability of smoked THC is approximately 25%, with large intra- and intersubject variability due to many factors including smoking topography.
- Smoked THC is rapidly absorbed from the lungs reaching peak plasma concentration (C_{max}) prior to the end of smoking, in about 6–10 min (Fig. 16.1).
- Peak plasma THC concentrations are only slightly lower after smoking compared to after intravenous (i.v.) administration.
- After 16 and 30 mg smoked THC doses, respective mean ± SD plasma THC concentrations are 7.0 ± 8.1 and 18.1 ± 12.0 micrograms/L following one inhalation with mean (range) C_{max} of 84.3 (range 50–129) and 162.2 micrograms/L (76–267).
- Mean THC concentrations are approximately 60% and 20% of peak concentrations 15 and 30 min after initiation of smoking, respectively, and within 2 h, at or below 5 micrograms/L.
- The smoked route of administration permits a user to titrate his/her dose by adjusting smoking topography or manner in which they smoke.
- THC metabolizes to equipotent 11-hydroxy-THC (11-OH-THC) and inactive 11-nor-9-carboxy-THC (THCCOOH) metabolites during cannabis smoking.

Schwope et al. (2011a, 2011b) developed the first liquid chromatography tandem mass spectrometry (LCMSMS) method to simultaneously measure six free and glucuronidated cannabinoids in blood and plasma with low detection limits (0.5–5 micrograms/L) and further characterized cannabinoid profiles following smoking. Ten participants (nine men, one woman) smoked one 6.8% THC cannabis cigarette and THC, 11-OH-THC, THCCOOH, cannabidiol (CBD), CBN, THC-glucuronide and THCCOOH-glucuronide were simultaneously quantified in blood and plasma within 24 h of collection (Fig. 16.2). Median whole blood (plasma) maximum concentrations in chronic daily cannabis smokers were 50 (76), 6.4 (10), 41 (67), 1.3 (2.0), 2.4 (3.6), and 89 (190) 0.25 h after smoking initiation for THC, 11-OH-THC, THCCOOH, CBD, CBN, and

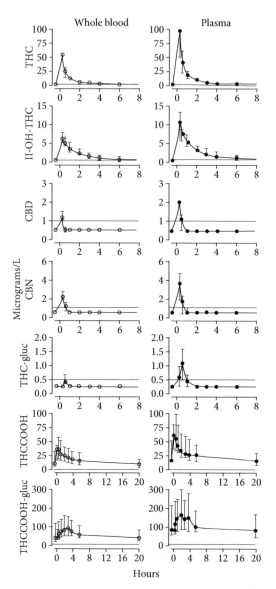

Fig. 16.2 Median (interquartile range) blood and plasma concentrations following smoking of a 6.8% THC cannabis cigarette. Samples collected at 0.5, 0.25, 0.5, 1.0, 2.0, 3.0, 4.0, 6.0, and 22 h after starting smoking. Dotted lines indicate limits of quantification: 1 microgram/L for THC; 11-OH-THC; THCCOOH; CBD; and CBN; 0.5 micrograms/L for THC-glucuronide; and 5 micrograms/L for THCCOOH-glucuronide.

Reproduced from David M. Schwope, Erin L. Karschner, David A. Gorelick, and Marilyn A. Huestis, Identification of Recent Cannabis Use: Whole-Blood and Plasma Free and Glucuronidated Cannabinoid Pharmacokinetics following Controlled Smoked Cannabis Administration, *Clinical Chemistry*, 57 (10), pp. 1406–1414 (c) 2011, American Association for Clinical Chemistry, with permission. doi: 10.1373/clinchem.2011.171777.

THCCOOH-glucuronide. At 0.5 h median THC-glucuronide blood (plasma) concentration was 0.7 (1.4) micrograms/L. At observed C_{max}, whole-blood (plasma) detection rates were 60% (80%), 80% (90%), and 50% (80%) for CBD, CBN, and THC-glucuronide, respectively. CBD and CBN were not found after 1 h in either matrix at a limit of quantification (LOQ) = 1.0 micrograms/L. The authors proposed that detection of CBD and CBN identifies recent intake.

More efficient THC delivery systems are being investigated. Van de Kooy et al. (2009) reported that mixing tobacco with cannabis increased volatility. Of course, the harmful side effects of tobacco smoking preclude employing this method for clinical treatment. The Volcano Vaporizer System (Storz & Bickel GmbH & Co., Tuttlingen, Germany) offers a more efficient delivery system reducing side stream smoke losses, and also reducing harmful by-products that do not volatilize at the lower temperatures utilized for cannabinoid vaporization (Pomahacova et al. 2009).

16.2.1.2 Oral administration

There are fewer THC and THC metabolite disposition data after oral administration. Studies of absorption following orally ingested THC are important since the licensed synthetic THC (dronabinol) medicine is taken orally and also because abuse by the oral route is common. THC is readily absorbed due to its high octanol/water coefficient, estimated at 6000 to 9 million. Absorption is slower when cannabinoids are ingested, with lower, delayed peak concentrations (Karschner et al. 2011a; Schwilke et al. 2009). Dose, route of administration, vehicle, and physiological factors such as absorption and metabolism and excretion rates influence drug concentrations. Early studies of oral THC bioavailability compared this route of administration to smoking (Huestis 2005). Some important characteristics are:

- Bioavailability is lower after oral ingestion compared to smoking, about 6%.
- Administering THC in sesame oil improves bioavailability.
- Time to plasma THC C_{max} after oral ingestion is about 2–6 h compared to minutes after smoking.
- Two peak THC concentrations after ingestion are possible due to enterohepatic recirculation.
- After a 20 mg dose in food (chocolate cookie) peak plasma THC concentrations are 4.4–11 micrograms/L 1–5 h after ingestion.
- Similar concentrations occur after 10 mg Marinol® (dronabinol).

Investigations after 2005 further characterized oral ingestion of THC. In a randomized, double-blind, within-subject, inpatient study of multiple 14.8 mg THC in hemp oil or 7.5 mg dronabinol doses, plasma THC and 11-OH-THC never exceeded 6.1 micrograms/L (Goodwin et al. 2006). Cannabinoids were always less than 0.5 micrograms/L 15.5 h after the last dose. THCCOOH concentrations exceeded 1.0 micrograms/L 1.5 h following the first dronabinol and 4.5 h after the first 14.8 mg hemp oil doses. THCCOOH peaked as high as 43 micrograms/L and always was 1.0 micrograms/L or less 39.5 h after the last dose. Cannabinoid concentrations were similar for 7.5 mg dronabinol and 14.8 mg hemp oil, demonstrating vehicle effect on absorption.

Schwilke et al. (2009) quantified free and conjugated cannabinoid plasma concentrations after multiple 20 mg oral THC doses to chronic daily cannabis smokers residing on a closed research unit. Twenty mg THC was administered every 4–8 h in escalating total daily doses (40–120 mg) for 7 days. Mean ± SE free plasma THC, 11-OH-THC, and THCCOOH concentrations 19.5 h after admission (before controlled oral THC dosing) were 4.3 ± 1.1, 1.3 ± 0.5, and 34.0 ± 8.4 micrograms/L, respectively. During oral dosing, free 11-OH-THC and THCCOOH increased steadily, whereas THC did not. Mean ± SE peak plasma free THC, 11-OH-THC, and THCCOOH 22.5 h after the last dose were 3.8 ± 0.5, 3.0 ± 0.7, and 196.9 ± 39.9 micrograms/L, respectively. Plasma THC concentrations remained greater than 1 microgram/L for at least 1 day after daily cannabis smoking and also after cessation of multiple oral THC doses. The authors commented that plasma THC concentrations greater than 1 microgram/L are often cited as evidence of recent cannabis intake but this may not be true following chronic frequent cannabis smoking or ingestion.

16.2.1.3 Rectal administration

THC-hemisuccinate had the highest (13.5%) THC bioavailability in monkeys among different suppository formulations maximizing bioavailability and reducing first-pass hepatic THC metabolism (Huestis 2005). Following 10–15 mg oral Marinol® for spasticity, plasma THC concentrations peaked after 1–8 h at 2.1–16.9 micrograms/L. Rectal 2.5–5 mg THC hemisuccinate suppositories produced maximum 1.1–4.1 micrograms/L plasma concentrations in 2–8 h. Rectal bioavailability was approximately twice that of the oral route.

16.2.1.4 Sublingual and dermal administration

Cannabis sativa plant extracts containing different cannabinoids with different effects are available or being developed as pharmacotherapies (see section 16.6). These preparations are administered by the sublingual route to reduce toxicity associated with smoked cannabis, and to reduce first-pass metabolism. Extract efficacy is being evaluated for analgesia, migraine relief, and spasticity among other indications.

Low (5.4 mg THC and 5.0 mg CBD) and high (16.2 mg THC and 15.0 mg CBD) oromucosal Sativex® (GW Pharma, Salisbury, England) was compared to 5 and 15 mg synthetic oral THC in a randomized, controlled, double-blind study in nine occasional cannabis smokers (Karschner et al. 2011a, 2011b). CBD, THC, 11-hydroxy-THC, and THCCOOH were quantified in plasma by two-dimensional gas chromatography mass spectrometry (2D-GCMS). There were significant differences (p <0.05) in the plasma THC C_{max} and areas under the curve (AUC) from 0–10.5 h postdose for all analytes between low and high doses for both medications. Similar absorption occurred with mean ± SE relative bioavailabilities of 92.6 ± 13.1% for 5 and 15 mg oral THC and 98.8 ± 11.0% for low- and high-dose Sativex®, respectively. This study demonstrated similar bioavailabilities for Sativex® and oral THC. In addition, there were no significant differences in THC effects with or without equivalent CBD and no significant pharmacokinetic interactions between THC and CBD at the administered doses and 1:1 THC:CBD ratio.

16.2.2 **Distribution**

THC concentrations decrease rapidly after smoking due to distribution into tissues, hepatic metabolism, and urinary and fecal excretion. THC is highly lipophilic and rapidly taken up by highly perfused tissues, such as lung, heart, brain, and liver. It is estimated that 2–22 mg THC is necessary to produce pharmacological effects in humans (Huestis 2005). Assuming 10–25% smoked THC bioavailability, 0.2–4.4 mg THC is the required smoked dose, with about 1% or 2–44 micrograms THC in brain at peak concentration. Equilibration between blood and tissue THC occurred approximately 6 h after an i.v. THC dose. When 200 micrograms/kg intrajugular THC was administered to pigs, blood terminal half-life was 10.6 h and volume of distribution (V_d) 32 L/kg, much larger than found in humans (Brunet et al. 2006). The authors observed that the pig had a higher percentage of body fat which may contribute to the larger V_d but believed the model yielded valuable data to assist in interpretation of human cannabinoid results. THC concentrations 0.5 h after 200 micrograms/kg intrajugular THC were blood 24, kidney 272, heart 178, lung 1888, muscle 55, spleen 34, fat 91, liver 155, brain 49, bile 0.4, and vitreous humor 1.2 micrograms/kg. THC was eliminated fastest from liver and was unmeasureable after 6 h (<5 micrograms/kg). THC concentrations decreased more slowly in brain than blood, but at 6 h were only 9% of those at 0.5 h. Fat had the highest THC retention, with detection beyond 24 h. 11-OH-THC was only found in liver, and THCCOOH was less than or equal to 5 micrograms/kg in most tissues.

In a study of 25 frequent, long-term cannabis smokers (12 males, 13 females), investigators found that blood THC concentrations persisted for multiple days after cannabis discontinuation (Karschner et al. 2009). Blood was collected during 7 days of monitored cannabis abstinence. Nine subjects (36%) had no measurable THC; 16 had at least one positive THC of at least 0.25 micrograms/L, but not necessarily on the first day. On day 7, six participants still had detectable THC concentrations (mean ± SD, 0.3 ± 0.7 micrograms/L) and all 25 had measurable THCCOOH

(6.2 ± 8.8 micrograms/L). Five participants, all female, had THC-positive blood specimens over all 7 days. The authors re-emphasize that THC distributed to lipid stores in chronic cannabis users can be released into blood over many days.

THC metabolism to 11-OH-THC, THCCOOH, and phase II metabolites also contributes to THC reduction in blood. When tritiated i.v. THC and 11-OH-THC pharmacodynamics and pharmacokinetics were compared, equal doses produced equal psychoactive effects, but the onset of effects and removal from the intravascular compartment was more rapid for 11-OH-THC (Huestis 2005). The earlier results suggest that 11-OH-THC diffuses into human brain more readily than THC and that plasma protein binding of 11-OH-THC is lower than for THC. Additional information about THC distribution from earlier studies include:

- Steady state V_d is about 3.4 L/kg.

- Less highly perfused tissues accumulate THC more slowly and release it over a longer period of time.

- THC stored in fat in chronic frequent cannabis smokers can be released into blood for days.

Because the degree of tolerance development following chronic frequent cannabis administration and the underlying mechanisms for tolerance were unclear, Gorelick et al. (2012) studied the development of tolerance following around-the-clock (every 3.5–6 h) 20 mg oral synthetic THC in 13 male daily cannabis smokers: 40 mg day 1; 100 mg days 2–4; and 120 mg days 5–7. Systolic and diastolic blood pressure, heart rate, and symptoms of subjective intoxication (100 mm visual analogue scales) were assessed on the morning of day 1 (before oral THC), and on days 2, 4, and 6, every 30 min for 3 h after the first THC dose. Morning subjective intoxication ratings increased from days 1 to 2, and then declined on days 4 and 6. The morning THC dose increased intoxication ratings on day 2, but had less effect on days 4 and 6, a pattern consistent with tolerance. THC lowered blood pressure and increased heart rate over 6 days. Plasma THC and 11-OH-THC increased significantly over the first 5 dosing days reaching mean C_{max} of 30 and 15 micrograms/L on day 5. Six days of around-the-clock, oral THC produced tolerance to subjective intoxication, but not to cardiovascular effects.

THC rapidly crosses the placenta, although concentrations are lower in fetal blood and tissues than in maternal plasma and tissues (Huestis 2005). THC metabolites, 11-OH-THC and THCCOOH, cross the placenta much less efficiently, and it is probable that THCCOOH does not pass from mother to fetus by placental transfer. THC in human umbilical cord blood is three to six times lower than in maternal blood, with greater transfer to the fetus early in pregnancy. THC also concentrates into breast milk from maternal plasma due to its high lipophilicity.

16.2.3 **Metabolism**

THC metabolizes primarily to 11-OH-THC, THCCOOH and glucuronide conjugates. THC hydroxylation at C9 by hepatic cytochrome P450 2C9, 2C19, and 3A4 enzymes produces the equipotent metabolite, 11-OH-THC, originally thought to be the true psychoactive analyte. More than 100 di- and tri-hydroxy, ketone, aldehyde, and carboxylic acid THC metabolites have been identified. Significant 8β-OH-THC and lower 8α-OH-THC concentrations also have been detected. Some important facts (Huestis 2005) regarding THC metabolism are:

- Plasma concentrations of 11-OH-THC following smoking are about 10% those of THC.

- Plasma concentrations of 11-OH-THC after oral ingestion are approximately equal to those of THC.

- THCCOOH-glucuronide is the principal Phase II metabolite.

- Plasma THCCOOH concentrations are greater than those of THC 30–45 min after smoking and 1 h after oral ingestion (dronabinol) for occasional cannabis users.
- There is no significant difference in metabolism between men and women.
- There is large intra- and intersubject variability in the concentration profile of plasma THC and metabolites.
- THC is primarily metabolized in the liver but additional drug is metabolized in other tissues including brain, intestine and lung.
- After occasional cannabis users smoked 16 and 30 mg THC cigarettes, mean (range) plasma THCCOOH C_{max} were 24.5 micrograms/L (15–54) and 54.0 micrograms/L (22–101), respectively (Huestis et al. 1992).

The previously cited study by Schwope et al. (2011a, 2011b) described blood and plasma concentration time profiles for THC, 11-OH-THC, THCCOOH, CBD, CBN, THC-glucuronide and THCCOOH-glucuronide following smoking of a 6.8% THC cigarette (Fig. 16.2). This study demonstrated that within hours THCCOOH-glucuronide, a more water soluble metabolite that is more readily excreted, is the major metabolite in blood and plasma. THCCOOH-glucuronide can be detected in blood for many hours, but can dissociate into free THCCOOH, especially when stored in blood outside the body at room temperature (Skopp and Potsch 2004).

16.2.4 Elimination

Within 5 days, 80–90% of a THC dose is excreted, primarily as hydroxylated and carboxylated metabolites (Huestis 2005). More than 65% is excreted in feces, with approximately 25% in urine. Of the many acidic urinary metabolites, THCCOOH glucuronide is primary, while 11-OH-THC predominates in feces. Some important facts (Huestis 2005) about THC elimination from the human body include the following:

- Elimination half-life for THC is nonlinear with a terminal half-life of about 4.1 days.
- Plasma THCCOOH and THCCOOH-glucuronide terminal elimination half-lives in frequent cannabis smokers were, respectively, 5.2 and 6.8 days and 6.2 and 3.7 days in occasional smokers.
- Urinary THCCOOH concentrations drop rapidly until approximately 20–50 micrograms/L, then are eliminated with a terminal half-life of about 3–4 days.
- The percent of a smoked THC dose excreted in urine over 7 days is about 0.54%.
- Detection times in urine after smoking a 3.55% THC cigarette with a 15 micrograms/L urine THCCOOH cutoff concentration is 2–5 days for occasional cannabis smokers but can extend to weeks in chronic daily cannabis smokers.

There is much less THC elimination data for chronic compared to occasional cannabis smokers. In view of this limitation, Lowe et al. (2009) monitored 33 chronic, daily cannabis smokers who abstained from drug use and resided on a secure unit under 24 h/day continuous medical surveillance for up to 30 days. Urine specimens were quantified for total THC, 11-OH-THC, and THCCOOH (LOQ = 0.25 micrograms/L) after tandem *Escherichia coli* β-glucuronidase and alkaline hydrolysis. This method efficiently hydrolyzes ester THCCOOH glucuronide linkages; enzymatic methods do not completely hydrolyze THCCOOH glucuronides in urine, yielding only about 50% free drug, while a combination of *Escherichia coli* β-glururonidase followed by 10N NaOH hydrolysis produced the most effective release of THC, 11-OH-THC and THCCOOH from their glucuronides (Abraham et al. 2007). Conversion of THC glucuronide to THC in urine was 90.4% but the tandem hydrolysis method in plasma produced poor chromatography and could not be utilized (Schwilke et al. 2009). Extended THC and 11-OH-THC excretion was observed by Lowe et al. (2009); 14 participants had measurable urine THC for at least 24 h after abstinence initiation. Seven of these were THC-positive for more than 3 days, 5 of these positive for 3–7 days, one for 12 days, and one for 24 days. 11-OH-THC and THCCOOH were detected in urine from one chronic frequent cannabis smoker for at least 24 days. These data document long detection windows for THC and 11-OH-THC in urine, as well as THCCOOH in urine from chronic cannabis smokers. Our new LCMSMS methods circumvent hydrolysis by directly quantifying THC, 11-OH-THC, THCCOOH, CBD, CBN, THC-glucuronide and THCCOOH-glucuronide in 1.0 mL whole blood or plasma (Schwope et al. 2011a) and 0.5 mL of urine (Scheidweiler et al. 2012). These methods should facilitate investigations of the disposition and identity of urinary cannabinoids.

16.3 Cannabinoids in oral fluid

OF is a suitable specimen for monitoring cannabinoid exposure and has applications in driving under the influence of drugs (DUID) investigations, drug treatment, workplace, pain management and forensic drug testing, and in clinical trials (Bosker and Huestis 2009). OF is easily and noninvasively collected, is gender neutral for a directly observed collection reducing adulteration potential, and basic drugs are present in OF in higher concentrations than in blood due to ion trapping in the more acidic OF environment. These characteristics provide advantages over blood and urine testing. Limitations include small sample volume, dry mouth after stimulant intake, potential contamination from smoking, and the need for high sensitivity analytical instrumentation. The Substance Abuse Mental Health Services Administration (SAMHSA) in the US is currently evaluating OF for federally mandated workplace drug testing (Substance Abuse and Mental Health Services Administration 2011). The European Union Roadside Testing Assessment (ROSITA) and DRUID studies demonstrated that OF was an acceptable matrix and identified collection devices that performed well (Houwing et al. 2013; Langel et al. 2008; Steinmeyer et al. 2001); currently, many European countries and Australia routinely utilize OF for DUID testing (Chu et al. 2012; Verstraete 2005).

Cannabinoid presence in OF primarily derives from THC depots in the mouth created by THC absorbed from THC-laden cannabis smoke (Huestis 2005). The first OF specimen collected immediately after smoking contains large amounts of THC (approximately 5800 micrograms/L) that fell to concentrations near 80 micrograms/L by 0.3 h. Initially, investigators believed that cannabis smoke was the only source of OF THC because cannabinoid metabolites could not be identified in studies using radiolabeled-THC or GCMS with an LOQ of 0.5 micrograms/L. As scientists developed methods for THCCOOH at ng/L detection limits, THCCOOH concentrations were 10–142 ng/L in 21 of 26 OF specimens previously reported THC-positive (Day et al. 2006). In the same year, Moore et al. (2006a, 2006b) validated the Quantisal™ collection device reporting 80% THCCOOH recovery, and examined 143 OF specimens previously THC-positive. Ninety-five (66.4%) were positive for THC and THCCOOH, 14 (9.7%) for THCCOOH only, and 27 (18.8%) for THC only (THC LOQ = 1 micrograms/L; THCCOOH LOQ = 2 ng/L). The physicochemical properties of THC and THCCOOH result in adherence of these cannabinoids to collection devices (Huestis et al. 2011). THC recovery from nine collection devices ranged from 12.5–85.4% (Langel et al. 2008). Addition of elution buffers to collection devices improved recoveries to greater than 90% in some collectors and stabilized labile OF analytes, potentially explaining inconsistencies in earlier reports (Bosker and Huestis 2009).

OF collection and analytical procedures improved over time. A series of controlled cannabinoid administration studies characterized OF cannabinoids pharmcokinetics (Bosker and Huestis 2009; Coulter et al. 2012; Desrosiers et al. 2012; Lee et al. 2012a; Milman et al. 2010). We measured THC, CBD, CBN, and THCCOOH disposition in ten chronic cannabis smokers' OF collected with a Quantisal™ device after each smoked a 6.8% THC cigarette (Lee et al. 2012a). Cannabinoids were quantified by 2D-GCMS (LOQ = 0.5, 0.5, 1, 0.0075 micrograms/L, respectively). OF samples (n = 86) were examined 0.5 h before and 0.25, 0.5, 1, 2, 3, 4, 6, and 22 h after smoking initiation. Before smoking, four and nine participants' OF samples were positive for THC and THCCOOH, respectively, but none were CBD or CBN positive. Maximum THC, CBD, and CBN concentrations occurred within 0.5 h, with medians of 644, 30.4, and 49.0 micrograms/L, respectively. All samples were THC positive at 6 h (2.1–44.4 micrograms/L), and four of six were positive at 22 h. CBD and CBN were positive only up to 6 h in three (0.6–2.1 micrograms/L) and four (1.0–4.4 micrograms/L) participants, respectively. Median OF THCCOOH C_{max} was 115 ng/L, with all samples positive to 6 h (14.8–263 ng/L) and five of six positive at 22 h. By quantifying multiple cannabinoids and evaluating eight alternative cutoff concentrations, windows of drug detection were determined, markers of recent smoking suggested, and passive contamination minimized.

Passive contamination of OF may occur when individuals are exposed to cannabis smoke. Identifying and quantifying THCCOOH in OF would rule out passive contamination, since it is not present in cannabis smoke. To investigate this issue, OF was collected from ten nonsmokers in a Dutch coffee shop where others smoked (Moore et al. 2011). THC was positive in all OF specimens collected 3 h after passive exposure to smoke (LOQ = 0.5 micrograms/L), with five subjects' OF THC exceeding 4 micrograms/L, the current recommended cutoff concentration for immunoassay screening. Seventy percent (70%) of specimens exceeded 2 micrograms/L THC, the recommended confirmation cutoff concentration. No THCCOOH was found at an LOQ = 2 ng/L.

Around-the-clock escalating 20 mg oral THC doses (40–120 mg/day) were administered for 8 days to ten daily cannabis smokers (Milman et al. 2011a, 2011b). Expectorated and Quantisal™ OF samples (n = 440 each) were analyzed by 2D-GCMS with a 7.5 ng/L THCCOOH LOQ and 0.5 micrograms/L for other cannabinoids (Milman et al. 2010). For Quantisal™ specimens, THCCOOH was the most prevalent analyte in 432 samples (98.2%), with concentrations up to 1117.9 ng/L. 11-OH-THC was not identified in any sample, while CBD and CBN were in three and eight samples, respectively, with maximum concentrations of 2.1 and 13 micrograms/L. THC was present in only 20.7% of samples, with highest concentrations near admission (median 4.2 micrograms/L, range 0.6–481.9), as was true for expectorated OF from previously self-administered smoked cannabis. Expectorated specimens gave similar results in specimens analyzed within 24 h to reduce analyte instability.

OF and plasma THC and THCCOOH concentrations in these chronic daily cannabis smokers were compared (Fig. 16.3) (Milman et al. 2011a). THC and THCCOOH plasma LOQs were 0.25 micrograms/L, and 0.5 micrograms/L for 11-OH-THC. Despite multiple oral THC administrations each day and increasing plasma THC concentrations, OF THC concentrations generally decreased over time, reflecting primarily, previously self-administered smoked cannabis. Log THC concentrations in OF and plasma were not significantly correlated (r = −0.10; P = 0.065). OF and plasma THCCOOH concentrations, albeit with 1000-fold higher concentrations in plasma, increased throughout dosing. Log OF and plasma THCCOOH concentrations were significantly correlated (r = 0.63; P <0.001), but there was high interindividual variation. A high OF/plasma THC ratio and a high OF THC/THCCOOH ratio indicated recent cannabis smoking. These data document that OF does not reliably detect oral THC ingestion and OF THC concentrations do not predict concurrent plasma concentrations after oral THC.

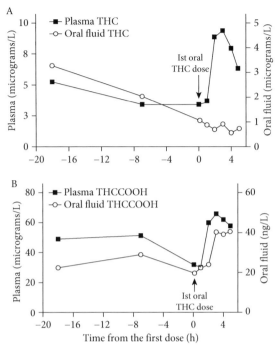

Fig. 16.3 Median (n = 10) (A) Δ^9-tetrahydrocannabinol (THC) in plasma (■) and oral fluid (○) and (B) 11-nor-9-carboxy-THC (THCCOOH) in plasma (■) and oral fluid (○) time course following previously self-administered smoked cannabis and the first 20 mg oral THC dose. Times are based on first THC administration.

Reproduced from Garry Milman, David M. Schwope, Eugene W. Schwilke, William D. Darwin, Deanna L. Kelly, Robert S. Goodwin, David A. Gorelick, and Marilyn A. Huestis, Oral Fluid and Plasma Cannabinoid Ratios after Around-the-Clock Controlled Oral Δ9-Tetrahydrocannabinol Administration, *Clinical Chemistry*, 57 (11), pp. 1597–1606 (c) 2011, American Association for Clinical Chemistry, with permission. doi: 10.1373/clinchem.2011.169490.

OF THC, CBD, CBN, and THCCOOH for up to 10.5 h following 5 and 15 mg synthetic oral THC and low- (5.4 mg THC, 5.0 mg CBD) and high-doe (16.2 mg THC, 15.0 mg CBD) Sativex® were determined in 14 occasional cannabis smokers (Fig. 16.4) (Lee et al. 2013). After oral THC, OF THC concentrations decreased over time from baseline, reflecting residual THC excretion from previously self-administered smoked cannabis. Also, CBD and CBN were rarely detected. After Sativex®, THC, CBD and CBN increased greatly, peaking at 0.25–1 h. Median CBD/THC and CBN/THC ratios were 0.82–1.34 and 0.04–0.06, respectively, reflecting the cannabinoid composition of Sativex®. THCCOOH/THC ratios within 4.5 h post Sativex® were 1.6 ng/mg or lower, always lower than after oral THC. THCCOOH/THC ratios increased throughout each session. Cannabinoid concentrations and ratios were compared to those following smoking of a 6.8% THC cigarette. This study demonstrated that OF could monitor compliance with Sativex® therapy.

OF is the most promising biological matrix for roadside DUID testing (Huestis et al. 2011); however, onsite tests previously lacked the sensitivity to detect cannabis smoking. This was a major problem, as cannabis is the primary illicit drug reported in DUID surveys, and motor vehicle accidents and fatalities (Drummer et al. 2004; Lacey et al. 2009; Mann et. al. 2008). Recently, the Draeger DrugTest® 5000 OF device was evaluated with OF samples collected 0.5 h before and

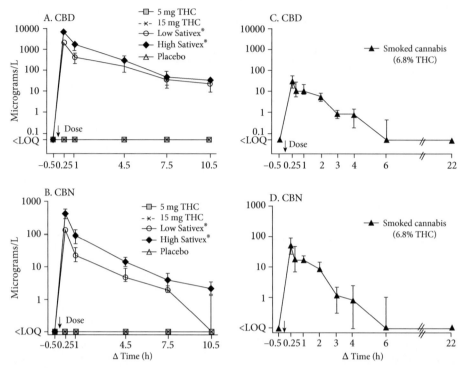

Fig. 16.4 Median cannabidiol (CBD; A) and cannabinol (CBN; B) oral fluid concentrations after 5 and 15 mg Δ^9-tetrahydrocannabinol (THC), low-dose (5.4 mg THC + 5 mg CBD) and high-dose (16.2 mg THC + 15 mg CBD) oromucosal Sativex®, and placebo. Panels C and D show median CBD and CBN time courses, respectively, after smoking one cannabis cigarette with 6.8% THC for comparison. Error bars indicate interquartile ranges.

Reprinted from *Drug and Alcohol Dependence*, 130 (1–3), Dayong Lee, Erin L. Karschner, Garry Milman, Allan J. Barnes, Robert S. Goodwin, Marilyn A. Huestis, Can oral fluid cannabinoid testing monitor medication compliance and/or cannabis smoking during oral THC and oromucosal Sativex administration?, pp. 68–76, Copyright (2013), with permission from Elsevier.

up to 22 h after ten chronic cannabis users smoked a 6.8% THC cigarette (Desrosiers et al. 2012). 2D-GCMS was utilized to quantify THC, THCCOOH, CBD, and CBN concentrations in simultaneously collected Quantisal™ OF samples (Lee et al. 2012). Diagnostic sensitivity, specificity, and efficiency at the DrugTest® 5000's 5 micrograms/L screening cutoff and various THC confirmation cutoffs were 86.2–90.7, 75.0–77.8, and 84.8–87.9%, respectively. Last detection times were greater than 22 h at the LOQ, longer than previously suggested. THCCOOH confirmation minimized the potential for passive OF contamination and provided 22 h windows of detection. These data document that an onsite OF testing device can sensitively and specifically identify cannabis smoking at the roadside and in the workplace.

OF THC concentrations generally correlate with plasma concentrations and with pharmacodynamic effects; however, inter- and intrasubject variability precludes calculating a blood or plasma concentration from an OF concentration (Milman et al. 2011a). Enforcement of drugged driving legislation with OF testing should be supported by laws that specifically permit OF specimens for screening and confirmation of drug use, or define OF screening, followed by confirmation of presumptive positive tests with blood collection and analysis.

It is important to compare OF testing to established urine testing methods. OF results (Intercept®) collection) were compared to urine results from ten subjects who smoked a 20–25 mg THC cannabis cigarette (Huestis 2005). Specimens were screened by enzyme immunoassay with a 1.0 microgram/L cutoff and confirmed for THC by gas chromatography tandem mass spectrometry (GCMSMS) at 0.5 micrograms/L. OF specimens were not analyzed for THCCOOH due to technology limitations. Urine specimens were tested for THCCOOH by enzyme immunoassay at 50 micrograms/L and confirmed by GCMS at 15 micrograms/L. With these cutoffs, OF THC was consistently positive for approximately 13 h (1–24) by GCMSMS, followed by interspersed negative and positive specimens. Mean THC detection times for the last positive OF specimen were 34 ± 11 (1–72) h. By comparison, THCCOOH appeared much later, after 4 h, in urine with mean detection times of 58 ± 6 (16–72) h. A subsequent study of 77,218 OF specimens tested for drugs of abuse in a commercial laboratory with immunoassay screening and confirmation cutoff concentrations of 3 and 1.5 micrograms/L THC, respectively, reported a 3.2% cannabinoids detection rate. This positive rate was similar to that of urine specimens tested from different donors with SAMHSA screening and confirmation cutoff concentrations of 50 micrograms/L and 15 micrograms/L THCCOOH (Cone et al. 2002).

16.4 **Cannabinoids in sweat**

To date, there are no published data on cannabinoids excretion in sweat following controlled THC or cannabis administration. Sweat testing monitors cannabis use in drug treatment, criminal justice, workplace drug testing, and clinical programs (Huestis 2005). Currently, there is a single commercially available sweat collection device, the PharmCheck patch, offered by PharmChem Laboratories, Inc. (Fort Worth, Texas, US). The patch is exchanged for a new one once each week during treatment or parole officer visits. As for OF testing, this is a developing new technology with much to be learned about cannabinoid sweat excretion pharmacokinetics, potential THC reabsorption by the skin, possible THC degradation on the patch, and THC adsorption onto the patch collection device. THC is the primary analyte detected in sweat, with little 11-OH-THC or THCCOOH. THC (4–38 ng/patch) was identified in 20 known heroin abusers who wore the PharmChek patch for 5 days during detoxification (Huestis 2005). Forehead swipes with cosmetic pads monitored sweat cannabinoids in motorists suspected of DUID. THC, but no 11-OH-THC or THCCOOH, was detected (4–152 ng/pad) in the sweat of 16 of 22 individuals testing positive for urine cannabinoids. Cannabinoids were quantified in sweat from 11 chronic daily cannabis smokers during 4 weeks of monitored sustained abstinence (Huestis et al. 2008). Sweat patches worn the first week had THC at least 1 ng/patch with a mean ± SE of 3.9 ± 0.9 ng/patch. In week 2, eight of 11 had negative weekly patches; one subject produced THC positive patches (>0.4 ng/patch) for 4 weeks. After oral 14.8 mg THC/day doses for 5 days, no patches were THC-positive, while THC in concurrently collected plasma samples were positive but with concentrations less than 6.1 micrograms/L.

16.5 **Cannabinoids in hair**

Multiple mechanisms contribute to cannabinoid incorporation into hair including diffusion from capillaries surrounding the hair bulb, from sebum secreted onto the hair shaft, from sweat excreted onto hair above the skin surface, and from environmental drug contamination. Cannabis is primarily smoked, providing an opportunity for environmental contamination of hair with THC in cannabis smoke. Basic drugs such as cocaine and methamphetamine concentrate in hair due to ionic bonding to melanin, the pigment in hair that determines hair color. The more neutral and lipophilic THC is not highly bound to melanin, resulting in much lower THC concentrations in hair compared to other drugs of abuse. Usually THC is present in hair at higher concentrations than THCCOOH (Huestis 2005). Despite the low concentrations, the advantage of measuring THCCOOH in hair is the same as for OF testing, THCCOOH is not present in cannabis smoke, avoiding the issue of passive exposure from the environment. Analysis of cannabinoids in hair is challenging due to the high analytical sensitivity required to quantify femtograms to picograms THCCOOH per mg hair; GCMSMS provides acceptable sensitivity.

It is difficult to conduct controlled studies on cannabinoid disposition in hair because of the inability to differentiate administered from previously self-administered cannabis. One solution would be administration of isotopically labeled drug but to date there have been no such studies. Hair testing advantages include a wide window of drug detection (months), a less invasive specimen collection procedure, and the ability to collect a later second specimen. However, one of the weakest aspects of cannabinoids hair testing is the low sensitivity of drug detection in this alternative matrix. Only about one-third of nondaily smokers and two-thirds of daily smokers had positive GCMSMS cannabinoid hair tests with LOD = 1 microgram/g for THC and 0.1 micrograms/g for THCCOOH (Huestis et al. 2007). All participants had positive urine cannabinoid tests at the time of hair collection.

In another study of 12 daily cannabis smokers and ten nonsmokers, at least one of the cannabinoids, THC, CBN, CBD (LOQ = 0.1 micrograms/g), was found in daily smokers' hair and none in nonsmokers' head hair (Skopp et al. 2007). THC concentrations did not correlate with self-reported dose, but the sum of THC, CBD, and CBN correlated with estimated total cannabis dose over 3 months (r = 0.71, p = 0.014).

Hair from 412 self-reported cannabis smokers contained THCCOOH 0.06–33.4 ng/g hair (LOQ = 0.05 ng/g) for those with a positive urine cannabinoid test and 0.05–7.2 ng/g for those whose urine was negative (Han et al. 2011a, 2011b, 2011c). The hair root bulb had higher THCCOOH concentrations than the hair shaft, and pubic hair had higher concentrations than head hair. Cannabinoids remain in hair for months to years, although decreasing concentrations are usually noted farther from the scalp, due to normal hygiene and ultraviolet degradation of drugs.

16.6 Cannabidiol pharmacokinetics

CBD is a nonpsychoactive natural constituent of *Cannabis sativa* that possesses pharmacological activity of interest for therapeutic applications. CBD has neuroprotective, analgesic, sedating, antiemetic, antispasmodic, and anti-inflammatory effects (Huestis 2005). In addition, CBD reportedly blocks anxiety produced by THC and is useful in autoimmune disease treatment. CBD pharmacokinetic studies are warranted by these potential therapeutic applications and needed resolution of the controversy over whether CBD alters THC pharmacokinetics.

CBD metabolism is similar to THC's, with primary oxidation of C9 to the hydroxy and carboxylic acid moieties and side chain oxidation. Like THC, CBD is subjected to a significant first-pass effect; however, unlike THC a large proportion is excreted unchanged in the feces. Most in vitro studies support that CBD does not affect THC pharmacokinetics (Huestis 2005).

Sativex®, the prescription drug derived from cannabis-based medicinal extracts, contains approximately 1:1 THC and CBD. Sativex® effectiveness is being evaluated in Phase 3 trials as an adjunct to opioid therapy for cancer pain. Few adverse side effects were observed. A controlled administration study comparing Sativex® to oral THC administration confirmed that CBD did not modulate THC effects through pharmacokinetic mechanisms, except for a slightly slower conversion of 11-OH-THC to THCCOOH (Fig. 16.5) (Karschner et al. 2011a, 2011b). CBD coadministration did not significantly affect total clearance, V_d and THC metabolites' terminal

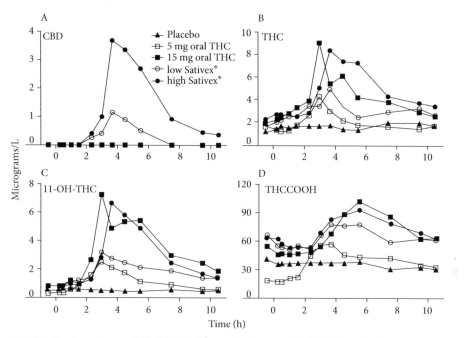

Fig. 16.5 Median (n = 9) cannabidiol (CBD), Δ^9-tetrahydrocannabinol (THC), 11-hydroxy-THC (11-OH-THC), and 11-nor-9-carboxy-THC (THCCOOH) plasma concentrations following controlled administration of placebo, 5 and 15 mg oral THC and low-dose (5.4 mg THC + 5 mg CBD) and high-dose (16.2 mg THC + 15 mg CBD) oromucosal Sativex®.

Reproduced from Erin L. Karschner, W. David Darwin, Robert S. Goodwin, Stephen Wright and Marilyn A. Huestis, Plasma Cannabinoid Pharmacokinetics following Controlled Oral Δ9-Tetrahydrocannabinol and Oromucosal Cannabis Extract Administration, *Clinical Chemistry*, 57 (1), pp. 66–75 (c) 2010, American Association for Clinical Chemistry, with permission. doi: 10.1373/clinchem.2010.152439.

elimination half-lives at this 1:1 ratio. CBD bioavailability following smoking averaged 31% (range 11–45%) as compared to intravenously administered drug (Huestis 2005).

Similar results were obtained when comparing sublingual administration of 25 mg THC to a combination of 25 mg THC and 25 mg CBD in cannabis-based medicinal extracts (Huestis 2005). There were no statistically significant differences in mean THC C_{max}, half-life, AUC for THC, and 11-OH-THC when CBD was coadministered with THC. The only statistically significant difference was a later time for maximum THC concentration. Despite administration of equivalent THC and CBD amounts, lower plasma CBD concentrations were always observed. In a separate evaluation of 10 mg THC and 10 mg CBD from a cannabis-based medicine extract, THC, 11-OH-THC and CBD pharmacokinetics were determined after sublingual, buccal, and oropharyngeal and oral administration. All three analytes were measurable 30 min after dosing, with higher THC than CBD concentrations. 11-OH-THC generally exceeded THC concentrations within 45 min. Mean THC, CBD, and 11-OH-THC C_{max} values were less than 5, less than 2, and less than 7 micrograms/L across all administration routes. High intra- and intersubject variability was noted.

CBD and CBN C_{max} in blood (1.3, 2.4 micrograms/L) and plasma (2.0, 3.6 micrograms/L) were determined in ten subjects after smoking 6.8% THC cigarettes containing 0.25% CBD and 0.21% CBN; these analytes were not detectable (LOQ = 1.0 micrograms/L) 1 h post dose (Schwope et al.

2011a). CBD and CBN in blood identified recent cannabis smoking, but were inclusionary, not exclusionary, as these analytes were not present in some subjects at all after cannabis smoking. Simultaneous OF maximum THC, CBD, and CBN concentrations occurred within 0.5 h of smoking initiation, with medians of 644, 30.4, and 49.0 micrograms/L, respectively (Lee et al. 2012b).

16.7 **Cannabinol pharmacokinetics**

CBN is a natural constituent of *Cannabis sativa* with approximately 10% of THC's activity (Huestis 2005). CBN metabolism is similar to THC's with hydroxylation of C9 as the primary mode of metabolism. Due to one additional aromatic ring, CBN is metabolized less extensively and slower than THC. The average bioavailability of a smoked CBN dose, as compared to i.v. administration, was 41% with a range of 8–77%.

16.8 **Interpretation of cannabinoid concentrations in biological fluids**

16.8.1 **Prediction models using blood and plasma for estimation of cannabis exposure**

There continues to be controversy in the interpretation of blood cannabinoid results but some general concepts have wide support. There is a dose–concentration relationship for smoked THC and THC plasma concentrations (Huestis 2005). It is well established that peak effects appear rapidly after smoking initiation, that plasma THC concentrations decline prior to the time for peak effects, and that THC and THCCOOH concentrations reach equivalency within 30–45 min after smoking initiation. Recent exposure (6–8 h) and possible impairment are linked to plasma THC concentrations in excess of 2–3 micrograms/L in occasional cannabis smokers. Interpretation is complicated by intra- and intersubject variability, variation in blood/plasma ratios (usually about 0.5), and by residual THC and THCCOOH concentrations found in blood of frequent cannabis smokers (Karschner et al. 2009).

Accurate prediction of time of last cannabis exposure provides valuable information in establishing the role of cannabis as a contributing factor to events under investigation. Two mathematical models were developed for prediction of time of last cannabis use from analysis of a single plasma specimen for cannabinoids (Huestis 2005). Model I is based on THC concentrations and Model II on the ratio of THCCOOH to THC in plasma. Both correctly predict exposure times within a 95% confidence interval (CI) for more than 90% of specimens evaluated. The models were validated following different routes of administration, smoking multiple cannabis cigarettes and plasma concentrations as low as 0.5 micrograms/L (Huestis 2005; Huestis et al. 2005, 2006). Each model predicted the range of time when cannabis was smoked or otherwise ingested with 95% CI established by a calculated upper and lower time. An important finding was that a more accurate prediction of time of last cannabis use was obtained by using the time interval defined by the lowest and highest times from both Models I and II. Also, inaccurate predictions were all overestimates of the actual time interval; there were no underestimates which might adversely affect the blood donor by falsely determining that he was impaired.

The models' accuracy in predicting time of last cannabis use in blood and plasma samples from ten chronic daily cannabis smokers receiving escalating doses of THC (40–120 mg) daily for 8 days was examined (Karschner et al. 2012). Predictive models accurately estimated last cannabis exposure in 96% and 100% of specimens collected within 1–5 h after a single oral THC dose and throughout multiple dosing, respectively. However, the models were only 60% and 12.5% accurate

12.5 and 22.5h after the last THC dose, respectively, in chronic daily cannabis smokers who had large residual THCCOOH concentrations.

Trying to predict time of last cannabis use for chronic daily cannabis smokers is a special challenge, and an important one, for example, when individuals are in cannabis dependence treatment, or when they are involved in motor vehicle or occupational accidents. Early studies found THC, 11-OH-THC, and THCCOOH plasma concentrations in frequent cannabis users of 0.86 $\pm$ 0.22, 0.46 $\pm$ 0.17 and 45.8 $\pm$ 13.1 micrograms/L, respectively, a minimum of 12 h after the last smoked dose (Huestis 2005). We recently had the opportunity to investigate cannabinoid excretion in chronic daily cannabis smokers during monitored sustained abstinence, required prior to administering rimonabant, the first CB_1 cannabinoid receptor antagonist. In this inpatient study, of 25 chronic daily cannabis smokers, we quantified THC in blood for 7 days of cannabis abstinence (Karschner et al. 2009). Surprisingly, blood THC concentrations decreased after 24 h, but then in some individuals remained fairly constant for 7 days, while in others negative and positive THC concentrations fluctuated over the 7 days. All five participants who were THC-positive for 7 days were females. More recently, THC, 11-OH-THC and THCCOOH (LOQ = 0.25 micrograms/L for THC and THCCOOH; 0.5 micrograms/L for 11-OH-THC) were quantified in daily blood specimens collected from 30 daily cannabis smokers during sustained abstinence over 30 days (Bergamaschi et al. 2013). Of the 30 participants, 27 were THC-positive on admission, with a median (range) concentration of 1.4 micrograms/L (0.3–6.3). THC decreased gradually; only one of 11 participants was negative at 26 days, two of five remained THC-positive (0.3 micrograms/L) for 30 days, and 5.0% of participants had THC 1.0 micrograms/L or higher for 12 days. Median 11-OH-THC concentrations were 1.1 micrograms/L on admission, with no results greater than or equal to 1.0 micrograms/L 24 h later. THCCOOH detection rates were 96.7% on admission, decreasing slowly to 95.7% and 85.7% on days 8 and 22, respectively; four of five participants remained THCCOOH positive (0.6–2.7 micrograms/L) after 30 days, and one remained positive on discharge at 33 days.

16.8.2 Interpretation of urinary cannabinoid concentrations

Urine is a popular matrix for detecting prior cannabis use because it is relatively easy to analyze and offers long detection times of days to weeks. Most current workplace drug testing, treatment, and judicial programs identify total THCCOOH in urine to detect prior cannabis ingestion. The principal question asked by those administering these programs is whether or not the worker, patient, or parolee smoked cannabis in the preceding days. However, more challenging questions arise in cannabis dependence treatment such as "Can urine cannabinoid concentrations identify smoked cannabis relapse?" One in ten individuals that smokes cannabis develops problematic cannabis usage, and as the most commonly used illicit drug, this results in cannabis treatment admissions being higher than for all other drugs of dependence except alcohol. As residual cannabinoid excretion can be more than 30 days in chronic, frequent smokers, it becomes critical to differentiate excretion following new cannabis use from residual excretion.

A model exists to answer this question based on creatinine-corrected THCCOOH concentrations (Huestis 2005). Creatinine normalization is necessary to reduce the variability in sequential urine THCCOOH concentrations due to intrinsic dilution. The model evaluates the ratio between creatinine normalized THCCOOH concentrations for a urine specimen and any preceding specimen. The original study found that the most accurate (85.4%) specimen ratio for differentiating new use from residual excretion was 0.5, i.e., a ratio higher than this value indicated new use

(Huestis 2005). This ratio provided 80.1% sensitivity, 90.2% specificity, and 5.6% false-positive and 7.4% false-negative predictions. Program managers can select a specimen ratio to obtain acceptable false-positive and false-negative results.

This model was further improved by also considering the time interval between specimens (Smith et al. 2009). A table with maximum, 95% below, and median THCCOOH/creatinine ratios was developed. For the time interval between two specimens and selected level of certainty desired, a ratio above the value in the table indicates new use.

These models were not accurate for detecting new cannabis use in daily cannabis smokers due to extended THC excretion from body stores. Since daily smokers are frequently those in treatment programs, new models were needed. Schwilke et al. (2011) developed a model with creatinine normalized THCCOOH concentrations in 48 daily cannabis smokers who resided on a closed research unit during abstinence for up to 30 days. More than 120,000 urine excretion pairs were included to develop the model. The model was validated with urine results from 67 different daily smokers who provided specimens each day for 30 days. The model developed was exponential with two parameters, initial urine specimen creatinine normalized THCCOOH concentration and the time interval between collections. Subjects were placed in groups based on their initial normalized urine THCCOOH concentration. Prediction intervals provided upper ratio limits for any urine specimen pair at a program selected probability level between 80% and 99%. Ratios above these limits suggest new use. Two additional rules were necessary to achieve high sensitivity and specificity for predicting new cannabis use. The first rule took into account that the donor may have smoked just prior to the first specimen collection, and THCCOOH urine concentrations may not have peaked, and the second rule accounted for the 8% of daily cannabis smokers whose THCCOOH/creatinine ratio was 800 ng/mg or higher in the first specimen (see Schwilke et al. 2011, for details on implementing these rules and models). The models for predicting time of cannabis ingestion that are important for interpretation of results in workplace drug testing, treatment, and judicial programs were made possible by the many thorough studies of cannabis pharmacokinetics.

16.9 **Conclusions**

Controlled cannabinoid administration studies simultaneously collecting pharmacodynamic and pharmacokinetic data provide the scientific basis for understanding mechanisms of drug action, interpreting cannabinoid results, and developing evidence-based drug policy and legislation. Current research focuses on alternative body fluids and tissues as each provides unique data about an individual's drug use history, and each offers advantages and limitations for drug testing in the many different monitoring programs. Characterizing human cannabinoid pharmacokinetics enables us to better understand the onset, peak, and duration of pharmacodynamic effects, the mechanism of drug–drug interactions, develop models that aid our interpretation of results, and comprehend the differences between acute and chronic cannabis exposure. Expanding the number of cannabinoid analytes quantified and applying different cutoff concentrations for these analytes in different alternative matrices can define windows of drug detection appropriate for achieving the goals of the drug monitoring program. For instance, workplace and pain management testing programs want the longest possible detection windows, while driving under the influence of cannabis testing would like a detection window that best matches the window of drug impairment. Treatment programs need to identify cannabis relapse between visits usually occurring between one and three times per week, so an intermediate detection window is ideal, and for antidoping monitoring, cannabis intake is only prohibited "in competition" requiring a different set of parameters. Controlled cannabinoid administration studies following different routes of drug administration to different populations of cannabis users, and monitoring the spectrum of cannabinoids present within the cannabis plant and their metabolic products provide the data required to understand cannabinoid effects, to accurately interpret cannabinoid results and to optimize cannabinoid monitoring.

Acknowledgments

Author's contribution to the Work was done as part of the Author's official duties as an NIH employee and is a Work of the United States Government. Therefore, copyright may not be established in the United States.

References

Abraham, T.T., Lowe, R.H., Pirnay, S.O., Darwin, W.D., and Huestis, M.A. (2007). Simultaneous GC-EI-MS determination of delta9-tetrahydrocannabinol, 11-hydroxy-delta9-tetrahydrocannabinol, and 11-nor-9-carboxy-delta9-tetrahydrocannabinol in human urine following tandem enzyme-alkaline hydrolysis. *Journal of Analytical Toxicology*, **31**, 477–485.

Bergamaschi, M.M., Karschner, E.L., Goodwin, R.S., *et al.* (2013). Impact of prolonged cannabinoid excretion in chronic daily cannabis smokers' blood on per se drugged driving laws. *Clinical Chemistry*, **59**, 519–526.

Bosker, W.M. and Huestis, M.A. (2009). Oral fluid testing for drugs of abuse. *Clinical Chemistry*, **55**, 1910–1931.

Brunet, B., Doucet, C., Venisse, N., *et al.* (2006). Validation of large white pig as an animal model for the study of cannabinoids metabolism: application to the study of THC distribution in tissues. *Forensic Science International*, **161**, 169–174.

Chu, M., Gerostamoulos, D., Beyer, J., Rodda, J., Boorman, M., and Drummer, O.H. (2012). The incidence of drugs of impairment in oral fluid from random roadside testing. *Forensic Science International*, **215**, 28–31.

Cone, E.J., Presley, L., Lehrer, M., *et al.* (2002). Oral fluid testing for drugs of abuse: positive prevalence rates by Intercept immunoassay screening and GC-MS-MS confirmation and suggested cutoff concentrations. *Journal of Analytical Toxicology*, **26**, 541–546.

Coulter, C., Garnier, M., and Moore, C. (2012). Analysis of tetrahydrocannabinol and its metabolite, 11-nor-delta(9)-tetrahydrocannabinol-9-carboxylic acid, in oral fluid using liquid chromatography with tandem mass spectrometry. *Journal of Analytical Toxicology*, **36**, 413–417.

Day, D., Kuntz D.J., Feldman, M., and Presley, L. (2006). Detection of THCA in oral fluid by GC-MS-MS. *Journal of Analytical Toxicology*, **30**, 645–650.

Desrosiers, N.A., Lee, D., Schwope, D.M., *et al.* (2012). On-site test for cannabinoids in oral fluid. *Clinical Chemistry*, **58**, 1418–1425.

Drummer, O.H., Gerostamoulos, J., Batziris, H., *et al.* (2004). The involvement of drugs in drivers of motor vehicles killed in Australian road traffic crashes. *Accident Analysis & Prevention*, **36**, 239–248.

Goodwin, R.S., Gustafson, R.A., Barnes, A., Nebro, A., Moolchan, E.T., and Huestis, M.A. (2006). Delta(9)-tetrahydrocannabinol, 11-hydroxy-delta(9)-tetrahydrocannabinol and 11-nor-9-carboxy-delta(9)-tetrahydrocannabinol in human plasma after controlled oral administration of cannabinoids. *Therapeutic Drug Monitoring*, **28**, 545–551.

Gorelick, D.A., Goodwin, R.S., Schwilke, E., *et al.* (2013). Tolerance to effects of high-dose oral delta9-tetrahydrocannabinol and plasma cannabinoid concentrations in male daily cannabis smokers. *Journal of Analytical Toxicology*, **37**, 11–16.

Han, E., Choi, H., Lee, S., Chung, H., and Song, J.M. (2011a). A study on the concentrations of 11-nor-delta(9)-tetrahydrocannabinol-9-carboxylic acid (THCCOOH) in hair root and whole hair. *Forensic Science International*, **210**, 201–205.

Han, E., Choi, H., Lee, S., Chung, H., and Song, J.M. (2011b). A comparative study on the concentrations of 11-nor-delta-9-tetrahydrocannabinol-9-carboxylic acid (THCCOOH) in head and pubic hair. *Forensic Science International*, **212**, 238–241.

Han, E., Park, Y., Kim, E., *et al.* (2011c). Simultaneous analysis of delta(9)-tetrahydrocannabinol and 11-nor-9-carboxy-tetrahydrocannabinol in hair without different sample preparation and derivatization by gas chromatography-tandem mass spectrometry. *Journal of Pharmaceutical and Biomedical Analysis*, **55**, 1096–1103.

Houwing, S., Hagenzieker, M., Mathissen, R.P., *et al.* (2013). Random and systematic errors in case-control studies calculating the injury risk of driving under the influence of psychoactive substances. *Accident Analysis & Prevention*, **52**, 144–153.

Huestis, M.A. (2005). Pharmacokinetics and metabolism of the plant cannabinoids. In: R.G. Pertwee (ed.). *Cannabinoids. Handbook of Experimental Pharmacology*. Vol. 168. Heidelberg: Springer-Verlag, pp. 657–690.

Huestis, M.A., Barnes, A., and Smith, M.L. (2005). Estimating the time of last cannabis use from plasma delta9-tetrahydrocannabinol and 11-nor-9-carboxy-delta9-tetrahydrocannabinol concentrations. *Clinical Chemistry*, **51**, 2289–2295.

Huestis, M.A., ElSohly, M., Nebro, W., Barnes, A., Gustafson, R.A., and Smith, M.L. (2006). Estimating time of last oral ingestion of cannabis from plasma THC and THCCOOH concentrations. *Therapeutic Drug Monitoring*, **28**, 540–544.

Huestis, M.A., Gustafson, R.A., Moolchan, E.T., *et al.* (2007). Cannabinoid concentrations in hair from documented cannabis users. *Forensic Science International*, **169**, 129–136.

Huestis, M.A., Henningfield, J.E., and Cone, E.J. (1992). Blood cannabinoids. I. Absorption of THC and formation of 11-OH-THC and THCCOOH during and after smoking marijuana. *Journal of Analytical Toxicology*, **16**, 276–282.

Huestis, M.A., Scheidweiler, K.B., Saito, T., *et al.* (2008). Excretion of delta9-tetrahydrocannabinol in sweat. *Forensic Science International*, **174**, 173–177.

Huestis, M.A., Verstraete, A., Kwong, T.C., Morland, J., Vincent, M.J., and de la Torre, R. (2011). Oral fluid testing: promises and pitfalls. *Clinical Chemistry*, **57**, 805–810.

Karschner, E.L., Darwin, W.D., Goodwin, R.S., Wright, S., and Huestis, M.A. (2011a). Plasma cannabinoid pharmacokinetics following controlled oral delta9-tetrahydrocannabinol and oromucosal cannabis extract administration. *Clinical Chemistry*, **57**, 66–75.

Karschner, E.L., Darwin, W.D., McMahon, R.P., *et al.* (2011b). Subjective and physiological effects after controlled Sativex® and oral THC administration. *Clinical Pharmacology and Therapeutics*, **89**, 400–407.

Karschner, E.L., Schwilke, E.W., Lowe, R.H., *et al.* (2009). Do delta 9-tetrahydrocannabinol concentrations indicate recent use in chronic cannabis users? *Addiction*, **104**, 2041–2048.

Karschner, E.L., Schwope, D.M., Schwilke, E.W. *et al.* (2012). Predictive model accuracy in estimating last delta9-tetrahydrocannabinol (THC) intake from plasma and whole blood cannabinoid concentrations in chronic, daily cannabis smokers administered subchronic oral THC. *Drug and Alcohol Dependence*, **125**, 313–319.

Lacey, J.H., Kelley-Baker, T., Furr-Holden, D., *et al.* (2009). *2007 National Roadside Survey of Alcohol and Drug Use by Drivers: Drug Results.* Report DOT HS 811 249. Washington, DC: National Highway Traffic Safety Administration Office of Behavioral Safety Research.

Langel, K., Engblom, C., Pehrsson, A., Gunnar, T., Ariniemi, K., and Lillsunde, P. (2008). Drug testing in oral fluid-evaluation of sample collection devices. *Journal of Analytical Toxicology*, **32**, 393–401.

Lee, D., Karschner, E.L., Milman, G., Barnes, A.J., Goodwin, R.S., and Huestis, M.A. (2013). Can oral fluid cannabinoid testing monitor medication compliance and/or cannabis smoking during oral THC and oromucosal Sativex® administration? *Drug Alcohol Dependence*, **130**(1–3), 68–76.

Lee, D., Milman, G., Schwope, D.M., Barnes, A.J., Gorelick, D.A., and Huestis, M.A. (2012a). Cannabinoid stability in authentic oral fluid after controlled cannabis smoking. *Clinical Chemistry*, **58**(7), 1101–1109.

Lee, D., Schwope, D.M., Milman, G., Barnes, A.J., Gorelick, D.A., and Huestis, M.A. (2012b). Cannabinoid disposition in oral fluid after controlled smoked cannabis. *Clinical Chemistry*, **58**(4), 748–756.

Lowe, R.H., Abraham, T.T., Darwin, W.D., Herning, R., Cadet, J.L., and Huestis, M.A. (2009). Extended urinary delta 9-tetrahydrocannabinol excretion in chronic cannabis users precludes use as a biomarker of new drug exposure. *Drug and Alcohol Dependence*, **105**(1–2), 24–32.

Mann, R.E., Stoduto, G., Macdonald, S., and Brands, B. (2008). Cannabis use and driving: implications for public health and transport policy. *European Monitoring Centre for Drugs and Drug Addiction (EMCDDA)*, **2**, 171–198.

Milman, G., Barnes, A.J., Lowe, R.H., and Huestis, M.A. (2010). Simultaneous quantification of cannabinoids and metabolites in oral fluid by two-dimensional gas chromatography mass spectrometry. *Journal of Chromatography A*, **1217**, 1513–1521.

Milman, G., Barnes, A.J., Schwope, D.M., *et al.* (2011b). Cannabinoids and metabolites in expectorated oral fluid after 8 days of controlled around-the-clock oral THC administration. *Analytical and Bioanalytical Chemistry*, **401**(2), 599–607.

Milman, G., Schwope, D.M., Schwilke, E.W., *et al.* (2011a). Oral fluid and plasma cannabinoid ratios after around-the-clock controlled oral delta9-tetrahydrocannabinol administration. *Clinical Chemistry*, **57**(11), 1597–1606.

Moore, C., Coulter, C., Rana, S., Vincent, M., and Soares, J. (2006a). Analytical procedure for the determination of the marijuana metabolite 11-nor-delta9-tetrahydrocannabinol-9-carboxylic acid in oral fluid specimens. *Journal of Analytical Toxicology*, **30**, 409–412.

Moore, C., Coulter, C., Uges, D., *et al.* (2011). Cannabinoids in oral fluid following passive exposure to marijuana smoke. *Forensic Science International*, **212**, 227–230.

Moore, C., Ross, W., Coulter, C., *et al.* (2006b). Detection of the marijuana metabolite 11-nor-delta9-tetrahydrocannabinol-9-carboxylic acid in oral fluid specimens and its contribution to positive results in screening assays. *Journal of Analytical Toxicology*, **30**, 413–418.

Pomahacova, B., Van der Kooy, F., and Verpoorte, R. (2009). Cannabis smoke condensate III: the cannabinoid content of vaporised *Cannabis sativa*. *Inhalation Toxicology*, **21**(13), 1108–1112.

Scheidweiler, K.B., Desrosiers, N.A., and Huestis, M.A. (2012). Simultaneous quantification of free and glucuronidated cannabinoids in human urine by liquid chromatography tandem mass spectrometry. *Clinica Chimica Acta*, **413**(23–24), 1839–1847.

Schwilke, E.W., Gullberg, R.G., Darwin, W.D., *et al.* (2011). Differentiating new cannabis use from residual urinary cannabinoid excretion in chronic, daily cannabis users. *Addiction*, **106**, 499–506.

Schwilke, E.W., Schwope, D.M., Karschner, E.L., *et al.* (2009). Delta9-tetrahydrocannabinol (THC), 11-hydroxy-THC, and 11-nor-9-carboxy-THC plasma pharmacokinetics during and after continuous high-dose oral THC. *Clinical Chemistry*, **55**, 2180–2189.

Schwope, D.M., Scheidweiler, K.B., and Huestis, M.A. (2011a). Direct quantification of cannabinoids and cannabinoid glucuronides in whole blood by liquid chromatography–tandem mass spectrometry. *Analytical and Bioanalytical Chemistry*, **401**, 1273–1283.

Schwope, D.M., Karschner, E.L., Gorelick, D.A., and Huestis, M.A. (2011b). Identification of recent cannabis use: whole-blood and plasma free and glucuronidated cannabinoid pharmacokinetics following controlled smoked cannabis administration. *Clinical Chemistry*, **57**, 1406–1414.

Skopp, G. and Potsch, L. (2004). An investigation of the stability of free and glucuronidated 11-nor-delta9-tetrahydrocannabinol-9-carboxylic acid in authentic urine samples. *Journal of Analytical Toxicology*. **28**, 35–40.

Skopp, G., Strohbeck-Kuehner, P., Mann, K., and Hermann, D. (2007). Deposition of cannabinoids in hair after long-term use of cannabis. *Forensic Science International*. **170**, 46–50.

Smith, M.L., Barnes, A.J., and Huestis, M.A. (2009). Identifying new cannabis use with urine creatinine-normalized THCCOOH concentrations and time intervals between specimen collections. *Journal of Analytical Toxicology*, **33** (4), 185–189.

Steinmeyer, S., Ohr, H., Maurer, H. J., and Moeller, M.R. (2001). Practical aspects of roadside tests for administrative traffic offences in Germany. *Forensic Science International*, **121**, 33–36.

Substance Abuse and Mental Health Services Administration. (2011). Mandatory guidelines for federal workplace drug testing programs; request for information regarding specific issues related to the use of the oral fluid specimen for drug testing. *Federal Register*, **76**(112), 34086–34087.

Van der Kooy, F., Pomahacova, B., and Verpoorte, R. (2009). Cannabis smoke condensate II: influence of tobacco on tetrahydrocannabinol levels. *Inhalation Toxicology*, **21**(2), 87–90.

Verstraete, A.G. (2005). Oral fluid testing for driving under the influence of drugs: history, recent progress and remaining challenges. *Forensic Science International*, **150**, 143–150.

Part 3

Medicinal Cannabis and Cannabinoids: Clinical Data

Ethan B. Russo

Part 3 Overview

In Chapter 17, Hazekamp and Pappas examine self-medication with cannabis and its various controversies, methods of administration, pros and cons, pitfalls, and political fallout.

Chapter 18 by Reiman probes the legal gray areas of cannabis dispensaries, compassion clubs, and coffee shops and their psychosocial and medical implications.

In Chapter 19, Thomson and Langfield summarize the seemingly Byzantine paths that cannabis-based medicines must take to attain regulatory approval as full-fledged pharmaceuticals in Europe and North America, serving as a practical blueprint for any such endeavor.

Wright and Guy bring their experience in pharmaceutical development to an elucidation of the benefits and pitfalls of cannabis-based medicines in the modern arena in Chapter 20.

In Chapter 21, Ware details the history and development of synthetic cannabinoids, specifically nabilone, a tetrahydrocannabinol (THC) analogue, and Marinol®, a synthetically-derived THC.

Notcutt and Clarke provide in Chapter 22 a British perspective on prescription cannabinoids that offers a practical guide to their usage.

Chapter 17

Self-Medication with Cannabis

Arno Hazekamp and George Pappas

17.1 Introduction

The medicinal use of cannabis is slowly gaining a more general acceptance worldwide. Canada (since 2001) and the Netherlands (since 2003) have government-run programs, in which quality-controlled herbal cannabis is supplied by specialized and licensed companies. Several other countries are now setting up their own programs (Israel, Czech Republic, Switzerland) or import products from the Dutch program (Italy, Finland, Germany, Switzerland). In the US, despite strong opposition by the federal government, so far 18 states including the District of Columbia have introduced laws to permit "medical marijuana use" (Americans for Safe Access 2012). In these states, patients grow it on their own or collectively, or obtain it from larger growers that act as caregivers for groups of patients. In some states, large-scale operations are licensed to supply the entire demand, but almost no official quality control standards have been released so far. But no matter how cannabis is supplied in all of these different programs, it is usually left up to patients themselves to decide how to administer the herb. Self-medication with cannabis is therefore probably the most common way of using cannabinoids medicinally. Consequently, there may be a lot to learn from the actual experiences of patients self-medicating with cannabis products worldwide.

Self-medication is inherently difficult to study, as it does not happen in the convenient and controlled setting of a laboratory or hospital. Currently, little published data is available on the extent of medicinal cannabis use and the characteristics of patients involved in it. The limited survey data, case reports, and other "soft" means of gathering information that exist make it hard to draw firm quantitative conclusions that can inform clinical practice on how to prescribe cannabis adequately. Fortunately, there is a growing interest in performing scientific studies (Hazekamp and Heerdink 2013; Janichek and Reiman 2012) and large-scale surveys (Hazekamp et al. 2013) on these patient populations, to contribute to the understanding of cannabinoid-based medicine by asking self-medicating patients detailed questions about their experiences.

At the same time, the policy developments that are designed to accommodate legitimate and qualified users are fiercely debated by medical authorities, law enforcement agencies, and politicians around the world, and sometimes with good reason. Although cannabis seems to fill some urgent medical needs, many current systems leave enough incentive for recreational users to act as pseudopatients in order to obtain legal protection for using cannabis. Furthermore, while safety of cannabis is generally accepted to be within the range often deemed to be acceptable for other medications, clinical trials have not yet been able to supply a clear answer on what are supposed to be the "real" medical indications for cannabis use. Finally, there is still much to learn about the risks of potential contaminations with pesticides, growth-enhancing chemicals, microbes, or heavy metals, especially in the absence of quality control. For all these reasons, physicians are often hesitant to play the role of prescriber or "gatekeeper," even in the official government programs of Canada (Sullivan 2012) and the Netherlands (Hazekamp and Heerdink 2013).

Unfortunately, on both sides of this discussion, arguments are all too often based on personal experiences, political intentions, and emotions, rather than on the growing scientific understanding we have of the cannabis plant. As a result, both the beneficial and harmful aspects of cannabis use may have become somewhat inflated, ranging from "cannabis cures cancer" and "it never killed anyone" to "cannabis will make you psychotic and addicted." The chemical diversity of the hundreds of varieties of cannabis that are in use today certainly does little to bring certainty to this discourse. Therefore, an important goal in the discussion on the pros and cons of self-medication with cannabis should be to find a sustainable supply model that can fulfil the requirements of medical authorities and policymakers (e.g., standardization, quality control, safety), as well as those of patients and their physicians (e.g., choice of variety and administration form, whole plant preparations), while making a strong but balanced effort to minimize diversion and abuse. Finding balance is crucial, and ensuring that we advance our scientific understanding of cannabis use is the key.

This chapter summarizes some important aspects of the medicinal use of cannabis, including clinical data, administration forms, quality control, dosing, and differences between cannabis varieties. The perspective of the self-medicating patient will be covered by discussing relevant issues such as typical user characteristics, cost, and the social aspects of self-medication. Although the term "medicinal/medical cannabis" is often used, we prefer to use the phrasing "medicinal *use* of cannabis" in this book chapter instead. While this difference is only subtle, it signifies that cannabis is not inherently medicinal, because the therapeutic effects depend on the variety used, the medical condition it is used for, and a range of other choices such as administration form and dosing regimen. In addition, the term "medicinal cannabis" may imply that the product used is of medical quality (quality controlled, standardized, etc.) which is often not the case with self-medication. We consider it therefore more correct to refer to the use of cannabis with the *intention* of creating therapeutic effects. Hence, the term: medicinal use of cannabis.

17.2 **Cannabis and medicine: an uneasy combination**

According to some, herbal cannabis, also known as marijuana, is a substance whose abuse potential is well documented, but whose benefits are poorly characterized. However, this view overlooks the fact that the harmfulness of cannabis abuse is not as widely accepted as often assumed (Nutt et al. 2007), and that some therapeutic effects claimed by patients are, in fact, clinically supported and sometimes even produced by registered medicines. On the other hand, there is indeed still much we need to learn about topics such as differences between cannabis varieties, synergy of cannabis components, and the sociocultural role of medicinal cannabis.

Unlike opioids, another class of controlled substances with a long history of debate, cannabis and cannabinoid are rarely discussed in medical school or residency. Even the existence or function of the ubiquitous endocannabinoid system seems largely unknown among medical professionals. As a result, it seems hard to reach any comfortable consensus on where the line may be drawn between the appropriate medical use and the abuse of this plant. Instead, what we observe is an interesting polarization of opinions on cannabis (Ware 2012). Addiction workers, concerned on the one hand by increases in problematic cannabis use, have on the other hand also reported that cannabis has been used successfully in harm-reduction programs targeting more addictive substances, such as opiates (heroin), cocaine, or alcohol (e.g., Reiman 2009). Psychiatrists, alerted about adolescent cannabis use and psychosis, are also aware of positive effects of cannabinoids on posttraumatic stress (Passie et al. 2012) and depression (Mikale et al. 2013). Pain specialists, intrigued by the effects of cannabis on pain, sleep, and anxiety, are equally concerned about drug-seeking behavior and functional impairment. And parents, worried about the dangerous interest children show toward cannabis, are simultaneously interested in the genuine pain relief that the drug may offer loved ones who need it.

While the reductionist approach of modern medicine has already been applied to cannabis for decades, the subsequent development of cannabinoid-based medication—mainly based on delta-9-tetrahydrocannabinol (Δ^9-THC) and cannabidiol (CBD)—has not been able to significantly reduce the worldwide use of cannabis as a medicine. Cannabis seems stuck in the middle; on the one hand too potent to be regulated as an herbal (or alternative) medicine, on the other hand too herbal to be regarded as conventional medicine. In general, there are multiple reasons that can explain why people choose self-medication over more conventional therapy, such as cost issues, distrust in modern healthcare, or an interest in "green" medicine. But in the case of cannabis we may add some less common reasons: a wide choice of chemical variety among cannabis strains, unconventional administration forms, and even interest in the underlying cannabis subculture. After all, a vast network of knowledge on cannabis exists, offering specialized magazines, extensive websites, and even international fairs and conferences. So despite the fact that cannabis and modern medicine have an uneasy relationship with each other, it seems that the medicinal use of cannabis is here to stay.

17.3 **Defining self-medication**

In the literature, self-medication generally refers to one of two behaviors: (1) the conscious use of nonprescribed medication (over-the-counter drugs, alternative treatments, etc.) to treat a diagnosed or undiagnosed condition, or (2) the use of a (often illicit) drug to consciously or subconsciously treat a physical or psychological condition, as presented in Khantzian's self-medication hypothesis (Suh et al. 2008). While the former suggests a conscious effort to target a specific disease state, the latter is often used as an explanation for the onset of a substance abuse disorder. Both of these definitions of self-medication have relevance when discussing the medicinal use of cannabis.

Self-medication is seen by some as a positive way to empower patients to take greater control over their care, and to increase healthcare efficiency by reducing doctor visits. This has been a justification for efforts to make some prescription medications for conditions such as diabetes, asthma, migraines, and hypertension, available over the counter (Woodward et al. 2012). Some countries that allow for medicinal use of cannabis simply require an "authorization" signed by a physician to receive protection from legal penalties. The patients are essentially left to use the cannabis on their own, assessing for themselves many of the treatment conditions that are normally assured by the formal healthcare infrastructure, such as the quality and/or reliability of the source, proper dosage, routes of administration, and efficacy in disease progress. The "hands-off" approach to medicinal cannabis use that defines these programs offers self-medication as the only option for participants. Evidence-based monitoring of the efficacy of cannabis on the indications for which it is used, and even whether it is being used effectively and responsibly, is almost entirely lacking. Greater inclusion of the physician in patients' cannabis use, such as through an actual prescription, could help to fill that gap in knowledge.

In contrast, in addiction psychology, self-medication may refer to recreational drug use that results in unexpected or unacknowledged improvements to an existing condition. In this context, this pattern of drug use may be the basis for a developing addiction (Hall and Queener 2007). Additionally, studies have shown that medicinal use of cannabis is often related to the treatment of a psychiatric condition (Lynch et al. 2006; Prentiss et al. 2004; Reinarman et al. 2011). As cannabis is by far the most widely used illicit drug in Western cultures, some people may initially use cannabis recreationally but then discover, consciously or subconsciously, an improvement of psychiatric symptoms of a diagnosed or undiagnosed condition. If the initial intent of drug use is not to treat a medical condition, but rather for other reasons (social acceptance, coping, etc.) then the unsupervised use can eventually become problematic (Henwood and Padgett 2007).

"Self-medication" in both of these contexts elucidates the importance of an educated physician being present and guiding patients in their medicinal use of cannabis, in order to determine the most efficacious pattern of use, and avoid problems associated with overuse and/or addiction. Because of the potentially fine line between proper self-medicating of a medical condition and using cannabis in situations where it may do more harm than good, a better understanding of the choices, preferences, and motivations of patients is a good starting point in our exploration of self-medicating with cannabis (section 17.4).

17.4 **Who and when: characterizing self-medicating patients**

There are an estimated 119–224 million frequent users of cannabis worldwide (United Nations Office on Drugs and Crime 2012) but it is presently unclear how many of them could be considered, or consider themselves, as medicinal users. Research from Canada suggests that 1.6–1.8% of the total population may be self-defined medical users, which could indicate a medical-use rate of 10% or more among the total cannabis-using population (Ogborne et al. 2000). Still, although a lot may be learned from the experiences of actual medicinal users of cannabis, there are remarkably few data available on this topic. Currently, most information available on the effects of cannabis use comes from studies on the abuse of cannabis as a recreational drug. As a result, new medical users and their physicians are often concerned about the risk of addiction, overdosing, and intoxication (feeling "high"). But although such studies indeed focus on the same drug (cannabis), it is important to recognize there may be large differences between medicinal and recreational users, for example, in terms of the intention for use (see section 17.1), frequency and size of dosing, and route of administration.

Randomized, placebo-controlled, and blinded clinical trials (RCTs) are the current gold standard for efficacy and safety, helping us to decide where and when the use of a medicinal substance is medically appropriate. However, the therapeutic effects of herbal cannabis have been directly compared to pharmaceutical products in only a few RCTs. Most of these studies compared an unregistered oral cannabis extract (Cannador®) to Marinol® (Freeman et al. 2006; Killestein et al. 2002; Strasser et al. 2006; Zajicek et al. 2003, 2005), while a few others compared smoked cannabis to Marinol® (Haney et al. 2005,2007). Clearly, other approaches may be needed, at least in the short term, to characterize self-medicating patients and better understand their choices and preferences.

For this reason, the International Association for Cannabinoid Medicines (IACM) performed a cross-sectional survey on the subjective preferences of patients for different administration forms of cannabinoids, comparing self-medication to pharmaceutical products such as Marinol®, Nabilone®, and Sativex®. Moreover, a recent evaluation of the Dutch medicinal cannabis program revealed a wealth of data on user characteristics in a more objective manner, by analyzing prescriptions for cannabis dispensed by Dutch pharmacies over multiple years. Both studies are discussed in the following sections (sections 17.4.1 and 17.4.2). Finally, the clinical data supporting the medicinal effects of cannabis may be limited, but they are certainly not absent. A short overview is therefore given of the studies supporting some of the various claims made by patients (section 17.4.3).

17.4.1 **IACM international survey**

The IACM survey was able to capture the experiences and opinions of 953 patients, making it the largest *international* study on users having experience with *multiple* cannabinoid-based medicines (CBMs) performed so far (Hazekamp et al. 2013). Although the authors warn of the limitations of self-selected participation, and point out a potential bias toward herbal cannabis, the study indicated a strong preference of those surveyed for herbal cannabis products and the inhaled route of administration, as opposed to oral pharmaceutical products.

On average, participants of the survey had experience with three to four different CBMs; were current users who had a health professional involved in the management of their illness; and had been using CBMs for at least several years. The average daily use, based on estimates by subjects, ranged from 2.4 g for tea, and 3.0 g for smoking and for vapourizing, up to 3.4 g for edibles or tincture. The top five symptoms that subjects intended to treat with CBMs were chronic pain (29.2% of participants), anxiety (18.3%), loss of appetite and/or weight (10.7%), depression (5.2%), and insomnia or sleeping disorder (5.1%). Interestingly, there seemed to be no apparent correlation of the preferred method of intake with the medical condition or symptoms under treatment. Several other studies have identified the same symptoms, particularly chronic pain, as leading reasons for using CBMs (Canadian Centre on Substance Abuse 2004; Clark 2004; Coomber et al. 2003; Hathaway and Rossiter 2007; Lucas 2012; Ogborne et al. 2000). It should be noted that some studies focused on the ability of cannabis products to ameliorate *symptoms*, while others were more concerned with the medical *indications* of those taking these products, which may somewhat complicate the comparison of different studies.

When the survey compared the advantages of pharmaceutical products to herbal preparations on many different aspects (side effects, onset and duration of effects, dosing, etc.), the latter were preferred in most cases. Pharmaceutical products were preferred only for their "ease of preparation and intake," although it should be noted that only a small number of surveyed subjects reported actual experience with these products. Indeed, herbal cannabis products are generally lacking convenient, reliable, and standardized administration forms, in contrast to conventional medicines. It is clear that the obtained user characteristics are in stark contrast with conventional medicine, which is mainly focused on prescribing oral single-compound drugs. Perhaps that is why, according to the survey, home-growing of cannabis remained widely popular even among those patients who had access to pharmaceutical cannabinoid drugs on prescription.

17.4.2 **The Dutch medicinal cannabis program**

The medicinal cannabis program of the Netherlands offers pharmaceutical-grade cannabis on prescription to chronically ill patients (OMC 2013). Although patients are advised to administer the product by using a vaporizer or by preparing it as a tea (Hazekamp et al. 2006, 2007), they are essentially free to choose their own preferred method of intake. Presently, most Dutch health insurance companies reimburse medicinal cannabis to some extent, and some now even cover the Volcano Medic vaporizer for medical use (NCSM 2012).

A recent study by Hazekamp and Heerdink (2013), making use of the prescriptions database of the Dutch Foundation for Pharmaceutical Statistics, was first to use objective data to evaluate consumption patterns of prescribed cannabis use. Covering the period 2003–2010, the study evaluated approximately 35,000 prescriptions for medicinal cannabis by Dutch physicians. Of the 5540 (anonymous) patients identified in the study, more females (56.8%) than males (42.7%) used medicinal cannabis on prescription. The mean (median) age of the study population was 55.6 (55) years, with a range of 14–93 years. The studied population received on average 6.4 prescriptions of medicinal cannabis with a median of 10 g dispensed per prescription. Overall, medicinal cannabis was prescribed for an average duration of 251 days. Interestingly, this contrasts with other studies that found cannabis was used medicinally more commonly over a period of years and even over a decade (Lucas 2012; Swift et al. 2005).

Although the route of administration could not be evaluated from the available prescription data, the average daily use of 0.68 g was significantly lower than the 3–4 g found in the IACM survey. These data point to a low potential of misuse, and a seeming absence of widespread development of tolerance to cannabis prescribed by a physician. By comparison, an average Dutch cannabis cigarette used for recreational purposes contains about 0.26 g of cannabis mixed with tobacco (Van der Pol et al. 2013). Interestingly, the relative use of different cannabis varieties remained quite stable over the years 2007–2010: about 60% of prescriptions were for variety Bedrocan®, with high THC (19%); 25% for Bedrobinol®, with lower THC (12%); and 15% for Bediol®, containing both THC (6%) and CBD (7.5%).

By analyzing the medication prescribed in the period right before first onset of cannabis use, the study was able to identify some medical indications correlated with cannabis use of the Dutch patients. It was found that pain medication was used by 53.6% of all prescribed cannabis users. Medication prescribed to treat nausea was used by 15.5% of all subjects. Although cancer, glaucoma, and HIV/AIDS are often mentioned in popular media in relation to medicinal cannabis use, oncolytics (2.7%), eye pressure medication (2.2%), and HIV medication (0.9%) were only used by a small proportion of subjects.

Because the study did not cover the entire Dutch general population, and a significant proportion of patients is believed to consume cannabis obtained from nonofficial sources, the calculated prevalence rate of 5–8 per 100,000 should be considered a very conservative estimate. Prevalence rates (unofficially) reported in some other countries where medicinal cannabis use is registered by national authorities are 35 (per 100,000) for Canada and 80 for Israel, while in some US states prevalence rates of well over 100 are claimed (IACM 2012). However, these numbers may be significantly inflated with recreational users posing as medicinal users (Nussbaum et al. 2011).

17.4.3 Clinical research in support of herbal cannabis

Clinical studies with single cannabinoids (natural or synthetic) or whole plant preparations (e.g., smoked cannabis, encapsulated extract) have often been inspired by positive anecdotal experiences of patients using crude cannabis products for self-treatment. For example, the antiemetic, appetite enhancing, analgesic, and muscle relaxant effects, and the therapeutic use of cannabinoids in Tourette's syndrome, were all discovered or rediscovered in this manner (Hazekamp et al. 2010). This clearly speaks to the critical role that collecting data on current patient behaviors has played—and may continue to play – in an evolving understanding of cannabis efficacy.

A comprehensive summary of clinical trials performed with cannabinoid-based medicines was given by two complementary review papers (Ben Amar 2006; Hazekamp and Grotenhermen 2010). In the period from 1975–2009, at least 109 controlled clinical studies were published, assessing well over 6500 patients suffering from a wide range of illnesses. Based on the data available, it is possible to confirm that cannabinoids, also in the form of herbal cannabis, exhibit a therapeutic potential mainly as analgesics in chronic neuropathic pain, as appetite stimulants and antiemetics in debilitating diseases (e.g., cancer, AIDS, hepatitis C), and for the treatment of various symptoms of multiple sclerosis. Additionally, cannabinoids may have potential in the symptomatic treatment of spinal cord injuries, intestinal dysfunction, Tourette's syndrome, hyperactivity and anxiety disorders, allergies, epilepsy, and glaucoma. Perhaps one of the most exciting recent findings is that cannabinoids may be effective in the treatment of some forms of cancer, by not just ameliorating symptoms but actually attacking and killing cancer cells (Velasco et al. 2012).

Nowadays it is better understood that cannabis constituents other than the psychoactive Δ^9-THC may play a role in therapeutic effects. Plant cannabinoids such as CBD and tetrahydro-cannabivarin (THCV), or the abundantly present terpenes, may influence the expected thera-peutic effects in a myriad of ways, including synergy, enhancement of uptake or penetration of the blood–brain barrier, and influencing receptor binding or metabolism (Izzo et al. 2009; Russo 2011). Unfortunately, such new insights are hardly reflected yet in our clinical understanding of cannabis. Moreover, clinical trials typically focus on isolated cannabinoids given orally, while self-medicating patients mainly use herbal cannabis in inhaled or edible forms. Those RCTs per-formed with cannabis often show significant limitations, including a limited choice of cannabis varieties (restricted to a few official sources of research-grade cannabis worldwide), dosing range (fear of overdosing), and administration form (smoking is strongly underpresented in clinical data). In contrast, self-medicating patients can choose from an almost endless range of varieties, from which they pick the optimal variety, dosing regimen, and administration form by a process of trial and error.

17.5 Why: reasons for self-medication

Since the United Nations adopted the Single Convention on Narcotic Drugs in 1961, cannabis and its products have been defined as "narcotics with a high potential for abuse and no accepted medicinal value." This strict legal classification has effectively delayed their progression into modern medicine, by not only keeping cannabis and cannabinoids out of the hands of medical users, but also by depriving researchers of the materials needed for scientific investigation. But despite its illegality, large numbers of patients have continued to push for the right to use cannabis, including for self-medication. Patient-driven lawsuits against their governments have been the basis for the availability of cannabis in Canada, Germany, and Finland, while voter initiatives have resulted in the legalizing of medical marijuana use in multiple US states. Even in situations where they have access to legal sources of herbal cannabis, patients frequently choose to grow their own cannabis (Hazekamp et al. 2013). Besides the (perceived) superior efficacy of self-medication, we will explore a few potential reasons why this may be the case in section 17.5.1.

17.5.1 Choice of varieties

As a result of extensive efforts in cannabis breeding and selection, an impressive range of culti-vated varieties (cultivars, also known as strains) has been developed worldwide. These are com-monly distinguished, by plant breeders, recreational users, and cannabis patients alike, through the use of fascinating names such as White Widow, Northern Lights, Amnesia, or Haze. Already, over 700 different varieties have been described (Snoeijer 2001) and many more are thought to exist. An important reason for patients to keep purchasing materials from illicit markets is the fact that, often by trial and error, they claim to have found particular strains that work optimally for treatment of their specific symptoms.

In the context of self-medicating, an obvious question is how the chemical constituents found in various cannabis cultivars reflect differential medicinal properties, and what types of cannabis should consequently be made available to patients. In Canada, a recent review of the national medical marijuana program indicated access to multiple cannabis varieties to be an important issue for patients (Health Canada 2011). The most common way currently used to classify canna-bis cultivars is through plant morphology (phenotype) with two main classes typically recognized:

Cannabis sativa and *Cannabis indica*. Most modern cultivars are, however, genetically a blend of both types. It is therefore unclear whether this classification reflects any relevant differences in chemical composition.

Clearly, a better understanding of chemical differences between cannabis cultivars could help bridge the gap between the vast knowledge on cannabis that exists within the community of recreational users, and the information needed by medicinal users and health professionals. However, it is becoming increasingly clear that components in cannabis beyond Δ^9-THC and CBD, such as other minor plant-cannabinoids and volatile secondary metabolites called terpenoids, are involved in the drug's overall effect (Russo 2011). This high number of (potential) active components significantly complicates a conventional reductionist approach using analytical chemistry, animal studies, and clinical trials, where typically a single active ingredient is identified before further study is possible.

An alternative approach to this multiple component problem may be to simultaneously identify and quantify all major components present in various cannabis types, and then use powerful statistical tools such as principal component analysis (PCA) to classify cultivars in a smaller number of chemically distinct groups. With this approach it may be possible to move away from cannabis *cultivars*, with often vague and unsubstantiated characteristics, toward a new classification using *chemovars* with a complex, but nevertheless well-defined chemical "fingerprint." This methodology has already been successfully applied to cannabis for differentiation of cultivars (Hazekamp and Fischedick 2012) as well as quality control (Fischedick et al. 2010).

Using a comprehensive *chemovar* approach may help medicinal users and their physicians to successfully switch from a beneficial cannabis variety obtained through illicit markets, to a similar strain that is available through official state-run programs. It may also help these national programs to narrow down the search for beneficial cannabis varieties to be standardized and introduced as an official medicine. Exchange of cultivars and analytical data between the various cannabis programs worldwide may greatly facilitate such a transition.

17.5.2 The role of the physician

Because physicians are the main gatekeepers to the legal and medically supervised use of cannabis, their role and attitudes deserve some further examination. With a rising interest in, and media coverage of, medicinal use of cannabis, patients may turn toward self-medication when their primary caregiver refuses to discuss the topic, or displays a clear lack of knowledge about it. Unfortunately, physicians often do not see themselves properly equipped for their gatekeeper role. A survey among US physicians regarding their attitudes toward legal prescription of cannabis as medical therapy found that only one-third of surveyed US physicians thought cannabis might have therapeutic value, versus nearly two-thirds of all Americans (Charuvastra et al. 2005). Safety concerns included the harms associated with smoking, psychological dependence, and risks of injury due to acute intoxication. Respondents made a clear call for more research to establish the risks and benefits of cannabis use in specific patient populations.

Also a survey by the Canadian Medical Association (CMA) showed that physicians have major concerns about the lack of rigorous research into the drug and about their own role prescribing it (Sullivan 2012). Respondents mainly worried that patients who requested medical cannabis actually wanted it for recreational purposes, and that medical doctors did not have enough information on the risks and benefits or on the appropriate use of cannabis for medicinal purposes. The CMA advised to improve scientific knowledge about cannabis, but also to develop compulsory education and licensing programs for physicians based on the knowledge already available. A survey among family physicians in Colorado (Kondrad and Reid 2013), the state with the highest recorded incidence of medicinal use of cannabis in the US, showed that most physicians believed cannabis use, even medicinal, carries risks, and almost half said that physicians should not recommend marijuana as a medical therapy at all. But understanding that medicinal use was already a reality in the state of Colorado, nearly all agreed on the need for further medical education and formal training (e.g., though the continuing medical education (CME) system) before prescribing or recommending it.

Since it is neither approved nor standardized according to Food and Drug Administration (FDA) standards or their equivalent in other countries, physicians who recommend cannabis ought to be especially scrupulous in their diagnosis and consequent recommendations. As a result, physicians ask for clear, definitive guidelines for medicinal use, which should come from the relevant authorities and medical associations in different countries. However, this requires at least some understanding of self-medicating patients, including choice of varieties, administration forms, dosage, and the main medical conditions it is used for. Physicians have some genuine concerns about self-medication with herbal cannabis, and it is important to make sure that these concerns are heard. If unaddressed, the impact may be noticed as physician frustration or even avoidance of situations where their care is critical for patient health. The main goal of these efforts should be to minimize diversion, misuse, and abuse potential while providing adequate treatment to all those who have a legitimate need. Recent opinions released by various medical associations are a significant step in that direction (American Medical Association 2009; Sullivan 2012).

17.5.3 Social aspects of self-medication

A common link between those who use cannabis medicinally seems to be that they suffer from conditions that are chronic and ongoing, and they are discontented with allopathic treatments (Hathaway and Rossiter 2007). So although the discussion on self-medicating with cannabis is primarily focused on therapeutic benefits versus pharmacological side effects, additional factors may be involved. A meta-analysis on the subjective effects of cannabis found that the most frequently reported effects were: improved mood (i.e., feeling good, content), enhanced relaxation, increased insight into self and others, and improved perceptions (Green et al. 2003). This indicates that establishing medical efficacy through clinical means alone overlooks a myriad of psychosocial factors.

The right to medicate with cannabis, as a social justice issue, is one that increasing numbers of North Americans and Europeans seem to support. However, employing mainly biomedical and technical approaches, public health agencies have not historically learned to incorporate such ideas and find it difficult to provide a clear answer to this development. Preconceived notions about cannabis are ubiquitous, and definitions of cannabis as a *natural* herb remedy as opposed to a *synthetic* pharmaceutical drug may also influence perceptions in favor of its use (Reiman 2008, 2009; Reinarman et al. 2011). As a result, those who self-medicate often do so on their own terms, without government approval or the guidance of physicians. In this unregulated climate, compassion clubs, coffee shops, dispensaries, and other sorts of collectives have emerged outside the law to play a vital role in the provision of safe access to, and therapeutic knowledge of, cannabis. Operating on the margins of society, these outlets fulfil an important role in creating a community among persons who are often highly marginalized themselves. Club membership may provide group identity, empowerment, and restorative supports over and above the cannabis use itself (Janichek and Reiman 2012).

In a study (Feldman and Mandel 1998) looking at the benefits of membership of "cannabis buyers' clubs" in the US, the authors concluded that such clubs were the soundest option—compared to doctors, pharmacists, police, and the black market—for providing access to cannabis as medicine. They argue that the clubs afford the best therapeutic setting, a healing environment that often offers an ethos of love, compassion, and emotional support in addition to health benefits of cannabis itself. The same message was echoed in a study by Hathaway and Rossiter (2007), where interviewed members contrasted their compassion clubs with treatments they received at the hands of doctors, welfare agencies, employers, authorities, and government officials. A common theme recorded was that "chronic illness stigmatizes and subjects those who suffer to shame and institutionalized abuse." So perhaps the greatest strength of medicinal cannabis use is in the holistic approach that cannot be found alongside the treatment with conventional drugs today.

Dispensaries can also help to decrease the gaps in substance education that many physicians have left open (see section 17.5.2) and fulfil unmet clinical desires by providing an opportune therapeutic setting to offer other services beneficial to patients. For example, in a study by Reiman (2008), 66% of the patients surveyed reported to make use of the holistic services in San Francisco Bay Area medical cannabis facilities including massage therapy, nutritional and herbal consultations, peer groups, and acupuncture. On the downside, few dispensaries currently offer clinical services related to the potential downsides of cannabis use, such as substance misuse, dependence, and mental health services (Janichek and Reiman 2012).

17.5.4 Costs and reimbursement

Because chronically ill patients, as a result of disability and unemployment, are often living on a small budget, the reason for choosing to self-medicate may simply be related to the cost. Indeed, when asked to rate ten different aspects of CBM use on a satisfaction scale ranging from 0–10, the factor *cost* scored lowest overall, indicating that the cost involved with using cannabinoid-based drugs, whether herbal or pharmaceutical, is a major issue for patients of all backgrounds. Of course, this may not be surprising as most healthcare systems in the world do not (yet) provide for reimbursement or health insurance coverage of CBMs.

The cost factor might have had substantial influence on available data on self-medication, as it may be a reason for patients to grow their own cannabis, or to choose poorer-quality products jeopardizing their health. Perhaps patients preferring herbal cannabis are simply those who need a very high dose of cannabinoids, which cannot be covered by the currently available pharmaceutical cannabinoid preparations, both practically and economically. The US Institute of Medicine already commented on this issue in 1999, stating that for patients without health insurance marijuana might be cheaper than an official source of Marinol® (Joy et al. 1999).

However, some promising changes are under way. In 2011, Sativex® was granted national reimbursement in Spain from the Spanish Ministry of Health (GW Pharmaceuticals 2011). And in the Netherlands a recent survey showed that 11 out of 15 major Dutch health insurance companies evaluated provided at least some form of reimbursement for medicinal cannabis (NCSM 2012). So although the need for more clinical data remains, a fair and complete comparison on total costs and benefits of different cannabinoids treatments may be another approach to this complex issue.

17.6 How: administration forms and quality control

The often cited report *Marijuana and Medicine: Assessing the Science Base* by the US Institute of Medicine (Joy et al. 1999) pointed out the need for effective administration forms for cannabinoids, stating that scientific data indicate the potential therapeutic value of cannabinoid drugs, primarily Δ^9-THC, for multiple indications, but that smoked cannabis is a crude cannabinoid delivery system that also delivers harmful substances. The report concluded that what is needed for optimal use of medicinal cannabinoids is a feasible, nonsmoked, rapid-onset delivery system.

Self-medication, almost by definition, is not driven by scientific insights, and may even actively oppose opinions expressed by institutional scientists or by companies seen as "Big Pharma." As a result, it is possible that self-medicating patients have, by trial and error, discovered particular cannabis varieties containing active components that only recently have attracted the interest of scientists, such as CBD (http://www.projectCBD.org), THCV (Izzo et al. 2009), certain types of terpenes (Hazekamp and Fischedick 2012), etc. And perhaps they simultaneously have discovered suitable administration forms for efficient delivery of these compounds. Indeed, multiple unconventional administration forms have been developed by the self-medicating population, including concentrated extracts known as cannabis oils, raw juiced buds, pot-brownies, and a range of vaporizer devices.

Although these remedies are sometimes used by large groups of patients, there is virtually nothing in the published literature about them in terms of cannabinoid/terpene composition, presence of contaminants, standardization of dose, or even their exact preparation methods. The following sections will discuss some common administration forms, and comment on important quality and safety aspects associated with them (sections 17.6.1–17.6.5).

17.6.1 The biochemistry of administration forms

Depending on the administration form, many changes to the original profile of compounds present in the fresh plant material may occur. A common, and often overlooked, function of most administration forms of (herbal) cannabis is a heating step, which is essential for conversion of the acidic cannabinoids into their, pharmacologically more active, neutral counterparts. If sufficient heat is applied, acidic cannabinoids such as THC-acid (THCA) and CBD-acid (CBDA) will turn into their neutral counterparts by losing the unstable carboxylic acid group. When cannabis is burned for smoking, baked for cookies, or boiled for tea, nonpsychoactive THCA turns into Δ^9-THC, CBDA turns into CBD, and so forth for all other cannabinoids. This conversion process, known as decarboxylation, also spontaneously takes place in aging cannabis samples, although at a much slower rate (Veress et al. 1990).

Besides the extent of decarboxylation, other aspects related to administration form may have a significant impact on therapeutic effects. For example, overheating, as well as exposure to light or air, may lead to the formation of degradation products such as cannabinol (CBN) and Δ^8-THC, with potential pharmacological properties of their own (Izzo et al. 2009). Fragile components such as the terpenes may get lost by evaporation as a result of long-term storage, or preparation methods that apply heat before consumption (e.g., boiling for tea, evaporating solvents for making extracts). Moreover, each administration form comes with its own set of specific metabolites formed upon consumption. As a result of all these factors combined, a different spectrum of compounds is finally entering the bloodstream, and consequently a different type and duration of effects may be observed for each cannabis medicine. The following sections (17.6.2–17.6.5) give a short overview of considerations related to the most common administration forms.

17.6.2 The inhaled route: smoking and vaporizing

Worldwide, smoking is by far the most commonly used method of consuming cannabis. The few studies that have directly compared the two forms of THC delivery show smoking to be comparable (Haney et al. 2005, 2007) or more effective (Chang et al. 1979; Hepler and Petrus 1976;

Vinciguerra et al. 1988) in achieving adequate blood concentrations than oral administration. Inhaling is about equal in efficiency to intravenous injection, while considerably more practical (Agurell et al. 1986; Ohlsson et al. 1980). A dose of 2–5 mg of Δ^9-THC consumed through smoking reliably produces blood concentrations above the effective level within a few minutes (Mattes et al. 1994; Wall and Perez-Reyes 1981). As a result, cannabis smoking is generally appreciated by self-medicating patients as a convenient method of administration, allowing accurate self-titration of the desired effects (Hazekamp et al. 2013), although many therapeutic studies using smoked or vaporized administration of cannabis reported at least some psychoactivity as a side effect (Hazekamp and Grotenhermen 2010). Although use of tobacco should obviously not be encouraged, it may be relevant to further study whether the addition of tobacco to cannabis cigarettes is merely a matter of taste or habit, or has an actual therapeutic function in combination with cannabis. At least one study has suggested that the presence of tobacco releases relatively more THC from cannabis when smoked (Van der Kooy et al. 2009).

Despite the absence of a clear association between cannabis use and lung cancer in clinical epidemiological studies (Aldington et al. 2008; Hashibe et al. 2006), inhalation of toxic compounds during cannabis smoking can pose serious health hazards (Mehra et al. 2006), probably even more so for chronically ill and weakened patients. This risk is not thought to be due to cannabinoids, but rather to noxious pyrolytic by-products such as tar, carbon monoxide, and ammonia (Hiller et al. 1984; Matthias et al. 1997). Consequently, the shortcomings of smoked cannabis have been widely viewed as a major obstacle for approval of crude (herbal) cannabis as a medicine by public health authorities (Joy et al. 1999).

Cannabis vaporization, or volatilization, is a technique aimed at suppressing irritating respiratory toxins by heating cannabis to a temperature where active cannabinoid vapors are formed, but below the point of combustion where pyrolytic toxic compounds are released. Vaporization offers the advantages of the pulmonary route of administration, i.e., rapid delivery into the bloodstream, ease of self-titration and concomitant minimization of the risk of over- and underdosing, while avoiding the respiratory disadvantages of smoking. Several studies have been performed in recent years showing that vaporizing can be considered an efficient way of cannabinoid administration (Hazekamp et al. 2006; Zuurman et al. 2008) with a bioavailability comparable to smoking (Abrams et al. 2007). Because of the temperatures used for vaporizing (typically in the range of 180–210°C), the whole range of terpenes present in herbal cannabis is efficiently inhaled, maximizing therapeutic potential.

17.6.3 The oral route: tea and edibles

Herbal cannabis can be consumed in the form of a decoction, also referred to as "cannabis tea." Although only a few standardized studies have been performed with tea preparations of cannabis (De Jong et al. 2005; Hazekamp et al. 2007; Steinagle and Upfal 1999), cannabis tea was found to be a relatively popular method of intake among patients who reported to have experience with the oral use of cannabis medicine (Hazekamp et al. 2013). Main advantages associated with its use included its relatively long duration of effects, and low occurrence of side effects.

Actual methods used for cannabis tea preparation by patients are largely unknown, and many variations may exist. In the Netherlands, patients are advised to prepare cannabis tea by adding 1.0 g of cannabis to 1 L of boiling water, letting it simmer for 15 min, and finally filtering out solid parts by using a wire-mesh tea-strainer (OMC 2013). Despite the fact that cannabinoids are notoriously insoluble in water (Hazekamp and Verpoorte 2006) it was found that cannabis tea prepared in this way yielded significant amounts of cannabinoids in a reproducible manner (Hazekamp et al. 2007). Considerably more THCA than Δ^9-THC (ratio about 5:1) was detected, which may be explained by the relatively higher water solubility of THCA compared to Δ^9-THC, combined with a relatively slow decarboxylation rate of acidic cannabinoids in boiling water (Hazekamp et al. 2007). In addition, several other cannabinoids were found in their acidic form, including cannabigerolic acid (CBGA) and tetrahydrocannabivarinic acid (THVA). This may be of particular interest, as most other administration forms are largely devoid of acidic cannabinoids. Although in general not much is known about biological activities of acidic cannabinoids, CBDA was reported to have a potent antimicrobial activity (Leizer et al. 2000) and to show promising anti-inflammatory effects (Takeda et al. 2008), while THCA was found to have a considerable effect on the human immune system (Verhoeckx et al. 2006).

Self-medication with cannabis in ingested form, such as cookies, brownies, or candies, seems to be particularly popular among North American patients (75.6% of survey participants; Hazekamp 2013) compared to other nationalities (46.5% of survey participants). As far as we know, there currently are no validated methods available for the analysis of cannabinoids and/or terpenes in edibles containing herbal cannabis or extracts. Indeed, preparing a neat analytical sample suitable for chromatographic analysis may be challenging in the presence of ingredients such as butter, flour, sugars, etc. As a result, no published data seem to be available on the composition or consistency of edibles. Theoretically, issues that are likely to occur with such products include homogenization (ensuring one cookie has the same potency as the next), consistent decarboxylation (a large brownie is baked longer than a smaller one), and shelf-life stability. Consequently, the use of standardized recipes and procedures may be even more important for edibles than for any other administration form discussed here.

17.6.4 **New kids on the block: tinctures, concentrates, and raw juice**

According to the IACM survey discussed in section 17.4.1, the most common issues regarding CBMs that patients are concerned with included bad taste, drowsiness, uncontrollable appetite (munchies), and mental effects (getting high). It was also suggested that different administration forms may be preferred in the privacy of one's home and in public (Hazekamp et al. 2013). In order to address such issues, self-medicating patients frequently experiment with new administration forms, some of which may then gather significant popularity. Not surprisingly, most of these new and unconventional administration forms have never been tested for any form of quality or safety.

When patients were asked what new cannabis-based product should be made legally available (besides herbal cannabis itself), tincture based on whole cannabis was found to be the most popular choice (Hazekamp et al. 2013). The main advantage cited was the variability of its use: as oral drops, in baked goods and in tea, and even for vaporizing or smoking, allowing for maximal flexibility of using cannabinoids throughout the day. Indeed, a standardized and quality-controlled cannabis tincture would be relatively easy to produce, and would connect the modern use of cannabis directly to the historical use of tinctures as described in older pharmacopoeia (Zuardi 2006). In order to "activate" the acidic cannabinoids, the tincture, or the plant material used to prepare it, should be heated at some point of the preparation process.

Cannabis oil is a concentrated extract obtained by solvent extraction of the buds or leaves of the cannabis plant, deriving its name from its sticky and viscous appearance. Various nonpolar solvents have been recommended for this purpose, including petroleum ether, naphtha, alcohol, and olive oil. The most well-known cannabis oil preparation is also known as "Rick Simpson" oil (Simpson 2008, 2013). Part of the self-medicating population firmly believes that these products are capable of curing cancer, a claim that is backed up by numerous anecdotal patient stories.

However, a recent study comparing five commonly used preparation methods found significant differences in cannabinoid and terpene composition of the resulting extracts. Also, the presence of residual solvent was found to be a significant concern, particularly in the case of using naphtha as the extraction solvent. The final conclusion of the study was to prepare extracts directly in olive oil, heated in a boiling water bath, for highest recovery of active compounds, and no risk of organic solvent residues (Romano and Hazekamp 2013).

Finally, the use of raw cannabis buds and leaves, prepared by juicing them in a blender with water or fruit juice, or by eating them directly as a salad, deserves some attention. The claimed, but unsubstantiated, therapeutic effects of these products include prevention of seizures, diabetes, and even curing brain tumors in infants (Cannabis International 2013). Different from the other administration forms mentioned earlier, this preparation does not undergo any form of heating, and therefore contains all cannabinoids in their native (acidic) form (Lee 2013).

17.6.5 Quality and safety

Because the intention of self-medication products is often to treat seriously ill, or even immune-compromised, patients, issues regarding chemical composition, quality, and safety should be of the highest priority. In the absence of clear guidelines for preparation or chemical characterization, medicinal users of cannabis may inadvertently purchase a product that has unexpected effects on their health and/or psyche. Changes in chemical composition may not only be derived from genetic differences between cannabis varieties, but could also be caused by variations in, for example, cultivation conditions, drying, processing, and storage. These factors may differ between different suppliers (coffee shop, dispensary, compassion club), and even between different batches of the same cannabis strain (Hazekamp and Fischedick 2012).

For conventional medicines, independent and certified quality control labs play a key role in ensuring quality and safety by performing a detailed analysis of the composition of these products. In the national cannabis programs of Canada and the Netherlands, products are independently tested for general appearance (i.e., color, bud shape, etc.), cannabinoid profile, terpene profile (the Netherlands only), and water content. Furthermore, the absence of heavy metals, pesticides, bacteria, molds, and fungal toxins is established. Because self-administration of cannabis most often takes place outside the realm of legal medicine, certified labs are wary of getting involved in the analysis of anything cannabis related. By necessity, this void is then often filled by unregulated labs that are set up from within the cannabis community, most notably in the US and Canada. However, cannabis is a complex phytomedicine with a wide profile of (potential) bioactive components, which may change in many ways depending on the administration form chosen (as discussed earlier in sections 17.6.1–17.6.4). As a result, each type of administration form needs its own properly validated methods for chemical analysis. Because these tests are costly, they are only affordable in the case of large batch sizes. As a result, smaller production sites may have an inherent problem with quality control. All these factors complicate the setting up of a reliable system for quality control, as was recently shown by a comparative test among ten different California-based labs (Gieringer and Hazekamp 2011).

Apart from THC overdosing, multiple case-studies have identified the consumption of unsafe cannabis as the cause for hospitalization, or even death. Among others, cannabis products were found to contain fungal spores of, e.g., *Aspergillus* or *Penicillium* species, or harmful bacteria such as *E. coli* (Hazekamp et al. 2006; McLaren et al. 2008), lead particles for added weight (cannabis is sold by weight) (Busse et al. 2008), or ground-up glass or talcum to mimic the presence of glandular hairs ("crystals") thereby suggesting higher potency (Scheel et al. 2012; Van Amsterdam et al. 2007). In the case of pesticides it is unclear which, if any, pose a threat to the health of consumers. As yet, no studies have been conducted on the safety of pesticides as applied to inhaled or ingested cannabis. Pesticides with known chemistry may be altered, destroyed, or rendered more or less toxic in the process of combustion or cooking. Although this may not be a major concern for recreational users who mainly seek intoxication by their own free will, patients cannot afford to be exposed to such risks. Cannabis products from a standardized and quality-controlled source, if available, may therefore be the safer choice for medicinal users preferring self-medication with herbal cannabis.

17.7 **Conclusion**

Self-medication with cannabis seems to be prominent currently, and rising in popularity. The emerging interest in studying this phenomenon has already provided important insight into several aspects regarding the medicinal use of cannabis that patients find effective and desirable. Such data are important in finding how to increase positive health outcomes regarding cannabis use, by bringing it progressively into the realm of modern medicine. Ultimately, as official and federally regulated medicinal cannabis programs continue to increase in prevalence and size, those who have been pushed into self-medication linked with the illicit market may get the opportunity to bring their medicinal use into the scope of a regular patient–physician relationship. In the ideal setting, physicians should have the information at hand to offer the same care with cannabis as they do with other pharmaceutical preparations. Self-medication with cannabis may then become strictly a matter of choice, rather than necessity.

References

Abrams, D.I., Vizoso, H.P., Shade, S.B., Jay, C., Kelly, M.E., and Benowitz, N.L. (2007). Vaporization as a smokeless cannabis delivery system: a pilot study. *Clinical Pharmacology & Therapeutics*, **82**(5), 572–578.

Agurell, S., Halldin, M., Lindgren, J.E., *et al.* (1986). Pharmacokinetics and metabolism of delta-1-tetrahydrocannabinol and other cannabinoids with emphasis on man. *Pharmacological Reviews*, **38**, 21–43.

Aldington, S., Harwood, M., Cox, B., *et al.* Cannabis and Respiratory Disease Research Group (2008). Cannabis use and risk of lung cancer: a case-control study. *European Respiratory Journal*, **31**, 280–286.

American Medical Association. (2009). *Report 3 of the Council on Science and Public Health (I-09) – Use of Cannabis for Medicinal Purposes*. [Online] Available at: http://www.ama-assn.org/resources/doc/csaph/csaph-report3-i09.pdf (accessed April 4, 2013).

Americans for Safe Access. (2012). *Connecticut Becomes 17th Medical Marijuana State in the Face of Ongoing Federal Intimidation*. [Online] Press release of June 1 2012. Available at: http://www.safeaccessnow.org/connecticut_becomes_17th_medical_marijuana_state_in_the_face_of_ongoing_federal_intimidation (accessed April 4, 2013).

Ben Amar, M. (2006). Cannabinoids in medicine: a review of their therapeutic potential. *Journal of Ethnopharmacology*, **105**(1–2), 1–25.

Busse, F., Omidi, L., Leichtle, A., Windgassen, M., Kluge, E., and Stumvoll, M. (2008). Lead poisoning due to adulterated marijuana. *New England Journal of Medicine*, **358**, 1641–1642.

Canadian Centre on Substance Abuse. (2004). *Canadian Addiction Survey 2004*. [Online] Ottawa: Canadian Centre on Substance Abuse. Available at: http://www.ccsa.ca/Eng/Priorities/Research/CanadianAddiction/Pages/CanadianAddictionSurveyReleaseofMicrodataFiles.aspx (accessed April 4, 2013).

Cannabis International. (2013). *Official website of Dr. Courtney.* [Online] Available at: http://www. cannabisinternational.org (accessed April 4, 2013).

Chang, A.E., Shiling, D.J., Stillman, R.C., et al. (1979). Delta-9-tetrahydrocannabinol as an antiemetic in cancer patients receiving high dose methotrexate: a prospective randomized evaluation. *Annals of Internal Medicine,* **91,** 819–824.

Charuvastra, A., Friedmann, P.D., and Stein, M.D. (2005). Physician attitudes regarding the prescription of medical marijuana. *Journal of Addictive Diseases,* **24**(3), 87–93.

Clark, A.J., Ware, M.A., Yazer, E., Murray, T.J., and Lynch, M.E. (2004). Patterns of cannabis use among patients with multiple sclerosis. *Neurology,* **62**(11), 2098–2100.

Coomber, R., Oliver, M., and Morris, C. (2003). Using cannabis therapeutically in the UK: a qualitative analysis. *Journal of Drug Issues,* **33**(2), 325–356.

De Jong, F.A., Engels, F.E., Sparreboom, A., et al. (2005). Influence of medicinal cannabis (MC) on the pharmacokinetics (PK) of docetaxel (DOC) andirinotecan (CPT-11). *Proceedings of the American Association for Cancer Research,* **46,** 938c–939c.

Feldman, H.W. and Mandel, R.J. (1998). Providing medical marijuana: the importance of cannabis clubs. *Journal of Psychoactive Drugs,* **30,** 179–186.

Fischedick, J.T., Hazekamp, A., Erkelens, T., Choi, Y.H., and Verpoorte, R. (2010). Metabolic fingerprinting of *Cannabis sativa* L., cannabinoids and terpenoids for chemotaxonomic and drug standardization purposes. *Phytochemistry,* **71**(17–18), 2058–2073.

Freeman, R.M., Adekanmi, O., Waterfield, M.R., Waterfield, A.E., Wright, D., and Zajicek, J. (2006). The effect of cannabis on urge incontinence in patients with multiple sclerosis: a multicentre, randomised placebo-controlled trial (CAMS-LUTS). *International Urogynecology Journal and Pelvic Floor Dysfunction,* **17**(6), 636–641.

Gieringer, D. and Hazekamp, A. (2011). How accurate is potency testing? *O'Shaughnessy's,* 17. Autumn issue. [Online] Available at: http://www.projectcbd.org/news/the-ring-test-oshaughnessys/ (accessed April 4, 2013).

Green, B., Kavanagh, D., and Young, R. (2003). Being stoned: a review of self-reported cannabis effects. *Drug and Alcohol Review,* **22**(4), 453–460.

GW Pharmaceuticals. (2011). *Sativex Granted National Reimbursement in Spain.* [Press release, February 17] [Online] Available at: http://www.gwpharm.com/Sativex%20granted%20reimbursement%20in%20Spain. aspx (accessed April 4, 2013).

Hall, D.H. and Queener, J.E. (2007). Self-medication hypothesis of substance use: testing Khantzian's updated theory. *Journal of Psychoactive Drugs,* **39**(2), 151–158.

Haney, M., Gunderson, E.W., Rabkin, J., et al. (2007). Dronabinol and marijuana in HIV-positive marijuana smokers. Caloric intake, mood, and sleep. *Journal of Acquired Immune Deficiency Syndromes,* **45**(5), 545–554.

Haney, M., Rabkin, J., Gunderson, E., and Foltin, R.W. (2005). Dronabinol and marijuana in HIV(+) marijuana smokers: acute effects on caloric intake and mood. *Psychopharmacology (Berlin),* **181**(1), 170–178.

Hashibe, M., Morgenstern, H., Cui, Y., et al. (2006). Marijuana use and the risk of lung and upper aerodigestive tract cancers: results of a population-based case-control study. *Cancer Epidemiology Biomarkers and Prevention,* **15,** 1829–1834.

Hathaway, A.D. and Rossiter, K. (2007). Medical marijuana, community building, and Canada's compassionate societies. *Contemporary Justice Review,* **10**(3), 283–296.

Hazekamp, A., Bastola, K., Rashidi, H., Bender, J., and Verpoorte, R. (2007). Cannabis tea revisited: a systematic evaluation of the cannabinoid composition of cannabis tea. *Journal of Ethnopharmacology,* **113,** 85–90.

Hazekamp, A. and Fischedick, J.T. (2012). Cannabis – from cultivar to chemovar. Towards a better definition of cannabis potency. *Drug Testing and Analysis*, **4**, 660–667.

Hazekamp, A., Fischedick, J.T., Diez, M.L., Lubbe, A., and Ruhaak, R.L. (2010). Chemistry of cannabis. In: L. Mander and H.-W. Lui (eds.). *Comprehensive Natural Products II Chemistry and Biology*. Vol. No. **3**. Oxford: Elsevier, pp. 1033–1084.

Hazekamp, A. and Grotenhermen, F. (2010). Review on clinical studies with cannabis and cannabinoids 2005-2009. *Cannabinoids*, **5**(special issue), 1–21.

Hazekamp, A. and Heerdink, E.R. (2013). The prevalence and incidence of medicinal cannabis on prescription in the Netherlands. *European Journal of Clinical Pharmacology*, **69**, 1575–1580.

Hazekamp, A., Ruhaak, R., Zuurman, L., van Gerven, J., and Verpoorte, R. (2006). Evaluation of a vaporizing device (Volcano®) for the pulmonary delivery of tetrahydrocannabinol. *Journal of Pharmaceutical Sciences*, **95**(6), 1308–1317.

Hazekamp, A. and Verpoorte, R. (2006). Structure elucidation of the tetrahydrocannabinol complex with randomly methylated-beta-cyclodextrin. *European Journal of Pharmaceutical Sciences*, **29**(5), 340–347.

Hazekamp, A., Ware, M.A., Muller-Vahl, K.R., Abrams, D., and Grotenhermen, F. (2013) The medicinal use of cannabis and cannabinoids; an international cross-sectional survey on administration forms. *Journal of Psychoactive Drugs*, **45**, 199–210.

Health Canada. (2011). *Medical Use of Marihuana; Latest Updates*. [Online] Available at: http://www.hc-sc.gc.ca/dhp-mps/marihuana/index-eng.php (accessed April 4, 2013).

Henwood, B. and Padgett, D.K. (2007). Reevaluating the self-medication hypothesis among the dually diagnosed. *The American Journal on Addictions*, **16**(3), 160–165.

Hepler, R.S. and Petrus, R. (1976). Experiences with administration of marijuana to glaucoma patients. In: S. Cohen and R. Stillman (eds.). *The Therapeutic Potential of Marihuana*. New York: Plenum Medical Book Company, pp. 63–76.

Hiller, F.C., Wilson, F.J.J., Mazumder, M.K., Wilson, J.D., and Bone, R.C. (1984). Concentration and particle size distribution in smoke from marijuana cigarettes with different delta9-tetrahydrocannabinol content. *Fundamental and Applied Toxicology*, **4**, 451–454.

IACM (International Association for Cannabinoid Medicine). (2012). *Increasing numbers of patients use cannabis for medicinal purposes*. [Online] Electronic newsletter of 08 April 2012. Available at: http://blog.norml.org/2012/04/11/estimate-worldwide-population-of-lawful-medical-marijuana-patients/ (accessed April 4, 2013).

Izzo, A.A., Borrelli, F., Capasso, R., Di Marzo, V., and Mechoulam, R. (2009). Non-psychotropic plant cannabinoids: new therapeutic opportunities from an ancient herb. *Trends in Pharmacological Sciences*, **30**(10), 515–527.

Janichek, J.L. and Reiman, A. (2012). Clinical service desires of medical cannabis patients. *Harm Reduction Journal*, **9**, 12–17.

Joy, J.E., Watson, S.J., and Benson, J.A. (eds.). (1999) *Marijuana and Medicine: Assessing the Science Base*. Washington, DC: Institute of Medicine, National Academy Press.

Killestein, J., Hoogervorst, E.L.J., Reif, M., *et al.* (2002). Safety, tolerability, and efficacy of orally administered cannabinoids in MS. *Neurology*, **58**(9), 1404–1407.

Kondrad, E. and Reid, A. (2013). Colorado family physicians' attitudes toward medical marijuana. *Journal of the American Board of Family Medicine*, **26**(1), 52–60.

Lee, M.A. (2013). Juicing raw cannabis. *O'Shaughnessy's*, 27. Winter/Spring issue. [Online] Available at: http://www.beyondthc.com/wp-content/uploads/2013/03/Juicing-33.pdf (accessed April 4, 2013).

Leizer, C., Ribnicky, D., Poulev, A., Dushenkov, S., and Raskin, I. (2000). The composition of hemp seed oil and its potential as an important source of nutrition. *Journal of Nutraceuticals, Functional & Medical Foods*, **2**(4), 35–53.

Lucas, P. (2012). It can't hurt to ask; a patient-centered quality of service assessment of Health Canada's medical cannabis policy and program. *Harm Reduction Journal*, **9**, 2.

Lynch, M., Young, J., and Clark, A.J. (2006). A case series of patients using medicinal marihuana for management of chronic pain under the Canadian marihuana medical access regulations. *Journal of Pain and Symptom Management*, **32**(5), 497–501.

Mattes, R.D., Engelman, K., Shaw, L.M., and Elsohly, M.A. (1994). Cannabinoids and appetite stimulation. *Pharmacology Biochemistry and Behavior*, **49**, 187–195.

Matthias, P., Tashkin, D.P., Marques-Magallanes, J.A., Wilkins, J.N., and Simmons, M.S. (1997). Effects of varying marijuana potency on deposition of tar and delta9-THC in the lung during smoking. *Pharmacology Biochemistry and Behaviour*, **58**, 1145–1150.

McLaren, J., Swift, W., Dillon, P., and Allsop, S. (2008). Cannabis potency and contamination: a review of the literature. *Addiction*, **103**, 1100–1109.

Mehra, R., Moore, B.A., Crothers, K., Tetrault, J., and Fiellin, D.A. (2006). The association between marijuana smoking and lung cancer: a systematic review. *Archives of Internal Medicine*, **166**, 1359–1367.

Micale, V., Di Marzo, V., Sulcova, A., Wotjak, C.T., and Drago, F. (2013). Endocannabinoid system and mood disorders: priming a target for new therapies. *Pharmacology & Therapeutics*, **138**(1), 18–37.

NCSM (Dutch foundation for legal cannabis and its constituents as medicine). (2012). *Survey Among Major Health Insurance Companies* [In Dutch]. [Online] Available at: http://www.ncsm.nl/cfsystem/userData/pdf/1358352476__document__ncsm-vergoeding-medicinale-cannabis-2012.doc.pdf (accessed April 4, 2013).

Nussbaum, A.M., Boyer, J.A., and Kondrad, E.C. (2011). "But my doctor recommended pot": medical marijuana and the patient-physician relationship. *Journal of General Internal Medicine*, **26**(11), 1364–1367.

Nutt, D., King, L.A., Saulsbury, W., and Blakemore, C. (2007). Development of a rational scale to assess the harm of drugs of potential misuse. *Lancet*, **369**(9566), 1047–1053.

Ogborne, A.C., Smart, R.G., Weber, T., and Birchmore-Timney, C. (2000). Who is using cannabis as a medicine and why: an exploratory study. *Journal of Psychoactive Drugs*, **32**, 435–443.

Ohlsson, A., Lindgren, J.E., A Wahlen,A., Agurell, S., Hollister, L.E., and Gillespie, H.K. (1980). Plasma delta-9-THC concentrations and clinical effects after oral and intravenous administrations and smoking. *Clinical Pharmacology & Therapeutics*, **28**, 409–416.

OMC (Office of Medicinal Cannabis). (2013). Department of Health, official website. [Online] Available at: http://www.cannabisbureau.nl (accessed April 4, 2013).

Passie, T., Emrich, H.M., Karst, M., Brandt, S.D., and Halpern, J.H. (2012). Mitigation of post-traumatic stress symptoms by *Cannabis* resin: a review of the clinical and neurobiological evidence. *Drug Testing & Analysis*, **4**(7–8), 649–659.

Prentiss, D., Power, R., Balmas, G., Tzuang, G., and Israelski, D.M. (2004). Patterns of marijuana use among patients with HIV/AIDS followed in a public health care setting. *Journal of Acquired Immune Deficiency Syndromes*, **35**(1), 38–45.

Reiman, A.E. (2008). Self-efficacy, social support and service integration at medical cannabis facilities in the San Francisco Bay Area of California. *Health & Social Care in the Community*, **16**(1), 31–41.

Reiman, A.E. (2009). Cannabis as a substitute for alcohol and other drugs. *Harm Reduction Journal*, **6**, 35.

Reinarman, C., Nunberg, H., Lanthier, F., and Heddleston, T. (2011). Who are medical marijuana patients? Population characteristics from nine California assessment clinics. *Journal of Psychoactive Drugs*, **43**(2), 128–135.

Romano, L.L. and Hazekamp, A. (2013). Cannabis oil, chemical evaluation of an upcoming cannabis-based medicine. *Cannabinoids*, **1**(1), 1–11.

Russo, E.B. (2011). Taming THC: potential cannabis synergy and phytocannabinoid-terpenoid entourage effects. *British Journal of Pharmacology*, **163**, 1344–1364.

Scheel, A.H., Krause, D., Haars, H., Schmitz, I., and Junker, K. (2012). Talcum induced pneumoconiosis following inhalation of adulterated marijuana, a case report. *Diagnostic Pathology*, **7**, 26.

Simpson, R. (2008). *Run from the Cure*. [Documentary film] [Online] Available at: http://www.youtube.com/watch?v=0psJhQHk_GI (accessed April 4, 2013).

Simpson, R. (2013). Rick Simpson official website. [Online] Available at: http://phoenixtears.ca/ (accessed April 4, 2013).

Snoeijer, W. (2001). *A Checklist of Some Cannabaceae Cultivars. Part 1: Cannabis*. Leiden: Div. Pharmacognosy, Leiden/Amsterdam Centre for Drug Research.

Steinagle, G.C. and Upfal, M. (1999). Concentration of marijuana metabolites in the urine after ingestion of hemp seed tea. *Journal of Occupational & Environmental Medicine*, **41**, 510–513.

Strasser, F., Luftner, D., Possinger, K., et al. (2006). Comparison of orally administered cannabis extract and delta-9-tetrahydrocannabinol in treating patients with cancer-related anorexia-cachexia syndrome: a multicenter, phase III, randomized, double-blind, placebo-controlled clinical trial from the Cannabis-In-Cachexia-Study-Group. *Journal of Clinical Oncology*, **24**(21), 3394–3400.

Suh, J.J., Ruffins, S., Robins, C.E., Albanese, M.J., and Khantzian, E.J. (2008). Self-medication hypothesis – connecting affective experience and drug choice. *Psychoanalytic Psychology*, **25**(3), 518–532.

Sullivan, P. (2012). *MD Role in Use of Medical Marijuana Baffles Many Doctors: Survey*. [Online] [Canadian Medical Association, news item released on October 11, 2012.] Available at: http://www.cma.ca/md-role-medical-marijuana-baffles (accessed April 4, 2013).

Swift, W., Gates, P., and Dillon, P. (2005). Survey of Australians using cannabis for medical purposes. *Harm Reduction Journal*, **2**, 18.

Takeda, S., Misawa, K., Yamamoto, I., and Watanabe, K. (2008). Cannabidiolic acid as a selective cyclooxygenase-2 inhibitory component in cannabis. *Drug Metabolism and Disposition*, **36**(9), 1917–1921.

United Nations Office on Drugs and Crime. (2012). *World Drug Report*. New York: United Nations Publishing.

Van Amsterdam, J.G.C., Van Marle, J., Van Dijk, P., Niesink, R., and Opperhuizen, A. (2007). *Electronenmicroscopisch onderzoek van vervuilde wietmonsters* [Electron-microscopic evaluation of polluted cannabis samples; study in Dutch]. Bilthoven: RIVM (Dutch National Institute for Health and the Environment).

Van der Kooy, F., Pomahacova, B., and Verpoorte, R. (2009). Cannabis smoke condensate II: influence of tobacco on tetrahydrocannabinol levels. *Inhalation Toxicology*, **21**(2), 87–90.

Van der Pol, P., Liebregts, N., De Graaf, R., Korf, D.J., Van den Brink, W., and Van Laar, M. (2013). Validation of self-reported cannabis dose and potency: an ecological study. *Addiction*, **108**(10), 1801–1808.

Velasco, G., Sánchez, C., and Guzmán, M. (2012). Towards the use of cannabinoids as antitumour agents. *Nature Reviews Cancer*, **12**(6), 436–444.

Veress, T., Szanto, J.I., and Leisztner, L. (1990). Determination of cannabinoid acids by high-performance liquid chromatography of their neutral derivatives formed by thermal decarboxylation in an open reactor. *Journal of Chromatography*, **520**, 339–347.

Verhoeckx, K.C., Korthout, H.A., Van Meeteren-Kreikamp, A.P., et al. (2006). Unheated Cannabis sativa extracts and its major compound THC-acid have potential immuno-modulating properties not mediated by CB1 and CB2 receptor coupled pathways. *International Immunopharmacology*, **6**(4), 656–665.

Vinciguerra, V., Moore, T., and Brennan, E. (1988). Inhalation of marijuana as an antiemetic for cancer chemotherapy. *New York State Journal of Medicine*, **85**, 525–527.

Wall, M.E. and Perez-Reyes, M. (1981). The metabolism of delta-9-tetrahydrocannabinol and related cannabinoids in man. *Journal of Clinical Pharmacology*, **21**, 178S–189S.

Ware, M. (2012). *Moving ahead on the medical use of cannabis.* [Online] Opinion paper sent to the Montreal Gazette. December 18, 2012. Available at: http://www.montrealgazette.com/Opinion+Moving+ahead+medical+cannabis/7710533/story.html#ixzz2GvABWL00 (accessed April 4, 2013).

Woodward, C. (2012). A move toward self-medication in the United States. *Canadian Medical Association Journal*, **184**(10), 1130–1131.

Zajicek, J., Fox, P., Sanders, H., *et al.* (2003). Cannabinoids for treatment of spasticity and other symptoms related to multiple sclerosis (CAMS study): multicentre randomised placebo-controlled trial. *Lancet*, **362**(9395), 1517–1526.

Zajicek, J.P., Sanders, H.P., Wright, D.E., *et al.* (2005). Cannabinoids in multiple sclerosis (CAMS) study: safety and efficacy data for 12 months follow up. *Journal of Neurology, Neurosurgery and Psychiatry*, **76**(12), 1664–1669.

Zuardi, A.W. (2006). History of cannabis as a medicine: a review. *Revista Brasileira De Psiquiatria*, **28**(2), 153–157.

Zuurman, L., Roy, C., Schoemaker, R., *et al.* (2008). Effect of intrapulmonary THC administration in humans. *Journal of Psychopharmacology*, **22**(7), 707–716.

Chapter 18

Cannabis Distribution: Coffee Shops to Dispensaries

Amanda Reiman

18.1 Introduction

The formal distribution of non-medical cannabis is only allowed in one nation, Uruguay. However, through policy loopholes and the increasing allowance of cannabis for medical purposes, cannabis distribution centers exist. Their existence most often takes the form of a coffee shop in the Netherlands, or a medical cannabis dispensary in the US and Canada. Coffee shops, often touted as a tourist attraction, assist in the separation of drug markets in the Netherlands (MacCoun and Reuter 2001), while dispensaries, collectives, or compassion centers as they are sometimes called, require proper documents from a physician to gain entry. Regardless of the context, the distribution of cannabis is a contentious issue, mostly due to assumptions about criminal activity and potential threats to the surrounding community, even though these fears have not been supported by research (Kepple and Freisthler 2012; Kintz 2010). This chapter will review the history of cannabis distribution through coffee shops and dispensaries, and the current models of distribution and related policies. Then, the current models of distribution will be defined. Next, the research on cannabis distribution will be discussed in relation to how dispensaries function as health service providers for medical marijuana patients, the impact, if any, distribution centers have on cannabis use, and the assumed connection between cannabis distribution and crime. Finally, recent developments in cannabis policy and their implications for the growing medical cannabis industry and future research will be discussed.

18.2 History

Establishments that allow for the community use of a psychoactive substance are common. From coffee shops to bars, to the once popular opium den, communal spaces for sharing psychoactive experiences have been a part of various cultures around the globe. Cannabis coffee shops in Amsterdam and dispensaries in the US and Canada have become these centers for those who consume cannabis. While the birth of these two models was under different circumstances, they share in how they function within their communities.

18.2.1 The birth of the cannabis distribution center: the Amsterdam coffee shop

A common misperception is that cannabis is legal in the Netherlands. In fact, cannabis is not legal, but is allowed via de facto legalization. This means that it is not explicitly legal, but not explicitly illegal. In an effort to curb serious drug use in the 1970s, the government decided to focus its efforts on eradicating the use of drugs such as heroin and cocaine and letting drugs like cannabis become less of a priority for law enforcement (Monshouwer et al. 2011). This gray area has allowed for an informal network of cannabis coffee shops where patrons can purchase and consume cannabis and cannabis products such as hashish. One of the drug policy aspects of the cannabis coffee shop is the resulting separation of markets. This phenomenon refers to a reduction in "harder" drug use (heroin, methamphetamine, etc.) as a result of readily available "soft" drugs (cannabis, hashish, mushrooms, etc.). The theory is that, by bringing the soft drugs into a quasi-licit market, consumers do not have to interact with purveyors of harder drugs, therefore reducing the likelihood of use (MacCoun and Reuter 2001). Officials in the Netherlands decided that, in order to address the public health issue of substance use, they would concentrate their policing efforts on hard drug use, and ease up on soft drugs. This policy decision spawned the birth of coffee shops such as Mellow Yellow, The Melkweg, Rusland, and The Bulldog, a former brothel in the red-light district. The Netherlands government saw no reason to disrupt this practice, as long as it was not causing a public health nuisance, which it had not (Bancroft 2010). The law officially changed in 1976 with the revision of the Opium Act. Since that time, various regulations have emerged, such as the decision in 1996 to raise the age of consumption from 16 to 18 years and to allow municipalities to decide whether to license coffee shops, and in 1999 to allow mayors to close coffee shops in violation of stated municipal codes (Monshouwer et al. 2011). The small-scale sales and possession of cannabis are regulated and recognized in Dutch law; however, commercial production in the Netherlands remains a point of legal intervention. In the Netherlands in 2005–2006, approximately 6000 cannabis nurseries were destroyed and in 2006 the penalty for large-scale cultivation was raised from 4 to 6 years, making it increasingly difficult to supply the coffee shops with cannabis, and there is concern that cutting off the supply will expand the underground market. Seventy percent of the cannabis purchases in the Netherlands are done via coffee shops. In 2007, there were approximately 700 coffee shops in the Netherlands which has steadily decreased since 1997, when there were 1179. In 2011, regulations surfaced regarding the proximity of one coffee shop to other coffee shops and to secondary schools, echoing similar concerns in the US about the impact that cannabis distribution has on a community (Monshouwer et al. 2011). In 2012, there was a proposal to prohibit out-of-towners or foreigners from patronizing the coffee shops by requiring a "weed pass" in order to enter. These passes were not given to nonresidents. However, the program was scrapped and local jurisdictions were tasked with enforcement. Another recent policy change prohibits the 220 currently licensed coffee shops from selling cannabis with a tetrahydrocannabinol level above 15% (Corder 2012). Amsterdam remains a popular destination for those around the globe eager to sit in a relaxed atmosphere, calmly select a strain of cannabis, and enjoy a smoke, free from the threat of criminal prosecution.

18.2.2 **Medical cannabis comes to the United States**

Although the first medical cannabis dispensaries in the US were modeled after the coffee shops in Amsterdam as a community-based, public health approach to cannabis distribution, actual cannabis distribution in the US began through a tightly controlled medical program. Modern US medical cannabis distribution began in 1976 through the Investigational New Drug compassionate access research program. Robert Randall had been diagnosed with glaucoma and found cannabis to be helpful in relieving intraocular pressure. Claiming medical necessity, Randall went to court over his right to use cannabis since, in his and his physician's opinions, available medical treatments had not been successful. Randall won the case and became the first federal medical cannabis patient in 1978 (Russo et al. 2002).

This new federal program accepted seriously ill participants and gave them access to up to nine pounds of cannabis per year. The program did not grow quickly as the application process was quite complicated. As such, only six patients were accepted into the program between 1976 and 1988. However, as HIV continued to spread across the US in the 1980s, the compassionate access program began receiving high volumes of applications from AIDS patients who had heard about the benefits of using cannabis for the pain, depression, and wasting syndromes that accompanied the disease. In 1989 alone, 34 new patients were granted access into the program. Then, in 1991 the program was suspended due to the contradiction between access to medical cannabis and then-President George H.W. Bush's stance on drug prevention. A year later in 1992, the program was discontinued. Today, only three patients from the compassionate access program survive. They continue to get medical cannabis from the federal government (Americans for Safe Access 2004; Pro-con.org 2013).

18.2.3 Medical cannabis dispensaries are born

Outside of the US government's own cannabis distribution program, medical cannabis dispensaries opened in conjunction with the passing of the first state medical cannabis law. Voters in California passed Proposition 215 in November 1996 allowing ill Californians to use cannabis for medical purposes with a doctor's recommendation. But Proposition 215 produced an immediate backlash with regard to implementation. One month later, then-Drug Czar Barry McCaffrey threatened to arrest any doctor who recommended cannabis to their patients (McCaffrey 1996). A group of physicians sued the federal government claiming that preventing them from recommending or even discussing cannabis with their patients violated their First Amendment rights and infringed on the doctor–patient relationship and their promise of confidentiality (Annas 1997). They won the case (*Conant v McCaffrey* 1997). Now that doctors were free to recommend cannabis to their patients, those with a recommendation needed a place to go and obtain their cannabis. What started out as an informal exchange system out of the home of one man would grow to become a billion-dollar industry.

Dennis Peron, the initiator of Proposition 215, developed the first medical cannabis dispensaries in San Francisco. Peron's activism was driven by his partner's experiences with AIDS and using medical cannabis to relieve the symptoms associated with his disease. Soon, Peron was distributing cannabis to HIV/AIDS patients out of his San Francisco home. Worried that the police would discover him and end his program, Peron championed Proposition P in 1992. Proposition P directed the San Francisco Police Department to make cannabis arrests its lowest priority (O'Brien 2004), which gave Peron some protection as he continued to distribute medical cannabis from his home. Peron's vision was to create a space not only to distribute cannabis to ill people, but a space for patients to support each other and benefit from contact with others in similar situations. For many HIV/AIDS patients in San Francisco and elsewhere in the 1990s, isolation and stigma were common and community became vital for survival. What grew from this vision has been described as "a combination of a community center and settlement house, a hospice, a friendly café, and—given the illegal nature of it prior to Proposition 215—a kind of speakeasy which had the approval and public support of San Francisco's Board of Supervisors, Mayors Frank Jordan and Willie Brown, its Department of Health, its District Attorney's Office, and the administration of the San Francisco Police Department" (Feldman and Mandel 1998, p. 181).

After Proposition 215 was passed in 1996 and medical cannabis became the law of the state, Peron formalized his distribution by opening the San Francisco Cannabis Buyers Club (SF CBC) on Market Street in San Francisco. Because they had the support of the local government, the SF CBC erroneously thought it had license to operate under the new law. However, although Proposition 215 protects those with a doctor's recommendation from prosecution for cannabis possession, it does not establish a licensure system for cannabis distribution. The law does allow for "caregivers" to provide cannabis to patients who cannot cultivate it themselves (Proposition 215 1996). Dispensaries such as the SF CBC designated itself a caregiver to all the patients that came in to purchase cannabis. The purchase was viewed as a "reimbursement" for cultivation costs rather than a retail sale. This issue was brought before the California Supreme Court in December 1997, where they ruled, 2 to 1, that Proposition 215 did not protect cannabis buyers' clubs because they were not considered caregivers. After the SF CBC was raided and closed in 1997, additional dispensaries decided to test the new law and began to open up in San Francisco and other "cannabis friendly" locations across California, such as Santa Cruz and Oakland. By the end of 1997 when the Supreme Court made their ruling, at least 17 other dispensaries had opened in California. Furthermore, several local municipalities supported the facilities, making the Supreme Court's ruling less relevant to the opening and operation of dispensaries in California (Daley 1997). While they were fighting for their right to exist, what began dividing dispensaries was what model of service to follow. Peron supported what is now referred to as the "social club" model and is similar to the coffee shop in Amsterdam (Grinspoon 2004). This model includes the ability to use cannabis on site (although most local regulations now prohibit this), and encourages patients to socialize and utilize each other as a support system, mainly through organized recreational activities. This type of dispensary often offers treatments in addition to cannabis, such as holistic health services and counseling. In 1997, in the city of San Jose, CA, however, a second model was brewing. More like a pharmacy than a community center, the Santa Clara Medical Cannabis Center, founded by Peter Baez, resembled a doctor's office and was the first municipally licensed dispensary in the US (Daley 1997). Along with the support of San Jose officials came regulation requirements for the dispensary. Previously, San Francisco had taken a hands-off approach when it came to regulating dispensaries within its own municipality. Included in the San Jose regulations were rules regarding how far dispensaries could be from schools and churches and requiring the facilities to keep records including patients' names, photographs, telephone numbers, addresses, ailments, and doctors' recommendations. Also, police were allowed to inspect a dispensary's records and premises at any time without a warrant, patients could not purchase more than one ounce of cannabis per week, all cannabis had to be grown on site, and the facility had to be protected by an alarm system (Gaura 1997). These were among the first cannabis distribution regulations in the US.

While other municipalities were maintaining full involvement in the development and regulation of medical cannabis dispensaries, San Francisco took a different approach. Thus, although local officials supported the notion of dispensaries and medical cannabis, the city did not impose regulations as had some of their neighboring communities. The result was that, by 2005, there were 43 medical cannabis dispensaries in San Francisco. This proliferation of dispensaries finally compelled the Board of Supervisors to develop regulations for facilities operating within the city (Argetsinger 2005). Those who managed the dispensaries, as well as advocates in the community, supported the idea of developing regulations, as long as patient and dispensary input was welcomed and considered. In July 2005, the city of San Francisco declared a 6-month moratorium on the opening of new dispensaries until regulations could be developed and implemented. This decision occurred around the same time as a federal raid on three dispensaries in San Francisco accused of drug-trafficking and money laundering. City Supervisor Ross Mirkarimi started the process of regulation development, including a call for annual licensing, limits on the number of dispensaries and where they could operate, and how much profit they could earn, which were requests very similar to those made in San Jose in 1997. There was concern that major city involvement might lead to a more pharmacy-style distribution system co-opted by the city or state. Social model clubs were revered by the patient population in San Francisco because they encouraged community and patient interaction. Dispensary managers echoed this concern and requested that the city require dispensary operators to be medical cannabis patients themselves in order to increase the comfort level of their clients and to increase the feeling of security and quality protection at the dispensary (Argetsinger 2005). The moratorium on new dispensaries in San Francisco expired November 20, 2005. Public hearings were held to allow public discussion concerning the regulations (Goodyear 2005). At the end of November, 2005, San Francisco drew up regulations for its estimated 35 medical cannabis dispensaries. Included in the regulations were the following:

♦ Dispensaries must apply for business permits which include criminal and employment background checks.

♦ Dispensary owners must pay $6610 per year for a permit in addition to $3100 for a business license (this was changed to an $8549 application fee and the implementation of an 8.5% sales tax in 2010).

♦ Zoning regulations, including no dispensaries in industrial or residential areas as well as a minimum of 500 feet from schools or daycare centers, 1000 feet if cannabis is used on the premises (Leff 2005).

18.2.4 Medical cannabis distribution in the Netherlands

While the US was struggling to define its medical cannabis distribution program, other nations developed their own medical cannabis policies and practices regarding distribution. Beginning in September 2003, the Netherlands required every pharmacy to keep cannabis in stock and dispense it to those with a doctor's prescription. Pharmacists were instructed to provide advice on use and reducing the harm associated with inhaling a smoked substance. Unlike the product sold in coffee shops, the Ministry of Health regulates the medical cannabis obtained at pharmacies in the Netherlands, which is grown in a medical grade facility, for quality. There were, however, still those critical of the move from small, personally owned medical cannabis operations to the larger, government-run pharmacy model. The worry was that the patients would pay with higher prices for cannabis and receive impersonal care (Conway 2003).

18.2.5 Pharmacy versus social model of care

While the pharmacy model is viewed as easier to control due to its centralized nature, the social model might be more appropriate for both the cannabis plant and those who consume it. Research suggests that the social support garnered by patients in a dispensary environment and the impact of service availability can be beneficial to those with serious and/or chronic illness (Reiman 2007, 2008a, 2008b). However, with the growth of complex local regulations, changes, such as the ability to use cannabis at the dispensary and the desire to keep spaces small, standardized, and nondescript, have moved the distribution system away from the social model and toward the pharmacy model. As more dispensaries started opening in California in the early 2000s, more cities decided to be proactive and institute a variety of regulations including: obtaining a business license from the city and operating as a nonprofit organization, limits on the number of dispensaries in a city, restrictions on dispensary location, limits on the amount of cannabis that can be bought and/ or possessed by patients, limits on the number of cannabis plants on site, and the prohibition of cannabis consumption on premises (Richie 2004). Not included in these early regulations were rules to protect the patients and the medical care process. For example, regulations did not include protocols for collecting and storing patient information or a declaration of patient protection in the case of federal interference. Furthermore, regulations did not mandate that dispensary workers have any special training or knowledge of cannabis or illnesses for which cannabis is used. This is starting to change, as Washington, DC has become the first jurisdiction to require training for all those working in the medical cannabis distribution industry. In addition to completing 4 hours of training, participants must pass an exam (Americans for Safe Access 2012).

Regulation of medical cannabis dispensaries is complicated. On the one hand, regulations can help distinguish and legitimize medical cannabis dispensaries as health service providers instead of drug dealing operations. This might be a protective factor against federal interference. Furthermore, in the case of federal interference, adhering to local regulations might ensure the support of local government and law enforcement on the side of dispensaries. On the other hand, adaptation of the dispensing of medical cannabis into the larger system of public healthcare might be the end of the social club model that was the vision of Dennis Peron in 1992, as limited funds and staffing might affect the level of personalized care a large, centralized health program can provide. Satisfaction with the federal program in Canada is extremely low and most Canadian patients obtain their cannabis from small, community-based distribution centers (Lucas 2012). The coffee shops in Amsterdam emerged out of a desire to address the most serious public health concerns in the Netherlands. Left to their own devices, coffee shops became cultural icons and tourist destinations. Ironically, although emerging from a more restrictive medical model in the US, the first medical cannabis dispensaries in the US looked very similar to the most famous of Amsterdam's coffee shops, enshrining the original distribution system in what would become modern-day cannabis provision in the US.

18.3 Current models and policies

California was the first state to formalize a medical cannabis distribution system on the local level. But, as more states began to pass medical cannabis legislation, the question arose of whether regulation was better made at the local or state level. While local regulations allow dispensaries to reflect the needs and desires of citizens at the community level, state-wide regulation may provide more protection from federal interference, and provides uniform rules for all involved in the industry in that state to comply with, thereby cutting down on confusion and potential law suits. Sections 18.3.1–18.3.3 will review the various models of cannabis distribution that have been developed and the policies around distribution that have been adopted by different states in the US that allow the use of medical cannabis.

18.3.1 Models of cannabis distribution

To date, four types of medical cannabis distribution have emerged, shaped by local and state regulation: storefronts, direct from garden to patient (caregiver model), delivery, and growing co-op. Some issues related to distribution, such as how cannabis is obtained for distribution and physical space requirements, will differ based on the model. The various models are defined as follows:

18.3.1.1 Storefront

A storefront is what is most often thought of when someone pictures a dispensary or coffee shop. A storefront is a physical location where qualified individuals (medical cannabis patients in the US, those over 18 years in the Netherlands, and those over 21 years in the US states of Washington and Colorado) can obtain cannabis. Usually, cannabis is brought to the storefront by a cannabis cultivator or wholesaler, and patients then purchase the product at the storefront location. Social model dispensaries are most often storefronts, as patients are encouraged to stay and socialize. Oftentimes, additional services, such as healthcare and counseling are offered in store front locations. Those who operate storefronts might obtain cannabis from a third-party grower, or they might produce the cannabis themselves in another location or at the same location as the storefront. Some states, such as Colorado, New Mexico, and Maine, have policies concerning who can provide cannabis to a storefront. These policies will be discussed later in the chapter. An example of a storefront that primarily cultivates their own cannabis at another location is the San Francisco Patients Resource Center (SPARC) (Fig. 18.1).

The storefront model of a dispensary is similar to the coffee shop in Amsterdam. In fact, one of the first storefront dispensaries in Oakland, CA, was named The Bulldog, after the iconic Amsterdam coffee shop. Furthermore, when several dispensaries settled in one area in Oakland, the area became known as Oaksterdam, a moniker that has stuck and is now the neighborhood that houses Oaksterdam University, the first trade school for those working in the medical cannabis industry (Oaksterdam University 2012).

18.3.1.2 Direct from garden to patient (caregiver model)

In this model, patients obtain cannabis directly from the cultivator either at the garden or through an ancillary location. While the cannabis is primarily grown by the distributor in this model, some states, such as New Mexico, allow licensed distributors to trade cannabis products with each other, although the majority of what is provided through the garden must be produced by its purveyor. Referred to as "vertical integration," the act of requiring a closed-loop system from cultivation to distribution is popular in modern cannabis regulation because of the belief that

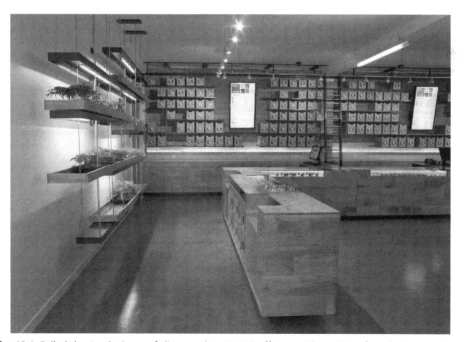

Fig. 18.1 Called the Apple Store of dispensaries, SPARC offers a wide variety of products as well as music, trivia and other social events for their patients.

Photo courtesy of SPARC.

vertical integration allows for better oversight and less diversion. Some patients prefer this model because they feel the product is fresher, similar to obtaining produce at a farmer's market versus the grocery store.

18.3.1.3 Delivery service

Although not permitted in all states that allow medical cannabis, in the delivery model, patients place an order via phone or online. Delivery services most often do not have a storefront but a center of operations from which orders are received and vehicles are dispatched. Some dispensaries operate both a storefront and delivery service. Sometimes this is in an effort to expand service and reach patients who are homebound or receiving hospice care. Sometimes delivery services are started because storefront locations are shut down by the federal government. Such was the case when Berkeley Patients Group, located in Berkeley, CA, was shuttered. The dispensary ran a delivery service while securing a new storefront location so as not to disrupt service to their patients. The delivery service continued even after a new storefront was secured (Berkeley Patients Group 2012). While some are skeptical about delivery services because of the ease of obtaining cannabis, concerns about driving while intoxicated are quelled by this model compared to the social model where consumption might be allowed at the dispensary. However, while delivery services are helpful for patients who are homebound and too ill to travel, they remove the social interaction that Peron and others involved early in dispensary creation felt was so important.

18.3.1.4 Growing co-op

A co-op model might be considered by some to be what voters in California had in mind when they approved Proposition 215. In this model, a group of patients gets together and grows cannabis collectively on property belonging to the entire group or a member of the group. Members of the co-op share in the harvest and their share is earned by contributing to the cultivation process. Duties can vary based on ability and are decided upon by the group. The growing co-op is a closed-loop system in that patients who are not members of the co-op may not obtain cannabis from the co-op. Recently, a court decision in California ruled that all members of a co-op do not have to actively participate in the cultivation process to obtain product grown by the co-op. This was an important decision because it finally clarified that a dispensary *can* be designated a caregiver, which was a point of contention in early California dispensary development (*People v Jackson* 2012). One of the most well-known growing co-ops is WAMM (Wo/men's Alliance for Medical Marijuana). Run by longtime cannabis activist Valerie Corral and located in Santa Cruz, CA, WAMM currently serves about 250 patients and was the subject of the book, *Dying to Get High* by Wendy Chapkis in 2008 (WAMM 2012).

18.3.2 Current policies: California and beyond

Since California passed Proposition 215 in 1996, 21 other states, plus Washington, DC, have also passed laws allowing for the use of cannabis with a doctor's recommendation. However, not all of these states have established programs for distributing cannabis to patients. The next section will review the current cannabis distribution policies in the US and Canada. Various types of regulation will be discussed, as well as the move from a federal to private distribution program that has recently been proposed in Canada.

18.3.2.1 Locally regulated: California

As previously discussed, California does not currently impose state-level regulations on the distribution of medical cannabis. Rather, local cities and counties have developed their own regulations.

There have been attempts to develop a state-level regulatory system, most recently in 2014 with two bills, Assembly Bill 1894 introduced by Assembly member Tom Ammiano, and Senate Bill 1262 introduced by Senator Lou Correa. Both bills are currently being considered by the California legislature. As it stands today, California is a patchwork of regulation, with some localities banning dispensaries all together, and others creating a complex system of regulation. In those localities that have chosen to impose regulations, there are some commonalities that hold across jurisdictions: a city licensure process, a limit on total number of dispensaries in the city, establishment of an oversight committee, strict zoning laws that dictate where dispensaries can be located, and flexible regulations that allow for the ever-changing cannabis regulatory landscape. In cities that have been slow to regulate, the proliferation of dispensaries has soured some on the idea of cannabis as medicine. Los Angeles, is currently trying to implement voter approved Measure D which allows only dispensaries licensed before 2007 to stay open. This was a reaction to the constant scrutiny of the free-market impact that a lack of regulation has had. In the absence of regulation, there were an estimated 1000 dispensaries in Los Angeles and the city council had thus far taken a hands-off approach to regulation, insisting that it is the job of the state, not the city to create such a structure (Onishi 2012). Another outcome of a lack of clear regulation is lawsuits. Attempts by cities to ban dispensaries or be selective concerning which dispensaries can open have led to lawsuits which have both slowed and clarified the distribution system in California (*City of Riverside v Inland Empire Patient's Health and Wellness Center*; *People v Jackson*; *Pack v City of Long Beach*). The lack of structure in California's cannabis distribution program has encouraged other medical cannabis states to either avoid the issue completely and continue with a system of informal distribution, or develop tightly controlled, state-level regulations regarding distribution.

18.3.2.2 Informal distribution: Oregon and Washington

Oregon and Washington passed medical cannabis legislation shortly after California (1998). However, neither state law describes a state-level distribution program, although both state laws protect patients and their caregivers from criminal prosecution for cannabis. In Washington, medical cannabis patients may create and participate in collective gardens for the purpose of producing, processing, transporting, and delivering cannabis. The law stipulates that no more than ten qualifying patients may participate in a single collective garden at any time and regulates how many plants can be grown at one time and stored at the garden. Furthermore, no useable cannabis from the collective garden can be delivered to anyone other than one of the participating patients. Cannabis distribution in Washington follows a true co-op model, which requires that patients share responsibility for acquiring and supplying the resources are required to produce and process the cannabis. Members are responsible for securing a location for a collective garden; equipment, supplies, and labor necessary to plant, grow, and harvest the cannabis. Patients may also grow their own cannabis for their own personal use (Washington State Legislature 2012). In Oregon, patients can cultivate their own cannabis, or designate a caregiver to grow it for them. Caregivers can grow for more than one patient. As in Washington, there are limits to the number of plants that can be grown by each patient/caregiver and the amount of dried cannabis that can be at the grow site or possessed by the patient/caregiver (Oregon Medical Marijuana Act 1998). Just like California's law, Oregon and Washington's policies do not establish a state-level structure for the creation, development, and oversight of cannabis distribution. Concerns over access for patients and the ability to institute quality control and oversight into the burgeoning cannabis industry led states such as Colorado, New Mexico, and Maine to institute tightly controlled, vertically integrated distribution systems.

18.3.2.3 **Vertical integration: New Mexico, Maine, and Colorado**

Perhaps in response to the ambiguity of distribution policies in California, Washington, and Oregon, states were soon looking to rein in cannabis distribution via tight regulatory models focused on vertical integration. Vertical integration refers to the attempt by a state to regulate every aspect of medical cannabis cultivation, manufacturing, and distribution by creating closed-loop systems which involve the fewest players possible. Three states that have adopted regulations in the context of vertical integration are New Mexico, Maine, and Colorado. Table 18.1 describes the variations in the three state programs regarding distribution and the aspects of each that fall under vertical integration.

The complex regulatory structures developed by these states rely on a sophisticated cannabis industry able to fulfill the obligations set by the states for compliance. As such, organizations such as the National Cannabis Industry Association (http://thecannabisindustry.org/) have developed to organize the industry, help set the standards for future cannabis distribution, and address issues of federal interference around banking, taxation, and labor. Advances in packaging and product

Table 18.1 Vertical integration in cannabis distribution programs: New Mexico, Maine, and Colorado

	New Mexico	**Maine**	**Colorado**
Distribution	Done via the state licensed producers. In a garden to patient model, cannabis is distributed by the producer	Done via the state licensed producers. Dispensaries must produce their own cannabis	Done through state licensed centers. 70% of cannabis dispensed through a dispensary must be grown by that dispensary
For/non profit	**Non-profit**	**Non-profit**	**Can be for profit**
Vertical integration	Licensed producers may obtain plants, seeds, and/or other usable cannabis from other licensed producers only	Patients may only belong to one dispensary. Dispensaries may cultivate up to 6 mature plants per registered patient. Dispensaries must cultivate their own cannabis. Cannabis may be donated to a dispensary from a caregiver who has extra. This may be given to low-income patients, but cannot be resold	70% of product distributed must be produced by that dispensary. Licensed dispensaries may contract with licensed infused product makers. A licensee may purchase up to 30% of its total inventory from another licensed dispensary. Infused product licensees, may not use cannabis from more than 5 licensed dispensaries
Zoning	Personal grow sites and nonprofit dispensing entities may not be located within 300 feet of any school, church, or day-care center. In addition, the applicant must demonstrate that the cannabis is not visible from streets or public areas	A dispensary or its grow site if cannabis is not grown at the retail dispensary site may not locate within 500 feet of the property line of a preexisting public or private school	Must be 1000 feet from other licensed facilities, schools, alcohol and drug treatment centers, principal campus of a university, or seminary, or residential child care facility. Localities may adjust this distance or choose not to allow medical cannabis businesses in their city

development, security requirements, dispensary pay rolls, insurance and retirement plans, and ever-changing restrictions on advertising have spawned an ancillary cannabis industry. In the US, the cannabis industry has relied heavily on private investment given the refusal of the federal government to engage with the program, except to try and stop it. This has not been the case elsewhere. Canada has had a federal medical cannabis distribution program since 1999 (Lucas 2012). However, a recent decision to shift the program from federal to private control has raised questions.

18.3.3 A shift from government program to private industry: Canada

Canada's medical cannabis distribution program was similar in nature to the informal systems in Oregon and Washington. The federal government oversees the registry of patients, and patients can obtain a permit from the government to cultivate their own medicine. Informal dispensaries popped up in more progressive areas of the country as a clearinghouse for patients to bring cannabis they had grown for redistribution among other patients. In 2010, these community-based dispensaries served over 30,000 Canadian patients, while the federal program only registered 4884 people. This was due to the complicated registration process and quality and safety concerns over the product produced by the one government licensed cultivator, Prairie Plant Systems (Lucas 2012). The lack of satisfaction with the federal program has led more Canadians to obtain personal cultivation licenses, 26,000 being issued between 2000 and 2010. As a result, in 2012, the decision was made to stop the country's federal program, including the personal cultivation licenses, in favor of vertical integration, for which a handful of cultivators will be chosen to produce and distribute cannabis to those in the federal program. Personal cultivation will not be allowed. The government plans to implement the new program by March 31, 2014 (Burgmann 2012).

Once states began to pass laws removing criminal penalties for those using cannabis with a doctor's recommendation, they had no choice but to address how patients were to obtain the cannabis. Various distribution systems, from local regulation, to informal distribution to vertical integration have created a naturally occurring experiment that has made it possible to obtain information about various aspects of cannabis distribution and its impact the health and well-being not only of patients, but also of the communities in which they exist.

18.4 Research

Medical cannabis dispensaries in the US and Canada are a fairly new phenomenon even though coffee shops in Amsterdam have existed since the 1970s. Concerns about those who patronize these facilities, the impact that these facilities have on their communities, and the cannabis-using behavior of those in proximity have spawned a flurry of research in recent years in an attempt to better understand the implications and outcomes associated with cannabis distribution. Sections 18.4.1–18.4.3 will review the research on cannabis distribution from coffee shops and dispensaries in the context of alternative healthcare, cannabis use by those in proximity to distribution centers, and the relationship between dispensaries and crime.

18.4.1 Dispensaries as alternative health service providers

Part of Dennis Peron's vision of a dispensary was its role as an alternative health service provider. Beliefs about the relationship between health, socialization, medicine, and community helped shape the first dispensaries to be part pharmacy, part community center, and part alternative medicine sanctuary. Feldman and Mandel (1998) provided the first exploratory and ethnographic study of a dispensary via their examination of the SF CBC that included interviews and participant observation. At the time of this study, the SF CBC was a four-story building on Market Street in San Francisco. Participants reported positive benefits from the support-group atmosphere of the facility. Furthermore, for those dealing with a terminal illness, the dispensary was a place for support and grief when friends and fellow medical cannabis patients died. After 2 years of interviews and observation, the authors concluded that the social club model of cannabis dispensary was the preferred method of distribution. Another early study of medical cannabis dispensaries in the US was one that focused on 57 medical cannabis patients at the SF CBC (Mikuriya 1995). Although the purpose of the study was to generate demographic data and information on the use of cannabis as self-medication, it included a colorful description of the SF CBC:

> Several doors away from a busy street corner is a nondescript door with a peep lens. Pressing the door-bell between the hours of 10 am and 7 pm weekdays, the door is opened by a doorman who asks to see the numbered club card . . . Entering midway into a large old former dime-a-dance hall above the bar below. The room is well lit from clerestory windows. The ceiling is covered by a huge rainbow flag. The walls are covered with local artists' work and political posters . . . A large old dining room table dominates the center of the room, a semi-circle of sofas at the left, and smaller tables against the wall on the right accommodate the buyers. Joints are rolled, pipes and water pipes are filled and shared from medium grade cannabis furnished by the house on small trays. The dealers measure out the cannabis from behind a "bar" where buyers inspect and purchase cannabis . . . In addition to smoked cannabis, baked goods for oral use are sold . . . On the periphery, tables with diverse health and informational literature provide reading materials for the buyers. Stationary, postage and lists of politicians provide other activities for buyers, staff and visitors. (Mikuriya 1995, p. 2)

Early dispensaries such as the SF CBC often offered a myriad of alternative health services in addition to cannabis, such as acupuncture, massage, and harm reduction groups. Rarely given the chance to participate in some of these services outside the dispensary (services were often free for patients), many patients viewed their dispensary as not only a place to obtain cannabis, but a place to engage in other methods of healing and self-awareness. Reiman's (2008a) study of 130 medical cannabis patients showed 66% of the sample using social services at their dispensary once or twice per week, 22% using life services such as food and housing help once or twice per week, and 46% using entertainment services once or twice per week. Dispensary familiarity, staff, and a feeling of comfort and security were listed as the most important reasons patients choose a particular dispensary. A more recent survey of 303 medical cannabis patients at a dispensary in California in 2011 revealed that 62% reported a desire to participate in free clinical services at the dispensary, 34% desired more information about substances and use, and 41% wanted to learn more about reducing harms from substance use. About one-quarter of the participants "would" or "likely would" participate in individual services such as consultation, psycho-educational forums, harm reduction information-sharing sessions, online support groups, and coping, life, and social skills groups (Janichek and Reiman 2012). In a qualitative report developed for a dispensary in Berkeley, CA, in-depth patient interviews revealed that, for many patients, alternative health services provided by their dispensary act as a bridge for times when they cannot afford those treatments on their own accord. Patients reported that these services allow them to continually improve, without lapses in care (Reiman 2008b). Although the public is generally supportive of increasing access to healthcare, there has been concern expressed in the US and the Netherlands as to how the increased access to cannabis through distribution centers has impacted the use rates of those who live in proximity to these facilities, especially young people.

18.4.2 **Distribution centers and cannabis use**

Most of the research on the impact of cannabis distribution and related policies on cannabis use has come from the Netherlands, save for research on youth use in the US. The Netherlands, like the US, conducts a general population survey aimed at assessing the prevalence of drug use. When looking at the Netherlands compared to other European nations without cannabis distribution, use is relatively low. The European average for recent use among those aged 15–64 is 6.8%, compared to the Dutch rate of 5.4%. This difference remains when looking at 15–34-year-olds (12.5% vs. 9.5%). The highest prevalence is in Spain (24.3% and 20.3% respectively for both age groups) and the lowest is in Greece (3.6% and 3.2% respectively). Furthermore, cannabis use among Dutch teens aged 12–17 has been on a steady decline since 1996, which some feel might be due to policies increasing the age of consumption from 16 to18 and the decline in the number of coffee shops between 1997 and 2007 (Monshouwer et al. 2011). The separation in markets referred to earlier can also be assessed by looking at Dutch drug use rates. According to a study by Craig Reinarman (2009), hard drug rates are higher in San Francisco than Amsterdam although cannabis access is greater in Amsterdam and cannabis use rates for the two cities are similar. A concern over the tightening of regulations in the Netherlands and the reduction in the number of coffee shops is an increase in underground purchases where hard drugs may be more available (Monshouwer et al. 2011). There are several complications in comparing cannabis use in the Netherlands to use in the US. First, use in both countries seems to occur in waves, fueled by cultural occurrences. Secondly, general population surveys do not always employ the same methodology and can therefore yield noncomparable results (Korf 2002). In the US, there has been particular concern about the impact of dispensaries on youth use. This concern is primarily based on the assumption that proximity to cannabis distribution impacts use. This theory was tested in Amsterdam in a 2012 study that concluded that proximity to coffee shops was not associated with frequency or intensity of cannabis use or harder drug use (Wouters et al. 2012). Research on the cannabis use patterns of medical cannabis patients in the US who utilize dispensaries reveals that most patients report no change in their cannabis use over the past 6 months. Furthermore, many patients report using cannabis as a substitute for alcohol and harder drugs (Lucas et al. 2013; Reiman 2007 and 2009). Concerns over dispensaries and access to medical cannabis encouraging teen use spawned a 2011 report which assessed changes in youth use in medical cannabis states after laws were passed Of the 13 states with medical cannabis laws at the time of the study, all but the two most recent states to pass laws (Michigan and New Mexico) showed declines in teen cannabis use after medical cannabis laws went into effect (O'Keefe and Earleywine 2011). In both the Netherlands and the US, cannabis distribution does not seem to be related to an increase in cannabis use.

18.4.3 **Dispensaries and crime**

One of the most common concerns surrounding cannabis distribution is the risk of crime. Both concerns over the patrons of the dispensary and the risk of burglary, has spawned tight security regulations for dispensaries and NIMBY ("not in my backyard") arguments against cannabis distribution. However, these concerns are largely unfounded. A recent study by Kepple and Freisthler (2012) employed an ecological design to examine the relationship between dispensary density, property, and violent crime in Los Angeles, California. The authors found no relationship between dispensary density and property or violent crime. Another study (Kintz 2010) looked at the 2010 census data for 189 census tracts in San Francisco to assess the relationship between dispensaries and neighborhood criminal activity. The author found no relationship between dispensaries and community crime. Furthermore, a 2009 analysis by the Denver Police Department found that dispensaries were robbed at lower rates than both banks and liquor stores (Ingold 2010). Similar findings surfaced in Los Angeles in 2009 when the police chief announced that the Los Angeles Police Department received reports of 71 robberies at the more than 350 banks in the city, compared with 47 robberies at medical cannabis dispensaries which, at the time, numbered at least 800 (Castro 2010). Despite this evidence, most medical cannabis distribution centers are required to be a certain number of feet from sensitive areas such as schools, churches and day care centers.

As the regulation of cannabis distribution in the US, Canada, and the Netherlands continues to evolve, more research will be required to determine the best practices for cannabis distribution. There are several recent developments that will impact how this practice looks in the years to come.

18.5 **Conclusion: the expansion and formalization of cannabis distribution**

Since the first coffee shops appeared in Amsterdam in the 1970s, cannabis distribution has continued to evolve. The California dispensaries that paved the way for 17 other states plus Washington, DC, borrowed their models of distribution from the coffee shops in Amsterdam. Today, the Netherlands, Canada, and the US contain a variety of cannabis distribution models, from social clubs to pharmacies. So, what is the next frontier for cannabis distribution in the US and elsewhere? That question was answered on Election Day 2012, when Colorado and Washington became the first US states to legalize cannabis for anyone aged 21 and over, even without a doctor's recommendation. While simple possession became legal in those states shortly after the election, both states have a period of time to develop a distribution system. Colorado, given the existence of a tightly regulated medical cannabis distribution system, is planning on expanding that system to include all adults, not just medical cannabis patients, while Washington, with its informal distribution network, will most likely develop a brand new system for distributing cannabis. Differences in the laws exist. In Colorado, persons are allowed to cultivate up to six cannabis plants. In Washington, personal cultivation is not allowed, unless a person is a medical cannabis patient. The federal government in the US has yet to announce how it will approach the idea of cannabis distribution. Other states likely to consider legalization for adult use in the near future include Maine, Rhode Island, California, and Oregon (Dickinson 2012).

Although this chapter has focused on the Netherlands, US, and Canada, other nations are beginning to experiment with their marijuana policies as well, although none but Israel has developed sophisticated distribution methods for medical marijuana. In 2001, Portugal became the first European nation to decriminalize possession of all drugs, resulting in a steep decline in HIV infection, illicit drug use, and addiction (Szalavitz 2009). Belize is also considering decriminalizing marijuana, while other nations, such as Mexico are considering the legalization of marijuana, along with establishing a system of distribution within the country (Cave 2012; Torres 2012; Williams 2012). In 2013, Uruguay became the first nation in the world to fully legalize marijuana.

Along with policy changes in the US and abroad, formal organizations and institutions are taking on the task of determining the best practices for cannabis distribution. Although not a formal government organization, the American Herbal Products Association (AHPA) is responsible for the regulation of herbal vitamins and supplements that are sold in stores by not regulated by the Food and Drug Administration (e.g., hemp products, herbal supplements, and remedies). The AHPA has a cannabis committee that has been working with the medical cannabis patient advocacy group, Americans for Safe Access, since 2011 on the development of regulatory guidelines for the cultivation, analysis, manufacturing and distribution of cannabis in the US. These guidelines, developed by experts from the cannabis industry, and the dietary supplement regulation industry are meant to guide regulators in how to create protocols in line with how other herbal products are currently regulated in the US (McGuffin 2012). Additionally, Humboldt State University in Northern California has recently instituted the Humboldt Interdisciplinary Institute for Marijuana Research (HIIMR) which will bring together scientists across fields to study the environmental, economic and public health aspects of cannabis and cannabis regulation. It is the first institute of its kind in the US. (http://www.humboldt.edu/hiimr/).

Cannabis distribution is a complex issue. In the 35 short years since Amsterdam saw its first coffee shop, cannabis policies and public attitudes have swung in both directions. Currently, with the fast-growing cannabis movement in the US and elsewhere, there is greater interest than ever in effective methods of distributing cannabis. Those with vested interests disagree as to the best model of delivery and the level of control that must exist to protect both access to cannabis and public safety. What has resulted is a naturally occurring experiment of various models of distribution and methods of regulation. Eventually, and with proper research, it can be determined what aspects of regulation and distribution models will meet the needs of a rapidly changing cannabis market and consumer population.

References

Americans for Safe Access. (2004). *Patients in the Crossfire.* Berkeley, CA: Americans for Safe Access.

Americans for Safe Access. (2012). *Medical Marijuana Patient Group Gets D.C. Department of Health Contract to Train Dispensary, Cultivation Center Staff.* [Online] Available at: http://americansforsafeaccess.org/medical-marijuana-patient-group-gets-dc-department-of-health-contract-to-train-dispensary-cultivation-center-staff.

Annas, G. (1997). Reefer madness: the federal response to California's medical marijuana law. *New England Journal of Medicine*, **337**, 435–439.

Argetsinger, A. (2005). Pot-club owners seek regulation; medical marijuana is falling into the wrong hands, proprietors fear. *Washington Post*, July 1, A3.

Bancroft, S. (2010). The history of Amsterdam's coffee shops. *Suite101.com*, September 23. [Online] Available at: http://suite101.com/article/the-history-of-amsterdams-coffee-shops-a289211.

Berkeley Patients Group. (2012). *Delivery Service Information.* [Online] Available at: http://www.berkeleypatientsgroup.com/delivery.html.

Burgmann, T. (2012). Medical marijuana delivery to go private. *Huffington Post* (Canada), December 17. [Online] Available at: http://www.huffingtonpost.ca/2012/12/16/medical-marijuana-delivery-private_n_2312600.html

Castro, T. (2010). Pot clinics draw fewer robberies than banks: chief says LAPD study disproves commonly held belief about dispensaries. *L.A. Daily News*, January 17, A1.

Cave, D. (2012). Uruguay: a vote for marijuana. *New York Times*, November 15. [Online] Available at: http://www.nytimes.com/2012/11/16/world/americas/uruguay-a-vote-for-marijuana.html?_r=0.

Chapkis, W. (2008). *Dying to Get High: Marijuana as Medicine.* New York: NYU Press.

Colorado Department of Public Health and Environment (2012). *Colorado Medical Marijuana Registry Home Page.* [Online] Available at: http://www.colorado.gov/cs/Satellite/CDPHE-CHEIS/CBON/1251593016680.

Conant v MacCaffrey (1997). No. C 97-00139 WHA. Filed in the United States District Court of Northern California.

Conway, I. (2003). Medical marijuana goes on sale in Dutch pharmacies. *The Independent (London)*, Foreign News, September 1, 9.

Corder, M. (2012). Amsterdam's pot-selling coffee shops remain open to tourists. *Huffington Post*, November 20. [Online] Available at: http://www.huffingtonpost.com/2012/11/20/amsterdam-tourists-will-still-visit-pot-coffee-shops_n_2164926.html.

Daley, Y. (1997). California marijuana clubs under fire; Court says they aren't dispensaries. *Boston Globe*, December 21, A8.

Dickenson, T. (2012). The next seven states to legalize pot. *Rolling Stone*, December, 18. [Online] Available at: http://www.rollingstone.com/politics/news/the-next-seven-states-to-legalize-pot-20121218.

Feldman, H. and Mandel, J. (1998). Providing medical marijuana: the importance of cannabis clubs. *Journal of Psychoactive Drugs*, **30**, 179–186.

Gaura, M. (1997). San Jose is first to regulate medical marijuana clubs; rules require photo ID, on site pot cultivation. *San Francisco Chronicle*, May 16, A14.

Goodyear, C. (2005). Supervisors working on new rules for pot clubs; regulations could include waiting lists, distance regulations. *San Francisco Chronicle*, October 7, B5.

Grinspoon, L. (2004). Medical marihuana in a time of prohibition. In: J. Inciardi and K. McElrath (eds.). *The American Drug Scene: An Anthology*. 4th ed. Los Angeles, CA: Roxbury Publishing Company, pp.121 –130.

Ingold, J. (2010). Cops: pot shop robbery rate is below banks. *Denver Post*, January 27, B01.

Janichek, J. and Reiman, A. (2012). Clinical service desires of medical cannabis patients. *Harm Reduction Journal*, 9, 12.

Kepple, N. and Freisthler, B. (2012). Exploring the ecological association between crime and medical marijuana dispensaries. *Journal on the Study of Alcohol and Drugs*, **73**, 523–530.

Kintz, M. (2010). *Smoke and Mirrors? Examining the relationship between medical cannabis dispensaries and crime*. Completed as part of the requirements for a Master's Degree in Public Policy from the Goldman School of Public Policy, University of California, Berkeley.

Korf, D. (2002). Dutch coffee shops and trends in cannabis use. *Addictive Behaviors*, **27**, 851–866.

Leff, L. (2005). San Francisco adopts rules for pot clubs. *The Washington Post*, November 16.

Lucas, P. (2012). It can't hurt to ask: a patient-centered quality of service assessment of health Canada's medical cannabis policy and program. *Harm Reduction Journal*, 9, 2.

Lucas, P., Reiman, A., Earleywine, M., *et al.* (2013). Cannabis as a substitute for alcohol and other drugs: a dispensary-based survey of substitution effect in Canadian medical cannabis patients. *Addiction Research and Theory*, **21**, 435–442.

McCaffrey, B. (1996). *The Administration's response to the passage of California Proposition 215 and Arizona's Proposition 200*. Statement released by Barry McCaffrey, Director of the Office of National Drug Control Policy, December 30. Washington, DC: Executive Office of the President.

McGuffin, M. (2012). Personal communication regarding the development of cannabis distribution guidelines with Michael McGuffin, President of the American Herbal Products Association.

MacCoun, R. and Reuter, P. (2001). *Drug War Heresies: Learning from Other Vices, Places and Times*. Cambridge, MA: Cambridge University Press.

Maine Department of Health and Human Services. (2012). *Maine's Medical Marijuana Law*. [Online] Available at: http://www.maine.gov/legis/lawlib/medmarij.html.

Mikuriya, T. (1995). *Medicinal Cannabis Users at a "Buyers" Club*. [Online] Available at: http://safeaccessnow.org/article.php?id=2830.

Monshouwer, K., Van Laar, M., and Vollebergh, W. (2011). Buying Cannabis in 'coffee shops'. *Drug and Alcohol Review*, **30**, 148–156.

New Mexico Department of Health. (2012). *Medical Cannabis Program*. [Online] Available at: http://nmhealth.org/mcp/.

O'Brien, M. (2004). *Regarding Medical Marijuana*. [Documentary] United States: MoFilms.

O'Keefe, K. and Earleywine, M. (2011). *Marijuana Use by Young People: The Impact of State Medical Marijuana Laws*. Washington, DC: Marijuana Policy Project.

Oaksterdam University. (2012). *Quality Training for the Cannabis Industry*. [Online] Available at: http://www.oaksterdamuniversity.com/#.

Onishi, N. (2012). *Marijuana Only for the Sick? A Farce, Some Angelenos Say. Los Angeles Times*, October 7. http://www.nytimes.com/2012/10/08/us/california-fight-to-ensure-marijuana-goes-only-to-sick.html?_r=0.

Oregon Medical Marijuana Act. (1998). [Online] Available at: http://public.health.oregon.gov/DiseasesConditions/ChronicDisease/MedicalMarijuanaProgram/Documents/statutes.pdf.

People v Jackson (2012). D058988. San Diego County Superior Court. SCD222793.

Pro-Con.Org (2013). *Medical Marijuana: Who are the patients receiving medical marijuana through the federal government's Compassionate IND program?* [Online]. Available at: http://medicalmarijuana.procon.org/view.answers.php?questionID=000257.

Proposition 215. (1996). *Compassionate Use Act of 1996*.

Reiman, A. (2007). Patient profiles: medical cannabis patients and health care utilization patterns. *Complementary Health Practice Review*, **12**(1), 31–50.

Reiman, A. (2008a). Self-efficacy, social support and service integration at medical cannabis facilities in the San Francisco Bay area of California. *Health and Social Care in the Community*, **16**(1), 31–41.

Reiman, A. (2008b). *A Social Model of Cannabis Care: Berkeley Patients Group*. Berkeley, CA: Berkeley Patients Group.

Reiman, A. (2009). Cannabis as a substitute for alcohol and other drugs. *Harm Reduction Journal*, 6, 35.

Reinarman C. (2009). Cannabis policies and user practices: market separation, price, potency, and accessibility in Amsterdam and San Francisco. *International Journal of Drug Policy*, **20**, 28–37.

Richie, D. (2004). Council restricts medical pot sale. Citrus Heights would still allow the city's first cannabis shop to open on Auburn Boulevard. *Sacramento Bee*, April 18, N1.

Russo, E., Mathre, M., Byrne, A., Velin, R., Bach, P., Sanchez-Ramos, J., and Kirlin, K. (2002). Chronic cannabis use in the Compassionate Investigational New Drug Program: an examination of benefits and adverse effects of legal clinical cannabis. *Journal of Cannabis Therapeutics*, **2**(1), 3–57.

Szalavitz, M. (2009). Drugs in Portugal: did decriminalization work? *Time*, April 26. [Online] Available at: http://www.time.com/time/health/article/0,8599,1893946,00.html.

Torres, N. (2012). Mexico Marijuana Legalization Bill introduced by lawmaker. *Huffington Post*, November 15. [Online] Available at: http://www.huffingtonpost.com/2012/11/15/mexico-marijuana-legalization_n_2140116.html.

WAMM (Wo/men's Alliance for Medical Marijuana). (2012). *About WAMM*. [Online] Available at: http://www.wamm.org/aboutus.php.

Washington State Legislature. (2012). *Chapter 69.51A: Medical Cannabis*. [Online] Available at: http://apps.leg.wa.gov/RCW/default.aspx?cite=69.51A

Williams, A. (2012). Legal marijuana debated as Belize joins regional push on drugs. *Bloomberg Business Week*, July 17. [Online] Available at: http://www.businessweek.com/news/2012-07-17/legal-marijuana-debated-as-belize-joins-regional-push-on-drugs.

Wouters, M., Benschop, A., van Laar M., and Korf, D. (2012). Cannabis use and proximity to coffee shops in the Netherlands. *European Journal of Criminology*, **9**, 337–353.

Chapter 19

Development of Cannabis-Based Medicines: Regulatory Hurdles/Routes in Europe and the United States

Alison Thompson and Verity Langfield

19.1 A new class of medicine: acknowledgment by the authorities

Following many years of discussion, by physicians and patients, of anecdotal evidence of the benefits of using cannabis in managing many and varied medical conditions, the UK House of Lords set up a Scientific Committee in 1998. Health professionals, patients, medical scientists, and pharmacists were all called to give evidence on whether cannabis could indeed have a place in medicine. It became clear that even though nabilone, a synthetic analogue of delta-9-tetrahydrocannabinol (THC) was licensed in the UK in 1982 for prescription-only, hospital-only use against nausea arising from chemotherapy, it was not widely used either for nausea or, for example, multiple sclerosis (MS). However, patients with MS were particularly supportive of the use of cannabis in some form for alleviating their MS symptoms (House of Lords 1998).

The House of Lords Committee recommended:

1 Clinical trials of cannabis for the treatment of MS and chronic pain should be mounted as a matter of urgency.

2 Research should be promoted into alternative modes of administration (e.g., inhalation, sublingual, rectal) which would retain the benefit of rapid absorption offered by smoking, without the adverse effects.

A medicinal product for which quality, safety, and efficacy data were available would have to be approved by the UK Medicines and Healthcare products Regulatory Agency (MHRA) (then the Medicines Control Agency) before it could be available as a prescription medicine to patients. And so the journey of the first pharmaceutical company to develop a truly cannabis-based pharmaceutical product began.

19.2 The development program: assembling the evidence

The extensive documented research and anecdotal evidence on the usefulness of cannabis for medicinal use would not be sufficient to support its legal use as a medicine. A full pharmaceutical development program, meeting the stringent conditions laid down in law, would have to be followed before a cannabis-based medicine could be approved and marketed.

Medicines have been controlled in some manner for many centuries. Use of pharmacopoeias began in the sixteenth century. In the nineteenth century, the emerging life sciences supported more sophisticated control of medicines. Poisoning of more than one hundred people by diethylene glycol used as a solvent in a medicine in the US resulted in the introduction of the Federal Food, Drugs and Cosmetic Act in 1938. In the UK, the effect of thalidomide (a hypnotic and sedative) on the human fetus, resulting in deformity, propelled the introduction of a Committee on Safety of Drugs which began its work in 1964. The European Community introduced a Directive in 1965 (EEC/65/65) laying down the law, regulation, and administrative action relating to medicinal products.

As the knowledge of, and experience with, medicines increases, the regulatory framework for controlling them increases in its stringency and complexity.

Different countries (or regions, e.g., European Union) have their own laws for controlling medicine production, sale, and use. In the European Union, Directive 2001/83/EC consolidates many Directives issued between 1965 and 2001, laying out the law concerning placement of medicines on the market. Initially, countries or regions developed their own standards and control methods for medicines. However, with globalization, a common approach emerged for drug development and control, through written guidance. This common guidance is through the International Conference on Harmonisation of Technical Requirements for Registration of Pharmaceuticals for Human Use (ICH). The European Union, the US, and Japan all participate; other countries observe and follow (e.g., Canada); others observe, e.g., the World Health Organization.

The ICH guidance describes the collation of evidence of, initially, the quality and safety of a drug and provision of sufficient reassurance that early studies in humans can be carried out.

19.2.1 Pharmaceutical development

Most medicines have a single main active ingredient that provides the therapeutic action. In the case of a medicine that has been prepared by extraction from plant material, it is likely that several of its components are important in its action. Williamson and Evans (2000) observe that, in the case of cannabis, not all the observed effects can be ascribed to THC, and the other constituents may also modulate its action; for example, cannabidiol (CBD) reduces anxiety induced by THC. All the extracted components need to be shown to be consistently controlled during the active substance and finished product preparation. It also needs to be shown that despite the complexity of the product, that it is a stable and acceptable formulated medicine. *Cannabis sativa* L. contains more than 400 chemical compounds of which more than 100 are cannabinoids (ElSohly and Slade 2005). Cannabis is very complex in its chemistry due to the vast number of its constituents and their possible interaction with one another; almost all of the chemical classes, e.g., mono- and sesquiterpenes, sugars, hydrocarbons, steroids, flavonoids, nitrogenous compounds, and amino acids, among others are present (ElSohly and Slade 2005). Although the use of extracted plant material is challenging as it needs to be standardized for consistency in effect, and simple medicines do not present this challenge, they may not have the overall therapeutic effect of the extracted medicine (Williamson and Evans 2000).

As the starting point for an extracted cannabis medicine is the cannabis plant, consistency demands that plants carefully chosen for their particular cannabinoid levels must be maintained as a genetically stable population that is always available as the raw material for the medicine. These plants must be maintained through vegetative propagation and in a pest-free environment.

The cannabinoids in fresh cannabis are present in their acid form (e.g., delta-9-tetrahydrocannabinolic acid (THCA) and cannabidiolic acid (CBDA)). Raw cannabis must be heated to convert the cannabinoids to their usefully active forms (e.g., THC and CBD). The heated, dried plants are then processed (e.g., by liquid carbon dioxide extraction), to produce the extracted "active substance" which is likely to be a very complex mixture of many plant components, high in cannabinoids. The active substance must then be "formulated" as a medicine.

The bioavailability of cannabinoids administered by the gastrointestinal route is poor unless accompanied by a lipid carrier, particularly because of a high rate of first-pass metabolism, and is highly variable between subjects (Pertwee 1999).

In order to reduce the impact of first-pass metabolism, several other routes of administration are available: pulmonary, nasal, oromucosal, and rectal. A nonsmoked, acceptable oral form, administrable in small quantities would enable titration to effect. In the case of Sativex® (MHRA 2010; and the Sativex® Summary of Product Characteristics (SmPC) (Electronic Medicines Compendium 2012)), the first whole cannabis-based medicine to be approved in the European Union, the medicine is a solution to be used as an oromucosal spray. There are two principal cannabinoids in Sativex®, present in an approximately 1:1 ratio (THC, 27 mg/mL, and CBD, 25mg/mL). It is provided in small vials each with a pump actuator that delivers 100 microliters per spray. Cannabinoids are virtually insoluble in water, so organic solvents such as ethanol and propylene glycol are helpful as excipients in the formulation. Ethanol level would have to be below the recommended maximum intake of ethanol within a medicine, including for children. The European guideline (EMEA/HMPC/85114/2008) provides this guidance.

The specifications that are given for each of the stages of the preparation of a medicine produced using extracted cannabis (botanical raw material, active ingredient, and for the finished medicine) are likely to be very complex.

They include a measure of the content of principal and other cannabinoids, and of noncannabinoid fractions such as carotenoids. To ensure quality and safety, testing for the presence of microbes and of substances such as aflatoxin and heavy metals should also be considered. The development of the analytical methodology for both cannabinoids and noncannabinoids, using thin-layer chromatography, high-performance liquid chromatography, and gas chromatography have been crucial in showing the consistency of the medicine in all its stages of manufacture as well as in supporting the stability testing of the medicine. Hazekamp (2005) describes cannabinoid analytical methodology.

19.2.2 Documenting safety for early studies in humans

Cannabis has, in its various forms, been in widespread use for over 5000 years (see Russo, Chapter 2, this volume). The effect of the drug in humans is therefore very well documented though the discovery in the late 1980s (Pertwee 2000) of specific cannabinoid receptors gave an impetus to cannabinoid research. The endogenous cannabinoid system in animals and humans is clearly of major physiological and pharmacological significance.

The House of Lords Science and Technology Report collated evidence on the toxicology of cannabis in 1998 and summarized the evidence: "the acute toxicity of cannabis and the cannabinoids is very low; no-one has ever died as a direct and immediate consequence of recreational or medical use; animal studies have shown a very large separation (by a factor of more than 10,000) between pharmacologically effective and lethal doses." However, other effects of cannabis need to be taken into account when developing a cannabis-based medicine. These include the short-term effect on the heart and vascular system which can lead to significant increases in heart rate and a lowering of the blood pressure; the short-term "high," a state of euphoric intoxication, leading to a slight impairment of psychomotor and cognitive function; in some instances cannabis use may lead to a longer-lasting toxic psychosis involving delusions and hallucinations that can be misdiagnosed as schizophrenic illness; exacerbation of the symptoms of those already suffering from schizophrenic illness (though there is little evidence that cannabis use can precipitate schizophrenia or other mental illness in those not already predisposed to it); untoward long-term effects on cognitive performance, i.e., the performance of the brain, particularly in heavy users. The Report notes that animal experiments have shown that cannabinoids cause alterations in both male and female sexual hormones; but there is no evidence that cannabis adversely affects human fertility, or that it causes chromosomal or genetic damage; and that the consumption of cannabis by pregnant women may, however, lead to significantly shorter gestation and lower birth-weight babies in mothers smoking cannabis six or more times a week. The Report also outlines the potential problems of tolerance and dependence.

The House of Lords summary showed the challenge to medical researchers to produce a cannabis-based medicine that either eliminated or massively reduced the negative effects of the use of cannabinoids, yet ensured benefit.

When a new active substance has been identified, through standard pharmaceutical screening procedures, there will be much to learn about its action(s) and its absorption, distribution, metabolism, and excretion. ICH lays down the requirements for toxicology testing as a medicine proceeds in its development program in "Guidance on Nonclinical Safety Studies for the Conduct of Human Clinical Trials and Marketing Authorisation for Pharmaceuticals." This guidance describes the step-wise approach that must be taken in first carrying out nonclinical studies at a range of doses and duration to enable choice of an appropriate starting dose in humans. The effects elicited in the nonclinical studies must provide guidance on the type of adverse clinical effects that might be seen. Effects that are potentially clinically relevant can be sufficiently characterized using either doses up to the maximum tolerated dose (MTD), doses that achieve large exposure multiples or doses that use the maximum feasible dose. Acute, subchronic, and chronic toxicity studies must be carried out step-wise; however, the ICH guidance also encourages the use of as few test animals as possible.

These early studies give crucial guidance on the amount of active substance that is likely to provide the required effect. They also begin to inform of the likely safety margin there is between deleterious and efficacious effect.

Safety pharmacology and pharmacodynamic studies are described in another ICH guidance ("ICH S7A Guideline: Safety Pharmacology Studies for Human Pharmaceuticals," November 2000).

The endocannabinoid system and the existence of cannabinoid receptors have been described elsewhere in this book. So extensive is cannabinoid pharmacology research that the documentation of pharmacology for cannabinoid medicines can, to some extent, rely on the literature, particularly primary pharmacodynamic studies. However, a battery of safety pharmacology studies must be carried out once the cannabis extract has been fully characterized. The core battery of safety pharmacology studies includes the assessment of effects on cardiovascular, central nervous system (CNS), and respiratory systems and should generally be conducted before human exposure.

Information on pharmacokinetics (PK) (e.g., absorption, distribution, metabolism, and excretion) in laboratory animals must be available and studies must be carried out to identify potential drug interactions before large groups of human subjects are exposed. The literature on the PK of cannabinoids is extensive. The PK profile of THC administered intravenously (i.v.) was examined in dogs by Garrett and Hunt (1977), in rabbits by Leuschner et al. (1986), and in Large White pigs by Brunet et al. (2006). Uptake following oral administration of THC is erratic because of degradation of the drug by stomach acids and extensive first-pass metabolism (Food and Drug Administration (FDA), Marinol Summary Basis of Approval (SBA), 1985) however, absorption of THC following sublingual mucosal administration increases plasma bioavailability relative to oral administration due to the avoidance of first-pass metabolism. Mannila et al. (2006) explored the comparative bioavailabilities of THC after sublingual administration of a solid

THC/β-cyclodextrin complex, oral administration of an ethanolic THC solution and i.v. administration of an aqueous THC solution. The plasma profiles of THC after i.v. administration implied first-order PK with an elimination half-life of 66.6 ± 3.1 min. The absolute bioavailability (F) of THC after sublingual administration was higher than after oral administration; F = 16.0 ± 7.5% compared to F = 1.3 ± 1.4% respectively, a result most likely due to the avoidance of first-pass metabolism in the case of sublingual administration.

Huestis (2005) has reviewed the PK of plant cannabinoids and interpreted the cannabinoid concentrations in biological fluids.

The PK profiles of CBD were studied in dogs (Samara et al. 1988) and rats (Siemens et al. 1980) following i.v. and oral administration. In rats, CBD was absorbed and distributed into tissues very rapidly. Terminal half-lives after i.v. and oral administration were found to be about 11 h (Siemens et al. 1980). In dogs, CBD administered i.v. was also rapidly absorbed into tissues and plasma levels declined in a triphasic fashion with mean terminal half-lives ranging from 7–9 h. In three of six dogs administered CBD orally, CBD could not be detected in the plasma. In the other three, the oral bioavailability ranged from 13% to 19%. The results of this study show that CBD has low bioavailability after oral administration to dogs and this has been attributed to extensive first-pass hepatic metabolism (Samara et al. 1988).

Due to the extensive cannabinoid pharmacology and PK literature, it is unlikely that extensive development work would be required in this respect for a new cannabinoid medicine.

19.2.3 Phase 1 and Phase 2 studies

"First-in-human" or Phase 1 clinical studies can only be undertaken when there is sufficient reassurance from early short-term toxicology studies with the test active substance, and from a knowledge of the active substance pharmacology, that under the restricted and controlled conditions of a Phase 1 study, the active substance will not be harmful. Further than that, it must be justifiable, based on the current evidence, to undertake the study. Phase 1 studies are carried out in healthy volunteers and seek to establish the pharmacokinetic profile and tolerability of a proposed new medicine. Very early Phase 1 studies may compare different formulations using the same active substance but different excipients. They may compare different modes of administration. They will provide information on the appropriate dose range which can then be used in planning the first studies in patients with the target indication.

Due to the known CNS effects of smoked cannabis, first-in-human studies with cannabinoid medicines are likely to be cautious. A highly characterized, consistent medicinal product will be needed to ensure successful Phase 1 studies that provide the required pharmacokinetic data.

While the Phase 2 studies are being planned (having been informed by the Phase 1 studies) and started, some further Phase 1 studies might be carried out on extrinsic factors such as drug/food interaction and interaction with other specified medicines. A study in healthy volunteers to assess the cardiovascular effects of multiple doses of the active substance may be required. Drug abuse potential studies are mandatory in some countries (e.g., US). The US FDA also requires studies of the effect of the medicine on certain aspects of heart activity and dedicated studies in humans with hepatic impairment before New Drug Application (NDA) approval.

19.2.4 Obtaining approval for carrying out clinical trials

In the European Union, a Clinical Trial Application (CTA) must be made to each individual country, though the process is based on a harmonized set of documents and a common form—the EudraCT form. A CTA consists of an application form, the protocol, an Investigator

Brochure (IB) summarizing the quality, safety, and clinical information (if any) so far, the investigational medicinal product (IMP) dossier (IMPD), which is a precursor to a full quality section described later in section 19.3.1, and a copy of the authorization of the IMP manufacturer to prepare the IMP. In addition, a justification or risk:benefit review of the proposal may be needed.

In the US, usually following a formal "pre-IND" meeting with the FDA, the regulatory process towards approval of a medicine begins with an "Investigational New Drug" (IND) submission. The IND consists of a general investigational plan (for product development), the IB, protocol(s), a comprehensive "chemistry, manufacture, and controls" section (which, again, is a precursor to a full quality section described later in section 19.3.1), pharmacology/toxicology data, a summary of previous human experience and any additional relevant information. Once the IND has been submitted to the FDA and approval of an Institutional Review Board (as for Ethics Committee review in the UK) has been received, then 30 days after receipt by the FDA of the IND, it is permissible to start the proposed clinical trial.

19.2.5 **Controlled drug specific requirements**

In the case of cannabinoid IMPs, not only the legislation concerning clinical trials must be adhered to, but also the laws governing drugs that might potentially be abused.

An IMP derived from *Cannabis sativa* L. and containing cannabinoids is a controlled drug under international law. In the case of cannabis extracts and tinctures, the movement of these across international borders is governed by the 1961 Single Convention on Narcotic Drugs (International Narcotics Control Board (INCB) Yellow list).

Under the Single Convention, cannabis extracts and tinctures are listed in Schedule I, the schedule that applies to most prescription narcotic drugs.

The 1961 Single Convention stresses that the use of psychoactive substances for legitimate medical and scientific purposes is indispensable and their availability for such purposes should not be unduly restricted. National Authorities are thereby encouraged to accept that such IMPs may be useful and that they can be legally marketed once the Authorities have been provided with all the evidence and the medicine is approved.

However, local national law and its implementation of international law will vary considerably. There will be rules governing the import, possession, movement, and storage of medicines that are also controlled drugs. It is possible that a medicine that is a controlled drug cannot be imported unless it would serve an unmet medical need.

In the UK, cannabis is regulated under the Misuse of Drugs Act 1971; Schedule 2 to the Act classifies cannabis itself, and cannabis resin, as Class B controlled drugs. The position in practice is therefore that cannabis and most of its derivatives may not be used in medicine, and may be possessed for research only under Home Office license. Therefore, Home Office licences must be obtained prior to any activity involving growing of cannabis, manufacturing an IMP, distributing the IMP, and use at research centers by subjects.

19.2.6 **The evidence of efficacy**

The House of Lords Report lists the many conditions that physicians and patients felt were alleviated by the use of cannabis either smoked or taken orally. These included MS, spinal injury, back pain, arthritis, epilepsy, myalgic encephalomyelitis, pain, antiemetic after chemotherapy, cerebral palsy, and glaucoma.

The Report documents a statement made on July 2, 1997 by Tessa Jowell MP, the then-Minister of State for Health: "At present the evidence is inconclusive. The key point is that a cannabis-based medicine has not been scientifically demonstrated to be safe, efficacious and of suitable quality."

19.3 The Marketing Authorisation Application

All the data produced during a medicine's development is assembled as an internationally accepted set of evidence called the Common Technical Document (CTD). Each country or region may also have additional guidance that must be followed in order to prepare the collated evidence (the Marketing Authorisation Application (MAA)) that must be submitted to the local authority for approval before a drug can be marketed.

19.3.1 Documenting quality (chemistry, manufacturing, and controls)

The quality section of a pharmaceutical dossier consists of two main parts: information about the active substance and about the finished product. The aim of the development process is to produce a consistent product that reliably performs as intended. A typical pharmaceutical will consist of the active substance, teamed with appropriate excipients to result in a medicine that is both stable in storage and, when taken by the patient, performs the necessary function and is bioavailable.

Cannabinoid medicines that are based only on delta-9-tetrahydrocannabinol are typically simple preparations of only THC and excipients in an acceptable medicinal form (e.g., a capsule). However, a medicine that reflected "whole cannabis" would be an enormous project due to the complex nature of a whole plant.

In the European Union a new Directive, "Directive 2004/24/EC of the European Parliament and of the Council amending, as regards traditional herbal medicinal products, Directive 2001/83/EC on the Community code relating to medicinal products for human use" describes herbal products. It allows for a simplified procedure to be followed "where the applicant can demonstrate by detailed references to published scientific literature that the constituent or the constituents of the medicinal product has or have a well-established medicinal use with recognized efficacy and an acceptable level of safety within the meaning of Directive 2001/83/EC, he/she should not be required to provide the results of preclinical tests or the results of clinical trials."

However, although a medicine derived from cannabis might be described as herbal, the fact that it would not have "well-established medicinal use" would mean that it would not fall within this Directive. In the US, the FDA has produced a draft "botanical guidance" (FDA 2004), which similarly calls for a herbal medicine to have had a "marketing history" for a simplified procedure for approval to be used.

For a medicine derived from cannabis to be made available, it would not only have to be manufactured in a controlled manner, but unlike a traditional "herbal" medicine, a complete program of safety testing and clinical trials would have to be undertaken.

The chemistry, manufacture, and controls for both the active substance and for the finished product (the medicine) require extensive work that provides documented evidence on the following matters:

Active substance: chemical structure, general properties, control of starting materials, manufacturing process, detailed description of the active substance, analytical procedures, validation of analytical procedures, batch data, description of the reference standards used in the analytical methods, container description, and stability.

Finished product: description and composition, pharmaceutical development, manufacture process, the specification for identification and control purposes, analytical procedures (and their validation), batch analyses, reference standards, container, and stability.

19.3.2 The MAA: nonclinical studies—safety testing

In the case of cannabinoids, there is much information in the literature on the nonclinical pharmacology. It is therefore unlikely that a full preclinical pharmacology program would need to be undertaken as so much reference can be made to the literature. However, pharmacology studies that are models for the proposed indication are likely to be necessary to support a MAA.

However, when it comes to toxicology, that is a different matter. As has already been mentioned, to ensure that a cannabis extract acts consistently, there must be a detailed, highly characterized specification for the active substance (cannabis extract). The full program of toxicology testing must be undertaken once the required active substance has been characterized and is known to be consistent batch after batch. The full program includes safety pharmacology to investigate the effects of the test substance on the CNS, the cardiovascular, and the respiratory systems. As far as absorption, distribution, metabolism, and excretion studies are concerned, for cannabinoids, the literature is likely to indicate whether there are any particular concerns that may be specific to particular cannabinoids. Investigations into the effects of cannabinoids on cytochrome P450 enzymes are informative. With nonclinical studies, another set of validated analytical methods must be developed to investigate the test material levels in plasma and tissue in the test species.

The following toxicology studies would be required to provide sufficient toxicological and pharmacokinetic data to provide the reassurance of safety required for a MAA:

- Single and repeat dose studies.
- In vitro genotoxicology studies: e.g., bacterial reverse mutation test (Ames test) and mouse lymphoma studies.
- In vivo gentoxicology studies: e.g., micronucleus test and unscheduled DNA synthesis.
- Two-year carcinogenicity study.
- Reproductive studies to cover fertility and early embryonic development, embryo-fetal development, and prenatal and postnatal development including maternal function.

19.3.3 The MAA: discussion with the national authorities and clinical data

As has been stated, ICH provides comprehensive guidance on what studies need to be undertaken and what information needs to be provided to the Authorities in a MAA before a medicine can be placed on the market. Regional authorities (e.g., European Medicines Agency (EMA)) or national (e.g., the US FDA) can be approached for scientific guidance meetings to ensure that the product developmental plan is likely to provide the data expected in the MAA. The timing of the meetings and the need for meetings with the Authorities depends on the type of product (e.g., established active ingredient or novel), the indication, and whether there is an established methodology for investigation.

In the European Union, although it is possible to request meetings with the authorities in individual Member States (e.g., the MHRA in the UK), as it is likely that the product will be marketed in several European Union countries, it is advisable to request scientific advice through the EMA. This is particularly true for advice on clinical protocols, where a consensus is important for future Europe-wide success.

In the US, the development, submission, review, and approval process can be guided each step of the way by the FDA. Contact with the FDA usually starts with a "Pre-Investigational New Drug" meeting within the FDA. This is the opportunity for the company to present the product and development plan to the FDA and receive initial opinions and guidance. The part of the FDA that is involved in reviewing and approving drugs is the Center of Drug Evaluation and Research (CDER). CDER is divided into "Offices," e.g., the Office of Pharmaceutical Science. Each "Office" may have several Divisions with different specialities, e.g., the Division of Pharmaceutical Analysis, the Division of Neurology products. When meeting with the FDA, it is likely that FDA expertise from several Divisions will be assembled to provide guidance.

19.3.4 MAA preparation

Once all the quality, safety, and the proof of efficacy data is available, the MAA can be assembled. ICH describes the international CTD dossier for provision to global authorities. The CTD consists of three levels: Modules 3, 4, and 5 (Quality, Nonclinical, and Clinical documentation respectively) are at the bottom of the "pyramid." Above this are Module 2.2 (CTD Summary), Module 2.3 (Quality Overall Summary), Modules 2.4 and 2.6 (Nonclinical Overview and Summaries), and Modules 2.5 and 2.7 (Clinical Overview and Summaries). Module 2 summarizes all the information in Modules 3, 4, and 5.

At the top of the pyramid is Module 1 (country or regional) containing local administrative information, local Product Information, information about the experts (authors of the overviews), pharmacovigilance summaries, information on studies in the pediatric population and any other country or region-specific information.

The local Product Information provides the guidance to the treating physician in summarizing all the information relevant to the safe and beneficial treatment of the patient and the culmination of the many years for development of the medicinal product.

The final step, of course, is a review by the national authority to determine if there is sufficient evidence of quality, safety, and efficacy and that a positive benefit:risk decision can be made and the medicine can be approved.

19.4 Regulatory aspects of the clinical development of Sativex® as a medicine

Following the Phase 1 clinical trials in healthy subjects, the IMP can be used in studies with patients who have the condition for which it is hoped the IMP will be helpful. There is considerable guidance from the EMA and from the US FDA on how to carry out the clinical trials given on their websites.

Phase 2 trials are usually with hundreds of patients, during which early proof of efficacy and the likely dose requirement is sought. Phase 3 studies, usually with thousands of patients, is when efficacy is hopefully proven and the safety profile of the IMP better understood.

As shown by the House of Lords Report, and not surprisingly given the existence of the endocannabinoid system, the variety and extent of conditions for which medicinal cannabis might be used is enormous.

The House of Lords Report had concluded: "Clinical trials of cannabis for the treatment of MS and chronic pain should be mounted as a matter of urgency." GW Pharma Ltd. focused on this as a starting point for clinical development in these conditions.

19.4.1 **Clinical trials with Sativex® in pain**

Some of the earliest clinical trials with cannabis-based medicines, including Sativex® were performed by Wade et al. (2003, 2004). Wade et al. (2003) reported a consecutive series of double blind, randomized, placebo-controlled, single-patient, cross-over trials with 2-week treatment periods with 24 patients with MS, four with spinal cord injury, one with brachial plexus damage, and one with limb amputation due to neurofibromatosis. Patients self-titrated with Sativex®, THC extract, CBD extract, or placebo. The results were encouraging, showing that cannabis extracts improved neurogenic symptoms unresponsive to standard treatments and that unwanted effects were predictable and generally well tolerated.

The objective of the study reported by Wade et al. (2004) was to determine whether a cannabis-based medicinal extract (CBME) benefits a range of symptoms due to MS. The primary objective of the study was to investigate the use of Sativex® compared with placebo in the alleviation of key symptoms of MS (pain, spasticity, spasms, bladder problems, tremor) in subjects with MS. At the time of inclusion in the study, subjects were asked to identify their single primary target symptom from among the five symptoms listed. A total of 160 patients were randomized in this multicenter, 6-week parallel group study and given either Sativex® or placebo. The primary objective of the study was achieved by comparing the change from baseline in the severity of the primary symptom after 6 weeks of therapy on Sativex®, with that on placebo. The severity scores were recorded using a 0–100 mm visual analogue scale (VAS), completed at the clinic visits, and also by subjects in a daily diary. For the primary endpoint of the study, the primary symptom score changes were aggregated across the entire study population. A secondary analysis looked at each of the five symptoms separately. The maximum permitted dose of study medication was eight actuations (21.6 mg THC and 20.0 mg CBD) in any 3 h period, and 48 actuations (129.6 mg THC and 120 mg CBD) in any 24 h period. Subjects titrated to their optimal dose based on efficacy, tolerability, and the maximum permitted dose. The adjusted mean change from baseline for the composite primary impairment VAS score at the end of Part 1 showed a decrease of 25.29 mm for the Sativex® treatment group and 19.35 mm for the placebo group. The estimated treatment difference did not reach statistical significance ($p = 0.124$; 95% confidence interval (CI): –13.52, 1.65 mm).

However, the treatment difference of 22.79 mm in the 39 subjects who recorded spasticity as their primary impairment was statistically significant in favor of the Sativex® treatment group ($p = 0.001$; 95% CI: –35.52, –10.07 mm). A responder analysis of those subjects with a 30% or greater improvement in primary spasticity symptoms (measured by diary card) found an odds ratio of 7.20 ($p = 0.029$) in favor of Sativex® treatment. The efficacy data indicated positive effects for spasticity in MS.

Berman et al. (2004) investigated the effectiveness of cannabis-based medicines including Sativex®, for the treatment of chronic pain associated with brachial plexus root avulsion. A reason for choosing this patient population is that they are an unusually homogeneous group in terms of anatomical location of injury, pain descriptions, and demographics; they therefore represent an excellent human model of central neuropathic pain. In this study, patients were given either placebo, Sativex®, or a cannabis extract containing mainly THC. Patients were allowed to titrate freely within the following limits according to subjective symptom relief and adverse events. The maximum permitted dose was eight sprays into the mouth (THC 21.6 mg or THC 21.6 mg/ CBD 20 mg or placebo) at any one time or within a 3 h period and 48 sprays within any 24 h period. A self-titration dosing schedule was chosen for several reasons; data from human volunteer studies showed a high intersubject variability in the bioavailability of Sativex®; self-titration enabled patients, most of whom were working and driving, to achieve their individual optimum therapeutic dose by balancing any analgesia against possible side effects and allowing them to vary the dose depending on their levels of pain, and to fit in with their lifestyle. The primary outcome measure was the mean pain severity score during the last 7 days of treatment. Secondary measures included pain-related quality of life assessments. The primary measure failed to fall by the two points defined in the proposed hypothesis. However, both this measure and measures of sleep showed statistically significant improvements. Eighty percent of the patients considered the study drugs of sufficient benefit to warrant continuing into an open-extension study. This put into context the clinical relevance of the modest drop in pain scores in a condition that is long-lasting, difficult to treat, and that had already proven refractory to the standard methods of treatment by both nerve repair and oral analgesics.

Nurmikko et al. (2007) investigated the effect of Sativex® on the severity of pain and allodynia and associated sleep disturbance, mental distress, and disability in patients with peripheral neuropathic pain, saying that there is a well-recognized need for better pain relief than is currently available. Sixty-three patients were randomized to take Sativex® and 62 placebo in this 5-week trial. Concomitant analgesia was maintained at a stable dosage regimen for the duration of the study. A self-titration regimen was used to optimize drug administration. The mean reduction in pain intensity scores was greater in patients receiving Sativex® than placebo (mean adjusted scores −1.48 points versus −0.52 points on a 0–10 numeric rating scale (NRS); p = 0.004; 95% CI: −1.59, 0.32). Improvements in Neuropathic Pain Scale composite score (p = 0.007), sleep NRS (p = 0.001), dynamic allodynia (p = 0.042), punctate allodynia (p = 0.021), Pain Disability Index (p = 0.003), and Patients' Global Impression of Change (p <0.001) were similarly greater on Sativex® vs. placebo. This study demonstrated that Sativex® is effective in the relief of peripheral neuropathic pain when given in addition to existing medication. Greater than 30% improvement in pain intensity, generally considered as clinically meaningful, was reported by 26% of subjects receiving Sativex® compared with 15% of patients taking placebo. When patients entered the study, they had not been experiencing any benefit from their existing treatment so pain reduction following Sativex® was particularly encouraging. Once titrated to effect, patients did not increase their Sativex® dose, even though they were free to do so; and nor did those patients who entered the 52-week open-extension study.

Rog et al. (2005) reported a 5-week, randomized, double-blind, placebo-controlled parallel group study in 66 adult patients with central neuropathic pain syndromes due to MS. Central pain for which a nociceptive cause appeared unlikely was required to be of at least 3 months' duration and expected to remain otherwise stable during the study. A stable neuropathic pain medication regimen was maintained during the 2 weeks immediately before screening and throughout the study. Pain and sleep were recorded daily on an 11-point NRS. Cannabis-based medicine (Sativex®) was superior to placebo in reducing the mean intensity of pain (Sativex® mean change −2.7, 95% CI: −3.4, −2.0; placebo −1.4, 95% CI: −2.0, −0.8, comparison between groups, p = 0.005) and sleep disturbance (Sativex® mean change −2.5, 95% CI: −3.4, −1.7; placebo −0.8, 95% CI: −1.5, −0.1, comparison between groups, p = 0.003). It was concluded that Sativex® was effective in reducing pain and sleep disturbance in patients with multiple sclerosis-related central neuropathic pain and is mostly well tolerated.

As can be seen from the studies outlined, these early clinical studies with Sativex® confirmed the range of clinical conditions that might be eased by cannabinoids. An early submission by GW Pharma Ltd. of efficacy data on Sativex® to the UK Authorities led to the publication of a Public Assessment Report summarizing that although results were encouraging, that there was insufficient proof of efficacy in a well-defined indication, to support a Marketing Authorisation (MA).

The encouraging results for the relief of spasticity in MS led GW Pharma Ltd. to focus further clinical trials on this condition in order to assemble sufficient efficacy data to support a MA. However, in the meantime, a MA was sought in Canada. Health Canada support a system where "promising medicines that meet unmet medical need" may be authorized if there are sufficient quality and safety data, though the clinical data are positive, but not the full set normally required for a submission. Such an approval is termed a "Notification of Compliance with Conditions." The use of Sativex® for the relief of neuropathic pain in MS was just such a case. Health Canada gave the first ever approval for a cannabis-based medicine, Sativex®, in April 2005. This was not only important to patients in Canada, but also to patients globally where a national authority, if the local legislation permitted, was able to refer to this approval in Canada and then support supply of its own patients where the patient's physician requested such treatment.

19.4.2 Clinical trials with Sativex® in MS

Typically, two positive clinical studies in the specified indication are required to provide evidence of efficacy in a MA application (MAA). Further studies were carried out with Sativex® specifically in patients with spasticity in MS.

Collin et al. (2007) reported a double blind, randomized, parallel group comparison of Sativex® with placebo in the treatment of spasticity associated with MS, involving 189 subjects with a post-randomization treatment period of 6 weeks. Patients had a clinical diagnosis of MS with spasticity not wholly relieved by their current therapy, experienced at least 3 months' stable disease prior to study entry, and had significant spasticity in at least two muscle groups defined as a score of two or more on the Ashworth Scale (where zero represents no increase in muscle tone and four represents limb rigid in flexion or extension). Subjects continued to take their antispasticity medication during the study, but were required to maintain a stable dose meaning that any improvement seen on the study was in addition to that already obtained on concomitant antispasticity medication.

The primary efficacy analysis was the comparison of the change from baseline in the severity of spasticity between the Sativex® and placebo treatment groups, as assessed by an 11-point NRS score for spasticity. In addition, responder analyses were performed. Of the 189 randomized subjects, 124 were in the Sativex® treatment group and 65 were in the placebo treatment group.

The adjusted mean change in NRS scores for spasticity for the Sativex® treatment group at the end of treatment was 1.18 points from a mean baseline period score of 5.49 points. For the corresponding period, the placebo group showed an adjusted mean decrease of 0.59 points from a mean baseline period score of 5.39 points. The estimated treatment difference of 0.52 points, in favor of the Sativex® treatment group was statistically significant ($p = 0.048$; 95% CI: -1.029, -0.004).

The responder analysis showed that in the Sativex® group 48 (40.0%) patients had a $\geq$30% reduction in NRS spasticity over the study as compared to 14 (21.9%) on placebo (difference in favor of Sativex® = 18.1%; 95% CI: 4.73, 31.52; $p = 0.014$). The change in Motricity Index score for affected legs from baseline to end of treatment (Visit 4) showed a treatment difference of 3.86 points in favor of Sativex®, which approached statistical significance ($p = 0.054$). There was an improvement in Ashworth score in the Sativex® population from a baseline score of 2.41 to a final visit score of 1.77; the placebo group improved from 2.44 to 1.92, however, the difference of 0.11 units in favor of Sativex® was not statistically significant.

This study has shown, via the primary efficacy analysis of the NRS spasticity scores, that Sativex® is an effective treatment in relieving spasticity in subjects with MS, who have failed to respond adequately to existing treatments. Of additional note in the interpretation of this study is the observation that more than 90% of subjects in both treatment groups were taking concomitant medication, which remained at a stable dose during the study. Thus the improvements seen on Sativex® are providing a benefit which was otherwise unavailable to these subjects.

Collin et al. (2010) reported a further double blind, randomized, placebo controlled, parallel group study, with a post randomization treatment period of 14 weeks, to evaluate the efficacy of Sativex® in subjects with symptoms of spasticity due to MS. Patients had at least a 3-month history of spasticity due to MS which was not wholly relieved with current therapy and they remained on their current therapy throughout the study. A total of 337 subjects were randomized and analyzed; 167 received Sativex® and 170 received placebo. Analysis of the change from baseline of the adjusted mean NRS spasticity scores for Sativex® showed a treatment difference of –0.23 points in favor of Sativex® that did not reach statistical significance ($p = 0.219$; 95% CI: –0.59, 0.14 points). However, a responder analysis in the per protocol (PP) set showed that 36% of subjects achieved at least a 30% improvement in spasticity NRS with an odds ratio of 1.74 ($p = 0.040$; 95% CI: 1.024, 2.960). Additional retrospective analysis suggested that the large difference in mean doses of study medication taken by the study groups may have been a significant contributor to the large placebo effect seen in this study.

The two studies just described were combined in a preplanned pooled analysis, which showed that Sativex® was statistically significantly superior to placebo for the change in spasticity NRS, for a responder analysis and for Subject Global Impression of Change (SGIC). These studies also showed, in post hoc analyses, that the response to treatment after 4 weeks was highly predictive of the response in longer-term treatment. These analyses suggested that a suitable approach to treatment with Sativex® was the "therapeutic trial" approach, in which subjects are first exposed to treatment, and their ability to respond determined. Subsequently, only those subjects who have shown the ability to respond are then randomized to the double-blind, placebo-controlled phase of the study.

The two studies described, along with the meta-analysis, were reviewed by the UK Authorities as the "Reference Member State" during a Decentralised Procedure. The concept of "responders" to Sativex® was also discussed with the Authorities during this procedure and it was decided that the Sativex® MAA would be withdrawn and a further study carried out that incorporated a 4-week therapeutic trial.

The study design for a further study was based on scientific advice from the National Competent Authorities in the UK and in Spain. Novotna et al. (2011) describes the two-phase Phase 3 study of the safety and efficacy of Sativex®, in the symptomatic relief of spasticity in subjects with spasticity due to multiple sclerosis where Phase A was a single-blind response assessment and Phase B was a double blind, randomized, placebo controlled, parallel group study. Patients had been diagnosed with any disease subtype of MS of at least 6 months' duration and with at least moderate spasticity of at least 3 months' duration, which was not adequately relieved with current antispasticity therapy. Patients maintained their antispasticity and disease-modifying therapy at a stable dose throughout the study. Patients entered a single blind, 4-week period of treatment with Sativex®. At the end of 4 weeks, those subjects who achieved at least a 20% improvement on the NRS were randomized to either Sativex® or placebo, maintaining the same dose they were taking at the end of Phase A. Five hundred and seventy-two patients enrolled in the study, 272 patients achieved a ≥20% improvement after 4 weeks of single-blind treatment and 241 were randomized (as not all were eligible, for other reasons, to continue). The primary endpoint of the difference between treatments in the mean spasticity NRS in Phase B showed a highly significant difference in favor of Sativex® ($p = 0.0002$). Most secondary endpoints were also significantly in favor of Sativex®.

This study design enabled those patients who could be helped by Sativex® to be identified. This approach was carried through to the SmPC for Sativex® (Electronic Medicines Compendium 2012) where the indication is:

> Sativex® is indicated as treatment for symptom improvement in adult patients with moderate to severe spasticity due to multiple sclerosis (MS) who have not responded adequately to other anti-spasticity medication *and who demonstrate clinically significant improvement in spasticity related symptoms during an initial trial of therapy.*

19.4.3 Long-term efficacy

In addition to all the studies already outlined, most studies were followed up by patients being able to enter an open-label, long-term safety extension. These have been summarized by Wade et al. (2006), Rog et al. (2007), and Serpell et al. (2013). However, for the MAA, a placebo controlled, parallel group, randomized withdrawal study of patients with symptoms of spasticity due to MS who are receiving long-term Sativex® was carried out (Notcutt et al. 2012). Patients who were already taking Sativex® for the relief of spasticity entered a 1-week period during which their spasticity was assessed. They were then randomized to either Sativex® or placebo for 28 days. Thirty-six patients were randomized. The patients had been using Sativex® for a mean duration of 3.6 years, and were taking a mean daily dose of 8.25 sprays of Sativex®. The primary outcome of time to treatment failure was significantly in favor of Sativex® ($p = 0.013$). Amongst the secondary endpoints, Subject's Global Impression of Change and the Carer Global Impression of Change of Functional Ability were significantly in favor of Sativex®. This study provided the necessary confirmatory evidence that Sativex® provides long-term benefit.

19.4.4 Validity of the NRS in assessing spasticity in MS

During the development of Sativex® it became clear that existing measures of spasticity were not sufficiently robust or clinically relevant. Therefore results obtained in the early studies with Sativex® that used the NRS were used to assess the validity of this scale as a measure of spasticity (Farrar et al. 2008). In addition, evidence was provided by Anwar and Barnes (2009). The MHRA in the Public Assessment Report (PAR) of Sativex® concluded (MHRA 2010):

> the company has provided reasonable demonstration of the validity of the NRS as a measure of symptoms related to spasticity for the purpose of supporting an indication for the symptomatic treatment of spasticity in this patient population.

19.4.5 Blinding of study medication

It had been suggested that cannabis-based medicines would be recognized in clinical trials by subjects that had previously used cannabis. However, although the psychoactive cannabinoid THC in Sativex® is also in street cannabis, Sativex® is not the same as smoked/inhaled street cannabis. Sativex® is an oromucosal spray of consistent content and has a very different pharmacokinetic profile to street cannabis. It also contains the nonpsychoactive cannabinoid, CBD. Plasma levels of THC increase much more when it is inhaled in smoke than when Sativex® is sprayed into the mouth (MHRA Public Assessment Report 2010, p. 12), indicating the different potential that smoked cannabis and oromucosal Sativex® have for inducing psychoactivity and therefore unblinding during a clinical trial. In the long-term Sativex® study reported by Wade (2006), patient-reported intoxication scores were consistently low throughout the study.

Assessments of mood would help to indicate if there had been unblinding in studies. In the studies described earlier (Novotna et al. 2011; Wade et al. 2004), there were no statistically significant or clinically relevant differences between the Beck Depression Index scores for Sativex®- and placebo-treated patients. In the studies described by Collin et al. (2010) and Novotna et al. (2011) there were no statistically significant or clinically relevant Sativex®-placebo differences in the change in subject-recorded anxiety depression scale from the EuroQol 5-D (EQ-5D) health status. In the study described by Rog et al. (2005) there was no evidence of widespread or substantial changes in anxiety or depression ratings in subjects with MS taking Sativex® compared with those taking placebo.

When reviewing the assembled efficacy data, the MHRA summarized in the PAR (2010):

> The presented analyses are not able to refute the possibility of bias arising as a result but at least there is no evidence of a major problem. The smaller the differences between active and placebo, the greater is the concern that a relevant contribution of that apparent difference may not be real. This still needs to be considered in the overall evidence of efficacy but if a compelling treatment effect can be shown the possibility of unblinding might not represent a major concern.

The two most recent studies with Sativex® in patients with spasticity in MS did indeed show a compelling treatment effect, thus the possibility of unblinding was of no concern.

19.4.6 Evidence of safety

In accordance with international guidance (ICH) all adverse events experienced by subjects during all clinical trials were recorded, collated, reviewed, and reported to all authorities where clinical trials were being carried out. All safety data were summarized in the Sativex® Investigator Brochure provided to all Investigators carrying out clinical trials with Sativex®. The safety profile for Sativex® was established during the early years of clinical trials. Once the product was approved and marketed, a Periodic Safety Update Report was prepared every 6 months starting with the first one submitted to Health Canada at 8 months after the "international birth date" for Sativex® of April 15, 2005. The Sativex® SPC summarizes the safety profile of Sativex®.

For controlled drugs, it is likely that studies that provide a thorough understanding of the abuse potential of a new medicine will be required. An abuse liability study carried out with Sativex® is described by Schoedel et al. (2011).

19.5 Conclusions

The development of any new medicine presents great challenges in the production and documentation of sufficient quality, safety, and efficacy data that show a positive benefit:risk ratio for the new medicine. However, for a complex botanical medicine the challenge in showing consistency and repeatability is far greater. The development and authorization of Sativex® in over 20 countries has shown that a cannabis-based medicine is beneficial in healthcare.

References

Anwar, K. and Barnes, M. (2009). A pilot study of a comparison between a patient scored numeric rating scale and clinician scored measures of spasticity in multiple sclerosis. *NeuroRehabilitation*, **24**(4), 333–340.

Berman, J.S., Symonds, C., and Birch, R. (2004). Efficacy of two cannabis based medicinal extracts for relief of central neuropathic pain from brachial plexus avulsion: results of a randomised controlled trial. *Pain*, **112**, 299–306.

Brunet, B., Doucet, C., Venisse, N., *et al.* (2006). Validation of the Large White Pig as an animal model for the study of cannabinoids metabolism: application to the study of THC distribution in tissues. *Forensic Science International*, **161**, 169–174.

Collin, C., Davies, P., Mutiboko, I.K., and Ratcliffe, S. (2007). Randomized controlled trial of cannabis-based medicine in spasticity caused by multiple sclerosis. *European Journal of Neurology*, **14**, 290–296.

Collin, C., Ehler, E., Waberzinek, G., *et al.* (2010). A double-blind, randomized, placebo-controlled, parallel group study of Sativex, in subjects with symptoms of spasticity due to multiple sclerosis. *Neurological Research*, **32**, 451–459.

Electronic Medicines Compendium. (2012). *Sativex Summary of Product Characteristics.* Available at: http://www.medicines.org.uk/emc/.

ElSohly, M.A. and Slade, D. (2005). Chemical constituents of marijuana: the complex mixture of natural cannabinoids. *Life Sciences*, **78**(5), 539–548.

Farrar, J.T., Troxel, A.B., Stott, C., Duncombe, P., and Jensen, M.P. (2008). Validity, reliability and clinical importance of change in a 0-10 numeric rating scale measure of spasticity: a post hoc analysis of a randomized, double-blind placebo-controlled trial. *Clinical Therapeutics*, **30**(5), 974–985.

Food and Drug Administration. (2004). *Guidance for Industry, Botanical Drug Products.* Washington, DC: US Department of Health and Human Services.

Garrett, E.R. and Hunt, C.A. (1977). Pharmacokinetics of Δ^9-tetrahydrocannabinol in dogs. *Journal of Pharmaceutical Sciences*, **66**(3), 395–407.

Hazekamp, A., Giroud, C., Peltenburg, A., and Verpoorte, R. (2005). Chromatographic and Spectroscopic data of cannabinoids from *Cannabis sativa*. *Journal of Liquid Chromatography and Related Technologies*, **28**(15), 2361–2382.

House of Lords. (1998). *Science and Technology; Cannabis – the Scientific Evidence; Session 1997–98, Ninth Report.* London: HMSO.

Huestis, M.A. (2005). Pharmacokinetics and metabolism of the plant cannabinoids Δ-9 tetrahydrocannabinol, cannabidiol and cannabinol. *Handbook of Experimental Pharmacology*, **168**, 657–690.

Leuschner, J.T.A., Harvey, D.J., Bullingham, R.E.S., and Paton, W.D.M. (1986). Pharmacokinetics of Δ^9-tetrahydrocannabinol in rabbits following single or multiple intravenous doses. *Drug Metabolism and Disposition*, **14**(2), 230–238.

Mannila, J., Jarvinen, T., and Jarvinen, K. (2006). Sublingual administration of Delta-9-tetrahydrocannabinol/Beta-cyclodextrin complex increase the bioavailability of delta-9-tetrahydrocannabinol in rabbits. *Life Sciences*, **78**, 1911–1914.

MHRA Public Assessment Report. (2010). *Decentralised Procedure, Sativex Oromucosal Spray, UK/H/2462/001/DC, UK licence no: PL 18024/0009, GW Pharma Ltd.* London: MHRA.

Notcutt, W., Langford, R., Davies, P., Ratcliffe, S., and Potts, R. (2012). A placebo-controlled, parallel-group, randomized withdrawal study of subjects with symptoms of spasticity due to multiple sclerosis who are receiving long-term Sativex (nabiximols). *Multiple Sclerosis*, **18**(2), 219–228.

Novotna, A., Mares, J., and Ratcliffe, S. (2011). A randomized, double-blind, placebo-controlled, parallel-group, enriched-design study of nabiximols (Sativex), as add-on therapy, in subjects with refractory spasticity caused by multiple sclerosis. *European Journal of Neurology*, **18**, 1122–1131.

Nurmikko, T.J., Serpell, M.G., Hoggart, B., Toomey, P.J., Morlion, B.J., and Haines, D. (2007). Sativex successfully treats neuropathic pain characterised by allodynia: a randomised, double-blind, placebo-controlled clinical trial. *Pain*, **133**, 210–220.

Pertwee, R. (1999). Prescribing cannabinoids for multiple sclerosis: current issues. *CNS Drugs*, **11**(5), 327–334.

Pertwee, R.G. (2000). Neuropharmacology and therapeutic potential of cannabinoids. *Addiction Biology*, **5**, 37–46.

Rog, D.J., Nurmikko, T.J., Friede, T., and Young, C.A. (2005). Randomized, controlled trial of cannabis-based medicine in central pain in multiple sclerosis. *Neurology* **65**, 812–819.

Rog, D.J., Nurmikko, T.J., and Young, C.A. (2007). Oromucosal delta-9-tetrahydrocannabinol/cannabidiol for neuropathic pain associated with multiple sclerosis: an uncontrolled, open-label, 2-year extension trial. *Clinical Therapeutics*, **29**(9), 2068–2079.

Samara, E., Bialer, M., and Mechoulam, R. (1988). Pharmacokinetics of cannabidiol in dogs. *Drug Metabolism and Disposition*, **16**(3), 469–472.

Schoedel, K.A., Chen, N., Hilliard, A., *et al.* (2011). A randomized, double-blind, placebo-controlled, crossover study to evaluate the subjective abuse potential and cognitive effects of nabiximols oromucosal spray in subjects with a history of recreational cannabis use. *Human Psychopharmacology: Clinical and Experimental*, **26**, 224–236.

Serpell, M.G., Notcutt, W., and Collin, C. (2013). Sativex long-term use: an open-label trial in patients with spasticity due to multiple sclerosis. *Journal of Neurology*, **260**, 285–295.

Siemens, A.J., Walczak, D., and Buckley, F.E. (1980). Characterization of blood disappearance and tissue distribution of tritiated cannabidiol. *Biochemical Pharmacology*, **29**(3), 462–464.

Wade, D.T., Makela, P.M., House, H., Bateman, C., and Robson, P. (2006). Long-term use of a cannabis-based medicine in the treatment of spasticity and other symptoms in multiple sclerosis. *Multiple Sclerosis*, **12**, 639–645.

Wade, D.T., Makela, P., Robson, P., House, H., and Bateman, C. (2004). Do cannabis-based medicinal extracts have general or specific effects on symptoms in multiple sclerosis? A double-blind, randomized, placebo-controlled study on 160 patients. *Multiple Sclerosis*, **10**, 434–441.

Wade, D.T., Robson, P., House, H., Makela, P., and Aram, J. (2003). A preliminary controlled study to determine whether whole-plant cannabis extracts can improve intractable neurogenic symptoms. *Clinical Rehabilitation*, **17**, 21–29.

Williamson, E.M. and Evans, F.J. (2000). Cannabinoids in clinical practice. *Drugs*, **60**(6), 1303–1314.

Chapter 20

Licensed Cannabis-Based Medicines: Benefits and Risks

Stephen Wright and Geoffrey Guy

20.1 Introduction

This chapter will review the clinical trials evidence for those cannabinoids which have achieved regulatory approval in some part of the world during the post-World War II era. This review will include those cannabinoids which are wholly synthetic, but based on naturally occurring compounds (which some might argue are not "cannabis based"). This has been a time during which the regulatory framework within which medicines have been approved has changed substantially, and it is apparent that the regulatory standards that applied when the first cannabis-based medicine was approved in the US in 1985 have changed very considerably. This chapter will make reference to the changing regulatory environment and then place the licensed cannabinoid medicines within that framework, although the reader is also referred to Thompson and Langfield (Chapter 19, this volume) where this regulatory context is described in detail. As the title suggests, we will describe and discuss the benefit/risk profile of each of the licensed medicines, concentrating firstly on those indications for which the cannabinoids are licensed, and then casting an eye over other, nonlicensed indications where there exists some evidence of a benefit of and/or a risk to their use.

20.2 Which cannabis-based medicines are licensed?

There are only three medicines which can be described as "cannabis based" and which are currently licensed for human use. Two of them, nabilone and dronabinol, are wholly synthetic—while the third, Sativex®, is a plant extract. The chronology of their approval carries with it an interesting slant on the relationship between social movements and the status of new medicines, and has to be seen in the context of sociopolitical attitudes to the use of cannabis as a medicine, which have been discussed eloquently earlier in this book (see section 20.1, and Thompson and Langfield, Chapter 19, this volume). This chapter aims to summarize the evidence of efficacy and safety for each of these approved medicines, and to discuss the key differences in risk/benefit between them. We will also try and look at the clinical development and regulatory processes which apply to the approval of a synthetic cannabinoid, although recognize that this has been done to a more detailed extent by Thompson and Langfield (Chapter 19, this volume).

20.3 Dronabinol (Marinol®)

The nomenclature of medicinal cannabinoids can be confusing, especially with regard to the relationship between the licensed medicine, the active pharmaceutical ingredient, and the status of each of them under the US Controlled Substances Act (CSA) of 1970. These scheduling complexities have been discussed earlier in the book, and here we will only repeat that dronabinol is not approved as a medicine except in the form of Marinol® (or a generic alternative). It is the finished product which is recognized to have medicinal value, and not the active pharmaceutical ingredient; the consequence of this distinction, which may seem to be a very fine distinction to some readers, is that dronabinol remains in Schedule 1 (meaning that it has a high abuse potential and no medicinal use) while Marinol® resides in Schedule 3 within the CSA. Marinol® is fully synthetic dronabinol, formulated in sesame oil, with colorings and preservatives, and supplied as soft gelatin capsules.

20.3.1 Regulatory history

Marinol® was approved by the US Food and Drug Administration (FDA) [NDA 18-651/S-021] on May 31, 1985, for nausea and vomiting associated with cancer chemotherapy that had failed to respond adequately to conventional antiemetic treatments. It is of interest to note that the New Drug Application (NDA) had first been filed in 1981, so that the approval process was not without its problems. The subsequent re-scheduling process took almost exactly a year, so Marinol® was first marketed in 1986. On December 22, 1992, Marinol® was approved for the relief of anorexia associated with weight loss in patients with HIV-AIDS (human immunodeficiency virus-acquired immunodeficiency syndrome). Since then, despite a number of published clinical studies, there have been no further indications approved. At the time of approval, it was well recognized and acknowledged by the FDA that dronabinol (delta-9-tetrahydrocannabinol (THC)) was considered the psychoactive component of marijuana. The reader may consider it ironic that the first cannabis-based medicine to be licensed in the modern era contained the only psychoactive component of marijuana, yet was immediately scheduled to be in a less restrictive schedule of the CSA than the parent plant. Since its first approval in the US, Marinol® has also been licensed for use in some other countries, such as Canada and Germany. Generic forms of dronabinol have now (first approved in 2011) been approved in the US.

20.3.2 Clinical trials

20.3.2.1 Chemotherapy-induced nausea and vomiting

20.3.2.1.1 **Background** Because THC had been placed into Schedule 1 following the CSA of 1970, clinical trials were severely restricted, despite significant interest. Not only were there few effective antiemetic agents available at the time, those that were available carried a significant safety burden. Metoclopramide, for example, widely used, carried the risk of tardive dyskinesia. At the same time, there was a well-publicized belief that smoking cannabis provided relief from the nausea and vomiting induced by chemotherapy. Anticancer cytotoxic agents may cause nausea and vomiting, and may be usefully classified into highly emetogenic or moderately emetogenic agents (Hesketh et al. 1997). The former include cisplatin, dacarbazine, and cyclophosphamide at doses in excess of 1500 mg/m^2 and carmustine at doses in excess of 250 mg/m^2 of body surface area. Of these agents, cisplatin is probably the most highly emetogenic agent, and although its structure had been described by Peyrone in 1844, it was first approved by the US FDA for the treatment of testicular cancer in 1978. The wider use of this highly emetogenic agent may have led to a wider recognition of the need for effective antiemetic agents, and hastened the development of Marinol®. Moderately emetogenic cytotoxics include doxorubicin, methotrexate, docetaxel, paclitaxel, and etoposide. Studies using dronabinol were initiated by the National Cancer Institute (NCI), and in a number of cases, compared dronabinol with smoked cannabis or placebo. There were a number of state-sponsored clinical studies in the late 1970s, all of which used smoked cannabis, and some of which used dronabinol, and which may have formed the experience base in which a number of US states subsequently deregulated herbal cannabis for medicinal use. In itself, this is an interesting observation, since it illustrates quite how long individual US states have been interested in the use of cannabis for therapeutic purposes. These six separate state-sponsored study results remained unpublished, except as technical reports, until 2001 when Musty and Rossi (2001) published a review of 748 patients exposed to smoked marijuana in these studies, in some of which oral THC was used as a compararator. Detailed results of these studies is beyond the scope of this chapter, but the studies all showed smoked marijuana to be variably effective, although all were open-label studies, using marijuana that did not seem to have been well standardized. In general, oral THC showed similar or lower efficacy than smoked marijuana. Assessing the extent to which there was a wave of political support behind the wish to develop a form of cannabis that was licensed for prescription use by the FDA is more or less impossible—however, the National Cancer Institutes (NCI) licensed the Marinol® patent to Unimed in 1981, who then filed an NDA more or less immediately in the indication, (and successfully defended a loss of patent action immediately following rescheduling). FDA approval then took 4 years, suggesting that there remained some significant issues during the review of the application, either related to quality concerns, abuse liability concerns, or perhaps that the efficacy and safety data in support of approval were not overwhelming. Studies of smoked marijuana more or less ceased after the approval of Marinol®.

In assessing the results of clinical trials, it is relevant to know with which cytotoxic the patients had been treated—highly emetogenic cytotoxics may produce chemotherapy-induced nausea and vomiting (CINV) which is more resistant to therapy. Furthermore, CINV can be acute—occurring within 24 h of chemotherapy, or delayed, when it may occur up to 5 days following chemotherapy. Clinical trials of Marinol® have looked very much at acute CINV.

Prior to approval, relatively small numbers of patients had been included in clinical trials, especially when compared with those included in the clinical trials showing the efficacy of the 5-HT$_3$ receptor antagonists such as ondansetron, palosetron, and granisetron, agents which have since become the "gold standard" of antiemetic therapy. In the latest update to the American Society for Clinical Oncology antiemetic guidelines, cannabinoids are relegated to agents of lower therapeutic index, and only recommended for use when all other agents (including corticosteroids) have failed.

20.3.2.1.2 **Efficacy of Marinol® in CINV** There seems no doubt that initial studies of THC in the treatment of CINV were encouraged by the observation that younger patients who smoked marijuana during their chemotherapy reported less nausea and vomiting (Gralla 1984). Early studies used doses of between 2.5 mg and 10 mg every 3–4 h, although a clear relationship between dose, dose schedule, and efficacy has never been established. The efficacy of dronabinol (THC) in CINV was reviewed by Gralla et al. in 1984, and again by Tramer et al. in 2001, and the conclusions of those reviews are similar. The former review identified 11 controlled clinical studies, and concluded that metoclopramide, corticosteroids, and butyrophenones offered greater efficacy than dronabinol, but that dronabinol was effective. Chang et al. (1979) found THC to be superior to placebo, as did Frytak et al. (1979) and Orr et al. (1980). Sallan et al. (1980) and Frytak et al. (1979) found THC to be superior to prochlorperazine. Gralla et al. (1984) found intravenous metoclopramide to be more effective than oral THC in a double-blind double-dummy study. The variability of trial designs, of the methods of reporting efficacy and of the emetogenic agent used makes clear statements of the quantitative efficacy of dronabinol difficult, although Gralla et al. (1984) concluded that THC was more effective when used with moderately emetogenic cytotoxics. Tramer et al. (2001) identified those comparative studies where control event rates (vomiting) were defined as "medium" (25–75%) and noted that cannabinoids were superior to comparators (most commonly prochlorperazine or metoclopramide). However, in patients with more extreme or less severe (>75% or < 25%, respectively) CINV, superiority has not been demonstrated. This would seem to support the earlier conclusions of Gralla et al. One small study (n = 64) showed dronabinol to be equally as effective as ondansetron in delayed CINV (Meiri et al. 2007), although each agent was effective in a higher proportion of subjects than the combination. Regrettably there do not appear to be any well-controlled studies comparing dronabinol with the 5-HT$_3$ receptor antagonists which have become the standard first-line therapy in acute CINV, and dronabinol was only ever approved for medicinal use in this indication in the US, Canada, and South Africa.

20.3.2.1.3 **Safety of Marinol® in CINV** The dominant side effects of dronabinol in the clinical trials investigating its place in the treatment of acute CINV are those which relate to its activity at the type 1 cannabinoid receptor (CB$_1$). There was a high rate of a "high" sensation, of drowsiness, somnolence, and sedation. Within the psychiatric or neurologic body systems, dizziness occurred in up to 50% of patients, and hallucination and paranoia in 6% and 5% respectively. Despite this, in those crossover studies where patients were asked to express a preference, the difference in favor of dronabinol over placebo was significant, and in active controlled studies, patient preference was generally in favor of dronabinol. Furthermore, relatively few (10%) patients withdrew from studies due to adverse events. This suggested to the authors (Tramer et al. 2001) either that these adverse effects were deemed to be minor compared with the benefit, or perhaps, that the "high" might be a positive experience for the patients. An insight into this might come from the NCI sponsored study by Ungerleider et al. (1985), who explored the reasons for patient preference in a crossover study of THC versus prochlorperazine in 139 patients undergoing a variety of chemotherapy regimens. Briefly they found that patient preference was closely related to efficacy—that the patients preferred the agent that gave them greatest symptom relief. THC-related side effects were also associated with a positive preference, and the authors suggested that somnolence might be a desirable part of the therapeutic profile in this indication. In an earlier controlled study in more than 200 patients, Ungerleider et al. (1982) separated spontaneously reported adverse effects into several categories: 45% of patients reported somnolence, 36% reported "physiological effects" (dizziness, headache, tachycardia, chills), while 34% reported "psychological effects" (mental clouding, short-term memory loss, and dissociative reactions).

20.3.2.2 AIDS-associated anorexia and weight loss

20.3.2.2.1 **Background** In 1992, Marinol® was approved by the FDA for the orphan indication of anorexia in AIDS patients. This approval seems to have been based largely on two studies by Beal et al. (1995, 1997). As a consequence of this approval, the market for Marinol® increased very substantially, with AIDS patients accounting for around 80% of sales. This approval was a time of very active lobbying by medicinal marijuana proponents who, in 1991, publicized the FDA's earlier decision to grant an IND to marijuana for a Compassionate Access Program as a no-cost supply of marijuana cigarettes for AIDS patients. This IND enabled individuals to receive a legal supply of marijuana cigarettes contingent upon a recommendation from their physicians, and was followed rapidly by the FDA approval of Marinol®. How much these events were coincidence, and how much driven by federal (or even Presidential) will is entirely unclear, but the reader will see that the normal requirements for a demonstration of efficacy and safety appear to have been generously interpreted by the FDA for this approval.

20.3.2.2.2 **Efficacy** The clinical studies that led to the approval of Marinol® in this indication comprised a single 6-week placebo-controlled randomized study in 139 patients, followed by an open-label extension study. In the placebo-controlled study, only 99/139 patients had data at 4 weeks and 91 at 6 weeks. The dose of dronabinol used was 2.5 mg twice daily, substantially lower than that used in CINV. There was a significant difference in a hunger Visual Analog Scale (VASH) between Marinol® and placebo, without any significant difference in weight. On Marinol® there was a 16-point increase in hunger compared with an 8-point improvement on placebo. Leaving aside the question of whether hunger is synonymous with appetite, this seems to have been the extent of the placebo-controlled data that persuaded the FDA of the efficacy of Marinol® in this indication. In long-term use (Beal 1997) the improvements in appetite were sustained, although drop-out rates were high, with 36/94 patients having withdrawn by 3 months. The mean duration of treatment was 5.8 months (standard deviation = 4.4 months). In retrospect, it seems out of the ordinary that the FDA would approve a new indication based on such limited efficacy data, and there must inevitably be speculation that other factors may have played a role.

20.3.2.2.3 **Safety** The dose of Marinol® used to stimulate appetite in AIDS patients is lower than the doses used in the antiemetic indication, and most likely because of this, the frequency of typical adverse events is less. In the former indication, a dose of 2.5 mg twice daily was used in the clinical studies, whereas in the latter indication, the dose was variable, but ranged from 2.5 mg up to 40 mg per day, usually taken every 3–4 h for 24 h. As a consequence of this, the Product Monograph (Canada) identifies the following adverse effects as being more common in the antiemetic indication: amnesia, ataxia, and hallucination. The US package insert identifies the phenomenon of getting "high" to occur in 24% of patients in the emesis indication, compared to 8% of patients with HIV-AIDS, taking the smaller dose (http://www.fda.gov/ohrms/dockets/dockets/05n0479/05N-0479-emc0004-04.pdf). Importantly, there do not appear to have been any unexpected long-term consequences of the continued use of Marinol®, to the extent that the WHO reported in its 2007 assessment (WHO 2007 p. 19) that:

> The US responded that, although its susceptibility (sic) for abuse can vary with the dosage form, the pharmaceutical product containing Marinol is associated with low levels of diversion and abuse. The US is not aware of any drug related deaths, drug dependence or addiction associated with Marinol.

20.4 **Nabilone**

20.4.1 **Background**

Nabilone (dl-3-(1,1-dimethylheptyl)-6,6ab 7,8,10,10a alpha-hexahydro-1-hydroxy-6,6-dimethyl-9H dibenzo [b,d] pyran-9-one) is a synthetic analogue of THC, which was developed in the 1970s (Lemberger and Rowe 1975) well before the target receptor was identified. It has low nanomolar affinity for the CB_1 receptor, and somewhat less at the CB_2 receptor.

20.4.2 **Regulatory history**

The regulatory history of nabilone (Cesamet®) mirrors to some extent that of dronabinol. Although the initial FDA approval for CINV was granted in 1985 (the same year as Marinol®) for the indication of CINV that has not responded to conventional antiemetics (the same indication as Marinol®), the drug was not marketed in the US until 2006. By this time, newer antiemetic agents had been developed, notably the $5\text{-}HT_3$ receptor antagonists and the Substance P (NeuroKinin 1) antagonists.

20.4.3 **Efficacy of nabilone in CINV**

The antiemetic efficacy of nabilone has been extensively reviewed by Tramer et al. (2001) and Ware et al. (2008). Herman et al. (1977, 1979) published two controlled studies comparing nabilone with prochlorperazine. The authors quoted an 80% success rate on nabilone, compared with a 32% response rate on prochlorperazine, and the effectiveness of nabilone was maintained over the 5-day treatment period. Subsequently, Einhorn et al. (1981) and others (Ahmedazai et al. 1983; Niiranen and Mattson 1985) found similar results in patients treated predominantly with the highly emetic cisplatin. The relevance of this finding to current treatment options is limited, since prochlorperazine is not regarded as a first-line antiemetic agent. So much have new treatment options come to dominate the therapeutic landscape that the place of nabilone or of prochlorperazine as a treatment option in CINV is not even discussed in the latest guidelines published by the American Society of Clinical Oncology (Basch et al. 2012).

20.4.4 **Safety of nabilone in CINV**

The activity that nabilone displays at the CB_1 receptor more or less predicts the safety profile. Overall, adverse events are seen in around twice as many patients as are seen in patients taking prochlorperazine in controlled studies, and were more often severe; despite this, patient preference remained in favor of nabilone, as was the case with dronabinol. Other reports make it apparent that the nature of the question may determine the answer, at least in part. For example, Ahmedzai et al. (1983) reported that patient preference was in favor of nabilone over prochlorperazine, but that far fewer patients wished to take it again than stated their preference for it over prochlorperazine. In short, while patients recognized the effectiveness of nabilone, this did not necessarily mean that they would like to take it again. Although the frequency of the most common adverse events varied between studies, the numbers reported in their controlled study by Ahmedzai et al. (1983) seem typical. They describe the adverse event of drowsiness in more than 50% of patients, and dizziness and light-headedness in 35% and 18% respectively. Euphoria was reported in 14%, and 7% reported getting "high." Jones et al. (1982) reported dizziness in 65% and drowsiness in 51% of patients. It was unusual for these events to provoke withdrawal from treatment.

20.5 **Nabiximols (Sativex®)**

20.5.1 **Background**

Despite the availability of synthetic THC in the form of dronabinol, it remained the case that large numbers of people with chronic symptomatic conditions, particularly those associated with chronic pain and/or spasticity associated with multiple sclerosis (MS), turned to the use of herbal cannabis for symptom relief. On both sides of the Atlantic, this phenomenon provoked government-sponsored reviews of what was seen as a problem for society as a whole, for the criminal justice system, and for the medical system as well. It is a reasonable conclusion that the synthetic cannabinoids were not apparently providing a legitimate medical alternative to the illegitimate herb. In the late 1990s, the House of Lords Science and Technology Select Committee in the UK, together with the British Medical Association, urged the development of a medicinal form of cannabis. The Ninth Report of the Select Committee concluded (1998, Para 8.22) "We therefore recommend that clinical trials of cannabis for the treatment of MS and chronic pain should be mounted as a matter of urgency." In the US, the Office of National Drug Control Policy (ONDCP) asked the Institute of Medicine to review the subject; among their recommendations was that clinical studies of cannabinoids should be done to establish medicinal value, and that smoking was not likely to be an acceptable method of delivery.

Sativex® is distinct from the other licensed cannabinoids insofar as it comprises an extract of the cannabis plant, formulated as a sublingual/oromucosal spray. Each 100 microliters of the spray delivers 2.7 mg of THC and 2.5 mg of cannabidiol (CBD).

20.5.2 Regulatory history

Sativex® received its first approvals in Canada in 2005 under legislation that permits conditional approval of a new medicine in areas of high unmet medical need, and in the presence of highly promising clinical data; approval in EU was delayed until late 2010 and early 2011, when Sativex® was approved in the UK and Spain following a decentralized procedure. As such, it became the first full plant extract to be approved as a prescription medicine in the modern era. The rocky regulatory path is described in more detail by Thompson and Langfield (Chapter 19, this volume). Since then, Sativex® has been approved across most of Europe, in Australia and New Zealand, in Canada, and in Israel. By the time this book reaches print, it seems likely that Sativex® will also have received approval in several other territories. While it is licensed as second-line therapy for the relief of spasticity in MS in all those countries where it is approved, in some countries it also can be prescribed for the treatment of neuropathic pain in people with MS, and for the treatment of cancer-related pain, where it is used as an adjunct to opioids. The pharmacology supporting each of these indications has been described in other chapters in this volume, but it is important to note that while the mechanism of action of dronabinol and nabilone is undoubtedly primarily based on their effect at the cannabinoid receptors, this is unlikely to be the case with Sativex®, where there may be an array of pharmacological actions which contribute to its efficacy. In particular, the recently described effects of CBD on the vanilloid receptor system (Bisogno et al. 2001), on the uptake of nucleosides (Carrier et al. 2006) and on the chemotaxis of immune active cells (Sacerdote et al. 2005) all provide a coherent reason why this cannabinoid is likely to contribute to the therapeutic effects of Sativex®. This observation alone should be enough to indicate that it is not appropriate to lump all cannabinoids together with regard to their risk/benefit, any more than it would be appropriate to lump together all beta-blockers or 3-hydroxy-3-methylglutaryl-coenzyme A (HMG-CoA) reductase inhibitors, or any class of medicine for that matter. Nonetheless, as we shall see, there is a considerable tendency to do so.

20.5.3 Spasticity in multiple sclerosis

MS is one of the most common neurological diseases of young adults. It is characterized by the development of inflammatory plaques in the central nervous system (CNS), including the brain, spinal cord, and optic nerves. The primary process is inflammatory damage to the myelin of the CNS, which may be reversible, but axonal damage may also occur and this leads to increasing permanent disability. MS also has a degenerative component, and is associated with progressive brain atrophy.

Spasticity is a common symptom in MS, but it may occur in any condition that damages the upper motor pathways of the CNS (Fig. 20.1), and it is also commonly seen in stroke and spinal cord injuries. The hallmark of spasticity is an increase in muscle tone and disinhibition of muscle stretch reflexes, but the upper motor neuron syndrome, of which spasticity is a part, is more complex in its manifestations. Because of this, the choice of clinically relevant endpoints in clinical trials is critical, and in the view of the Cochrane review (Shakespeare et al. 2003) "must reflect the patient daily experience of their spasticity." It is not adequate to use only one component of the phenomenon of spasticity in order to determine therapeutic responses, and efforts to do so have usually resulted in failure.

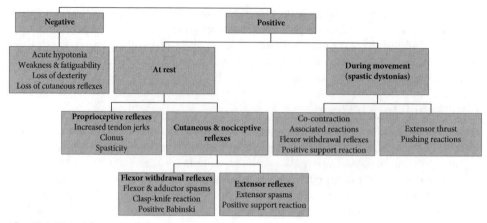

Fig. 20.1 Clinical features of the upper motor neuron syndrome.

Characteristically, spasticity leads to exaggerated flexor tone and extensor weakness in the upper limbs, and exaggerated extensor tone and flexor weakness in the lower limbs, so that patients with spasticity tend to have flexed upper limbs and stiff, extended lower limbs. This leads to gait difficulties with poor knee bending and poor toe clearance, and may greatly increase the effort of walking beyond the problems caused by weakness alone, because flexor muscle groups may have to overcome the unwanted activity in antagonistic extensor muscle groups. Some spasticity may be useful, however, because it may keep the legs stiff enough to support body weight when voluntary power alone may be inadequate. Hence assessing the clinical relevance of an intervention in spasticity, whether it be pharmacological or physical (i.e., physical therapy), must make an effort to incorporate the effect of the intervention on the way the patient feels or functions.

20.5.4 Clinical trials with Sativex®

20.5.4.1 Efficacy in the treatment of spasticity in MS

The clinical development of Sativex® followed a more "conventional" course than that of Marinol®, insofar as it comprised a series of Phase 1 studies, aimed at determining the pharmacokinetics of the cannabinoids (and metabolites) within the botanical medicine, followed by Phase 2 studies aimed at better defining the efficacy, and a series of Phase 3 studies aimed at investigating the benefit/risk in people with MS and spasticity. These studies have been reviewed elsewhere (Oreja-Guevara 2012), but essentially comprise five placebo-controlled, randomized studies, in all of which Sativex® was added to existing oral antispasticity agents, in patients who were experiencing at least moderately severe spasticity, despite the use of optimal conventional therapy, such as baclofen, tizanidine, gabapentin, and benzodiazepines. The baseline characteristics of the patients included in the studies were similar: the history of MS was greater than 10 years in all studies, the Expanded Disability Status Scale (EDSS) at baseline was between 5.5 and 6, and all patients had tried and failed at least one line of oral antispasticity therapy. In chronological order, the first study was that of Wade et al. (2004), in which patients identified their most troublesome symptom out of five possible symptoms—spasticity, pain, bladder disturbance, tremor, or spasms, using a 0–100 Visual Analogue Scale. Those who identified spasticity as their primary symptom showed a highly significant improvement on Sativex® compared with placebo, which was not seen with the other symptoms. This study, along with previously published Phase 2 studies (Wade et al. 2003), suggested that spasticity was the optimal target for the product. Collin et al. (2007) studied 189 patients with spasticity due to MS, using a 0–10 Numeric Rating Scale (NRS) as the primary outcome measure, and found a statistically significant difference between Sativex® and placebo in improving the patient-rated outcome of spasticity severity, over a 6-week treatment period. Of the secondary efficacy measures, only the motricity index approached significance in favor of Sativex®. This may be important, because that index can be regarded as a measure of voluntary muscle power, and reduction in muscle power, with the consequence of an increased risk of falls, is a recognized problem with existing antispasticity agents. The fact that Sativex® showed a quantitative improvement in the motricity index compared with placebo, suggests that it may be unlikely to cause muscle weakness, and may not therefore be associated with an increased risk of falls.

The same lead investigator (Collin et al. 2010) published a larger study (n = 337), with a 12-week post-randomization treatment period, in which the intent-to-treat analysis showed no significant difference between Sativex® and placebo, although the per-protocol analysis did so. The three studies were then reported as a meta-analysis (Wade et al. 2010), which used a responder analysis as the key efficacy assessment. This showed that 35% of patients on Sativex® achieved an improvement of at least 30% from baseline—which is equivalent to feeling "much improved" (Farrar 2008) compared with 24% of patients on placebo. While this difference between drug and placebo may seem relatively small, it is very much in line with many medicines used in neuropsychiatry. The meta-analysis also showed significant differences in spasm scores and in global impression of change.

These studies illustrated one of the recurring difficulties in analyzing studies of medicines aimed at treating chronic symptomatic conditions, such as pain and spasticity. It is clear from clinical practice that patients do not all respond to such medicines. To include a proportion of nonresponders in clinical studies will mask the effect of a medicine in those patients who are capable of mounting a response, and thus bias the study against the drug under investigation. From a statistical point of view, there is an implicit assumption in sample size calculations that all patients are capable of responding, so that when a condition is encountered where this is not the case, sample size calculations may be wrong. One method of overcoming this bias is to randomize only those patients who are capable of responding to treatment—a maneuver which is becoming increasingly common in oncology studies using targeted therapies, and has been used in cardiovascular medicine for many years. McQuay et al. (2008) have recently discussed the merits of using an enriched study design, and guidance regarding how to design such studies can be found on the US FDA website (http://www.fda.gov/).

The final two published randomized studies of Sativex® in MS spasticity both used a form of enriched study design. Novotna et al. (2011) first exposed patients to a 4-week, single blind treatment period with Sativex®, then randomized only those patients who showed a clinically meaningful improvement. In this way, the only patients exposed to the Sativex® versus placebo comparison were those who were capable of improvement, and who would have continued with the medicine in a setting of "real-world" clinical practice. In this way, this study may be said to have had more external validity than the conventional clinical study, since it better reflected the way that the drug would be used in the clinic. This study firstly showed that 47% of patients show a meaningful response to Sativex®, and that there was a highly significant difference in outcomes between Sativex® and placebo, when such patients were exposed over a 13-week period. This study also showed highly significant differences in sleep quality, spasm scores, patient, carer, and physician global impression of function, and perhaps most notably in the Barthel Activities of Daily Living Index—confirming functional improvement.

Notcutt et al. (2012) reported a modification of the enriched study design by randomizing a cohort of patients who had been receiving long-term benefit from Sativex® to either continue on Sativex® or to switch, blind, to placebo. This type of study is termed an enriched enrolment, randomized withdrawal study, and is especially suited to showing whether the efficacy of a medicine is maintained in long-term use. This study showed that patients were significantly more likely to fail treatment on placebo than on Sativex®. It reinforced the conclusions of long-term open-label safety studies which also showed efficacy on Sativex® to be maintained in long-term use.

Following the first regulatory approval of Sativex®, several other studies have been published which add to the body of information available to prescribers. Notcutt (2012) conducted a questionnaire survey of long-term Sativex® users and found a reduced frequency of visits to the doctor, a reduced rate of accidents requiring medical attention, and continued improvement in spasticity and sleep in particular. Carers reported in this questionnaire survey that their own quality of life had improved, even to the extent that they were able to get back to work. Slof et al. (2012) published a pharmacoeconomic evaluation of Sativex® that confirmed its pharmacoeconomic benefit, although this has been questioned by others.

20.5.4.2 The use of a patient-reported outcome measure

In general, health outcomes may be either physician based or patient reported. Physician-based measures generally address the pathological basis of disease, and evaluate health in terms of quantity. They do not provide a picture of disease impact, and in the case of the Ashworth Scale in particular, may also bear little or no relation to the functional abilities of the patient. The Ashworth Scale is a widely used scale for the clinical assessment of spasticity from all causes (Skold 2000). It mainly assesses one component of spasticity, movement-provoked spastic muscle resistance (tonic stretch reflex). This is only one part of the spasticity syndrome, which includes increased tendon reflexes (phasic stretch reflex), increased exteroceptive reflexes (flexor reflex) and pathologic radiation of reflexes between spinal segments over time (see Fig. 20.1). The syndrome causes stiffness, a reduced range of movement, painful spasms, contractures, and a consequent range of functional disabilities.

Evidence validating the Ashworth Scale as a measure of increased tone (especially in the lower limbs, and especially in MS) is lacking, and many careful studies have confirmed its lack of validity.

Hobart et al. (2004) have commented:

> Patient-based outcomes are the consequences of disease and treatment that are considered important to patients. Patients are the best source of information about therapeutic benefit defined in terms of function and well-being. As patients, their caregivers and their physician differ in their interpretation of the impact of illness, it is important to elicit information from patients about which outcomes are important. This is supported by irrefutable evidence that patients can provide reliable and valid judgements of health status and the benefits of treatment.

In assessing the clinical relevance of an intervention, whether it be pharmacologic, or physiotherapy, for example, it is important to use a measure that reflects therapeutic benefit. Patient report has been described as the ultimate measure of health status (Ware 1993).

EU Guidelines (E9) make clear that the primary variable of a clinical study (i.e., primary endpoint) should be the variable capable of providing the most clinically relevant and convincing evidence directly related to the primary objective of the trial to provide scientific evidence regarding efficacy of the product. The selection of the primary endpoint should reflect the accepted norms and standards in the field of research to which the product pertains. The use of a reliable and validated variable with which experience has been gained either in earlier studies or in published literature is recommended. The guidance goes on to say that there should be sufficient evidence that the primary variable can provide a valid and reliable measure of some clinically relevant and important treatment benefit in the target patient population.

Robert Temple is the Head of the Office of Medical Policy at the FDA's Center for Drug Evaluation and Response. In a detailed discussion of the value of disease markers, he has expressed very clearly his view of what constitutes a clinically relevant endpoint for clinical studies. It is "a direct measure of how a patient feels, functions or survives" (Temple 1999).

With specific reference to spasticity in people with MS the Cochrane reviewers (Shakespeare et al. 2003, p. 11) concluded:

> The variability of spasticity and the lack of a sensitive, reliable, functionally- and symptomatically-relevant assessment tool for spasticity have contributed to the inconclusive results of placebo-controlled trials attempting to document the efficacy of anti-spasticity agents which are in widespread use.

They go on to make their view clear on what constitutes an appropriate primary outcome measure.

> Such measures must correspond to the daily patient experience of spasticity.

This view has also been expressed very clearly by Sneed et al. (2006, p. 79), who summarized the debate as follows:

> Ultimately what is overlooked in tone/spasticity measures is that it is not the score but how the person functions that matters to the person. One is not interested in one's Ashworth Score first thing in the morning, but whether one can comb one's hair or cook one's breakfast.

For these reasons, and also because of the shortcomings of the Ashworth Scale, and because of the expert consensus in favor of a patient-reported outcome measure, the Sativex® studies used the NRS. However, and recognizing the importance of the independence of the physician, the studies also used a Physician Global Impression of change in the severity of spasticity as an independent and objective assessment of the patient's function. In the protocol for the study reported by Novotna et al. (2011), the physician was asked to ensure that his or her assessment was a measure of the general functional capacity of the patients as it related to the severity of their spasticity. As well as this, the use of a caregiver's assessment of the functional capacity of the patient adds to the reliability of the results. Both of these scales provide independent verification of the patients' reports of the severity of their spasticity-associated symptoms. The validity of the NRS has also been confirmed in a longitudinal validation study, in which the correlation between the NRS and a basket of physician assessments of spasticity was tracked over time in a cohort of MS patients with stable spasticity, attending a neurorehabilitation clinic (Anwar and Barnes 2009), and in a transverse study in which the change in NRS with treatment was correlated with the change in a series of other assessments of the severity of spasticity (Farrar et al. 2008).

20.5.4.3 Maintaining the blind-to-treatment allocation

There is a perceived danger that patients exposed to a medicine with a typical adverse event profile might become aware of their treatment allocation and become unreliable in their reports of the effects of the drug. This was investigated in the Sativex® studies using an interesting methodology whereby the interaction between the occurrence of typical adverse events, or the presence of prior experience of cannabis, and the efficacy of Sativex®, was explored using a series of statistical models (Wright et al. 2012). These analyses showed no evidence of any impact of the presence of typical adverse events on efficacy, nor any effect of prior experience of cannabis. This provides reassurance that the results of the studies were not likely to have been confounded by unblinding to treatment allocation.

20.5.4.4 Safety of Sativex®

The safety profile of Sativex® appears to compare favorably with that of dronabinol and nabilone, and has been recently reviewed (Wade 2012). The most common unwanted effects are dizziness fatigue, and somnolence, although these do not commonly lead to treatment cessation. Euphoria is present at a much lower rate than that published for dronabinol and nabilone, suggesting that there is something in the composition or mode of administration of Sativex® which reduces this effect. In the published clinical studies with Sativex®, the mean daily dose was persistently around eight sprays, containing 21.6 mg of THC and 20 mg of CBD. At similar daily doses of dronabinol, rates of dizziness are much higher than those seen with Sativex®, and adverse events within the psychiatric body system were also notably higher. For example, in the body of data submitted in support of the approval of Marinol® in CINV, the rate of euphoria was reported as between 3% and 10%. In Sativex® studies in patients with cancer pain, a similar population of patients, the rate of euphoria was 0.3%. Hallucinations, paranoia, and abnormal thinking all occurred at a greater incidence in the Marinol® studies, even though the dose of THC was similar. It may be that the presence of CBD is responsible for this lower frequency of psychiatric adverse events, since CBD has been shown to reduce the psychoactivity of THC (see McPartland and Russo, Chapter 15, this volume). Equally, the delivery of Sativex® by the oromucosal route has the potential to reduce the extent of first-pass metabolism, and there is some evidence that the proportion of the first metabolite of THC—11-OH-THC—is reduced in patients using Sativex® compared with those using Marinol® (Karschner et al. 2011). This metabolite is active at the CB_1 receptor, and there is evidence that it may give rise to a dysphoric, rather than euphoric, effect.

20.5.4.5 Effects on cognition

The adverse event data suggest that Sativex® may have an adverse effect on short-term memory, at least as perceived by the subject, but formal placebo-controlled studies show no effect in tests of cognition. A Phase 1 study showed that the cannabidiol present in Sativex® is able to reduce the cognitive impairment associated with THC (Nicholson et al. 2004). A recent placebo-controlled crossover study examined the effect of Sativex® versus placebo on the Paced Auditory Serial Addition Task (PASAT) in a series of 18 subjects with spasticity due to MS. PASAT is a serial addition task used to assess the rate of information processing, sustained attention, and working memory. This study showed no significant differences in cognitive function between Sativex® and placebo (Aragona et al. 2008).

A human abuse liability study assessed the effect of substantial single doses of Sativex® on various aspects of cognitive performance. At doses of four, eight, and 16 sprays taken all at once, Sativex® was not significantly different from placebo with regard to its effect on cognition (Schoedel et al. 2011). Nonetheless, there is significant concern expressed in the literature about the long-term effects of cannabinoids on cognition, and it will be interesting to see whether the increasingly widespread use of Sativex® results in any new findings in this area. While Marinol® has been used in the US since 1986, there have been no significant findings of long-term cognitive impairment, and while the short-term adverse effects of the licensed cannabinoids are particularly targeted towards the CNS, there seems little evidence of long-term effects.

20.5.5 Abuse liability

Cannabis as herbal material, or derivatives thereof, are classed as having a high level of abuse liability, and are therefore included in Schedule 1 in the US. Cannabis is easily the most widely used illicit drug in the world with estimates of up to 200 million current consumers. Prevalence rates in the UK and US are around 10% of the adult population as a whole, two-thirds of which are accounted for by individuals between the ages of 16 and 29 years. Cannabis is approximately equivalent to alcohol in its ability to produce psychological dependence, but only half as likely to produce physical dependence (Nutt et al. 2007). Between 4% and 9% of those who try cannabis eventually become dependent upon it, and in the UK it now represents the primary drug problem for around 7% of admissions to drug dependency programs. The euphoric effects of cannabis and its dependence potential are the result of the interaction of the cannabinoid, THC, with CB_1 receptors in the CNS, where it acts as a partial agonist (Devane et al. 1988; Mechoulam 1970). These effects are enhanced when THC reaches high levels quickly (Busto et al. 1986).

Therefore the manufacturer and developer of any medicine based on cannabis, and in particular any medicine containing components of the cannabis plant, has the responsibility of determining the abuse liability of their medicine. This has become an increasing preoccupation of regulatory agencies and governments, as the abuse of prescription medicines, and in particular prescription opioids, has become more and more widespread. The determination of abuse liability may depend on postapproval investigation, as was the case with Marinol®. Its abuse potential has been reviewed by Calhoun and colleagues (1998). They found no evidence of significant abuse or diversion, "scrip-chasing," or a street market for the drug. Marijuana users do not value its effects since the onset of action is slow and gradual, it is at most only weakly reinforcing, and most people find its effects are dysphoric and unappealing. The authors concluded that the evidence suggest that dronabinol has a very low abuse potential. An evaluation of the abuse potential of nabilone reached similar conclusions, with cases of abuse or diversion "rare or isolated" (Ware 2008). The World Health Organization, in their 2006 report, noted that "the pharmaceutical product containing Marinol is associated with low levels of diversion and abuse. The US is not aware of any drug related deaths, drug dependence or addiction associated with Marinol" (World Health Organization 2006).

The abuse liability of Sativex® has been compared with that of Marinol® in a formal human abuse liability study (Schoedel et al. 2011). This study was conducted as a randomized, double-blind, 6-period crossover study with six treatment sessions. Sativex® was administered at four, eight, and 16 sprays (containing 10.8, 21.6, and 43.2 mg THC and 10, 20, and 40 mg CBD) and compared with two doses of Marinol® (20 mg and 40 mg THC), and placebo in active recreational marijuana users.

The three primary study endpoints were: Drug Liking Visual Analogue Scale (DL VAS), Subjective Drug Value (SDV), and Addiction Research Center Inventory Morphine Benzedrine Subscale (ARCI MBG; a measure of euphoria).

Secondary endpoints included (Choice Reaction Time (CRT), Divided Attention (DA) and Sternberg Short-Term Memory (STM) tests). Serial pharmacodynamic evaluations (taken at each treatment session) in this study consisted of various Addiction Research Center Inventory (ARCI) subscales (marijuana, LSD, etc.), Overall Drug Liking and other subjective effects VASs ("High", "Stoned" "Drowsiness", "Good / Bad effects," etc.).

On a dose-for-dose basis, virtually all primary variables produced higher scores on Marinol® than for Sativex® containing the corresponding THC dose. Of specific interest is that two of the three Drug Liking parameters were significantly higher for dronabinol 20 mg than for Sativex®, with the third parameter approaching significance. There were no significant differences between the products in any of the parameters at the high (40 mg) dose. In addition, with regard to secondary variables, there appear to be significant differences between eight sprays of Sativex® and an approximate dose equivalent of Marinol® containing 20 mg THC. Dronabinol produced significantly higher values on a number of key secondary variables, whereas for the 16 sprays of Sativex® and an approximate dose equivalent of Marinol® containing 40 mg THC, no such difference appeared to exist.

The study concluded that, at a dose of four sprays (10.8 mg THC), Sativex® in subjects with a history of recreational marijuana use had no significant abuse potential compared to placebo (primary endpoints). As for any THC-containing medication taken at larger doses, Sativex® at doses of 21.6 mg THC and 43.2 mg THC in subjects with a history of recreational marijuana use had statistically significant abuse potential compared to placebo. Marinol® at doses of 20 mg and 40 mg in such subjects also has statistically significant abuse potential compared to placebo.

The authors concluded:

> The study was valid for detecting abuse-related effects of cannabinoid compounds, and the results demonstrated that Marinol® has significant abuse potential. Sativex® (21.6 mg and 43.2 mg) also had significant abuse potential compared with placebo, but on a dose-per-dose basis, less abuse potential compared with Marinol®. Although this was statistically significant primarily for the 21.6 mg versus 20 mg doses, the overall pattern of results suggest that Sativex® is subjectively different from Marinol®. Therefore, it can be concluded that the risk for abuse associated with Sativex® should be no higher and possibly lower than Marinol®, a Schedule III drug that does not appear to be significantly abused.

One of the key features of abuse liability is the presence of physical dependence and withdrawal symptoms. Budney and colleagues (2004) have reviewed the validity and significance of the cannabis withdrawal syndrome, and concluded: "Converging evidence from basic laboratory and clinical studies indicates that a withdrawal syndrome reliably follows discontinuation of chronic heavy use of cannabis or tetrahydrocannabinol. Common symptoms are primarily emotional and behavioural, although appetite change, weight loss, and physical discomfort are also frequently reported." They went on to propose that the syndrome be defined by the presence of at least four of the following symptoms accompanied by "evidence that these symptoms produced clinically significant distress or dysfunction": anger or aggression; decreased appetite or weight loss; irritability; nervousness/anxiety; restlessness; sleep difficulties, including strange dreams; chills; depressed mood; stomach pain; shakiness; sweating.

The possibility that abrupt cessation of Sativex® treatment might produce a withdrawal syndrome has been explored systematically. Notcutt et al. (2012) studied 36 MS patients receiving long-term Sativex® (median exposure 3.6 years) who were randomly allocated either to continue Sativex® or switch to identical placebo for 4 weeks. No withdrawal syndrome was reported in the latter group. Langford et al. (2013) studied 42 MS patients who had received at least 12 weeks of treatment with Sativex® and were randomized to continue the drug or switch to placebo over a 4-week treatment period. Again, no withdrawal syndrome was apparent in the placebo recipients.

20.5.6 **Other approved indications**

Neither dronabinol nor nabilone have been licensed for use in other indications, although there have been a series of clinical studies published in other conditions, notably neuropathic pain. Results of these studies have been variable, and are shown in Table 20.1. On the other hand, Sativex® has been approved in certain geographies for the relief of central neuropathic pain in patients with MS (Canada, Israel) and in Canada for the relief of persistent (as opposed to breakthrough) cancer-related pain, in patients with advanced cancer. In each of these settings, Sativex® has been used as an adjunct, illustrating the fact that cannabinoids appear to enhance the efficacy of other agents, particularly where those other agents have not been able to confer adequate relief. The specific positive interaction between cannabinoids and opioids has been described in more detail elsewhere in this book (see Costa and Comelli, Chapter 25, this volume).

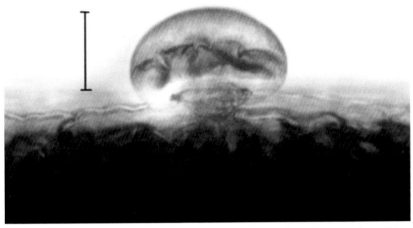

Fig. 4.1 A capitate sessile trichome observed on the edge of one of the first pair of true leaves of a cannabis seedling. (Scale bar = 25μm.)

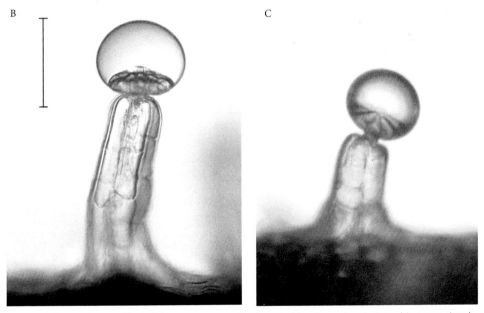

B

C

Fig. 4.2 (B) A capitate stalked trichome, temporarily mounted in glycerol and viewed in transmitted light. (C) A glandular trichome with partly abscised resin head.

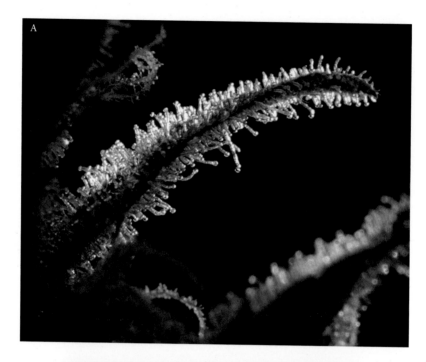

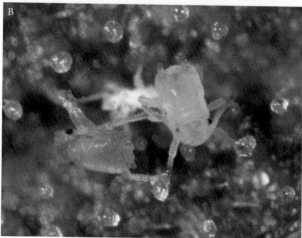

Fig. 4.3 (A) A dense pubescence of glandular stalked trichomes on a bract within a cannabis female inflorescence. The orange/brown structures are senesced stigmas. (B) Two young cotton-melon aphids (*Aphis gossypii*) irreversibly adhered to the resin heads of capitate stalked trichomes.

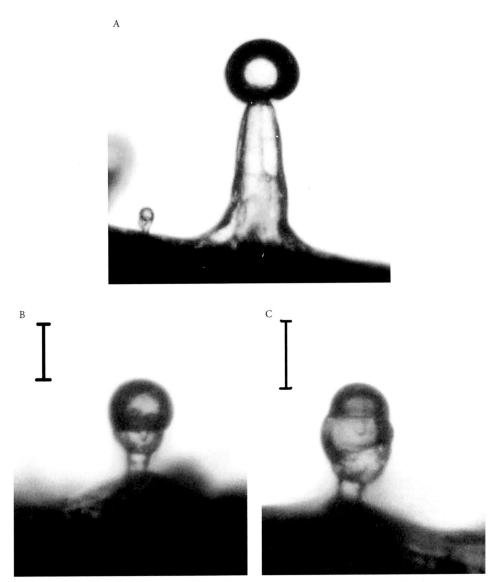

Fig. 4.4 (A) A small bulbous trichome alongside a fully developed glandular stalked trichome. The contrast in resin head diameter (10 μm vs. 100 μm) is clear. (B) A simple bulbous trichome and (C) a complex bulbous trichome. These are 10–15 μm in diameter.

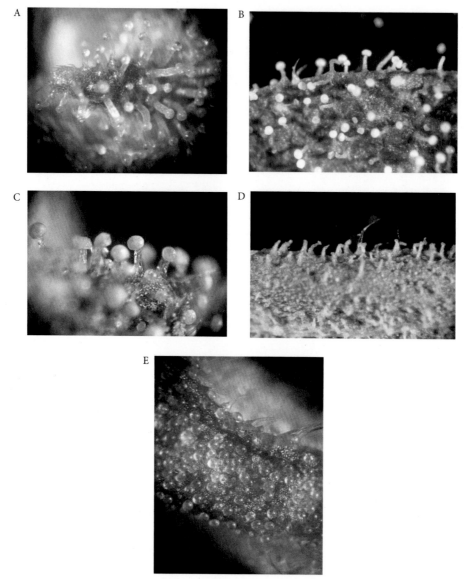

Fig. 5.3 Glandular trichomes associated to different chemotypes. (A) CBDA- and/or THCA-predominant plants carry stalked trichomes with large transparent heads. CBGA-predominant clones with underlying $B_{D0}{}^2/B_{D0}{}^2$ (B) and B_{T0}/B_{T0} (C) genotype both show white opaque trichome heads. (D) Cannabinoid-free chemotypes carry trichomes with shriveled heads. (E) Optimized CBCA predominant clones lack stalked trichomes and show a high density of sessile trichomes.

© T.J. Wilkinson.

A

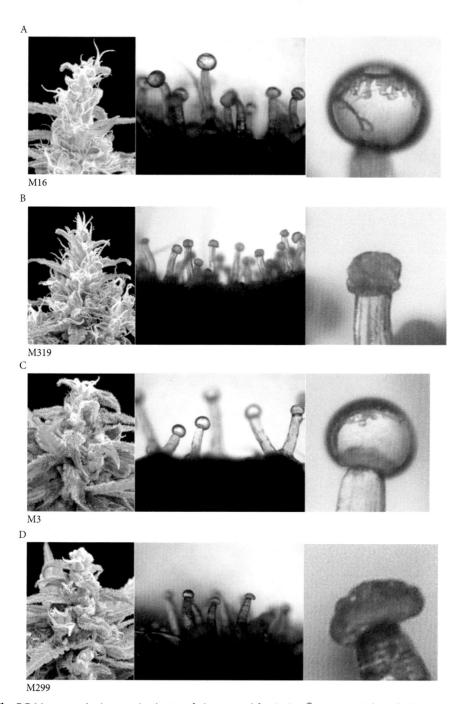

M16

B

M319

C

M3

D

M299

Fig. 5.5 Macro- and microscopic photos of clones used for Sativex® raw material production, M16 (CBD) and M3 (THC), and their respective cannabinoid-free homologues M319 and M299. The homologues were selected from backcross progenies (e.g., M299 = M3 × (M3 × (M3 × knockout progenitor))) and share 87.5% genetic identity with the corresponding "original."

© T.J. Wilkinson.

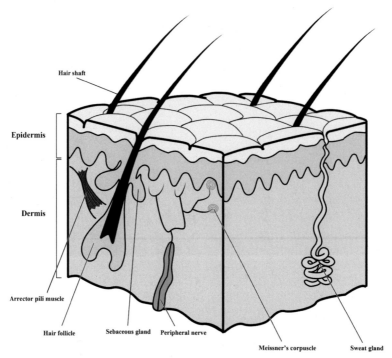

Fig. 32.1 Schematic representation of the skin. See text for details.

Hair shaft

Epidermis

Dermis

Arrector pili muscle

Hair follicle   Sebaceous gland   Peripheral nerve

Meissner's corpuscle   Sweat gland

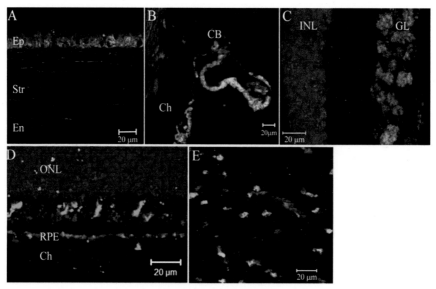

Fig. 33.1 CB$_1$ receptor expression in mouse eye. Eye sections from a 3-month-old mouse were stained for CB$_1$ receptor (green) and propidium iodide (red), and observed by confocal microscopy. (A) cornea, (B) ciliary body, (C) inner retina, (D) outer retina; (E) optic nerve. CB, ciliary body; Ch, choroid; En, endothelia; Ep, epithelia; GL, ganglion layer; INL, inner nuclear layer; ONL, outer nuclear layer; RPE, retinal pigment epithelia; Str, stroma.

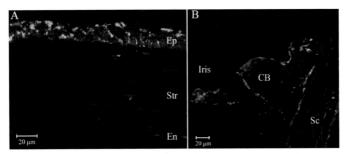

Fig. 33.2 CB$_2$ receptor expression in mouse cornea and ciliary body. Eye sections from a 3-month-old mouse were stained for CB$_2$ receptor (green) and propidium iodide (red), and observed by confocal microscopy. (A) cornea, (B) ciliary body. CB, ciliary body; En, endothelia; Ep, epithelia; Sc, sclera; Str, stroma.

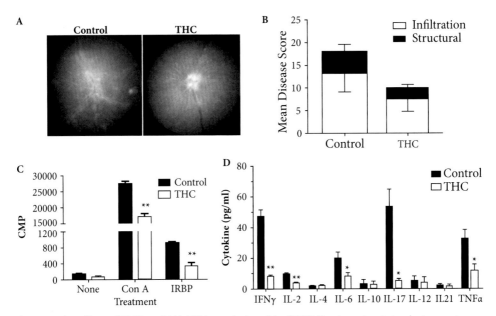

Fig. 33.4 The effect of THC on EAU. EAU was induced in C57BL/6 mice using interphotoreceptor retinoid binding protein (IRBP) peptide 1–20 immunization. Mice were treated with THC (i.p., daily 5 mg/kg) from day 1–20 post-immunization. Control mice were treated with the vehicle (Tween-20). (A) Fundus images from control and THC-treated EAU mice. (B) Histological investigation showing the retinal structural score and infiltration score. (C) T-lymphocyte proliferation in response to con-canavalin A (Con A) or IRBP1-20 peptide stimulation. (D) Cytokine production by splenocytes from control and THC treated EAU mice. *P < 0.05; **P < 0.01 compared to control group (n ≥ 5).

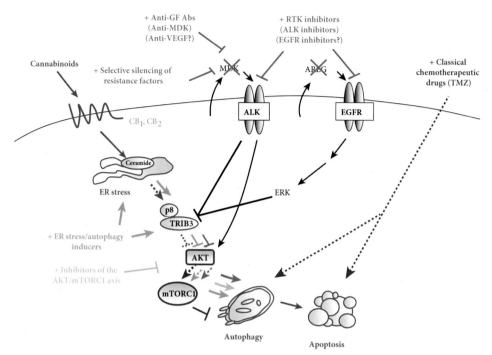

Fig. 35.2 Possible strategies aimed at optimizing cannabinoid-based therapies against gliomas. Glioblastoma is highly resistant to current anticancer therapies (Lonardi et al. 2005; Nieder et al. 2006; Purow et al. 2009). Specifically, resistance of glioma cells to cannabinoid-induced cell death relies, at least in part, on the enhanced expression of the growth factor midkine (MDK) and the subsequent activation of the anaplastic lymphoma receptor tyrosine kinase (ALK) (Lorente et al. 2011). Likewise, enhanced expression of the heparin-bound EGFR-ligand amphiregulin (AREG) can promote resistance to THC antitumor action via ERK stimulation (Lorente et al. 2009). Combination of THC with pharmacological inhibitors of ALK (or genetic inhibition of MDK) enhances cannabinoid action in resistant tumors, which provides the rationale for the design of targeted therapies capable of increasing cannabinoid antineoplastic activity (Lorente et al. 2011). Combinations of cannabinoids with classical chemotherapeutic drugs such as the alkylating agent temozolomide (TMZ; the benchmark agent for the management of glioblastoma (Lonardi et al. 2005; Stupp et al. 2005)) have been shown to produce a strong anticancer action in animal models (Torres et al. 2011). Combining cannabinoids and TMZ is thus a very attractive possibility for clinical studies aimed at investigating cannabinoids antitumor effects in glioblastoma. Other potentially interesting strategies to enhance cannabinoid anticancer action (still requiring additional experimental support from data obtained using preclinical models) could be combining cannabinoids with endoplasmic reticulum (ER) stress and/or autophagy inducers or with inhibitors of the AKT–mechanistic target of rapamycin C1 (mTORC1) axis. Abs: antibodies; EGFR: epidermal growth factor receptor; ERK: extracellular signal-regulated kinase; GF: growth factors; RTK: receptor tyrosine kinase; TRIB3: tribbles 3; VEGF: vascular endothelial growth factor.

Table 20.1 Randomized controlled clinical trials of approved cannabis-based medicines in pain states

Cannabinoid	Indication	Study design	Reference
Dronabinol	Cancer pain	RCT (crossover)	Noyes et al. 1975a, 1975b
Intravenous THC	Dental pain	RCT (crossover)	Raft et al. 1977
Dronabinol	Postoperative pain	RCT	Buggy et al. 2003
Dronabinol	Experimental pain	RCT (crossover)	Naef et al. 2003
Dronabinol	Spinal cord injury	N of 1	Maurer et al. 1990
Dronabinol	Neuropathic pain in MS	RCT (crossover)	Svendsen et al. 2004
Nabilone	Postoperative pain	RCT—1-day dosing	Beaulieu 2006
Nabilone	Chronic neuropathic pain	RCT vs. dihydrocodeine	Frank et al. 2008
Nabilone	Pain in spasticity	RCT	Wissel et al. 2006
Nabilone	Fibromyalgia	RCT	Skrabek et al. 2008
Sativex®	Neuropathic pain due to MS	RCT	Rog et al. 2005
Sativex®	Peripheral neuropathic pain	RCT	Nurmikko et al. 2007
Sativex®	Neuropathic pain due to MS	RCT with randomized withdrawal phase	Langford et al. 2013
Sativex®	Neuropathic pain due to brachial plexus avulsion	RCT (crossover)	Berman et al. 2004
Sativex®	Neuropathic pain	RCT (crossover)	Notcutt et al. 2004
Sativex®	Chronic cancer-related pain	RCT	Johnson et al. 2010
Sativex®	Chronic cancer-related pain	RCT	Portenoy et al. 2012

Abbreviation: RCT, randomized controlled trial.

20.5.6.1 Neuropathic pain

The approval of Sativex® in neuropathic pain is based on two published Phase 3 studies, and long-term open-label safety data. Rog et al. (2005) studied 66 patients with central neuropathic pain due to MS, and found a highly significant reduction in pain, as assessed both by the 0–10 NRS, and by the Neuropathic Pain Scale, significant improvement in sleep and in the patient global impression of change. In their study of long-term use of Sativex® in this indication, they found that efficacy was maintained over a 1-year period, in the 34 of 63 patients who completed 1 year of follow-up. Langford et al. (2013) conducted an interesting study with two phases. Phase A comprised a parallel-group, randomized, placebo-controlled study of Sativex® as an add-on treatment in patients with neuropathic pain due to MS, who had failed to gain adequate relief from existing analgesics. Phase B comprised a 13-week open-label treatment of a cohort of the patients who completed Phase A, followed by a randomized withdrawal phase. This latter phase served not only to explore the maintenance of efficacy in a controlled setting, but also allowed for the investigation of any cannabis withdrawal syndrome, using previously published criteria (Budney et al. 2004).

While the placebo-controlled parallel group phase of the study did not show a significant difference in pain relief between Sativex® and placebo, the randomized withdrawal phase did, thus confirming maintenance of efficacy in a population of patients who had shown efficacy in short-term use. One explanation for this is that the randomized withdrawal phase included only those patients who had previously responded to Sativex®, whereas the initial parallel group phase included all comers—including a proportion of nonresponders. The presence of a significant proportion of nonresponders in a study of an analgesic may introduce bias into the study, by masking any treatment effect in background "noise." In this setting, the mean improvement seen in the active treatment group includes the nonresponders, thus telling us little about the size of the response in responding patients. This phenomenon has been discussed by McQuay et al. (2008), who mention study designs which may help avoid this negative bias. More recently, a discussion about the value of enriched study designs, where nonresponders are excluded from the randomization process, has appeared on the US FDA website. We suspect that there will be an increasing number of enriched study designs appearing in the literature in the coming years.

20.5.6.2 Cancer-related pain

Preclinical data show analgesic synergy between THC and opioids active at the μ-opioid receptor (Cox et al. 2007), so the investigation of cannabinoid-based medicines in patients with cancer-related pain makes sense. There have been two large placebo-controlled studies published, including more than 530 patients, using Sativex® as an adjunct to opioids, in patients who have not been able to gain optimum analgesia from strong (Step 3) opioids. Both studies have shown that Sativex® can bring a significant reduction in pain to patients with advanced cancer in these patients with a clear unmet medical need (Johnson et al. 2010; Portenoy et al. 2012). The earlier study also looked at THC alone, and found no difference in pain relief from placebo, providing the best clinical evidence that CBD is contributing to the analgesic efficacy of THC.

Neither of the two synthetic cannabis-based medicines is approved in any pain indication, although a number of studies have been reported (see Table 20.1).

20.6 Conclusions

The two synthetic cannabinoids so far approved as medicines—dronabinol and nabilone—are distinguished by the fact that they were developed prior to the discovery of the cannabinoid receptors, and of the endogenous cannabinoid system. Their development therefore was not based in any way on an understanding of their pharmacology, and they were essentially designed to be substitutes for medicinal marijuana. Sativex®, on the other hand, was developed in the light of the developing understanding of the endocannabinoid system, and it has become known as an "endocannabinoid system modulator." A review of the evidence makes it clear that there is a more substantial body of good quality clinical trials data supporting the clinical utility of Sativex® than of Marinol® or Cesamet®. The synthetic cannabinoids have shown longevity as marketed products, indicating that their safety profile is acceptable in both long-term and short-term use, even though their efficacy has been limited. The apparently greater efficacy of Sativex®, together with its good tolerability, and our understanding of the endocannabinoid system, suggest that the future will see the development of more cannabis-based medicines.

References

Ahmedzai, S., Carlyle, D.L., Calder, I.T., *et al.* (1983). Anti-emetic efficacy and toxicity of nabilone, a synthetic cannabinoid, in lung cancer chemotherapy. *British Journal of Cancer*, **48**, 657–663.

Anwar, K. and Barnes, M.P. (2009). A pilot study of a comparison between a patient scored numeric rating scale and clinician scored measures of spasticity in multiple sclerosis. *NeuroRehabilitation*, **24**, 333–340.

Aragona, M., Onesti, E., and Tomassini, V., *et al.* (2008). Psychopathological and cognitive effects of therapeutic cannabinoids in multiple sclerosis: a double blind, placebo controlled, crossover study. *Clinical Neuropharmacology*, **32**, 41–47.

Basch, E., Prestrud, A.A., Hesketh, P.J., *et al.* (2011) Antiemetics: American Society of Clinical Oncology Clinical Practice Guideline Update. *Journal of Clinical Oncology*, **29**, 4189–4198.

Beal, J.E., Olson, R., Laubenstein, L., *et al.* (1995). Dronabinol as a treatment for anorexia associated with weight loss in patients with AIDS. *Journal of Pain and Symptom Management*, **10**, 89–97.

Beal, J.E., Olson, R., Lefkowitz, L., *et al.* (1997). Long-term efficacy and safety of dronabinol for acquired immunodeficiency syndrome-associated anorexia. *Journal of Pain and Symptom Management*, **14**, 7–14.

Beaulieu, P. (2006) Effects of nabilone, a synthetic cannabinoid, on postoperative pain: Les effets de la nabilone, un cannabinoide synthetique, sur la douleur postoperatoire. *Canadian Journal of Anaesthesiology*, **53**, 769–75.

Berman, J.S., Symonds, C., and Birch, R. (2004). Efficacy of two cannabis based medicinal extracts for relief of central neuropathic pain from brachial plexus avulsion: results of a randomised controlled trial. *Pain*, **112**, 299–306.

Bisogno, T., Hanus, L., De Petrocellis, L., *et al.* (2001). Molecular targets for cannabidiol and its synthetic analogues: effect on vanilloid VR1 receptors and on the cellular uptake and enzymatic hydrolysis of anandamide. *British Journal of Pharmacology*, **134**, 845–852.

Budney, A.J., Hughes, J.R., Moore, B.A., and Vandrey, R. (2004). Review of the validity and significance of cannabis withdrawal syndrome. *American Journal of Psychiatry*, **161**, 1967–1977.

Buggy, D.J., Toogood, L., Maric, S., Sharpe, P., Lambert, D.G., and Rowbotham, D.J. (2003). Lack of analgesic efficacy of oral delta-9-tetrahydrocannabinol in post-operative pain. *Pain*, **106**, 169–172.

Busto, U. and Sellers, E.M. (1986). Pharmacokinetic determinants of drug abuse and dependence. A conceptual perspective. *Clinical Pharmacokinetics*, **11**, 144–153.

Calhoun, S.R., Galloway, G.P., and Smith, D.E. (1998). Abuse potential of dronabinol (Marinol). *Journal of Psychoactive Drugs*, **30**, 187–196.

Carrier, E.J., Auchampach, J.A., and Hillard, C.J., (2006). Inhibition of an equilibrative nucleoside transporter by cannabidiol: a mechanism of cannabinoid immunosuppression. *Proceedings of the National Academy of Sciences of the United States of America*, **103**, 7895–7900.

Chang, A.E., Shiling, D.J., Stillman, R.C., *et al.* (1979). Delta-9-tetrahydrocannabinol as an antiemetic in cancer patients receiving high-dose methotrexate. A prospective, randomized evaluation. *Annals of Internal Medicine*, **91**, 819–824.

Collin, C., Davies, P., Mutiboko, I.K., and Ratcliffe, S. (2007). Randomized controlled trial of cannabis-based medicine in spasticity caused by multiple sclerosis. *European Journal of Neurology*, **14**, 290–296.

Collin, C., Ehler, E., Waberzinek, G., *et al.* (2010). A double-blind, randomized, placebocontrolled, parallel-group study of Sativex, in subjects with symptoms of spasticity due to multiple sclerosis. *Neurological Research*, **32**, 451–459.

Cox, M.L., Haller, V.L., and Welch, S.P. (2007). Synergy between Δ9-tetrahydrocannabinol and morphine in the arthritic rat. *European Journal of Clinical Pharmacology*, **567**, 125–130.

Devane, W.A., Dysarz, F.A., Johnson, M.R., Melvin, L.S, and Howlett, A.C. (1988) Determination and characterization of a cannabinoid receptor in rat brain. *Molecular Pharmacology*, **34**, 605–613.

Einhorn, L.H., Nagy, C., Furnas, B., and Williams, S.D. (1981). Nabilone: an effective antiemetic in patients receiving cancer chemotherapy. *Journal of Clinical Pharmacology*, **21**(Suppl.), 64–69.

Farrar, J.T., Troxel, A.B., Stott, C., Duncombe, P., and Jensen, M.P. (2008). Validity, reliability and clinical importance of change in a 0-10 numeric rating scale measure of spasticity: a post hoc analysis of a randomized, double-blind placebo-controlled trial. *Clinical Therapeutics*, **30**, 974–985.

Frank, B., Serpell, M.G., Hughes, J., Matthews, J.N., and Kapur, D. (2008). Comparison of analgesic effects and patient tolerability of nabilone and dihydrocodeine for chronic neuropathic pain: randomised, crossover, double blind study. *British Medical Journal*, **336**, 199–201.

Frytak, S., Moertel, C.G., O'Fallon, J., *et al.* (1979). Delta-9-tetrahydrocannabinol as an anti-emetic in patients treated with cancer chemotherapy: a double comparison with prochlorperazine and a placebo. *Annals of Internal Medicine*, **91**, 825–830.

Gralla, R.J., Tyson, L.B., Bordin, L.A., *et al.* (1984). Anti-emetic therapy: a review of recent studies and a report of a random assigned trial comparing metoclopramide with delta-9-tetrahydrocannabinol. *Cancer Treatment Reports*, **68**, 163–172.

Herman, T.S., Einhorn, L.H., Jones, S.E., *et al.* (1979). Superiority of nabilone over prochlorperazine as an antiemetic in patients receiving cancer chemotherapy. *New England Journal of Medicine*, **300**, 1295–1297.

Herman, T.S., Jones, S.E., Dean, J., *et al.* (1977). Nabilone: a potent antiemetic cannabinol with minimal euphoria. *Biomedicine*, **27**, 331–334.

Hesketh, P.J., Kris, M.G., and Grunberg, S.M. (1997). Proposal for classifying the acute emetogenicity of cancer chemotherapy. *Journal of Clinical Oncology*, **15**,103–109.

Hobart, J.C., Riazi, A., Lamping, D.L., Fitzpatrick, R., and Thompson, A.J. (2004). Improving the evaluation of therapeutic interventions in multiple sclerosis: development of a patient-based measure of outcome. *Health Technology Assessment*, **8**(9).

House of Lords Science and Technology Ninth Report (Session 1997–1998). *Cannabis: The Scientific and Medical Evidence.* Available at: http://www.parliament.the-stationery-office.co.uk/pa/ld199798/ldselect/ldsctech/151/15101.htm.

Johnson, J.R., Burnell-Nugent, M., Lossignol, D., Ganae-Motan, E.D., Potts, R., and Fallon, M.T. (2010). Multicenter, double-blind, randomized, placebo-controlled, parallel-group study of the efficacy, safety, and tolerability of THC:CBD extract and THC extract in patients with intractable cancer-related pain. *Journal of Pain and Symptom Management*, **39**, 167–179.

Jones, S.E., Durant, J.R., Greco, F.A., and Robertone, A. (1982). A multi-institutional Phase III study of nabilone vs. placebo in chemotherapy-induced nausea and vomiting. *Cancer Treatment Reviews*, **9**, (Suppl. 2), 45–48.

Karschner, E.L., Darwin, W.D., McMahon, R.P., *et al.* (2011). Subjective and physiological effects after controlled Sativex and oral THC administration. *Clinical Pharmacology and Therapeutics*, **89**, 400–407.

Langford, R.M., Mares, J., Novotna, A., *et al.* (2013). A double-blind, randomized, placebo-controlled, parallel-group study of THC/CBD oromucosal spray in combination with the existing treatment regimen, in the relief of central neuropathic pain in patients with multiple sclerosis. *Journal of Neurology*, **260**, 984–997.

Lemberger, L. and Rowe, H. (1975). Clinical pharmacology of nabilone, a cannabinol derivative. *Clinical Pharmacology and Therapeutics*, **18**, 720–26.

Maurer, M., Henn, V., Dittrich, A., and Hoffmann, A. (1990). Delta-9-tetrahydrocannabinol shows antispastic and analgesic effects in a single case double-blind trial. *European Archives of Psychological and Clinical Neurosciences*, **240**, 1–4.

McQuay, H.J., Derry, S., Moore, R.A., Poulain, P., and Legout, V. (2008) Enriched enrolment with randomized withdrawal (EERW): time for a new look at clinical trial design in chronic pain. *Pain*, **135**, 217–220.

Mechoulam, R. (1970). Marihuana chemistry. *Science*, **168**, 1159–1166.

Meiri, E., Jhangiani, H., Vredenburgh, J.J., *et al.* (2007). Efficacy of dronabinol alone and in combination with ondansetron versus ondansetron alone for delayed chemotherapy-induced nausea and vomiting. *Current Medical Research and Opinion*, **23**, 533–543.

Musty, R.E. and Rossi, R. (2001). Effects of smoked cannabis and oral Δ9-tetrahydrocannabinol on nausea and emesis after cancer chemotherapy: A review of state clinical trials. *Journal of Cannabis Therapeutics*, **1**, 29–54.

Naef, M., Curatolo, M., Petersen-Felix, S., Arendt-Nielsen, L., Zbinden, A., and Brenneisen, R. (2003). The analgesic effect of oral delta-9-tetrahydrocannabinol (THC), morphine, and a THC-morphine combination in healthy subjects under experimental conditions. *Pain*, **105**, 79–88.

Nicholson, A.N., Turner, C., Stone, B.M., and Robson, P.J. (2004). Effect of delta-9-tetrahydrocannabinol and cannabidiol on nocturnal sleep and early-morning behavior in young adults. *Journal of Clinical Psychopharmacology*, **24**, 305–313.

Niiranen, A. and Mattson, K. (1985). A cross-over comparison of nabilone and prochlorperazine for emesis induced by cancer chemotherapy. *American Journal of Clinical Oncology*, **8**, 336–340.

Notcutt, W., Langford, R., Davies, P., Ratcliffe, S., and Potts, R. (2012). A placebo-controlled, randomised withdrawal study of subjects with symptoms of spasticity due to multiple sclerosis who are receiving long-term Sativex (nabiximols). *Multiple Sclerosis Journal*, **18**, 219–228.

Notcutt, W., Price, M., Miller, R., et al. (2004). Initial experiences with medicinal extracts of cannabis for chronic pain: results from 34 'N of 1' studies. *Anaesthesia*, **59**, 440–452.

Novotna, A., Mares, J., and Ratcliffe, S. (2011). A randomized, double-blind, placebo-controlled, parallel-group, enriched-design study of nabiximols* (Sativex®), as add-on therapy, in subjects with refractory spasticity caused by multiple sclerosis. *European Journal of Neurology*, **18**, 1122–1131.

Noyes, R., Brunk, S.F., Avery, D.H., and Canter, A. (1975a). The analgesic properties of delta-9-tetrahydrocannabinol and codeine. *Clinical Pharmacology and Therapeutics*, **18**, 84–89.

Noyes, R.Jr., Brunk, S.F., Baram, D.A., and Canter, A. (1975b). Analgesic effect of delta-9-tetrahydrocannabinol. *Journal of Clinical Pharmacology*, **15**, 139–143.

Nurmikko, T.J., Serpell, M.G., Hoggart, B., Toomey, P.J., Morlion, B.J., and Haines, D. (2007). Sativex successfully treats neuropathic pain characterised by allodynia: a randomised, double-blind, placebo-controlled clinical trial. *Pain*, **133**, 210–220.

Oreja-Guevara, C. (2012). Clinical efficacy and effectiveness of Sativex®, a combined cannabinoid medicine, in multiple sclerosis-related spasticity. *Expert Review of Neurotherapeutics*, **12**(4 Suppl. 1), 3–8.

Orr, L.E., McKernan, J.F., and Bloome, B. (1980). Antiemetic effect of tetrahydrocannabinol, compared with placebo and prochlorperazine in chemotherapyassociated nausea and emesis. *Archives of Internal Medicine*, **140**, 1431–1433.

Peyrone, M. (1844). Ueber die Einwirkung des Ammoniaks auf Platinchlorür. *Annalen der Chemie und Pharmacie*, **51**, 1–29.

Portenoy, R.K., Ganae-Motan, E.D., Allende, S., et al. (2012). Nabiximols for opioid-treated cancer patients with poorly-controlled chronic pain: a randomized, placebo-controlled, graded-dose trial. *Journal of Pain*, **13**, 438–449.

Raft, D., Gregg, J., Ghia, J., and Harris, L. (1977). Effects of intravenous tetrahydrocannabinol on experimental and surgical pain. Psychological correlates of the analgesic response. *Clinical Pharmacology and Therapeutics*, **21**, 26–33.

Rog, D.J., Nurmikko, T.J., Friede, T., and Young, C.A. (2005). Randomized, controlled trial of cannabis-based medicine in central pain in multiple sclerosis. *Neurology*, **65**, 812–819.

Sacerdote, P., Martucci, C., Vaccani, A., et al. (2005). The non-psychoactive component of marijuana cannabidiol modulates chemotaxis and IL-10 and IL-12 production of murine macrophages both in vivo and in vitro. *Journal of Neuroimmunology*, **159**, 97–105.

Sallan, S.E., Cronin, C., Zelen, M., and Zinberg, N.E. (1980). Antiemetics in patients receiving chemotherapy for cancer: a randomized comparison of delta9tetrahydrocannabinol and prochlorperazine. *New England Journal of Medicine*, **302**, 135–138.

Schoedel, K.A., Chen, N., Hilliard A., et al. (2011). A randomized, double-blind, placebo-controlled, crossover study to evaluate the subjective abuse potential and cognitive effects of nabiximols oromucosal spray in subjects with a history of recreational cannabis use. *Human Psychopharmacology*, **26**, 224–236.

Shakespeare, D.T., Boggild, M., and Young, C. (2003) Anti-spasticity agents for multiple sclerosis. *Cochrane Database of Systematic Reviews*, **4**, CD001332.

Skold, C. (2000). Spasticity in spinal cord injury: self- and clinically rated intrinsic fluctuations and intervention-induced changes. *Archives of Physical Medicine and Rehabilitation*, **81**, 144–149.

Skrabek, R.Q., Galimova, L., Ethans, K., and Perry, D. (2008). Nabilone for the treatment of pain in fibro-myalgia. *Journal of Pain*, **9**, 164–173.

Slof, J. and Gras, A. (2012). Sativex® in multiple sclerosis spasticity: a cost–effectiveness model. *Expert Reviews in Pharmacoeconomic Outcomes Research*, **12**, 1–14.

Sneed, R.C., Manning, E.L., and Hansen, C.F. (2006). Pediatric neurologic and rehabilitation rating scales. In: R.M. Herndon (ed.). *Handbook of Neurologic Rating Scales*. New York: Demos Medical Publishing, p. 79.

Svendsen K.B, Jensen T.S, and Bach F.W. (2004) Does the cannabinoid dronabinol reduce central pain in multiple sclerosis? Randomised double blind placebo controlled crossover trial. *British Medical Journal*, **329**, 253–257.

Temple, R. (1999). Are surrogate markers adequate to assess cardiovascular disease drugs? *Journal of the American Medical Association*, **282**, 790–795.

Tramer, M.R., Carroll, D., Campbell, F.A., *et al.* (2001). Cannabinoids for control of chemotherapy induced nausea and vomiting: quantitative systematic review. *British Medical Journal*, **323**, 1–8.

Ungerleider, J.T., Andrysiak, T., Fairbanks, L.A., Goodnight, J., Sarna, G., and Jamison, K. (1982). Cannabis and cancer chemotherapy. A comparison of oral delta-9-THC and prochlorperazine. *Cancer*, **50**, 636–645.

Ungerleider, J.T., Sarna, G., Fairbanks, L.A., Goodnight, J., Andrysiak, T., and Jamison, K. (1985). THC or compazine for the cancer chemotherapy patient—the UCLA study. Part II: patient drug preference. *American Journal of Clinical Oncology*, **8**, 142–147.

Wade, D.T. (2012). Evaluation of the safety and tolerability profile of Sativex®: is it reassuring enough? *Expert Review of Neurotherapeutics*, **12**(4 Suppl. 1), 9–14.

Wade, D.T., Collin, C., Stott, C., and Duncombe, P. (2010). Meta-analysis of the efficacy and safety of Sativex (nabiximols), on spasticity in people with multiple sclerosis. *Multiple Sclerosis*, **16**, 701–714.

Wade, D.T., Makela, P., Robson, P., House, H., and Bateman, C. (2004). Do cannabis-based medicinal extracts have general or specific effects on symptoms in multiple sclerosis? A double-blind, randomized, placebo-controlled study on 160 patients. *Multiple Sclerosis*, **10**, 1–8.

Wade, D.T., Robson, P. House, H., Makela, P., and Aram, J. (2003). A preliminary controlled study to determine whether whole-plant cannabis extracts can improve intractable neurogenic symptoms. *Clinical Rehabilitation*, **17**, 21–29.

Ware, J.E. (1993). Measuring patients' views: the optimum outcome measure. *British Medical Journal*, **306**, 1429–1430.

Ware, M.A., Daeninck, P., and Maida, V. (2008). A review of nabilone in the treatment of chemotherapy-induced nausea and vomiting. *Therapeutics and Clinical Risk Management*, **4**, 99–107

Wissel, J., Haydn, T., Muller, J., *et al.* (2006). Low dose treatment with the synthetic cannabinoid nabilone significantly reduces spasticity related pain: a double-blind placebo-controlled cross-over trial. *Journal of Neurology*, **253**, 1337–1341.

World Health Organization. (2007). Assessment of dronabinol and its stereoisomers. In: *Who Expert Committee on Drug Dependence: Thirty-Fourth Report*. Geneva: World Health Organization.

Wright, S., Duncombe, P.D., and Altman, D.G. (2012). Assessment of blinding to treatment allocation in studies of a cannabis-based medicine (Sativex®) in people with multiple sclerosis: a new approach. *Trials*, **13**, 189.

Chapter 21

Synthetic Psychoactive Cannabinoids Licensed as Medicines

Mark A. Ware

21.1 Introduction

Since the identification of the primary psychoactive ingredient of cannabis, delta-9-tetrahydrocannabinol (THC) in 1964, and the recognition of the therapeutic potential of cannabinoids in general, there has been an extensive search for synthetic molecules that mimic the therapeutic actions of cannabinoids. The goal of such drug development has been guided by several motives: to avoid the psychoactive and abuse potential of the plant-derived cannabinoids; to develop and protect intellectual property and therefore develop novel and profitable pharmaceutical drugs; and to improve on the pharmacological properties of the plant-based cannabinoids. While several synthetic cannabinoids have been put into clinical trials in recent years, notably ajulemic acid (CT-3) (Burstein 2000), levonantradol (Diasio et al. 1981), dronabinol hemisuccinate ester (Mattes et al. 1993), and dexanabinol (Maas et al. 2006), none of these compounds has been approved for clinical use outside of research protocols and will not be discussed further. In addition, the recent emergence of the synthetic cannabinoids "spice" and "K-2" as drugs of abuse are not going to be discussed here as they have neither been developed nor studied for clinical use.

This chapter explores the trajectory of the synthetic cannabinoids nabilone and dronabinol from the first published clinical use to modern trials. The source of the material comes exclusively from available publications indexed and listed on PubMed under the drug name(s) and from cited reference searches.

21.2 Nabilone: the first synthetic cannabinoid

Early attempts to characterize and modify THC to develop more acceptable clinical formulation were spearheaded by Louis Lemberger, professor of pharmacology at Indiana University School of Medicine and Director of Clinical Pharmacology at the Eli Lilly Laboratory for Clinical Research. An early candidate, delta-6a,10a-dimethyl heptyl tetrahydrocannabinol (DMHP) was found to have significant cardiovascular effects including tachycardia and postural hypotension (Lemberger et al. 1973, 1974). Nabilone (dl-3-(1,1-dimethylheptyl)-6,6ab 7,8,10,10a alpha-hexahydro-1-hydroxy-6,6-dimethyl-9H dibenzo [b,d] pyran-9-one) was first reported in 1975 as a novel psychoactive crystalline benzopyran cannabinoid that was not a tetrahydrocannabinol (Stark 1975) (Fig. 21.1). Following preclinical development work in which the analgesic, anxiolytic, and antipsychotic effects of nabilone were demonstrated, the clinical pharmacology was described in 1975 (Lemberger and Rowe 1975). The drug was administered to healthy male volunteers in single and ascending doses of 0.1–5 mg. Doses of 3–5 mg showed euphoric effects similar to cannabis, with most common side effects being dizziness, drowsiness, and dry mouth.

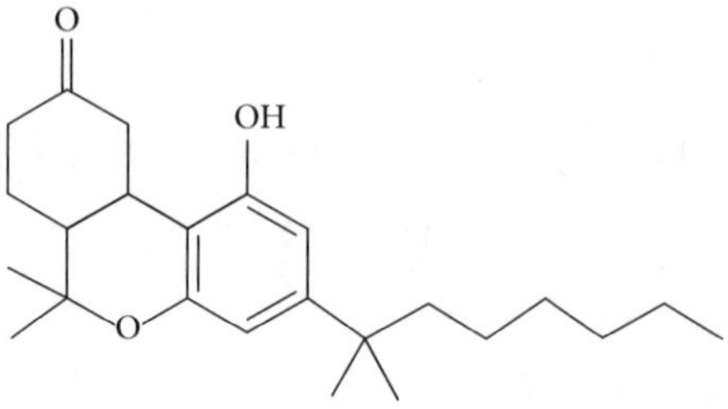

Fig. 21.1 Chemical structure of nabilone.

Subjects felt less anxious and more relaxed. No effects on routine blood chemistry or hematology were noted. Tachycardia and postural hypotension were seen but no arrhythmias. Repeated administration of doses up to 5 mg twice daily (b.i.d.) for 7 days showed some tolerance developing to side effects (including euphoric effects) while reduced anxiety and relaxation were noted.

21.2.1 Clinical pharmacology

Nabilone is a partial cannabinoid receptor types 1 and 2 (CB_1 and CB_2) agonist that is well absorbed from the gastrointestinal tract, metabolized to a carbinol with predominantly fecal (65%) and urinary (20%) excretion (Rubin et al. 1977). The half-life of nabilone is 2 h, while that of the metabolite was noted to be as long as 20 h.

21.2.2 Clinical effects

Early considerations for the clinical use of nabilone included antiemetic and anxiolytic effects. The following section (21.2.2.1) outlines the major clinical studies for these effects, including comparative trials, and describes additional exploratory trials of nabilone in other clinical conditions. Table 21.1 summarizes the clinical conditions for which nabilone has been investigated in clinical trials to date.

21.2.3 Antiemetic effects

The observed antiemetic effects of nabilone in animals led to clinical studies in humans. Nabilone has been evaluated in a range of clinical conditions associated with nausea including chemotherapy, radiation, surgery, and human immunodeficiency virus (HIV)/acquired immunodeficiency syndrome (AIDS).

In the earliest published exploratory study, nausea and vomiting induced by cancer chemotherapy was reduced in ten of 13 treatment refractory patients, with adverse effects of dizziness, postural hypotension, impaired concentration, but minimal euphoric effects (Herman et al. 1977). Nabilone was subsequently shown to be a superior antiemetic to prochlorperazine in a randomized controlled trial (RCT) of 113 subjects with chemotherapy-induced nausea and vomiting (CINV) in terms of episodes of nausea and vomiting and also for subject preference (Herman et al. 1979); adverse events were expected and consistent with earlier studies. Antiemetic effects were confirmed in subsequent studies, one consisting of 37 subjects in a crossover design RCT (Steele et al. 1980), and another in which the same design was used and which enrolled 80 subjects (Einhorn et al. 1981). Subsequent studies reported similar effects (Johansson et al. 1982; Jones et al. 1982; Levitt 1982; Wada et al. 1982). Further uncontrolled reports continued to support a possible antiemetic role for nabilone (Cone et al. 1982; Einhorn 1982). However, despite confirming the superiority of the antiemetic effects of nabilone compared to prochlorperazine, concerns for the unpredictability of the adverse effects of nabilone were raised (Ahmedzai et al. 1983). An RCT

Table 21.1 Clinical syndromes for which the use of synthetic cannabinoids has been reported (includes case reports; not all studies have been positive; see text for details and references)

Condition	Nabilone	Dronabinol
Acute pain	✓	✓
Antiemesis	✓	✓
Anxiety	✓	✓
Appetite		✓
Asthma	✓	
Blepharospasm		✓
Cancer pain	✓	✓
Cannabis dependency	✓	✓
Chronic noncancer pain	✓	
Cluster headaches		
Dementia-related agitation	✓	✓
Fibromyalgia	✓	
Glaucoma	✓	✓
Huntington's chorea	✓	
Idiopathic intracranial hypertension		✓
Irritable bowel syndrome		✓
Isaac's syndrome		✓
Medication overuse headache	✓	
Multiple sclerosis	✓	✓
Neuropathic pain	✓	✓
Night vision		✓
Obsessive–compulsive disorder		✓
Obstructive sleep apnea		✓
Schizophrenia		✓
Sexual dysfunction		✓
Spinal cord injury	✓	
Parkinson's associated tardive dyskinesia	✓	
Posttraumatic stress disorder	✓	
Primary dystonia	✓	
Pruritus		✓
Tremor		✓
Tourette's syndrome		✓
Trichotillomania		✓
Upper motor neuron disease	✓	

comparing nabilone (3 mg b.i.d. for 3 days) to chlorpromazine in cisplatin-induced nausea and vomiting did not show superiority for nabilone although patients preferred nabilone (George et al. 1983). Side effects were also a concern in a trial of 24 cancer patients undergoing chemotherapy, including loss of coordination and hallucinations (Niiranen and Mattson 1985), and no difference between nabilone and metoclopramide was noted in another RCT of 32 subjects on cisplatin (Crawford and Buckman 1986). Further studies confirmed the antiemetic effects of nabilone in patients with testicular cancer on cisplatin (Niederle et al. 1986) and compared it to domperidone (Pomeroy et al. 1986). In an attempt to specify the effects of different approaches to different chemotherapeutic regimens, a large trial of 80 subjects with first-episode cisplatin or carboplatin chemotherapy showed that metoclopramide plus dexamethasone was better for cisplatin therapy while nabilone plus prochlorperazine was better for carboplatin (Cunningham et al. 1988).

A pilot study suggested that nabilone may have effects on radiation-induced nausea and vomiting, after subjects had failed to respond to metoclopramide (Priestman and Priestman 1984), though a subsequent RCT of 40 subjects found that nabilone was no different to metoclopramide in this disorder (Priestman et al. 1987).

Nabilone was compared to domperidone in 23 children (aged 10 months to 17 years) with CINV, and showed fewer vomiting episodes, reduced nausea, and patient preference (Dalzell et al. 1986). Nabilone was found to be superior to prochlorperazine in children (aged 3.5–17.8 years) with CINV (Chan et al. 1987). Coadministration of nabilone with dexamethasone was shown to improve antiemetic effects and patient preference compared to nabilone alone (Niiranen and Mattson 1987).

Nabilone has been evaluated for postoperative nausea and vomiting; in an RCT of preoperative nabilone administration in 60 patients undergoing total abdominal hysterectomy, no difference was noted between nabilone 2 mg and metoclopramide 10 mg when given 90 min before induction of anesthesia (Lewis et al. 1994).

Case reports have suggested the antiemetic effect of nabilone may also extend to HIV/AIDS (Flynn and Hanif 1992; Green et al. 1989).

21.2.4 Anxiolytic effects

Twenty subjects with high trait anxiety were subjected to the anxiety-provoking Stroop test and to mirror drawing tests, and when the effects of single doses of nabilone (2 mg) and diazepam (5 mg) on anxiety were compared it was found that diazepam had more anxiolytic properties (Nakano et al. 1978) which was explored in further studies (Glass et al. 1979). Anxiolytic effects of nabilone were not observed in one study of four anxious volunteers undergoing a continuous avoidance procedure (Glass et al. 1980), in which doses of 4–5 mg were associated with hypotension, tachycardia, and sedation. Another uncontrolled study of eight anxious subjects (an extension of their earlier study) also failed to note any anxiolytic effects (Glass et al. 1981). The first published placebo-controlled trial to evaluate the effects of nabilone on clinical anxiety enrolled 25 subjects and showed "dramatic" anxiolytic effects of nabilone, with expected side effects and no reported "altered state" experiences (Fabre and McLendon 1981).

21.2.5 Open-angle glaucoma

In an open-label study, administration of 0.5–2 mg of nabilone was shown to reduce intraocular pressure (IOP) by an average of 28% (Newell et al. 1979).

21.2.6 Asthma

Nabilone was compared to terbutaline in a study involving six healthy and six asthmatic subjects and found to have no effect on bronchodilation in the asthmatic patients (Gong et al. 1983).

21.2.7 **Multiple sclerosis**

The potential for nabilone to be used in patients with multiple sclerosis (MS) was first described in a patient who first reported benefit with herbal cannabis (Martyn et al. 1995). In an n-of-1 study, a 45-year-old male was given either nabilone (2 mg on alternate days) or placebo, alternating weekly for 4 weeks; improvements in painful muscle spasm, nocturia, and general well-being were noted. Mild sedation but not euphoria was reported. In a separate report, the analgesic effects of nabilone in MS were not blocked by naloxone (Hamann and Di Vadi 1999).

21.2.8 **Movement disorders**

A single-dose open-label study of 1 mg nabilone in a patient with Huntingdon's disease showed increase in choreiform movements (Muller-Vahl et al. 1999), while a subsequent case report noted improvement in chorea in a cannabis-responsive patient (Curtis and Rickards 2006). A pilot RCT randomized 22 subjects to 5-week crossover blocks of nabilone (1 or 2 mg) or placebo. Nabilone significantly decreased chorea scores (Curtis et al. 2009b). A placebo-controlled RCT of nabilone in seven patients with Parkinson's disease showed significant reduction in levodopa-induced dyskinesia (Sieradzan et al. 2001). No effect of nabilone was noted in an RCT evaluating effects of the cannabinoid in generalized and segmental primary dystonia (Fox et al. 2002).

21.2.9 **Acute pain**

In 41 patients undergoing a variety of general surgical procedures, nabilone at two dose levels (1 and 2 mg) was compared to ketoprofen and placebo given 8-hourly for 24 h postoperatively. There was no difference in morphine consumption or other secondary outcomes, but pain at rest and on movement was significantly increased in those receiving 2 mg nabilone compared to the other groups (Beaulieu 2006).

In an experimental model of heat pain, nabilone at single doses of 0.5 and 1 mg was not found to be analgesic, and reduced temporal summation was only noted in women (Redmond et al. 2008). Similar negative analgesia and antihyperalgesic effects were reported following administration of nabilone to healthy volunteers in a capsaicin-induced pain paradigm (Kalliomaki et al. 2012).

21.2.10 **Chronic pain**

An early case series of 20 patients with a variety of chronic noncancer pain syndromes found that nabilone was used for pain, sleep, and nausea (Berlach et al. 2006). This was subsequently confirmed in a crossover trial of 30 patients with treatment refractory pain in which nabilone was added on to existing therapy (Pinsger et al. 2006). In chronic neuropathic pain, nabilone (up to 2 mg daily) was found to be inferior to dihydrocodeine (up to 240 mg daily) with more side effects (Frank et al. 2008).

21.2.11 **Fibromyalgia**

Nabilone has been shown to significantly reduce pain intensity at doses of up to 1 mg b.i.d. compared to placebo in a 4-week crossover trial in 40 patients with fibromyalgia (Skrabek et al. 2008). In an active control crossover RCT, nabilone (0.5–1.0 mg at night) was compared to low-dose amitriptyline (10–20 mg at night) for 2 weeks in 31 fibromyalgia patients with severe insomnia, with the main outcome being sleep quality measured using the Insomnia Severity Index. While both drugs improved sleep, nabilone was found to result in superior sleep quality compared to amitriptyline (Ware et al. 2010).

21.2.12 Upper motor neuron disease

A small RCT of 13 patients with painful spasticity associated with upper motor neuron disease (including MS) found that nabilone, given initially as 0.5 mg daily for 1 week then 1 mg daily for 3 weeks, was superior to placebo in terms of spasticity-related pain (Wissel et al. 2006).

21.2.13 Cancer pain and symptom management

A case series of four patients with paraneoplastic night sweats reported beneficial effects (Maida 2008). In a novel retrospective study using propensity analysis, nabilone was found to improve pain, nausea, anxiety, and distress and was associated with lower daily morphine equivalents (Maida et al. 2008).

21.2.14 Dementia-related agitation

Nabilone was reported to successfully reduce severe agitation and aggressive behavior in an institutionalized 77-year-old male in whom other treatments had been unsuccessful; the patient was discharged on 0.5 mg b.i.d. (Passmore 2008).

21.2.15 Posttraumatic stress disorder

The early work on nabilone as an anxiolytic drug resurfaced in the late 2000s in research investigating its potential for the treatment of posttraumatic stress disorder. In a retrospective case series of 47 combat veterans with severe refractory nightmares, nabilone therapy resulted in either cessation of nightmares, or reduction in intensity, in 77%, with concomitant improvements in sleep quality (Fraser 2009).

21.2.16 Spinal cord injury

The antispasmodic effects of nabilone in patients with spinal cord injury were evaluated in a crossover RCT of 12 subjects comparing nabilone (0.5 mg once or twice daily) to placebo for 4 weeks on each. The primary outcome, the Ashworth score (total and most affected muscle group) was significantly reduced in the nabilone group, with mild to moderate adverse effects (Pooyania et al. 2010).

21.2.17 Peripheral neuropathic pain

Increasing awareness of the potential for cannabinoids to be useful in neuropathic pain conditions led to a series of clinical trials. In a 6-month, open-label nonrandomized study, nabilone or gabapentin either alone or added to existing therapy were found to reduce pain in patients with peripheral neuropathy (Bestard and Toth 2011). Sleep, anxiety, and quality of life were also improved, with sleep particularly improved under the nabilone condition. The same team further evaluated the efficacy of nabilone in painful diabetic neuropathy in an enriched enrollment, placebo-controlled RCT involving 26 subjects and found improvements in pain, anxiety, sleep, and quality of life (Toth et al. 2012).

21.2.18 Medication-overuse headache

Nabilone (0.5 mg/day) was compared to ibuprofen (400 mg/day) in an 8-week randomized crossover trial including 30 patients with medication overuse headache; nabilone was superior to ibuprofen in terms of pain intensity and daily analgesic intake and was well tolerated (Pini et al. 2012).

21.2.19 **Cannabis dependence**

Nabilone was found to have similar behavioral effects in cannabis users to pure THC (Lile et al. 2010). The reliability and availability of nabilone as a slow release CB_1 agonist has given rise to considerations of the use of nabilone in the treatment of cannabis dependence (Bedi et al. 2013).

21.2.20 **Adverse events of nabilone**

Adverse effects of nabilone are almost always more common than the comparator in clinical trials, but for the most part they are mild, self-limited, do not require additional treatment, and in spite of them, patients consistently reported preference for nabilone in most trials where they were asked. The most commonly reported adverse effects are dry mouth, dizziness, drowsiness, postural hypotension, and tachycardia. There are no known clinically important drug–drug interactions, and neither nabilone nor its metabolites test positive in urine drug tests for THC.

21.2.21 **Endocrine effects**

No effect of nabilone on prolactin levels has been noted (Mendelson et al. 1984).

21.2.22 **Visual effects**

Nabilone has been show to impair binocular depth inversion, a model of impaired perception in psychotic states (Leweke et al. 2000).

21.2.23 **Abuse liability**

While early studies found no suggestion of reinforcing effects of nabilone (Mendelson and Mello 1984) increases in prescriptions and off-label use of nabilone in the 2000s, coupled with concerns about opioid abuse, led to investigations about whether nabilone was emerging as a drug of abuse. A series of media and Internet searches and interviews with major law enforcement, pain management, and addictions experts in 2009 were unable to find any evidence of systematic nabilone abuse, or that nabilone had any street value (Ware and St Arnaud-Trempe 2010).

21.2.24 **Cognitive effects**

No effect of nabilone (2 mg/day) was noted on five parameters of psychomotor performance (reaction time, working memory, divided attention, psychomotor speed, and mental flexibility) in an RCT involving six patients with MS for whom nabilone was used for 4 weeks for pain and spasticity (Kurzthaler et al. 2005). Nabilone at doses of 1–3 mg in healthy male volunteers produced cognitive effects including deficits in attention, working and episodic memory, and self-ratings of alertness (Wesnes et al. 2010).

21.3 **Dronabinol: synthetic THC**

21.3.1 **Introduction**

Since first being characterized by Mechoulam and Gaoni in 1964 (Gaoni and Mechoulam 1964) the pure form of THC (the pharmacological name is dronabinol) has been studied in humans since the late 1960s (Isbell et al. 1967) (Fig. 21.2). Initial studies set out mainly to describe its pharmacological properties in various forms and investigate its effects on human cognition and behavior. Recent reviews of the pharmacokinetics of dronabinol suggest that following oral administration, psychotropic and clinical effects appear within 30–90 min, reach their maximum

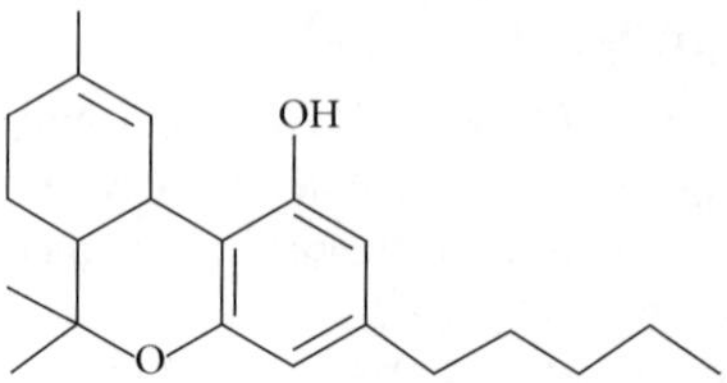

Fig. 21.2 Chemical structure of dronabinol.

after 2–3 h, and last for about 4–12 h (Goodwin et al. 2006; Grotenhermen 2003, 2004; McGilveray 2005). Dronabinol is metabolized by the liver and metabolites are excreted in the feces and urine; one of these metabolites, THC-COOH, is the primary compound detected in urinary drug testing (Gustafson et al. 2003) and plasma (Ferreiros et al. 2013).

Dronabinol administered by vaporization has been investigated and found to mimic smoked cannabis THC pharmacokinetics (Hazekamp et al. 2006); attempts to increase speed of absorption following oral administration have also been explored (Klumpers et al. 2012).

21.3.2 Analgesia

The first attempts to investigate analgesic effects began in 1975 with small studies showing analgesic properties of dronabinol in patients with cancer pain but dose-limiting side effects were noted (Noyes et al. 1975a, 1975b). Studies of dronabinol for postoperative pain have not demonstrated analgesic or opioid-sparing effects (Seeling et al. 2006). However a single- and multiple-dose study comparing dronabinol (10 and 20 mg) to placebo in patients with severe low back pain despite stable opioid therapy showed significant additive analgesic effects of dronabinol (Narang et al. 2008).

21.3.3 Antiemetic effects

Antiemetic properties of dronabinol were noted early on in patients with CINV (Ekert et al. 1979; Sallan et al. 1975), with concerns about dose-related adverse events (Colls et al. 1980). The antiemetic effects of dronabinol were confirmed in an RCT of 84 subjects that, despite high dropout rates, suggested that dronabinol was superior to prochlorperazine in refractory chemotherapy-induced (methotrexate) nausea and vomiting (Sallan et al. 1980). While it was suggested that the antiemetic effects were restricted to certain types of chemotherapy (Chang et al. 1981), further studies showed equivalence to haloperidol in other emetic paradigms (Neidhart et al. 1981) as well as to prochlorperazine (Orr and McKernan 1981; Ungerleider et al. 1982). In light of these trials, dronabinol was considered at that time to represent "a major advance in antiemetic therapy" (Poster et al. 1981).

These studies led to the approval of dronabinol by the US Food and Drug Administration (FDA) in 1985 for CINV. Further confirmatory evidence emerged in the 1990s (Lane et al. 1990). A systematic review in 2001 concluded "cannabinoids . . . may be useful as mood-enhancing adjuvants for controlling chemotherapy related sickness" (Tramer et al. 2001); this conclusion is supported by a meta-analysis conducted in 2008 (Machado Rocha et al. 2008).

A combination of prochlorperazine (25 mg rectally) and dronabinol (5 mg orally) given prophylactically has been found to reduce postoperative nausea and vomiting in a retrospective study of women undergoing breast surgery (Layeeque et al. 2006). In a placebo-controlled RCT of 66 patients, dronabinol has been shown to be as effective as ondansetron in the treatment of CINV (Meiri et al. 2007).

21.3.4 **Appetite**

Orexigenic effects were not seen in an early small study of dronabinol in 11 women with primary anorexia nervosa (Gross et al. 1983). However the appetite-stimulating effects of cannabis, and its use by anorexic patients during the emerging epidemic of HIV/AIDS, led to further studies (Beal et al. 1995; Gorter et al. 1992; Struwe et al. 1993) and a second FDA approval for this indication in the early 1990s. Longer-term studies suggested the appetite-stimulating effects could be maintained for up to 1 year (Beal et al. 1997). Comparative studies with megestrol acetate did not show superiority of dronabinol (Jatoi et al. 2002; Timpone et al. 1997). Increases in food intake have been noted following dronabinol use in HIV-positive marijuana smokers (Haney et al. 2005). A retrospective study of patients living with HIV/AIDS receiving dronabinol reported an association between dronabinol use and improved appetite and weight gain (Dejesus et al. 2007), which was supported in a subsequent trial (Haney et al. 2007). A small RCT of seven HIV-positive marijuana smokers confirmed that 10 mg dronabinol given four times daily over a 16-day period resulted in increased caloric intake (and improved sleep) over the first 8 days, but it was suggested that cannabis-experienced patients required higher doses of dronabinol to achieve this effect and that tolerance to these effects developed in the second 8 days of the study (Bedi et al. 2010).

Appetite-stimulating effects of dronabinol have also been noted in case series of patients with cancer-induced anorexia (Walsh et al. 2005) and metastatic melanoma (Zutt et al. 2006). In addition, a trial comparing dronabinol (2.5 mg b.i.d.) to placebo in 21 patients with advanced cancer, poor appetite, and chemosensory alterations found that dronabinol improved chemosensory perception along with protein caloric intake and pre-meal appetite over an 18-day period (Brisbois et al. 2011).

Anorexia associated with aging has also been shown to increase weight in long-term care elderly patients; intriguingly, a lack of response to dronabinol (weight gain) was associated with increased risk of death (Wilson et al. 2007).

21.3.5 **Asthma**

Bronchodilatory effects of oral dronabinol were not found in asthmatic patients (Abboud and Sanders 1976) although such effects of inhaled THC had been shown (Tashkin et al. 1975; Williams et al. 1976).

21.3.6 **Blepharospasm**

There is a single case report of a woman whose painful intractable blepharospasm (painful contractions of the periorbital muscles) was relieved by 25 mg dronabinol daily over several weeks, and was well tolerated (Gauter et al. 2004).

21.3.7 **Cannabis dependence**

The use of dronabinol as a treatment for cannabis dependence has been suggested following a report of two cases (Levin and Kleber 2008), but a subsequent large (n = 156) 12-week RCT found no difference between dronabinol at doses of 20 mg b.i.d. and placebo in rates of cannabis abstinence in cannabis-dependent subjects, though improved retention and fewer withdrawal symptoms were noted in the dronabinol group (Levin et al. 2011). It has been suggested, however, that nabilone may be superior to dronabinol for this purpose because of its superior bioavailability (Bedi et al. 2013). Doses of up to 120 mg/day of dronabinol have been used to treat cannabis withdrawal symptoms (Vandrey et al. 2013).

21.3.8 **Cluster headaches**

There has been one report of successful treatment of cluster headaches with 5 mg doses of dronabinol (Robbins et al. 2009).

21.3.9 **Dementia**

Open-label studies of patients with severe dementia have reported that doses of 2.5 mg dronabinol daily can reduce nighttime motor activity and agitation (Mahlberg and Walther 2007; Walther et al. 2006). These findings were not supported by a recent Cochrane review which found no evidence to support the use of cannabinoids in dementia or related symptoms (Krishnan et al. 2009); however case reports of the successful use of dronabinol for agitation in dementia continue to appear (Walther et al. 2011).

21.3.10 **Gastrointestinal effects**

Dronabinol (5 mg b.i.d.) has been shown to reduce gastric emptying in healthy subjects, particularly in females, though fasting gastric volumes were increased in males on dronabinol (Esfandyari et al. 2006). Dronabinol (single dose of 7.5 mg) has also been shown to reduce postprandial colonic mobility and tone in healthy human volunteers (Esfandyari et al. 2007). In irritable bowel syndrome (IBS), studies are mixed: at doses of 5–10 mg, dronabinol did not result in changes in visceral perception of rectal distension in one small trial of patients (n = 10) with IBS and healthy volunteers (n = 12) (Klooker et al. 2011), but a second placebo-controlled trial found that 2.5–5 mg dronabinol did reduce fasting colonic motility in 75 patients with IBS (Wong et al. 2011); these authors also suggested that CB_1 receptor and fatty acid amide hydroxylase genetic polymorphisms could explain interindividual differences (Wong et al. 2012).

21.3.11 **Glaucoma**

There have been reports that neither oral (Tiedeman et al., 1981) nor topical (Jay and Green 1983) dronabinol appears to reduce IOP, though another study of eight healthy volunteers administered with 7.5 mg dronabinol did show reduced IOP and increased retinal hemodynamics (Plange et al. 2007).

21.3.12 **Intracranial hypertension**

A single case report has been published of complete resolution of symptoms and signs in a woman with idiopathic intracranial hypertension following treatment with dronabinol 10 mg b.i.d. followed by 5 mg b.i.d. (Raby et al. 2006).

21.3.13 **Movement disorders**

Dronabinol was reportedly effective in reducing a hyperkinetic movement disorder in a pregnant woman (Farooq et al. 2009). Use of dronabinol from 2.5 mg titrated up to 20 mg/day resulted in dramatic and sustained benefit in a patient with Isaac's syndrome, a peripheral motor nerve hyperactivity syndrome (Meyniel et al. 2011).

21.3.14 **Neuropathic pain**

Strong preclinical evidence of the antinociceptive properties of dronabinol have led to several investigations of this drug in the management of central and peripheral neuropathic pain. Two adolescents with intractable neuropathic pain were treated short term with dronabinol (5–25 mg/day) with improvements in pain, function, mood, and sleep (Rudich et al. 2003). The first RCT of dronabinol for neuropathic pain was conducted in 24 patients with central neuropathic pain due to MS; the study found dronabinol (maximum dose 10 mg/day) was superior to placebo with respect to pain intensity and quality of life (Svendsen et al. 2004). Dronabinol at a dose of 5–20 mg/day was compared to diphenhydramine in seven patients with spinal cord injury; there was no difference found between the effects of the two drugs on pain intensity (Rintala et al. 2010).

21.3.15 Obsessive–compulsive disorder

There is one report suggesting that a patient with refractory obsessive–compulsive disorder responded to oral dronabinol (Schindler et al. 2008).

21.3.16 Obstructive sleep apnea

A small open-label proof-of-concept study suggested that dronabinol 2.5–10 mg once daily over 3 weeks improved the Apnea/Hypoapnea Index in 17 adults with obstructive sleep apnea without affecting sleep architecture (Prasad et al. 2013).

21.3.17 Pruritus

The itch (pruritus) caused by cholestatic liver disease was found to respond to 2.5–5 mg doses of dronabinol in three patients with intractable pruritus who had failed to respond to other therapies (Neff et al. 2002).

21.3.18 Schizophrenia

Despite the known association between cannabis and the onset of psychosis in predisposed adolescents, dronabinol has been used in patients with schizophrenia who report improvement of psychotic symptoms with smoked cannabis; oral dronabinol reduced core psychotic symptoms in three of four subjects (Schwarcz et al. 2009). Additional case reports of improvement in refractory psychosis following dronabinol therapy (Schwarcz and Karajgi 2010) suggest that this issue is not a straightforward one.

21.3.19 Spasticity

In very small preliminary studies, the effects of dronabinol on spasticity associated with MS were first reported in 1981 (Petro and Ellenberger 1981), and on tremor in 1983 (Clifford 1983). Antispasmodic effects were confirmed in patients with refractory MS-associated spasticity (Ungerleider et al. 1987). Initial reports suggested dronabinol may have antispasmodic effects in patients with spinal cord injury (Kogel et al. 1995) and other disorders (Brenneisen et al. 1996).

21.3.20 Tourette's syndrome

A small RCT of 24 subjects with intractable tics due to Tourette's syndrome found that oral doses of dronabinol given over 6 weeks was superior to placebo in reducing tic frequency (Muller-Vahl 2003), but a recent Cochrane review suggests that despite two small positive trials, the evidence base is not yet strong enough to support the use of dronabinol for tics and obsessive–compulsive behavior in people with Tourette's syndrome (Curtis et al. 2009a).

21.3.21 **Trichotillomania**

Compulsive hair-pulling behavior refractory to conventional treatment was shown to respond to dronabinol (2.5–15 mg/day) in a 12-week open-label trial involving 14 women, and did not result in negative cognitive effects (Grant et al. 2011).

21.3.22 **Sexual dysfunction**

There has been one case report of dronabinol improving sexual dysfunction secondary to pharmacotherapy for bipolar disorder; use of 10 mg dronabinol by a 43-year-old woman 1 h before sex improved all aspects of sexual function and effectiveness was sustained over a 2-year period of follow-up (Salerian 2004).

21.3.23 **Adverse events of dronabinol**

Most clinical reports of dronabinol conclude with a cautionary message about adverse events. It is clear that side effects of dronabinol are consistent and dose dependent, to a large part expected, and that these effects may be the limiting factor in patient compliance. It appears that rewarding, euphoric properties of dronabinol are uncommon in clinical practice, and that, like nabilone, it is not a drug with street value and likelihood of diversion.

21.3.24 **Abuse liability**

Concerns regarding the abuse potential of dronabinol led to an investigation of dronabinol as a street drug or abused substance, through both a search of multiple sources including literature reviews, and the conducting of interviews with law enforcement, addictions specialists, and others. No evidence for the abuse or diversion of dronabinol was found (Calhoun et al. 1998). Modest reinforcing effects of dronabinol have been shown in laboratory paradigms of choice (Hart et al. 2005). Dronabinol (at a single dose of either 20 or 40 mg) was compared to the cannabis-based medicine, nabiximols, and placebo in 23 healthy cannabis-experienced volunteers, and showed some evidence of abuse liability on psychomotor and cognitive tests after 24 h compared to placebo (Schoedel et al. 2011).

21.3.25 **Drug interactions**

Short-term use of dronabinol (14 days) has not been found to have clinically meaningful effects on plasma levels of the antiretroviral drugs indinavir and nelfinavir (Kosel et al. 2002).

21.3.26 **Effects on driving**

Studies of oral dronabinol intake suggest that there are impairing effects on roadside and tracking tests at medium (16.5 mg) and high (45.7 mg) doses of dronabinol in healthy volunteers, though volunteers under these conditions had reduced willingness to drive (Menetrey et al. 2005). Driving test measures such as standard deviation of lateral position (SDLP; weaving) have been shown to be worsened by dronabinol (10–20 mg); in light cannabis users but not in heavy users; the standard field sobriety test (SFST) was not sensitive to dronabinol effects (Bosker et al. 2012).

21.3.27 **Gynecomastia**

Enlargement of the breasts has been reported in a male patient prescribed dronabinol 5 mg daily for severe intractable nausea; prolactin levels and other endocrine test data were normal (Allen et al. 2007).

21.3.28 **Immunosuppressive effects**

Despite concerns about the potential immunosuppressive effects of cannabinoids from in vivo and in vitro studies, no significant differences have been observed between dronabinol, smoked cannabis, and placebo in a study evaluating the immunological effects of these drugs in HIV-positive patients on highly active antiretroviral therapy (HAART). These included results obtained from assays of immune phenotype (including flow cytometric quantitation of T-cell subpopulations, B cells, and natural killer (NK) cells) and immune function (including assays for induced cytokine production, NK-cell function, and lymphoproliferation) (Bredt et al. 2002). Neither smoked cannabis nor oral dronabinol (2.5 mg three times daily) had negative effects on viral load, plasma levels of antiretroviral drugs, $CD4^+$ or $CD8^+$ cell counts in HIV-infected adults in an RCT of 67 subjects (22 randomized to dronabinol) over a 21-day period (Abrams et al. 2003).

21.3.29 **Pediatric use**

Reports of dronabinol use in pediatric cases have not resulted in major safety concerns; in eight adolescents with a variety of spastic and epileptic conditions dronabinol at doses of 0.04–0.12 mg/kg were generally well tolerated (Lorenz 2004).

21.3.30 **Visual effects**

Dronabinol, like nabilone, has been shown to impair binocular depth inversion, a visual process requiring top-down processing of visual sensory data (Leweke et al. 1999). Oral dronabinol (up to 20 mg) has been shown to improve dark adaptometry and scotopic sensitivity (Russo et al. 2004).

21.4 **Discussion**

A number of observations can be made from this review of 40 years of published clinical experience with the synthetic cannabinoids nabilone and dronabinol. The number of clinical syndromes in which both drugs have been used and reported to be effective, either in case reports, case series, or clinical trials, goes far beyond their indications as antiemetics (both) and appetite stimulant (dronabinol). The range of symptoms and disorders that are listed in Table 21.1 can only be explained by the effects of a drug class on a ubiquitous substrate, the endocannabinoid system, which is discussed in detail elsewhere in this book. The range of conditions also reflects reports by patients' use of herbal cannabis for similar purposes (Ware et al. 2005) and lists of conditions for which cannabis is approved for medical purposes in US states (Hoffmann and Weber 2010).

Nabilone and dronabinol are old compounds, no longer protected by patents, and are available on prescription in the UK, Canada, US, and elsewhere. Generic formulations are now available which has reduced the price of these medications making them more accessible. However, in the ongoing debate about medical marijuana, the potential utility of these synthetic cannabinoids is rarely mentioned. It is worth reflecting on why this might be.

The side effect profile of the synthetic cannabinoids continues to be a major barrier to widespread use, and it is widely reported that patients prefer herbal cannabis to the synthetic versions. This may be a difference of mode of administration (herbal cannabis is most often smoked) but may also be a result of the complex botanical composition of herbal cannabis giving differing pharmacological effects to single synthetic agents (Russo 2011; Russo and Guy 2006). Clinical experience suggests that if starting doses of synthetic cannabinoids are low, and dose escalation is handled carefully, tolerance may develop to many of the early mild and moderate adverse effects.

As with many cannabinoids, the side effect of drowsiness may be harnessed to improve sleep, and dosing is often initiated at night for this purpose.

In conclusion, synthetic cannabinoids are accessible and relatively safe drugs with 40 years of therapeutic history. Side effects are predictable, dose related, and typically mild to moderate. While these oral agents have not been approved with formal indications beyond antiemesis and appetite stimulation, the large number of conditions for which they have been investigated and the existence of these compounds on many national formularies suggests that for many clinicians treating intractable chronic and debilitating diseases and symptoms, synthetic cannabinoid agents remain a potential therapeutic option provided patients are informed of potential side effects and are carefully monitored.

References

Abboud, R.T. and Sanders, H.D. (1976). Effect of oral administration of delta-tetrahydrocannabinol on airway mechanics in normal and asthmatic subjects. *Chest*, **70**, 480–485.

Abrams, D.I., Hilton, J.F., Leiser, R.J., *et al.* (2003). Short-term effects of cannabinoids in patients with HIV-1 infection: a randomized, placebo-controlled clinical trial. *Annals of Internal Medicine*, **139**, 258–266.

Ahmedzai, S., Carlyle, D.L., Calder, I.T., and Moran, F. (1983). Anti-emetic efficacy and toxicity of nabilone, a synthetic cannabinoid, in lung cancer chemotherapy. *British Journal of Cancer*, **48**, 657–663.

Allen, R.C., Wallace, A.M., and Royce, M. (2007). Marinol-induced gynecomastia: a case report. *American Journal of Medicine*, **120**, e1.

Beal, J.E., Olson, R., Laubenstein, L., *et al.* (1995). Dronabinol as a treatment for anorexia associated with weight loss in patients with AIDS. *Journal of Pain and Symptom Management*, **10**, 89–97.

Beal, J.E., Olson, R., Lefkowitz, L., *et al.* (1997). Long-term efficacy and safety of dronabinol for acquired immunodeficiency syndrome-associated anorexia. *Journal of Pain and Symptom Management*, **14**, 7–14.

Beaulieu, P. (2006). Effects of nabilone, a synthetic cannabinoid, on postoperative pain. *Canadian Journal of Anaesthesia*, **53**, 769–775.

Bedi, G., Cooper, Z.D., and Haney, M. (2013). Subjective, cognitive and cardiovascular dose-effect profile of nabilone and dronabinol in marijuana smokers. *Addiction Biology*, **18**, 872–881.

Bedi, G., Foltin, R.W., Gunderson, E.W., *et al.* (2010). Efficacy and tolerability of high-dose dronabinol maintenance in HIV-positive marijuana smokers: a controlled laboratory study. *Psychopharmacology (Berlin)*, **212**, 675–686.

Berlach, D.M., Shir, Y., and Ware, M.A. (2006). Experience with the synthetic cannabinoid nabilone in chronic noncancer pain. *Pain Medicine*, **7**, 25–29.

Bestard, J.A. and Toth, C.C. (2011). An open-label comparison of nabilone and gabapentin as adjuvant therapy or monotherapy in the management of neuropathic pain in patients with peripheral neuropathy. *Pain Practitioner*, **11**, 353–368.

Bosker, W.M., Kuypers, K.P., Theunissen, E.L., *et al.* (2012). Medicinal delta(9) -tetrahydrocannabinol (dronabinol) impairs on-the-road driving performance of occasional and heavy cannabis users but is not detected in Standard Field Sobriety Tests. *Addiction*, **107**, 1837–1844.

Bredt, B.M., Higuera-Alhino, D., Shade, S.B., *et al.* (2002). Short-term effects of cannabinoids on immune phenotype and function in HIV-1-infected patients. *Journal of Clinical Pharmacology*, **42**, 82S–89S.

Brenneisen, R., Egli, A., Elsohly, M.A., Henn, V., and Spiess, Y. (1996). The effect of orally and rectally administered delta 9-tetrahydrocannabinol on spasticity: a pilot study with 2 patients. *International Journal of Clinical Pharmacology and Therapeutics*, **34**, 446–452.

Brisbois, T.D., De Kock, I.H., Watanabe, S.M., *et al.* (2011). Delta-9-tetrahydrocannabinol may palliate altered chemosensory perception in cancer patients: results of a randomized, double-blind, placebo-controlled pilot trial. *Annals of Oncology*, **22**, 2086–2093.

Burstein, S.H. (2000). Ajulemic acid (CT3): a potent analog of the acid metabolites of THC. *Current Pharmaceutical Design*, **6**, 1339–1345.

Calhoun, S.R., Galloway, G.P., and Smith, D.E. (1998). Abuse potential of dronabinol (Marinol). *Journal of Psychoactive Drugs*, **30**, 187–196.

Chan, H.S., Correia, J.A., and Macleod, S.M. (1987). Nabilone versus prochlorperazine for control of cancer chemotherapy-induced emesis in children: a double-blind, crossover trial. *Pediatrics*, **79**, 946–952.

Chang, A.E., Shiling, D.J., Stillman, R.C., *et al.* (1981). A prospective evaluation of delta-9-tetrahydrocannabinol as an antiemetic in patients receiving adriamycin and cytoxan chemotherapy. *Cancer*, **47**, 1746–1751.

Clifford, D.B. (1983). Tetrahydrocannabinol for tremor in multiple sclerosis. *Annals of Neurology*, **13**, 669–671.

Colls, B.M., Ferry, D.G., Gray, A.J., Harvey, V.J., and McQueen, E.G. (1980). The antiemetic activity of tetrahydrocannabinol versus metoclopramide and thiethylperazine in patients undergoing cancer chemotherapy. *New Zealand Medical Journal*, **91**, 449–451.

Cone, L.A., Greene, D.S., and Helm, N.A. (1982). Use of nabilone in the treatment of chemotherapy-induced vomiting in an outpatient setting. *Cancer Treatment Reviews*, **9**(Suppl. B), 63–70.

Crawford, S.M. and Buckman, R. (1986). Nabilone and metoclopramide in the treatment of nausea and vomiting due to cisplatinum: a double blind study. *Medical Oncology and Tumor Pharmacotherapy*, **3**, 39–42.

Cunningham, D., Bradley, C.J., Forrest, G.J., *et al.* (1988). A randomized trial of oral nabilone and prochlorperazine compared to intravenous metoclopramide and dexamethasone in the treatment of nausea and vomiting induced by chemotherapy regimens containing cisplatin or cisplatin analogues. *European Journal of Cancer and Clinical Oncology*, **24**, 685–689.

Curtis, A., Clarke, C.E., and Rickards, H.E. (2009a). Cannabinoids for Tourette's syndrome. *Cochrane Database of Systematic Reviews*, **4**, CD006565.

Curtis, A., Mitchell, I., Patel, S., Ives, N., and Rickards, H. (2009b). A pilot study using nabilone for symptomatic treatment in Huntington's disease. *Movement Disorders*, **24**, 2254–2259.

Curtis, A. and Rickards, H. (2006). Nabilone could treat chorea and irritability in Huntington's disease. *Journal of Neuropsychiatry and Clinical Neurosciences*, **18**, 553–554.

Dalzell, A.M., Bartlett, H., and Lilleyman, J.S. (1986). Nabilone: an alternative antiemetic for cancer chemotherapy. *Archives of Diseases in Childhood*, **61**, 502–505.

Dejesus, E., Rodwick, B.M., Bowers, D., Cohen, C.J. and Pearce, D. (2007). Use of dronabinol improves appetite and reverses weight loss in HIV/AIDS-infected patients. *Journal of the International Association of Physicians in AIDS Care (Chicago)*, **6**, 95–100.

Diasio, R.B., Ettinger, D.S., and Satterwhite, B.E. (1981). Oral levonantradol in the treatment of chemotherapy-induced emesis: preliminary observations. *Journal of Clinical Pharmacology*, **21**, 81S–85S.

Einhorn, L. (1982). Nabilone: an effective antiemetic agent in patients receiving cancer chemotherapy. *Cancer Treatment Reviews*, **9**(Suppl. B), 55–61.

Einhorn, L.H., Nagy, C., Furnas, B., and Williams, S.D. (1981). Nabilone: an effective antiemetic in patients receiving cancer chemotherapy. *Journal of Clinical Pharmacology*, **21**, 64S–69S.

Ekert, H., Waters, K.D., Jurk, I.H., Mobilia, J., and Loughnan, P. (1979). Amelioration of cancer chemotherapy-induced nausea and vomiting by delta-9-tetrahydrocannabinol. *Medical Journal of Australia*, **2**, 657–659.

Esfandyari, T., Camilleri, M., Busciglio, I., *et al.* (2007). Effects of a cannabinoid receptor agonist on colonic motor and sensory functions in humans: a randomized, placebo-controlled study. *American Journal of Physiology: Gastrointestinal and Liver Physiology*, **293**, G137–G145.

Esfandyari, T., Camilleri, M., Ferber, I., *et al.* (2006). Effect of a cannabinoid agonist on gastrointestinal transit and postprandial satiation in healthy human subjects: a randomized, placebo-controlled study. *Neurogastroenterology and Motility*, **18**, 831–838.

Fabre, L.F. and McLendon, D. (1981). The efficacy and safety of nabilone (a synthetic cannabinoid) in the treatment of anxiety. *Journal of Clinical Pharmacology*, **21**, 377S–382S.

Farooq, M.U., Ducommun, E., and Goudreau, J. (2009). Treatment of a hyperkinetic movement disorder during pregnancy with dronabinol. *Parkinsonism and Related Disorders*, **15**, 249–251.

Ferreiros, N., Labocha, S., Walter, C., Lotsch, J., and Geisslinger, G. (2013). Simultaneous and sensitive LC-MS/MS determination of tetrahydrocannabinol and metabolites in human plasma. *Analytical and Bioanalytical Chemistry*, **405**, 1399–1406.

Flynn, J. and Hanif, N. (1992). Nabilone for the management of intractable nausea and vomiting in terminally staged AIDS. *Journal of Palliative Care*, **8**, 46–47.

Fox, S.H., Kellett, M., Moore, A.P., Crossman, A.R., and Brotchie, J.M. (2002). Randomised, double-blind, placebo-controlled trial to assess the potential of cannabinoid receptor stimulation in the treatment of dystonia. *Movement Disorders*, **17**, 145–149.

Frank, B., Serpell, M.G., Hughes, J., Matthews, J.N., and Kapur, D. (2008). Comparison of analgesic effects and patient tolerability of nabilone and dihydrocodeine for chronic neuropathic pain: randomised, crossover, double blind study. *British Medical Journal*, **336**, 199–201.

Fraser, G.A. (2009). The use of a synthetic cannabinoid in the management of treatment-resistant nightmares in posttraumatic stress disorder (PTSD). *CNS Neuroscience and Therapeutics*, **15**, 84–88.

Gaoni, Y. and Mechoulam, R. (1964). Isolation, structure and partial synthesis of an active constituent of hashish. *Journal of the American Chemistry Society*, **86**, 1646–1647.

Gauter, B., Rukwied, R., and Konrad, C. (2004). Cannabinoid agonists in the treatment of blepharospasm – a case report study. *Neuroendocrinology Letters*, **25**, 45–48.

George, M., Pejovic, M.H., Thuaire, M., Kramar, A., and Wolff, J.P. (1983). [Randomized comparative trial of a new anti-emetic: nabilone, in cancer patients treated with cisplatin]. *Biomedicine and Pharmacotherapy*, **37**, 24–27.

Glass, R.M., Uhlenhuth, E.H., and Hartel, F.W. (1979). The effects of nabilone, a synthetic cannabinoid, on anxious human volunteers [proceedings]. *Psychopharmacology Bulletin*, **15**, 88–90.

Glass, R.M., Uhlenhuth, E.H., Hartel, F.W., Schuster, C.R., and Fischman, M.W. (1980). A single dose study of nabilone, a synthetic cannabinoid. *Psychopharmacology (Berlin)*, **71**, 137–142.

Glass, R.M., Uhlenhuth, E.H., Hartel, F.W., Schuster, C.R., and Fischman, M.W. (1981). Single-dose study of nabilone in anxious volunteers. *Journal of Clinical Pharmacology*, **21**, 383S–396S.

Gong, H., Jr., Tashkin, D.P., and Calvarese, B. (1983). Comparison of bronchial effects of nabilone and terbutaline in healthy and asthmatic subjects. *Journal of Clinical Pharmacology*, **23**, 127–133.

Goodivin, R.S., Gustafson, R.A., Barnes, A., et al. (2006). Δ^9-tetrahydrocannabinol, 11-hydroxy-Δ^9-tetrahydrocannabinol and 11-nor-9-carboxy-Δ^9-tetrahydrocannabinol in human plasma after controlled oral administration of cannabinoids. *Therapeutic Drug Monitoring*, **28**, 545–551.

Gorter, R., Seefried, M., and Volberding, P. (1992). Dronabinol effects on weight in patients with HIV infection. *AIDS*, **6**, 127.

Grant, J.E., Odlaug, B.L., Chamberlain, S.R., and Kim, S.W. (2011). Dronabinol, a cannabinoid agonist, reduces hair pulling in trichotillomania: a pilot study. *Psychopharmacology (Berlin)*, **218**, 493–502.

Green, S.T., Nathwani, D., Goldberg, D.J., and Kennedy, D.H. (1989). Nabilone as effective therapy for intractable nausea and vomiting in AIDS. *British Journal of Clinical Pharmacology*, **28**, 494–495.

Gross, H., Ebert, M.H., Faden, V.B., et al. (1983). A double-blind trial of delta 9-tetrahydrocannabinol in primary anorexia nervosa. *Journal of Clinical Psychopharmacology*, **3**, 165–71.

Grotenhermen, F. (2003). Pharmacokinetics and pharmacodynamics of cannabinoids. *Clinical Pharmacokinetics*, **42**, 327–360.

Grotenhermen, F. (2004). Pharmacology of cannabinoids. *Neuroendocrinology Letters*, **25**, 14–23.

Gustafson, R.A., Levine, B., Stout, P.R., et al. (2003). Urinary cannabinoid detection times after controlled oral administration of delta9-tetrahydrocannabinol to humans. *Clinical Chemistry*, **49**, 1114–1124.

Hamann, W. and Di Vadi, P.P. (1999). Analgesic effect of the cannabinoid analogue nabilone is not mediated by opioid receptors. *Lancet*, **353**, 560.

Haney, M., Gunderson, E.W., Rabkin, J., *et al.* (2007). Dronabinol and marijuana in HIV-positive marijuana smokers. Caloric intake, mood, and sleep. *Journal of the Acquired Immune Deficiency Syndrome*, **45**, 545–554.

Haney, M., Rabkin, J., Gunderson, E., and Foltin, R.W. (2005). Dronabinol and marijuana in HIV(+) marijuana smokers: acute effects on caloric intake and mood. *Psychopharmacology (Berlin)*, **181**, 170–178.

Hart, C.L., Haney, M., Vosburg, S.K., Comer, S.D., and Foltin, R.W. (2005). Reinforcing effects of oral delta9-THC in male marijuana smokers in a laboratory choice procedure. *Psychopharmacology (Berlin)*, **181**, 237–243.

Hazekamp, A., Ruhaak, R., Zuurman, L., Van Gerven, J., and Verpoorte, R. (2006). Evaluation of a vaporizing device (Volcano) for the pulmonary administration of tetrahydrocannabinol. *Journal of Pharmaceutical Sciences*, **95**, 1308–1317.

Herman, T.S., Einhorn, L.H., Jones, S.E., *et al.* (1979). Superiority of nabilone over prochlorperazine as an antiemetic in patients receiving cancer chemotherapy. *New England Journal of Medicine*, **300**, 1295–1297.

Herman, T.S., Jones, S.E., Dean, J., *et al.* (1977). Nabilone: a potent antiemetic cannabinol with minimal euphoria. *Biomedicine*, **27**, 331–334.

Hoffmann, D.E. and Weber, E. (2010). Medical marijuana and the law. *New England Journal of Medicine*, **362**, 1453–1457.

Isbell, H., Gorodetzsky, C.W., Jasinski, D., *et al.* (1967). Effects of (–)delta-9-trans-tetrahydrocannabinol in man. *Psychopharmacologia*, **11**, 184–188.

Jatoi, A., Windschitl, H.E., Loprinzi, C.L., *et al.* (2002). Dronabinol versus megestrol acetate versus combination therapy for cancer-associated anorexia: a North Central Cancer Treatment Group study. *Journal of Clinical Oncology*, **20**, 567–573.

Jay, W.M. and Green, K. (1983). Multiple-drop study of topically applied 1% delta 9-tetrahydrocannabinol in human eyes. *Archives of Ophthalmology*, **101**, 591–593.

Johansson, R., Kilkku, P., and Groenroos, M. (1982). A double-blind, controlled trial of nabilone vs. prochlorperazine for refractory emesis induced by cancer chemotherapy. *Cancer Treatment Reviews*, **9**(Suppl. B), 25–33.

Jones, S.E., Durant, J.R., Greco, F.A., and Robertone, A. (1982). A multi-institutional Phase III study of nabilone vs. placebo in chemotherapy-induced nausea and vomiting. *Cancer Treatment Reviews*, **9**(Suppl. B), 45–48.

Kalliomaki, J., Philipp, A., Baxendale, J., *et al.* (2012). Lack of effect of central nervous system-active doses of nabilone on capsaicin-induced pain and hyperalgesia. *Clinical and Experimental Pharmacology and Physiology*, **39**, 336–342.

Klooker, T.K., Leliefeld, K.E., Van Den Wijngaard, R.M., and Boeckxstaens, G.E. (2011). The cannabinoid receptor agonist delta-9-tetrahydrocannabinol does not affect visceral sensitivity to rectal distension in healthy volunteers and IBS patients. *Neurogastroenterology and Motility*, **23**, 30–35, e2.

Klumpers, L.E., Beumer, T.L., Van Hasselt, J.G., *et al.* (2012). Novel Δ^9-tetrahydrocannabinol formulation Namisol® has beneficial pharmacokinetics and promising pharmacodynamic effects. *British Journal of Clinical Pharmacology*, **74**, 42–53.

Kogel, R.W., Johnson, P.B., Chintam, R., Robinson, C.J., and Nemchausky, B.A. (1995). Treatment of spasticity in spinal cord injury with dronabinol, a tetrahydrocannabinol derivative. *American Journal of Therapeutics*, **2**, 799–805.

Kosel, B.W., Aweeka, F.T., Benowitz, N.L., *et al.* (2002). The effects of cannabinoids on the pharmacokinetics of indinavir and nelfinavir. *AIDS*, **16**, 543–550.

Krishnan, S., Cairns, R., and Howard, R. (2009). Cannabinoids for the treatment of dementia. *Cochrane Database of Systematic Reviews*, 2, CD007204.

Kurzthaler, I., Bodner, T., Kemmler, G., *et al.* (2005). The effect of nabilone on neuropsychological functions related to driving ability: an extended case series. *Human Psychopharmacology*, 20, 291–293.

Lane, M., Smith, F.E., Sullivan, R.A., and Plasse, T.F. (1990). Dronabinol and prochlorperazine alone and in combination as antiemetic agents for cancer chemotherapy. *America Journal of Clinical Oncology*, 13, 480–484.

Layeeque, R., Siegel, E., Kass, R., *et al.* (2006). Prevention of nausea and vomiting following breast surgery. *American Journal of Surgery*, 191, 767–772.

Lemberger, L., McMahon, R.E., Archer, R.A., Matsumoto, K., and Rowe, H. (1973). The in vitro and in vivo metabolism of delta 6a,10a dimethyl heptyl tetrahydrocannabinol (DMHP). *Journal of Pharmacology and Experimental Therapeutics*, 187, 169–175.

Lemberger, L., McMahon, R., Archer, R., Matsumoto, K. and Rowe, H. (1974). Pharmacologic effects and physiologic disposition of delta 6a,10a dimethyl heptyl tetrahydrocannabinol (DMHP) in man. *Clinical Pharmacology and Therapeutics*, 15, 380–386.

Lemberger, L. and Rowe, H. (1975). Clinical pharmacology of nabilone, a cannabinol derivative. *Clinical Pharmacology and Therapeutics*, 18, 720–726.

Levin, F.R. and Kleber, H.D. (2008). Use of dronabinol for cannabis dependence: two case reports and review. *America Journal of Addiction*, 17, 161–164.

Levin, F.R., Mariani, J.J., Brooks, D.J., *et al.* (2011). Dronabinol for the treatment of cannabis dependence: a randomized, double-blind, placebo-controlled trial. *Drug and Alcohol Dependence*, 116, 142–150.

Levitt, M. (1982). Nabilone vs. placebo in the treatment of chemotherapy-induced nausea and vomiting in cancer patients. *Cancer Treatment Reviews*, 9(Suppl. B), 49–53.

Leweke, F.M., Schneider, U., Radwan, M., Schmidt, E. and Emrich, H.M. (2000). Different effects of nabilone and cannabidiol on binocular depth inversion in man. *Pharmacology, Biochemistry and Behaviour*, 66, 175–181.

Leweke, F.M., Schneider, U., Thies, M., Munte, T.F. and Emrich, H.M. (1999). Effects of synthetic delta9-tetrahydrocannabinol on binocular depth inversion of natural and artificial objects in man. *Psychopharmacology (Berlin)*, 142, 230–235.

Lewis, I.H., Campbell, D.N., and Barrowcliffe, M.P. (1994). Effect of nabilone on nausea and vomiting after total abdominal hysterectomy. *British Journal of Anaesthesia*, 73, 244–246.

Lile, J.A., Kelly, T.H., and Hays, L.R. (2010). Substitution profile of the cannabinoid agonist nabilone in human subjects discriminating delta9-tetrahydrocannabinol. *Clinical Neuropharmacology*, 33, 235–242.

Lorenz, R. (2004). On the application of cannabis in paediatrics and epileptology. *Neuroendocrinology Letters*, 25, 40–44.

Maas, A.I., Murray, G., Henney, H., 3rd, *et al.* (2006). Efficacy and safety of dexanabinol in severe traumatic brain injury: results of a phase III randomised, placebo-controlled, clinical trial. *Lancet Neurology*, 5, 38–45.

Machado Rocha, F.C., Stefano, S.C., De Cassia Haiek, R., Rosa Oliveira, L.M., and Da Silveira, D.X. (2008). Therapeutic use of *Cannabis sativa* on chemotherapy-induced nausea and vomiting among cancer patients: systematic review and meta-analysis. *European Journal of Cancer Care (England)*, 17, 431–443.

Mahlberg, R. and Walther, S. (2007). Actigraphy in agitated patients with dementia. Monitoring treatment outcomes. *Zeitschrift für Gerontologie und Geriatrie*, 40, 178–184.

Maida, V. (2008). Nabilone for the treatment of paraneoplastic night sweats: a report of four cases. *Journal of Palliative Medicine*, 11, 929–934.

Maida, V., Ennis, M., Irani, S., Corbo, M., and Dolzhykov, M. (2008). Adjunctive nabilone in cancer pain and symptom management: a prospective observational study using propensity scoring. *Journal of Supportive Oncology*, 6, 119–124.

Martyn, C.N., Illis, L.S., and Thom, J. (1995). Nabilone in the treatment of multiple sclerosis. *Lancet*, **345**, 579.

Mattes, R.D., Shaw, L.M., Edling-Owens, J., Engelman, K., and Elsohly, M. A. (1993). Bypassing the first-pass effect for the therapeutic use of cannabinoids. *Pharmacology, Biochemistry and Behaviour*, **44**, 745–747.

McGilveray, I.J. (2005). Pharmacokinetics of cannabinoids. *Pain Research and Management*, **10**(Suppl. A), 15A–22A.

Meiri, E., Jhangiani, H., Vredenburgh, J.J., *et al.* (2007). Efficacy of dronabinol alone and in combination with ondansetron versus ondansetron alone for delayed chemotherapy-induced nausea and vomiting. *Current Medical Research and Opinion*, **23**, 533–543.

Mendelson, J.H., Ellingboe, J., and Mello, N.K. (1984). Acute effects of natural and synthetic cannabis compounds on prolactin levels in human males. *Pharmacology, Biochemistry and Behaviour*, **20**, 103–106.

Mendelson, J.H. and Mello, N.K. (1984). Reinforcing properties of oral delta 9-tetrahydrocannabinol, smoked marijuana, and nabilone: influence of previous marijuana use. *Psychopharmacology (Berlin)*, **83**, 351–356.

Menetrey, A., Augsburger, M., Favrat, B., *et al.* (2005). Assessment of driving capability through the use of clinical and psychomotor tests in relation to blood cannabinoids levels following oral administration of 20 mg dronabinol or of a cannabis decoction made with 20 or 60 mg Delta9-THC. *Journal of Analytical Toxicology*, **29**, 327–338.

Meyniel, C., Ollivier, Y., Hamidou, M., Pereon, Y., and Derkinderen, P. (2011). Dramatic improvement of refractory Isaacs' syndrome after treatment with dronabinol. *Clinical Neurology and Neurosurgery*, **113**, 323–324.

Muller-Vahl, K.R. (2003). Cannabinoids reduce symptoms of Tourette's syndrome. *Expert Opinion in Pharmacotherapy*, **4**, 1717–1725.

Muller-Vahl, K.R., Schneider, U., and Emrich, H.M. (1999). Nabilone increases choreatic movements in Huntington's disease. *Movement Disorders*, **14**, 1038–1040.

Nakano, S., Gillespie, H.K., and Hollister, L.E. (1978). A model for evaluation of antianxiety drugs with the use of experimentally induced stress: comparison of nabilone and diazepam. *Clinical Pharmacology and Therapeutics*, **23**, 54–62.

Narang, S., Gibson, D., Wasan, A.D., *et al.* (2008). Efficacy of dronabinol as an adjuvant treatment for chronic pain patients on opioid therapy. *Journal of Pain*, **9**, 254–264.

Neff, G.W., O'Brien, C.B., Reddy, K.R., *et al.* (2002). Preliminary observation with dronabinol in patients with intractable pruritus secondary to cholestatic liver disease. *American Journal of Gastroenterology*, **97**, 2117–2119.

Neidhart, J.A., Gagen, M.M., Wilson, H.E., and Young, D.C. (1981). Comparative trial of the antiemetic effects of THC and haloperidol. *Journal of Clinical Pharmacology*, **21**, 38S–42S.

Newell, F.W., Stark, P., Jay, W.M., and Schanzlin, D.J. (1979). Nabilone: a pressure-reducing synthetic benzopyran in open-angle glaucoma. *Ophthalmology*, **86**, 156–160.

Niederle, N., Schutte, J., and Schmidt, C.G. (1986). Crossover comparison of the antiemetic efficacy of nabilone and alizapride in patients with nonseminomatous testicular cancer receiving cisplatin therapy. *Klinische Wochenschrift*, **64**, 362–365.

Niiranen, A. and Mattson, K. (1985). A cross-over comparison of nabilone and prochlorperazine for emesis induced by cancer chemotherapy. *American Journal of Clinical Oncology*, **8**, 336–340.

Niiranen, A. and Mattson, K. (1987). Antiemetic efficacy of nabilone and dexamethasone: a randomized study of patients with lung cancer receiving chemotherapy. *American Journal of Clinical Oncology*, **10**, 325–329.

Noyes, R., Jr., Brunk, S.F., Avery, D.A., and Canter, A.C. (1975a). The analgesic properties of delta-9-tetrahydrocannabinol and codeine. *Clinical Pharmacology and Therapeutics*, **18**, 84–89.

Noyes, R., Jr., Brunk, S.F., Baram, D.A., and Canter, A. (1975b). Analgesic effect of delta-9-tetrahydrocannabinol. *Journal of Clinical Pharmacology*, **15**, 139–143.

Orr, L.E. and McKernan, J.F. (1981). Antiemetic effect of delta 9-tetrahydrocannabinol in chemotherapy-associated nausea and emesis as compared to placebo and compazine. *Journal of Clinical Pharmacology*, **21**, 76S–80S.

Passmore, M.J. (2008). The cannabinoid receptor agonist nabilone for the treatment of dementia-related agitation. *International Journal of Geriatric Psychiatry*, **23**, 116–117.

Petro, D.J. and Ellenberger, C., Jr. (1981). Treatment of human spasticity with delta 9-tetrahydrocannabinol. *Journal of Clinical Pharmacology*, **21**, 413S–416S.

Pini, L.A., Guerzoni, S., Cainazzo, M.M., et al. (2012). Nabilone for the treatment of medication over-use headache: results of a preliminary double-blind, active-controlled, randomized trial. *Journal of Headache Pain*, **13**, 677–684.

Pinsger, M., Schimetta, W., Volc, D., et al. (2006). [Benefits of an add-on treatment with the synthetic cannabinomimetic nabilone on patients with chronic pain – a randomized controlled trial]. *Wiener klinische Wochenschrift*, **118**, 327–335.

Plange, N., Arend, K.O., Kaup, M., et al. (2007). Dronabinol and retinal hemodynamics in humans. *American Journal of Ophthalmology*, **143**, 173–174.

Pomeroy, M., Fennelly, J.J., and Towers, M. (1986). Prospective randomized double-blind trial of nabilone versus domperidone in the treatment of cytotoxic-induced emesis. *Cancer Chemotherapy and Pharmacology*, **17**, 285–288.

Pooyania, S., Ethans, K., Szturm, T., Casey, A., and Perry, D. (2010). A randomized, double-blinded, crossover pilot study assessing the effect of nabilone on spasticity in persons with spinal cord injury. *Archives of Physical Medicine and Rehabilitation*, **91**, 703–707.

Poster, D.S., Penta, J.S., Bruno, S., and MacDonald, J.S. (1981). delta 9-tetrahydrocannabinol in clinical oncology. *Journal of the American Medical Association*, **245**, 2047–2051.

Prasad, B., Radulovacki, M.G., and Carley, D.W. (2013). Proof of concept trial of dronabinol in obstructive sleep apnea. *Frontiers in Psychiatry*, **4**, 1.

Priestman, S.G., Priestman, T.J., and Canney, P.A. (1987). A double-blind randomised cross-over comparison of nabilone and metoclopramide in the control of radiation-induced nausea. *Clinical Radiology*, **38**, 543–5444.

Priestman, T.J. and Priestman, S.G. (1984). An initial evaluation of nabilone in the control of radiotherapy-induced nausea and vomiting. *Clinical Radiology*, **35**, 265–266.

Raby, W.N., Modica, P.A., Wolintz, R.J., and Murtaugh, K. (2006). Dronabinol reduces signs and symptoms of idiopathic intracranial hypertension: a case report. *Journal of Ocular Pharmacology and Therapeutics*, **22**, 68–75.

Redmond, W.J., Goffaux, P., Potvin, S., and Marchand, S. (2008). Analgesic and antihyperalgesic effects of nabilone on experimental heat pain. *Current Medical Research and Opinion*, **24**, 1017–1024.

Rintala, D.H., Fiess, R.N., Tan, G., Holmes, S.A., and Bruel, B.M. (2010). Effect of dronabinol on central neuropathic pain after spinal cord injury: a pilot study. *American Journal of Physical Medicine and Rehabilitation*, **89**, 840–848.

Robbins, M.S., Tarshish, S., Solomon, S., and Grosberg, B.M. (2009). Cluster attacks responsive to recreational cannabis and dronabinol. *Headache*, **49**, 914–916.

Rubin, A., Lemberger, L., Warrick, P., et al. (1977). Physiologic disposition of nabilone, a cannabinol derivative, in man. *Clinical Pharmacology and Therapeutics*, **22**, 85–91.

Rudich, Z., Stinson, J., Jeavons, M., and Brown, S.C. (2003). Treatment of chronic intractable neuropathic pain with dronabinol: case report of two adolescents. *Pain Research and Management*, **8**, 221–224.

Russo, E. and Guy, G.W. (2006). A tale of two cannabinoids: the therapeutic rationale for combining tetrahydrocannabinol and cannabidiol. *Medical Hypotheses*, **66**, 234–246.

Russo, E.B. (2011). Taming THC: potential cannabis synergy and phytocannabinoid-terpenoid entourage effects. *British Journal of Pharmacology*, **163**, 1344–1364.

Russo, E.B., Merzouki, A., Mesa, J.M., Frey, K.A., and Bach, P.J. (2004). Cannabis improves night vision: a case study of dark adaptometry and scotopic sensitivity in kif smokers of the Rif mountains of northern Morocco. *Journal of Ethnopharmacology*, **93**, 99–104.

Salerian, A.J. (2004). Successful treatment of sexual dysfunction with dronabinol: a case report. *Journal of Clinical Psychiatry*, **65**, 1146–1147.

Sallan, S.E., Cronin, C., Zelen, M., and Zinberg, N.E. (1980). Antiemetics in patients receiving chemotherapy for cancer: a randomized comparison of delta-9-tetrahydrocannabinol and prochlorperazine. *New England Journal of Medicine*, **302**, 135–138.

Sallan, S.E., Zinberg, N.E., and Frei, E., 3rd (1975). Antiemetic effect of delta-9-tetrahydrocannabinol in patients receiving cancer chemotherapy. *New England Journal of Medicine*, **293**, 795–797.

Schindler, F., Anghelescu, I., Regen, F., and Jockers-Scherubl, M. (2008). Improvement in refractory obsessive compulsive disorder with dronabinol. *American Journal of Psychiatry*, **165**, 536–537.

Schoedel, K.A., Chen, N., Hilliard, A., *et al.* (2011). A randomized, double-blind, placebo-controlled, crossover study to evaluate the subjective abuse potential and cognitive effects of nabiximols oromucosal spray in subjects with a history of recreational cannabis use. *Human Psychopharmacology*, **26**, 224–236.

Schwarcz, G. and Karajgi, B. (2010). Improvement in refractory psychosis with dronabinol: four case reports. *Journal of Clinical Psychiatry*, **71**, 1552–153.

Schwarcz, G., Karajgi, B., and McCarthy, R. (2009). Synthetic delta-9-tetrahydrocannabinol (dronabinol) can improve the symptoms of schizophrenia. *Journal of Clinical Psychopharmacology*, **29**, 255–258.

Seeling, W., Kneer, L., Buchele, B., *et al.* (2006). Δ^9-tetrahydrocannabinol and the opioid receptor agonist piritramide do not act synergistically in postoperative pain. *Anaesthesist*, **55**, 391–400.

Sieradzan, K.A., Fox, S.H., Hill, M., *et al.* (2001). Cannabinoids reduce levodopa-induced dyskinesia in Parkinson's disease: a pilot study. *Neurology*, **57**, 2108–2111.

Skrabek, R.Q., Galimova, L., Ethans, K., and Perry, D. (2008). Nabilone for the treatment of pain in fibromyalgia. *Journal of Pain*, **9**, 164–173.

Steele, N., Gralla, R.J., Braun, D.W., Jr., and Young, C.W. (1980). Double-blind comparison of the antiemetic effects of nabilone and prochlorperazine on chemotherapy-induced emesis. *Cancer Treatment Reports*, **64**, 219–224.

Struwe, M., Kaempfer, S.H., Geiger, C.J., *et al.* (1993). Effect of dronabinol on nutritional status in HIV infection. *Annals of Pharmacotherapy*, **27**, 827–831.

Svendsen, K.B., Jensen, T.S., and Bach, F.W. (2004). Does the cannabinoid dronabinol reduce central pain in multiple sclerosis? Randomised double blind placebo controlled crossover trial. *British Medical Journal*, **329**, 253.

Tashkin, D.P., Shapiro, B.J., Lee, Y.E., and Harper, C.E. (1975). Effects of smoked marijuana in experimentally induced asthma. *American Review of Respiratory Disorders*, **112**, 377–386.

Tiedeman, J.S., Shields, M.B., Weber, P.A., *et al.* (1981). Effect of synthetic cannabinoids on elevated intraocular pressure. *Ophthalmology*, **88**, 270–277.

Timpone, J.G., Wright, D.J., Li, N., *et al.* (1997). The safety and pharmacokinetics of single-agent and combination therapy with megestrol acetate and dronabinol for the treatment of HIV wasting syndrome. The DATRI 004 Study Group. Division of AIDS Treatment Research Initiative. *AIDS Research and Human Retroviruses*, **13**, 305–315.

Toth, C., Mawani, S., Brady, S., *et al.* (2012). An enriched-enrolment, randomized withdrawal, flexible-dose, double-blind, placebo-controlled, parallel assignment efficacy study of nabilone as adjuvant in the treatment of diabetic peripheral neuropathic pain. *Pain*, **153**, 2073–2082.

Tramer, M.R., Carroll, D., Campbell, F.A., *et al.* (2001). Cannabinoids for control of chemotherapy induced nausea and vomiting: quantitative systematic review. *British Medical Journal*, **323**, 16–21.

Ungerleider, J.T., Andrysiak, T., Fairbanks, L., *et al.* (1982). Cannabis and cancer chemotherapy: a comparison of oral delta-9-THC and prochlorperazine. *Cancer*, **50**, 636–645.

Ungerleider, J.T., Andyrsiak, T., Fairbanks, L., Ellison, G.W., and Myers, L.W. (1987). Delta-9-THC in the treatment of spasticity associated with multiple sclerosis. *Advances in Alcohol and Substance Abuse*, **7**, 39–50.

Vandrey, R., Stitzer, M.L., Mintzer, M.Z., *et al.* (2013). The dose effects of short-term dronabinol (oral THC) maintenance in daily cannabis users. *Drug and Alcohol Dependence*, **128**, 64–70.

Wada, J.K., Bogdon, D.L., Gunnell, J.C., *et al.* (1982). Double-blind, randomized, crossover trial of nabilone vs. placebo in cancer chemotherapy. *Cancer Treatment Reviews*, **9** Suppl. B, 39–44.

Walsh, D., Kirkova, J., and Davis, M.P. (2005). The efficacy and tolerability of long-term use of dronabinol in cancer-related anorexia: a case series. *Journal of Pain and Symptom Management*, **30**, 493–495.

Walther, S., Mahlberg, R., Eichmann, U., and Kunz, D. (2006). Delta-9-tetrahydrocannabinol for night-time agitation in severe dementia. *Psychopharmacology (Berlin)*, **185**, 524–528.

Walther, S., Schupbach, B., Seifritz, E., Homan, P., and Strik, W. (2011). Randomized, controlled crossover trial of dronabinol, 2.5 mg, for agitation in 2 patients with dementia. *Journal of Clinical Psychopharmacology*, **31**, 256–258.

Ware, M.A., Adams, H., and Guy, G.W. (2005). The medicinal use of cannabis in the UK: results of a nationwide survey. *International Journal of Clinical Practice*, **59**, 291–295.

Ware, M.A., Fitzcharles, M.A., Joseph, L., and Shir, Y. (2010). The effects of nabilone on sleep in fibromyalgia: results of a randomized controlled trial. *Anesthesia and Analgesia*, **110**, 604–610.

Ware, M.A. and St Arnaud-Trempe, E. (2010). The abuse potential of the synthetic cannabinoid nabilone. *Addiction*, **105**, 494–503.

Wesnes, K.A., Annas, P., Edgar, C.J., *et al.* (2010). Nabilone produces marked impairments to cognitive function and changes in subjective state in healthy volunteers. *Journal of Psychopharmacology*, **24**, 1659–1669.

Williams, S.J., Hartley, J.P., and Graham, J.D. (1976). Bronchodilator effect of delta1-tetrahydrocannabinol administered by aerosol of asthmatic patients. *Thorax*, **31**, 720–723.

Wilson, M.M., Philpot, C., and Morley, J.E. (2007). Anorexia of aging in long term care: is dronabinol an effective appetite stimulant? – a pilot study. *Journal of Nutrition, Health and Aging*, **11**, 195–198.

Wissel, J., Haydn, T., Muller, J., *et al.* (2006). Low dose treatment with the synthetic cannabinoid Nabilone significantly reduces spasticity-related pain: a double-blind placebo-controlled cross-over trial. *Journal of Neurology*, **253**, 1337–1341.

Wong, B.S., Camilleri, M., Busciglio, I., *et al.* (2011). Pharmacogenetic trial of a cannabinoid agonist shows reduced fasting colonic motility in patients with nonconstipated irritable bowel syndrome. *Gastroenterology*, **141**, 1638–1647 e1–7.

Wong, B.S., Camilleri, M., Eckert, D., *et al.* (2012). Randomized pharmacodynamic and pharmacogenetic trial of dronabinol effects on colon transit in irritable bowel syndrome-diarrhea. *Neurogastroenterology and Motility*, **24**, 358–e169.

Zutt, M., Hanssle, H., Emmert, S., Neumann, C., and Kretschmer, L. (2006). [Dronabinol for supportive therapy in patients with malignant melanoma and liver metastases]. *Der Hautarzt*, **57**, 423–427.

Chapter 22

Cannabinoids in Clinical Practice: A UK Perspective

William Notcutt and Emily L. Clarke

22.1 Introduction

Mechoulam's discovery of delta 9-tetrahydrocannabinol (THC) was the starting point in the late 1960s of basic science research into cannabinoids. This led to the exploration of their therapeutic potential and finally 30 years later, to modern scientific investigation into their clinical use. However, unlike most other medicines, the journey has been difficult and complex, principally due to the association with the recreational use of the drug and the inevitable opprobrium from politicians and the media.

Opiates did not encounter this problem since they became well established in medical practice prior to both the modern era of medicine evaluation and the concerns over the potential for dependency. Consider the difficulty of introducing morphine these days, an analgesic with a narrow therapeutic range and major side effects (sedation, respiratory depression, addiction, nausea, vomiting, constipation, etc.). Would morphine ever get past a Phase 1 trial? Many patients find their pain easier to tolerate than the side effects of this opiate and yet morphine remains a cornerstone of analgesic therapy.

Research into the basic science of cannabinoids has informed the growing interest in the clinical potential, but movement from the laboratory to the bedside has been a long, slow process for a number of reasons:

1 There has been a lack of appropriate medicinal-grade materials.

2 The delivery systems have needed to be developed beyond the established methods used recreationally.

3 There is little widespread, accurate, basic knowledge of cannabinoid therapy amongst medical practitioners.

4 There is still a widespread societal concern regarding cannabis amongst patients, the media, and politicians, which is both the cause and consequence of the Schedule 1 status for cannabis and the Schedule 2 status for cannabinoid medicines (from 2010). It is notable that both nabilone and Sativex® (nabiximols) were originally prescribed as Schedule 4 medicines until 2010 in the UK, and then Sativex® was returned to Schedule 2 in 2013!

5 The variable legal and regulatory frameworks in different nations make the widespread international introduction of medicinal cannabinoids very difficult. Similar problems continue to affect the use of medicinal opiates.

6 Currently the cost of recently developed medicinal cannabinoids is high, primarily due to the cost of research and development and low usage. Illicit cannabis is generally much cheaper, leading to the bizarre situation of it being less expensive to commit a criminal act and purchase one's medicine on the "street."

Meek (1994) stated that 75% of doctors wished to be able to prescribe medicinal cannabinoids, but until recently very few physicians have been able to do so. Furthermore, many doctors have found themselves in the situation of having to discuss with their patient the use of "street" cannabis as a medicine, and potentially having to give advice on various aspects of its use alongside other pharmaceutical agents. There is not only a lack of accurate and basic knowledge of cannabinoids and their therapeutic use, but also a large amount of unscientific ignorance and mythology surrounding cannabis. Regretfully many patients and doctors find the idea of discussing the use of an illicit substance as a medicine very difficult and uncomfortable, particularly as possession of cannabis still remains a criminal act as defined by its Class B status in the UK. In addition, the majority of the general public believe that the potential side effects of medicinal cannabinoids are very similar to those associated with recreational materials.

As cannabinoid therapy starts to be incorporated into medical practice there is a need for dissemination of the current clinical knowledge, both the effectiveness data and the real-life experience, to the wider medical and lay worlds. This chapter aims to fulfil that contemporary need through a discussion of the management of patients undergoing cannabinoid therapy which is based on current peer-reviewed evidence and on the growing clinical experiences of one of the authors, Willy Notcutt (WN), and other cannabinoid prescribers in the UK and elsewhere (Grotenhermen and Müller-Vahl 2012).

22.2 Medicinally available cannabinoids and their administration

The delivery method of cannabinoid medicines has presented a challenge. Most patients who want to take a medicine for pain or similar symptoms wish to be made more comfortable so that they can participate in activities of daily living (ADLs). It is of no great benefit to exchange a state of immobility because of pain, spasticity, or nausea for one caused by excessive plasma levels of cannabinoid. Controlling the intake of cannabinoid into the body presents problems. Currently the only two routes formally accepted by regulators in the UK are oral and oromucosal (sublingual and buccal). However, we will comment on the other established routes of delivery of cannabis that may be used by patients presenting to the doctor.

22.2.1 Smoking

Whilst smoking cannabis has been the traditional method of administering the drug recreationally, this is not an acceptable method of use as a medicine to most patients, to doctors, to regulators, or to the law. Undoubtedly some patients can inhale smoke or vapor accurately and control their intake without overloading (Grotenhermen 2003). In many respects this mimics a patient-controlled analgesia device (inhale a small quantity, wait a short time, and assess the benefit before deciding on a further intake of the drug). However, unless one is an experienced smoker, high plasma levels of THC can easily be generated, risking the onset of psychoactive effects. In general, the experienced cannabis smokers are those who are frequent recreational users. The other drawbacks of smoking are the harm from potentially carcinogenic combustion products (Hall 1998; Henry et al. 2003), the inconvenience of use, particularly in public, and social unacceptability due to association with recreational use.

22.2.2 Vaporizing

Vaporizing the drug into a gas by the controlled electrical heating of plant material avoids burning and the production of smoke. However, the same problems arise: the potential for high initial plasma levels, the risk from the inhalation of hot gas, and the significant inconvenience of administration. Again, as with smoking, it can be used with a reasonable level of patient control of the intake.

Unfortunately, unlike water-soluble medicines, cannabinoids cannot easily be nebulized into the small droplet size suitable to penetrate the lower airways; larger droplets irritate the respiratory tract and induce coughing.

22.2.3 **Oral**

The oral route is regarded as the most appropriate form of analgesic drug delivery for opioids with a predictable onset in 20–30 min for an immediate-release preparation. Two licensed cannabinoid-based medications employ this route of administration. Nabilone (Cesamet®) is a synthetic THC analogue developed in 1984 and is licensed in the UK for chemotherapy-induced nausea and vomiting (CINV). It is given orally in capsule form. Dronabinol (Marinol®), a synthetic form of THC, is licensed in the US (but unavailable in the UK) for CINV and anorexia.

Unfortunately, oral cannabinoids have a slow, variable absorption and 80% of ingested THC converts to the possibly more psychoactive 11-hydroxy-THC during first-pass metabolism (Russo and Guy 2006). Consequently, it is difficult to titrate to an individual optimum dose, thereby increasing the risk of the common side effects. In the UK, titration is made more difficult because of the lack of a range of capsule strengths for nabilone (1 mg only), whereas in the US, dronabinol is supplied in 2.5, 5, and 10 mg strengths.

In Europe outside the UK, cannabis plant material in a standardized strength and in an uncontaminated and defined form is available as a pharmaceutical product and delivered via a vaporizer or made into a tea (e.g., Bedrocan®, Netherlands). However, the patient then has the problem of finding the most convenient and predictable method of administration. Finally, Cannador®, a German preparation comprised of an oral capsule-containing plant extract, has been used in some clinical trials (Holdcroft et al. 2006; Zajicek et al. 2003). However, it is not available for clinical use in the UK.

22.2.4 **Sublingual/oromucosal**

In order to avoid some of the problems of the oral route, the oromucosal method of administration was developed. Sativex® is a sublingual spray combining THC with cannabidiol (CBD), and was licensed in 2010 in the UK for spasticity and spasms in multiple sclerosis (MS). This route of administration enables efficient and accurate delivery of active agent. The sublingual administration combining THC and CBD as primary ingredients has improved the ability of the patient to control dosing and has a reasonably fast speed of onset whilst probably lowering the side effect potential (Lynch 2011; Pertwee 2004). Also, through the addition of CBD, Sativex® possesses analgesic, antispasmodic, anticonvulsant, anxiolytic, and anti-inflammatory properties, as well as being neuroprotective and antipsychotic (Jiang et al. 2005; Roser and Haussleiter 2012) most of which may be valuable in the management of pain. Recently, Robson (2011) reported that Sativex® achieved far fewer reported psychotropic effects (2.2%) than nabilone.

Clinical research into cannabinoid therapy is still in its infancy and the most appropriate routes of administration of these agents are still to be determined. It may be that different preparations will be needed for different uses in order to strike a balance between the benefits and drawbacks, as with opioids. It has been suggested that a background oral dose may be used alongside a more rapidly acting and patient-controlled sublingual or vaporized dose to help maintain symptomatic control for acute changes in symptoms (Grotenhermen 2001). Within the clinical setting it is essential to customize the prescription of cannabinoids on a patient-by-patient basis, which may involve multiple agents, preparations, or timings rather than following a rigid dose regimen. This parallels the way in which an opioid would be used in managing chronic pain. As yet there are no cannabinoid preparations available that are delivered rectally, transdermally, or parenterally, but these are future possibilities.

22.2.5 Illicit sources of plant material

Many patients are desperate enough to use illicit supplies of cannabis as a medicine, smoked or orally ingested. The physician needs to be aware of this when managing such a patient as they may also be using other prescribed medication. Understanding the speed of onset of effect, the endpoint of titration that the patient uses, the pattern of use, and the duration of action is important and can usually be obtained from careful history taking. It is almost impossible to do anything more than guess the strength or composition of the illicit material, although assessing the reported effects and side effects may be a guide.

22.3 Cannabinoids and clinical use

Cannabis has been used therapeutically for some 5000 years and like many other plant-based medicines (opiates, salicylic acid, digoxin, senna, hyoscine, taxol, curare, quinine, chilli, etc.), its use has been explored for a wide range of ailments. Many of the uses being evaluated today with modern research techniques have appeared in observational studies dating back to the late 1800s. Clinicians experimented with cannabis in a variety of different situations, largely intractable to the medical practice of those days. Had cannabis not been perceived to be addictive (principally because of the commercial corruption and the Reefer Madness campaigns in the US in the 1930s) it is likely that it would have become well established in clinical practice. As we have subsequently learnt, cannabis is equivalent to benzodiazepines and most other commonly used psychoactive drugs in the harm potential for the individual (Nutt et al. 2010).

Whereas opiates and benzodiazepines have narrowly defined uses (nociceptive pain and anxiolysis respectively), the physiological action and the clinical potential of cannabinoids appears much broader. This reflects the ubiquitous nature of the endocannabinoid system. Sometimes one can almost hear the marketing hype of the nineteenth-century snake oil salesman selling his wares, when one hears a patient describing the benefit gained. Yet all those symptomatic improvements were described by one, very sensible, woman with MS (Box 22.1).

Currently, the major clinical trials of medicinal-grade cannabinoids have been directed towards developing licenses for clinical use, which now include CINV, spasticity and spasms in multiple sclerosis (MS), neuropathic and cancer pain, and acquired immunodeficiency syndrome (AIDS)-related anorexia. Furthermore, the use is only advocated when symptoms remain refractory to all other agents.

Now that the safety of medicinal-grade cannabinoids has been demonstrated, other uses are emerging. There is still a wide range of chronic clinical problems with distressing and intractable

---

Box 22.1 A patient of the author WN describes her benefit

The fatigue goes. The migraine attacks are reduced; sleep is better. The spasms and cramps are cured, night-time visits to the toilet are less; balance is improved. The strange sensations in the legs are improved; I am able to move and dress more easily.

symptoms that modern medicine is unable to relieve. Therefore clinicians are sometimes resorting to prescribing "off label" in order to respond to patient need.

22.3.1 Chemotherapy-induced nausea and vomiting and appetite stimulation

In 1984, CINV became the first indication for the use of nabilone (Cesamet®) in the UK through exploitation of THC's antiemetic properties. More recently, dronabinol (Marinol®), synthetic THC, was licensed for the same purpose in the US, but it remains unavailable in the UK. Despite nabilone being superseded by 5-HT$_3$ antagonists for CINV in the UK, Meiri et al. (2007) concluded that the antinausea properties of dronabinol (71%) had similar efficacy to ondansetron (64%) and both drugs were well tolerated.

Appetite stimulation by THC when used recreationally is a well-known side effect and so the possibility of use to treat anorexia has been suggested, especially in AIDS. Haney et al. (2007) concluded that both oral dronabinol and smoking cannabis caused an increase in caloric intake and weight in patients taking antiretroviral therapy. The benefit of cannabinoids to patients with AIDS may extend much further than merely appetite stimulation as several studies have shown that cannabinoid therapy also reduces HIV-associated pain (Abrams et al. 2007; Ellis et al. 2009), nausea (Flynn and Hanif 1992) and vomiting, whilst increasing adherence to antiretroviral therapy (de Jong et al. 2005).

22.3.2 Spasticity and spasms

In the UK, patients with MS championed the use of cannabis as a medicine in the 1990s. The advent of a purified extract (Sativex®) allowing precise titration of intake allowed the development of a series of placebo-controlled randomized controlled trials with ongoing observational extension studies and other associated investigations. The trials were difficult and complex due to the heterogeneous nature of the symptomatology of MS and the variety of responses that patients may experience. The symptoms known to be improved by the drug include spasticity, spasms, neuropathic pain, and bladder dysfunction, whilst also sometimes helping with fatigue, sleep disturbance, and dysesthesia (Brady et al. 2004; Collin et al. 2010; Novotna et al. 2011; Rog et al. 2005; Vermersch 2011; Wade et al. 2010) (Box 22.1). Consequently, the new combination cannabinoid therapy, Sativex® was eventually licensed in 2010 in the UK for spasticity and spasms in sufferers of MS.

The Cannabis in Multiple Sclerosis (CAMS) randomized controlled trial by Zajicek et al. (2003), assessed patient spasticity with a cannabis extract, THC, and placebo. They concluded that while there was no improvement to be found when assessing spasticity on the Ashworth scale, cannabinoids did improve some subjective secondary outcomes. In 2012, however, the Multiple Sclerosis and Extract of Cannabis (MUSEC) trial (Zajicek et al. 2012) concluded that the rate of relief of muscle stiffness in MS patients after 12 weeks of therapy was doubled with cannabis extract compared to placebo.

22.3.3 Long-term use in spasticity and spasms

Following on from many of the Sativex® studies, patients have had the option to enter extension studies to evaluate long-term effects. This has all been open-label primarily assessing the maintenance of benefit alongside the possible emergence of side effects (Serpell et al. 2013).

Additionally, Notcutt et al. (2012a) evaluated the ability of Sativex® to provide long-term relief from spasticity by assessing the impact of sudden medicine withdrawal after its use for at least

12 weeks, demonstrating the ongoing benefit patients were receiving. An observational study (Notcutt 2012b) reviewed the benefits that patients continued to get with long-term use: spasticity, pain, sleep, ADLs. This study also showed the improvements that the patient's carers were experiencing.

Despite many patients stating that cannabis has altered their disease progression and not just merely their symptoms, no human trials have so far proved this. However, data from animal trials have suggested some disease-modifying activity and so in time cannabinoids may prove useful in this respect.

22.3.4 Neuropathic pain

Neuropathic pain, pain secondary to nerve damage, is a further indication for the use of Sativex® in Canada. It is a type of pain that is commonly difficult to treat and is least satisfied by available analgesics. A systematic review by Lynch and Campbell (2011) and a case series by Notcutt et al. (2004) found that cannabinoids were an efficacious treatment option. There is also evidence to suggest that long-term use does not diminish the effects (Nurmikko et al. 2007).

22.3.5 Emerging uses

The history of cannabis use has thrown up evidence of the ability of cannabis to treat a wide range of intractable problems and this is supported by knowledge emerging from basic science.

Use as an analgesic agent is an emerging indication for cannabinoids that has been reviewed by Campbell et al. (2001) and Lynch and Campbell (2011). Early studies showed that THC has similar analgesic efficacy to codeine in short-term use in acute pain (Campbell et al. 2001). However, Cichewicz et al. (1999) and Karst et al. (2010) stated that cannabinoids employ a different mechanism of action to opiates and therefore could augment an opiate effect and be a good possibility as an adjuvant choice for those with intractable pain. This would be similar to the way tricyclic antidepressants are used in chronic pain management.

Cannabinoids may also be of great use in patients who suffer sleep disturbance as a consequence of chronic pain since cannabinoids have been shown to aid sleep (Vermersch 2011). Furthermore, it is well documented that opiates and tricyclic antidepressants may disrupt sleep architecture which can exacerbate perceived pain.

Postoperative pain may also be an area that could benefit from cannabinoid therapy since opiates are known to cause nausea, vomiting, respiratory depression, and basal atelectasis, which may delay wound healing and cause patient distress. Cannabinoids, by contrast, are antiemetic and therefore would both augment the analgesic effect of the opiate, whilst ameliorating the nauseating effects. Although this may theoretically seem like a winning formula, Seeling et al. (2006) found no improvement when using opiate and cannabinoid combination therapy for postoperative prostatectomy patients as compared to opiates alone. However, this was an unusual model for studying postoperative pain.

Fibromyalgia and chronic fatigue syndrome are two diseases that are not well understood and have very limited treatment options. One theory regarding the pathophysiology of these diseases is a disruption of sleep—again this may be helped with cannabinoid therapy as nabilone has been used for sleep disturbance with some success (Ware et al. 2010). However, Skrabek et al. (2008) and Russo (2004) suggest that the etiology of fibromyalgia may also be based on an endocannabinoid deficiency syndrome, thereby benefitting from therapy with exogenous cannabinoids.

Psychotic disorders may also be aided by using cannabidiol. Unlike all other emerging uses, different cannabinoids have different effects on psychotic disorders. THC worsens the state of schizophrenic patients (D'Souza et al. 2005), but cannabidiol is antipsychotic (Leweke et al. 2007) and therefore may be of use in this field.

There has also been some investigation into the effect of Sativex® on rheumatoid arthritis, with promising indications of significant analgesic effects and suppressed disease activity (Blake et al. 2006; Dunn et al. 2012).

In addition, diarrheal disease such as irritable bowel syndrome may be attenuated through use of THC; Esfandyari et al. (2006, 2007) have demonstrated that this cannabinoid relaxes the colon and reduces postprandial colonic motility.

Cannabis has been used since the nineteenth century for the treatment of epilepsy and is currently licensed for this purpose in 14 US states (Hoffman and Weber 2010). It has been theorized that cannabidiol may be responsible as it has been found to have anticonvulsant effects (Jones et al. 2010). However, a recent Cochrane review (Gloss and Vickrey 2012) on this topic did not draw any reliable conclusions due to lack of evidence. It is possible that cannabidiol could be explored for use against treatment-resistant epilepsy.

As with most other up-and-coming fields of research, anecdotal evidence usually precedes any formal studies. There are many other hypothesized usages of cannabinoids but few have been investigated formally. A small example of these other potential uses for cannabinoids includes treatment of: Crohn's disease (Naftaeli et al. 2011), posttraumatic stress disorder (Ganon-Elazar and Akirav et al. 2009), amyotrophic lateral sclerosis (Scotter et al. 2010), cancer pain (Portenoy et al. 2010), acute brain injury, and adjunctive use in palliative care (Grotenhermen et al. 2012), with further studies into cancer pain already underway (GW Pharmaceuticals).

It is clear that cannabinoids may be effective at treating a wide range of different disorders and intractable symptoms unmanaged by established treatment options.

22.4 Side effects and contraindications

22.4.1 General points

Most drugs that cross the blood–brain barrier have a range of adverse effects, with some medicines presenting more of a problem than others. Fortunately, cannabinoids seem to be remarkably benign in terms of their side effects and there seem to be very few contraindications. However, many patients may already be using other drugs that act on the central nervous system (CNS), thereby potentially increasing the risk of side effects.

It is important to realize that care should be taken in the elderly and the frail. Also, since there has been no significant research into the effect of cannabinoids in children (<18 years old), or in pregnant or lactating women, the use in these patient groups is not advocated unless benefits outweigh the risks.

Patient and doctors are commonly concerned about the side effects and contraindications of cannabinoids. Therefore these are presented here in the form of frequently asked questions (FAQs) based on questions often asked.

22.4.2 FAQs

Are there specific physical contraindications to using medicinal cannabinoids?

Long-term clinical trials have not identified any absolute contraindications as a result of any organic disease. However, it would be wise to exercise caution in use in severe cardiovascular, liver, kidney, and immunological disease, especially in acute illness. Conversely, if a prescribed cannabinoid is controlling severe pain or spasticity etc., then stopping it suddenly may cause the patient to be plunged into a severe exacerbation of their symptoms, adding to the burden of their other medical problems.

No problems have been experienced by WN in managing patients who use medicinal cannabinoids, through some acute illnesses and anesthesia. Naturally, in time some problems may eventually be observed.

What are the common side effects of cannabinoids?

Dizziness, drowsiness, and fatigue are common side effects of using cannabinoids and they may be due to poor titration. Gastrointestinal effects of diarrhea, nausea, and dry mouth sometimes occur. More specifically, Sativex® can cause hypersalivation, unpleasant taste, and a stinging sensation as it is delivered sublingually (oromucosally). Hypotonia is also an important side effect that should be highlighted to MS patients.

Although nabilone is licensed in the US for anorexia associated with AIDS, there is no indication that it causes weight gain in human immunodeficiency virus (HIV) negative patients (Strasser et al. 2006). Similarly, the evidence from the Sativex® studies suggests that weight gain is not a significant side effect.

Can you become addicted to a cannabis medicine?

At therapeutic levels it has been shown that the abuse potential of the clinical cannabinoids is very low (Calhoun et al. 1998; Nutt et al. 2010; Schoedel et al. 2011; Ware and St Arnaud-Trempe 2010). The addiction potential of cannabinoids is also low and there is no significant withdrawal syndrome from medicinal use (Nutt et al. 2010). No evidence of tolerance to the effects of Sativex® with subsequent increased dose requirements has emerged in clinical trials to date (Robson 2011; Wade 2012).

Is previous recreational cannabis usage a contraindication?

Cannabis use is widespread. If the patient has a significant history of recreational cannabis use then the author WN will not prescribe cannabinoids. This is principally due to lack of data on prescribing in this group of patients who may continue to access illicit sources. This may render the medicinal cannabinoids less effective, since patients may look to find an endpoint of therapy in the range of the levels needed for recreational effects. Therefore the risk of misuse of a medicinal cannabinoid may be greater in this group and so this represents a strong contraindication currently.

Many patients with MS have tried using illicit cannabis, especially those with severe symptoms. Other patients have used it for a range of chronic pain problems reflecting the failure of modern medicines to provide adequate relief. Therefore if the illicit source is not suitable or is unavailable to them, then WN will consider them for a trial of treatment if they have previously obtained benefit.

Is euphoria or a "high" possible?

Euphoria is a common side effect of smoked cannabis due to high plasma levels rapidly generated by inhaling it as a vapor. Oral and oromucosal cannabinoids have a much slower onset time and plasma levels are much lower. Therefore the likelihood of a euphoric effect is also low when using these routes (Wade 2012). However, the nature of the cannabinoid used is also important and one may be more likely to see psychoactive effects when cannabidiol is not a constituent. Incautious titration may lead to a relative overload for an individual, thereby generating euphoric, dysphoric, or intoxicating effects.

What about psychosis or paranoia?

Whilst it is widely accepted that there is a modest increase in the risk of psychosis associated with the regular recreational user of cannabis (Degenhardt and Hall 2002; Henquet et al. 2005), this has not been demonstrated to be a problem for users of the medicinal preparations (Aragona et al. 2009). The likely important factors in this differentiation are the combination of much lower dosages, slower titration, and the presence of cannabidiol, alongside the different usage aims, patient age range (non-child or adolescent), and personality profiles. Even so, it is still advised that medicinal cannabinoids should be avoided in patients with significant psychiatric disorders (e.g., psychosis, substance misuse disorders, personality disorders) until further data becomes available.

However, it should be remembered that patients with MS can develop psychotic symptoms that are unrelated to their cannabinoid therapy. Psychosis is not only a well-documented feature of the disease, but is also a consequence of a urinary sepsis secondary to long-term catheter use.

What about less severe mental health problems?

Anxiety and depression are very commonly associated with chronic pain and other neurological disorders. The effective treatment of the underlying symptoms with cannabinoids may significantly improve their mental health. Panic and anxiety are side effects following overdose of cannabinoids and are therefore preventable with correct titration. These side effects are common features of uncontrolled recreational use.

Is memory affected?

Cognitive decline and amnesia are possible side effects of cannabinoids especially for the high-dose, long-term recreational user. Johns (2001) stated that acute recreational cannabis use may cause confusion and chronic use has been associated with amotivation syndrome. There is no evidence that this is a feature of medicinal cannabinoid use. It is not uncommon for patients with chronic pain to complain of an impaired memory, but this probably reflects the dominating and distracting effects of such symptoms on mental processes.

Can you become allergic to cannabinoids? Are there any drug interactions?

Allergy to cannabinoid medicines is very rare. Moreover Liu et al. (2010) has demonstrated that CBD attenuates hypersensitivity.

No evidence of significant drug interactions has emerged in the studies on medicinal cannabinoids. However, the potential for additive sedative effects when used alongside other CNS depressants is always a possibility, particularly in the frail.

Can you drive when using medicinal cannabinoids?

Different countries will have different attitudes and laws concerning driving and the use of cannabis (whether used recreationally or medicinally). Most will have yet to produce appropriate advice to patients. In the UK, it is for patients to determine their own fitness to drive and it may be the disease itself or the therapy or other medication that hinders this. Most patients manage this decision satisfactorily. Therefore the rest of this section refers to advice given to UK drivers (by author WN).

From studies of smoked cannabis in volunteers in driving simulators it has been shown (UK Transport Research Lab 2000) that the main effects of cannabis on driving are that:

- the ability to steer and maneuver may be mildly impaired
- reaction times to sudden events may be increased
- the car is driven at a slower speed as the driver is aware of impairment, which may offset any slowing of reaction times.

A good example to give to patients is for them to consider their ability to stop if a child were to run out into the street in front of them. Are they confident in their ability to stop?

Whilst it is reasonable to recognize that acute recreational cannabis consumption may increase the risk of a collision resulting in serious injury or death (Asbridge et al. 2012; Sexton et al. 2000), the likelihood of problems occurring with driving whilst using therapeutic doses is probably low. The intoxication levels in studies of therapeutic Sativex® show that these are little different from placebo (Wade 2012). However, it also seems likely that any impairment is probably well within the range of (or lower than) what is currently produced by other pharmaceutical agents which are commonly used for similar conditions (including opiates, benzodiazepines, tricyclic antidepressants, baclofen, etc.). WN cautions patients on driving not only within 4 h of cannabinoid ingestion but also if their symptoms are uncontrolled (e.g., pain, spasticity, spasms etc.).

As yet there is no roadside test of cannabis use, but unlike alcohol, any measure of the presence of cannabis within the body is not an indication that it is having a psychomotor effect. At present there is no specific information on the effect of the use of medicinal cannabis on the insurance status of the driver.

Will I put on weight?

Whilst recreational cannabis use may lead to an increased appetite, no significant problems with weight gain in clinical trials have been seen (Strasser et al. 2006).

Are cannabinoids dangerous if overdosed?

Overdose is likely to cause dizziness, drowsiness, and hypotonia. It is reassuring that in over 5,000 years there have been no recorded deaths directly due to cannabis use, even at recreational doses. It is estimated from rat studies that the lethal dose of cannabis is the equivalent of 30,000 cigarettes (Yassa et al. 2010), all smoked at the same time.

In conclusion, the side effect profile of medicinal cannabinoids is well within the spectrum of problems seen with other psychoactive medicines used in neurology, psychiatry and pain management.

22.5 **Prescribing medicinal cannabinoids**

22.5.1 **General points**

Cannabinoids are new medicines to doctors and patients alike and careful instruction in their use is essential.

The most important principle in administering cannabinoids is gradual dose titration to ensure optimum benefit with minimum side effects. It is impossible to predict the dose at which benefit or side effects will start to emerge for an individual patient and this is particularly important when other psychoactive medicines are already being used. The commonest side effects that determine dosage are drowsiness and dizziness although sometimes these will lessen over time allowing for further small dose increases.

A further valuable principle is to start dosing at nighttime, unless the patient is only symptomatic during the day. Many patients, particularly those with spasticity or pain problems, do not sleep well. Therefore the benefit to spasticity and pain may be supplemented by drowsiness at night leading to improved sleep with less fatigue and drowsiness during the day.

It is important to advise patients on the safe storage of their medicine in a similar way to opioids, especially if there are young people in the house. It is also wise for patients not to broadcast their use of medicinal cannabinoids too widely to avoid becoming a target for thieves.

22.5.2 **Nabilone**

The manufacturers of nabilone recommend a dosing of 1 or 2 mg twice a day 1–3 h before initiation of chemotherapy to try and prevent CINV. Nabilone can be given for the entire course of each chemotherapy cycle, if required. However, the side effects have limited its use and consequently it is rarely used in oncology since the introduction of 5-HT$_3$ receptor antagonists.

The awareness of the potential benefits of cannabinoids has led some clinicians from the early 1990s to explore its use, particularly for pain and spasticity. From experience, the usual starting dose has been 1 mg, the only capsule strength. However, this is often poorly tolerated due to dizziness and dysphoria, with perhaps half the patients who get benefit deciding that the side effects are not sufficiently tolerable to continue treatment (Notcutt et al. 1997).

As experience regarding the use of nabilone has grown, an approach to patient management has emerged. The use of nabilone initially only at night normally avoids the problem of drowsiness and dysphoria, with clinical benefit lasting into the day. Some patients, who obtain benefit but seem very sensitive to developing side effects, cut open the capsule and split the powder into quarters in order to be able to take a lower dose. From a pharmaceutical point of view, this practical solution is unsatisfactory and a 0.25 mg capsule would make slow and flexible titration much more accurate and acceptable.

22.5.3 **Dronabinol**

Dronabinol is not available in the UK. The principles of administration are similar to nabilone with the benefit of a range of capsule strengths (2.5, 5, 10 mg capsules) making titration easier along with the ability to customize the dose more flexibly across the 24 h period.

22.5.4 **Sativex® (nabiximols)**

The oromucosal route was developed to provide a simple alternative to oral administration which would avoid the irregularities of absorption and the "first-pass" effect of the liver, thereby enabling more convenient and accurate titration. Principally the sublingual area is recommended but some patients find this area too sensitive for the alcohol in Sativex® spray. Therefore, the buccal mucosa on the inside of the cheek is suggested as a suitable alternative. As Sativex® may stimulate salivation it is advised not to apply more than one or two sprays at a time and ideally the spray should be held in the mouth for at least 5 min or more to enable adequate absorption before swallowing or having a drink. A period of 15 min should elapse between sprays and a maximum of 12 sprays per day is advised as the limit.

To guide the initial titration of Sativex®, a simple scheme has been developed (Table 22.1). Some may consider this too slow but it has emerged as optimal to establish benefit, whilst minimizing side effects, especially if the patient is being managed as an outpatient. A faster titration is feasible if the patient is in a hospital under close supervision.

Occasionally patients find the taste of Sativex® too unpleasant and even nauseating. In these instances, swallowing it with milk or food may be a suitable compromise, although the onset of effect may be slower and a retitration is necessary.

Table 22.1 A schedule for starting Sativex® dosing. Initially the night and then the morning are targeted. However, this can be adjusted to include dosing at other times to customize according to the timing and severity of the symptoms being treated. Overall the total daily dose should not increase by more than one spray/day

Day	Morning	Evening	Total/day
1	0	1	1
2	0	1	1
3	0	2	2
4	0	2	2
5	1	2	3
6	1	3	4
7	1	4	5
8	2	4	6
9	2	5	7
10	3	5	8
11	3	6	9
12	4	6	10
13	4	7	11
14	5	7	12

22.5.5 Comparative doses

There have been no "head-to-head" studies comparing the effectiveness or dosing of the available medicinal cannabinoids. From clinical experience, 2 mg of nabilone seems to be approximately equivalent to eight sprays of Sativex®. In comparing Sativex® and dronabinol at equal THC levels the side effect profile is better with Sativex®, probably due to the presence of cannabidiol (Johnson et al. 2010). How different the therapeutic effects are from symptom to symptom may vary and also depend on the disease process.

From clinical experience (WN), it is recommended that careful titration should be undertaken when switching from one cannabinoid to another, especially if the patient is moving from illicit plant material to the medicinal.

22.5.6 Breakthrough pain, spasms

Some patients may have significant fluctuations in their symptoms, and as with slow release opiate therapy, a breakthrough dose may be required. The oral preparations are slow in onset, and nabilone is particularly difficult to use in this way because of the lack of a range of doses. Sativex® has a faster onset and is therefore more flexible. It should not be assumed that the breakthrough pain from an unrelated disease process should be treated in this way.

22.5.7 Overdose/overload

Whilst patients need to realize the importance of careful titration, significant side effects may occur. Therefore they should be informed that if dizziness, drowsiness, dysphoria, or hypotonia are a problem then lying down and resting is the best immediate treatment and symptoms will almost always resolve in 2–3 h. A subsequent dose reduction of about 25% is advised and physician guidance may need to be sought.

22.5.8 Assessing outcomes

For most patients starting to use cannabinoids for the symptoms of a chronic disease, an assessment of outcomes should occur between 2 and 4 weeks (Wade 2012). By this time a clear indication as to whether the patient is benefitting from this therapy can normally be established. For those who benefit, further "fine tuning" may be necessary to determine the optimum pattern in terms of dosing and timing across a 24 h period. For Sativex®, this may include increasing the number of uses of the spray at other times of day to establish a suitable maintenance regimen.

Those who fail to get any benefit should discontinue and no withdrawal phenomena would be expected. Sometimes a patient discovers after discontinuation that they were indeed getting benefits and these may be different to the original therapeutic targets. A retrial of therapy may therefore be justified with adjusted parameters.

Currently cannabinoids are (1) expensive and (2) still controversial (especially to non-clinicians), and therefore formal assessment of benefits is very important. Unfortunately doctors are notorious for undertaking only minimal symptom assessment often focusing more on disease progression or on side effects.

The principal scientific studies have generally focused on showing effectiveness for a single parameter (e.g., spasticity, pain, etc.). However, in practice there are often improvements across a number of different symptoms many of which may be of significant value to the patient (Box 22.1). Therefore the assessment needs to be customized to the individual.

Some have suggested that a patient should only continue with Sativex® if a 20% improvement in spasticity has been obtained. However, it can be difficult to quantify the improvement in spasticity clinically over a period of time with the same degree of accuracy achieved in clinical trials. The impact of other benefits such as a reduction in the number of spasms, an improvement in sleep, and a benefit to the partner in a reduction of their work load in caring for the patient, should all be included (Notcutt 2012b). A preliminary study on the use of nabilone and ongoing assessment showed a poor standard of evaluation of dosing, benefit, and side effects (Notcutt et al. 2011). Therefore a schedule of parameters to guide the physician/nurse evaluating the patient using a cannabinoid is being developed so that a better standard of information collection is available in ordinary clinical practice (Table 22.2). Whether one uses a numeric rating score, widely used in the formal studies of effectiveness for spasticity and pain, or simple verbal rating scores or patient and carer impressions of change, may vary according to the circumstances of cannabinoid use. To note that a patient stops screaming out in pain whenever they are being washed, is a suitable measure (patient of WN).

22.5.9 Discontinuation of cannabinoids

Patients who have been using cannabinoids on a long-term basis may wish or need to discontinue their cannabinoid either permanently or on a temporary basis to assess their symptom control. In general a short downward titration period of a few days would seem reasonable although cannabinoids may take several weeks to be completely eliminated from the body. Patients may experience a return of their symptoms but a withdrawal syndrome is very unlikely, although sleep and mood may be upset temporarily (Notcutt et al. 2012a).

Table 22.2 A schedule of potential parameters for routine clinical assessment of effects of cannabinoid therapy

Cannabinoid assessment	
Pattern of dosing	**Patient's ADLs**
Morning dose	Sleep
Midday dose	Walking
Evening dose	Transferring
Night dose	Dressing
Total/day (sprays or mg)	Washing
	Sex
	Other
Target symptom assessment (numerical rating score 0–10, verbal rating or similar)	**Carer's ADLs**
Spasticity	Sleep (carer)
Spasms	Dressing/washing (patient)
Pain problems	Transferring
Sleep	Other
Bladder dysfunction	
Other	
Side effect assessment	**Changes to other medications**
Oral mucosa (Sativex® only)	Baclofen, tizanidine
Drowsiness	Antidepressants
Dizziness	Gabapentin, pregabalin, carbamazepine, etc.
Hallucinations, dysphoria	Opioids
Other	
Unexpected benefits	**Other comments**

22.5.10 Emergency or elective admission to hospital

If a patient is admitted for an unrelated emergency condition or elective surgery then limited experience so far suggests it is acceptable to continue with cannabinoid treatment unless there is an absolute contraindication. However, this needs to be assessed on an individual basis, recognizing that symptoms of spasticity or pain may rapidly get worse thereby adding to the burden of the disease process.

Unrelated pain from an injury or disease should be treated in the normal way using conventional analgesics and the usual pain management strategies.

22.5.11 Travel abroad

If patients wish to travel abroad, they will need advice on the regulations for carrying cannabinoids into another country. An embassy should be able to provide information about the local regulations and the legality. In the UK, a Home Office license is not needed for users when leaving the country. Patients should always carry a letter detailing their travel arrangements, medical condition, and the medicines they will be carrying. A contact telephone number for the patient's general practitioner is also useful.

22.5.12 Long-term use

The long-term studies on Sativex® and the clinical experience from patients using cannabinoids for several years have indicated that the dose of cannabinoid remains relatively stable once an optimum dose has been established. Therefore any reasons for increasing the dose need to be carefully evaluated.

So far there is no evidence of long-term side effects emerging (e.g., dependency, tolerance, and mental health effects) and therefore careful assessment of any apparent new problem is essential to determine etiology. It should be remembered that new CNS symptoms may not be caused by the patient's cannabinoid therapy, but by their underlying disease.

Sativex® has been evaluated as an add-on therapy for intractable symptoms, uncontrolled by established therapies. Therefore, once the overall benefit is established, the value of any other medicines needs to be reviewed to ensure optimum management and avoid ineffective medication.

22.6 **Summary**

Although the use of cannabis as a medicine has a long history, its formal use in modern medicine is still in its infancy. Whilst there is still very little research into this class of medicines in comparison to other established medicines, the safety profile is impressive. The development of medicinal-grade products has allowed high-quality research, especially in the field of neurological disease, particularly when set against previous studies on medicines for spasticity (Shakespeare et al. 2003).

As with any new class of medicine, it takes time to establish a widespread clinical experience. This needs to start with an understanding of the basic science but sadly, teaching on the endocannabinoid system is still sparse, despite 20 years of knowledge of the system. Undoubtedly there will be more to learn on the practical use of medicinal cannabinoids as confidence in their medicinal use develops and new therapeutic areas emerge.

References

Abrams, D.I., Jay, C.A., Shade, S.B., *et al.* (2007). Cannabis in painful HIV-associated sensory neuropathy: a randomized placebo-controlled trial. *Neurology*, **68**, 515–521.

Aragona, M., Onesti, E., Tomassini, V., *et al.* (2009). Psychopathological and cognitive effects of therapeutic cannabinoids in multiple sclerosis: a double-blind, placebo controlled, crossover study. *Clinical Neuropharmacology*, **32**, 41–47.

Asbridge, M., Hayden, J.A., and Cartwright, J.L. (2012). Acute cannabis consumption and motor vehicle collision risk: systematic review of observational studies and meta-analysis. *British Medical Journal*, **344**, e536.

Blake, D.R., Robson, P., Ho, M., Jubb, R.W., and McCabe, C.S. (2006). Preliminary assessment of the efficacy, tolerability and safety of a cannabis-based medicine (Sativex) in the treatment of pain caused by rheumatoid arthritis. *Rheumatology*, **45**, 50–52.

Brady, C.M., DasGupta, R., Dalton, C., *et al.* (2004). An open-label pilot study of cannabis-based extracts for bladder dysfunction in advanced multiple sclerosis. *Multiple Sclerosis*, **10**, 425–433.

Calhoun, S.R., Galloway, G.P., and Smith, D.E. (1998). Abuse potential of dronabinol (Marinol). *Journal of Psychoactive Drugs*, **30**, 187–196.

Campbell, F.A., Tramer, M.R., Carroll, D., *et al.* (2001). Are cannabinoids an effective and safe treatment option in the management of pain? A qualitative systematic review. *British Medical Journal*, **323**, 13–16.

Cichewicz, D.L., Martin, Z.L., Smith, F.L., and Welch, S.P. (1999). Enhancement mu opioid antinociception by oral delta9-tetrahydrocannabinol: dose-response analysis and receptor identification. *Journal of Pharmacology and Experimental Therapeutics*, **289**, 859–867.

Collin, C., Ehler, E., Waberzinek, G., *et al.* (2010). A double-blind, randomized, placebo controlled, parallel-group study of Sativex, in subjects with symptoms of spasticity due to multiple sclerosis. *Neurological Research*, **32**, 451–459.

D'Souza, D.C., Abi-Saab, W.M., Madonick, S., *et al.* (2005). Delta-9-tetrahydrocannabinol effects in schizophrenia: implications for cognition, psychosis, and addiction. *Biological Psychiatry*, **57**, 594–608.

de Jong, B.C., Prentiss, D., McFarland, W., Machekano, R., and Israelski, D.M. (2005). Marijuana use and its association with adherence to antiretroviral therapy among HIV-infected persons with moderate to severe nausea. *Journal of Acquired Immune Deficiency Syndromes*, **38**, 43–46.

Degenhardt, L., and Hall, W. (2002). Cannabis and psychosis. *Current Psychiatric Reports*, **4**, 191–196.

Dunn, S.L., Wilkinson, J.M., Crawford, A., Le Maitre, C.L., and Bunning, R.A. (2012). Cannabinoids: novel therapies for arthritis? *Future Medicinal Chemistry*, **4**, 713–725.

Ellis, R.J., Toperoff, W., Vaida, F., *et al.* (2009). Smoked medicinal cannabis for neuropathic pain in HIV: a randomized, crossover clinical trial. *Neuropsychopharmacology*, **34**, 672–680.

Esfandyari, T., Camilleri, M., Busciglio, I., *et al.* (2007). Effects of a cannabinoid receptor agonist on colonic motor and sensory functions in humans: a randomized, placebo-controlled study. *American Journal of Physiology – Gastrointestinal and Liver Physiology*, **293**, 137–145.

Esfandyari, T., Camilleri, M., Ferber, I., *et al.* (2006). Effect of a cannabinoid agonist on gastrointestinal transit and postprandial satiation in healthy human subjects: a randomized, placebo-controlled study. *Neurogastroenterology and Motility*, **18**, 831–838.

Flynn, J. and Hanif, N. (1992). Nabilone for the management of intractable nausea and vomiting in terminally staged AIDS. *Journal of Palliative Care*, **8**, 46–47.

Ganon-Elazar, E. and Akirav, I. (2009). Cannabinoid receptor activation in the basolateral amygdala blocks the effects of stress on the conditioning and extinction of inhibitory avoidance. *Journal of Neuroscience*, **29**, 11078–11088.

Gloss, D. and Vickrey, B. (2012). Cannabinoids for epilepsy. *Cochrane Database of Systematic Reviews*, **6**, CD009270.

Grotenhermen, F. (2001). Harm reduction associated with inhalation and oral administration of cannabis and THC. *Journal of Cannabis Therapy*, **1**, 133–152.

Grotenhermen, F. (2003). Pharmacokinetics and pharmacodynamics of cannabinoids. *Clinical Pharmacokinetics*, **42**, 327–360.

Grotenhermen F. and Müller-Vahl, K. (2012). The therapeutic potential of cannabis and cannabinoids. *Deutsches Arzteblatt International*, **109**, 495–501.

Hall, W. (1998). The respiratory risks of cannabis smoking. *Addiction*, **93**, 1461–1463.

Haney, M., Gunderson, E.W., Rabkin, J., *et al.* (2007). Dronabinol and marijuana in HIV-positive marijuana smokers. Caloric intake, mood, and sleep. *Journal of Acquired Immune Deficiency Syndromes*, **45**, 545–554.

Henquet, C., Krabbendam, L., Spauwen, J., *et al.* (2005). Prospective cohort study of cannabis use, predisposition for psychosis, and psychotic symptoms in young people. *British Medical Journal*, **330**, 11.

Henry, J.A., Oldfield, W.L.G., and Kon, O.M. (2003). Comparing cannabis with tobacco. *British Medical Journal*, **326**, 942–943.

Hoffman, D.E. and Weber, E. (2010). Medical marijuana and the law. *New England Journal of Medicine*, **362**, 1453–1456.

Holdcroft, A., Mervyn, M., Dore, C., Tebbs, S., and Thompson, S. (2006). A multicenter dose-escalation study of the analgesic and adverse effects of an oral cannabis extract (cannador) for postoperative pain management. *Anesthesiology*, **104**, 1040–1046.

Jiang, W., Zhang, Y., Xiao, L., *et al.* (2005). Cannabinoids promote embryonic and adult hippocampus neurogenesis and produce anxiolytic and antidepressant-like effects. *Journal of Clinical Investigation*, **115**, 3104–3116.

Johns, A. (2001). Pyschiatric effects of cannabis. *The British Journal of Psychiatry*, **178**, 116–122.

Johnson, J.R., Burnell-Nugent, M., Lossignol, D., *et al.* (2010). Multicenter, double-blind, randomized, placebo-controlled, parallel-group study of the efficacy, safety, and tolerability of THC: CBD extract and

THC extract in patients with intractable cancer-related pain. *Journal of Pain and Symptom Management*, **39**, 167–179.

Jones, N.A., Hill, A.J., Smith, I., *et al.* (2010). Cannabidiol displays antiepileptiform and antiseizure properties in vitro and in vivo. *Journal of Pharmacology and Experimental Therapeutics*, **332**, 569–577.

Karst, M., Wippermann, S., and Ahrens, J. (2010). Role of cannabinoids in the treatment of pain and (painful) spasticity. *Drugs*, **70**, 2409–2438.

Leweke, F.M., Giuffrida, A., Koethe, D., *et al.* (2007). Anandamide levels in cerebrospinal fluid of first-episode schizophrenic patients: impact of cannabis use. *Schizophrenia Research*, **94**, 29–36.

Liu, D.Z., Hu, C.M., Huang, C.H., Wey, S.P., and Jan, T.R. (2010). Cannabidiol attenuates delayed-type hypersensitivity reactions via suppressing T-cell and macrophage reactivity. *Acta Pharmacoligica Sinica*, **31**, 1611–1617.

Lynch, M.E. and Campbell, F. (2011). Cannabinoids for treatment of chronic non-cancer pain; a systematic review of randomized trials. *British Journal of Clinical Pharmacology*, **72**, 735–744.

Meek, C. (1994). Doctors want cannabis prescriptions allowed. *British Medical Association News Review*, **15** February, 15.

Meiri, E., Jhangiani, H., Vredenburgh, J.J., *et al.* (2007). Efficacy of dronabinol alone and in combination with ondansetron versus ondansetron alone for delayed chemotherapy-induced nausea and vomiting. *Current Medical Research and Opinion*, **23**, 533–543.

Naftali, T., Bar Lev, L., Yablekovitz, D., Half, E., and Konikoff, F.M. (2011). Treatment of Crohn's disease with cannabis: an observational study. *Israel Medical Association Journal*, **13**, 455–458.

Notcutt, W., Langford, R., Davies, P., Ratcliffe, S., and Potts, R. (2012a). A placebo-controlled, parallel-group, randomized withdrawal study of subjects with symptoms of spasticity due to multiple sclerosis who are receiving long-term Sativex® (nabiximols). *Multiple Sclerosis*, **18**, 219–228.

Notcutt, W., Price, M., and Chapman, G. (1997). Clinical experience with nabilone for chronic pain. *Pharmaceutical Sciences*, **3**, 551–555.

Notcutt, W., Price, M., Miller, R., *et al.* (2004). Initial experiences with medicinal extracts of cannabis for chronic pain: results from 34 'N of 1' studies. *Anaesthesia*, **59**, 440–452.

Notcutt, W.G. (2012b). A questionnaire survey of patients and carers of patients prescribed Sativex as an unlicensed medicine. *Primary Health Care Research and Development*, **12**, 1–8.

Notcutt, W.G., Rocket, M., Zajicek, J., and Muthusamy, K. (2011). A retrospective description of the use of nabilone in UK clinical practice. *British Pain Society Annual Scientific Meeting, Poster Presentation*.

Novotna, A., Mares, J., Ratcliffe, S., *et al.* (2011). A randomized, double-blind, placebo-controlled, parallel-group, enriched-design study of nabiximols (Sativex), as add-on therapy, in subjects with refractory spasticity caused by multiple sclerosis. *European Journal of Neurology*, **18**, 1122–1131.

Nurmikko, T.J., Serpell, M.G., Hoggart, B., *et al.* (2007). Sativex successfully treats neuropathic pain characterised by allodynia: a randomised, double-blind, placebo-controlled clinical trial. *Pain*, **133**, 210–220.

Nutt, D.J., King, L.A., and Phillips, L.D., Independent Scientific Committee on Drugs. (2010). Drug harms in the UK: a multicriteria decision analysis. *Lancet*, **376**, 1558–1565.

Pertwee, R.G. (2004). The pharmacology and therapeutic potential of cannabidiol. In: V. Di Marzo (ed.). *Cannabinoids*. New York: Kluwer Academic/Plenum Publishers, pp. 32–83.

Portenoy, R.K., Ganae-Motan, E.D., Allende, S., *et al.* (2012). Nabiximols for opioid-treated cancer patients with poorly-controlled chronic pain: a randomized, placebo-controlled, graded-dose trial. *The Journal of Pain*, **13**, 438–449.

Robson, P. (2011). Abuse potential and psychoactive effects of d-9-tetrahydrocannabinol and cannabidiol oromucosal spray (Sativex), a new cannabinoid medicine. *Expert Opinion on Drug Safety*, **10**, 675–685.

Rog, D.J., Nurmikko, T.J., Friede, T., and Young, C.A. (2005). Randomized, controlled trial of cannabis based medicine in central pain in multiple sclerosis. *Neurology*, **65**, 812–819.

Roser, P. and Haussleiter, I.S. (2012). Antipsychotic-like effects of cannabidiol and rimonabant: systematic review of animal and human studies. *Current Pharmaceutical Design*, **32**, 5141–5155.

Russo, E. (2004). Clinical endocannabinoid deficiency (CECD): can this concept explain therapeutic benefits of cannabis in migraine, fibromyalgia, irritable bowel syndrome and other treatment-resistant conditions? *Neuroendocrinology Letters*, **25**, 31–39.

Russo, E. and Guy, G.W. (2006). A tale of two cannabinoids: the therapeutic rationale for combining tetrahydrocannabinol and cannabidiol. *Medical Hypotheses*, **66**, 234–246.

Schoedel, K.A., Chen, N., Hilliard, A., *et al.* (2011). A randomized, double blind, placebo controlled, crossover study to evaluate the subjective abuse potential and cognitive effects of nabiximols oromucosal spray in subjects with a history of recreational cannabis use. *Human Psychopharmacology: Clinical and Experimental*, **26**, 224–236.

Scotter, E.L., Abood, M.E., and Glass, M. (2010). The endocannabinoid system as a target for the treatment of neurodegenerative disease. *British Journal of Pharmacology*, **160**, 480–498.

Seeling, W., Kneer, L., Büchele, B., *et al.* (2006). Delta(9)-tetrahydrocannabinol and the opioid receptor agonist piritramide do not act synergistically in postoperative pain. *Anaesthesist*, **55**, 391–400.

Serpell, M., Notcutt, W., and Collin, C. (2013). Sativex long-term use: an open-label trial in patients with spasticity due to multiple sclerosis. *Journal of Neurology*, **260**, 285–295.

Sexton, B.F., Tunbridge, R.J., Brook-Carter, N., *et al.* (2000). *The Influence Of Cannabis On Driving*. Report 477. London: UK Department of the Environment. Available at: http://www.erowid.org/plants/cannabis/cannabis_driving6.pdf.

Shakespeare, D.T., Boggild, M., and Young, C. (2003). Anti-spasticity agents for multiple sclerosis. *Cochrane Database of Systematic Reviews*, **4**, CD001332.

Skrabek, R.Q., Galimova, L., Ethans, K., and Perry, D. (2008). Nabilone for the treatment of pain in fibromyalgia. *Journal of Pain*, **9**, 164–173.

Strasser, F., Luftner, D., Possinger, K., *et al.* (2006). Comparison of orally administered cannabis extract and delta-9-tetrahydrocannabinol in treating patients with cancer-related anorexia-cachexia syndrome: a multicenter, phase III, randomized, double-blind, placebo-controlled clinical trial from the Cannabis-In-Cachexia-Study-Group. *Journal of Clinical Oncology*, **24**, 3394–400.

Vermersch, P. (2011). Sativex® (Tetrahydrocannabinol + cannabidiol), an endocannabinoid system modulator: basic features and main clinical data. *Expert Review of Neurotherapeutics*, **11**, 15–19.

Wade, D. (2012). Evaluation of the safety and tolerability profile of Sativex: is it reassuring enough? *Expert Review of Neurotherapeutics*, **12**, 9–14.

Wade, D.T., Collin, C., Stott, C., and Duncombe, P. (2010). Meta-analysis of the efficacy and safety of Sativex (nabiximols), on spasticity in people with multiple sclerosis. *Multiple Sclerosis*, **16**, 707–714.

Ware, M.A., Fitzcharles, M.A., Joseph, L., and Shir, Y. (2010). The effects of nabilone on sleep in fibromyalgia: results of a randomized controlled trial. *Anesthesia and Analgesia*, **110**, 604–610.

Ware, M.A. and St Arnaud-Trempe, E. (2010). The abuse potential of the synthetic cannabinoid nabilone. *Addiction*, **105**, 494–503.

Yassa, H.A., Dawood Ael, W., Shehata, M.M., Abdel-Hady, R.H., and Aal, K.M. (2010). Subchronic toxicity of cannabis leaves on male albino rats. *Human and Experimental Toxicology*, **29**, 37–47.

Zajicek, J., Fox, P., Sanders, H., *et al.* (2003). Cannabinoids for treatment of spasticity and other symptoms related to multiple sclerosis (CAMS study): multicentre randomised placebo-controlled trial. *Lancet*, **362**, 1517–1526.

Zajicek, J.P., Hobart, J.C., Slade, A., Barnes, D., and Mattison, P.G. (2012). Multiple sclerosis and extract of cannabis: results of the MUSEC trial. *Journal of Neurology, Neurosurgery and Psychiatry*, **83**, 1125–1132.

Part 4

Approved Therapeutic Targets for Phytocannabinoids: Preclinical Pharmacology

Marnie Duncan

Part 4 Overview

In Chapter 23, Rock, Sticht, and Parker review the effects of cannabinoids on nausea and vomiting. The authors highlight nausea as an area of the unmet medical need. They review the preclinical data for phytocannabinoids such as cannabidiol (CBD), cannabidiolic acid (CBDA), tetrahydrocannabinolic acid (THCA), and cannabidivarin (CBDV), which show efficacy in preclinical models of nausea and vomiting.

In Chapter 24, Cristino and Di Marzo provide an extensive review of the endocannabinoid system in the homeostatic regulation of food intake. They describe the effects of cannabinoids on appetite and suggest that these compounds may represent therapeutic candidates for the treatment of cachexia and anorexia.

In Chapter 25, Costa and Comelli review the large body of literature on the analgesic actions of THC and cover the possible interaction between the opioid and cannabinoid systems. The authors also present preclinical evidence that the non-psychoactive phytocannabinoids CBD, tetrahydrocannabivarin (THCV), cannabigerol (CBG), and cannabichromene (CBC) may be possible candidates for the treatment of pain.

In Chapter 26, Pryce and Baker provide an extensive overview of the disease progression of the various types of multiple sclerosis (MS) and the underlying pathologies. The authors describe the body of clinical evidence of cannabinoids in MS and highlight the difficulties in measuring beneficial effects in clinical trials.

Chapter 23

Effect of Phytocannabinoids on Nausea and Vomiting

Erin M. Rock, Martin A. Sticht, and Linda A. Parker

23.1 Introduction

As has been reviewed elsewhere, *Cannabis sativa* has been used as a medicine for over 5000 years (see Hanus and Mechoulam 2005; Iversen 2008). Only much more recently was the psychoactive cannabinoid, delta-9-tetrahydrocannabinol (Δ^9-THC), discovered (Gaoni and Mechoulam 1964a). Since this discovery, over 60 unique terpeno-phenols have been derived from the cannabis plant, which Mechoulam (2007) describes as a "neglected pharmacological treasure trove." There has been little investigation of these neglected compounds until very recently. In this chapter, recent findings on the potential of phytocannabinoids to reduce nausea and vomiting are reviewed. First, however, we present the history of current treatments for chemotherapy-induced nausea and vomiting, which is currently in need of specific treatments for nausea. In order to evaluate treatments for nausea, preclinical models are required. Currently available models are described here. Finally, the current status of phytocannabinoids as treatments for nausea and vomiting is reviewed, with links to more recent work on the role of the endocannabinoid (eCB) system in the regulation of nausea and vomiting.

23.2 Chemotherapy-induced nausea and vomiting

The treatment of chemotherapy-induced nausea and vomiting has been revolutionized by the discovery that antagonism of the 5-hydroxytryptamine-3 ($5\text{-}HT_3$) receptor suppresses acute vomiting induced by cisplatin in the ferret and the shrew (e.g., Costall et al. 1986; Miner and Sanger 1986; Torii et al. 1991). Treating human patients with $5\text{-}HT_3$ receptor antagonists combined with the corticosteroid, dexamethasone, has reduced the incidence of acute vomiting (within 18–24 h post treatment) by 70% (e.g., Hickok et al. 2003). The $5\text{-}HT_3$ receptor antagonists are less effective at suppressing acute nausea (e.g., only 18% reported nausea relief) than they are at suppressing acute vomiting and they are ineffective in reducing delayed (over 24 h later, e.g., Hesketh et al. 2003) and anticipatory (conditioned) nausea and vomiting (e.g., Ballatori and Roila 2003; Hickok et al. 2003; Morrow and Dobkin 1988; Nesse et al. 1980) when they occur. The development of the Neurokinin 1 (NK_1) receptor antagonists (e.g., aprepitant) has further aided in the suppression of acute vomiting, and decreased delayed vomiting resulting from cisplatin-based chemotherapy (e.g., Van Belle et al. 2002). Still however, even combined treatment with a $5\text{-}HT_3$ receptor antagonist, a NK_1 receptor antagonist and dexamethasone is essentially ineffective in reducing acute and delayed nausea (e.g., Hickok et al. 2003; Poli-Bigelli et al. 2003), which are the symptoms reported to be the most distressing to cancer patients undergoing chemotherapy together with $5\text{-}HT_3$ receptor antagonist treatment (de Boer-Dennert et al. 1997). None of these treatments are effective in reducing anticipatory nausea when it occurs. Therefore, nausea (acute, delayed, and anticipatory) continues to be a challenge for available pharmacotherapies.

Patients report that nausea is more distressing than vomiting (e.g., de Boer-Dennert et al. 1997; Foubert and Vaessen 2005). Indeed, this continuous distressing symptom associated with chemotherapy treatment (even when vomiting is pharmacologically controlled) can become so severe that as many as 20% of patients discontinue their treatment (Jordan et al. 2005). Furthermore, several studies have found that both physicians and nurses tend to underestimate the prevalence of nausea, particularly the delayed nausea, following chemotherapy over several days (e.g., Grunberg et al. 2004; Liau et al. 2005). Therefore, new treatments for nausea are needed.

23.3 **Animal models of nausea**

Animal models of vomiting have been valuable in elucidating the neural mechanisms of the emetic reflex (e.g., Hornby 2001); however, the central mechanisms regulating nausea are still not well understood (e.g., Andrews and Horn 2006). Considerably greater progress has been made toward the control of vomiting than the control of nausea. One reason is that nausea is much more difficult to quantify than is vomiting, and therefore, preclinical model development has been challenging. Although vomiting is a gastrointestinal event under control of brainstem structures (e.g., Hornby 2001), it is generally agreed that activation of central forebrain structures is required to produce the distinct sensation of nausea. The gastrointestinal visceral inputs to the brain are well characterized (Cechetto and Saper 1987), but the way in which they are processed in the forebrain, leading to the sensation of nausea, is only beginning to be understood. The major route for visceral afferent information from the nucleus of the solitary tract (NTS) to the parabrachial nucleus (PBN) in the brainstem projects to the granular insular cortex via routes including the parvicellular thalamic nucleus (VPpc) (Cechetto and Saper 1987). Indeed the insular cortex (IC) has been termed the 'interoceptive cortex" and work in both animals (Contreras et al. 2007; Fiol et al.; Kaada 1951; Kiefer and Orr 1992; Limebeer et al. 2012; Tuerke et al. 2012a) and humans (e.g., Aziz et al. 2000; Catenoix et al. 2008; Penfield and Faulk 1955) suggests that the sensation of nausea is generated in this cortical region.

One limitation in the preclinical screening of the nauseating side effect of compounds and the potential of compounds to treat nausea has been the lack of a reliable preclinical rodent model of nausea. In the following sections we describe the current models used to determine the nauseating potential of compounds and to determine the potential of antinausea agents that reverse nausea. These models do not rely upon the use of an animal capable of vomiting and have been primarily employed in rodents, which lack an emetic reflex. Although rodents lack an emetic reflex, their gastric afferents respond in the same manner to physical and chemical (intragastric copper sulfate and cisplatin) stimulation that precedes vomiting in ferrets, presumably resulting in nausea that precedes vomiting (Billig et al. 2001; Hillsley and Grundy 1998). Indeed, 5-HT$_3$ receptor antagonists that block vomiting in ferrets also disrupts this preceding neural afferent reaction in rats, suggesting that the rat detects nausea, but that the vomiting reaction may be absent in this species.

23.3.1 **Pica**

Consumption of non-nutritive kaolin clay, an example of pica (the eating of a nonfood substance), is a putative direct indicator of nausea in rodents. This consumption may ameliorate the effects of toxins in the diet (e.g., Mitchell et al. 1976; Rudd et al. 2002). Pica has been reported in several strains of rats and mice exposed to emetic compounds (e.g., Stern et al. 2011); however, in emetic species, such as the *Suncus murinus*, pica has not been demonstrated (Liu et al. 2005; Stern et al. 2011; Yamamoto et al. 2004). Pica has the advantage of being a measure of unconditioned nausea, but it has poor temporal resolution. In addition, it may be difficult to apply to a species when intake is small, and it can be produced by factors other than nausea, such as stress or pain (Burchfield et al. 1977); therefore it may not be selectively produced by nausea.

23.3.2 Lying on belly

Lying on belly (LOB) in rats (e.g., Parker et al. 1984) or flopping in ferrets (Stern et al. 2011) is another behavior that has been characterized as a nausea-induced response. In rats, this behavior has only been evaluated as a measure of lithium chloride (LiCl)-induced nausea (e.g., Bernstein et al. 1992; Contreras et al. 2007; Tuerke et al. 2012b). No other emetic agents have been evaluated using this measure. Both area postrema (AP) lesions (Bernstein et al. 1992) and visceral insular cortex (VIC) lesions (Contreras et al. 2007) reduce LiCl-induced LOB. As well, pretreatment with the 5-HT$_3$ receptor antagonist, ondansetron, reduces LiCl-induced LOB in rats (Tuerke et al. 2012b). A major limitation in this measure of nausea-induced behavior, however, is the difficulty in discriminating LOB from nonspecific locomotor suppression (e.g., Tuerke et al. 2012b); therefore, this measure may not be a specific model of nausea-induced behavior.

23.3.3 Conditioned taste avoidance

Another commonly employed rodent measure of nausea is conditioned taste avoidance learning (e.g., Garcia et al. 1974). This is not a direct measure of nausea, but relies upon a rodent's reluctance to consume flavors of foods that have been previously paired with nausea-inducing treatments. However, conditioned flavor avoidance is not a selective measure of conditioned nausea, because in the nonemetic rat, even drugs that are rewarding (such as amphetamine and cocaine) produce conditioned taste avoidance (e.g., Berger 1972; Parker 1995 for review). As well, antiemetic drugs do not necessarily prevent the establishment of conditioned taste avoidance produced by a nausea-inducing drug, such as LiCl (Limebeer and Parker 2000; Rudd et al. 1998). In the nonemetic rat, the conditioned taste avoidance measure may reflect a process more similar to conditioned fear of any treatments that change the rat's hedonic state following consumption of a novel flavored solution (see Parker et al. 2008, 2009a).

23.3.4 Conditioned gaping

23.3.4.1 Conditioned gaping to a nausea-paired flavor

Considerable recent evidence indicates that conditioned disgust (gaping) reactions elicited by exposure to a flavor previously paired with an emetic agent, such as LiCl, is a selective and sensitive rodent model of nausea (see Grill and Norgren 1978; Parker et al. 2008). Unlike conditioned taste avoidance, only drugs which produce emetic reactions in species capable of vomiting produce conditioned gaping reactions in rats when paired with a flavor. As well, antiemetic drugs consistently suppress the establishment of conditioned gaping reactions, without modifying conditioned taste avoidance (see Parker et al. 2009a). Suppression of the establishment of nausea-induced conditioned gaping reactions by the antiemetic treatment serves as a model to evaluate the potential of a treatment in reducing acute nausea. Most of the work on the effects of phytocannabinoids on nausea employs this model.

23.3.4.2 Conditioned gaping to a nausea-paired context

Interestingly, rats not only display conditioned gaping reactions when re-exposed to a flavor previously paired with a nausea-inducing drug, but they also display conditioned gaping reactions when re-exposed to a context previously paired with a nausea-inducing drug (e.g., Chan et al. 2009; Limebeer et al. 2008; Rock et al. 2008). As well, *Suncus murinus* also displays conditioned retching when re-exposed to a context previously paired with toxin-induced vomiting (Parker and Kemp 2001; Parker et al. 2006). These contextually elicited conditioned gaping or retching reactions represent animal models of anticipatory nausea analogous to that experienced by human chemotherapy patients, which can be produced following three to four conditioning trials. In human chemotherapy patients, when anticipatory nausea develops, the classic antiemetic agent ondansetron is ineffective in reducing this symptom (Hickok et al. 2003); likewise rats and shrews pretreated with ondansetron do not show a suppression of anticipatory nausea (gaping and retching reactions, respectively; Limebeer et al. 2006; Parker and Kemp 2001; Parker et al. 2006; Rock et al. 2008).

The conditioned gaping model provides a tool for evaluating the potential of a treatment to reduce both acute nausea (suppressed establishment of gaping during conditioning to a flavor) and anticipatory nausea (suppressed expression of gaping during testing to a context) in rats. This tool has the potential to reveal new treatments for these distressing symptoms that persist in human chemotherapy patients, even with the development of highly effective treatments to control vomiting.

23.4 Effects of synthetic and plant cannabinoids on nausea and vomiting

As already mentioned, there is clearly a need of treatments for acute, delayed, and anticipatory nausea in chemotherapy treatment. As well, although vomiting is well controlled by the first-line therapy, not all patients are responsive (Poli-Bigelli et al. 2003). One of the first recognized medicinal benefits of cannabis was for the treatment of nausea and vomiting (e.g., Iversen 2008). The most investigated compound has been Δ^9-THC, however, other nonpsychoactive compounds in the cannabis plant have recently been reported to also have benefits in preclinical models of nausea and vomiting. This research is reviewed here.

23.4.1 Delta-9-tetrahydrocannabinol

Δ^9-THC, the major psychoactive component in cannabis (Mechoulam et al. 1970), identified by Gaoni and Mechoulam (1964a), effectively interferes with nausea and vomiting in nonhumans (e.g., Parker et al. 2011) and in human cancer patients (see Cotter 2009 for review).

23.4.1.1 Δ^9-THC and chemotherapy-induced nausea and vomiting

Nabilone (Cesamet®) an orally active, synthetic analogue of Δ^9-THC, was licensed for management of chemotherapy-induced nausea and vomiting in 1985, but is only prescribed after conventional antiemetics fail (i.e., nabilone is not a first-line treatment). To our knowledge, studies have only compared nabilone with dopamine receptor 2 (D_2) receptor antagonists for their antiemetic/antinausea effects in chemotherapy patients. When compared with D_2 receptor antagonists, such as metoclopramide, nabilone treatment resulted in fewer vomiting episodes (Ahmedzai et al. 1983; Herman et al. 1979; Pomeroy et al. 1986; Steele et al. 1980) and reports of nausea (Ahmedzai et al. 1983; Dalzell et al. 1986; Herman et al. 1979) in patients taking moderately toxic chemotherapy treatments; however, when given to cancer patients receiving cisplatinum chemotherapy, nabilone was only as effective as the D_2 receptor antagonist in reducing vomiting (Crawford and Buckman 1986). Therefore, nabilone is superior to D_2 receptor antagonists for the treatment of moderate emesis but probably not for the treatment of severe emesis.

Another orally active, synthetic Δ^9-THC known as dronabinol (Marinol®), has also been used as an antiemetic and was later used as an appetite stimulant (Pertwee 2009). When compared with prochlorperazine (a D_2 receptor antagonist) or a combination of dronabinol and the D_2 receptor antagonist, those patients given the combination treatment had less severe nausea and the duration was significantly shorter than with either agent alone, when they were being treated with moderately emetogenic chemotherapy (Lane et al. 1991). Most recently, Namisol®, a tablet containing pure Δ^9-THC, was designed to improve absorption after ingestion. Evidence in healthy adults indicates its rapid onset may be beneficial for rapid therapeutic effects, but no clinical trials have yet been completed to demonstrate its clinical efficacy (Klumpers et al. 2012).

In cancer patients, administration of oral Δ^9-THC has been shown to significantly suppress the experience of nausea and vomiting, in comparison to placebo controls (Chang et al. 1979; Frytak et al. 1979; Orr et al. 1980; Sallan et al. 1975; Sweet et al. 1981) and when compared to the D_2 receptor antagonists available at the time, Δ^9-THC was at least as effective (Carey et al. 1983; Crawford and Buckman 1986; Cunningham et al. 1988; Frytak et al. 1979; Tramèr et al. 2001; Ungerleider et al. 1984) if not *more* effective (Ekert et al. 1979; Orr and McKernan 1981) at reducing nausea and vomiting. Only one published clinical trial has directly compared the antiemetic and antinausea effects of a cannabinoid with a $5\text{-}HT_3$ receptor antagonist. Meiri et al. (2007) compared dronabinol, ondansetron, or their combination, for efficacy in reducing delayed chemotherapy-induced nausea and vomiting. Dronabinol and ondansetron alone were equally effective in reducing nausea and vomiting, but the combined therapies were no more effective than either agent alone. When assessing severity of nausea alone, dronabinol was more effective than ondansetron for mildly to moderately severe nausea produced by chemotherapy treatments, but not for severe emetogenic treatments. However, there has been no report of a direct comparison of Δ^9-THC and the current first-line treatment of $5\text{-}HT_3$ receptor antagonist/dexamethasone/ NK_1 receptor antagonist on acute or delayed chemotherapy-induced nausea or vomiting in human chemotherapy patients.

23.4.1.2 Δ^9-THC and vomiting in animal models

The potential of Δ^9-THC to reduce toxin-induced vomiting has been demonstrated in cats, dogs, ferrets, and shrews. Early work revealed that nabilone reduced cisplatin-induced vomiting in cats (London et al. 1979; McCarthy and Borison 1981). On the other hand, neither nabilone nor Δ^9- THC suppressed cisplatin- or apomorphine-induced vomiting in dogs (Gylys et al. 1979; Shannon et al. 1979). In the ferret, Δ^9-THC (0.5–1 mg/kg, intraperitoneally (i.p.)) and the synthetic CB_1 receptor agonist, WIN55,212-2, effectively suppressed vomiting produced by both morphine- 6-glucuronide and cisplatin (Van Sickle et al. 2001, 2003) and these effects were reversed by CB_1 receptor antagonism.

The insectivorous shrews are also capable of vomiting in response to toxins. Two species recently used to evaluate the potential of Δ^9-THC and other CB_1 receptor agonists to reduce vomiting are the house musk shrew, or *Suncus murinus* (30–60 g body weight), and the much smaller least shrew, or *Cryptotis parva* (4–6 g body weight). In the house musk shrew, Δ^9-THC reduces cisplatin- (Kwiatkowska et al. 2004), LiCl- (Parker et al. 2004), and motion-induced vomiting (Cluny et al. 2008). Interestingly, when combined, subthreshold doses (those that were ineffective alone) of Δ^9-THC and ondansetron completely abolished cisplatin-induced vomiting in the house musk shrew (Kwiatkowska et al. 2004). In the tiny least shrew, Δ^9-THC (>2.5 mg/kg, i.p.) reduces acute cisplatin- (Darmani 2001a), rimonabant- (SR141716, a CB_1 receptor antagonist, Darmani 2001b), radiation- (Darmani et al. 2007) and 5-hydroxytryptophan- (an indirect 5-HT receptor agonist, Darmani and Johnson 2004) induced vomiting. Similarly, the potent CB_1 agonists, CP55,940 and

HU-210, have also been shown to suppress cisplatin-induced vomiting in least shrews (Darmani et al. 2003). As reported by Kwiatkowska et al. (2004), and more recently by Wang et al. (2009), the combination of low doses of Δ^9-THC (0.25 and 0.5 mg/kg, i.p.) and a 5-HT$_3$ receptor antagonist (ondansetron (0.025 mg/kg, i.p.) or tropisetron (0.025–0.25 mg/kg, i.p.)) respectively were more efficacious in reducing the frequency of emesis than each dose given individually, but higher doses failed to show this interaction. Since Δ^9-THC suppresses serotonin (5-HT)-induced vomiting it is possible that Δ^9-THC may be acting at CB$_1$ receptors located presynaptically on serotonergic neurons (Haring et al. 2007), possibly inhibiting 5-HT release (Darmani and Johnson 2004; Howlett et al. 2002; Schlicker and Kathmann 2001) to exert its antiemetic effects.

The antiemetic properties of CB$_1$ receptor agonists, including Δ^9-THC, are subsequently reversed by selective antagonism of CB$_1$ receptors and these effects are typically mediated by emetic brainstem structures located in the dorsal vagal complex (DVC) (see Horn 2008). For example, Darmani et al. (2003) reported that CB$_1$ receptor localization and activation following administration of CP55,940 occurred in DVC structures such as the NTS. In ferrets, cannabinoid-induced suppression of vomiting was linked to activation of CB$_1$ receptors in the DVC (Van Sickle et al. 2001), such that CB$_1$ receptor agonism reduced subsequent neuronal activation within the DVC in response to an emetic stimulus (Van Sickle et al. 2003). Taken together, CB$_1$ receptor agonists appear to exert their antiemetic effects within brainstem emetic structures of the DVC.

23.4.1.3 Δ^9-THC and acute nausea in animal models

Δ^9-THC, has also been evaluated for its potential to interfere with nausea in animal models. Although Δ^9-THC has not been specifically evaluated for its antinausea effects in the pica model of increased intake of kaolin, the synthetic CB$_1$ receptor agonist, WIN 55,212-2 did not modify pica produced by chronic administration of cisplatin (Vera et al. 2007). Using the conditioned gaping measure, Δ^9-THC (0.5 mg/kg, i.p.) and the CB$_1$ receptor agonist, HU-210 (0.001–0.1 mg/kg, i.p.) interfere with both the establishment and expression of cyclophosphamide- (Limebeer and Parker 1999) and LiCl-induced conditioned gaping (Parker and Mechoulam 2003; Parker et al. 2003), and this effect of Δ^9-THC is reversed by CB$_1$ receptor antagonists (rimonabant or AM251), indicating a CB$_1$ receptor mediation of Δ^9-THC's antinausea effects.

23.4.1.4 Δ^9-THC and anticipatory nausea in animal models

Although pretreatment with ondansetron is ineffective in reducing contextually elicited conditioned gaping, Δ^9-THC (0.5 mg/kg, i.p.) does reduce this kind of gaping in rats (Limebeer et al. 2006). Additionally, Δ^9-THC (3 mg/kg, i.p.) pretreatment prior to re-introduction to a context previously associated with LiCl-induced vomiting, suppresses the expression of conditioned retching in *Suncus murinus*, a shrew model of anticipatory nausea (Parker and Kemp 2001; Parker et al. 2006).

23.4.2 Cannabidiol

Another chemical compound in cannabis, cannabidiol (CBD), was first isolated in 1940 from Mexican marihuana by Roger Adams and from Indian charas by Alexander Todd. It was not until 1963 that Mechoulam isolated CBD from Lebanese hashish and established its structure (see Mechoulam and Hanus 2002). This nonpsychoactive cannabinoid is now available as a sublingual spray called Nabidiolex® (GW Pharmaceuticals). There are no reports of any specific evaluation of CBD alone to reduce nausea and vomiting in human chemotherapy patients.

23.4.2.1 CBD and vomiting in animal models

In the house musk shrew, CBD produces a biphasic effect, at low doses (5 and 10 mg/kg, subcutaneously (s.c.)) suppressing acute cisplatin- and LiCl induced vomiting (Rock et al. 2011, 2012), but at high doses (40 mg/kg, i.p.) potentiating (Kwiatkowska et al. 2004) or having no effect (Darmani et al. 2007) on the production of such vomiting. CBD does not attenuate motion-induced vomiting (Cluny et al. 2008), but its acid precursor (CBDA) is highly effective (Bolognini et al. 2013). The suppression of LiCl-induced vomiting was not reversed by the CB_1 receptor antagonist rimonabant (Parker et al. 2004), but was reversed by the 5-hydroxytryptamine-1A (5-HT_{1A}) receptor antagonist WAY100135 (Rock et al. 2012).

23.4.2.2 CBD and acute nausea in animal models

In rats, CBD (5 mg/kg, i.p. or s.c.) has been shown to reduce acute nausea produced by LiCl (Parker and Mechoulam 2003: Parker et al. 2002; Rock et al. 2011, 2012). The CBD-induced suppression of acute nausea is reversed by administration of the 5-HT_{1A} antagonists WAY100135 and WAY100635 (Rock et al. 2012). In addition, when administered directly to the dorsal raphe nucleus (DRN), CBD (10 micrograms) completely abolished LiCl-induced conditioned gaping and this effect was blocked by systemic administration of WAY100635. Conversely, systemic administration of CBD was blocked by intra-DRN administration of WAY100635, but not when WAY100635 was administered outside of the DRN. Furthermore, combined subthreshold doses of CBD and 8-hydroxy-2-(di-n-propylamino) tetralin (8-OH-DPAT, a 5-HT_{1A} receptor agonist) enhanced suppression of acute nausea, above that of either agent alone. CBD also displayed significant potency (with a bell shaped dose-response curve) at enhancing the ability of 8-OH-DPAT to stimulate [^{35}S]GTPγS binding to rat brainstem membranes in vitro. Taken together, these results indicate a 5-HT_{1A} receptor-linked mechanism of action for CBD's antinausea properties. More specifically, it seems that CBD may be acting at somatodendritic 5-HT_{1A} autoreceptors located in the DRN to reduce the release of 5-HT in forebrain regions (e.g., possibly the interoceptive insular cortex (Tuerke et al. 2012a)) to ultimately suppress toxin-induced nausea and vomiting.

23.4.2.3 CBD and anticipatory nausea in animal models

In addition, low doses of CBD (5 mg/kg, i.p.) but not ondansetron, have also been shown to suppress anticipatory nausea in shrews when administered prior to placement in a context previously paired with vomiting (Parker et al. 2006). In rats, CBD at low doses (1 and 5 mg/kg, i.p.) also interfered with the expression of conditioned gaping to a context previously paired with LiCl, while a higher dose (10 mg/kg, i.p.) did not (Rock et al. 2008). Therefore, CBD may be a nonpsychoactive alternative to Δ^9-THC as a treatment for anticipatory nausea in human chemotherapy patients; however, its narrow range of dose efficacy may be problematic.

23.4.3 Combined Δ^9-THC and CBD

Interestingly, there have been no reports of the evaluation of combined Δ^9-THC and CBD on emesis or nausea in animal models. However in humans, a phase II clinical trial evaluated Sativex® (an oromucosally administered cannabis-based medicine containing Δ^9-THC and CBD in a 1:1 ratio), taken in conjunction with standard antiemetic therapies (5-HT_3 receptor antagonists), for its ability to control delayed chemotherapy-induced nausea and vomiting (Duran et al. 2010). When compared with placebo, Sativex® reduced the incidence of delayed nausea and vomiting and was well tolerated by patients. Fifty-seven percent of Sativex® patients experienced no delayed nausea compared to 22% in the placebo group. In terms of emesis, 71% of Sativex® patients versus

22% of placebo patients experienced no delayed emesis. These results indicate that Δ^9-THC and CBD in combination may be useful in managing delayed nausea and vomiting in human patients.

23.4.4 Cannabidiolic acid

The nonpsychoactive carboxylic acidic precursor of CBD, cannabidiolic acid (CBDA), is present in the fresh cannabis plant and slowly loses its acidic function (decarboxylates) in the plant in response to heating (e.g., when cannabis is smoked). Recent evidence indicates that CBDA (0.1 and/or 0.5 mg/kg, i.p.) potently interferes with motion-, LiCl-, and cisplatin-induced vomiting in *Suncus murinus* (Bolognini et al. 2013). CBDA also reduced acute nausea produced by LiCl, an effect that was prevented by pretreatment with the 5-HT$_{1A}$ receptor antagonist, WAY100635, and not by rimonabant. CBDA also increased the ability of the 5-HT$_{1A}$ receptor agonist, 8-OH-DPAT, to potently stimulate [^{35}S]GTPγS binding to rat brainstem membrane, again without activating CB$_1$ receptors in vitro or in vivo. More recently, CBDA has been shown to reduce acute nausea at a dose as low as 0.5 microgram/kg (Rock and Parker 2013). As well, a subthreshold dose of CBDA (0.1 micrograms/kg, i.p.) enhanced the ability of a mildly effective dose of ondansetron (1 microgram/kg) to reduce LiCl-induced acute nausea in the rat flavor-induced gaping model.

CBDA also suppressed contextually elicited conditioned gaping in the rodent model of anticipatory nausea and this effect was also reversed by the 5-HT$_{1A}$ receptor antagonist, WAY100635 (Bolognini et al. 2013). CBDA potently suppresses nausea and vomiting in a 5-HT$_{1A}$ receptor dependent manner, suggesting that CBDA could be developed as a potent and selective treatment for nausea and vomiting, perhaps particularly for the treatment of anticipatory nausea, as there is no current therapeutic available once anticipatory nausea does develop. CBDA is also promising for development as a treatment for acute nausea, because unlike CBD, it does not potentiate nausea and/or vomiting at high doses. It is active at much lower doses than CBD, but at high doses is merely ineffective.

23.4.5 Tetrahydrocannabinolic acid

The carboxylic acidic precursor of Δ^9-THC is tetrahydrocannabinolic acid (THCA) (Gaoni and Mechoulam 1964a). In the fresh plant, THCA is decarboxylated to THC by heating or burning. Interestingly, no psychotomimetic activity was observed when THCA was administered to: rhesus monkeys at doses up to 5 mg/kg (intravenously, i.v.), mice at doses up to 20 mg/kg (i.p.), and dogs at doses up to 7 mg/kg (Grunfeld and Edery 1969).

Recent results from our laboratory (Rock et al. 2013a) indicate that THCA (0.5 and 0.05 mg/kg, i.p.) reduced LiCl-induced vomiting in *Suncus murinus*, an effect that was reversed with rimonabant pretreatment. THCA (0.5 and 0.05 mg/kg i.p.) also reduced conditioned gaping elicited by a flavor, with no effect on conditioning hedonics or conditioned taste avoidance. When administered at the lower of these two doses (0.05 mg/kg, i.p.), Δ^9-THC did not suppress conditioned gaping to a LiCl-paired flavor, or have an effect on conditioning hedonics or conditioned taste avoidance. In the anticipatory nausea paradigm, THCA (0.05 mg/kg, i.p.) suppressed conditioned gaping elicited by a context previously paired with LiCl-induced illness, while an identical low dose of Δ^9-THC (0.05 mg/kg, i.p.) did not reduce conditioned gaping to a LiCl-paired context. The effect of THCA on anticipatory nausea was reversed by pretreatment with rimonabant (2.5 mg/kg, i.p.), but not by the 5-HT$_{1A}$ receptor antagonist, WAY100635 (0.1 mg/kg, i.p.), suggesting a CB$_1$ receptor dependent mechanism of action. Thus, THCA appears to be a more potent antinausea treatment than Δ^9-THC, and to lack Δ^9-THC-like psychoactive properties.

Although our in vivo results suggest a CB_1 receptor-mediated mechanism for THCA's effects, the few published in vitro studies to date do not seem to support this finding. In vitro studies have revealed that THCA's ability to inhibit the tumor necrosis factor alpha (TNF-α) in culture supernatants from U937 macrophages was not blocked by administration of the CB_1 receptor antagonist AM281, or the cannabinoid receptor type 2 (CB_2) receptor antagonist AM630 (Verhoeckx et al. 2006). In addition, binding assays indicate that THCA is not active at the CB_1 receptor (Ahmed et al. 2008). Further studies about THCA's mechanism of action are needed. These latest results indicate that THCA may also be a better therapeutic treatment for nausea and vomiting than Δ^9-THC.

23.4.6 Tetrahydrocannabivarin

Tetrahydrocannabivarin (THCV), identified in the 1970s (Gill et al. 1970; Merkus 1971) was initially described as sharing the ability of Δ^9-THC to produce signs of catalepsy in the mouse ring mobility test (Gill et al. 1970) and to produce mild Δ^9-THC-like effects in humans (Hollister 1974). More recently, synthetic THCV (0–4394) at doses greater than 10 mg/kg i.v., was shown to resemble the effects of Δ^9-THC on catalepsy, and to induce antinociception in the tail-flick test (Pertwee et al. 2007); this latter effect was reversed with rimonabant (3 mg/kg, i.p.).

THCV effects are dose dependent, with lower doses (2.5 mg/kg, i.v.) of THCV acting as a CB_1 receptor antagonist (Pertwee et al. 2007). At low doses, THCV blocks the effects of Δ^9-THC. More specifically, 0–4394 attenuates Δ^9-THC induced hypothermia at 0.3 and 3 mg/kg, i.v. and Δ^9-THC-induced antinociception in the tail-flick test at 3 mg/kg, i.v. (Pertwee et al. 2007). There is also evidence that THCV shares the ability of AM251 to reduce food intake and body weight of nonfasted and fasted nonobese mice (Riedel 2009).

The low-dose THCV (0–4394) effects of CB_1 receptor antagonism, in contrast to rimonabant, are devoid of inverse agonist activity in the $[^{35}S]$GTPγS-binding assay in mouse whole-brain membranes (Pertwee et al. 2007). Indeed, unlike rimonabant, THCV is also devoid of anxiogenic activity in the light/dark immersion test and does not reduce saccharin palatability in the taste reactivity test (O'Brien et al. 2012). Interestingly, the CB_1 receptor neutral antagonists, AM6545 and AM6527, also do not modify saccharin palatability in the taste reactivity test, unlike AM251 (Limebeer et al. 2010). Furthermore, THCV (2.5–20 mg/kg, i.p.), unlike rimonabant (10 mg/kg, i.p.) did not produce nausea in the gaping model.

Evaluation of the effects of THCV and rimonabant on the establishment of LiCl-induced conditioned gaping (Rock et al. 2013b) revealed that unlike rimonabant (2.5 mg/kg, i.p.), which enhances LiCl-induced conditioned gaping reactions, THCV (10 or 20 mg/kg, but not 2.5 mg/kg, i.p.) reduces LiCl-induced conditioned gaping, as does the CB_1 receptor agonist, Δ^9-THC (Limebeer and Parker 1999). This finding supports previous research suggesting that THCV may act as a CB_1 receptor agonist at high doses (Pertwee et al. 2007; Thomas et al. 2005). At a low dose of 2.5 mg/kg, i.p., THCV did not potentiate LiCl-induced acute nausea, unlike rimonabant, again providing evidence that this phytocannabinoid does not act as a CB_1 receptor inverse agonist. The CB_1 receptor inverse agonists, rimonabant and AM251, potentiate LiCl-induced nausea at doses below those that produce nausea on their own, unlike the CB_1 receptor neutral antagonists, AM4113, AM6545, or AM6527 (Cluny et al. 2010; Limebeer et al. 2010; McLaughlin et al. 2005; Sink et al. 2008). Therefore, at low doses, THCV acts as a neutral CB_1 receptor antagonist, but at high doses it may act as a CB_1 receptor agonist, reducing nausea like a low dose of Δ^9-THC (0.5 mg/kg, i.p.). Future studies need to further examine the dose-dependent effects of THCV on nausea and vomiting in animal models.

23.4.7 **Cannabidivarin**

In the cannabis plant, cannabidivarin (CBDV) is the precursor of THCV, and under acidic conditions, CBDV isomerizes into THCV (Deiana et al. 2012). Recent evidence from our laboratory (Rock et al. 2013b) shows that CBDV (10 or 200 mg/kg, i.p.) attenuated LiCl-induced gaping reactions and does not act as a CB_1 receptor inverse agonist; that is it neither produced gaping on its own, nor potentiated LiCl-induced gaping reactions (Rock et al. 2013b). Therefore it seems that this phytocannabinoid may be a promising therapeutic, devoid of symptoms associated with CB_1 receptor inverse agonism.

23.4.8 **Cannabigerol**

Cannabigerol (CBG) is another nonpsychoactive component found in cannabis (Gaoni and Mechoulam 1964b; Mechoulam et al. 1970), but little work has focused on this agent. Recently, in vitro (Cascio et al. 2010) and in vivo (Rock et al. 2011) data have indicated that CBG may be acting as a $5\text{-}HT_{1A}$ receptor antagonist because CBG (5 mg/kg, i.p.) blocked the CBD- (5 mg/kg, i.p.) and 8-OH-DPAT- (0.01 mg/kg, s.c.) induced suppression of LiCl-induced gaping (Rock et al. 2011). Furthermore, CBG (5 mg/kg, i.p.) also reversed the CBD- (5 mg/kg, i.p.) induced suppression of LiCl-induced vomiting in house musk shrews. Therefore, it seems that CBG and CBD can both target $5\text{-}HT_{1A}$ receptors, although with opposite actions, to modulate the effects of these receptors on nausea and vomiting.

23.5 **Endocannabinoids and nausea and vomiting**

Endogenously produced cannabinoids, or endocannabinoids (eCBs) have also been shown to have antiemetic and antinausea effects. The eCBs consist of the lipid messengers N-arachidonoylethanolamine, or anandamide (Devane et al. 1992), and 2-arachidonoylglycerol (2-AG) (Mechoulam et al. 1995), which are synthesized in an activity-dependent manner from N-arachidonoyl phosphatidylethanolamine and 1, 2-diacylglycerol, respectively (Piomelli 2003). Once released, endocannabinoids bind to metabotropic CB_1 or CB_2 receptors located on presynaptic axon terminals, resulting in inhibition of neurotransmitter release (Piomelli 2003), followed by carrier-mediated transport into the postsynaptic cell and enzymatic hydrolysis (Deutsch and Chin 1993; Di Marzo et al. 1994). Anandamide is hydrolyzed by the enzyme fatty acid amide hydrolase (FAAH) (Cravatt et al. 1996), whereas 2-AG is degraded primarily by monoacylglycerol-lipase (MAGL) (Dinh et al. 2002).

23.5.1 **Endocannabinoids as endogenous modulators of emesis**

Much like the antiemetic and antinausea properties of synthetic and plant-based cannabinoids, endocannabinoids also suppress emesis in a number of animal models. Administration of exogenous anandamide has been shown to reduce toxin-induced vomiting in ferrets (Sharkey et al. 2007; Van Sickle et al. 2005) and suppress vomiting in least shrews (Darmani 2002), along with its stable analogue, methanandamide (Darmani 2002; Van Sickle et al. 2001). Similarly, by prolonging the action of endogenously released anandamide, the FAAH inhibitor, URB597, has been shown to interfere with cisplatin- and nicotine-induced vomiting in *Suncus murinus* (Parker et al. 2009b), and in ferrets (Sharkey et al. 2007; Van Sickle et al. 2005). In all cases, the antiemetic effects were blocked by a CB_1 receptor antagonist/inverse agonist indicating a CB_1 receptor-dependent mechanism of action of anandamide in suppressing vomiting. Unlike anandamide, however, the role of 2-AG in emesis remains less clear.

The earliest reports of exogenous 2-AG administration suggested that this particular endocannabinoid played a functionally opposite role in modulating emesis compared to that of anandamide. Specifically, Darmani and colleagues (2002) reported that administration of exogenous 2-AG alone dose-dependently (0.25–10 mg/kg, i.p.) produced vomiting among least shrews, an effect that was blocked by the CB_1 receptor antagonist/inverse agonist, rimonabant, and in a subsequent study revealed that brain 2-AG levels were increased following cisplatin-induced vomiting (Darmani et al. 2005). Interestingly, pretreatment with anandamide partially blocked the emetic effects of 2-AG (Darmani 2002). Thus, among least shrews, 2-AG appears to be a highly emetogenic endocannabinoid.

However, opposite effects have been reported in other animal models. Van Sickle et al. (2005) found that a low dose of 2-AG (0.5 mg/kg, i.p.) attenuated toxin-induced vomiting in ferrets when combined with the cannabinoid re-uptake inhibitor, VDM11, while higher doses (1–2 mg/kg, i.p.) were capable of blocking vomiting alone (Sharkey et al. 2007; Van Sickle et al. 2005). Interestingly, the antiemetic effects of 2-AG were reversed not only by CB_1 receptor blockade, but also by a CB_2 receptor antagonist (Van Sickle et al. 2005), which is particularly interesting given that the effects of anandamide are not reversed by CB_2 receptor antagonism (Van Sickle et al. 2005). More recently, Sticht et al. (2012) demonstrated similar antiemetic effects associated with increased endogenous 2-AG levels. Administration of the selective MAGL inhibitor, JZL184, dose-dependently suppressed LiCl-induced vomiting in *Suncus murinus*, whereby the suppression of vomiting was mediated through a CB_1 receptor-dependent mechanism of action (Sticht et al. 2012). Although it is unclear whether exogenous 2-AG administration leads to similar antiemetic effects in house musk shrews, or precisely how higher doses of 2-AG modulate toxin-induced vomiting in ferrets, the conflicting reports regarding the effects of 2-AG on vomiting may point to important species differences in emesis.

23.5.2 Role of the endocannabinoid system in nausea

In addition to their powerful antiemetic properties, eCBs are equally effective in reducing conditioned nausea in rats. Inhibition of FAAH-mediated hydrolysis of anandamide has been shown to suppress LiCl-induced conditioned gaping in rats, with an even greater suppressive effect upon coadministration with exogenous anandamide (Cross-Mellor et al. 2007). Similarly, URB597 was found to interfere with both the establishment and expression of conditioned gaping to an illness-paired context in the rat model of anticipatory nausea (Rock et al. 2008). In either model, the effects of anandamide on conditioned gaping were CB_1 receptor mediated as pretreatment with a CB_1 receptor antagonist reversed the antinausea effects of increased anandamide levels.

The endocannabinoid, 2-AG, like anandamide, also appears to reduce nausea in rats. Specifically, pretreatment with exogenous 2-AG was shown to dose-dependently suppress the establishment of conditioned gaping (Sticht et al. 2012). However, unlike the antinausea effects of anandamide, those of 2-AG do not seem to be entirely dependent on CB_1 receptors since they can be reversed by the cyclooxygenase (COX) inhibitor, indomethacin (Sticht et al. 2012), but not by the CB_1 or CB_2 receptor antagonists, AM-251 and AM630, respectively. Interestingly, the suppression of conditioned gaping following concomitant pretreatment with the MAGL inhibitor, JZL184, and exogenous 2-AG was partially reversed by a CB_1 receptor antagonist (Sticht et al. 2012), suggesting that decreased 2-AG turnover reduces nausea, in part, through an action at CB_1 receptors. Nonetheless, the finding that COX inhibition blocks the antinausea effects of 2-AG serves to highlight the dynamic nature of eCB suppression of nausea, such that 2-AG acts through several potential mechanisms to modulate this sensation. Further research will likely clarify the precise role of downstream eCB metabolites in the suppression of nausea.

Whereas the antinausea effects of cannabinoids are reversed by relatively low doses of CB_1 receptor antagonists/inverse agonists, higher doses alone are sufficient to produce nausea. For example, high doses of AM251 were found to not only suppress food intake in rats, but also induce conditioned gaping upon re-exposure to the AM251-paired taste (McLaughlin et al. 2005). More recently, Limebeer et al. (2010) reported that compared to controls, rats pretreated with a low dose of AM251 (2.5 mg/kg, i.p.) displayed a greater frequency of conditioned gaping upon re-exposure to LiCl-paired saccharin, whereas rats treated with AM251 alone did not display conditioned gaping. That is, a low dose of AM251 (2.5 mg/kg, i.p.) potentiated the illness-inducing effects of LiCl in rats, albeit without producing conditioned gaping on its own (Limebeer et al. 2010). A similar potentiation of LiCl-induced conditioned gaping was demonstrated with the CB_1 receptor antagonist/inverse agonist, rimonabant, as well (Parker et al. 2003). It is important to point out that a mere blockade of CB_1 receptors is not sufficient to produce nausea on its own; the neutral CB_1 receptor antagonist, AM4113, alone did not produce conditioned gaping in rats when paired directly with saccharin in the taste reactivity test (Sink et al. 2008), nor did the peripherally restricted drug, AM6545, or the central/peripheral neutral receptor antagonist, AM6527, potentiate conditioned gaping either (Limebeer et al. 2010). Therefore, CB_1 receptor antagonism alone is not sufficient to produce nausea in rats, but rather inverse agonism of this receptor is associated with malaise.

23.5.3 Endocannabinoids in human nausea and vomiting

Investigations surrounding the role of the eCB system in nausea and vomiting have typically relied on a number of animal models, and, therefore, human data concerning eCB involvement has been rather scarce. However, recent research by Schelling and colleagues suggests that the eCB system, indeed, acts to modulate nausea and vomiting in humans. Specifically, Choukèr et al. (2010) reported that motion sickness corresponded with lower blood eCB levels among participants undergoing parabolic flight maneuvers (PFs), whereas anandamide and 2-AG levels were higher among participants who did not experience motion sickness. Moreover, CB_1 receptor expression was reduced among participants experiencing motion sickness compared to those unaffected by PFs, who did not show any change in CB_1 receptor expression from baseline values. Interestingly, anandamide increases were observed early on during PFs, whereas 2-AG levels were highest following the in-flight maneuvers, suggesting that eCBs may play different roles in reducing both motion sickness and stress induced by PFs (Choukèr et al. 2010).

23.6 Conclusion

Only recently have the potential therapeutic benefits of phytocannabinoids, other than psychoactive Δ^9-THC, been scientifically evaluated, yet the cannabis plant has been used medicinally for centuries. Here we provide evidence that several nonpsychoactive phytocannabinoids (CBD, CBDA, THCA, and CBDV) possess therapeutic potential for the treatment of nausea and vomiting.

Acknowledgments

We would like to thank NSERC (Grant #92057) and GW Pharmaceuticals for their support of this work, and, in particular GW Pharmaceuticals for access to several compounds that we have evaluated in the experiments reviewed here.

References

Ahmed, S.A., Ross, S.A., Slade, D., *et al.* (2008). Cannabinoid ester constituents from high-potency *Cannabis sativa*. *Journal of Natural Products*, **71**, 536–542.

Ahmedzai, S., Carlyle, D.L., Calder, I.T., and Moran, F. (1983). Anti-emetic efficacy and toxicity of nabilone, a synthetic cannabinoid, in lung cancer chemotherapy. *British Journal of Cancer*, **48**, 657–663.

Allen, G.V., Saper, C.B., Hurley, K.M., and Cechetto, D.F. (1991). Organization of visceral and limbic connections in the insular cortex of the rat. *The Journal of Comparative Neurology*, **311**, 1–16.

Andrews, P.L. and Horn, C.C. (2006). Signals for nausea and emesis: implications for models of upper gastrointestinal diseases. *Autonomic Neuroscience: Basic & Clinical*, **125**, 100–15.

Aziz, Q., Schnitzler, A., and Enck, P. (2000). Functional neuroimaging of visceral sensation. *Journal of Clinical Neurophysiology*, **17**, 604–612.

Ballatori, E. and Roila, F. (2003). Impact of nausea and vomiting on quality of life in cancer patients during chemotherapy. *Health and Quality of Life Outcomes*, **1**, 46.

Berger, B.D. (1972). Conditioning of food aversions by injections of psychoactive drugs. *Journal of Comparative and Physiological Psychology*, **81**, 21–26.

Bernstein, I.L., Chavez, M., Allen, D., and Taylor, E.M. (1992). Area postrema mediation of physiological and behavioral effects of lithium chloride in the rat. *Brain Research*, **575**, 132–137.

Billig, I., Yates, B.J., and Rinaman, L. (2001). Plasma hormone levels and central c-Fos expression in ferrets after systemic administration of cholecystokinin. *American Journal of Physiology. Regulatory Integrative and Comparative Physiology*, **281**, R1243–1255.

Bolognini, D, Rock, E.M., Cluny, N.L., *et al.* (2013). Cannabidiolic acid prevents vomiting in *Suncus murinus* and nausea-induced behavior in rats by enhancing 5-HT1A receptor activation. *British Journal of Pharmacology*, **168**, 1456–1470.

Burchfield, S.R., Elich, M.S., and Woods, S.C. (1977). Geophagia in response to stress and arthritis. *Physiology & Behavior*, **19**, 265–267.

Carey, M.P., Burish, T.G, and Brenner, D.E. (1983). Delta-9-tetrahydrocannabinol in cancer chemotherapy: research problems and issues. *Annals of Internal Medicine*, **99**, 106–114.

Cascio, M.G., Gauson, L.A., Stevenson, L.A., Ross, R.A., and Pertwee, R.G. (2010). Evidence that the plant cannabinoid cannabigerol is a highly potent alpha2-adrenoceptor agonist and moderately potent 5HT1A receptor antagonist. *British Journal of Pharmacology*, **159**, 129–141.

Catenoix, H., Isnard, J., Guénot, M., Petit, J., Remy, C., and Mauguière, F. (2008). The role of the anterior insular cortex in ictal vomiting: a stereotactic electroencephalography study. *Epilepsy & Behavior*, **13**, 560–563.

Cechetto, D.F. and Saper, C.B. (1987). Evidence for a viscerotopic sensory representation in the cortex and thalamus in the rat. *The Journal of Comparative Neurology*, **262**, 27–45.

Chan, M.Y., Cross-Mellor, S.K., Kavaliers, M., and Ossenkopp, K.P. (2009). Lipopolysaccharide (LPS) blocks the acquisition of LiCl-induced gaping in a rodent model of anticipatory nausea. *Neuroscience Letters*, **450**, 301–305.

Chang, A.E., Shiling, D.J., Stillman, R.C., *et al.* (1979). Delata-9-tetrahydrocannabinol as an antiemetic in cancer patients receiving high-dose methotrexate. A prospective, randomized evaluation. *Annals of Internal Medicine*, **91**, 819–824.

Choukèr, A., Kaufmann, I., Kreth, S., *et al.* (2010). Motion sickness, stress and the endocannabinoid system. *PLoS One*, **5**, e10752.

Cluny, N.L., Naylor, R.J., Whittle, B.A., and Javid, F.A. (2008). The effects of cannabidiol and tetrahydrocannabinol on motion-induced emesis in *Suncus murinus*. *Basic & Clinical Pharmacology & Toxicology*, **103**, 150–156.

Contreras, M., Ceric, F., and Torrealba, F. (2007). Inactivation of the interoceptive insula disrupts drug craving and malaise induced by lithium. *Science*, **318**, 655–658.

Costall, B., Domeney, A.M., Naylor, R.J., and Tattersall, F.D. (1986). 5-Hydroxytryptamine M-receptor antagonism to prevent cisplatin-induced emesis. *Neuropharmacology*, **25**, 959–961.

Cotter, J. (2009). Efficacy of crude marijuana and synthetic delta-9-tetrahydrocannabinol as treatment for chemotherapy-induced nausea and vomiting: a systematic literature review. *Oncology Nursing Forum*, **36**, 345–352.

Crawford, S.M. and Buckman, R. (1986). Nabilone and metoclopramide in the treatment of nausea and vomiting due to cisplatinum: a double blind study. *Medical Oncology and Tumor Pharmacotherapy*, **3**, 39–42.

Cravatt, B.F., Giang, D.K., Mayfield, S.P., Boger, D.L., Lerner, R.A., and Gilula, N.B. (1996). Molecular characterization of an enzyme that degrades neuromodulatory fatty-acid amides. *Nature*, **384**, 83–87.

Cross-Mellor, S.K., Ossenkopp, K.P., Piomelli, D., and Parker, L.A. (2007). Effects of the FAAH inhibitor, URB597, and anandamide on lithium-induced taste reactivity responses: a measure of nausea in the rat. *Psychopharmacology (Berlin)*, **190**, 135–143.

Cunningham, D., Bradley, C.J., Forrest, G.J., et al. (1988). A randomized trial of oral nabilone and prochlorperazine compared to intravenous metoclopramide and dexamethasone in the treatment of nausea and vomiting induced by chemotherapy regimens containing cisplatin or cisplatin analogues. *European Journal of Cancer & Clinical Oncology*, **24**, 685–689.

Dalzell, A.M., Bartlett, H., and Lilleyman, J.S. (1986). Nabilone: an alternative antiemetic for cancer chemotherapy. *Archives of Disease in Childhood*, **61**, 502–505.

Darmani, N.A. (2001a). Delta-9-tetrahydrocannabinol differentially suppresses cisplatin-induced emesis and indices of motor function via cannabinoid CB_1 receptors in the least shrew. *Pharmacology, Biochemistry, Behavior*, **69**, 239–249.

Darmani, N.A. (2001b). Delta(9)-tetrahydrocannabinol and synthetic cannabinoids prevent emesis produced by the cannabinoid CB_1 receptor antagonist/inverse agonist SR 141716A. *Neuropsychopharmacology*, **24**, 198–203.

Darmani, N.A. (2002). The potent emetogenic effects of the endocannabinoid, 2-AG (2-arachidonoylglycerol) are blocked by delta(9)-tetrahydrocannabinol and other cannnabinoids. *The Journal of Pharmacology and Experimental Therapeutics*, **300**, 34–42.

Darmani, N.A., Janoyan, J.J., Crim, J., and Ramirez, J. (2007). Receptor mechanism and antiemetic activity of structurally-diverse cannabinoids against radiation-induced emesis in the least shrew. *European Journal of Pharmacology*, **563**, 187–196.

Darmani, N.A. and Johnson, J.C. (2004). Central and peripheral mechanisms contribute to the antiemetic actions of delta-9-tetrahydrocannabinol against 5-hydroxytryptophan-induced emesis. *European Journal of Pharmacology*, **488**, 201–212.

Darmani, N.A., McClanahan, B.A., Trinh, C., Petrosino, S., Valenti, M., and Di Marzo, V. (2005). Cisplatin increases brain 2-arachidonoylglycerol (2-AG) and concomitantly reduces intestinal 2-AG and anandamide levels in the least shrew. *Neuropharmacology*, **49**, 502–513.

Darmani, N.A., Sim-Selley, L.J., Martin, B.R., et al. (2003). Antiemetic and motor-depressive actions of CP55,940: cannabinoid CB1 receptor characterization, distribution, and G-protein activation. *European Journal of Pharmacology*, **459**, 83–95.

De Boer-Dennert, M., de Wit, R., Schmitz, P.I., et al. (1997). Patient perceptions of the side-effects of chemotherapy: the influence of 5HT3 antagonists. *British Journal of Cancer*, **76**, 1055–1061.

Deiana, S., Watanabe, A., Yamasaki, Y., et al. (2012). Plasma and brain pharmacokinetic profile of cannabidiol (CBD), cannabidivarine (CBDV), Delta-tetrahydrocannabivarin (THCV) and cannabigerol (CBG) in rats and mice following oral and intraperitoneal administration and CBD action on obsessive-compulsive behaviour. *Psychopharmacology (Berlin)*, **219**, 859–873.

Deutsch, D.G. and Chin, S.A. (1993). Enzymatic synthesis and degradation of anandamide, a cannabinoid receptor agonist. *Biochemical Pharmacology*, **46**, 791–796.

Devane, W.A., Hanus, L., Breuer, A., et al. (1992). Isolation and structure of a brain constituent that binds to the cannabinoid receptor. *Science* (New York, N.Y.), **258**, 1946–199.

Di Marzo, V., Fontana, A., Cadas, H., *et al.* (1994). Formation and inactivation of endogenous cannabinoid anandamide in central neurons. *Nature*, 372, 686–691.

Dinh, T.P., Freund, T.F., and Piomelli, D. (2002). A role for monoglyceride lipase in 2-arachidonoylglycerol inactivation. *Chemistry and Physics of Lipids*, 121, 149–158.

Duran, M., Pérez, E., Abanades, S., *et al.* (2010). Preliminary efficacy and safety of an oromucosal standardized cannabis extract in chemotherapy-induced nausea and vomiting. *British Journal of Clinical Pharmacology*, 70, 656–663.

Ekert, H., Waters, K.D., Jurk, I.H., Mobilia, J., and Loughnan, P. (1979). Amelioration of cancer chemotherapy-induced nausea and vomiting by delta-9-tetrahydrocannabinol. *The Medical Journal of Australia*, 2, 657–659.

Fiol, M.E., Leppik, I.E., Mireles, R., and Maxwell, R. (1988). Ictus emeticus and the insular cortex. *Epilepsy Research*, 2, 127–131.

Foubert, J. and Vaessen, G. (2005). Nausea: the neglected symptom? *European Journal of Oncology Nursing*, 9, 21–32.

Frytak, S., Moertel, C.G., O'Fallon, J.R., *et al.* (1979). Delta-9-tetrahydrocannabinol as an antiemetic for patients receiving cancer chemotherapy. A comparison with prochlorperazine and a placebo. *Annals of Internal Medicine*, 91, 825–830.

Gaoni, Y. and Mechoulam, R. (1964a). Isolation, structure, and partial synthesis of an active constituent of hashish. *Journal of the American Chemical Society*, 86, 1646–1647.

Gaoni, Y. and Mechoulam, R. (1964b). The structure and synthesis of cannabigerol, a new hashish constituent. *Proceedings of Chemical Society*, 82.

Garcia, J., Hankins, W.G., and Rusiniak, K.W. (1974). Behavioral regulation of the milieu interne in man and rat. *Science*, 185, 824–831.

Gill, E.W., Paton, W.D.M., and Pertwee, R.G. (1970). Preliminary experiments on the chemistry and pharmacology of cannabis. *Nature*, 228, 134–136.

Grill, H.J. and Norgren, R. (1978). The taste reactivity test. I. Mimetic responses to gustatory stimuli in neurologically normal rats. *Brain Research*, 143, 263–279.

Grunberg, S.M., Deuson, R.R., Mavros, P., *et al.* (2004). Incidence of chemotherapy-induced nausea and emesis after modern antiemetics. *Cancer*, 100(10), 2261–2268.

Grunfeld, Y. and Edery, H. (1969). Psychopharmacological activity of the active constituents of hashish and some related cannabinoids. *Psychopharmacologia*, 14, 200–210.

Gylys, J.A., Doran, K.M., and Buyniski, P.J. (1979) Antagonism of cisplatin induced emesis in the dog. *Research Communications in Chemical Pathology and Pharmacology*, 23, 61–68.

Hanus, L.O., and Mechoulam, R. (2005). Cannabinoid chemistry: an overview. In: R. Mechoulam (ed.) *Cannabinoids as Therapeutics*. Basel: Birkhäuser, pp. 23–46.

Haring, M., Marsicano, G., Lutz, B., and Monory, K. (2007). Identification of the cannabinoid receptor type 1 in serotonergic cells of raphe nuclei in mice. *Neuroscience*, 146, 1212–1219.

Herman, T.S., Einhorn, L.H., Jones, S.E., *et al.* (1979). Superiority of nabilone over prochlorperazine as an antiemetic in patients receiving cancer chemotherapy. *The New England Journal of Medicine*, 300, 1295–1297.

Hesketh, P.J., Van Belle, S., Aapro, M., *et al.* (2003). Differential involvement of neurotransmitters through the time course of cisplatin-induced emesis as revealed by therapy with specific receptor antagonists. *European Journal of Cancer*, 39, 1074–1080.

Hickok, J.T., Roscoe, J.A., Morrow, G.R., King, D.K., Atkins, J.N., and Fitch, T.R. (2003). Nausea and emesis remain significant problems of chemotherapy despite prophylaxis with 5-hydroxytryptamine-3 antiemetics: a university of Rochester James P. Wilmot cancer center community clinical oncology program study of 360 cancer patients treated in the community. *Cancer*, 97, 2880–2886.

Hillsley, K. and Grundy, D. (1998). Serotonin and cholecystokinin activate different populations of rat mesenteric vagal afferents. *Neuroscience Letters*, 255, 63–66.

Hollister, L.E. (1974). Structure-activity relationships in man of cannabis constituents, and homologs and metabolites of delta9-tetrahydrocannabinol. *Pharmacology*, **11**, 3–11.

Horn, C.C. (2008). Why is the neurobiology of nausea and vomiting so important? *Appetite*, **50**, 430–434.

Hornby, P.J. (2001). Central neurocircuitry associated with emesis. *The American Journal of Medicine*, **111**, 106S–12S.

Howlett, A.C., Barth, F., Bonner, T.I., *et al.* (2002). International Union of Pharmacology. XXVII. Classification of cannabinoid receptors. *Pharmacological Reviews*, **54**, 161–202.

Iversen, L.L. (2008). *The Science of Marijuana*. 2nd ed. New York: Oxford University Press.

Jordan, K., Grothey, A., Kegel, T., Fibich, C., and Schöbert, C. (2005). Antiemetic efficacy of an oral suspension of granisetron plus dexamethasone and influence of quality of life on risk for nausea and vomiting. *Onkologie*, **28**, 88–92.

Kaada, B.R. (1951). Somato-motor, autonomic and electrocorticographic responses to electrical stimulation of rhinencephalic and other structures in primates, cat, and dog; a study of responses from the limbic, subcallosal, orbito-insular, piriform and temporal cortex, hippocampus-fornix and amygdala. *Acta Physiologica Scandinavica Supplementum*, **24**, 1–262.

Kiefer, S.W. and Orr, M.R. (1992). Taste avoidance, but not aversion, learning in rats lacking gustatory cortex. *Behavioral Neuroscience*, **106**, 140–146.

Klumpers, L.E., Beumer, T.L., van Hasselt, J.G., *et al.* (2012). Novel Δ(9)-tetrahydrocannabinol formulation Namisol® has beneficial pharmacokinetics and promising pharmacodynamic effects. *British Journal of Clinical Pharmacology*, **74**, 42–53.

Kwiatkowska, M., Parker, L.A., Burton, P., and Mechoulam, R. (2004). A comparative analysis of the potential of cannabinoids and ondansetron to suppress cisplatin-induced emesis in the *Suncus murinus* (house musk shrew). *Psychopharmacology (Berlin)*, **174**, 254–259.

Lane, M., Vogel, C.L., Ferguson, J., *et al.* (1991). Dronabinol and prochlorperazine in combination for treatment of cancer chemotherapy-induced nausea and vomiting. *Journal of Pain and Symptom Management*, **6**, 352–359.

Liau, C.T., Chu, N.M., Liu, H.E., Deuson, R., Lien, J., and Chen, J.S. (2005). Incidence of chemotherapy-induced nausea and vomiting in Taiwan: physicians' and nurses' estimation vs. patients' reported outcomes. *Supportive Care in Cancer*, **13**, 277–286.

Liu, Y.L., Malik, N., Sanger, G.J., Friedan, M.I., and Andrews, P.L. (2005). Pica--a model of nausea? Species differences in response to cisplatin. *Physiology & Behavior*, **85**, 271–217.

Limebeer, C.L., Hall, G., and Parker, L.A. (2006). Exposure to a lithium-paired context elicits gaping in rats: a model of anticipatory nausea. *Physiology & Behavior*, **88**, 398–403.

Limebeer, C.L., Krohn, J.P., Cross-Mellor, S., Litt, D.E., Ossenkopp, K.P., and Parker, L.A. (2008). Exposure to a context previously associated with nausea elicits conditioned gaping in rats: a model of anticipatory nausea. *Behavioural Brain Research*, **187**, 33–40.

Limebeer, C.L. and Parker, L.A. (1999). Delta-9-tetrahydrocannabinol interferes with the establishment and the expression of conditioned rejection reactions produced by cyclophosphamide: a rat model of nausea. *Neuroreport*, **10**, 3769–3772.

Limebeer, C.L. and Parker, L.A. (2000). The antiemetic drug ondansetron interferes with lithium-induced conditioned rejection reactions, but not lithium-induced taste avoidance in rats. *Journal of Experimental Psychology. Animal Behavior Processes*, **26**, 371–384.

Limebeer, C.L, Rock, E.M., Mechoulam, R., and Parker, L.A. (2012). The anti-nausea effects of CB_1 agonists are mediated by an action at the visceral insular cortex. *British Journal of Pharmacology*, **167**, 1126–1136.

Limebeer, C.L., Vemuri, V.K., Bedard, H., *et al.* (2010). Inverse agonism of cannabinoid CB_1 receptors potentiates LiCl-induced nausea in the conditioned gaping model in rats. *British Journal of Pharmacology*, **161**, 336–349.

London, S. W., McCarthy, L. E., and Borison, H. L. (1979). Suppression of cancer chemotherapy-induced vomiting in the cat by nabilone, a synthetic cannabinoid. *Proceedings of the Society for Experimental Biology and Medicine,* **160**, 437–440.

Lundy, R.F. Jr. and Norgren, R. (2004). Activity in the hypothalamus, amygdala, and cortex generates bilateral and convergent modulation of pontine gustatory neurons. *Journal of Neurophysiology,* **91**, 1143–1157.

McCarthy, L.E. and Borison, H.L. (1981). Antiemetic activity of N-methyllevonantradol and nabilone in cisplatin-treated cats. *Journal of Clinical Pharmacology,* **21**, 30S–37S.

McLaughlin, P.J., Winston, K.M., Limebeer, C.L., Parker, L.A., Makriyannis, A., and Salamone, J.D. (2005). The cannabinoid CB_1 antagonist AM 251 produces food avoidance and behaviors associated with nausea but does not impair feeding efficiency in rats. *Psychopharmacology (Berlin),* **180**, 286–293.

Mechoulam, R. (2007). Plant cannabinoids: a neglected pharamcological treasure trove. *British Journal of Pharamcology,* **146**, 913–915.

Mechoulam, R. and Hanus, L. (2002). Cannabidiol: an overview of some chemical and pharmacological aspects. Part I: chemical aspects. *Chemistry and Physics of Lipids,* **121**, 35–43.

Mechoulam, R., Ben-Shabat, S., Hanus, L., *et al.* (1995). Identification of an endogenous 2-monoglyceride, present in canine gut, that binds to cannabinoid receptors. *Biochemical Pharmacology,* **50**, 83–90.

Mechoulam, R., Shani, A., Edery, H., and Grunfeld, Y. (1970). Chemical basis of hashish activity. *Science,* **169**, 611–612.

Meiri, E., Jhangiani, H., Vredenburgh, J.J., *et al.* (2007). Efficacy of dronabinol alone and in combination with ondansetron versus ondansetron alone for delayed chemotherapy-induced nausea and vomiting. *Current Medical Research and Opinion,* **23**, 533–543.

Merkus, F.W. (1971). Cannabivarin and tetrahydrocannabivarin, two new constituents of hashish. *Nature.* **232**, 579–580.

Miner W.D., and Sanger, G.J. (1986). Inhibition of cisplatin-induced vomiting by selective 5-hydroxytryptamine M-receptor antagonism. *British Journal of Pharmacology,* **88**, 497–499.

Mitchell, D., Wells, C., Hoch, N., Lind, K., Woods, S.C., and Mitchell, L.K. (1976). Poison induced pica in rats. *Physiology & Behavior,* **17**, 691–697.

Morrow, G.R. and Dobkin, P.L. (1988). Behavioral approaches for the management of aversive side effects of cancer treatment. *Psychiatric Medicine,* **5**, 299–314.

Nesse, R.M., Carli, T., Curtis, G.C., and Kleinman P.D. (1980). Pretreatment nausea in cancer chemo-therapy: a conditioned response? *Psychosomatic Medicine,* **42**, 33–36.

O'Brien, L.D., Wills, K.L., Segsworth, B., *et al.* (2012). Effect of chronic exposure to rimonabant and phytocannabinoids on anxiety-like behavior and saccharin palatability. *Pharmacology, Biochemistry, Behavior,* **103**, 597–602

Orr, L.E. and McKernan, J.F. (1981). Antiemetic effect of delta 9-tetrahydrocannabinol in chemotherapy-associated nausea and emesis as compared to placebo and compazine. *Journal of Clinical Pharmacology,* **21**, 76S–80S.

Orr, L.E., McKernan, J.F., and Bloome, B. (1980). Antiemetic effect of tetrahydrocannabinol. Compared with placebo and prochlorperazine in chemotherapy-associated nausea and emesis. *Archives of Internal Medicine,* **140**, 1431–1433.

Parker, L.A. (1995). Rewarding drugs produce taste avoidance, but not taste aversion. *Neuroscience and Biobehavioral Reviews,* **19**, 143–157.

Parker, L.A., Hills, K., and Jensen, K. (1984). Behavioral CRs elicited by a lithium- or an amphetamine-paired contextual test chamber. *Animal Learning & Behavior,* **12**, 307–315.

Parker, L.A. and Kemp, S.W. (2001). Tetrahydrocannabinol (THC) interferes with conditioned retching in *Suncus murinus*: an animal model of anticipatory nausea and vomiting (ANV). *Neuroreport,* **12**, 749–751.

Parker, L.A., Kwiatkowska, M., Burton, P., and Mechoulam, R. (2004). Effect of cannabinoids on lithium-induced vomiting in the *Suncus murinus* (house musk shrew). *Psychopharmacology (Berlin)*, **171**, 156–161.

Parker, L.A., Kwiatkowska, M., and Mechoulam, R. (2006). Delta-9-tetrahydrocannabinol and cannabidiol, but not ondansetron, interfere with conditioned retching reactions elicited by a lithium-paired context in *Suncus murinus*: an animal model of anticipatory nausea and vomiting. *Physiology & Behavior*, **87**, 66–71.

Parker, L.A., Limebeer, C.L., and Rana, S.A. (2009a). Conditioned disgust, but not conditioned taste avoidance, may reflect conditioned nausea in rats. In: S. Reilly and T.R. Schachtman (eds.). *Conditioned Taste Aversions: Behavioral and Neural Processes*. New York: Oxford University Press, pp. 92–113.

Parker, L.A., Limebeer, C.L., Rock, E.M., Litt, D.L., Kwiatkowska, M., and Piomelli, D. (2009b). The FAAH inhibitor URB-597 interferes with cisplatin- and nicotine-induced vomiting in the *Suncus murinus* (house musk shrew). *Physiology & Behavior*, **97**, 121–124.

Parker, L.A. and Mechoulam, R. (2003). Cannabinoid agonists and antagonists modulate lithium-induced conditioned gaping in rats. *Integrative Physiological and Behavioral Science*, **38**, 133–145.

Parker, L.A., Mechoulam, R., and Schlievert, C. (2002). Cannabidiol, a non-psychoactive component of cannabis and its synthetic dimethylheptyl homolog suppress nausea in an experimental model with rats. *Neuroreport* **13**, 567–570.

Parker, L.A., Mechoulam, R., Schlievert, C., Abbott, L., Fudge, M.L., and Burton, P. (2003). Effects of cannabinoids on lithium-induced conditioned rejection reactions in a rat model of nausea. *Psychopharmacology (Berlin)*, **166**, 156–162.

Parker, L.A., Rana, S.A., and Limebeer, C.L. (2008). Conditioned nausea in rats: assessment by conditioned disgust reactions, rather than conditioned taste avoidance. *Canadian Journal of Experimental Psychology*, **62**, 198–209.

Parker, L.A., Rock, E.M., and Limebeer, C.L. (2011). Regulation of nausea and vomiting by cannabinoids. *British Journal of Pharmacology*, **163**, 1411–1422.

Penfield, W. and Faulk, M.E. (1955). The insula; further observations on its function. *Brain*, **78**, 445–470.

Pertwee, R.G. (2009). Emerging strategies for exploiting cannabinoid receptor agonists as medicines. *British Journal of Pharmacology*, **156**, 397–411.

Pertwee, R.G., Thomas, A., Stevenson, L.A., *et al.* (2007). The psychoactive plant cannabinoid, Delta9-tetrahydrocannabinol, is antagonized by Delta8- and Delta9-tetrahydrocannabivarin in mice in vivo. *British Journal of Pharmacology*, **150**, 586–594.

Piomelli, D. (2003). The molecular logic of endocannabinoid signalling. *Nature Reviews. Neuroscience*, **4**, 873–884.

Poli-Bigelli, S., Rodrigues-Pereira, J., Carides, A.D., *et al.* (2003). Addition of the neurokinin 1 receptor antagonist aprepitant to standard antiemetic therapy improves control of chemotherapy-induced nausea and vomiting. Results from a randomized, double-blind, placebo-controlled trial in Latin America. *Cancer*, **97**, 3090–3098.

Pomeroy, M., Fennelly, J.J., and Towers, M. (1986). Prospective randomized double-blind trial of nabilone versus domperidone in the treatment of cytotoxic-induced emesis. *Cancer Chemotherapy and Pharmacology*, **17**, 285–288.

Riedel, G., Fadda, P., McKillop-Smith, S., Pertwee, R.G., Platt, B., and Robinson, L. (2009). Synthetic and plant-derived cannabinoid receptor antagonists show hypophagic properties in fasted and non-fasted mice. *British Journal of Pharmacology*, **156**, 1154–1166.

Rock, E.M and Parker, L.A. (2013). Effect of low doses of cannabidiolic acid and ondansetron on LiCl-induced conditioned gaping (a model of nausea-induced behaviour) in rats. *British Journal of Pharmacology*, **169**, 685–92.

Rock, E.M., Bolognini, D., Limebeer, C.L., *et al.* (2012). Cannabidiol, a non-psychotropic component of cannabis, attenuates vomiting and nausea-like behaviour via indirect agonism of 5-HT(1A) somatodendritic autoreceptors in the dorsal raphe nucleus. *British Journal of Pharmacology*, **165**, 2620–2634.

Rock, E.M., Goodwin, J.M., Limebeer, C.L., *et al.* (2011). Interaction between non-psychotropic cannabinoids in marihuana: effect of cannabigerol (CBG) on the anti-nausea or anti-emetic effects of cannabidiol (CBD) in rats and shrews. *Psychopharmacology (Berlin)*, **215**, 505–512.

Rock, E.M., Kopstick, R.L., Limebeer, C.L., Parker, L.A. (2013a). Tetrahydrocannabinolic acid reduces nausea-induced conditioned nausea in rats and vomiting in *Suncus murinus*. *British Journal of Pharmacology*, **170**(3), 641–648.

Rock, E.M., Limebeer, C.L., Mechoulam, R., Piomelli, D., and Parker, L.A. (2008). The effect of cannabidiol and URB597 on conditioned gaping (a model of nausea) elicited by a lithium-paired context in the rat. *Psychopharmacology (Berlin)*, **196**, 389–395.

Rock, E.M., Sticht, M.A., Duncan, M. Stott, C., and Parker, L.A. (2013b). Evaluation of the potential of the phytocannabinoids, cannabidivarin (CBDV) and Δ^9-tetrahydrocannabivarin (THVC), to produce CB_1 receptor inverse agonism symptoms of nausea in rats. *British Journal of Pharmacology*, **170**, 671–678.

Rudd, J.A., Ngan, M.P., and Wai, M.K. (1998). 5-HT3 receptors are not involved in conditioned taste aversions induced by 5-hydroxytryptamine, ipecacuanha or cisplatin. *European Journal of Pharmacology*, **352**, 143–149.

Rudd, J.A., Yamamoto, K., Yamatodani, A., and Takeda, N. (2002). Differential action of ondansetron and dexamethasone to modify cisplatin-induced acute and delayed kaolin consumption ("pica") in rats. *European Journal of Pharmacology*, **454**, 47–52.

Sallan, S.E., Zinberg, N.E., and Frei, E., 3rd. (1975). Antiemetic effect of delta-9-tetrahydrocannabinol in patients receiving cancer chemotherapy. *New England Journal of Medicine*, **293**, 795–797.

Saper, C.B. (2004). Organization of cerebral cortical afferent systems in the rat. II. Magnocellular basal nucleus. *The Journal of Comparative Neurology*, **222**, 313–342.

Schlicker, E. and Kathmann, M. (2001). Modulation of transmitter release via presynaptic cannabinoid receptors. *Trends in Pharmacological Sciences*, **22**, 565–572.

Shannon, H.E., Martin, W.R., and Silcox, D. (1978) Lack of antiemetic effect of delta9-tetrahydrocannabinol in apomorophine-induced emesis in the dog. *Life Sciences*, **23**, 49–53.

Sharkey, K.A., Cristino, L., Oland, L.D., *et al.* (2007). Arvanil, anandamide and N-arachidonoyl-dopamine (NADA) inhibit emesis through cannabinoid CB1 and vanilloid TRPV1 receptors in the ferret. *The European Journal of Neuroscience*, **25**, 2773–2782.

Sink, K.S., McLaughlin, P.J., Wood, J.A., *et al.* (2008). The novel cannabinoid CB1 receptor neutral antagonist AM4113 suppresses food intake and food-reinforced behavior but does not induce signs of nausea in rats. *Neuropsychopharmacology*, **33**, 946–955.

Steele, N., Gralla, R.J., Braun, D.W.Jr., and Young, C.W. (1980). Double-blind comparison of the antiemetic effects of nabilone and prochlorperazine on chemotherapy-induced emesis. *Cancer Treatment Reports*, **64**, 219–224.

Stern, R.M., Koch, K.L., and Andrews, P.L.R. (2011). *Nausea: Mechanisms and Management*. New York: Oxford University Press.

Sticht, M.A., Long, J.Z., Rock, E.M., *et al.* (2012). Inhibition of monoacylglycerol lipase attenuates vomiting in *Suncus murinus* and 2-arachidonoyl glycerol attenuates nausea in rats. *British Journal of Pharmacology*, **165**, 2425–2435.

Sweet, D.L., Miller, N.J., Weddington, W., Senay, E., and Sushelsky, L. (1981). Delta 9-Tetrahydrocannabinol as an antiemetic for patients receiving cancer chemotherapy. A pilot study. *Journal of Clinical Pharmacology*, **21**, 70S–75S.

Thomas, A., Stevenson, L.A., Wease, K.N., *et al.* (2005). Evidence that the plant cannabinoid Delta9-tetrahydrocannabivarin is a cannabinoid CB_1 and CB_2 receptor antagonist. *British Journal of Pharmacology*, **146**, 917–926.

Torii, Y., Saito, H., and Matsuki, N. (1991). 5-Hydroxytryptamine is emetogenic in the house musk shrew, *Suncus murinus*. *Naunyn-Schmiedeberg's Archives of Pharmacology*, **344**, 564–567.

Tramèr, M.R., Carroll, D., Campbell, F.A., Reynolds, D.J., Moore, R.A., and McQuay, H.J. (2001). Cannabinoids for control of chemotherapy induced nausea and vomiting: quantitative systematic review. *British Medical Journal (Clinical Research ed.)*, **323**, 16–21.

Tuerke, K.J., Limebeer, C.L., Fletcher, P.J., and Parker, L.A. (2012a). Double dissociation between regulation of conditioned disgust and taste avoidance by serotonin availability at the 5-HT3 receptor in the posterior and anterior insular cortex. *The Journal of Neuroscience*, **32**, 13709–13717.

Tuerke, K.J., Winters, B.D., and Parker, L.A. (2012b). Ondansetron interferes with unconditioned lying-on belly and acquisition of conditioned gaping induced by LiCl as models of nausea-induced behaviors in rats. *Physiology & Behavior*, **105**, 856–860.

Ungerleider, J.T., Andrysiak, T.A., Fairbanks, L.A., Tesler, A.S., and Parker, R.G. (1984). Tetrahydrocannabinol vs. prochlorperazine. The effects of two antiemetics on patients undergoing radiotherapy. *Radiology*, **150**, 598–599.

Van Belle, S., Lichinitser, M.R., Navari, R.M., *et al.* (2002). Prevention of cisplatin-induced acute and delayed emesis by the selective neurokinin-1 antagonists, L-758,298 and MK-869. *Cancer*, **94**, 3032–3041.

Van Sickle, M.D., Duncan, M., Kingsley, P.J., *et al.* (2005). Identification and functional characterization of brainstem cannabinoid CB_2 receptors. *Science*, **310**, 329–332.

Van Sickle, M.D., Oland, L.D., Ho, W., *et al.* (2001). Cannabinoids inhibit emesis through CB_1 receptors in the brainstem of the ferret. *Gastroenterology*, **121**,767–774.

Van Sickle, M.D., Oland, L.D., Mackie, K., Davison, J.S., and Sharkey, K.A. (2003). Delta9-tetrahydrocannabinol selectively acts on CB_1 receptors in specific regions of dorsal vagal complex to inhibit emesis in ferrets. *American Journal of Physiology. Gastrointestinal and Liver Physiology*, **285**, G566–G576.

Vera, G., Chiarlone, A., Cabezos, P.A., Pascual. D., Martin, M.I., and Abalo, R. (2007). WIN 55,212-2 prevents mechanical allodynia but not alterations in feeding behaviour induced by chronic cisplatin in the rat. *Life Sciences*, **81**, 467–479.

Verhoeckx, K.C., Korthout, H.A., van Meeteren-Kreikamp, A.P., *et al.* (2006). Unheated *Cannabis sativa* extracts and its major compound THC-acid have potential immuno-modulating properties not mediated by CB_1 and CB_2 receptor coupled pathways. *International Immunopharmacology*, **6**, 656–665.

Wang, Y., Ray, A.P., McClanahan, B.A., and Darmani, N.A. (2009). The antiemetic interaction of Delta-9-tetrahydrocannabinol when combined with tropisetron or dexamethaone in the least shrew. *Pharmacology, Biochemistry and Behavior*, **91**, 367–373.

Yamamoto, K., Ngan, M.P., Takeda, N., Yamatodani, A., and Rudd, J.A. (2004). Differential activity of drugs to induce emesis and pica behavior in *Suncus murinus* (house musk shrew) and rats. *Physiology & Behavior*, **83**, 151–156.

Chapter 24

Established and Emerging Concepts of Cannabinoid Action on Food Intake and their Potential Application to the Treatment of Anorexia and Cachexia

Luigia Cristino and Vincenzo Di Marzo

24.1 A little bit of history: cannabis, Δ^9-tetrahydrocannabinol, and appetite

The capability of cannabis preparations to stimulate appetite, especially for palatable foods, has been documented as far back as 300 AD (Chopra and Chopra 1939). Therefore, it is surprising that, in modern times and when it was understood that this orexigenic action of cannabis was mainly due to its major psychotropic constituent, Δ^9-tetrahydrocannabinol (Δ^9-THC), this well-known phenomenon has been only sparsely supported by empirical evidence, with few detailed human studies and even fewer well-controlled investigations in experimental models. In an early report, Hollister (1971) demonstrated that a single oral dose of marijuana (containing 0.35 mg/kg Δ^9-THC) increased the intake of milkshakes in healthy unfasted volunteers. Foltin and colleagues showed that subjects given marijuana cigarettes (containing 1.84% w/w Δ^9-THC) showed a marked increase in food intake (1500 kcal), primarily attributable to an increase in "snack" food consumption (Foltin et al. 1986, 1988). In animals, the first full dose–response analysis of Δ^9-THC-induced hyperphagia was documented in the late 1990s (Williams et al. 1998); a range of Δ^9-THC doses were administered orally to satiated rats and hyperphagia was seen at doses of 0.5 mg/kg and above. Later, the hyperphagic action of Δ^9-THC was shown to: (1) be mediated by stimulation of type 1 cannabinoid receptors (CB_1) (see section 24.2), which are widely distributed throughout the brain (Beal et al. 1997; Herkenham et al. 1990), as this effect was blocked by administration of the selective CB_1 receptor antagonist, N-piperidino-5-(4-chlorophenyl)-1-(2,4-dichlorophenyl)-4-methylpyrazole-3-carboxamide (SR141716, or rimonabant), which is effective against other effects of Δ^9-THC also in human volunteers (Huestis et al. 2001); and (2) occur through a marked reduction in the latency to begin a new meal (Williams and Kirkham 2002a, 2002b). In agreement with Foltin's human study, the action of the drug was stronger when rats were fed a palatable, high-fat diet (HFD) (Koch 2001). Together with an apparently preferential suppression of palatable ingesta in animals by the CB_1 antagonist rimonabant, when administered alone, observed in the studies by Arnone et al. (1997) and Simiand et al. (1998), these data led to the initial hypothesis that CB_1 receptor activation by Δ^9-THC may promote feeding by amplifying the incentive or rewarding value of food. Indeed, CB_1 involvement in general reward processes is supported by a number of different studies showing, for example, that rimonabant reduces the sensitivity of rats to rewarding electrical brain stimulation (Deroche-Gamonet et al. 2001), and prevents the acquisition of drug- or food-induced place preferences (Chaperon et al. 1998). Nevertheless, given the paucity of data in humans, it is possible that CB_1-induced hyperphagia may involve also other aspects of feeding regulation. For example, it may result from the inhibition of any of the satiety signals that have been proposed to regulate appetite (Clapham et al. 2001) (see section 24.2).

Therapeutically, appetite stimulation by Δ^9-THC and cannabis has been studied for several decades, particularly in relation to the cachexia associated with cancer, acquired immunodeficiency syndrome (AIDS), and anorexia nervosa. Cachexia is a term derived from Greek *kakos*, meaning bad, and *hexis*, meaning condition, and describes the progressive loss of adipose tissue and lean body mass subsequent of several chronic wasting disorders. Increased proteolysis, decreased protein synthesis, and accelerated lipolysis due to high energy demands all contribute to a dramatic decline in lean body mass and fat mass and increased mortality in this setting (O'Gorman et al. 2000; Tisdale 2009). Anorexia, instead, is defined as the loss of the desire to eat despite caloric deprivation, and, apart from anorexia nervosa, is also frequently seen in patients with advanced chronic illness (Walsh et al. 2000). Caloric restriction per se induces a less severe degree of weight loss and a different metabolic pattern from cachexia, being characterized by decreased energy expenditure and preservation of lean at the expense of fat mass. This indicates that anorexia alone does not cause the extreme weight loss seen in cachexia. Accordingly, nutritional support is not sufficient to reverse this latter condition (Tisdale 2002).

Synthetic Δ^9-THC (dronabinol) has been used in the clinic for a number of years to combat a reduction in appetite and consequent weight reduction and wasting, as observed in conditions that can significantly affect appetite and alter psychological responses to food and eating, such as AIDS, cancer, and related drug or radiation treatments (Kirkham 2005; Mechoulam et al. 1998). In a pilot study, dronabinol caused weight gain in the majority of subjects (Plasse 1991). A relatively low oral dose of dronabinol, 2.5 mg twice daily, enhanced appetite and stabilized body weight in patients with AIDS suffering from anorexia (Beal et al. 1997) for at least 7 months. Interestingly, in a pilot double-blind study conducted in AIDS patients with HIV-associated neuropathic pain, compared to placebo, cannabis administration was associated with significant increases in plasma levels of the orexigenic hormones, ghrelin and leptin (see section 24.2), and decreases in the levels of the anorectic mediator, peptide YY (PYY), with no influence on insulin levels (Riggs et al. 2012). In another study on patients with AIDS, however, no weight gain was reported over the course of 12 weeks of dronabinol administration (2.5 mg twice a day), whereas a dose of 750 mg/day of megestrol acetate (a synthetic progestational drug) produced significant weight gain (Timpone et al. 1999). In a more recent study, carried out with 243 patients with cancer-related cachexia, treated twice daily with either placebo, a cannabis extract or Δ^9-THC (in both latter cases the dose of this cannabinoid was 2.5 mg), again no difference in patient appetite or quality of life assessment was found among groups, although both the extract and the pure compound were very well tolerated (Strasser et al. 2006). Nevertheless, treatments with Δ^9-THC or its synthetic derivative, nabilone, devised in a way that higher, more effective and otherwise not tolerated doses of these compounds could be used (see later), may still have benefits, and beyond mere stimulation of appetite. Patients may lose enjoyment of, or interest in, food due to changes in taste perception produced by chemotherapy or through the acquisition of conditioned taste aversions following the nausea or vomiting accompanying many radical treatments. Indeed, wasting in the elderly is accompanied by decreased taste and smell acuity, whereas, in subjects with dementia, these factors are aggravated by the inability of patients to feed themselves, or even by food refusal. Cannabinoid preparations that stimulate appetite by enhancing the attractiveness and enjoyment of food, or reduce the negative effects of other therapeutic interventions on feeding behaviors, may be beneficial under these circumstances.

Indeed, cannabis has long been known to possess antiemetic properties (Loewe 1946; O'Shaugnessy 1843), and Δ^9-THC was shown to exert antinausea and antiemetic effects in the 1970s, that is, even before CB_1 receptors were discovered and found to be widely expressed in the brainstem dorsal vagal complex associated with the triggering of emetic responses (Herkenham et al. 1990; McCarthy and Borison 1984; Van Sickle et al. 2001). In particular, cannabinoids may be useful as pretreatments to avoid the establishment of conditioned nausea and anticipatory emesis associated with chemotherapy (Andrykowski 1988; Morrow et al. 1996). Patients who experience nausea or vomiting with chemotherapy treatments often experience anticipatory, conditioned retching or nausea that impairs their ability to tolerate subsequent medication as well as to feed properly. In animal models, Δ^9-THC and the potent CB_1 receptor agonist HU210 can prevent conditioned rejection (disgust) responses to flavors, usually associated with illness or the corresponding drug treatments (Limebeer and Parker 1999; Parker et al. 2004). A complicating issue, however, is the association of cannabinoid therapy with side effects, most commonly euphoria, sedation, dizziness, and ataxia. It is likely that these unwanted effects may be attenuated by improved formulations, or by coadministration with other cannabinoids that allow for self-titration of Δ^9-THC up to more efficacious and still well-tolerated doses. This strategy is used for Sativex®, which contains, in the form of a botanical extract administered as oromucosal spray, an approximately 1:1 ratio of Δ^9-THC and cannabidiol (CBD). CBD is an abundant and nonpsychotropic plant cannabinoid, which can counteract some of the central unwanted effects of Δ^9-THC (Russo 2011). On the other hand, the euphoric effects of cannabinoids are not always an obstacle to their effective administration. Mood elevation, or even actual antidepressant actions of chronic Δ^9-THC, may be an important component of its effectiveness in patients with cancer or AIDS. Alternatively, it may be possible to use cannabinoids that lack the psychotropic potency of Δ^9-THC. For example, a nonpsychotropic, CB_1-inactive, synthetic cannabinoid, HU-211, was found to provide almost complete protection against emesis produced by one of the most emetogenic cytotoxins, cisplatin (Feigenbaum et al. 1989). Additionally, the earlier mentioned CBD prevents nausea induced by lithium chloride or conditioned nausea elicited by a flavor paired with the toxin in rats (Parker et al. 2002).

24.2 **The endocannabinoid system in food intake: regulation of appetite and reward**

Investigations into the biological bases of the multiple effects of cannabis have yielded important breakthroughs in recent years: the discovery of two cannabinoid receptors in the brain and peripheral organs, and of endogenous ligands (endocannabinoids) for these receptors. These recent advances in cannabinoid pharmacology may lead to improved treatments for cachexia and/or anorexia conditions or, conversely, for combating excessive appetite and body weight, for example, by using CB_1 receptor antagonists as antiobesity medications.

The endocannabinoid system (ECS) is composed of two $G_{i/o}$ protein-coupled receptors for Δ^9-THC, known as "cannabinoid" receptor types 1 (CB_1) and 2 (CB_2), their lipid ligands (i.e., the endocannabinoids, ECs), and the enzymatic machinery for EC (endocannabinoid) synthesis and degradation. The most studied ECs, N-arachidonoyl-ethanolamide (anandamide, AEA) and 2-arachidonoylglycerol (2-AG), are produced from cell membrane phospholipids following cell stimulation, before being released by cells to target CB_1 and CB_2 receptors (reviewed in Di Marzo 2011). Within the central nervous system, ECs, and 2-AG in particular, usually signal in a retrograde manner, i.e., they are produced, at least to some extent, by postsynaptic neurons and act on CB_1 in presynaptic terminals to inhibit excitatory or inhibitory neurotransmitter

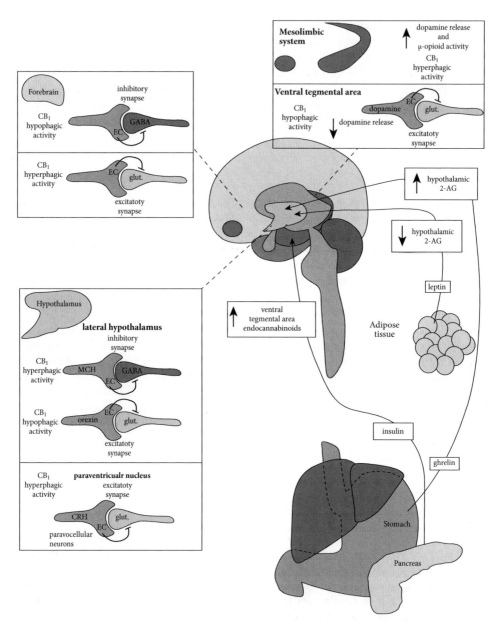

Fig. 24.1 Local effects of endocannabinoids and CB$_1$ receptors on the neural mechanisms regulating food intake from either the homeostatic or hedonic standpoint, and their regulation by peripheral hormones.

release. EC release is believed to occur immediately after biosynthesis from phospholipid precursors, with no intermediate storage in vesicles. Within a neuronal network, EC "tone" is the result not only of the expression and functional coupling to G-proteins of CB$_1$ and CB$_2$ receptors, but also of the regulation of EC levels as determined by different enzymatic biosynthetic and catabolic cascades (reviewed in Kano et al. 2009). Thus, ECs are ideal mediators for responding in real-time to the ever changing feeding state of an organism. They regulate appetite and food intake in a local manner, by modulating, via activation of CB_1 receptors, the activity of hypothalamic neurons, and subsequently the release of orexigenic and anorexigenic neuropeptides, as well as the function of mesolimbic and brainstem neurons, and by translating input information from peripherally derived hormones, such as leptin, ghrelin, and glucocorticoids, to these neurons. Thus, ECs regulate energy balance and food intake by affecting basal functions, including the hedonic evaluation of foods at the mesolimbic level, and integrative functions both at central (hypothalamus and hindbrain) and peripheral (intestinal system and adipose tissue) levels (Fig. 24.1).

24.2.1 ECs, CB_1, and the homeostatic regulation of food intake

The hypothalamus plays a key role in integrating the multiple biochemical and behavioral components of feeding and weight regulation. It is the most extensively interconnected area of the brain, and through its wide web of neural circuits it controls a variety of essential autonomic and somatomotor functions. Neuroanatomical studies have demonstrated direct projections to and from hypothalamic areas of several brain regions, e.g., cortical/limbic areas and the autonomic and motor system of the brainstem. Such extensive connectivity is thought to represent the anatomical basis supporting sleep–wake regulation, energy homeostasis, and cognitive and reward-related functions (Morton et al. 2006). Hormonal and nutrient signals are processed in the hypothalamus and inform the brain about the free and stored levels of fuel available for the organism (Cota et al. 2007). In turn, the hypothalamic neuronal circuits use this information to regulate caloric intake, energy consumption, and peripheral lipid and glucose metabolism. Because of their intrinsic functional activities, and the necessity to adapt to often dramatic changes in the nutritional status, these neural feeding circuitries are endowed with plasticity modulated by neurotransmitters and hormones. Among the chemical mediators involved in this integration, ECs are master regulators of the fast (i.e., mostly nongenomic) and stress-related fine-tuning of energy intake. Indeed, administration of CB_1 agonists and ECs into hypothalamic nuclei induces eating (Jamshidi and Taylor 2001; Kirkham and Williams 2001a), and EC levels in the hypothalamus vary according to changes in nutritional status. The levels of 2-AG are increased in the hypothalamus after 24 h of food deprivation in rats (Kirkham et al. 2002) and mice (Hanus et al. 2003), and decline as animals eat, returning to control levels with the onset of satiety (Kirkham et al. 2002). These changes are compatible with the behavioral actions of Δ^9-THC and CB_1 agonists in laboratory animals, whose enhanced motivation to eat largely reflects that observed after fasting in untreated healthy individuals. However, Hanus et al. (2003) also reported that hypothalamic 2-AG levels decrease after 12 days of food restriction. This finding was elegantly explained by the authors to reflect adaptive behavioral strategies in response to acute or chronic food deprivation. Thus, during short-term starvation, it is beneficial to produce high levels of the appetite-inducing 2-AG to compel the animal to actively seek food. Conversely, during imposed long-term deprivation, when no food can be found, it may aid survival to conserve energy by reducing the motivation to engage in food seeking—perhaps by reducing the conscious experience of hunger—also via reduced production of 2-AG in the hypothalamus (Hanus et al. 2003).

The hormone leptin, which originates in adipose tissue and affects a number of appetite-related factors in the hypothalamus, is a core component in the regulation of food intake and weight control (Lawrence et al. 1999; Schwartz et al. 2000). It is therefore of great interest that a strong functional relationship between ECs and leptin has been demonstrated (Di Marzo et al. 2001; also see Mechoulam and Fride 2001), and that EC biosynthesis and inactivation can be regulated by this hormone. Thus, leptin administration, which exerts an anorectic action, suppresses hypothalamic EC levels in healthy rats, whereas in the hypothalamus of obese and hyperphagic rodents lacking leptin, such as *ob/ob* (obese/obese, leptin mutant) mice, or with defective leptin signaling, i.e., *db/db* (diabetes/diabetes, leptin receptor mutant) mice and Zucker[fa/fa] (leptin receptor mutant) rats, EC levels are significantly increased (Di Marzo et al. 2001). Careful studies of food intake, appetite, and fat mass of CB_1 knockout mice showed that these animals display a lean phenotype throughout their lifetime and are resistant to the obesigenic effect of HFDs. This is different from the effects of simultaneous deletion of neuropeptide Y (NPY) and Agouti-related protein, transmitters heavily implicated in food intake, which does not result in a lean phenotype (Qian et al. 2002). This comparison may indicate that the EC system is more important for the regulation of energy balance than either of these orexigenic neuropeptides (McNay et al. 2012).

However, based on the absence of a change in hypothalamic CB_1 receptors as well as a lack of correlation between receptor density and plasma leptin under conditions of diet-induced obesity (Harrold et al. 2002), Harrold and Williams suggested that hypothalamic CB_1 receptors do not play a role in driving appetite during dietary obesity, but may stimulate hunger under different conditions such as starvation (Harrold and Williams 2003). This interpretation does not take into account the earlier mentioned effects of short- and long-term food deprivation on hypothalamic 2-AG concentrations, nor the inverse correlation between leptin and plasma AEA levels reported in healthy women and in women with anorexia nervosa (Monteleone et al. 2005). Indeed, the latter report, while explaining the observed increase in plasma AEA levels during this condition, which is well known to be characterized by low circulating leptin levels, is at odds with the observation of reduced hypothalamic EC tone during *imposed* long-term food deprivation. Based on the increasingly accepted role of the EC system in reward (see later), these other authors suggested that increased peripheral AEA levels during anorexia nervosa, if reflecting a similar scenario in the brain, might instead underlie the sense of reward that is often reported during this disorder and suggested to contribute to persistent *voluntary* food deprivation (Monteleone et al. 2005). At any rate, the leptin deficiency-mediated enhanced EC tone during anorexia nervosa might explain why no successful trial with Δ^9-THC has been reported yet for this eating disorder. Furthermore, the link existing between leptin anorectic actions and inhibition of EC signaling is strengthened by the recent finding that functional CB_1 receptor signaling within the hypothalamus is required by leptin to exert its effects on food intake and body weight, since selective genetic knock-out of CB_1 receptors in the hypothalamus abolishes the inhibition of food intake by leptin (Cardinal et al. 2012). Interestingly, the orexigenic actions of another peripheral hormone, stomach-derived ghrelin, also rely on EC signaling, since they are absent in CB_1 knockout mice (Kola et al. 2008).

Very little is presently known about the interaction of the EC system with other mediators involved in energy control and food intake. Cota and colleagues (Cota et al. 2003) have shown colocalization of CB_1 receptor with appetite regulating hormones in the paraventricular nucleus of the hypothalamus, i.e., the anorexigenic cocaine amphetamine regulated transcript and corticotropin-releasing hormone (CRH), and the orexigenic melanin concentrating hormone (MCH), while no colocalization was found with the orexigenic neuropeptide, NPY in the arcuate nucleus. There is also evidence for functional interactions between ECs and orexin-A, an orexigenic peptide that is selectively expressed in the lateral hypothalamus and linked to the stimulation of feeding (Dube et al.1999; Hilairet et al. 2003; Sweet et al. 1999). In an in vitro study, it was demonstrated that the coexpression of CB_1 and OX1 receptors results in a higher potentiation of ERK signaling, possibly due to heterodimerization/oligomerization of these two receptors (Ward et al. 2011). Recently, however, it was also shown that 2-AG can be produced and released through activation of OX1 receptor-mediated signaling, and act as a paracrine or autocrine messenger via

CB_1 receptors (Jäntti et al. 2013; Turunen et al. 2012), thus possibly explaining the potentiation of ERK phosphorylation that follows $OX1/CB_1$ receptor coexpression. CB_1 may also downregulate CRH signaling, since CB_1 receptor knockout mice show higher levels of mRNA for this hormone (Cota et al. 2003).

Interactions between cannabinoids and the melanocortin system have also been detected in relation to the observation that rimonabant facilitates the anorectic actions of alpha-melanocyte stimulating hormone (Verty et al. 2003), while an antagonist of the receptor for this peptide, the melanocortin receptor type 4, causes a late increase in hypothalamic EC levels concomitant to its long-term anorectic action in rats (Matias et al. 2008). Evidence was also provided suggesting that the expression of CB_1 receptors located in feeding-relevant hindbrain areas such as the dorsal motor nucleus of the vagus and the nucleus tractus solitarius may be subject to inhibition by the anorectic hormone, colecystokinin, or by food consumption (which elevates the levels of this hormone) (Burdyga et al. 2004). In an elegant study by Bellocchio et al. (2010) based on conditional CB_1 deletion in either glutamatergic or GABAergic forebrain neurons, the authors suggested that exogenous Δ^9-THC, as well as EC level elevation induced by fasting or exposure to palatable food, produced not only the expected hyperphagic effect, but also (and in the case of Δ^9-THC, at higher doses) a more surprising hypophagic effect, depending on the restriction of their action to CB_1 on excitatory or inhibitory terminals, respectively (Bellocchio et al. 2010). That CB_1 activation on different axon terminal populations could potentially produce opposing effects on food intake could have been surmised also from a previous in vitro study (Huang et al. 2007), although with conclusions seemingly opposite to those obtained by Bellocchio and colleagues. In fact, in the lateral hypothalamus, CB_1 activation was shown to result in retrograde inhibition of GABA or glutamate release from inputs onto MCH, or orexin-A releasing neurons, thereby resulting in disinhibition or inhibition of stimulation, respectively, of two orexigenic signals, and in potential orexigenic or anorexic effects. On the other hand, it was also found that presynaptic CB_1 activation inhibits glutamate release onto parvocellular neurons, resulting in inhibition of the release into the paraventricular nucleus of the anorexic hormone, CRH (Malcher-Lopes et al. 2006). At any rate, and regardless of these in vitro studies, it is clear that the hypophagic phenotype which occurs after global or conditioned deletion of CB_1 on glutamatergic neuronal inputs (Bellocchio et al. 2010) is similar to that following pharmacological CB_1 receptor antagonism by agents like the CB_1 antagonist, rimonabant. On this basis, it is reasonable to assume that the effect of CB_1 on glutamatergic signaling overall predominates over that on GABAergic signaling when it comes to explaining the hypophagic effects of CB_1 blockade, or the hyperphagic effects of low doses of Δ^9-THC, in wild-type mice.

24.2.2 ECs, CB_1, and orosensory reward

Increasing evidence supports the notion that the ECS plays a pivotal role in reward/reinforcement circuits of the mesolimbic system. In the striatum, the distribution of CB_1-expressing neurons exhibits a progressive dorsolateral-to-ventromedial reduction, with fewer CB_1-positive neurons in the nucleus accumbens (NAc) (Herkenham et al. 1990). However, although expression of CB_1 in the NAc is low, manipulation of CB_1 signaling within the NAc triggers robust emotional/motivational alterations related to food and drug addiction and other psychiatric disorders, and these effects cannot be exclusively attributed to CB_1 located at afferents to the NAc. Winters et al. (2012) demonstrated that CB_1-positive neurons within the NAc are exclusively fast-spiking interneurons (FSIs), electrically coupled with each other, and thus may help synchronize populations/ensembles of NAc neurons. These FSIs are not only electrically connected with each other but exert extensive inhibitory control over nearby medium spiny neurons, the principal neurons in the NAc, via monosynaptic connections. Furthermore, the membrane excitability of these neurons becomes significantly upregulated and influences the overall functional output of the NAc by modulating both dopaminergic and opioidergic pathways, thereby participating in reinforcing both the "liking" and "wanting" of highly palatable food.

In limbic forebrain sections containing the NAc, similar to the hypothalamus, short-term food deprivation and refeeding are accompanied by increased and decreased EC levels, respectively (Kirkham et al. 2002). On the other hand, injection into the shell of the NAc of 2-AG, AEA, and agents that inhibit EC inactivation stimulates food intake (Kirkham et al. 2002; Soria-Gómez et al. 2007) and increases the activity of hypothalamic neurons, particularly in the lateral hypothalamus, which also participates in reward (Soria-Gómez et al. 2007). These data, together with the well-known ability of CB_1 antagonists to reduce the rewarding effects of food as well as of drugs of abuse, confirm behavioral studies indicating that activation of CB_1 receptors by Δ^9-THC or endocannabinoids enhances food intake by reinforcing the motivational and hedonic aspects of feeding behavior. Indeed, studies carried out by injecting anandamide in the NAc identified a 1.6 mm^3 "hotspot" in the dorsal medial shell of this area, specifically responsible for the sensory pleasure induced by intraoral sucrose (Mahler et al. 2007). Furthermore, injection into the NAc of Δ^9-THC increases sucrose-induced hedonic activity and dopamine release (De Luca et al. 2012). On the other hand, CB_1 antagonists reduce the increase of extracellular dopamine release in the NAc provoked by novel highly palatable food (Melis et al. 2007), which is suggestive of a possible palatable food-induced activation of EC tone in this area. Harrold and colleagues (2002) have shown that NAc CB_1 receptors are downregulated in rats under a HFD. This effect is consistent with increased activation, and subsequent downregulation, of these receptors by ECs, and suggests that they mediate the hedonic evaluation of palatable foods. Furthermore, in mice made obese by a HFD, EC levels are upregulated in the hippocampus, which is another important anatomical substrate of hedonic eating, indicating that high-energy foods may be more satisfying under these conditions, resulting in a vicious circle leading to obesity (Massa et al. 2010). In the hypothalamus, which, as mentioned earlier, is involved in the control of reward through its lateral hypothalamus-originating connections with the mesolimbic system, 2-AG is transiently or permanently upregulated following acute or prolonged fat consumption, respectively, thus possibly participating in both the induction and maintenance stage of HFD preference (Higuchi et al. 2011).

EC signaling in both central and peripheral tissues might also modulate the way the sensory properties of food are perceived, in a manner that maximizes food intake. Thus, the levels of 2-AG are elevated in the olfactory epithelium of tadpoles following food deprivation and the subsequent activation of CB_1 in this tissue lowers odor detection thresholds, thus rendering olfactory neurons more sensitive and heightening food-seeking behavior (Breunig et al. 2010). CB_1 receptor activation by ECs in type II taste cells that also express the T1r3 sweet taste receptor, increases behavioral responses and electrophysiological responses of taste receptor cells to sweet compounds, without affecting responses to salty, sour, bitter, and umami compounds. Thus, opposite to leptin, the ECS also enhances the sensory properties of sweet foods (Yoshida et al. 2010). Furthermore, simple mouth exposure to fatty food in "sham-fed" rats leads to vagus nerve-mediated increases of EC levels in the small intestine, which then, by activating CB_1 in this gut region, may participate in stimulating fat food intake (DiPatrizio et al. 2011). Finally, also in the pontine parabrachial nucleus, a brainstem region associated with the gustatory properties of food and that receives inputs from the vagus and transmits these to higher centers for reward control, CB_1 stimulation by exogenous agonists or ECs enhances the consumption of palatable foods containing fat and/or sugar (DiPatrizio and Simansky 2008).

In healthy human volunteers, consumption of a favorite food, as compared to normal food, was recently shown to be accompanied by elevated 2-AG plasma levels, which in turn correlated positively with elevated ghrelin plasma levels (Monteleone et al. 2012). This effect might be due to direct or indirect (e.g., ghrelin-mediated) effects of palatable food consumption on central and peripheral EC levels, briefly mentioned earlier. However, the volunteers, who knew what type of food they would be given, exhibited higher 2-AG plasma levels also 10 min before consuming their favorite food. This might suggest that anticipatory mechanisms also trigger changes in peripheral EC levels, which might again participate in both the motivational and rewarding/sensory aspects of palatable food.

ECs may also have important functional relationships with the endogenous opioid system, which also mediates the rewarding properties of food (Kirkham 1991). Thus, in rats, the hyperphagic action of Δ^9-THC is reversed by the μ-opioid receptor antagonist, naloxone (Williams and Kirkham 2002b). Importantly, the facilitatory effects of a CB_1 agonist on responding for palatable solutions were reversed by both a CB_1 antagonist and naloxone (Gallate and McGregor 1999). Moreover, low doses of rimonabant and naloxone that are behaviorally inactive when administered alone, synergize to produce a profound anorectic action when coadministered (Kirkham and Williams 2001b; Rowland et al. 2001). Given the established ability of opioid antagonists to reduce the hedonic evaluation of foods and to reverse CB_1 agonist-stimulated ingestion, the potentiation of anorexia by combined CB_1 and opioid receptor blockade strengthens the proposition that ECs contribute to orosensory reward processes.

Finally, and in agreement with the hypothesis that ECs and CB_1 can also produce anorectic actions in a site-specific manner, a very recent study showed that the ECS mediates, through retrograde signaling, the inhibitory effect of insulin on excitatory (glutamatergic) axons which innervate dopaminergic neurons of the mouse ventral tegmental area (Labouèbe et al. 2013). As a result, the ECS is involved in insulin-induced reduction of motivation and preference for palatable food cues, and this seems to contradict the concept that activation of CB_1 receptors on glutamatergic neurons exclusively induces stimulatory effects on food intake (Bellocchio et al. 2010).

24.3 **Pharmacological effects of non-Δ^9-THC cannabinoids in relation to appetite**

The plant *Cannabis sativa* contains over 100 compounds derived from a diterpene structure, known as "cannabinoids" (ElSohly and Slade 2005; Mehmedic et al. 2010). The large number of cannabinoids present in the plant—and the low naturally occurring levels of some of them—rendered it difficult to obtain sufficient quantities of such pure chemical entities in the past, thus explaining in part the slow progress of our understanding of the pharmacology of most of these compounds. Among non-Δ^9-THC cannabinoids, the best characterized compounds are currently Δ^9-tetrahydrocannabivarin (Δ^9-THCV), CBD, and cannabinol (CBN) (Gaoni and Mechoulam 1964; Gill et al. 1970; Mechoulam and Shvo 1963). Given the ever-increasing number of reports on their effects on food intake and energy balance, it is possible that Δ^9-THCV and CBD have important and, as yet, unexplored clinical roles in cannabis (i.e., marijuana) consumption-induced changes in eating behavior.

However, prior to 2009, there were very few studies investigating the actions of individual non-Δ^9-THC "phytocannabinoids" on feeding, the majority of which have been either unreplicated or contradictory. More recent animal data indicate that these cannabinoids produce significant effects on the appetitive, but not consummatory, aspects of feeding behavior. Nevertheless, no detailed analysis of changes in feeding microstructure has yet been undertaken, which limits the extent to which these new findings can be interpreted.

24.3.1 Δ^9-tetrahydrocannabivarin

There is a broad literature implicating CB_1 receptor blockade as a potential antiobesity strategy; however, the recent withdrawal of inverse agonists such as rimonabant or taranabant, because of unwanted psychiatric side effects (i.e., anxiety and depression), has highlighted the need to develop safer alternatives (Izzo et al. 2009; Lee et al. 2009; Silvestri and Di Marzo 2012). In particular, neutral antagonists at CB_1 receptors have been recently suggested to be safer than inverse agonists because, whilst still efficacious at reducing food intake, they do not produce the anxiogenic actions of the latter, nor do they reduce motivation for reward, and hence are devoid of the potential anhedonic actions of agents like rimonabant (Meye et al. 2013; Silvestri and Di Marzo 2012). One compound with such neutral CB_1 antagonist action in vitro and in vivo, Δ^9-THCV (Pertwee et al. 2007; Thomas et al. 2005), is present in the *Cannabis* plant (Gill et al. 1970) and was recently subjected to further pharmacological characterization. In particular, Riedel et al. (2009) investigated the effects on feeding by lean mice of Δ^9-THCV (3, 10, and 30 mg/kg, intraperitoneally (i.p.)) and of a Δ^9-THCV SCE (standardized cannabis extract) also administered at a Δ^9-THCV dose of 3, 10, or 30 mg/kg, i.p. All doses of pure Δ^9-THCV significantly reduced food intake during the 12 h following treatment, whereas Δ^9-THCV SCE did not affect consumption. The authors suggested that future work should investigate effects of purified Δ^9-THCV and Δ^9-THCV SCE using conditions which would be expected to maximize food intake (e.g., during the dark phase of the light–dark cycle or following periods of deprivation), thus ensuring high baseline food intake and possibly unmasking stronger effects of these cannabinoid-based preparations on food intake. It must be pointed out, however, that other molecular targets, apart from CB_1 receptors, are emerging for Δ^9-THCV that might explain its anorectic effects, including CB_2 receptor agonism (Romero-Zerbo et al. 2012; Thomas et al. 2005) and transient receptor potential vanilloid type-1 (TRPV1) channel activation (De Petrocellis et al. 2008; Wang et al. 2005).

24.3.2 Cannabidiol and other phytocannabinoids

In 1976, Sofia and Knobloch examined the acute effects of two non-Δ^9-THC cannabinoids, CBD and CBN (both at 50 mg/kg, i.p.), on food and sucrose consumption. In this paradigm, animals were pretrained to consume their total daily food intake during a 6 h feeding period; water, 5% sucrose, or 20% sucrose solutions were also available during this period. Both CBN and CBD significantly reduced food intake, effects which persisted for 4–5 days post drug administration (Sofia and Knobloch 1976). However, the two compounds affected sucrose consumption to a significantly smaller extent, with a reduction that returned to pre-baseline levels by day 3–4 post drug administration. The authors interpreted these findings as suggestive that CBN and CBD produced a preference for sweet calories. It should also be noted that the Sofia and Knobloch (1976) study used doses of CBN and CBD between 200 and 1500 times greater than those used in more recent studies that have suggested that these non-Δ^9-THC phytocannabinoids stimulate feeding (Farrimond et al. 2010a, 2010b, 2012a, 2012b; see later). Much later, Wiley et al. (2005) showed that CBD (3–100 mg/kg, i.p.) failed to significantly alter food intake in mice; yet it should be noted that, in this study, doses of 3 and 10 mg/kg CBD showed a nonsignificant trend toward an increase in intake, suggesting that CBD may be worthy of further investigation. However, a recent study by Scopinho et al. (2011) showed that CBD (1, 10, or 20 mg/kg, i.p.) failed to alter feeding in rats and failed to replicate the nonsignificant trend toward an increase in feeding at low doses, and similar data, in mice, obtained using a dose of 10.0 mg/kg (i.p.), were also recently reported by Riedel et al. (2009). Nevertheless, Scopinho et al. (2011) did find that CBD could prevent the hyperphagic effects induced by the CB_1/CB_2 agonist, WIN55,212-2 ((R)-(+)-[2,3-dihydro-5-methyl-3-(4-morpholinylmethyl) pyrrolo[1,2,3-de]-1,4-benzoxazin-6-yl]-1-naphthalenylmethanone mesylate), and the $5-HT_{1A}$ (5-hydroxytryptamine subtype 1A) receptor agonist, 8-OH-DPAT (8-hydroxy-N,N-dipropyl-2-aminotetralin). Furthermore, CBD (2.5 and 5 mg/kg/day, i.p., for 14 days) was recently reported to produce significant decreases in body weight in rats, although no measures of food intake were taken in this study (Ignatowska-Jankowska et al. 2011); interestingly, CBD action was sensitive to coadministration of the CB_2 receptor selective antagonist, AM630 (6-iodopravadoline), suggesting that a CB_2 receptor-mediated mechanism may be critical to the action of this compound. However, CBD has very low affinity for CB_1 and CB_2 receptors, but exerts a wide array of other effects in vitro, including modulation of Ca^{2+} homeostasis (Ryan et al. 2009), TRPV1 channel activation (De Petrocellis et al. 2008), and inhibition of AEA cellular reuptake and enzymatic hydrolysis, and hence potential cannabinoid receptor "indirect" agonism (Bisogno et al. 2001; Izzo et al. 2009), whilst also exhibiting functional and "indirect" antagonism at CB_1 receptors (Thomas et al. 2007). In summary, although the data describing the effects of CBD on feeding have remained inconclusive for several decades, the overall impression, from reports published before 2012, is that this compound could affect food intake under certain circumstances. However, the molecular mechanisms by which CBD would exert this action and eventually influence body weight, remain to be established.

Indeed, very recently, Farrimond et al. (2012a) demonstrated that lower doses (up to 4.4 mg/kg) of CBD, when administered orally can induce significant reductions in chow consumption in mice over a 4 h period. Specifically, CBD oral administration induced only subtle, nonsignificant reductions in animal intake during any individual hour of the test; however, together, this led to a significant reduction in total chow intake over the test period due to significant reductions in intake during all meals. It is worthwhile mentioning that these apparent late-onset suppressive effects may reflect the relatively slow pharmacokinetic profile of CBD, since Deiana et al. (2012) have recently shown that brain levels of CBD continue to rise progressively for 4 h, following an admittedly much higher oral dose (120 mg/kg), in mice and rats. Despite these effects on hourly intakes, CBD administration had no significant effect on any other critical meal parameters linked to CB_1 receptor activation. Since CBD is unlikely to directly interact with CB_1 (Hill et al. 2012), these data may suggest that low-dose CBD can affect a feeding pathway which is unrelated to the ECS. Apart from the doses used, another difference between the study of Farrimond et al. (2012a, 2012b) and previous studies on the effects of CBD (see earlier) was that in none of these former investigations did the authors use prefed animals, i.e., a condition that may facilitate the finding of anorectic actions, although not when ECs are involved (rimonabant is usually more efficacious in fasted vs. ad lib fed rodents). This observation may again indicate that non-CB_1-mediated mechanisms are involved in the effect of CBD.

In conclusion, the short-term CBD-induced feeding reductions reported in the studies by Farrimond and colleagues suggest that relatively low oral doses of this cannabinoid can reduce consummatory behavior. However, given the pharmacological profile of CBD, such effects are unlikely to be CB_1 mediated. Finally, in agreement, instead, with the activity of CBN as a partial agonist at CB_1 receptors, these authors confirmed that this other cannabinoid, which is a degradation product formed from Δ^9-THC in cannabis preparations, can induce food intake in rats via significant reductions in the latency to feed and increases in consummatory behaviors, due to increases in meal size and duration, which is compatible with CB_1 activation. The other phytocannabinoid tested in this study, cannabigerol, produced instead no effect whatsoever on food intake (Farrimond et al. 2012a).

24.4 **Conclusions**

The stimulatory effect on food intake is one of the best known pharmacological actions of cannabis preparations used for recreational purposes. However, although over the last 25 years, and particularly after the discovery of CB_1 and CB_2 receptors, much progress has been made in the understanding of the mechanisms through which Δ^9-THC affects food intake and energy metabolism (Silvestri and Di Marzo 2013), the application of this knowledge to the development of novel, efficacious, and safe treatments for cachexia and, particularly, anorexia, has unfortunately lagged behind. In the former condition, which is a hallmark of several chronic wasting disorders, the lack of a truly efficacious cannabinoid-based therapy is probably also due to the fact that the use of Δ^9-THC has been limited by its central unwanted side effects, which narrow the therapeutic window for this compound. This problem might be solved by the use of botanical drugs such as Sativex® (Russo 2011), the presence of CBD in which allows for the administration of higher and otherwise not tolerated doses of Δ^9-THC. Given the slight inhibitory effects of CBD on food intake, it is possible that combinations of lower doses of this compound with higher doses of Δ^9-THC, rather than Sativex® itself, might do the trick. Given the potentially important role of lean mass, and hence skeletal muscle loss, in cachexia, it is also possible that the so far only partial knowledge of the role of the ECS in this tissue (see Heyman et al. 2012, for a recent review) may have hampered the development of EC-based therapies for this condition. In the case of anorexia nervosa, instead, it is possible to hypothesize, from the data available to date, that the ECS may be deregulated in different ways during the course of this eating disorder, and thus play opposing roles in its onset and progression. Therefore, it is still not clear whether interventions that enhance or reduce the activity of CB_1 receptors should be employed for its pharmacological treatment, again, perhaps, suggesting the clinical testing of Δ^9-THC and CBD combinations. The future development of more clinically relevant experimental models of anorexia nervosa is to be awaited to facilitate mechanistic studies in this direction. At any rate, the ever increasing understanding of EC roles in food intake and energy metabolism, and the discovery of the additional mechanisms of action that will likely follow future investigations of non-Δ^9-THC phytocannabinoids, are likely to provide us, in the not so distant future, with new weapons to combat the two so far untreatable and life-threatening conditions that are cachexia and anorexia.

References

Andrykowski, M.A. (1988). Defining anticipatory nausea and vomiting: differences among cancer chemotherapy patients who report pretreatment nausea. *Journal of Behavioral Medicine*, **11**, 59–69.

Arnone, M., Maruani, J., Chaperon, F., *et al.* (1997). Selective inhibition of sucrose and ethanol intake by SR 141716, an antagonist of central cannabinoid (CB1) receptors. *Psychopharmacology*, **132**, 104–106.

Beal, J.E., Olson, R., Lefkowitz, L., *et al.* (1997). Long-term efficacy and safety of dronabinol for acquired immunodeficiency syndrome-associated anorexia.*Journal of Pain Symptom Management*, **14**, 7–14.

Bellocchio, L., Lafenetre, P., Cannich, A., *et al.* (2010). Bimodal control of stimulated food intake by the endocannabinoid system. *Nature Neuroscience*, **13**, 281–283.

Bisogno, T., Hanus, L., De Petrocellis, L., *et al.* (2001). Molecular targets for cannabidiol and its synthetic analogues: effect on vanilloid VR1 receptors and on the cellular uptake and enzymatic hydrolysis of anandamide. *British Journal of Pharmacology*, **134**, 845–852.

Breunig, E., Czesnik, D., Piscitelli, F., Di Marzo,V., Manzini, I., and Schild, D. (2010). Endocannabinoid modulation in the olfactory epithelium. *Results and Problems in Cell Differentiation*, **52**, 139–145.

Burdyga, G., Lal, S., Varro, A., Dimaline, R., Thompson, D.G., and Dockray G.J. (2004). Expression of cannabinoid CB1 receptors by vagal afferent neurons is inhibited by cholecystokinin. *The Journal of Neuroscience*, **24**, 2708–2715.

Clapham, J.C., Arch, J.R.S., and Tadayyon, M. (2001). Anti-obesity drugs: a critical review of current therapies and future opportunities. *Pharmacology & Therapeutics*, **89**, 81–121.

Cardinal, P., Bellocchio, L., Clark, S., *et al.* (2012). Hypothalamic CB_1 cannabinoid receptors regulate energy balance in mice. *Endocrinology*, **153**, 4136–4143.

Chaperon, F., Soubrié, P., Puech, A.J., and Thiébot, M.H. (1998). Involvement of central cannabinoid (CB1) receptors in the establishment of place conditioning in rats. *Psychopharmacology*, **135**, 324–332.

Chopra, R.N. and Chopra, G.S. (1939). The present position of hemp drug addiction in India. *Indian Medical Research Memoirs*, **31**, 1–119.

Cota, D., Marsicano, G., Tschöp, M., *et al.* (2003). The endogenous cannabinoid system affects energy balance via central orexigenic drive and peripheral lipogenesis. *Journal of Clinical Investigation*, **112**, 423–431.

Cota, D., Proulx, K., and Seeley, R.J. (2007). The role of CNS fuel sensing in energy and glucose regulation. *Gastroenterology*, **132**, 2158–2168.

De Luca, M.A., Solinas, M., Bimpisidis, Z., Goldberg, S.R., and Di Chiara, G. (2012). Cannabinoid facilitation of behavioral and biochemical hedonic taste responses. *Neuropharmacology*, **63**, 161–168.

De Petrocellis, L., Vellani, V., and Schiano-Moriello, A. (2008). Plant-derived cannabinoids modulate the activity of transient receptor potential channels of ankyrin type-1 and melastatin type-8. *Journal of Pharmacology and Experimental Therapeutics*, **325**, 1007–1015.

Deiana, S., Watanabe A., Yamasaki Y., *et al.* (2012). Plasma and brain pharmacokinetic profile of cannabidiol (CBD), cannabidivarine (CBDV), Δ^9-tetrahydrocannabivarin (THCV) and cannabigerol (CBG) in rats and mice following oral and intraperitoneal administration and CBD action on obsessive-compulsive behaviour. *Psychopharmacology*, **219**, 859–873.

Deroche-Gamonet, V., Le Moal, M., Piazza, P.V., and Soubrié, P. (2001). SR141716, a CB1 receptor antagonist, decreases the sensitivity to the reinforcing effects of electrical brain stimulation in rats. *Psychopharmacology*, **157**, 254–259.

Di Marzo, V. (2011). Endocannabinoid signaling in the brain: biosynthetic mechanisms in the limelight. *Nature Neuroscience*, **14**, 9–15.

Di Marzo, V., Goparaju, S.K., Wang, L., *et al.* (2001). Leptin-regulated endocannabinoids are involved in maintaining food intake. *Nature*, **410**, 822–825.

DiPatrizio, N.V., Astarita, G., Schwartz, G., Li, X., and Piomelli, D. (2011). Endocannabinoid signal in the gut controls dietary fat intake. *Proceedings of the National Academy of Sciences of the United States of America*, **108**, 12904–12908.

DiPatrizio, N.V. and Simansky, K.J. (2008). Activating parabrachial cannabinoid CB_1 receptors *selectively* stimulates feeding of palatable foods in rats. *Journal of Neuroscience*, **28**, 9702–979.

Dube, M.G., Kalra, S.P., and Kalra, P.S. (1999). Food intake elicited by central administration of orexins/hypocretins: identification of hypothalamic sites of action. *Brain Research*, **842**, 473–477.

Elsohly, M.A. and Slade, D. (2005). Chemical constituents of marijuana: the complex mixture of natural cannabinoids. *Life Sciences*, **78**, 539–548.

Farrimond, J.A., Hill, A.J., Whalley, B.J., and Williams, C.M. (2010a). Cannabis constituents modulate Δ9-tetrahydrocannabinol-induced hyperphagia in rats. *Psychopharmacology*, **210**, 97–106.

Farrimond, J.A., Whalley, B.J., and Williams, C.M. (2010b). A low-Δ^9tetrahydrocannabinol cannabis extract induces hyperphagia in rats. *Behavioral Pharmacology*, **21**, 769–772.

Farrimond, J.A., Whalley, B.J., and Williams, C.M. (2012a). Cannabinol and cannabidiol exert opposing effects on rat feeding patterns. *Psychopharmacology*, **223**, 117–129.

Farrimond, J.A., Whalley, B.J., and Williams, C.M. (2012b). Non-Δ-9 tetrahydrocannabinol phytocannabinoids stimulate feeding in rats. *Behavioral Pharmacology*, **23**, 113–117.

Feigenbaum, J.J., Richmond, S.A., Weissman, Y., and Mechoulam, R. (1989). Inhibition of *cis* platin-induced emesis in the pigeon by a non-psychotropic synthetic cannabinoid. *European Journal of Pharmacology*, **169**, 159–165.

Foltin, R.W., Brady, J.V., and Fischman, M.W. (1986). Behavioral analysis of marijuana effects on food intake in humans. *Pharmacology Biochemistry & Behavior*, **25**, 577–582.

Foltin, R.W., Fischman, M.W., and Byrne, M.F. (1988). Effects of smoked marijuana on food intake and body weight of humans living in a residential laboratory. *Appetite*, **11**, 1–14.

Gallate, J.E. and McGregor, I.S. (1999). The motivation for beer in rats: effects of ritanserin, naloxone and SR 141716. *Psychopharmacology*, **142**, 302–308.

Gaoni, Y. and Mechoulam, R. (1964). Isolation, structure and partial synthesis of an active constituent of hashish. *Journal of the American Chemical Society*, **86**, 1646–1647.

Gill, E.W., Paton, W.D., and Pertwee, R.G. (1970). Preliminary experiments on the chemistry and pharmacology of cannabis. *Nature*, **228**, 134–136.

Hanus, L., Avraham, Y., Ben-Shushan, D., Zolotarev, O., Berry, E.M., and Mechoulam, R. (2003). Short-term fasting and prolonged semistarvation have opposite effects on 2-AG levels in mouse brain. *Brain Research*, **983**, 144–151.

Harrold, J.A., Elliott, J.C., King, P.J., Widdowson, P.S., and Williams, G. (2002). Downregulation of cannabinoid-1 (CB-1) receptors in specific extrahypothalamic regions of rats with dietary obesity: a role for endogenous cannabinoids in driving appetite for palatable food? *Brain Research*, **952**, 232–238.

Harrold, J.A. and Williams, G. (2003). The cannabinoid system: a role in both the homeostatic and hedonic control of eating? *British Journal of Nutrition*, **90**, 729–734.

Heyman, E., Gamelin, F.X., Aucouturier, J., and Di Marzo, V. (2012). The role of the endocannabinoid system in skeletal muscle and metabolic adaptations to exercise: potential implications for the treatment of obesity. *Obesity Reviews*, **13**, 1110–1124.

Herkenham, M., Lynn, A.B., Little, M.D., *et al.* (1990). Cannabinoid receptor localization in brain. *Proceedings of the National Academy of Sciences of the United States of America*, **87**, 1932–1936.

Higuchi, S., Ohji, M., Araki, M., *et al.* (2011). Increment of hypothalamic 2-arachidonoylglycerol induces the preference for a high-fat diet via activation of cannabinoid 1 receptors. *Behavioural Brain Research*, **216**, 477–480.

Hilairet, S., Bouaboula, M., Carriere, D., Le Fur, G., and Casellas, P. (2003). Hypersensitization of the orexin 1 receptor by the CB_1 receptor: evidence for cross-talk blocked by the specific CB_1 antagonist, SR141716. *Journal of Biological Chemistry*, **278**, 23731–23737.

Hill, A.J., Williams, C.M., Whalley, B.J., and Stephens G.J. (2012). Phytocannabinoids as novel therapeutic agents in CNS disorders. *Pharmacology & Therapeutics*, **133**, 79–97.

Hollister, L.E. (1971). Actions of various marihuana derivatives in man. *Pharmacological Reviews*, **23**, 349–357.

Huang, H., Acuna-Goycolea, C., Li, Y., Cheng, H.M., Obrietan, K., and van den Pol, A.N. (2007). Cannabinoids excite hypothalamic melanin-concentrating hormone but inhibit hypocretin/orexin neurons: implications for cannabinoid actions on food intake and cognitive arousal. Journal of Neuroscience, **27**, 4870–4881.

Huestis, M.A., Gorelick, D.A., Heishman, S.J., *et al.* (2001). Blockade of effects of smoked marijuana by the CB1-selective cannabinoid receptor antagonist SR141716. *Archives of General Psychiatry*, **58**, 322–328.

Ignatowska-Jankowska, B., Jankowski, M.M., and Swiergiel, A.H. (2011). Cannabidiol decreases body weight gain in rats: involvement of CB_2 receptors. *Neuroscience Letters*, **490**, 82–84.

Izzo, A., Borrelli, F., Capasso, R., Di Marzo, V., and Mechoulam, R. (2009). Non-psychotropic plant cannabinoids: new therapeutic opportunities from an ancient herb. *Trends in Pharmacological Sciences*, **30**, 515–527.

Jamshidi, N. and Taylor, D.A. (2001). Anandamide administration into the ventromedial hypothalamus stimulates appetite in rats. *British Journal of Pharmacology*, **134**, 1151–1154.

Jäntti, M.H., Putula, J., Turunen, P.M., *et al.* (2013). Autocrine endocannabinoid signaling through CB1 receptors potentiates OX1 orexin receptor signaling. *Molecular Pharmacology*, **83**, 621–632.

Kano, M., Ohno-Shosaku, T., Hashimotodani, Y., Uchigashima, M., and Watanabe, M. (2009). Endocannabinoid-mediated control of synaptic transmission. *Physiological Reviews*, **89**, 309–380.

Kirkham, T.C. (1991). Opioids and feeding reward. *Appetite*, **17**, 74–75.

Kirkham, T.C. (2005). Endocannabinoids in the regulation of appetite and body weight. *Behavioral Pharmacology*, **16**, 297–313.

Kirkham, T.C. and Williams, C.M. (2001a). Synergistic effects of opioid and cannabinoid antagonists on food intake. *Psychopharmacology (Berlin)*, **153**, 267–270.

Kirkham, T.C. and Williams, C.M. (2001b). Endocannabinoids: neuromodulators of food craving? In: M. Hetherington (ed.). *Food Cravings and Addiction*. Leatherhead: Leatherhead Publishing, pp. 85–120.

Kirkham, T.C., Williams, C.M., Fezza, F., and Di Marzo, V. (2002). Endocannabinoid levels in rat limbic forebrain and hypothalamus in relation to fasting, feeding and satiation: stimulation of eating by 2-arachidonoyl glycerol. *British Journal of Pharmacology*, **136**, 550–557.

Koch, J.E. (2001). Delta(9)-THC stimulates food intake in Lewis rats: effects on chow, high-fat and sweet high-fat diets. *Pharmacology Biochemistry & Behavior*, **68**, 539–543.

Kola, B., Farkas, I., Christ-Crain, M., *et al.* (2008). The orexigenic effect of ghrelin is mediated through central activation of the endogenous cannabinoid system. *Public Library of Science One*, **3**, 1797.

Labouèbe, G., Liu, S., Dias, C., *et al.* (2013). Insulin induces long-term depression of ventral tegmental area dopamine neurons via endocannabinoids. *Nature Neuroscience*, **16**, 300–308.

Lawrence, C.B., Turnbull, A.V., and Rothwell, N.J. (1999). Hypothalamic control of feeding. *Current Opinion in Neurobiology*, **9**, 778–783.

Lee, S., Kim, D.H., Yoon, S.H., and Ryu, J.H. (2009). Sub-chronic administration of rimonabant causes loss of antidepressive activity and decreases doublecortin immunoreactivity in the mouse hippocampus. *Neuroscience Letters*, **467**, 111–116.

Limebeer, C.L. and Parker, L.A. (1999). Delta-9-tetrahydrocannabinol interferes with the establishment and the expression of conditioned rejection reactions produced by cyclophosphamide: a rat model of nausea. *Neuroreport*, **10**, 3769–3772.

Loewe, S. (1946). Studies on the pharmacology and acute toxicity of compounds with marihuana activity. *Journal of Pharmacology Experimental Therapy*, **88**, 154–161.

Mahler, S.V., Smith, K.S., and Berridge, K.C. (2007). Endocannabinoid hedonic hotspot for sensory pleasure: anandamide in nucleus accumbens shell enhances 'liking' of a sweet reward. *Neuropsychopharmacology*, **32**, 2267–2278.

Malcher-Lopes, R., Di, S., Marcheselli, V.S., *et al.* (2006). Opposing crosstalk between leptin and glucocorticoids rapidly modulates synaptic excitation via endocannabinoid release. *The Journal of Neuroscience*, **26**, 6643–6650.

Massa, F., Mancini, G., Schmidt, H., *et al.* (2010). Alterations in the hippocampal endocannabinoid system in diet-induced obese mice. *The Journal of Neuroscience*, **30**, 6273–6281.

Matias, I., Vergoni, A.V., Petrosino, S., *et al.* (2008). Regulation of hypothalamic endocannabinoid levels by neuropeptides and hormones involved in food intake and metabolism: insulin and melanocortins. *Neuropharmacology*, **54**, 206–212.

McCarthy, L.E. and Borison, H.L. (1984). Cisplatin-induced vomiting eliminated by ablation of the area postrema in cats. *Cancer Treatement Reports*, **68**, 401–404.

McNay, D.E.G.,Briançon, N., Kokoeva, M.V., Maratos-Flier, E., and Flier, J.S. (2012). Remodeling of the arcuate nucleus energy-balance circuit is inhibited in obese mice. *Journal of Clinical Investigation*, **122**, 142–152.

Mechoulam, R. and Fride, E. (2001). Physiology. A hunger for cannabinoids. *Nature*, **410**, 763–765.

Mechoulam, R., Hanus, L., and Fride, E. (1998). Towards cannabinoid drugs revisited. *Progress in Medicinal Chemistry*, **35**, 199–243.

Mechoulam, R. and Shvo, Y. (1963). Hashish I. The structure of cannabidiol. *Tetrahedron*. **19**, 2073–2078.

Mehmedic, Z., Chandra, S., Slade, D., *et al.* (2010). Potency trends of Δ9-THC and other cannabinoids in confiscated cannabis preparations from 1993 to 2008. *Journal of Forensic Sciences*, **55**, 1209–1217.

Melis, T., Succu, S., Sanna, F., Boi, A., Argiolas, A., and Melis, M.R. (2007). The cannabinoid antagonist SR 141716A (Rimonabant) reduces the increase of extra-cellular dopamine release in the rat nucleus accumbens induced by a novel high palatable food. *Neuroscience Letters*, **419**, 231–235.

Meye, F.J., Trezza, V., Vanderschuren, L.J., Ramakers, G.M., and Adan, R.A. (2013). Neutral antagonism at the cannabinoid 1 receptor: a safer treatment for obesity. *Molecular Psychiatry*, **18**, 1294–1301.

Monteleone, P., Matias, I., Martiadis, V., De Petrocellis, L., Maj, M., and Di Marzo, V. (2005). Blood levels of the endocannabinoid anandamide are increased in anorexia nervosa and in binge-eating disorder, but not in bulimia nervosa. *Neuropsychopharmacology*, **30**, 1216–1221.

Monteleone, P., Piscitelli, F., Scognamiglio, P., *et al.* (2012). Hedonic eating is associated with increased peripheral levels of ghrelin and the endocannabinoid 2-arachidonoyl-glycerol in healthy humans: a pilot study. *Journal of Clinical Endocrinology & Metabolism*, **97**, 917–924.

Morrow, G.R., Hickok, J.T., Burish, T.G., and Rosenthal, S.N. (1996). Frequency and clinical implications of delayed nausea and delayed emesis. *American Journal of Clinical Oncology*, **19**, 199–203.

Morton, G.J., Cummings, D.E., Baskin, D.G., Barsh, G.S., and Schwartz, M.W. (2006). Central nervous system control of food intake and body weight. *Nature*, **443**, 289–295.

O'Gorman, P., McMillan, D.C., and McArdle, C.S. (2000). Prognostic factors in advanced gastrointestinal cancer patients with weight loss. *Nutrition and Cancer*, **37**, 36–40.

O'Shaugnessy, W. (1843). On the *Cannabis indica* or Indian hemp, *Journal of Pharmacology*, **2**, 594.

Parker, L.A., Kwiatkowska, M., Burton, P., and Mechoulam, R. (2004). Effect of cannabinoids on lithium-induced vomiting in the *Suncus murinus* (house musk shrew). *Psychopharmacology (Berlin)*, **171**, 156–161.

Parker, L.A., Mechoulam, R., and Schlievert, C. (2002). Cannabidiol, a non-psychoactive component of cannabis and its synthetic dimethylheptyl homolog suppress nausea in an experimental model with rats. *Neuroreport*, **13**, 567–570.

Pertwee, R.G., Thomas, A., Stevenson, L.A., *et al.* (2007). The psychoactive plant cannabinoid, Δ9-tetrahydrocannabinol, is antagonized by Δ8- and Δ9-tetrahydrocannabivarin in mice in vivo. *British Journal of Pharmacology*, **150**, 586–594.

Plasse, T.F. (1991). Clinical use of dronabinol. *Journal of Clinical Oncology*, **9**, 2079–2080.

Qian, S., Chen, H., Weingarth, D., *et al.* (2002). Neither agouti-related protein nor neuropeptide Y is critically required for the regulation of energy homeostasis in mice. *Molecular Cell Biology*, **22**, 5027–5035.

Riedel, G., Fadda, P., McKillop-Smith, S., Pertwee, R.G., Platt, B., and Robinson, L. (2009). Synthetic and plant-derived cannabinoid receptor antagonists show hypophagic properties in fasted and non-fasted mice. *British Journal of Pharmacology*, **156**, 1154–1166.

Riggs, P.K., Vaida, F., Rossi, S.S., *et al.* (2012). A pilot study of the effects of cannabis on appetite hormones in HIV-infected adult men. *Brain Research*, **1431**, 46–52.

Romero-Zerbo, S.Y., Garcia-Gutierrez, M.S., Suárez, J., *et al.* (2012). Overexpression of cannabinoid CB2 receptor in the brain induces hyperglycaemia and a lean phenotype in adult mice. *Journal of Neuroendocrinology*, **24**, 1106–1119.

Rowland, N.E., Mukherjee, M., and Robertson, K. (2001). Effects of the cannabinoid receptor antagonist SR 141716, alone and in combination with dexfenfluramine or naloxone, on food intake in rats. *Psychopharmacology*, **159**, 111–116.

Russo, E. (2011). Taming THC: potential cannabis synergy and phytocannabinoid-terpenoid entourage effects. *British Journal of Pharmacology*, **163**, 1344–1364.

Ryan, D., Drysdale, A.J., Lafourcade, C., Pertwee, R.G., and Platt, B. (2009). Cannabidiol targets mitochondria to regulate intracellular Ca^{2+} levels. *Journal of Neuroscience*, **29**, 2053–2063.

Schwartz, M.W., Woods, S.C., Porte, D. Jr., Seeley, R.J., and Baskin, D.G. (2000). Central nervous system control of food intake. *Nature*, **404**, 661–671.

Scopinho, A.A., Guimarães, F.S., Corrêa, F.M., and Resstel, L.B. (2011). Cannabidiol inhibits the hyper-phagia induced by cannabinoid-1 or serotonin-1A receptor agonists. *Pharmacology Biochemistry & Behavior*, **98**, 268–272.

Silvestri, C. and Di Marzo, V. (2012). Second generation CB1 receptor blockers and other inhibitors of peripheral endocannabinoid overactivity and the rationale of their use against metabolic disorders. *Expert Opinion on Investigational Drugs*, **21**, 1309–1322.

Silvestri, C. and Di Marzo, V. (2013). The endocannabinoid system in energy homeostasis and the aetiopa-thology of metabolic disorders. *Cell Metabolism*, **17**, 475–490.

Simiand, J., Keane, M., Keane, P.E., and Soubrié, P. (1998). SR 141716, a CB_1 cannabinoid receptor antag-onist, selectively reduces sweet food intake in marmoset. *Behavioural Pharmacology*, **9**, 179–181.

Sofia, R.D. and Knobloch, L.C. (1976). Comparative effects of various naturally occurring cannabi-noids on food, sucrose and water consumption by rats. *Pharmacology Biochemistry & Behavior*, **4**, 591–599.

Soria-Gómez, E., Matias, I., Rueda-Orozco, P.E., *et al.* (2007). Pharmacological enhancement of the endo-cannabinoid system in the nucleus accumbens shell stimulates food intake and increases c-Fos expres-sion in the hypothalamus. *British Journal of Pharmacology*, **151**, 1109–1116.

Strasser F., Luftner D., Possinger K., *et al.* (2006). Comparison of orally administered cannabis extract and delta-9-tetrahydrocannabinol in treating patients with cancer-related anorexia-cachexia syn-drome: a multicenter, phase III, randomized, double-blind, placebo-controlled clinical trial from the Cannabis-In-Cachexia-Study-Group. *Journal of Clinical Oncology*, **24**, 3394–3400.

Sweet, D.C., Levine, A.S., Billington, C.J., and Kotz, C.M. (1999). Feeding response to central orexins. *Brain Research*, **821**, 535–538.

Timpone, J., Wright, D., Li, N., *et al.* (1999). The safety and pharmacokinetics of single-agent and com-bination therapy with megestrol acetate and dronabinol for the treatment of HIV wasting syndrome. In: G.G. Nahas, K.M. Sutin, D. Harvey, and S. Agurell (eds.). *Marihuana and Medicine*. Totowa, NJ: Humana Press, pp. 701–716.

Tisdale, M.J. (2002). Cachexia in cancer patients. *Nature Reviews Cancer*, **2**, 862–871.

Tisdale, M.J. (2009). Mechanisms of cancer cachexia. *Physiological Reviews*, **89**, 381–410.

Thomas, A., Baillie, G.L., Phillips, A.M., Razdan, R.K., Ross, R.A., and Pertwee, R.G. (2007). Cannabidiol displays unexpectedly high potency as an antagonist of CB_1 and CB_2 receptor agonists in vitro. *British Journal of Pharmacology*, **150**, 613–623.

Thomas, A., Stevenson, L.A., Wease, K.N., *et al.* (2005). Evidence that the plant cannabinoid $\Delta 9$-tetrahydrocannabivarin is a cannabinoid CB_1 and CB_2 receptor antagonist. *British Journal of Pharmacology*, **146**, 917–926.

Turunen, P.M., Jäntti, M.H., and Kukkonen, J.P. (2012). OX1 orexin/hypocretin receptor signaling through arachidonic acid and endocannabinoid release. *Molecular Pharmacology*, **82**, 156–167.

Van Sickle, M.D., Oland, L.D., Ho, W., *et al.* (2001). Cannabinoids inhibit emesis through CB1 receptors in the brainstem of the ferret. *Gastroenterology*, **121**, 767–774.

Verty, A.N., Singh, M.E., McGregor, I.S., and Mallet, P.E. (2003). The cannabinoid receptor antagonist SR 141716 attenuates overfeeding induced by systemic or intracranial morphine. *Psychopharmacology (Berlin)*, **168**, 314–323.

Walsh, D., Donnelly, S., and Rybicki, L. (2000). The symptoms of advanced cancer: relationship to age, gender, and performance status in 1,000 patients. *Supportive Care in Cancer*, **8**, 175–179.

Wang, X., Miyares, R.L., and Ahern, G.P (2005). Oleoylethanolamide excites vagal sensory neurones, induces visceral pain and reduces short-term food intake in mice via capsaicin receptor TRPV1. *Journal of Physiology*, **564**, 541–547.

Ward, S.J. and Raffa, R.B. (2011). Rimonabant redux and strategies to improve the future outlook of CB_1 receptor neutralantagonist/inverse-agonist therapies. *Obesity*, **19**, 1325–1334.

Wiley, J.L., Burston, J.J., Leggett, D.C., *et al.* (2005). CB_1 cannabinoid receptor-mediated modulation of food intake in mice. *British Journal of Pharmacology*, **145**, 293–300.

Williams, C.M. and Kirkham, T.C. (2002a). Observational analysis of feeding induced by Delta9-THC and anandamide. *Physiology & Behavior*, **76**, 241–250.

Williams, C.M. and Kirkham, T.C. (2002b). Reversal of delta 9-THC hyperphagia by SR141716 and naloxone but not dexfenfluramine. *Pharmacology Biochemistry and Behavior*, **71**, 333–340.

Williams, C.M., Rogers, P.J., and Kirkham, T.C. (1998). Hyperphagia in pre-fed rats following oral delta9-THC. *Physiology & Behavior*, **65**, 343–346.

Winters, B.D., Krüger, J.M., Huang, X., *et al.* (2012). Cannabinoid receptor 1-expressing neurons in the nucleus accumbens. *Proceedings of the National Academy of Sciences of the United States of America*, **109**, E2717–E27125.

Yoshida, R., Ohkuri, T., and Jyotaki, M. (2010). Endocannabinoids selectively enhance sweet taste. *Proceedings of the National Academy of Sciences of the United States of America*, **107**, 935–939.

Chapter 25

Pain

Barbara Costa and Francesca Comelli

25.1 Introduction

Marijuana has been used to treat chronic pain for thousands of years (Burns and Ineck 2006; Murray et al. 2007). However, the widespread use of medical marijuana is still controversial because the plant produces both therapeutic and psychoactive effects. This chapter focuses on the antinociceptive properties of phytocannabinoids, with emphasis on chronic pathological pain, such as neuropathic pain. Indeed, acute pain is well controlled by actual therapies, whereas chronic pain is still often refractory to conventional pharmacotherapies, necessitating the development and validation of novel analgesics. The preclinical evidence obtained in well-characterized animal models of pathological pain, contributes to the hypothesis that one of the most promising therapeutic uses of phytocannabinoids in humans is their employment as pain killers.

25.2 Delta-9-tetrahydrocannabinol

Delta-9-tetrahydrocannabinol (THC) has been tested in a wide range of antinociceptive assays. It has been demonstrated as effective in producing antinociception in both phasic (e.g., tail-flick and hot-plate tests) and tonic (e.g., abdominal stretch test) nociceptive assays and, actually, there are a wide range of animal models of acute and tonic pain in which THC exhibits antinociceptive activity, when administered orally, systemically, or directly into the brain or spinal cord (see Costa 2007 for review and Table 25.1).

One of the major obstacles in developing THC as a medicine is its cannabimimetic side effect profile. Various approaches have been suggested in order to overcome this issue. One of these approaches is the addition of cannabidiol (CBD) as well as of other phytocannabinoids (see section 25.7). Also cannabinoids, which stimulate cannabinoid type 2 receptors (CB_2), can further separate analgesic activity from cannabimimetic psychotropic activity. Since THC is a mixed cannabinoid CB_1/CB_2 receptor agonist, some studies evaluated the effectiveness of this compound in pathological pain, in which the CB_2 receptor plays a pivotal role (it is distributed in peripheral tissues and inhibits the release of inflammatory mediators that excite nociceptors), such as chronic inflammatory pain. In the rat model of Freund's adjuvant-induced chronic arthritic pain (CFA), it was shown that, although THC is equipotent and equiefficacious in nonarthritic and arthritic rats, the antinociceptive effects of THC in arthritic rats are produced via activation of both cannabinoid CB_1 and CB_2 receptors, whereas in nonarthritic rats, THC appears to produce antinociception via cannabinoid CB_1 receptor activation only (Cox et al. 2007a). One might hypothesize from such data that chronic pain such as that experienced by arthritics has two distinct, but interacting components that involve both cannabinoid CB_1 and CB_2 receptors. Another possible strategy would be to induce antinociception with a peripherally restricted cannabinoid receptor agonist. Indeed, CT-3 (ajulemic acid), a synthetic analogue of a metabolite of THC, binds with

Table 25.1 Studies demonstrating the analgesic effect of THC in animal models (see Costa 2007 for review and references)

Acute pain	Tonic/chronic pain
Hot plate	Abdominal stretch test (phenylbenzoquinone into peritoneum)
Tail flick	Acetic or formic acid into peritoneum
Randall–Selitto paw pressure	Freund's adjuvant into hind paw
Flinch jump	Formalin into hind paw
Electrically stimulated sciatic nerve	Capsaicin
Tooth pulp	Loose ligation of sciatic nerve
Skin-twitch reflex	Stretching

high affinity to human CB_1 and CB_2 receptors and has potent antihyperalgesic activity in models of chronic neuropathic and inflammatory pain in the rat which is mediated only by the CB_1 receptor subtype (Dyson et al. 2005). Its weak psycho-activity is due to the pharmacokinetics of the compound which has a partially restricted entry into the central nervous system with brain levels reaching only 30–40% of peak plasma levels following oral administration (Dyson et al. 2005). These and other findings (Fox et al. 2001; Ibrahim et al. 2003) suggest: (1) that it is possible to induce a significant relief of chronic pain through the activation of peripheral CB_1 and (2) that the CB_2 contribution to chronic pain relief is essentially due to its expression on microglial cells within the spinal cord. Unexpectedly, concerning neuropathic pain, there is only one report showing an antihyperalgesic effect of THC, when it is administered intrathecally to rats with neuropathic pain (Mao et al. 2000). There is a more recent paper showing the ability of THC to alleviate diabetic neuropathy; THC showed a significantly higher antinociceptive effect at a dose of 50 mg/kg orally (p.o.) in diabetic mice versus nondiabetic mice (Williams et al. 2008). There is no doubt that THC is a potent analgesic, but the findings that THC-induced antinociception is mediated principally through the activation of CB_1 receptors accounts for the concomitant behavioral side effects that hinder its use. This is probably why the effectiveness of THC against neuropathic pain has been so little investigated. The obvious consequence has been the attempt to use low doses of THC, especially in combination with other analgesics. Consistent with this approach many studies explored the combination of THC in low, nonpsychoactive doses, with opioids. The idea is that, since THC acts synergistically with opioids as an opioid-sparing agent, combined low-dose administration of THC with an opioid would produce pain relief with fewer side effects than those produced by analgesic doses of each of these drugs when they are administered alone. Low doses of THC were found to significantly enhance morphine-induced antinociception in the tail-flick test in the mouse when both were administered intrathecally (Welch and Stevens 1992), and intracerebroventricular administration of both drugs resulted in an enhancement of morphine-induced antinociception (Welch et al. 1995). It was further established that THC enhanced the potency of morphine in any subcutaneous (s.c.)–p.o. combination in mice in the tail-flick test, and that both given s.c. enhanced the potency of morphine in mice for its inhibition of paw withdrawal to radiant heat (Smith et al. 1998). The enhancement of both morphine- and codeine-induced antinociception by THC, administered p.o., was found to be a synergistic rather than an additive interaction, as indicated by isobolographic analysis (Cichewicz and McCarthy 2003).

The clinical utility of such combinations has yet to be studied, but has the possibility of producing effective pain relief with a decrease in side effects, not the least of which is tolerance to both cannabinoids and opioids, as demonstrated in acute pain models utilizing the drugs in combination: tolerance to morphine was prevented in groups of animals receiving a daily cotreatment with a nonanalgesic dose of THC (Cichewicz and Welch 2003). Importantly, morphine-tolerant mice were more sensitive to the acute antinociceptive effects of THC, suggesting no cross-tolerance development (Cichewicz and Welch 2003). The same research group reported that morphine and THC exhibit synergy in the expression of antinociception in chronic pain models, too (Cox et al. 2007b). Particularly in chronic inflammatory pain a THC/morphine combination results both in a synergistic antinociceptive interaction in both normal and arthritic rats and in less tolerance development (Cox et al. 2007b). Also, morphine-induced antinociception is significantly enhanced by THC in both nondiabetic and diabetic mice, although the enhancement was found to be greatest in degree in diabetic mice (Williams et al. 2008). Interestingly, morphine was found to release both leu-enkephalin and β-endorphin in nondiabetic rats, but failed to release these endogenous opioids in diabetic rats, whereas THC did induce release of dynorphin and leu-enkephalin in diabetic rats (Williams et al. 2008), suggesting that diabetes itself may affect the ability of morphine to release endogenous opioids and produce analgesia in diabetic models of pain. In summary, many preclinical findings suggest that cannabinoid/opioid therapy may be able to produce long-term antinociceptive effects at doses devoid of substantial side effects, while avoiding production of the neuronal biochemical changes that give rise to tolerance. A critical future direction is the evaluation of the clinical utility of such a combination. In particular, the potential pharmacokinetics and the safety of the combination in humans are unknown.

25.3 **Cannabidiol**

Interest in exploiting the therapeutic properties of CBD was initially focused on its interactions with the main psychotropic constituent of *Cannabis sativa*, THC. However, the past several years have seen a growing interest in CBD per se because of the discovery of its antioxidant, anti-inflammatory, and neuroprotective effects, all of which are produced independently of the cannabinoid CB_1 and CB_2 receptors (Izzo et al. 2009; De Petrocellis and Di Marzo 2010). Concerning pain, the analgesic effectiveness of CBD was firstly assessed in mice using the acetic-induced writhing model and in rats submitted to hot-plate tests and the Randall–Selitto paw pressure test (Sofia et al. 1975). This study demonstrated no analgesic effect of CBD, and this lack of efficacy was then confirmed in the acetic acid abdominal constriction test (Sanders et al. 1979). Conversely, CBD was found effective in the phenylbenzoquinone (PBQ)-induced mouse writhing test (model of peripheral pain), when given orally 20 min before the intraperitoneal (i.p.) injection of PBQ (Formukong et al. 1988). These conflicting results suggested that CBD is ineffective against acute pain, but is effective against pathological pain. As a consequence, the analgesic properties of CBD were tested in models of persistent and inflammatory pain with conflicting results. In fact, Costa et al. (2004a) reported that in inflammatory conditions, CBD had potent antihyperalgesic activity; only 1 h after single, very low doses, CBD abolished the hyperalgesia which develops in the rat paw after carrageenan injection. In a subsequent paper, the same group showed that the antihyperalgesic effect of CBD in the carrageenan model of inflammatory pain was mediated by transient receptor potential (TRP)V1 and did not involve the cannabinoid receptor subtypes CB_1 and CB_2 (Costa et al. 2004b), highlighting: (1) the ability of CBD to target receptors different from CB_1 and CB_2 for which it displays poor affinity and (2) the effectiveness of CBD in relieving pain in pathological conditions. In the same year it was reported that CBD failed to reduce the first and second phases of formalin-evoked nociceptive behavior (Finn et al. 2004), and, in line with this finding, a more recent report by Booker et al. (2009) demonstrated that CBD did not affect abdominal stretching, a model of visceral pain, suggesting, again, that although CBD lacks antinociceptive activity in animal models of acute and tonic pain, it may have therapeutic use in chronic pathological pain, such as inflammatory and neuropathic hyperalgesia. The first report showing the effectiveness of CBD in pathological inflammatory and neuropathic pain was from our research group (Costa et al. 2007); in our hands CBD was able to reduce hyper-algesic responses to thermal and mechanical stimuli when repeatedly administered at 20 mg/kg to CFA-injected and to neuropathic rats via an oral route. Interestingly, the antihyperalgesic effect of CBD was prevented by the vanilloid antagonist capsazepine but not by cannabinoid receptor antagonists, indicating the pivotal role of the TRPV1 receptor in CBD-induced relief of neuro-pathic pain. Thereafter, CBD was also shown effective in relieving neuropathic pain induced in rats by the antineoplastic drug, paclitaxel, when administered i.p. daily at 5–10 mg/kg for 2 weeks (Ward et al. 2011). Of interest, CBD completely prevented the development of paclitaxel-induced cold and mechanical allodynia, with no latent neuropathy emerging after the cessation of CBD treatment (Ward et al. 2011). These authors didn't investigate the potential mechanisms underly-ing CBD's effectiveness, but did suggest that the effect could be related to the potency it displays at lowering the levels of key proinflammatory cytokines, because paclitaxel has been shown to increase the expression of such cytokines. Peripheral neuropathy is a common complication occurring during diabetes and its management is often inadequate and unsatisfactory. CBD was found to ameliorate neuropathic pain in streptozotocin-diabetic CD1 mice after intranasal dos-ing (Toth et al. 2010). In this experimental setting CBD administered at the onset of diabetes and prior to identified neuropathic pain, limited the development of later neuropathic pain and this effect was mediated by CB_2 receptors (Toth et al. 2010). Taken together, these findings have demonstrated broad-spectrum antinociceptive properties of CBD in different models of painful neuropathy. Concerning the mechanism of action, over the last years, several potential alternative pharmacological targets for CBD have been proposed, often based solely on pharmacological evi-dence obtained in vitro. Indeed, the most intriguing properties of CBD are related to its capability to interact pharmacologically with various receptors/systems, including those involved in pain modulation. Table 25.2 summarizes the molecular targets of CBD which could be responsible for the analgesic properties of this phytocannabinoid.

On the basis of these observations, a recent study has provided evidence suggesting that CBD and its analogue dehydroxyl-CBD (DH-CBD), suppress neuropathic pain in rats with spinal nerve ligation, by targeting the α3 glycine receptor (Xiong et al. 2012). Both CBD and DH-CBD-induced analgesic effects were significantly reduced in mice lacking the α3 glycine receptor but not in mice lacking CB_1 and CB_2 receptors. Furthermore, structural and functional analysis revealed that the magnitude of the CBD and DH-CBD-induced analgesic effects correlated with their potentiation of the α3 glycine receptor but not with their binding affinity for CB_1 and CB_2 recep-tors. Spinal α3 glycine receptors have been proposed as an important target for pain treatment. However, α3 glycine receptor-based therapeutic agents are not yet available for the treatment of chronic pain or other diseases. The preclinical data obtained by Xiong and colleagues, together with findings showing that several phytocannabinoids, including THC and CBD, can potentiate glycine currents (IGly) in native neurons isolated from the ventral tegmental area, amygdala, hippocampus, and spinal cord (Ahrens et al. 2009), suggest that "glycinergic phytocannabinoids" are ideal therapeutic agents for the treatment of neuropathic pain. It was also found that the CBD derivative O-1602, which is a GPR55 agonist, was able to reduce joint afferent mechanosensitiv-ity in an acute model of joint inflammation (Schuelert and McDougall 2011). The desensitizing

Table 25.2 Proposed molecular targets of CBD

Receptor/enzyme	Activity	Reference
CB$_1$	Antagonist	Thomas et al. 2007
CB$_2$	Agonist/inverse agonist	Thomas et al. 2007
Fatty acid amide hydrolase	Inhibition	Ligresti et al. 2006
GPR55	Antagonist	Ryberg et al. 2007
α1 and α1β glycine receptors	Positive allosteric modulator	Ahrens et al. 2009
μ and δ opioid receptor	Positive allosteric modulator	Kathmann et al. 2006
TRPA1	Agonist	De Petrocellis et al. 2008
TRPM8	Antagonist	De Petrocellis et al. 2008
TRPV1	Agonist	De Petrocellis et al. 2008
TRPV2	Agonist	Qin et al. 2008
5-HT$_{1A}$	Direct agonist Indirect agonist	Russo et al. 2005 Rock et al. 2012
Abnormal-CBD receptor	Antagonist	Walter et al. 2003

effect of O-1602 was abolished by coadministration of the abnormal cannabidiol receptor/GPR55 antagonist O-1918, while pretreatment with CB$_1$ and CB$_2$ receptor antagonists had no effect on O-1602 responses. Thus, O-1602 appears to act on GPR55 receptors to inhibit peripheral sensitization of joint nociceptors (Schuelert and McDougall 2011). A role for GPR55 in nociceptive signaling is corroborated by the finding that this receptor is highly expressed by mouse primary sensory neurons and by evidence indicating that GPR55 knockout mice do not develop mechanical hyperalgesia in response to inflammatory or neuropathic insults (Staton et al. 2008). While the investigation by Schuelert and McDougall indicates an antinociceptive role for GPR55, pain behavioral studies need to be carried out to ascertain whether activation of this receptor can truly produce analgesia. The capability of CBD to behave as a positive allosteric modulator of μ and δ opioid receptors (Kathmann et al. 2006) indicates that CBD could potentially enhance the analgesic effects of opiates. Even though this effect is produced only by high concentrations of CBD in vitro, it is possible that in neuropathic pain conditions in vivo, modulation of opioid receptor activity by CBD could contribute to its analgesic effect, a hypothesis that has, however, yet to be explored. Further molecular mechanisms that could explain CBD-induced relief of neuropathic pain include TRPA1/TRPV2/TRPV1 activation/desensitization (De Petrocellis et al. 2008; Qin et al. 2008), as well as TRPM8 antagonism. Many studies in mice deficient in TRP channels indicate that TRP channels may play a crucial role in the hypersensitivity to thermal, chemical and mechanical stimuli that is associated with neuropathies. The stimulating effects of CBD at TRPA1, TRPV1, and TRPV2 result in the desensitization of these channels (De Petrocellis et al. 2011). Desensitization might have important consequences for the potential use of CBD as a therapeutic agent in those disorders, such as chronic and inflammatory pain, in which these channels have been shown to be implicated and to play a permissive role. TRPA1, TRPV1, and TRPV2 antagonists are of course also effective against pain. However, the antinociception exerted through TRP channel desensitization should be devoid of the unwanted effects typically induced by TRP channel blockade (Vay et al. 2012; Wong and Gavva 2009). In addition, TRPM8 has emerged as a sensory transducer contributing to pain hypersensitivity associated with neuropathy since it is strongly expressed in C- and possibly Aδ-fibers (Kobayashi et al. 2005), and very probably in a subset of cells different from those expressing TRPV1 (Appendino et al. 2008). It is noteworthy, therefore, that CBD is a TRPM8 antagonist, since this action could contribute to its ability to induce antinociception. Finally, the functions of certain serotonin receptors, including 5-HT$_{2A}$, 5-HT$_{2B}$, 5-HT$_4$, and 5-HT$_{1A}$, are profoundly affected by neuropathic pain (Aira et al. 2010; Nitanda et al. 2005), and a selective 5-HT$_{1A}$ agonist has very recently been found to potently depress evoked field potentials in neuropathic rats (Aira et al. 2010), revealing another possible mechanism by which CBD might induce analgesia: direct or indirect activation of 5-HT$_{1A}$ receptors (Table 25.2). In addition, evidence for the involvement of adenosine A$_1$ receptors in CBD-induced antinociception was recently obtained in experiments with rats (Maione et al. 2011). Thus, injections of CBD directly into the ventrolateral periaqueductal gray (vl-PAG) produced antinociceptive responses in the tail-flick test accompanied, in this brain area, by a decrease in the ongoing activity of ON neurons, as expected, and also, paradoxically, by a decrease in the ongoing activity of OFF neurons, effects that were antagonized by selective antagonists of cannabinoid CB$_1$, adenosine A$_1$, and TRPA1 receptors, although not of TRPV1 receptors. That these effects of CBD on the vl-PAG were mediated by CB$_1$ and adenosine A$_1$ receptors, as well as by TRPA1 receptors could explain why this compound inhibited ongoing activity of both ON and OFF neurons. Importantly, neuropathic pain is associated with microglial activation in the spinal cord and brain and the subsequent release of proinflammatory cytokines, such as interleukin-6, interleukin-1β, and tumor necrosis factor α. The etiology of neuropathic pain, which is common in cancer, diabetes, multiple sclerosis, and peripheral nerve injury, is poorly understood, but recent evidence indicates that increased reactive oxygen species generation by microglial cells is a critical initiating factor. Thus, the antioxidant and anti-inflammatory properties of CBD could strongly contribute to its potent effect upon neuropathic pain. In fact, CBD was shown to inhibit activated microglial cell migration by antagonizing an abnormal cannabidiol-sensitive receptor (Walter et al. 2003). CBD is also a competitive inhibitor, with an IC$_{50}$ in the nanomolar range, of adenosine uptake by the equilibrative nucleoside transporter 1 of macrophages and microglial cells and it has been shown to have potent actions in attenuating oxidative and nitrosative stress (Carrier et al. 2006; Pan et al. 2009). Furthermore, the antinociceptive effects of CBD in diabetic mice were associated with a restriction in elevation of microglial density and p38 MAPK activity in the dorsal spinal cord (Toth et al. 2010). Altogether, these observations strongly suggest that CBD attenuates chronic pain not through a single mechanism, but rather by acting through several mechanisms on both neuronal and non-neuronal cells. This pharmacological profile, together with its lack of psychotropic side effects, makes this phytocannabinoid a strong candidate for pathological pain treatment.

25.4 **Tetrahydrocannabivarin**

Tetrahydrocannabivarin (THCV) is the propyl homolog of THC and behaves as a potent CB$_2$ receptor partial agonist in vitro and as an antagonist and/or inverse agonist of the CB$_1$ receptor both in vitro and in vivo (Pertwee 2008). This it does with relatively high potency and in a manner that is both tissue and ligand dependent. This peculiar pharmacological profile may be of great interest in the employment of THCV against pain for at least two reasons. The first is the evidence indicating that CB$_1$ antagonists/inverse agonists can reduce pain hypersensitivity as well as CB$_1$ agonists, even if only in chronic pathological conditions, characterized by altered endocannabinoid tone and by the presence of regulatory changes in cannabinoid receptors or in other related systems (vanilloid). In fact, it has been shown that repeated administration of the CB_1 antagonist/inverse agonist, rimonabant, is effective in alleviating thermal and mechanical hyperalgesia in two rat models of neuropathic pain (Comelli et al. 2010; Costa et al. 2005) and that this effectiveness could be due to its blockade of the constitutive activity of the CB_1 receptor which maintains the TRPV1 channel in a sensitized state responsive to noxious chemical stimuli (Fioravanti et al. 2008). The second is the emerging evidence for a role for the CB_2 receptor in chronic pain modulation. Thus, there have been reports that CB_2 receptor agonists are effective against many types of pain: inflammatory, neuropathic, postsurgical, and cancer pain (see Atwood and Mackie 2010 for review). It is still unclear as to where these CB_2 agonists exert their analgesic effects, one likely possibility being microglia, since it is currently not clear whether CB_2 receptors are expressed by neurons involved in the process of nociception. Accordingly, the effectiveness of THCV as pain killer could be due to its combined activation of CB_2 receptors and blockade of CB_1 receptors. It is noteworthy that THCV has been found to behave in vivo, although not in vitro, as a CB_1 receptor agonist at doses above those at which it produces signs of CB_1 receptor blockade (Pertwee et al. 2007). Thus, THCV displays antihyperalgesic activity in carrageenan and formalin models of inflammatory pain in mice, the first of these effects being significantly attenuated by SR144528, and the second not only by this CB_2 receptor-selective antagonist, but also by the CB_1 receptor-selective antagonist, rimonabant (Bolognini et al. 2010). On the basis of these findings it would also be of interest to explore the possibility that this compound can suppress chronic inflammatory, or indeed, neuropathic pain, conditions characterized by a strong CB_2 involvement. A further important property has been recently reported for THCV that augments the interest in testing this phytocannabinoid as a chronic pain reliever: THCV stimulated and desensitized TRPV1 and TRPV2 receptors (De Petrocellis et al. 2011) whose involvement in pain has been already discussed in section 25.3.

25.5 **Cannabigerol**

Cannabigerol (CBG) is a little-studied phytocannabinoid that was detected in cannabis in 1964 and subsequently found not to induce THC-like psychopharmacological effects in vivo. However, it does possess some ability to interact with the endocannabinoid system since it behaves as a CB_1 receptor antagonist at nanomolar concentrations (Cascio et al. 2010) and as an anandamide reuptake inhibitor at concentrations in the low micromolar range (Ligresti et al. 2006). The search for CBG targets led to the discovery that CBG can activate TRPA1 transient receptor potential channels and block the activation of TRPM8 transient receptor potential channels in vitro (De Petrocellis et al. 2008). A recent study directed at determining CBG affinity for a variety of receptors showed, in in vitro experiments, that CBG is a potent α_2-adrenoceptor agonist (Cascio et al. 2010). This was unexpected considering the structure of this phytocannabinoid and as no other cannabinoid has been reported to behave in this way. In the same study evidence was also obtained that CBG can block 5-HT_{1A} and cannabinoid CB_1 receptors, albeit with a potency lower than that with which it appears to activate α_2-adrenoceptors (Cascio et al. 2010). These observations open up the possibility that CBG, like established α_2-adrenoceptor agonists (for example, clonidine), could display significant efficacy as an antinociceptive agent when administered in vivo. We tested this hypothesis by assessing the antinociceptive properties of CBG in two different murine models of pain, the formalin and the λ-carrageenan tests. More specifically, we showed for the first time that CBG was able to reduce in a dose-dependent manner (1, 5, 10 mg/kg, i.p.) both the first and the second nocifensive phase associated with the intraplantar injection of formalin, and to reduce λ-carrageenan-evoked hypersensitivity. The antinociceptive effects of CBG were comparable with those evoked by clonidine and antagonism studies directed at investigating the mechanism of action underlying these effects suggested that α_2 receptors contributed to the antinociceptive effects evoked by CBG in both animal models (Comelli et al. 2012). However, it is possible that part of the CBG-induced relief of inflammatory and tonic pain is also due to its ability to decrease inactivation of the endocannabinoid, anandamide (Ligresti et al. 2006), thereby augmenting endogenous antinociceptive tone. In the light of the α_2-adrenoceptor-mediated mechanism for CBG-induced relief of pain, it is possible that CBG can synergistically interact with other cannabinoids. In fact, an interaction between synthetic cannabinoids, i.e., WIN55,212-2 and CP55,940, and α_2-adrenoceptor agonists has already been demonstrated. Particularly, spinal combination of WIN 55,212–2 with clonidine or neostigmine can augment the antinociceptive effect of each drug alone, in both an acute nociceptive state and a tissue-injury state evoked by for-malin stimulus (Yoon and Choi 2003). In addition, CP55,940 combined with an α_2-adrenoceptor agonist showed simple additivity in the tail flick assay, but synergy in the hot-plate assay, indicat-ing that the synergism may be specific to the spinal and supraspinal pathways involved in each type of acute pain stimulus (Tham et al. 2005). The ability of CBG to counteract chronic pain, including neuropathic pain, alone or in combination with other phytocannabinoids (i.e., THC, as already suggested (Pertwee 2009)), awaits investigation.

25.6 **Cannabichromene**

Despite the presence of cannabichromene (CBC) in certain marijuana strains, relatively few studies have investigated the pharmacological effects of this compound. CBC has been shown to have analgesic properties and to potentiate the analgesic effect of THC in the mouse tail-flick assay (Davis and Hatoum 1983). More recently it has been shown that CBC produced significant pharmacological effects only when administered at a high dose (i.e., 100 mg/kg, intravenously (i.v.)), which consistently produced locomotor suppression, catalepsy, and hypothermia, but only occasionally produced a small magnitude of antinociception (DeLong et al. 2010). Interestingly, administration of a threshold dose of THC produced leftward shifts in the CBC dose–response curve for antinociception, suggesting a possible synergism between these two phytocannabinoids. Additionally, CBC was comparable to mustard oil in stimulating TRPA1-mediated increases in intracellular Ca^{2+} in human embryonic kidney 293 cells (50–60 nM) (De Petrocellis et al. 2008). CBC recently proved to be a strong anandamide uptake inhibitor (De Petrocellis et al. 2011). Like CBD, CBC produced tail-flick-related antinociceptive responses accompanied by the expected decrease in ON cell ongoing activity and by a paradoxical decrease of OFF cell ongoing activity, in the rostral ventromedial medulla (RVM) after intra-vl-PAG injections (Maione et al. 2011), indicative of a supraspinal mechanism of action. These effects were antagonized not only by a CB_1 receptor antagonist, but also by the selective adenosine A_1 receptor antagonist DPCPX (Maione et al. 2011), suggesting that the antinociceptive effects of CBC might be the result of sequential or simultaneous activation of different targets. In light of its nonpsychotropic activity (El-Alfy et al. 2010), CBC is a good candidate for testing in combination with other phytocannabinoids for the relief of pain.

25.7 **Phytocannabinoid mixtures and cannabis extracts**

There is growing evidence supporting the therapeutic usage of whole extracts of cannabis for pain relief; these might offer a number of advantages over pure cannabinoids. The most notable examples are Sativex®, which contains THC/CBD in an approximately 1:1 ratio, and GW-2000-02, which contains primarily THC, for the relief of pain from brachial-plexus avulsion, a human model of central neuropathic pain, and of pain associated with multiple sclerosis (Berman et al. 2004; Rog et al. 2005). Whole-plant extracts contain a complex mixture of natural cannabinoids and other noncannabinoid compounds that may interact synergistically to provide a superior therapeutic profile over that of single pure components of cannabis. This may explain why a cannabis-based medicine made from whole-plant extracts may be more effective than single cannabinoid products (e.g., Sofia et al. 1975; Varvel et al. 2006). In addition to potentiating the pharmacological efficacy of cannabinoids, the use of standardized extracts could also decrease the adverse effects following in vivo administration. This could be true for many phytocannabinoid-induced effects, especially analgesia, since phytocannabinoids exert antinociceptive effects via different mechanisms, as described in this chapter. The first study exploring the potential of combining phytocannabinoids for pain relief dated from 1975 when the analgesic effectiveness of THC, a crude marijuana extract (CME), and cannabinol (CBN) following oral administration was directly compared in mice using the acetic-induced writhing and hot-plate tests and the Randall–Selitto paw pressure test in rats. In terms of THC content, CME was nearly equipotent in the hot-plate and Randall–Selitto tests, but was three times more potent in the acetic acid writing test. On the other hand, CBN was only effective in reducing writhing frequency in mice and raising the pain threshold of the inflamed hind paws of rats. The results of this investigation seem to suggest that CME possesses higher potency because it contains more than one active compound (Sofia et al. 1975). In spite of these early studies, further investigations in this area were not reported until a few years ago, when the contribution of CBD, other cannabinoids, terpenes, and flavonoids to the clinical effect of cannabis was espoused as an "entourage effect" (Russo and McPartland 2003), and, more recently, evidence has been presented indicating a potentiation of THC's antinociceptive effect by a high dose of CBD (Varvel et al. 2006). Particularly, this study showed that i.v. administered CBD (30 mg/kg) did potentiate the antinociceptive effect of a threshold dose of THC assessed in the mouse tail-flick test, suggesting there may be some therapeutic benefit of adding high doses of CBD to THC for pain management. However, effects of THC on locomotor activity, catalepsy, and hypothermia were also increased by CBD. In addition CBD was reported not to alter the antinociceptive effects of THC in the formalin test in rats (Finn et al. 2004). In our opinion, the ability of CBD to potentiate the antinociceptive effects of THC in animals may be sensitive to the particular pain model used and could be particularly relevant in chronic pathological pain; furthermore, we can suggest that other substances contained in the plant and not only the two main constituents (CBD and THC) can explain the overall therapeutic effect of the herb. This was demonstrated in a neuropathic pain model: a standardized extract of *Cannabis sativa*, containing a large quantity of CBD and a small percentage of THC and other minor cannabinoid and noncannabinoid components, evoked a total relief of thermal hyperalgesia, exceeding the effects of single cannabinoids (Comelli et al. 2008). Thus, repeated treatment with only CBD or only THC, administered at the same dose present in the extract, displayed only a partial effect and a lack of efficacy on nociceptive behavior, respectively. The difference between antinociceptive responses to the pure cannabinoids and to the extract prompted the hypothesis that this could be solely due to the combination of CBD and THC in the extract. Therefore, a mixture was tested which did not contain any noncannabinoid compounds or additional phytocannabinoids, apart from THC and CBD at the same doses as present in the extract; it evoked an antihyperalgesic effect lower than that elicited by the extract, suggesting that other constituents present in the plant account for the greater efficacy of the extract (Comelli et al. 2008). In the perspective of a possible future therapeutic employment of *Cannabis sativa* extracts, it will be crucial to characterize more completely their constituents, including THCV, CBG, and CBC, whose antinociceptive properties have been described previously in this chapter (sections 25.4–25.6). Although the spectrum of the antinociceptive effects of these compounds is largely unexplored, and, although they tend to be present both in different amounts in samples of marijuana of different origins and in lower amounts than THC, there is growing evidence that some of them constitute new and attractive tools for pain management, especially in combination. Another intriguing idea is that terpenoids present in the plant could be responsible for the greater antinociception produced by some cannabis plant extracts than by single phytocannabinoids (Russo 2011). Particularly, β-caryophyllene is generally the most common sesquiterpenoid encountered in cannabis and it is frequently the predominant terpenoid overall in cannabis extracts. It displays anti-inflammatory and analgesic activity, and selectively binds to the CB_2 receptor ($K_i = 155 \pm 4$ nM) behaving as a functional CB_2 agonist (Gertsch et al. 2008). Further research is required to better characterize synergistic pharmacological interactions between some of the constituents of cannabis, not least because this could lead to the discovery of improved new treatments for pain.

25.8 Conclusions and future directions

Together, the preclinical data on the antinociceptive properties of phytocannabinoids summarized in this chapter strongly suggest that the possibility exists of developing new effective medications for pain relief that contain one or more phytocannabinoids, alone or in combination with other constituents of cannabis, and that display favorable benefit-to-risk ratios. Thus, the rational use of cannabis-based medications for alleviating the suffering of patients caused by severe pain deserves serious consideration.

References

Ahrens, J., Demir, R., Leuwer, M., *et al.* (2009). The nonpsychotropic cannabinoid cannabidiol modulates and directly activates alpha-1 and alpha-1-Beta glycine receptor function. *Pharmacology*, **83**(4), 217–222.

Aira, Z., Buesa, I., Salgueiro, M., *et al.* (2010). Subtype-specific changes in 5-HT receptor-mediated modulation of C fibre-evoked spinal field potentials are triggered by peripheral nerve injury. *Neuroscience*, **168**(3), 831–841.

Appendino, G., Minassi, A., Pagani, A., and Ech-Chahad, A. (2008). The role of natural products in the ligand deorphanization of TRP channels. *Current Pharmaceutical Design*, **14**(1), 2–17.

Atwood, B.K. and Mackie, K. (2010). CB_2: a cannabinoid receptor with an identity crisis. *British Journal of Pharmacology*, **160**(3), 467–479.

Berman, J.S., Symonds, C., and Birch, R. (2004). Efficacy of two cannabis based medicinal extracts for relief of central neuropathic pain from brachial plexus avulsion: results of a randomised controlled trial. *Pain*, **112**(3), 299–306.

Bolognini, D., Costa, B., Maione, S., *et al.* (2010). The plant cannabinoid Delta9-tetrahydrocannabivarin can decrease signs of inflammation and inflammatory pain in mice. *British Journal of Pharmacology*, **160**(3), 677–687.

Booker, L., Naidu, P.S., Razdan, R.K., Mahadevan, A., and Lichtman, A.H. (2009). Evaluation of prevalent phytocannabinoids in the acetic acid model of visceral nociception. *Drug and Alcohol Dependence*, **105**(1–2), 42–47.

Burns, T.L. and Ineck, J.R. (2006). Cannabinoid analgesia as a potential new therapeutic option in the treatment of chronic pain. *The Annals of Pharmacotherapy*, **40**(2), 251–260.

Carrier, E.J., Auchampach, J.A., and Hillard, C.J. (2006). Inhibition of an equilibrative nucleoside transporter by cannabidiol: a mechanism of cannabinoid immunosuppression. *Proceedings of the National Academy of Sciences of the United States of America*, **103**(20), 7895–7900.

Cascio, M.G., Gauson, L.A., Stevenson, L.A., Ross, R.A., and Pertwee, R.G. (2010). Evidence that the plant cannabinoid cannabigerol is a highly potent alpha2-adrenoceptor agonist and moderately potent 5HT1A receptor antagonist. *British Journal of Pharmacology*, **159**(1), 129–141.

Cichewicz, D.L. and McCarthy, E.A. (2003). Antinociceptive synergy between delta(9)-tetrahydrocannabinol and opioids after oral administration. *Journal of Pharmacology and Experimental Therapeutics*, **304**(3), 1010–1015.

Cichewicz, D.L. and Welch, S.P. (2003). Modulation of oral morphine antinociceptive tolerance and naloxone-precipitated withdrawal signs by oral Delta 9-tetrahydrocannabinol. *Journal of Pharmacology and Experimental Therapeutics*, **305**(3), 812–817.

Comelli, F., Bettoni, I., Colombo, A., Fumagalli, P., Giagnoni, G., and Costa, B. (2010). Rimonabant, a cannabinoid CB1 receptor antagonist, attenuates mechanical allodynia and counteracts oxidative stress and nerve growth factor deficit in diabetic mice. *European Journal of Pharmacology*, **637**(1–3), 62–69.

Comelli, F., Filippi, G., Papaleo, E., De Gioia, L., Pertwee, R.G., and Costa, B. (2012). Evidence that the phytocannabinoid cannabigerol can induce antinociception by activating α2-adrenoreceptors: a computational and pharmacological study. *Proceedings 22nd Annual Symposium on the Cannabinoids*. International Cannabinoid Research Society: Freiburg, Germany, p. 44

Comelli, F., Giagnoni, G., Bettoni, I., Colleoni, M., and Costa, B. (2008). Antihyperalgesic effect of a *Cannabis sativa* extract in a rat model of neuropathic pain: mechanisms involved. *Phytotherapy Research*, **22**(8), 1017–1024.

Costa, B. (2007). On the pharmacological properties of Delta9-tetrahydrocannabinol (THC). *Chemistry & Biodiversity*, **4**(8), 1664–1677.

Costa, B., Colleoni, M., Conti, S., et al. (2004a). Oral anti-inflammatory activity of cannabidiol, a non-psychoactive constituent of cannabis, in acute carrageenan-induced inflammation in the rat paw. *Naunyn-Schmiedeberg's Archives of Pharmacology*, **369**(3), 294–299.

Costa, B., Giagnoni, G., Franke, C., Trovato, A.E., and Colleoni, M. (2004b). Vanilloid TRPV1 receptor mediates the antihyperalgesic effect of the nonpsychoactive cannabinoid, cannabidiol, in a rat model of acute inflammation. *British Journal of Pharmacology*, **143**(2), 247–250.

Costa, B., Trovato, A.E., Comelli, F., Giagnoni, G., and Colleoni, M. (2007). The non-psychoactive cannabis constituent cannabidiol is an orally effective therapeutic agent in rat chronic inflammatory and neuropathic pain. *European Journal of Pharmacology*, **556**(1–3), 75–83.

Costa, B., Trovato, A.E., Colleoni, M., Giagnoni, G., Zarini, E., and Croci, T. (2005). Effect of the cannabinoid CB_1 receptor antagonist, SR141716, on nociceptive response and nerve demyelination in rodents with chronic constriction injury of the sciatic nerve. *Pain*, **116**(1–2), 52–61.

Cox, M.L., Haller, V.L., and Welch, S.P. (2007a). The antinociceptive effect of Delta9-tetrahydrocannabinol in the arthritic rat involves the CB_2 cannabinoid receptor. *European Journal of Pharmacology*, **570**(1–3), 50–56.

Cox, M.L., Haller, V.L., and Welch, S.P. (2007b). Synergy between delta9-tetrahydrocannabinol and morphine in the arthritic rat. *European Journal of Pharmacology*, **567**(1–2), 125–130.

Davis, W.M. and Hatoum, N.S. (1983). Neurobehavioral actions of cannabichromene and interactions with delta 9-tetrahydrocannabinol. *General Pharmacology*, **14**(2), 247–252.

DeLong, G.T., Wolf, C.E., Poklis, A., and Lichtman, A.H. (2010). Pharmacological evaluation of the natural constituent of *Cannabis sativa*, cannabichromene and its modulation by Δ(9)-tetrahydrocannabinol. *Drug and Alcohol Dependence*, **112**(1–2), 126–133.

De Petrocellis, L. and Di Marzo, V. (2010). Non-CB_1, non-CB_2 receptors for endocannabinoids, plant cannabinoids, and synthetic cannabimimetics: focus on G-protein-coupled receptors and transient receptor potential channels. *Journal of Neuroimmune Pharmacology*, **5**(1), 103–21.

De Petrocellis, L., Ligresti, A., and Schiano-Moriello, A., et al. (2011). Effects of cannabinoids and cannabinoid-enriched Cannabis extracts on TRP channels and endocannabinoid metabolic enzymes. *British Journal of Pharmacology*, **163**(7), 1479–1494.

De Petrocellis, L., Vellani, V., Schiano-Moriello, A., *et al.* (2008). Plant-derived cannabinoids modulate the activity of transient receptor potential channels of ankyrin type-1 and melastatin type-8. *Journal of Pharmacology and Experimental Therapeutics*, **325**(3), 1007–1015.

Dyson, A., Peacock, M., Chen, A., *et al.* (2005). Antihyperalgesic properties of the cannabinoid CT-3 in chronic neuropathic and inflammatory pain states in the rat. *Pain*, **116**(1–2), 129–137.

El-Alfy, A.T., Ivey, K., Robinson, K., *et al.* (2010). Antidepressant-like effect of delta9-tetrahydrocannabinol and other cannabinoids isolated from *Cannabis sativa* L. *Pharmacology Biochemistry and Behavior*, **95**(4), 434–442.

Finn, D.P., Beckett, S.R., Roe, C.H., *et al.* (2004). Effects of coadministration of cannabinoids and morphine on nociceptive behaviour, brain monoamines and HPA axis activity in a rat model of persistent pain. *European Journal of Neuroscience*, **19**(3), 678–686.

Fioravanti, B., De Felice, M., Stucky, C.L., *et al.* (2008). Constitutive activity at the cannabinoid CB1 receptor is required for behavioral response to noxious chemical stimulation of TRPV1: antinociceptive actions of CB1 inverse agonists. *The Journal of Neuroscience*, **28**(45), 11593–11602.

Formukong, E.A., Evans, A.T., Evans, F.J. (1988). Analgesic and antiinflammatory activity of constituents of *Cannabis sativa* L. *Inflammation*, **12**(4), 361–371.

Fox, A., Kesingland, A., Gentry, C., *et al.* (2001). The role of central and peripheral cannabinoid 1 receptors in the antihyperalgesic activity of cannabinoids in a model of neuropathic pain. *Pain*, **92**(1–2), 91–100.

Gertsch, J., Leonti, M., Raduner, S., *et al.* (2008). Beta-caryophyllene is a dietary cannabinoid. *Proceedings of the National Academy of Sciences of the United States of America*, **105**(26), 9099–9104.

Ibrahim, M.M., Deng, H., Zvonok, A., *et al.* (2003). Activation of CB_2 cannabinoid receptors by AM1241 inhibits experimental neuropathic pain: pain inhibition by receptors not present in the CNS. *Proceedings of the National Academy of Sciences of the United States of America*, **100**(18), 10529–10533.

Izzo, A.A., Borrelli, F., Capasso, R., Di Marzo, V., and Mechoulam, R. (2009). Non-psychotropic plant cannabinoids: new therapeutic opportunities from an ancient herb. *Trends in Pharmacological Sciences*, **30**(10), 515–527.

Kathmann, M., Flau, K., Redmer, A., Trankle, C., and Schlicker, E. (2006). Cannabidiol is an allosteric modulator at mu- and delta-opioid receptors. *Naunyn-Schmiedeberg's Archives of Pharmacology*, **372**(5), 354–361.

Kobayashi, K., Fukuoka, T., Obata, K., *et al.* (2005). Distinct expression of TRPM8, TRPA1, and TRPV1 mRNAs in rat primary afferent neurons with adelta/c-fibers and colocalization with trk receptors. *Journal of Comparative Neurology*, **493**(4), 596–606.

Ligresti, A., Schiano-Moriello, A., Starowicz, K., *et al.* (2006). Antitumor activity of plant cannabinoids with emphasis on the effect of cannabidiol on human breast carcinoma. *Journal of Pharmacology and Experimental Therapeutics*, **318**(3), 1375–1387.

Maione, S., Piscitelli, F., Gatta, L., *et al.* (2011). Non-psychoactive cannabinoids modulate the descending pathway of antinociception in anaesthetized rats through several mechanisms of action. *British Journal of Pharmacology*, **162**(3), 584–596.

Mao, J., Price, D.D., Lu, J., Keniston, L., and Mayer, D.J. (2000). Two distinctive antinociceptive systems in rats with pathological pain. *Neuroscience Letters*, **280**(1), 13–16.

Murray, R.M., Morrison, P.D., Henquet, C., and Di Forti, M. (2007). Cannabis, the mind and society: the hash realities. *Nature Reviews Neuroscience*, **8**(11), 885–895.

Nitanda, A., Yasunami, N., Tokumo, K., Fujii, H., Hirai, T., and Nishio, H. (2005). Contribution of the peripheral 5-HT 2A receptor to mechanical hyperalgesia in a rat model of neuropathic pain. *Neurochemistry International*, **47**(6), 394–400.

Pan, H., Mukhopadhyay, P., Rajesh, M., *et al.* (2009). Cannabidiol attenuates cisplatin-induced nephrotoxicity by decreasing oxidative/nitrosative stress, inflammation, and cell death. *Journal of Pharmacology and Experimental Therapeutics*, **328**(3), 708–714.

Pertwee, R.G., Thomas, A., Stevenson, L.A., *et al.* (2007). The psychoactive plant cannabinoid, Delta9-tetrahydrocannabinol, is antagonized by Delta8- and Delta9-tetrahydrocannabivarin in mice in vivo. *British Journal of Pharmacology*, **150**(5), 586–594.

Pertwee, R.G. (2008). The diverse CB1 and CB2 receptor pharmacology of three plant cannabinoids: delta9-tetrahydrocannabinol, cannabidiol and delta9-tetrahydrocannabivarin. *British Journal of Pharmacology*, **153**(2), 199–215.

Pertwee, R.G. (2009). Emerging strategies for exploiting cannabinoid receptor agonists as medicines. *British Journal of Pharmacology*, **156**(3), 397–411.

Qin, N., Neeper, M.P., Liu, Y., Hutchinson, T.L., Lubin, M.L., and Flores, C.M. (2008). TRPV2 is activated by cannabidiol and mediates CGRP release in cultured rat dorsal root ganglion neurons. *Journal of Neuroscience*, **28**(24), 6231–6238.

Rock, E.M., Bolognini, D., and Limebeer, C.L., *et al.* (2012). Cannabidiol, a non-psychotropic component of cannabis, attenuates vomiting and nausea-like behaviour via indirect agonism of 5-HT1A somatodendritic autoreceptors in the dorsal raphe nucleus. *British Journal of Pharmacology*, **165**(8), 2620–2634.

Rog, D.J., Nurmikko, T.J., Friede, T., and Young, C.A. (2005). Randomized, controlled trial of cannabis-based medicine in central pain in multiple sclerosis. *Neurology*, **65**(6), 812–819.

Russo, E.B. (2011). Taming THC: potential cannabis synergy and phytocannabinoid-terpenoid entourage effects. *British Journal of Pharmacology*, **163**(7), 1344–1364.

Russo, E.B., Burnett, A., Hall, B., and Parker, K.K. (2005). Agonistic properties of cannabidiol at 5-HT1a receptors. *Neurochemical Research*, **30**(8), 1037–1043.

Russo, E.B. and McPartland, J.M. (2003). Cannabis is more than simply delta(9)-tetrahydrocannabinol. *Psychopharmacology (Berlin)*, **165**(4), 431–432.

Ryberg, E., Larsson, N., Sjögren, S., *et al.* (2007). The orphan receptor GPR55 is a novel cannabinoid receptor. *British Journal of Pharmacology*, **152**(7), 1092–1101.

Sanders, J., Jackson, D.M., and Starmer, G.A. (1979). Interactions among the cannabinoids in the antagonism of the abdominal constriction response in the mouse. *Psychopharmacology (Berlin)*, **61**(3), 281–285.

Schuelert, N. and McDougall, J.J. (2011). The abnormal cannabidiol analogue O-1602 reduces nociception in a rat model of acute arthritis via the putative cannabinoid receptor GPR55. *Neuroscience Letters*, **500**(1), 72–76.

Smith, F.L., Cichewicz, D., Martin, Z.L., and Welch, S.P. (1998). The enhancement of morphine antinociception in mice by delta9-tetrahydrocannabinol. *Pharmacology Biochemistry and Behavior*, **60**(2), 559–566.

Sofia, R.D., Vassar, H.B., and Knobloch, L.C. (1975). Comparative analgesic activity of various naturally occurring cannabinoids in mice and rats. *Psychopharmacologia*, **40**(4), 285–295.

Staton, P.C., Hatcher, J.P., Walker, D.J., *et al.* (2008). The putative cannabinoid receptor GPR55 plays a role in mechanical hyperalgesia associated with inflammatory and neuropathic pain. *Pain*, **139**(1), 225–236.

Tham, S.M., Angus, J.A., Tudor, E.M., and Wright, C.E. (2005). Synergistic and additive interactions of the cannabinoid agonist CP55,940 with μ opioid receptor and α_2-adrenoceptor agonists in acute pain models in mice. *British Journal of Pharmacology*, **144**(6), 875–884.

Thomas, A., Baillie, G.L., Phillips, A.M., Razdan, R.K., Ross, R.A., and Pertwee, R.G. (2007). Cannabidiol displays unexpectedly high potency as an antagonist of CB_1 and CB_2 receptor agonists in vitro. *British Journal of Pharmacology*, **150**(5), 613–623.

Toth, C.C., Jedrzejewski, N.M., Ellis, C.L., and Frey, W.H. 2nd (2010). Cannabinoid-mediated modulation of neuropathic pain and microglial accumulation in a model of murine type I diabetic peripheral neuropathic pain. *Molecular Pain*, **6**, 16.

Varvel, S.A., Wiley, J.L., Yang, R., *et al.* (2006). Interactions between THC and cannabidiol in mouse models of cannabinoid activity. *Psychopharmacology (Berlin)*, **186**(2), 226–634.

Vay, L., Gu, C., and McNaughton, P.A. (2012) The thermo-TRP ion channel family: properties and therapeutic implications. *British Journal of Pharmacology*, **165**(4), 787–801.

Walter, L., Franklin, A., Witting, A., *et al.* (2003). Nonpsychotropic cannabinoid receptors regulate microglial cell migration. *The Journal of Neuroscience*, **23**(4), 1398–1405

Ward, S.J., Ramirez, M.D., Neelakantan, H., and Walker, E.A. (2011). Cannabidiol prevents the development of cold and mechanical allodynia in paclitaxel-treated female C57BI6 mice. *Anesthesia and Analgesia*, **113**(4), 947–950.

Welch, S.P. and Stevens, D.L. (1992). Antinociceptive activity of intrathecally administered cannabinoids alone, and in combination with morphine, in mice. *Journal of Pharmacology and Experimental Therapeutics*, **262**(1), 10–18.

Welch, S.P., Thomas, C., and Patrick, G.S. (1995). Modulation of cannabinoid-induced antinociception after intracerebroventricular versus intrathecal administration to mice: possible mechanisms for interaction with morphine. *Journal of Pharmacology and Experimental Therapeutics*, **272**(1), 310–321.

Williams, J., Haller, V.L., Stevens, D.L., and Welch, S.P. (2008) Decreased basal endogenous opioid levels in diabetic rodents: effects on morphine and delta-9-tetrahydrocannabinoid-induced antinociception. *European Journal of Pharmacology*, **584**(1), 78–86.

Wong, G.Y. and Gavva, N.R. (2009) Therapeutic potential of vanilloid receptor TRPV1 agonists and antagonists as analgesics: Recent advances and setbacks. *Brain Research Reviews*, **60**(1), 267–277.

Xiong, W., Cui, T., Cheng, K., *et al.* (2012). Cannabinoids suppress inflammatory and neuropathic pain by targeting α3 glycine receptors. *Journal of Experimental Medicine*, **209**(6), 1121–1134.

Yoon, M.H. and Choi, J. (2003). Pharmacologic interaction between cannabinoid and either clonidine or neostigmine in the rat formalin test. *Anesthesiology*, **99**(3), 701–707.

Chapter 26

Cannabis and Multiple Sclerosis

Gareth Pryce and David Baker

26.1 Multiple sclerosis

26.1.1 Natural history and pathology

Multiple sclerosis (MS) is an inflammatory, demyelinating disease of the central nervous system (CNS) and is the most common cause of nontraumatic neurological disability in young adults of northern European descent (Compston and Coles 2002, 2008). This disease affects about 100,000 people within the UK. The absolute number of cases of MS around the world has steadily increased, possibly as a result of improved diagnosis amongst other factors and affects 2–3 million people worldwide (Kurtzke 1993). The incidence of MS is geographically restricted and occurs with high incidence in Northern Europe and in regions colonized by white Northern Europeans such as Canada and Northern US, Australia, and New Zealand with a gradient of higher incidence further from the equator (Compston and Coles 2002). MS is more common in females compared to males with an increasing ratio of 3:1, with a more pronounced female incidence in younger MS patients with relapsing-remitting disease (RRMS) (Runmarker and Andersen 1993). The highest incidence of MS reported is in the Orkney Isles with an incidence of 1 in 170 females (Visser et al. 2012).

Disease is influenced by genetics, as evidenced by an increased concordance of MS in monozygotic twins (~30%) compared to dizygotic twins (~5% concordance rate) and is polygenically controlled (Compston and Coles 2002, 2008). Disease is associated with the expression of certain MHC haplotypes such as human leukocyte antigen (HLA)-DRB1*1501 and is influenced by over 50 other immune-related, susceptibility genes (Prat et al. 2005; Sawcer et al. 2011). However the concordance of disease rate in identical twins demonstrates that other, environmental, factors may influence susceptibility. Migration studies from low- to high-incidence areas suggest that the environmental trigger is acquired before the age of 15 (Compston and Coles 2002). Some have suggested that it may relate to age of infection and there are thoughts that this could relate to Epstein–Barr virus infection (Ascherio and Munger 2010; Sumaya et al. 1980). The vast majority of people with MS are infected with Epstein–Barr virus compared to 90% of the general population and there is increased frequency of MS in people who developed glandular fever (Handel et al. 2010). This is indirectly supported by the geographic distribution of people with MS (Ebers and Savodnick 1993). Vitamin D levels can influence the immune response and may even be important in utero (Willer et al. 2005). Importantly a number of genes associated with MS, such as certain HLA haplotypes, contain vitamin D responsive elements in their promoter regions that can influence expression and may link environment and genetic susceptibility elements (Ramagopalan et al. 2009, 2010). MS most commonly (about 80%) presents as a series of relapsing-remitting episodes of loss of neurological function that eventually develops into a chronic, secondary progressive (SPMS) phase with no remission and increasing disability over time, which correlates with CNS atrophy and axonal loss, particularly in the spinal cord (Bjartmar et al. 2000). In about 10–15% of people, particularly in those with an onset later in life, the disease becomes progressive (primary progressive MS) from onset (Compston and Coles 2002, 2008). As such about 80% of people with MS will be severely disabled within 25 years from disease onset.

Disease is associated with blood–brain barrier dysfunction and mononuclear cell infiltration that arises around postcapillary venules, and leukocytes then invade the brain parenchyma leading to an expanding ring of macrophage-mediated myelin-destruction. This leads to the pathological hallmark of MS, which is demyelination of the white and gray matter, due to loss of oligodendrocytes and myelin. Although initially there is remyelination (shadow plaques), the capacity to repair eventually becomes exhausted and astrogliotic scars are formed within demyelinated plaques. Whilst lesion load is decreased following successful immunosuppressive treatment (Jones and Coles 2010; Polman et al. 2006), suggesting that leukocyte inflammation is the damaging force in MS, it has also been suggested that damage to the astrocyte or oligodendrocyte may be the primary event followed by infiltration of mononuclear cells (Barnett and Prineas 2004; Parratt and Prineas 2010).

As the disease evolves, inflammatory attacks increase the burden of demyelination and a dystrophic environment leads to eventual axonal loss, which impairs normal neurotransmission. This leads to the development of additional distressing symptoms such as incontinence, limb tremor, pain, spasms, fatigue, and spasticity, which have a major negative impact on quality of life indices (Compston and Coles 2002; Confavreux and Vukusic 2006). RRMS is the most common clinically presenting form of MS, with an incidence of approximately 85%, with the typical age of onset being the early third decade of life. RRMS is characterized by acute or subacute onset of neurological dysfunction lasting for more than 24 h, usually resolving within weeks to complete or partial recovery. The frequency of relapses varies over time but there appears to be a clear trend for relapses to be more common in the initial years of the disease and recovery from these early relapses to be more complete (Weinshenker et al. 1989). The time taken to convert to a secondary progressive neurodegenerative phenotype can vary widely between individuals and may reflect differences in an individual's ability to cope with episodes of neuronal insult, perhaps consistent with genetic control and heterogeneity of disease (Compston and Coles 2002). In approximately a quarter of cases, neurological disability does not reach a level where it impinges on daily living but conversely in around 15% of cases the progression to disability is rapid. The prognosis for patients is better in cases where sensory symptoms dominate the course of disease and there is a complete recovery from these symptoms at remission whereas the prognosis is poorer when there is motor involvement such as deficits of pyramidal, visual, sphincteric and cerebellar systems (Amato and Ponziani 2000). Frequent relapses and incomplete recovery plus a short time period between the initial neurological event and the subsequent relapse also have a poorer prognosis. There is also a poorer prognosis for the disease in older men who develop MS (Compston and Coles 2002; Weinshenker et al. 1989). However, once a threshold of disability has been reached, disability progression is remarkably uniform (Confavreux et al. 2000), and approximately 90% of RRMS patients will develop progressive disease after 25 years of clinical follow-up (Weinshenker et al. 1989). It may be that given enough time, all RRMS patients will eventually convert to the progressive phase of the disease. A recent study demonstrated that disability progression seems to follow a two-stage course. The first stage, corresponding to clinical disease onset to irreversible Kurztke expanded disability status scale (EDSS) 3 (moderate disability in one of eight functional systems, or mild disability in three or four functional systems), is dependent on ongoing focal neuroinflammation. There is a second stage, from irreversible disability scale 3 to irreversible disability scale 6 (intermittent or unilateral constant assistance (cane, crutch, brace) required to walk about 100 m with or without resting), which is independent of ongoing focal neuroinflammation and where neuroprotective strategies are indicated, rather than immunomodulatory therapies which are indicated for the phase one stage of MS (Leray et al. 2010).

Whilst immune-mediated conduction block and destruction of CNS myelin, followed by lesion resolution and limited myelin repair, may account for the relapsing-remitting nature of the disease, what is less clear are the mechanisms that account for the conversion to the chronic neurodegenerative secondary phase, which appears to be independent of, though worsened by, the accumulated neuronal dysfunction accompanying relapses (Bjartmar et al. 2003). A gradual degeneration of predominantly the pyramidal and cerebellar systems evolves which is often accompanied by sphincter and sexual dysfunction (Amato and Ponziani 2000). In addition, a subtype of MS, primary progressive MS (PPMS) presents as a progressive degenerative phenotype in 10–15% of patients after an initial bout of CNS inflammation, which along with secondary progressive MS is largely refractory to currently available MS therapies such as immunomodulation (Miller and Leary 2007), and where neuroprotective strategies are urgently indicated. Clinically, PPMS develops at a later age than RRMS, with onset in the fourth decade rather than the third decade as seen in RRMS (Andersson et al. 1999), and with a lower female preponderance.

26.1.2 **Symptoms and disability**

Over recent years, axonal pathology during MS has been re-examined and it has been established that CNS atrophy and axonal loss occurs, coincident with inflammatory lesion formation, early in the relapsing-remitting phase. This may be accommodated initially by remodeling of neuronal circuits (neural plasticity) or an increase in the number of neural precursors in some lesional areas contiguous with subventricular zones (Chang et al. 2008). However, as the disease continues, a threshold is reached, beyond which permanent impairment and increasing disability is established (Bjartmar et al. 2000, 2003; Confavreux and Vukusic 2006; Confavreux et al. 2000). This suggests that axonal loss rather than myelin damage is the key determinant of progressive disability in MS. In addition, a doubling in the levels of glutamate, an excitatory amino acid that has been shown to be neurotoxic in excess is seen in the CSF of MS patients undergoing an inflammatory episode (Stover et al. 1997).

In experimental allergic encephalomyelitis (EAE), an animal model of MS induced by the development of autoimmunity against myelin antigens, 15–30% of spinal cord axons can be lost before permanent locomotor impairment is noted (Bjartmar et al. 2000; Wujek et al. 2002). After a number of relapse events, permanent disability develops with significant axonal loss (40–80%, as also occurs in MS), in the spinal cord (Wujek et al. 2002) and the development of hind limb spasticity and tremor (Baker et al. 2000), which may reflect as the preferential loss of inhibitory circuits in certain locations of the spinal cord and their influence on signaling to skeletal muscles. Whilst inflammatory events are associated with axonal transections, chronic demyelination may contribute to a slow degenerative process.

As increasing numbers of axons are lost, this creates an extra burden on the remaining neurons and potential excitotoxicity due to increased activity on these neurons within the neural circuitry. Thus, a slow amplifying cascade of neuronal death may be triggered, which could occur independently of significant inflammation. This would be compatible with the slow progression in secondary progressive MS and the inability of potent immunosuppressive agents to inhibit this aspect of disease despite their efficacy in reducing blood–brain barrier dysfunction and the reduction of relapse rate (Coles et al. 1999; Confavreux and Vukusic 2006). During all neurodegenerative diseases, symptoms occur because homeostatic control of neurotransmission is lost, and may result from increased neurotransmission by excessive signaling of excitatory circuits or loss of inhibitory circuits or vice versa. As it appears that an important function of the cannabinoid system is the modulation of neurotransmitter release via cannabinoid receptor type 1 (CB_1) expression at presynaptic nerve terminals (Wilson and Nicoll 2002), this raises the possibility of therapeutic intervention in CNS events for symptom control by the manipulation of this system.

26.2 Cannabinoids and symptom management in MS

26.2.1 Historical studies

The primary area of investigation of the cannabinoids in MS so far has been that of symptom relief, in particular: bladder incontinence, tremor, and particularly limb spasticity, as patients claim that these particular symptoms are alleviated by cannabis (Consroe et al. 1997). Spasticity is one of the most common reported symptoms of MS and can affect approximately 50% of patients to some degree which has significant deleterious effects of quality of life and the ability to function in daily life (Barnes et al. 2003). A recent web-based survey of MS patients in Spain reported the presence of spasticity in 65% of patients with 40% rating this as moderate or severe with the severity increasing with the degree of disability (Oreja-Guevara et al. 2013). Current therapies for spasticity include the gamma-aminobutyric acid (GABA) receptor agonist baclofen, tinazidine, and benzodiazepines (Paisley et al. 2002). Intrathecal baclofen is commonly used for the treatment of severe refractory spasticity (Kita and Goodkin 2000). The anticonvulsant gabapentin and local administration of botulinum toxin have also shown efficacy in clinical trials (Kita and Goodkin 2000; Paisley et al. 2002). A recent German study has reported that 55% of physicians were dissatisfied with current treatment options for spasticity and the chief patient-reported negative effects were adverse side effects (92.5%) and poor efficacy (88%) with one-third of patients seeking relief by self-medication (Henze et al. 2013).

The pathophysiology of spasticity remains poorly understood but it may reflect a preferential loss of inhibitory circuitry in the spinal cord resulting in excessive levels of stimulatory signals. Under normal circumstances, inhibitory signals are sent via the corticospinal tract to the spinal cord, but following injury, damage to the corticospinal tract, a hallmark of MS, causes disinhibition of the stretch reflex leading to a reduction in the triggering threshold. This can result in excessive contraction of the muscles, sometimes even at rest (Adams and Hicks 2005; Brown 1994; Nielsen et al. 2007). The hypertonic mouse mutant *hyrt* (Gilbert et al. 2006), shows spastic signs in the hind limbs associated with a reduction in the level of inhibitory $GABA_A$ receptors in lower motor neurons. Loss of GABAergic inputs or GABA receptor-expressing neurons may produce the spasticity seen in MS as neurodegeneration progresses and explains the efficacy of GABA agonists such as baclofen. Improved treatment regimens for spasticity are required as agents that directly interfere with neurotransmitter activity are often associated with undesirable side effects such as cognitive impairment (Paisley et al. 2002).

26.2.2 Experimental evidence

Experimental data in MS models in mice have proved the antispastic and antitremor effects of cannabinoids and cannabinoid CB_1 receptor agonists (Baker et al. 2000, 2001; Pryce and Baker 2007) and any CB_1 agonist that reaches the CNS has the potential to inhibit spasticity. Furthermore and importantly, antagonism of the cannabinoid system by CB_1 receptor antagonists produces a worsening of these signs, indicating the presence of an endogenous cannabinoid tone, which is modulating these signs to some degree via the release of endocannabinoids in response to elevated neuronal excitation (Baker et al. 2000, 2001). The cannabis-derived medication Sativex®

consisting of an approximate 1:1 mixture of delta-9-tetrahydrocannabinol (THC) and cannabidiol has also demonstrated efficacy in the reduction of hind limb spasticity in an experimental model of MS (Hilliard et al. 2012). In addition, endocannabinoid (particularly anandamide) levels are raised in the spinal cords and brains of mice, which show hind limb spasticity, but not in animals, which have equivalent levels of neurodegeneration but without associated limb spasticity (Baker et al. 2001). This further indicates the presence of an endocannabinoid tone, which is elevated as a result of spasticity and tremor in these animals. Furthermore, administration of compounds which elevate endogenous anandamide levels, via inhibition either of re-uptake, or of enzymatic degradation by fatty acid amide hydrolase (FAAH), also reduces the level of spasticity in mice (Baker et al. 2001; Pryce et al. 2013). These observations provide objective evidence, to underpin patient perceptions of the efficacy of cannabis on MS symptoms.

26.2.3 Clinical evidence

In MS patients, it has been reported that a cannabis extract administered as a sublingual spray, showed efficacy in the treatment of bladder incontinence, showing both a decrease in emptying episodes and an increase in bladder retention volume (Brady et al. 2004). A second study as part of the Cannabis in Multiple Sclerosis (CAMS) study of patients, treated with a cannabis extract or THC, reported a significant reduction in episodes of urge incontinence compared to placebo (Freeman et al. 2006). This suggests that cannabinoids can compensate for the dysregulation of bladder neural circuitry that frequently accompanies disease progression in multiple sclerosis.

The first reports of the efficacy of cannabinoids for the alleviation of spasticity in MS were described in four small-scale studies (Brenneisen et al. 1996; Meinck et al. 1989; Petro and Ellenburger 1981; Ungerleider et al. 1987) all showing positive improvements. A number of larger controlled and blinded trials have since been undertaken on spasticity in MS (Collin et al. 2007; Killestein et al. 2002; Vaney et al. 2004; Wade et al. 2004, 2006; Zajicek et al. 2003, 2005). Although oral cannabis at doses that lack overt psychoactivity, showed no or marginal effects in treating spasticity as assessed by the Ashworth Scale (Killestein et al. 2002), there was an improvement in the time taken to complete a 10 m walk (Zajicek et al. 2003). Oral administration of cannabinoids is hampered compared to other routes due to variable absorption and metabolism including a significant first-pass effect through the liver which complicates dose-titration (Grotenhermen 2003). However, similar studies with a sublingual cannabis extract spray (Sativex®), has likewise had a minimal impact on objective outcomes such as the Ashworth Scale (Collin et al. 2007; Wade et al. 2003, 2004), but have had consistent, subjective patient-assessed, perceived improvements in spasms and spasticity. These apparently negative results may be largely due to the insensitivity of the Ashworth Scale in detecting positive effects of antispastic therapies where many of the currently prescribed drugs fail to show efficacy using this measure (Shakespeare et al. 2003).

As cannabis can affect cognitive processes (Curran et al. 2002), it can be argued that whilst patients feel subjectively improved due to mood modulation, these may not be objectively demonstrable at cannabinoid doses that do not induce significant cannabimimetic psychoactive effects (Killestein et al. 2002; Pertwee 2007; Wade et al. 2004, 2006; Zajicek et al. 2003, 2005). However, positive effects, with few exceptions (Killestein et al. 2002), have been reported following treatment with THC or medical cannabis extracts (Collin et al. 2007; Vaney et al. 2004; Wade et al. 2004, 2006; Zajicek et al. 2003). Importantly, patients on clinical trials suggest that only certain signs such as spasticity, pain, and sleep disturbances are improved, suggesting that these positive effects are unlikely to be simply due to a generalized perception of improvement following drug administration (Collin et al. 2007; Vaney et al. 2004; Wade et al. 2004, 2006;

Zajicek et al. 2003). This suggested some positive benefit of cannabinoids, and further evidence of the efficacy on MS-related spasticity following long-term administration of THC was reported showing a positive improvement on the Ashworth Scale in patients treated with THC for 1 year (Zajicek et al. 2005).

The apparently equivocal evidence in these studies of the efficacy of cannabis on spasticity in MS may reflect the poorly designed nature of many of the early trials, with subjective rather than quantitative outcome measures and insufficient appreciation of the pharmacokinetic problems such as first-pass effects via the liver with the oral route of administration (a clinically preferred route compared to smoking) (Agurell et al. 1986; Pertwee 2002). It would appear that routes of delivery, which facilitate rapid entry to the bloodstream and then to the CNS, are preferable to the orally administered route. Such routes are; aerosol inhalation, rectal suppository, or sublingual spray (Grotenhermen 2003). This may account for the claims that smoked cannabis, which is rapidly absorbed and has no first-pass effects, allowing the self-titration of the therapeutic effect, is preferable to orally administered THC, which is slowly absorbed and subjected to first-pass metabolism in the liver plus there is little chance of self-titration (Agurell et al. 1986; Consroe et al. 1997; Pertwee 2002). The biology of the cannabinoid system indicates that CB_1 mediates both the psychoactive and the majority of the potentially therapeutic effects of cannabis, and therefore its use will invariably be associated with side effects, which some people may find intolerable (Baker et al. 2003; Killestein et al. 2002; Pryce and Baker 2007). However, through individual dose-titration, these may be limited to achieve a therapeutic window where a benefit is achieved whilst unwanted side effects are limited. A study on cannabinoid-mediated control of tics associated with Tourette's syndrome suggests it is indeed possible to have a positive therapeutic outcome without significant cognitive impairment (Müller-Vahl et al. 2003).

Therefore, usage in any clinical indication will be a balance between treatment of a particular condition and the acceptability of side effects. In a recent small-scale study, the use of smoked or ingested street cannabis by MS patients was associated with a negative effect on cognitive function compared to a noncannabis using MS cohort, indicating the importance of defined doses of THC and dose titration (Honarmand et al. 2011). In contrast, in cannabis naïve MS patients treated with Sativex® (a 50:50 mixture of THC and CBD), there was no induction of psychopathology or cognitive impairment observed in the treatment group, further indicating the potential benefits of defined cannabis therapeutics versus street cannabis (Aragona et al. 2009).

26.2.4 Recent studies

More recent clinical trials with improved outcome measurements have reported positive effects of cannabinoid therapeutics in the treatment of spasticity which seem to have finally overcome the dubiety arising from previous studies. More weight has been given to a patient rated Numeric Rating Scale of improvements in spasticity as a result of treatment rather than relying on the unreliable Ashworth Scale as the primary outcome measure.

As previously mentioned, in the CAMS study (Zajicek et al. 2003), despite there being no significant improvement in spasticity as assessed by the Ashworth Scale, there was a significant improvement in a 10 m walking time test in Marinol® (synthetic THC)-treated patients. Patient-rated evaluations also reported significant improvements in spasticity and also quality of sleep and pain. In the extension study over a period of 12 months, a modest but significant improvement in spasticity assessed by observer-assessed Ashworth Scale was reported as well as patient-rated improvements in cannabinoid treated groups (Zajicek et al. 2005).

In light of the poor experience with the Ashworth Scale due to its limited ability to detect positive improvements in spasticity, a study investigating the effects of Sativex® on spasticity used a patient-assessed numerical rating scale (NRS) with a range of 1–10 as the primary endpoint (Collin et al. 2007). Sativex®-treated MS patients reported a significant decrease in their spasticity score of 1.18 compared to placebo. In comparison, the decrease assessed by the Ashworth Scale was not significant. Of the 40% of patients who responded to Sativex® a reduction of at least 30% in the NRS score was reported.

In a study which was enriched by the inclusion of early responding patients to treatment who were refractory to available antispastic medication (at least 20% reduction in NRS score compared to baseline after 4 weeks of treatment), in the second phase of the study (12 weeks) a significant reduction in NRS score was maintained compared to placebo over this period (Novotna et al. 2011).

The MUSEC (Multiple Sclerosis and Extract of Cannabis) trial recently reported the superiority of a standardized oral cannabis extract in the treatment of muscle stiffness also using a category rating scale (CRS) measuring patient-reported muscle stiffness from baseline. Cannabis extract to a maximum of 25 mg THC daily over 10 weeks demonstrated twice the amount of relief compared to placebo (Zajicek et al. 2012). Effective pain relief was also achieved by the cannabis extract particularly in those patients with high baseline scores.

This less equivocal and positive recent clinical evidence for the potential benefit of cannabis on MS-associated spasticity has led (June, 2010) to the approval for prescription in the UK and elsewhere of the cannabis extract Sativex® for the treatment of spasticity in MS. In addition, a small-scale Canadian study investigating the use of smoked cannabis for the treatment of spasticity in MS patients refractory to current medications reported highly significant reductions in spasticity as assessed by the modified Ashworth Scale (reduction of 2.74 points compared to placebo) and also significant reductions in pain scores (Corey-Bloom et al. 2012). The proviso here is that the patients smoking cannabis were significantly cognitively affected which will be a negative indication for many patients. Indeed it is likely that all patients reporting improvements in spasticity with cannabinoid therapeutics will have cognitive side effects to a greater or lesser degree due to the ubiquitous expression of the CB_1 receptor in the brain. That these patients showed a positive response on the Ashworth Scale in addition to side effects, would be consistent with the idea that CB_1 receptors mediate both the positive and negative aspects of cannabis, as shown in animals (Pryce and Baker 2007; Wilkinson et al. 2003). Furthermore, in cases where psychoactive side effects were not induced, as was the aim in most trials with oral and sublingual cannabis that failed to show influences on the Ashworth Scale, it is likely that treatment was suboptimal. This is because the biology dictates that cannabis has only a limited mechanism to target CNS centers controlling movement, whilst avoiding centers controlling cognitive functions. Thus cannabis has a narrow therapeutic window.

Thus whilst the data suggest that medicinal cannabis has benefit, a recent publication raises the concern that this medication will not be available to a large percentage of MS patients that could benefit from cannabinoid treatment of their spasticity (Lu et al. 2012). The study highlights that due to issues of pricing versus quality of life measurements, the authors state "Sativex® appears unlikely to be considered cost effective by UK funders of healthcare for spasticity in MS. This is unfortunate, since it appears that Sativex® use is likely to benefit some patients in the management of this common consequence of MS."

This is a concern for all those who have contributed greatly, over many years to the acceptance of the medicinal properties of cannabinoid-based medicine in MS in the face of great skepticism by some members of the medical/scientific profession and would seem to have the potential of driving MS patients back into the arms of their local illegal cannabis supplier to alleviate their symptoms, rather than being prescribed legal medication from their general practitioner.

26.3 **Cannabinoids as a neuroprotective therapy in MS**

26.3.1 **Experimental evidence**

The neurotoxic mechanisms during MS and experimental models are varied, with the potential agents of neuronal/axonal damage including; oxidative damage to mitochondria, release of inflammatory cytokines, nitric oxide release from activated macrophages/microglia and excitotoxicity due to excessive glutamate signaling leading to toxic levels of calcium ion influx. There is increasing evidence that elevated levels of glutamate are seen in both MS and EAE particularly during the active stages of disease (Marte et al. 2010; Stover et al. 1997; Sulkowski et al. 2009), accompanied by an increase in the level of expression of Group 1 metabotropic glutamate receptors and excitatory amino acid transporters (Sulkowski et al. 2009). Elevation of glutamate was also observed in the progressive phase of EAE concomitant with increased levels of neurodegeneration, further implicating glutamate excitotoxicity as a mechanism for neuronal degeneration in experimental MS (Marte et al. 2010). Modulation of the effects of elevated CNS glutamate levels has been reported to show disease amelioration in experimental and clinical studies (Bolton and Paul 2006; Pitt et al. 2000; Smith et al. 2000; Srinivasan et al. 2005). Elevated levels of glutamate may result from: the downregulation of enzymes responsible for the catabolism of glutamate (Hardin-Pouzet et al. 1997), the downregulation or reversal of the actions of neuronal and astrocytic glutamate transporters (Loría et al. 2010; Ohgoh et al. 2002) or the direct release of glutamate from activated Th17 cells forming direct synapse-like contact with neurons (Siffrin et al. 2010).

The ability of cannabinoids to downregulate the release of neurotransmitters such as glutamate is long established (Shen and Thayer 1999) leading to the hypothesis that they may have neuroprotective properties in neuroinflammatory disease.

The important role of the cannabinoid system in the protection against neurodegeneration was revealed in a mouse model of MS in mice where the CB_1 receptor had been genetically deleted. In these mice, neuroinflammation resulted in an accelerated accumulation of neurological deficits compared to wild-type animals (Jackson et al. 2005; Pryce et al. 2003). In addition, administration of exogenous cannabinoid agonists can significantly inhibit neurodegeneration due to neuroinflammation in acute and chronic disease models in the absence of any overt immunosuppression which would modify the level of neuronal insult (Croxford et al. 2008; Pryce et al. 2003). These observations would suggest that cannabinoid therapy may have a potential role in the slowing of neurodegeneration as a result of MS and may be considered as an adjunctive therapy to current disease-modifying therapies.

26.3.2 **Clinical evidence**

One clinical study to investigate the potential of cannabinoid therapy (THC) to slow the neurodegeneration that causes disease progression in MS has been undertaken. The Cannabinoid Use in Progressive Inflammatory brain Disease (CUPID) study was a multicenter based trial performed in the UK, coordinated by John Zajicek at Derriford Hospital, Plymouth (Zajicek et al. 2013). Four hundred and ninety-three MS patients with primary or secondary progressive MS were recruited to the study from 27 centers across UK between May 2006 and July 2008. It was a requirement for participants entering the trial that their walking was affected by their MS but that they could still walk, with aids if necessary. Participants were randomly assigned to receive THC capsules or placebo capsules, to be taken by mouth over a period of 3 years. Three hundred and twenty-nine people were allocated to receive the THC capsules and 164 were allocated to the placebo group. For each participant, the first 4 weeks of the trial were devoted to establishing the best tolerated dose of study treatment. For the remainder of the study period, participants remained on a stable dose of trial treatment, as far as possible, before the dose was gradually reduced to zero at the end of the treatment period. The study was "double-blind," meaning that neither the participants nor the doctors and nurses involved at the study sites knew which treatment group they were in. Despite the abundant experimental evidence that cannabinoid therapy has a neuroprotective role in a spectrum of neurological diseases, overall the study found no evidence that THC had an effect on MS progression in either of the main outcomes (the EDSS neurological assessments conducted by doctors at the study clinics or the Multiple Sclerosis Impact Scale (MSIS-29) questionnaire responses provided by the participants). The MSIS-29 is a new measure of the physical and psychological impact of MS from the patient's perspective (Hobart et al. 2001). The EDSS and MSIS-29 scores showed little change over the course of the study and no difference was found between the active and placebo groups. However, it was evident that the placebo group had not progressed as expected, which complicates assessing the value of the trial. However, and potentially importantly, there was some evidence that THC might have a significant (P <0.01) beneficial effect in participants at the lower end of the EDSS disability scale (<5.5 EDSS). As this benefit was only found in a small group of people rather than the whole study population, further studies will be needed to assess the robustness of this finding.

The interpretation of this study is that although the study found no evidence that THC has an effect on MS progression, most study participants were at the high end of the disability scale at the start of the study and as a whole did not exhibit much change in their MS. There was some evidence from the two main study assessments (EDSS and MSIS-29) that participants with less disability had some slowing of MS progression but the number of people in this category was too small (in statistical terms) to conclude with certainty that THC is effective in slowing MS progression. More research will be needed to investigate these findings and patients will need to be selected at the lower end of the disability spectrum before meaningful conclusions on the neuroprotective ability of cannabinoids to slow the rate of disease progression in MS can be drawn.

As was the case in clinical trials of cannabinoids for the treatment of spasticity in MS, early unsuccessful trials can point to the correct protocol being selected for later trials to provide a definitive conclusion (Zajicek et al. 2003, 2012) and the CUPID trial will be valuable in terms of what MS researchers across the world will learn about conducting trials in progressive disease, so that we can continue to improve study design and the accuracy with which outcomes can be measured in both clinical practice and research. However, because of the perceived failure of the study it is not yet clear whether subsequent studies will be performed with cannabinoids and it is possible that a useful therapeutic agent will be lost.

In summary, great strides have been made in recent years in the acceptance of cannabis as a medication for MS patients. Cannabis has proved its efficacy in spasticity and is now an approved medication for this in many countries. The jury is still out on the utility of cannabis as a neuroprotective therapy in MS but the overwhelming amount of experimental data suggests that with the correct clinical trial design, establishment of the case for its use in the slowing of neurodegeneration is only a matter of time with the proviso that funding can be found to conduct another study.

26.4 **Cannabis for chronic neuropathic pain in MS**

There is abundant evidence for the efficacy of cannabinoids in the reduction of pain in a number of experimental models (Lever and Rice 2007), and chronic pain is a frequent symptom in MS patients (Ehde et al., 2003, 2006). A recent Phase 3 clinical trial has investigated the ability of cannabis (Sativex®) to treat chronic neuropathic pain in MS patients (Langford et al. 2013). MS patients who had failed to gain adequate analgesia from existing medication were treated with THC/CBD spray or placebo as an add-on treatment, in a double-blind manner, for 14 weeks to investigate the efficacy of the medication in MS-induced neuropathic pain. This parallel-group phase of the study was then followed by an 18-week randomized-withdrawal study (14-week open-label treatment period plus a double-blind 4-week randomized-withdrawal phase) to investigate time to treatment failure and show maintenance of efficacy. The results of this investigation were equivocal, with conflicting findings in the two phases of the study. While there were a large proportion of responders to THC/CBD spray treatment during the phase A double-blind period, the primary endpoint was not met due to a similarly large number of placebo responders. In contrast, there was a marked effect in phase B of the study, with an increased time to treatment failure in the THC/CBD spray group compared to placebo. These findings suggest that further studies are required to explore the full potential of cannabis-based medication in MS patients.

26.5 Summary and future directions

The confirmation of the ability of cannabis and medications derived from cannabis to alleviate MS-related spasticity in both experimental and clinical settings is now well established, leading to the long overdue reintroduction of cannabis (Sativex®) into the list of prescribable medications around the world. This is encouraging but there are concerns that issues around pricing may mean that it will not be available to as many MS patients that could benefit from a new medication for this most distressing of symptoms. Time will tell whether these concerns have any credence although the decision to refuse to prescribe by many primary care trusts in the UK are not encouraging as a result of the absence of a recommendation so far by the UK National Institute for Health and Care Excellence (NICE). It is to be hoped that this situation may change in the foreseeable future.

With current cannabis medications, efficacy will always have to be balanced with the well-known side effects of cannabis that many patients find undesirable due to the global stimulation of cannabinoid receptors in the brain rather than just where stimulation is required and a degree of psychoactive effect will always be seen though this may be limited by dose titration. This has led to the hypothesis that spasticity in MS patients may be controlled by boosting the levels of endocannabinoids in the CNS by uptake inhibition or inactivation of enzymatic degradation of anandamide or 2-arachidonoyl glycerol by inhibitors of FAAH or monoacyl glycerol lipase, respectively. In the experimental setting, both these approaches have shown efficacy in the treatment of spasticity (Baker et al. 2001, 2012), indicating that they may be useful in the clinical setting with the added benefit that boosting of endocannabinoid levels does not have the same psychoactive side effects as conventional cannabinoid receptor agonists (Ligresti et al. 2006).

Another strategy may be to develop cannabinoid receptor agonists that are excluded from the brain and so unable to stimulate brain cannabinoid receptors yet may also have the ability to stimulate peripheral cannabinoid receptors, such as those at the neuromuscular junction to alleviate spasticity (Baker et al. 2012). These new experimental approaches may lead to the next generation of cannabinoid therapeutics for MS. The situation concerning the potential of cannabinoids as potential neuroprotective agents in MS is, despite abundant experimental evidence, currently lacking firm clinical evidence due to the paucity of clinical trial data.

It is to be hoped that rigorous clinical trials with better design capable of determining the neuroprotective benefits of cannabinoids in slowing disease progression in MS will be performed so that the potentially exciting potential of the cannabinoids in this situation are not lost to the medical community and MS patients.

References

Adams, M.M. and Hicks, A.L. (2005). Spasticity after spinal cord injury. *Spinal Cord*, **43**, 577–586.

Agurell, S., Halldin, M., Lindgren, J.E. (1986). Pharmacokinetics and metabolism of delta 1-tetrahydrocannabinol and other cannabinoids with emphasis on man. *Pharmacological Reviews*, **38**, 21–43.

Amato, M.P. and Ponziani, G. (2000). A prospective study on the prognosis of multiple sclerosis. *Neurological Sciences*, **21**, S831–838.

Andersson, P.B., Waubant, E., Gee, L., and Goodkin, D.E. (1999). Multiple sclerosis that is progressive from the time of onset: clinical characteristics and progression of disability. *Archives of Neurology*, **56**, 1138–1142.

Aragona, M., Onesti, E., Tomassini, V., *et al.* (2009). Psychopathological and cognitive effects of therapeutic cannabinoids in multiple sclerosis: a double-blind, placebo controlled, crossover study. *Clinical Neuropharmacology*, **32**, 41–47.

Ascherio, A. and Munger, K.L. (2010). Epstein-Barr virus infection and multiple sclerosis: a review. *Journal of Neuroimmune Pharmacology*, **5**, 271–277.

Baker, D., Pryce, G., Croxford, J.L., *et al.* (2000). Cannabinoids control spasticity and tremor in a multiple sclerosis model. *Nature*, **404**, 84–87.

Baker, D., Pryce, G., Croxford, J.L., *et al.* (2001). Endocannabinoids control spasticity in a multiple sclerosis model. *FASEB Journal*, **15**, 300–302.

Baker, D., Pryce, G., Giovannoni, G., and Thompson A.J. (2003). The therapeutic potential of cannabis. *Lancet Neurology*, **2**, 291–298.

Baker, D., Pryce, G., Jackson, S.J., Bolton, C., and Giovannoni, G. (2012). The biology that underpins the therapeutic potential of cannabis-based medicines for the control of spasticity in multiple sclerosis. *Multiple Sclerosis and Related Disorders*, **1**, 64–75.

Barnes, M.P., Kent, R.M., Semlyen, J.K., and McMullen, K.M. (2003). Spasticity in multiple sclerosis. *Neurorehabilitation Neural Repair*, **17**, 66–70.

Barnett, M.H. and Prineas, J.W. (2004). Relapsing and remitting multiple sclerosis: pathology of the newly forming lesion. *Annals of Neurology*, **55**, 458–468.

Bjartmar, C., Kidd, G., Mork, S., Rudick, R., and Trapp, B.D. (2000). Neurological disability correlates with spinal cord axonal loss and reduced N-acetyl aspartate in chronic multiple sclerosis patients. *Annals of Neurology*, **48**, 893–901.

Bjartmar, C., Wujek, J.R., and Trapp, B.D. (2003). Axonal loss in the pathology of MS: consequences for understanding the progressive phase of the disease. *Journal of the Neurological Sciences*, **206**, 165–171.

Bolton, C. and Paul, C. (2006). Glutamate receptors in neuroinflammatory demyelinating disease. *Mediators of Inflammation*, **2006**, 93684.

Brady, C.M., DasGupta, R., Dalton, C., Wiseman, O.J., Berkley, K.J., and Fowler, C.J. (2004). An open-label pilot study of cannabis-based extracts for bladder dysfunction in advanced multiple sclerosis. *Multiple Sclerosis*, **10**, 425–433.

Brenneisen, R., Egli, A., Elsohly, M.A., Henn, V., and Spiess, Y. (1996). The effect of orally and rectally administered delta 9-tetrahydrocannabinol on spasticity: a pilot study with 2 patients. *International Journal Clinical Pharmacology and Therapeutics*, **34**, 446–452.

Brown, P. (1994). Pathophysiology of spasticity. *Journal of Neurology, Neurosurgery and Psychiatry*, **57**, 773–777.

Chang, A., Smith, M.C., Yin, X., Fox, R.J., Staugaitis, S.M., and Trapp, B.D. (2008). Neurogenesis in the chronic lesions of multiple sclerosis. *Brain*, **131**, 2366–2375.

Coles, A.J., Wing, M.G., Molyneux, P., *et al.* (1999). Monoclonal antibody treatment exposes three mechanisms underlying the clinical course of multiple sclerosis. *Annals of Neurology*, **46**, 296–304.

Collin, C., Davies, P., Mutiboko, I.K., and Ratcliffe, S. (2007). Randomized controlled trial of cannabis-based medicine in spasticity caused by multiple sclerosis. *European Journal of Neurology*, **14**, 290–296.

Compston, A. and Coles, A. (2002). Multiple sclerosis. *Lancet*, **359**, 1221–1231.

Compston, A. and Coles, A. (2008). Multiple sclerosis. *Lancet*, **372**, 1502–1517.

Confavreux, C. and Vukusic, S. (2006). Accumulation of irreversible disability in multiple sclerosis: from epidemiology to treatment. *Clinical Neurology and Neurosurgery*, **108**, 327–332.

Confavreux, C., Vukusic, S., Moreau, T., and Adeleine, P. (2000). Relapses and progression of disability in multiple sclerosis. *New England Journal of Medicine*, **343**, 1430–1438.

Consroe, P., Musty, R., Rein, J., Tillery, W., and Pertwee, R. (1997). The perceived effects of smoked cannabis on patients with multiple sclerosis. *European Neurology*, **38**, 44–48.

Corey-Bloom, J., Wolfson, T. GamstA., *et al.* (2012). Smoked cannabis for spasticity in multiple sclerosis: a randomized, placebo-controlled trial. *Canadian Medical Association Journal*, **184**, 1143–1150.

Croxford, J.L., Pryce, G., Jackson, S.J., *et al.* (2008). Cannabinoid-mediated neuroprotection, not immunosuppression, may be more relevant to multiple sclerosis. *Journal of Neuroimmunology*, **193**, 120–129.

Curran, H.V., Brignell, C., Fletcher, S., Middleton, P., and Henry, J. (2002). Cognitive and subjective dose-response effects of acute oral delta 9-tetrahydrocannabinol (THC) in infrequent cannabis users. *Psychopharmacology (Berlin)*, **164**, 61–70.

Ebers, G.C. and Sadovnick, A.D. (1993). The geographic distribution of multiple sclerosis: a review. *Neuroepidemiology*, **12**, 1–5.

Ehde, D.M., Gibbons, L.E., Chwastiak, L., Bombardier, C.H., Sullivan, M.D., and Kraft, G.H. (2003). Chronic pain in a large community sample of persons with multiple sclerosis. *Multiple Sclerosis*, **9**, 605–611.

Ehde, D.M., Osborne, T.L., Hanley, M.A., Jensen, M.P., and Kraft, G.H. (2006). The scope and nature of pain in persons with multiple sclerosis. *Multiple Sclerosis*, **12**, 629–638.

Freeman, R.M., Adekanmi, O., Waterfield, M.R., Waterfield, A.E., Wright, D., and Zajicek, J. (2006). The effect of cannabis on urge incontinence in patients with multiple sclerosis: a multicentre, randomised placebo-controlled trial (CAMS-LUTS). *International Urogynecology Journal and Pelvic Floor Dysfunction*, **17**, 636–641.

Gilbert, S.L., Zhang, L., Forster, M.L., *et al.* (2006). Trak1 mutation disrupts GABA(A) receptor homeostasis in hypertonic mice. *Nature Genetics*, **38**, 245–250.

Grotenhermen, F. (2003). Pharmacokinetics and pharmacodynamics of cannabinoids. *Clinical Pharmacokinetics*, **42**, 327–360.

Handel, A.E., Williamson, A.J., Disanto, G., Handunnetthi, L., Giovannoni, G., and Ramagopalan, S.V. (2010). An updated meta-analysis of risk of multiple sclerosis following infectious mononucleosis. *PLoS One*, **2010**,5e12496.

Hardin-Pouzet, H., Krakowski, M., Bourbonniere, L., Didier-Bazes, M., Tran, E., and Owens, T. (1997). Glutamate metabolism is down-regulated in astrocytes during experimental allergic encephalomyelitis. *Glia*, **20**, 79–85.

Henze, T., Flachenecker, P., and Zettl, U.K. (2013). Importance and treatment of spasticity in multiple sclerosis: results of the MOVE 1 study. *Der Nervenarzt*, **84**, 214–222.

Hilliard, A., Stott, C., Wright, S., *et al.* (2012). Evaluation of the effects of Sativex (THC BDS: CBD BDS) on inhibition of spasticity in a chronic relapsing experimental allergic autoimmune encephalomyelitis: a model of multiple sclerosis. *ISRN Neurology*, **2012**, 802649.

Hobart, J., Lamping, D., Fitzpatrick, R., Riazi, A., and Thompson, A. (2001). The Multiple Sclerosis Impact Scale (MSIS-29): a new patient-based outcome measure. *Brain*, **124**, 962–973.

Honarmand, K., Tierney, M.C., O'Connor, P., and Feinstein, A. (2011). Effects of cannabis on cognitive function in patients with multiple sclerosis. *Neurology*, **76**, 1153–1160.

Jackson, S.L., Pryce, G., Diemel, D.T., and Baker, D. (2005). Cannabinoid receptor null mice are susceptible to neurofilament damage and caspase 3 activation. *Neuroscience*, **134**, 261–268.

Jones, J.L. and Coles, A.J. (2010). New treatment strategies in multiple sclerosis. *Experimental Neurology*, **225**, 34–39.

Killestein, J., Hoogervorst, E.L., Reif, M., *et al.* (2002). Safety, tolerability, and efficacy of orally administered cannabinoids in MS. *Neurology*, **58**, 1404–1407.

Kita, M., and Goodkin, D.E. (2000). Drugs used to treat spasticity. *Drugs*, **59**, 487–495.

Kurtzke, J.F. (1993). Epidemiologic evidence for multiple sclerosis as an infection. *Clinical Microbiology Reviews*, **6**, 382–427.

Langford, R.M., Mares, J., Novotna, A., *et al.* (2013). A double-blind, randomized, placebo-controlled, parallel-group study of THC/CBD oromucosal spray in combination with the existing treatment regimen, in the relief of central neuropathic pain in patients with multiple sclerosis. *Journal of Neurology*, **260**, 984–987.

Leray, E., Yaouanq, J., Le Page, E., *et al.* (2010). Evidence for a two-stage disability progression in multiple sclerosis. *Brain*, **133**, 1900–1913.

Lever, I.J. and Rice, A.S. (2007). Cannabinoids and pain. *Handbook of Experimental Pharmacology*, **177**, 265–306.

Ligresti, A., Cascio, M.G., Pryce, G., *et al.* (2006). New potent and selective inhibitors of anandamide reuptake with antispastic activity in a mouse model of multiple sclerosis. *British Journal of Pharmacology*, **147**, 83–91.

Loría, F., Petrosino, S., Hernangómez, M., *et al.* (2010). An endocannabinoid tone limits excitotoxicity in vitro and in a model of multiple sclerosis. *Neurobiology of Disease*, **37**, 166–176.

Lu, L., Pearce, H., Roome, C., Shearer, J., Lang, I.A., and Stein, K. (2012). Cost effectiveness of oromucosal cannabis-based medicine (Sativex®) for spasticity in multiple sclerosis. *Pharmacoeconomics*, **30**, 1157–1171.

Marte, A., Cavallero, A., Morando, S., Uccelli, A., Raiteri, M., and Fedele, E. (2010). Alterations of glutamate release in the spinal cord of mice with experimental autoimmune encephalomyelitis. *Journal of Neurochemistry*, **115**, 343–352.

Meinck, H.M., Schönle, P.W., and Conrad, B. (1989). Effect of cannabinoids on spasticity and ataxia in multiple sclerosis. *Journal of Neurology*, **236**, 120–122.

Miller, D.H. and Leary, S.M. (2007). Primary-progressive multiple sclerosis. *Lancet Neurology*, **6**, 903–912.

Müller-Vahl, K.R., Prevedel, H., Theloe, K., Kolbe, H., Emrich, H.M., and Schneider, U. (2003). Treatment of Tourette syndrome with delta-9-tetrahydrocannabinol (delta 9-THC): no influence on neuropsychological performance. *Neuropsychopharmacology*, **28**, 384–388.

Nielsen, J.B., Crone, C. and Hultborn, H. (2007). The spinal pathophysiology of spasticity – from a basic science point of view. *Acta Physiologica (Oxford)*, **189**, 171–180.

Notcutt, W., Langford, R., Davies, P., Ratcliffe, S. and Potts, R. (2012). A placebo-controlled, parallel-group, randomized withdrawal study of subjects with symptoms of spasticity due to multiple sclerosis who are receiving long-term Sativex® (nabiximols). *Multiple Sclerosis Journal*, **18**, 219–228.

Novotna, A., Mares, J., Ratcliffe, S., *et al.* (2011). A randomized, double-blind, placebo-controlled, parallel-group, enriched-design study of nabiximols* (Sativex®), as add-on therapy, in subjects with refractory spasticity caused by multiple sclerosis. *European Journal Neurology*, **18**, 1122–1131.

Ohgoh, M., Hanada, T., Smith, T., *et al.* (2002). Altered expression of glutamate transporters in experimental autoimmune encephalomyelitis. *Journal of Neuroimmunology*, **125**, 170–178.

Oreja-Guevara, C., González-Segura, D., and Vila, C. (2013). Spasticity in multiple sclerosis: results of a Spanish patient survey. *International Journal of Neuroscience*, **123**, 400–408.

Paisley, S., Beard, S., Hunn, A., and Wight, J. (2002). Clinical effectiveness of oral treatments for spasticity in multiple sclerosis: a systematic review. *Multiple Sclerosis*, **8**, 319–329.

Parratt, J.D. and Prineas, J.W. (2010). Neuromyelitis optica: a demyelinating disease characterized by acute destruction and regeneration of perivascular astrocytes. *Multiple Sclerosis*, **16**, 1156–1172.

Pertwee, R.G. (2002). Cannabinoids and multiple sclerosis. *Pharmacology and Therapeutics*, **95**, 165–174.

Pertwee, R.G. (2007). Cannabinoids and multiple sclerosis. *Molecular Neurobiology*, **36**, 45–59.

Petro, D.J. and Ellenberger, C. Jr. (1981). Treatment of human spasticity with delta 9-tetrahydrocannabinol. *Journal of Clinical Pharmacology*, **21**, (8–9 Suppl.), 413S–416S.

Pitt, D., Werner, P., and Raine, C.S. (2000). Glutamate excitotoxicity in a model of multiple sclerosis. *Nature Medicine*, **6**, 67–70.

Polman, C.H., O'Connor, P.W., Havrdova, E., *et al.* (2006). A randomized, placebo-controlled trial of natalizumab for relapsing multiple sclerosis. *New England Journal of Medicine*, **354**, 899–910.

Prat, E., Tomaru, U., Sabater, L., *et al.* (2005). HLA-DRB5*0101 and -DRB1*1501 expression in the multiple sclerosis-associated HLA-DR15 haplotype. *Journal of Neuroimmunoogy*, **167**, 108–119.

Pryce, G., Ahmed, Z., Hankey, D.J., *et al.* (2003). Cannabinoids inhibit neurodegeneration in models of multiple sclerosis. *Brain*, **126**, 2191–2202.

Pryce, G. and Baker, D. (2007). Control of spasticity in a multiple sclerosis model is mediated by CB_1, not CB_2 cannabinoid receptors. *British Journal of Pharmacology*, **150**, 519–525.

Pryce G., Cabranes A., Fernández-Ruiz J., *et al.* (2013). Control of experimental spasticity by targeting the degradation of endocannabinoids using selective fatty acid amide hydrolase inhibitors. *Multiple Sclerosis Journal*, **19**, 1896–1904.

Ramagopalan, S.V., Heger, A., Berlanga, A.J., *et al.* (2010). A ChIP-seq defined genome-wide map of vitamin D receptor binding: Associations with disease and evolution. *Genome Research*, **2**, 1352–1360.

Ramagopalan, S.V., Maugeri, N.J., Handunnetthi, L., *et al.* (2009). Expression of the multiple sclerosis-associated MHC class II Allele HLA-DRB1*1501 is regulated by vitamin D. *PLoS Genetics*, **5**, e1000369.

Runmarker, B. and Andersen, O. (1993). Prognostic factors in a multiple sclerosis incidence cohort with twenty-five years of follow-up. *Brain*, **116**, 117–134.

Sawcer, S., Hellenthal, G., Pirinen, M. *et al.*, *et al.* (2011). Genetic risk and a primary role for cell-mediated immune mechanisms in multiple sclerosis. *Nature*, **476**, 214–219.

Shakespeare, D.T., Boggild, M., and Young, C. (2003). Anti-spasticity agents for multiple sclerosis. *Cochrane Database of Systematic Reviews*, **4**, CD001332.

Shen, M. and Thayer, S.A. (1999). Delta9-tetrahydrocannabinol acts as a partial agonist to modulate glutamatergic synaptic transmission between rat hippocampal neurons in culture. *Molecular Pharmacology*, **55**, 8–13.

Siffrin, V., Radbruch, H., Glumm, R., *et al.* (2010). In vivo imaging of partially reversible th17 cell-induced neuronal dysfunction in the course of encephalomyelitis. *Immunity*, **33**, 424–436.

Smith, T., Groom, A., Zhu, B., and Turski, L. (2000). Autoimmune encephalomyelitis ameliorated by AMPA antagonists. *Nature Medicine*, **6**, 62–66.

Srinivasan, R., Sailasuta, N., Hurd, R., Nelson, S., and Pelletier, D. (2005). Evidence of elevated glutamate in multiple sclerosis using magnetic resonance spectroscopy at 3 T. *Brain*, **128**, 1016–1025.

Stover, J.F, Pleines, U.E, Morganti-Kossmann, M.C., Kossmann, T., Lowitzsch, K., and Kempski, O.S. (1997). Neurotransmitters in cerebrospinal fluid reflect pathological activity. *European Journal of Clinical Investigation*, **27**, 1038–1043.

Sulkowski, G., Dabrowska-Bouta, B., Kwiatkowska-Patzer, B., and Struzyńska, L. (2009). Alterations in glutamate transport and group I metabotropic glutamate receptors in the rat brain during acute phase of experimental autoimmune encephalomyelitis. *Folia Neuropathologica*, **47**, 329–337.

Sumaya, C.V., Myers, L.W., and Ellison, G.W. (1980). Epstein-Barr virus antibodies in multiple sclerosis. *Archives of Neurology*, **37**, 94–96.

Ungerleider, J.T., Andyrsiak, T., Fairbanks, L., Ellison, G.W., and Myers, L.W. (1987). Delta-9-THC in the treatment of spasticity associated with multiple sclerosis. *Advances in Alcohol and Substance Abuse*, **7**, 39–50.

Vaney, C., Heinzel-Gutenbrunner, M., Jobin, P., *et al.* (2004). Efficacy, safety and tolerability of an orally administered cannabis extract in the treatment of spasticity in patients with multiple sclerosis: a randomized, double-blind, placebo-controlled, crossover study. *Multiple Sclerosis*, **10**, 417–424.

Visser, E.M., Wilde, K., Wilson, J.F., Yong, K.K., and Counsell, C.E. (2012). A new prevalence study of multiple sclerosis in Orkney, Shetland and Aberdeen city. *Journal of Neurology Neurosurgery and Psychiatry*, **83**, 719–724.

Wade, D.T., Makela, P.M., House, H., Bateman, C., and Robson, P. (2006). Long-term use of a cannabis-based medicine in the treatment of spasticity and other symptoms in multiple sclerosis. *Multiple Sclerosis*, **12**, 639–645.

Wade, D.T., Makela, P., Robson, P., House, H., and Bateman, C. (2004). Do cannabis-based medicinal extracts have general or specific effects on symptoms in multiple sclerosis? A double-blind, randomized, placebo-controlled study on 160 patients. *Multiple Sclerosis*, **10**, 434–441.

Wade, D.T., Robson, P., House, H., Makela, P., and Aram, J. (2003). A preliminary controlled study to determine whether whole-plant cannabis extracts can improve intractable neurogenic symptoms. *Clinical Rehabilitation*, **17**, 21–29.

Weinshenker, B.G., Bass, B., Rice, G.P., *et al.* (1989). The natural history of multiple sclerosis: a geographically based study. I. Clinical course and disability. *Brain*, **112**, 133–146.

Wilkinson, J.D., Whalley, B.J.,Baker, D., *et al.* (2003). Medicinal cannabis: is delta9-tetrahydrocannabinol necessary for all its effects? *Journal of Pharmacy and Pharmacology*, **55**, 1687–1694.

Willer, C.J., Dyment, D.A., Sadovnick, A.D., Rothwell, P.M., Murray, T.J., and Ebers, G.C; Canadian Collaborative Study Group. (2005). Timing of birth and risk of multiple sclerosis: population based study. *British Medical Journal*, **330**, 120–123.

Wilson, R.I. and Nicoll, R.A. (2002). Endocannabinoid signalling in the brain. *Science*, **296**, 678–682.

Wujek, J.R., Bjartmar, C., Richer, E., *et al.* (2002). Axon loss in the spinal cord determines permanent neurological disability in an animal model of multiple sclerosis. *Journal of Neuropathology and Experimental Neurology*, **61**, 23–32.

Zajicek, J., Ball, S. and Wright, D., *et al.* on behalf of the CUPID investigator group. (2013). Effect of dronabinol on progression in progressive multiple sclerosis (CUPID): a randomised, placebo-controlled trial. *Lancet Neurology*, **12**, 857–865.

Zajicek, J., Fox, P., Sanders, H., *et al.* (2003). Cannabinoids for treatment of spasticity and other symptoms related to multiple sclerosis (CAMS study): multicentre randomised placebo-controlled trial. *Lancet*, **362**, 1517–1526.

Zajicek, J.P., Hobart, J.C., Slade, A., Barnes, D., Mattison, P.G., and MUSEC Research Group. (2012). Multiple sclerosis and extract of cannabis: results of the MUSEC trial. *Journal of Neurology Neurosurgery and Psychiatry*, **83**, 1125–1132.

Zajicek, J.P., Sanders, H.P., Wright, D.E., *et al.* (2005). Cannabinoids in multiple sclerosis (CAMS) study: safety and efficacy data for 12 months follow up. *Journal of Neurology, Neurosurgery and Psychiatry*, **76**, 1664–1669.

Part 5

Some Potential Therapeutic Targets for Phytocannabinoids

Marnie Duncan

Part 5 Overview

In Chapter 27, Fernández Ruiz and colleagues describe the neuroprotective actions of phytocannabinoids acting via components of the endocannabinoid system as well as noncannabinoid targets. The authors also provide an overview of preclinical work in Huntington's disease, Parkinson's disease, Alzheimer's disease, and amyotrophic lateral sclerosis.

In Chapter 28, Parolaro, Zamberletti, and Rubino present available data for the use of cannabinoids in psychosis. They review the preclinical models available for the positive and negative symptoms of schizophrenia and the actions of phytocannabinoids in these models. The authors then present the available clinical data for cannabidiol (CBD) and discuss putative mechanisms of action for CBD in psychosis.

In Chapter 29, Murillo-Rodríguez and colleagues review the physiology of sleep and provide an overview of sleep disorders. They present intriguing data for phytocannabinoids where tetrahydrocannabinol (THC) has sleep-inducing effects whereas CBD appears to promote alertness.

In Chapter 30, Williams, Jones, and Whalley provide an overview of anecdotal cannabis use and clinical trials of CBD in epilepsy patients. They also outline the various preclinical models of epilepsy and the actions of phytocannabinoids in these models.

In Chapter 31, Pacher and Kunos provide an in-depth review of the actions of CB_1 and CB_2 receptors in the cardiovascular system, metabolic system, liver and kidney, and describe the signalling pathways involved.

In Chapter 32, Oddi and Maccarrone describe the anatomy and physiology of the skin, and the expression of the endocannabinoid system within the skin. They present the pharmacological effects of phytocannabinoids in skin pathophysiology including psoriasis, skin tumours, dermatitis, scleroderma, and acne.

In Chapter 33, Xu and Azuara-Blanco provide an overview of the use of cannabinoids in glaucoma, summarizing the available preclinical and clinical data. The authors also review preclinical data generated in the research area of diabetic retinopathy, age-related macular degeneration, and uveoretinitis and discuss possible therapeutic potential.

In Chapter 34, Bab provides an in-depth overview of the skeletal cannabinoid system highlighting the possibility of targeting the CB_2 receptor in both osteoporosis and metastatic bone cancer.

In Chapter 35, Velasco, Sánchez, and Guzmán review the current preclinical literature for the actions of cannabinoids in a range of cancer cells, with a focus on glioma. They describe the signalling pathways targets by cannabinoids, and the ability of cannabinoids to inhibit tumor growth, angiogenesis, and invasion. The authors report the findings of a Phase 1 study, and speculate on the possibility of identifying biomarkers to determine if patients would be responsive to cannabinoid therapies.

Chapter 27

Neurodegenerative Disorders Other Than Multiple Sclerosis

Javier Fernández-Ruiz, Eva de Lago,
María Gómez-Ruiz, Concepción García,
Onintza Sagredo, and Moisés García-Arencibia

27.1 Introduction

Among the numerous cell and tissue functions assigned to the endocannabinoid system, the regulation of the cellular homeostasis, including the cellular decision of death/survival, appears to be one of the most basic. This explains the notable cytoprotective properties exerted by different phytocannabinoids, as well as by other related molecules that also target the endocannabinoid system, in different pathological conditions. This is particularly relevant to the central nervous system (CNS) (Fernández-Ruiz et al. 2010), as loss of neurons constitutes an extremely difficult problem because of the postmitotic characteristics of these cells and the present limitations of adult brain neurogenesis. There are already numerous preclinical studies that have addressed the ability of phytocannabinoids to protect not only neurons but also some glial cell subpopulations from different types of insults. This places these molecules in a promising position to become a novel form of therapy aimed at delaying/arresting disease progression in neurodegenerative disorders (Fernández-Ruiz et al. 2010). Phytocannabinoids appear to have a neuroprotective potential equivalent to those therapeutic strategies based on antiexcitotoxic agents (e.g., glutamate receptor antagonists), calcium channel blockers (e.g., nimodipine), antioxidant compounds (e.g., coenzyme Q10, N-acetylcysteine), anti-inflammatory substances (e.g., minocycline), and other neuroprotective pharmacotherapies used as individual treatments. The advantage of phytocannabinoids is that they can combine all these properties in a single molecule or in a mixture of two or more compounds. This is extremely important for the treatment of neurodegenerative disorders in which neuronal damage is the consequence of the progressive combination of different types of cytotoxic events—energy failure, excitotoxicity, mitochondrial dysfunction, inflammation, and oxidative stress—that therefore demand the development of therapies based on broad-spectrum compounds ("multitarget designed drugs") or on the combination of different therapeutic agents (Geldenhuys and Van der Schyf 2013).

There are three reasons why phytocannabinoids have this broad spectrum of neuroprotective properties. First, phytocannabinoids can target some components of the endocannabinoid signaling system, for example, cannabinoid receptors type 1 and 2 (CB_1 and CB_2), and the enzyme, fatty acid amide hydrolase (FAAH), which play a key role in neuroprotective responses (Hill et al. 2012). They can also act on other nonendocannabinoid molecular targets such as the nuclear receptors of the peroxisome proliferator-activated receptor (PPAR) family (O'Sullivan and Kendall 2010) and/or some transcription factors (Iuvone et al. 2009; Fernández-Ruiz et al. 2013), which are also key elements in the control of neuronal homeostasis and survival. Second, these molecular targets appear to have a specific location in different cell substrates within the CNS, i.e., neurons, astrocytes, resting and reactive microglia, perivascular microglial cells, oligodendrocytes, and neural progenitor cells, thus enabling phytocannabinoids to exert a selective control of the specific roles played by these cells in degenerative, protective and/or repair processes (Galve-Roperh et al. 2008). Lastly, by acting on the endocannabinoid system, some phytocannabinoids appear to be able to pharmacologically mimic the ability of different elements of this signaling system to oppose the effects of stimuli that damage the brain (Fernández-Ruiz et al. 2010; Pacher and Mechoulam 2011). This activation has been found in most neurodegenerative diseases, either acute episodes or chronic progressive disorders. For example, increased generation of endocannabinoids has been detected in some neurodegenerative conditions including brain trauma in neonatal (Hansen et al. 2001) or adult (Panikashvili et al. 2001) rats, experimental parkinsonism in rats (Gubellini et al. 2002), and kainate-induced excitotoxicity in mice (Marsicano et al. 2003). Upregulation of CB_1 receptors has been observed after experimental stroke (Jin et al. 2000), after excitotoxic stimuli in neonatal rats (Hansen et al. 2001), after lesions of the substantia nigra that induce parkinsonism in primates (Lastres-Becker et al. 2001), in the postmortem basal ganglia of Parkinson's disease (PD) patients (Lastres-Becker et al. 2001), and in the postmortem cerebellum of patients affected by spinocerebellar ataxias (SCAs) (Rodríguez-Cueto et al. 2014). However, given that CB_1 receptors are preferentially located in neurons within the CNS including those that degenerate in most neurodegenerative disorders, the expected response of these receptors is normally markedly reduced by the neuronal loss that occurs in these disorders. In those cases in which upregulation of CB_1 receptors was found, this response appears to occur only in surviving neurons (i.e., SCAs) or in neuronal subpopulations other than the one(s) affected by the disease (i.e., PD). This does not happen in the case of CB_2 receptors which display a marked upregulation that has been found in all neurodegenerative disorders in which effects on these receptors have been investigated, including Alzheimer's disease (AD), Huntington's disease (HD), amyotrophic lateral sclerosis (ALS), which is also known as motor neuron disease, and other disorders (Fernández-Ruiz et al. 2007, 2010). This also includes SCAs, which had not been investigated up to 2012 (Rodríguez-Cueto et al. 2014), as well as PD (García et al. 2011; Price et al. 2009), in which the identification of this response had remained elusive for various years. It is important to remark that CB_2 receptors are, in general, poorly concentrated in the brain in healthy conditions, being located preferentially in astrocytes (Fernández-Ruiz et al. 2010) and oligodendrocytes (Molina-Holgado et al. 2002), showing a relatively weak distribution in a few neuronal subpopulations (Atwood and Mackie 2010), and being apparently absent from quiescent microglial cells (Sagredo et al. 2009; Stella 2010) except some subpopulations of human perivascular microglial cells (Nuñez et al. 2004). As mentioned earlier, they upregulate in inflammatory, excitotoxic, infectious, traumatic, or oxidant insults occurring in most neurodegenerative disorders, and this upregulation is extremely intense in reactive microglial cells recruited at lesioned sites (Fernández-Ruiz et al. 2007, 2010).

This chapter aims to bring together all information generated so far that supports promising therapeutic applications of phytocannabinoids and related compounds for the treatment of conditions of acute or chronic neurodegeneration. To meet this objective, we have divided the chapter into two parts. First, we have reviewed the different cellular and molecular mechanisms underlying the neuroprotective effects of phytocannabinoids against neurodegenerative cellular events. Second, we have provided an overview of additional information about these neuroprotective effects in acute neurodegeneration, in particular in the two major accidental causes of this pathology, cerebral ischemia and traumatic brain injury, and also in four chronic neurodegenerative disorders, AD, HD, PD, and ALS, for which relevant information has been recently published, including clinical data.

27.2 Mechanisms involved in neuroprotection by phytocannabinoids

The molecular mechanisms underlying the neuroprotectant properties of phytocannabinoids are quite diverse and, frequently, complementary. This broad-spectrum activity represents their major advantage compared with other types of neuroprotective agents (a summary of all these mechanisms is given in Fig. 27.1). These mechanisms include actions that do not involve components of the endocannabinoid system, particularly cannabinoid receptors, for example, the ability

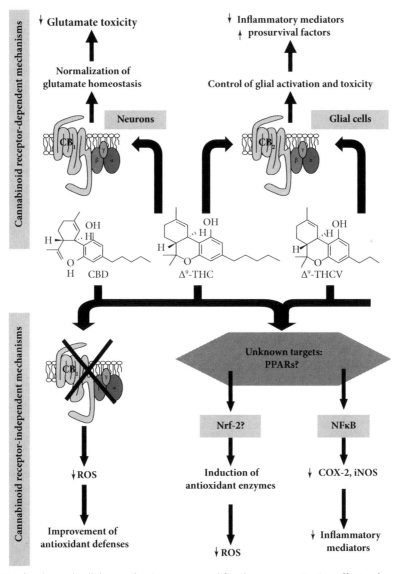

Fig. 27.1 Molecular and cellular mechanisms proposed for the neuroprotective effects of phytocannabinoids.

of certain cannabinoids to block N-methyl-D-aspartate (NMDA) receptors, the antioxidant properties of most phytocannabinoids, their ability to bind nuclear receptors of the PPAR family, and to affect some transcription factors (Iuvone et al. 2009; Fernández-Ruiz et al. 2013; O'Sullivan and Kendall 2010). By contrast, they also include some responses that are definitively mediated by either CB_1 or CB_2 receptors, for example, the ability of those phytocannabinoids targeting the CB_1 receptor to improve blood supply to the injured brain in ischemic conditions (Fernández-Ruiz et al. 2005) and, in particular, their ability to attenuate excitotoxic damage that occurs in most acute or chronic neurodegenerative disorders (Fernández-Ruiz et al. 2010). With regard to CB_2 receptors, their activation plays an important role in the processes of glial activation and neuroinflammation that occur in most neurodegenerative disorders (Fernández-Ruiz et al. 2007).

27.2.1 Neuroprotective effects of phytocannabinoids mediated by CB_1 receptors

The most important neuroprotective property of those phytocannabinoids targeting the CB_1 receptor is the normalization of glutamate homeostasis (Fernández-Ruiz et al. 2010). Alterations in this important excitatory neurotransmitter system in neurodegenerative disorders, a so-called excitotoxicity process, consist of excessive extracellular levels of glutamate and hyperactivation of glutamate receptors, mainly the ionotropic receptors, resulting in an intracellular accumulation of cytotoxic concentrations of calcium, which activate numerous destructive pathways, e.g., calpains, caspases, protein kinases, nitric oxide (NO) synthase, reactive oxygen species (ROS), and others, leading to severe cell swelling and death (Doble 1999).

The activation of CB_1 receptors opposes both glutamatergic cytotoxic events (Fernández-Ruiz et al. 2010). On the one hand, it reduces the excessive glutamate release through CB_1 receptors located at the presynaptic level in glutamatergic terminals. On the other hand, it reduces the excessive intracellular levels of calcium through postsynaptic CB_1 receptors (located on neurons containing NMDA receptors) that close voltage-dependent calcium channels, thereby reducing the overall calcium current and the overactivation of destructive pathways. This information has been collected both in vitro, e.g., from neuronal cultures (Abood et al. 2001; Shen and Thayer 1998), rat brain slices (Hampson et al. 1998a), and in vivo, e.g., from rodent models of ischemic damage (Nagayama et al. 1999) or neurotoxin lesions (Marsicano et al. 2003; van der Stelt et al. 2001). In all cases, the participation of CB_1 receptors has been strongly demonstrated by using either selective CB_1 receptor antagonists or mice genetically deficient in CB_1 receptors (Fernández-Ruiz et al. 2005, 2010).

Another CB_1 receptor-mediated neuroprotective effect of phytocannabinoids, particularly relevant in ischemia, is the improvement of blood supply to the injured brain, an effect that is related to the reduction in the levels of some vasoconstrictor factors (Fernández-Ruiz et al. 2005). Brain damage occurring during stroke or traumatic injuries is associated with the release of several endothelium-derived mediators (Madden 2012), in particular endothelin-1, which produces vasoconstriction, thus limiting the blood supply to the injured area and thereby aggravating brain damage (Schinelli 2002). Different cannabinoids, including the phytocannabinoid Δ^9-tetrahydrocannabinol (Δ^9-THC), are potent modulators of vascular tone (Wagner et al. 1998), and therefore might provide neuroprotection in ischemic conditions by reducing endothelin-1-induced vasoconstriction and by restoring blood supply to the injured brain (Mechoulam et al. 2002). This effect appears to be mediated by CB_1 receptors located in brain microvasculature (Hillard 2000), as it was reversed by rimonabant (Chen et al. 2000). However, recent findings also support an involvement of CB_2 receptors (see section 27.3).

27.2.2 Neuroprotective effects of phytocannabinoids mediated by CB$_2$ receptors

The key neuroprotective action of CB$_2$ receptors is the control of glial influences on neurons (Fernández-Ruiz et al. 2007, 2010). This does not exclude the possibility that CB$_1$ receptors may also be involved in some effects related to glial processes (de Lago et al. 2012; Molina-Holgado et al. 2003; Smith et al. 2000), but the major contribution is made by CB$_2$ receptors. The proliferation, recruitment, activation, and migration at lesioned sites of several glial subpopulations, i.e., astrocytes, microglia, is an important event in acute and chronic brain degenerative pathologies (Khandelwal et al. 2011). They have been associated with inflammatory processes that may induce or aggravate brain damage, although there are also positive effects associated with the proliferation of these glial cells (Wee Yong 2010). Classically, astrogliosis is regarded as being protective because of the positive influences exerted by astrocytes (e.g., trophic and metabolic support, generation of prosurvival and neurotrophic factors; see Allaman et al. 2011), whereas the proliferation and activation of microglial cells from their quiescent phenotype to a reactive state has been associated with greater neuronal injury (Cunningham 2013). However, there is also evidence that some reactive astrocytes may damage neuronal homeostasis (Singh et al. 2011), whereas activated microglial cells may also exert positive effects on neuronal survival (Czeh et al. 2011). The classic detrimental effects assigned to reactive microglial cells are exerted through the generation of numerous neurotoxic mediators, including tumor necrosis factor-alpha (TNF-α), interleukin (IL)-1β, IL-6, eicosanoids, NO, and ROS, that impact on neurons and produce neuronal damage (Liu and Hong 2003). They can also impact on other neural cells to promote demyelination, thrombosis, leukocyte infiltration, and blood–brain barrier disruption (Liu and Hong 2003).

As previously mentioned, targeting CB$_2$ receptors may serve to modulate glial events. This includes CB$_2$ receptors located in microglial cells, where these receptors play an important role in the proliferation and migration of these cells at lesion sites (Carrier et al. 2004; Walter et al. 2003). They also reduce the production by reactive microglial cells of a plethora of factors that damage neurons (Fernández-Ruiz et al. 2007, 2010). Of particular interest is the inhibitory effect on the production of TNF-α, as this is a major contributor to the pathophysiology of brain injury (Stella 2010). This inhibitory effect possibly involves the inhibition of the nuclear factor kappa B (NF-κB) (Oh et al. 2010), a transcription factor that is critically involved in proinflammatory responses. However, cannabinoids that do not activate the CB$_2$ receptor, for example, the phytocannabinoid cannabidiol (CBD) or the inactive synthetic cannabinoid dexanabinol (HU-211), are also able to inhibit this transcription factor (Jüttler et al. 2004; Kozela et al. 2010; Shohami and Mechoulam 2000), presumably because of their activity at nuclear receptors of the PPAR family (O'Sullivan and Kendall 2010; Stahel et al. 2008) that also control NF-κB signaling (Chung et al. 2008; Stahel et al. 2008).

The activation of CB$_2$ receptors, presumably located in astrocytes, may also serve to improve neuronal homeostasis, although this possibility remains controversial because of the possible participation of CB$_1$ receptors alone or even in combination with CB$_2$ receptors (Fernández-Ruiz et al. 2007, 2010; Stella 2010). Targeting CB$_2$ receptors in astrocytes would increase the supply of metabolic substrates (e.g., lactate, ketone bodies) or the generation of neurotrophins (e.g., GDNF), anti-inflammatory cytokines (e.g., IL-1 receptor antagonist) and other prosurvival molecules (e.g., transforming growth factor-beta) by astrocytes (Molina-Holgado et al. 2003; Fernández-Ruiz et al. 2007, 2010; Stella 2010). In addition, targeting CB$_2$ receptors also protects astrocytes and even oligodendrocytes from death, which is also beneficial for neurons (Gómez del Pulgar et al. 2002; Molina-Holgado et al. 2002).

27.2.3 **Neuroprotective effects of phytocannabinoids which are independent of CB$_1$ and CB$_2$ receptors**

The neuroprotective effects of phytocannabinoids also include some responses that are not medi-ated by classic targets within the endocannabinoid system, for example, the antioxidant prop-erties of most of them, their ability to bind nuclear receptors of the PPAR family and to affect some transcription factors (Iuvone et al. 2009; Fernández-Ruiz et al. 2013; O'Sullivan and Kendall 2010). An interesting compound is CBD, a phytocannabinoid with a broad spectrum of potential therapeutic applications, including neuroprotective effects, but poor affinity for CB$_1$ and CB$_2$ receptors (Fernández-Ruiz et al. 2013). Therefore, its neuroprotective effects cannot be attributed to the control of excitotoxicity via the direct activation of CB$_1$ receptors and/or to the control of microglial toxicity via the direct activation of CB$_2$ receptors. However, CBD is no less active against the brain damage produced by alterations in glutamate homeostasis (El-Remessy et al. 2003; Hampson et al. 2000), oxidative stress (Hampson et al. 1998b; Marsicano et al. 2002) and local inflammatory events (Martín-Moreno et al. 2011; Ruiz-Valdepeñas et al. 2011) than other cannabinoids that can activate these receptors. These effects of CBD may be explained by its abil-ity to inhibit endocannabinoid inactivation (Bisogno et al. 2001; Leweke et al. 2012), which may enhance the action of endocannabinoids at their different receptors. However, CBD has other properties that may contribute more to its neuroprotective effects. On the one hand, it is frequently assumed that the neuroprotective effects of CBD are related to its innate chemical properties, in particular the presence of two hydroxyl groups that enables CBD to have an important antioxi-dant activity, rather than due to pharmacodynamic events and/or activation of specific signaling pathways. The antioxidant activity of CBD is comparable, and, even superior, to classic dietary antioxidants such as ascorbate and α-tocopherol (Fernández-Ruiz et al. 2013). CBD works well against the accumulation of harmful oxidative products, which are highly produced in response to excitotoxicity and/or mitochondrial dysfunction (Lenaz 2012). This antioxidant capability seems also to be possessed by other structurally-similar compounds, e.g., Δ^9-THC, cannabinol (CBN), nabilone, levonantradol, and dexanabinol (Marsicano et al. 2002), presumably because it depends on the presence of phenolic groups and is cannabinoid receptor-independent (Fernández-Ruiz et al. 2013). In comparison with CBD, Δ^9-THC has an equivalent antioxidant activity. However, CBD is significantly superior to Δ^9-THC as a potential antioxidant medicine. Thus, since it lacks psychoactivity and tolerance to it does not develop, CBD can be used at higher doses and for longer times than those possible with Δ^9-THC (Malfait et al. 2000). In addition to this ROS scavenger action, phytocannabinoids may also be antioxidant by activating intracellular mechanisms that control the availability of endogenous antioxidant defenses, in particular the signaling triggered by the transcription factor nuclear factor-erythroid 2-related factor 2 (Nrf-2), which plays a major role in the control of antioxidant-response elements located in genes encoding for different phase II antioxidant enzymes. In this case, phytocannabinoids may to bind to an intracellular target, pres-ently unknown, linked to the regulation of this transcription factor (Fernández-Ruiz et al. 2013).

On the other hand, despite its lack of activity at CB$_2$ receptors, CBD elicits the same responses as CB$_2$ agonists, i.e., it reduces microglial cell migration (Walter et al. 2003) and the production of proinflammatory mediators by these cells (Esposito et al. 2007), like cannabinoid compounds tar-geting the CB$_2$ receptor (Fernández-Ruiz et al. 2007). A key element in this CBD effect is the inhibi-tory control of NFκB signaling and the control of those genes regulated by this transcription factor (e.g., inducible NO synthase) (Esposito et al. 2006a, 2007). This may be related to the ability of CBD (like other phytocannabinoids) to bind to the nuclear receptors of the PPAR family (Esposito et al. 2011; O'Sullivan and Kendall 2010) and to regulate their downstream signals, i.e., inhibition of NFκB leading to low expression of proinflammatory enzymes (cyclooxygenase-2, inducible NO synthase), proinflammatory cytokines, and metalloproteases.

27.3 **Phytocannabinoids in ischemia, brain trauma, and spinal injury**

Acute neurodegeneration, resulting from brain trauma, spinal cord injury, perinatal hypoxia-ischemia, or ischemic stroke, is associated with high morbidity and mortality. It is also a major cause of permanent disability, and thus it represents a significant socioeconomic challenge world-wide. The primary injury leads to secondary damage characterized by a complex of harmful pathways including neuroinflammation, glutamatergic excitotoxicity, calcium influx, caspase activation, vasoconstriction, and oxidative stress (Moskowitz et al. 2010). Various neuroprotective drugs acting through specific pathological mechanisms, including anti-inflammatory drugs, antiglutamatergic compounds, calcium-channel blockers, vasodilators, and antioxidants, have been tested for their ability to reduce this secondary damage. None of them have shown a significant effect (Beauchamp et al. 2008), and it is now accepted that therapeutic approaches must be aimed at finding drugs that can act on different cytotoxic pathways simultaneously, and this is why phytocannabinoids are considered good candidates and have been significantly studied in preclinical models over the last 15 years. In vivo, treatment with different cannabinoids, including the phytocannabinoids Δ^9-THC and CBD, reduced lesion expansion and neurological deficits in animal models of acute neurodegeneration: (1) rodents with global (Braida et al. 2000; Louw et al. 2000; Nagayama et al. 1999; Suzuki et al. 2012; Zani et al. 2007) or focal (Hayakawa et al. 2004; Leker et al. 2003; Mauler et al. 2003; Nagayama et al. 1999) ischemia, (2) rats with contusive spinal cord injury (Arévalo-Martin et al. 2010), (3) mouse models of close head injury (Panikashvili et al. 2001), and (4) newborn animals with hypoxia-ischemia (Alvarez et al. 2008; Lafuente et al. 2011; Pazos et al. 2012). These neuroprotective effects have been confirmed in different in vitro experiments using cultured neurons subjected to hypoxia and/or glucose deprivation, or exposed to excitotoxic stimuli, conditions that reproduce the key cytotoxic events involved in acute neurodegeneration, and in all cases cannabinoids, including the phytocannabinoids Δ^9-THC and CBD, were effective in preserving neuronal survival (Fernández-Ruiz et al. 2005; Hampson and Grimaldi 2001; Hampson et al. 1998b; Marsicano et al. 2002; Shen and Thayer 1998; Sinor et al. 2000; Skaper et al. 1996).

Despite a few articles showing the opposite (Nagayama et al. 1999; Sinor et al. 2000), most studies have indicated that CB_1 receptor-mediated reduction of excitotoxicity is the main mechanism by which cannabinoids provide protection in acute neurodegeneration, as CB_1 receptor antagonists attenuated most of these neuroprotective effects (Fernández-Ruiz et al. 2005). Further support has come from a study using CB_1 knockout mice, which showed increased mortality from permanent focal cerebral ischemia and larger infarcts after transient focal cerebral ischemia, compared with the wild-type mice (Parmentier-Batteur et al. 2002). However, there is also growing evidence for the involvement of CB_2 receptors, and even of receptor-independent mechanisms, in some of these effects, particularly with regard to glial-mediated effects of cannabinoids in ischemia or brain trauma (Capettini et al. 2012) or to the antioxidant activity of some phytocannabinoids like CBD (Fernández-Ruiz et al. 2013), respectively.

Cannabinoids may also help to protect the brain against ischemia and traumatic brain injury by attenuating blood–brain barrier damage (Amenta et al. 2012; Chi et al. 2012; Zhang et al. 2009) and by improving microcirculatory dysfunction (Zhang et al. 2009). These effects were initially attributed to the activation of CB_1 receptors (Chen et al. 2000), but CB_2 receptors are also now known to be involved (Amenta et al. 2012; Zhang et al. 2009). Lastly, as well as being neuroprotective, cannabinoids can also reduce acute neurodegeneration by improving neural repair. Thus, protection of oligodendrocyte precursor cells, promotion of oligodendrogenesis and enhancement of remyelination have been found in rat models of stroke (Sun et al. 2013a, 2013b) and also in neonatal hypoxia-ischemia (Fernández-López et al. 2010) with the non-selective CB_1/CB_2 cannabinoid receptor agonist WIN55,212-2, raising the possibility that some phytocannabinoids may act in this way as well to reduce neurodegeneration.

Therefore, this preclinical evidence appears promising and demands an urgent development of clinical studies in patients. Unfortunately, such clinical development is still poor and only dexanabinol has been tested in a Phase 3 clinical trial in patients affected by severe brain trauma (Maas et al. 2006), and this study could not confirm the beneficial effects shown by dexanabinol in animal models (Shohami et al. 1995) and in a previous Phase 2 clinical trial (Knoller et al. 2002). However, it should be noted that dexanabinol may be considered a cannabinoid because of its chemical structure rather than its pharmacological properties, as it acts as a noncompetitive NMDA receptor antagonist but displays negligible activity at cannabinoid receptors (Eshhar et al. 1995). Therefore novel clinical studies with stroke/brain trauma patients using the phytocannabinoid combination of Sativex® might be interesting, as would clinical studies conducted with neonatal ischemia patients using CBD alone in this case (Lafuente et al. 2011) (see Fig. 27.2).

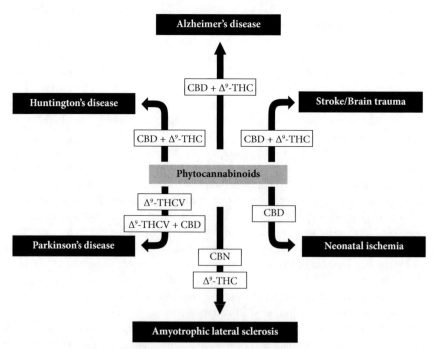

Fig. 27.2 Summary of phytocannabinoids and their combinations that appear to be most suitable for clinical evaluation as neuroprotective therapies in different neurodegenerative disorders.

27.4 **Phytocannabinoids in Huntington's disease**

Huntington's disease is an inherited chronic progressive neurodegenerative disorder caused by a mutation in the huntingtin gene (IT15), which consists of an excessive repetition of the CAG triplet (>35) resulting in an expansion of glutamines in the amino-terminal portion of the huntingtin protein (Arrasate and Finkbeiner 2012). Huntingtin is widely distributed throughout the body, in particular within the CNS, and its function seems to be related to intracellular vesicular trafficking (Caviston and Holzbaur 2009), mitochondrial energy metabolism (Cattaneo et al. 2005), transcription of key genes, e.g., brain-derived neurotrophic factor (BDNF) (Zuccato et al. 2001), and regulation of apoptosis (Luo and Rubinsztein 2009). Accordingly, the toxicity of the mutated huntingtin progresses through the aggregation of proteolytic fragments of mutant huntingtin, transcriptional dysregulation, mitochondrial dysfunction and energy depletion, occurrence of excitotoxic and oxidative events, and glial activation/local inflammatory episodes (Ross and Tabrizi 2011; Walker 2007). Despite its ubiquitous distribution, the mutant huntingtin affects preferentially the medium spiny GABAergic striatal neurons, an effect associated with the characteristic "choreic" movements that appear in early stages of the disease (Ross and Tabrizi 2011), and also the glutamatergic neurons that project from the cortex to the striatum and that are associated with the cognitive dysfunctions and psychiatric symptoms that also appear in HD (Walker 2007).

The first therapies investigated in HD attempted to alleviate the choreic movements, using antidopaminergic agents (Factor and Friedman 1997), although the only medicine approved is tetrabenazine, an inhibitor of the monoamine vesicular transporter, with modest effects in HD patients (Chen et al. 2012). There are still no approved therapies aimed at modifying the progression of HD, although antiglutamatergic agents were investigated for many years (Kieburtz et al. 1999). Recently, attempts have been made to inhibit the aggregation of mutant huntingtin (e.g., autophagy enhancers), to normalize transcriptional dysregulation (e.g., inhibitors of histone deacetylases), to reduce inflammatory (e.g., minocycline) and oxidative (e.g., cysteamine) events, to ameliorate energy depletion (e.g., coenzyme Q10, creatine), or to improve lipid dysregulation (e.g., unsaturated fatty acids). Some of these compounds have yielded promising results in preclinical studies and they are presently being investigated at the clinical level (Butler and Bates 2006; Ha and Fung 2012; Venuto et al. 2012).

Phytocannabinoids have also been proposed as candidates for a neuroprotective therapy in HD and this involves both CB_1 and CB_2 receptors and also receptor-independent mechanisms (Sagredo et al. 2012). In fact, there is evidence indicating that defects in CB_1 receptor signaling in the basal ganglia might trigger an imbalance in glutamate homeostasis and initiate excitotoxicity (Blázquez et al., 2011), so that the early stimulation of these receptors might reduce the progression of striatal degeneration associated with excitotoxicity (Blázquez et al., 2011; Pintor et al. 2006). By contrast, CB_2 receptors appear to be upregulated in astrocytes and reactive microglial cells recruited at the lesioned striatum (Bouchard et al. 2012; Palazuelos et al. 2009; Sagredo et al. 2009). Interestingly, targeting these receptors protects striatal projection neurons from death, presumably by enhancing the trophic support exerted by astrocytes and, in particular, by reducing the toxicity of reactive microglial cells (Palazuelos et al. 2009; Sagredo et al. 2009).

In addition to targeting CB_1 and/or CB_2 receptors, certain phytocannabinoids, particularly those devoid of activity at the classic cannabinoid receptors such as CBD, have been found to be highly active in animal models of HD (Sagredo et al. 2007, 2011; Valdeolivas et al. 2012). As has been outlined in section 27.2.3, these effects are directly linked to the control of oxidative stress, which is an important cytotoxic mechanism involved in the pathogenesis of HD. These experiments have been frequently conducted in rats lesioned with the irreversible mitochondrial complex II inhibitor, 3-nitropropionate, which damages the mitochondria and elevates the generation of ROS in parallel to the activation of the calcium-binding protein calpain. CBD was neuroprotective in this model, either in the form of pure compound (Sagredo et al. 2007) or as an enriched botanical extract, alone or combined with Δ^9-THC-enriched botanical extract (Sagredo et al. 2011). Δ^9-THC by itself was also active in both forms (Lastres-Becker et al. 2004; Sagredo et al. 2011).

Therefore, the evidence derived from these pharmacological studies suggests that a cannabinoid-based neuroprotective therapy in HD patients should be based on targeting both CB_1 (to reduce excitotoxicity) and CB_2 (to attenuate inflammation) receptors, as well as other cannabinoid receptor-independent processes (to decrease oxidative injury). With this idea in mind, a clinical study has been recently conducted in HD patients (NCT01502046) to determine the neuroprotective effect of the phytocannabinoid-based medicine Sativex® (see Fig. 27.2). This has been the first clinical study conducted in HD patients with cannabinoids that monitored their effects on HD progression: previous clinical studies focused only on the relief of symptoms such as chorea (Consroe et al. 1991; Curtis and Rickards 2006; Curtis et al. 2009; Müller-Vahl et al. 1999). The clinical trial with Sativex® demonstrated that this cannabinoid-based medicine was safe and well-tolerated in HD patients, but, unfortunately, there was no evidence of slower disease progression.

27.5 Phytocannabinoids in Parkinson's disease

Parkinson's disease is a chronic progressive neurodegenerative disorder characterized by the occurrence of bradykinesia, resting tremor, rigidity, and postural disturbances (Mazzoni et al. 2012). These symptoms are the consequence of the progressive degeneration of dopaminergic neurons of the substantia nigra pars compacta (Blandini et al. 2000) caused by oxidative stress, mitochondrial dysfunction, protein aggregation, and inflammatory stimuli, presumably triggered by genetic risk factors in combination with environmental factors (Surmeier and Sulzer 2013). Different therapeutic strategies have been investigated, and in some cases approved, for the treatment of PD patients, including: (1) stimulation of specific basal ganglia structures (e.g., bilateral stimulation of the subthalamic nucleus or the medial globus pallidus, deep brain stimulation), (2) replacement of degenerated neurons with dopamine-producing cells (e.g., chromaffin cells, embryonic neurons, differentiated stem cells), and (3) pharmacological treatments aimed at relieving specific motor symptoms (e.g., levodopa, dopamine agonists, MAO-B inhibitors), although they produce some unwanted side effects (Jankovic and Poewe 2012). The therapies investigated in PD patients also include neuroprotective strategies to slowdown the progression of striatal dopaminergic denervation and nigral degeneration (Santos 2012), although the evidence collected so far is controversial.

Phytocannabinoids have also been proposed as a promising disease-modifying therapy in PD (García-Arencibia et al. 2009), in particular CBD and delta-9-tetrahydrocannabivarin (Δ^9-THCV). Both phytocannabinoids were neuroprotective in 6-hydroxydopamine-lesioned rats due to their cannabinoid receptor-independent antioxidant properties (García et al. 2011; Lastres-Becker et al. 2005). Similar effects have also been described for other antioxidant phytocannabinoids such as Δ^9-THC (Lastres-Becker et al. 2005). The activation of CB_1 receptors may also provide neuroprotection in PD. In fact, mice lacking this receptor were more sensitive to 6-hydroxydopamine (Pérez-Rial et al. 2011), whereas targeting the CB_1 receptor preserved dopaminergic neurons in MPTP-lesioned mice (Chung et al. 2011). However, a neuroprotective strategy based on targeting the CB_1 receptor (e.g., with Δ^9-THC) might have some disadvantages in

PD, given that the activation of this receptor may worsen specific parkinsonian symptoms, e.g., bradykinesia (Garcia-Arencibia et al. 2009). By contrast, Δ^9-THCV, which is also antioxidant in 6-hydroxydopamine-lesioned rats (García et al. 2011), may be a better option for PD as it behaves as a CB_1 receptor antagonist (Hill et al. 2012) and these antagonists have shown benefits in the reduction of parkinsonian bradykinesia (Fernández-Ruiz 2009).

The anti-inflammatory efficacy of certain phytocannabinoids, dependent on the activation of CB_2 receptors, but also on NFκB signaling, extended to the neuroinflammatory component of PD. In fact, overexpresssion of CB_2 receptors in mice protected against 6-hydroxydopamine (Ternianov et al. 2012), and these receptors were particularly important in inflammatory models of PD (e.g., LPS-lesioned rodents) (Chung et al. 2012; García et al. 2011). Compounds activating these receptors, such as the CB_2-selective agonist HU-308 or the phytocannabinoid Δ^9-THCV, preserved dopaminergic neurons in LPS-lesioned mice, whereas CB_2 receptor-deficient mice were more vulnerable to LPS than wild-type animals (García et al. 2011). Similar effects were also found in MPTP-lesioned mice (Price et al. 2009).

Therefore, it seems obvious that phytocannabinoids constitute potential novel neuroprotective therapies for PD. The emphasis should be put on their antioxidant profile and/or their effects on CB_2 receptors, and on trying to minimize effects derived from the direct activation of CB_1 receptors. In this context, the phytocannabinoid Δ^9-THCV emerges as an interesting compound to be used alone or in combination with CBD, demanding a prompt investigation in patients (see Fig. 27.2).

27.6 Phytocannabinoids in Alzheimer's disease

Alzheimer's disease affects more than 25 million people worldwide and its incidence is expected to grow in years to come, given the increase in life expectancy in developed countries. AD is clinically defined by the progressive deterioration of cognition and memory (Minati et al. 2009). The pathological hallmarks of AD include deposition of β-amyloid protein in senile plaques, neurofibrillary tangles, and selective synaptic degeneration resulting in the neuronal loss preferentially in cortical and subcortical areas (Perl 2010). The majority of drugs currently in use for the treatment of AD act as inhibitors of acetylcholinesterase (e.g., tacrine, donepezil, rivastigmine) (Savonenko et al. 2012) or by blocking NMDA receptors (e.g., memantine) (Danysz and Parsons 2012). Strong efforts are being made to find new disease-modifying treatments based on inhibiting the aberrant processing leading to β-amyloid peptide generation, reducing β-amyloid peptide aggregation and deposition, or facilitating its brain clearance (Corbett et al. 2012), as well as on inhibiting the kinases involved in the hyperphosphorylation of tau protein (Medina et al. 2011).

Phytocannabinoids are also being investigated as a novel disease-modifying therapy in AD and, as in other disorders, their therapeutic advantage is based on their widespread effects against excitotoxicity, oxidative stress and inflammation (Gowran et al. 2011; Karl et al. 2012). However, certain phytocannabinoids may also affect the processing, aggregation and clearance of β-amyloid protein, which represents an additional target specific for AD. This is the case for Δ^9-THC which exhibits some ability to inhibit acetylcholinesterase activity (Eubanks et al. 2006). This additional action of Δ^9-THC is presently being exploited through the design of novel compounds that are capable of producing all of its likely AD-ameliorating actions (González-Naranjo et al. 2013). Another important phytocannabinoid for AD is CBD (Iuvone et al. 2009), which is active in the prevention of glutamate-induced toxicity, oxidative damage, and inflammatory responses induced by β-amyloid protein in vitro (Iuvone et al. 2004) and in vivo (Esposito et al. 2007; Martin-Moreno et al. 2011). CBD was also active against β-amyloid protein-induced tau protein hyperphosphorylation by glycogen synthase kinase-3β (Esposito et al. 2006b).

Based on the potential shown by Δ^9-THC and CBD in experimental AD, the combination of both phytocannabinoids (i.e., Sativex®) may be useful for the treatment of AD patients (see Fig. 27.2), even though the activation of CB_1 receptors by Δ^9-THC may worsen some symptoms such as memory deficits. However, no clinical investigation of this possibility has yet been made (Gowran et al. 2010; Karl et al. 2012). The only clinical studies performed so far have been a small number that used dronabinol, an oil-based solution of synthetic Δ^9-THC, which was found to ameliorate only some AD-related symptoms (Volicer et al. 1997; Walther et al. 2006).

27.7 **Phytocannabinoids in amyotrophic lateral sclerosis**

Amyotrophic lateral sclerosis, also known as motor neuron disease, is a fatal neurodegenerative disorder characterized by the selective injury and death of motor neurons in the spinal cord, brainstem, and motor cortex (Ferraiuolo et al. 2011). Most cases of ALS are sporadic (90%) with an etiology still unknown, but the disease also includes familial cases (10%) caused by mutations in specific genes (Ahmed and Wicklund 2011). This includes mutations in superoxide dismutase 1 (SOD-1), resulting in abnormal oxidative metabolism, as well as in the TAR DNA-binding protein-43 (TDP-43), leading to defects in RNA transcription, processing, and stability (Liscic and Beljak 2011). Even though the pathogenic process remains to be completely elucidated, pathological mechanisms that operate in other chronic neurodegenerative disorders, such as oxidative stress, excitotoxicity, neuroinflammation, protein aggregation and deposition, and dysregulation of RNA transcription and processing (Ferraiuolo et al. 2011) have also been found in ALS. Riluzol (Rilutek®) is the only therapy available for treatment of ALS patients. It is an antiglutamatergic agent that acts by blocking voltage-dependent sodium channels located in motor neurons, thereby reducing the activity of these neurons (Cheach et al. 2010). However, its effects are limited and there is an urgent need for novel compounds for the treatment of ALS.

Data obtained using the G93A transgenic mouse that overexpresses a mutated form of human SOD-1 support phytocannabinoids as a possible and promising therapeutic option for ALS (Carter et al. 2010; Rossi et al. 2010). The first studies were conducted by Abood and coworkers who observed that the administration of the phytocannabinoid Δ^9-THC delayed motor impairment and increased survival in these mice (Raman et al. 2004). Δ^9-THC was also effective in reducing oxidative damage and excitotoxicity in spinal cord neuronal cultures (Raman et al. 2004). Similar results were obtained with the less psychotrophic phytocannabinoid CBN (Weydt et al. 2005), and with synthetic cannabinoids (Bilsland et al. 2006; Kim et al. 2006; Shoemaker et al. 2007). These pharmacological experiments have been paralleled by other studies using mice deficient in specific endocannabinoid receptors or enzymes. Thus, the genetic ablation of the FAAH enzyme, which leads to a permanent elevation of endocannabinoid levels, also delayed the onset of the disease in SOD-1 mutant mice (observed in animals having the SOD-1 mutation and genetic ablation of FAAH in comparison with classic SOD-1 mutant mice) but it did not affect their survival (Bilsland et al. 2006). However, genetic ablation of the CB_1 receptor had no effect on the onset of the disease in SOD-1 mutant mice, although it did significantly extend life span (Bilsland et al. 2006).

This topic has also been investigated at the clinical level. However, too few clinical data have yet been generated to allow any firm conclusions to be drawn, prompting an urgent need for additional clinical investigation (Carter et al. 2010). A randomized, double-blind crossover trial conducted with oral Δ^9-THC detected no effect on cramp frequency or intensity (Weber et al. 2010). These results should, however, be interpreted with caution due to the small number of patients recruited and the dose used. Two additional studies indicated good tolerability to Δ^9-THC in ALS patients (Gelinas et al. 2002; Joerger et al. 2012), although a high interindividual variability was found in Δ^9-THC pharmacokinetics (Joerger et al. 2012).

27.8 Concluding remarks and future perspectives

Due to several of the pharmacological effects that they produce, phytocannabinoids have been found to be potentially useful and clinically promising neuroprotective molecules. In this chapter, we have reviewed the cellular and molecular mechanisms that might be involved in the neuroprotective effects of phytocannabinoids, putting emphasis on those effects induced by the activation of CB_1 receptors (e.g., reduction of excitotoxic stimuli produced either by inhibiting glutamate release or by reducing NMDA receptor-induced calcium influx), by the activation of CB_2 receptors (e.g., reduction of local inflammatory events resulting from the activation of glial elements), or through other, cannabinoid receptor-independent, mechanisms (e.g., reduction of oxidative injury by scavenging ROS or by inducing antioxidant defenses). Through one or more of these effects, phytocannabinoids may provide neuroprotection in conditions of acute pathological or accidental neurodegeneration, such as that occurring in ischemia, brain trauma, or spinal lesion. They might also come to be used to delay/arrest the progression of neurodegeneration in chronic diseases affecting cognitive processes, such as AD, or motor control or performance, such as PD, HD, and ALS. It is important to note that most of the studies so far carried out to investigate phytocannabinoids as potential medicines for the treatment of these diseases have been preclinical and that these studies have already provided sufficient solid evidence to justify the progression of these molecules, alone or in combination, from preclinical to clinical investigations.

Acknowledgments

This work has been supported by grants from CIBERNED (CB06/05/0089), MICINN (SAF2009/11847 and SAF2012/39173) and CAM (S2011/BMD-2308).

References

Abood, M.E., Rizvi, G., Sallapudi, N., and McAllister, S.D. (2001). Activation of the CB_1 cannabinoid receptor protects cultured mouse spinal neurons against excitotoxicity. *Neuroscience Letters*, **309**, 197–201.

Ahmed, A. and Wicklund, M.P. (2011). Amyotrophic lateral sclerosis: what role does environment play? *Neurologic Clinics*, **29**, 689–711.

Allaman, I., Bélanger, M., and Magistretti, P.J. (2011). Astrocyte-neuron metabolic relationships: for better and for worse. *Trends in Neurosciences*, **34**, 76–87.

Alvarez, F.J., Lafuente, H., Rey-Santano, M.C., *et al.* (2008). Neuroprotective effects of the nonpsychoactive cannabinoid cannabidiol in hypoxic-ischemic newborn piglets. *Pediatric Research*, **64**, 653–658.

Amenta, P.S., Jallo, J.I., Tuma, R.F., and Elliott, M.B. (2012). A cannabinoid type 2 receptor agonist attenuates blood–brain barrier damage and neurodegeneration in a murine model of traumatic brain injury. *Journal of Neuroscience Research*, **90**, 2293–2305.

Arévalo-Martin, A., García-Ovejero, D., and Molina-Holgado, E. (2010). The endocannabinoid 2-arachidonoylglycerol reduces lesion expansion and white matter damage after spinal cord injury. *Neurobiology of Disease*, **38**, 304–312.

Arrasate, M. and Finkbeiner, S. (2012). Protein aggregates in Huntington's disease. *Experimental Neurology*, **238**, 1–11.

Atwood, B.K. and Mackie, K. (2010). CB_2: a cannabinoid receptor with an identity crisis. *British Journal of Pharmacology*, **160**, 467–479.

Beauchamp, K., Mutlak, H., Smith, W.R., Shohami, E., and Stahel, P.F. (2008). Pharmacology of traumatic brain injury: where is the "golden bullet"? *Molecular Medicine*, **14**, 731–740.

Bilsland, L.G., Dick, J.R., Pryce, G., *et al.* (2006). Increasing cannabinoid levels by pharmacological and genetic manipulation delay disease progression in SOD1 mice. *FASEB Journal*, **20**, 1003–1005.

Bisogno, T., Hanus, L., De Petrocellis, L., *et al.* (2001). Molecular targets for cannabidiol and its synthetic analogues: effects on vanilloid VR1 receptors and on the cellular uptake and enzymatic hydrolysis of anandamide. *British Journal of Pharmacology*, **134**, 845–852.

Blandini, F., Nappi, G., Tassorelli, C., and Martignoni, E. (2000). Functional changes in the basal ganglia circuitry in Parkinson's disease. *Progress in Neurobiology*, **62**, 63–88.

Blázquez, C., Chiarlone, A., Sagredo, O., *et al.* (2011). Loss of striatal type 1 cannabinoid receptors is a key pathogenic factor in Huntington's disease. *Brain*, **134**, 119–136.

Bouchard, J., Truong, J., Bouchard, K., *et al.* (2012). Cannabinoid receptor 2 signaling in peripheral immune cells modulates disease onset and severity in mouse models of Huntington's disease. *Journal of Neuroscience*, **32**, 18259–18268.

Braida, D., Pozzi, M., and Sala, M. (2000). CP 55,940 protects against ischemia-induced electroencephalographic flattening and hyperlocomotion in Mongolian gerbils. *Neuroscience Letters*, **296**, 69–72.

Butler, R. and Bates, G.P. (2006). Histone deacetylase inhibitors as therapeutics for polyglutamine disorders. *Nature Reviews Neuroscience*, **7**, 784–796.

Capettini, L.S., Savergnini, S.Q., da Silva, R.F., *et al.* (2012). Update on the role of cannabinoid receptors after ischemic stroke. *Mediators of Inflammation*, **2012**, 824093.

Carrier, E.J., Kearn, C.S., Barkmeier, A.J., *et al.* (2004). Cultured rat microglial cells synthesize the endocannabinoid 2-arachidonylglycerol, which increases proliferation via a CB_2 receptor-dependent mechanism. *Molecular Pharmacology*, **65**, 999–1007.

Carter, G.T., Abood, M.E., Aggarwal, S.K., and Weiss, M.D. (2010). Cannabis and amyotrophic lateral sclerosis: hypothetical and practical applications, and a call for clinical trials. *American Journal of Hospice & Palliative Care*, **27**, 347–356.

Cattaneo, E., Zuccato, C., and Tartari, M. (2005). Normal huntingtin function: an alternative approach to Huntington's disease. *Nature Reviews Neuroscience*, **6**, 919–930.

Caviston, J.P. and Holzbaur, E.L. (2009). Huntingtin as an essential integrator of intracellular vesicular trafficking. *Trends in Cell Biology*, **19**, 147–155.

Cheah, B.C., Vucic, S., Krishnan, A.V., and Kiernan, M.C. (2010). Riluzole, neuroprotection and amyotrophic lateral sclerosis. *Current Medicinal Chemistry*, **17**, 1942–1949.

Chen, J.J., Ondo, W.G., Dashtipour, K., and Swope, D.M. (2012). Tetrabenazine for the treatment of hyperkinetic movement disorders: a review of the literature. *Clinical Therapeutics*, **34**, 1487–1504.

Chen, Y., McCarron, R.M., Ohara, Y., *et al.* (2000). Human brain capillary endothelium: 2-arachidonoglycerol (endocannabinoid) interacts with endothelin-1. *Circulation Research*, **87**, 323–327.

Chi, O.Z., Barsoum, S., Grayson, J., Hunter, C., Liu, X., and Weiss, H.R. (2012). Effects of cannabinoid receptor agonist WIN 55,212-2 on blood-brain barrier disruption in focal cerebral ischemia in rats. *Pharmacology*, **89**, 333–338.

Chung, E.S., Bok, E., Chung, Y.C., Baik, H.H., and Jin, B.K. (2012). Cannabinoids prevent lipopolysaccharide-induced neurodegeneration in the rat substantia nigra in vivo through inhibition of microglial activation and NADPH oxidase. *Brain Research*, **1451**, 110–116.

Chung, J.H., Seo, A.Y., Chung, S.W., *et al.* (2008). Molecular mechanism of PPAR in the regulation of age-related inflammation. *Ageing Research Reviews*, **7**, 126–136.

Chung, Y.C., Bok, E., Huh, S.H., *et al.* (2011). Cannabinoid receptor type 1 protects nigrostriatal dopaminergic neurons against MPTP neurotoxicity by inhibiting microglial activation. *Journal of Immunology*, **187**, 6508–6517.

Consroe, P., Laguna, J., Allender, J., *et al.* (1991). Controlled clinical trial of cannabidiol in Huntington's disease. *Pharmacology, Biochemistry and Behavior*, **40**, 701–708.

Corbett, A., Smith, J., and Ballard, C. (2012). New and emerging treatments for Alzheimer's disease. *Expert Review of Neurotherapeutics*, **12**, 535–543.

Cunningham, C. (2013). Microglia and neurodegeneration: the role of systemic inflammation. *Glia*, **61**, 71–90.

Curtis, A., Mitchell, I., Patel, S., Ives, N., and Rickards, H. (2009). A pilot study using nabilone for symptomatic treatment in Huntington's disease. *Movement Disorders*, **24**, 2254–2259.

Curtis, A. and Rickards, H. (2006). Nabilone could treat chorea and irritability in Huntington's disease. *Journal of Neuropsychiatry and Clinical Neurosciences*, **18**, 553–554.

Czeh, M., Gressens, P., and Kaindl, A.M. (2011). The yin and yang of microglia. *Developmental Neuroscience*, **33**, 199–209.

Danysz, W. and Parsons, C.G. (2012). Alzheimer's disease, β-amyloid, glutamate, NMDA receptors and memantine – searching for the connections. *British Journal of Pharmacology*, **167**, 324–352.

De Lago, E., Moreno-Martet, M., Cabranes, A., Ramos, J.A., and Fernández-Ruiz, J. (2012). Cannabinoids ameliorate disease progression in a model of multiple sclerosis in mice, acting preferentially through CB_1 receptor-mediated anti-inflammatory effects. *Neuropharmacology*, **62**, 2299–2308.

Doble, A. (1999). The role of excitotoxicity in neurodegenerative disease: implications for therapy. *Pharmacology & Therapeutics*, **81**, 163–221.

El-Remessy, A.B., Khalil, I.E., Matragoon, S., *et al.* (2003). Neuroprotective effect of (-)Δ⁹-tetrahydrocannabinol and cannabidiol in N-methyl-D-aspartate-induced retinal neurotoxicity: involvement of peroxynitrite. *American Journal of Pathology*, **163**, 1997–2008.

Eshhar, N., Striem, S., Kohen, R., Tirosh, O., and Biegon, A. (1995). Neuroprotective and antioxidant activities of HU-211, a novel NMDA receptor antagonist. *European Journal of Pharmacology*, **283**, 19–29.

Esposito, G., De Filippis, D., Carnuccio, R., Izzo, A.A., and Iuvone, T. (2006b). The marijuana component cannabidiol inhibits beta-amyloid-induced tau protein hyperphosphorylation through Wnt/beta-catenin pathway rescue in PC12 cells. *Journal of Molecular Medicine*, **84**, 253–258.

Esposito, G., De Filippis, D., Maiuri, M.C., De Stefano, D., Carnuccio, R., and Iuvone, T. (2006a). Cannabidiol inhibits inducible nitric oxide synthase protein expression and nitric oxide production in beta-amyloid stimulated PC12 neurons through p38 MAP kinase and NF-kappaB involvement. *Neuroscience Letters*, **399**, 91–95.

Esposito, G., Scuderi, C., Savani, C., *et al.* (2007). Cannabidiol in vivo blunts beta-amyloid induced neuroinflammation by suppressing IL-1β and iNOS expression. *British Journal of Pharmacology*, **151**, 1272–1279.

Esposito, G., Scuderi, C., Valenza, M., *et al.* (2011). Cannabidiol reduces Aβ-induced neuroinflammation and promotes hippocampal neurogenesis through PPARγ involvement. *PLoS One*, **6**, e28668.

Eubanks, L.M., Rogers, C.J., Beuscher, A.E., *et al.* (2006). A molecular link between the active component of marijuana and Alzheimer's disease pathology. *Molecular Pharmaceutics*, **3**, 773–777.

Factor, S.A. and Friedman, J.H. (1997). The emerging role of clozapine in the treatment of movement disorders. *Movement Disorders*, **12**, 483–496.

Fernández-López, D., Pradillo, J.M., García-Yébenes, I., Martínez-Orgado, J.A., Moro, M.A., and Lizasoain, I. (2010). The cannabinoid WIN55212-2 promotes neural repair after neonatal hypoxia-ischemia. *Stroke*, **41**, 2956–2964.

Fernández-Ruiz, J. (2009). The endocannabinoid system as a target for the treatment of motor dysfunction. *British Journal of Pharmacology*, **156**, 1029–1040.

Fernández-Ruiz, J., García, C., Sagredo, O., Gómez-Ruiz, M., and de Lago, E. (2010). The endocannabinoid system as a target for the treatment of neuronal damage. *Expert Opinion in Therapeutic Targets*, **14**, 387–404.

Fernández-Ruiz, J., González, S., Romero, J., and Ramos, J.A. (2005). Cannabinoids in neurodegeneration and neuroprotection. In: R. Mechoulam (ed.). *Cannabinoids as Therapeutics*. Milestones in Drug Therapy. Basel: Birkhaüser Verlag, pp. 79–109.

Fernández-Ruiz, J., Romero, J., Velasco, G., Tolón, R.M., Ramos, J.A., and Guzmán, M. (2007). Cannabinoid CB$_2$ receptor: a new target for controlling neural cell survival? *Trends in Pharmacological Sciences*, **28**, 39–45.

Fernández-Ruiz, J., Sagredo, O., Pazos, M.R., *et al.* (2013). Cannabidiol for neurodegenerative disorders: important new clinical applications for this phytocannabinoid? *British Journal of Clinical Pharmacology*, **75**, 323–333.

Ferraiuolo, L., Kirby, J., Grierson, A.J., Sendtner, M., and Shaw, P.J. (2011). Molecular pathways of motor neuron injury in amyotrophic lateral sclerosis. *Nature Reviews Neurology*, **7**, 616–630.

Galve-Roperh, I., Aguado, T., Palazuelos, J., and Guzmán, M. (2008). Mechanisms of control of neuron survival by the endocannabinoid system. *Current Pharmaceutical Design*, **14**, 2279–2288.

García, C., Palomo-Garo, C., García-Arencibia, M., Ramos, J.A., Pertwee, R.G., and Fernández-Ruiz, J. (2011). Symptom-relieving and neuroprotective effects of the phytocannabinoid Δ^9-THCV in animal models of Parkinson's disease. *British Journal of Pharmacology*, **163**, 1495–1506.

García-Arencibia, M., García, C., and Fernández-Ruiz, J. (2009). Cannabinoids and Parkinson's disease. *CNS & Neurological Disorders – Drug Targets*, **8**, 432–439.

Geldenhuys, W.J. and Van der Schyf, C.J. (2013). Rationally designed multi-targeted agents against neurodegenerative diseases. *Current Medicinal Chemistry*, **20**, 1662–1672.

Gelinas, D., Miller, R., and Abood, M. (2002). A pilot study of safety and tolerability of Δ^9-THC (Marinol) treatment for ALS. *Amyotrophic Lateral Sclerosis and Other Motor Neuron Disorders*, **3**, 23.

Gómez Del Pulgar, T., De Ceballos, M.L., Guzmán, M., and Velasco, G. (2002). Cannabinoids protect astrocytes from ceramide-induced apoptosis through the phosphatidylinositol 3-kinase/protein kinase B pathway. *Journal of Biological Chemistry*, **277**, 36527–36533.

González-Naranjo, P., Campillo, N.E., Pérez, C., and Páez, J.A. (2013). Multitarget cannabinoids as novel strategy for Alzheimer disease. *Current Alzheimer Research*, **10**, 229–239.

Gowran, A., Noonan, J., and Campbell, V.A. (2011). The multiplicity of action of cannabinoids: implications for treating neurodegeneration. *CNS Neuroscience & Therapeutics*, **17**, 637–644.

Gubellini, P., Picconi, B., Bari, M., *et al.* (2002), Experimental parkinsonism alters endocannabinoid degradation: implications for striatal glutamatergic transmission. *Journal of Neuroscience*, **22**, 6900–6907.

Ha, A.D. and Fung, V.S. (2012). Huntington's disease. *Current Opinion in Neurology*, **25**, 491–498.

Hampson, A.J., Bornheim, L.M., Scanziani, M., *et al.* (1998a). Dual effects of anandamide on NMDA receptor-mediated responses and neurotransmission. *Journal of Neurochemistry*, **70**, 671–676.

Hampson, A.J. and Grimaldi, M. (2001). Cannabinoid receptor activation and elevated cyclic AMP reduce glutamate neurotoxicity. *European Journal of Neuroscience*, **13**, 1529–1536.

Hampson, A.J., Grimaldi, M., Axelrod, J., and Wink, D. (1998b). Cannabidiol and (-) Δ^9-tetrahydrocannabinol are neuroprotective antioxidants. *Proceedings of the National Academy of Sciences of the United States of America*, **95**, 8268–8273.

Hampson, A.J., Grimaldi, M., Lolic, M., Wink, D., Rosenthal, R., and Axelrod, J. (2000). Neuroprotective antioxidants from marijuana. *Annals of the New York Academy of Science*, **899**, 274–282.

Hansen, H.H., Schmid, P.C., Bittgau, P., *et al.* (2001). Anandamide, but not 2-arachidonoylglycerol, accumulates during in vivo neurodegeneration. *Journal of Neurochemistry*, **78**, 1415–1427.

Hayakawa, K., Mishima, K., Abe, K., *et al.* (2004). Cannabidiol prevents infarction via the non-CB$_1$ cannabinoid receptor mechanism. *Neuroreport*, **15**, 2381–2385.

Hill, A.J., Williams, C.M., Whalley, B.J., and Stephens, G.J. (2012). Phytocannabinoids as novel therapeutic agents in CNS disorders. *Pharmacology & Therapeutics*, **133**, 79–97.

Hillard, C.J. (2000). Endocannabinoids and vascular function. *Journal of Pharmacology and Experimental Therapeutics*, **294**, 27–32.

Iuvone, T., Esposito, G., Esposito, R., Santamaria, R., Di Rosa, M., and Izzo, A.A. (2004). Neuroprotective effect of cannabidiol, a non-psychoactive component from *Cannabis sativa*, on beta-amyloid-induced toxicity in PC12 cells. *Journal of Neurochemistry*, **89**, 134–141.

Iuvone, T., Esposito, G., De Filippis, D., Scuderi, C., and Steardo, L. (2009). Cannabidiol: a promising drug for neurodegenerative disorders? *CNS Neuroscience & Therapeutics*, **15**, 65–75.

Jankovic, J. and Poewe, W. (2012). Therapies in Parkinson's disease. *Current Opinion in Neurology*, **25**, 433–447.

Jin, K.L., Mao, X.O., Goldsmith, P.C., and Greenberg, D.A. (2000). CB_1 cannabinoid receptor induction in experimental stroke. *Annals of Neurology*, **48**, 257–261

Joerger, M., Wilkins, J., Fagagnini, S., *et al.* (2012). Single-dose pharmacokinetics and tolerability of oral Δ^9-tetrahydrocannabinol in patients with amyotrophic lateral sclerosis. *Drug Metabolism Letters*, **6**, 102–108.

Jüttler, E., Potrovita, I., Tarabin, V., *et al.* (2004). The cannabinoid dexanabinol is an inhibitor of the nuclear factor-kappa B (NF-kappa B). *Neuropharmacology*, **47**, 580–592.

Karl, T., Cheng, D., Garner, B., and Arnold, J.C. (2012). The therapeutic potential of the endocannabinoid system for Alzheimer's disease. *Expert Opinion in Therapeutic Targets*, **16**, 407–420.

Khandelwal, P.J., Herman, A.M., and Moussa, C.E. (2011). Inflammation in the early stages of neurodegenerative pathology. *Journal of Neuroimmunology*, **238**, 1–11.

Kieburtz, K. (1999). Antiglutamate therapies in Huntington's disease. *Journal of Neural Transmission* **55**(Suppl.), 97–102.

Kim, K., Moore, D.H., Makriyannis, A., and Abood, M.E. (2006). AM1241, a cannabinoid CB_2 receptor selective compound, delays disease progression in a mouse model of amyotrophic lateral sclerosis. *European Journal of Pharmacology*, **542**, 100–105.

Knoller, N., Levi, L., Shoshan, I., *et al.* (2002). Dexanabinol (HU-211) in the treatment of severe closed head injury: a randomized, placebo controlled, phase II clinical trial. *Critical Care Medicine*, **30**, 548–554.

Kozela, E., Pietr, M., Juknat, A., Rimmerman, N., Levy, R., and Vogel, Z. (2010). Cannabinoids Δ^9-tetrahydrocannabinol and cannabidiol differentially inhibit the lipopolysaccharide-activated NF-kappaB and interferon-β/STAT proinflammatory pathways in BV-2 microglial cells. *Journal of Biological Chemistry*, **285**, 1616–1626.

Lafuente, H., Alvarez, F.J., Pazos, M.R., *et al.* (2011). Cannabidiol reduces brain damage and improves functional recovery after acute hypoxia-ischemia in newborn pigs. *Pediatric Research*, **70**, 272–277.

Lastres-Becker, I., Bizat, N., Boyer, F., Hantraye, P., Fernández-Ruiz, J., and Brouillet, E. (2004). Potential involvement of cannabinoid receptors in 3-nitropropionic acid toxicity *in vivo*: implication for Huntington's disease. *Neuroreport*, **15**, 2375–2379.

Lastres-Becker, I., Cebeira, M., de Ceballos, M., *et al.* (2001). Increased cannabinoid CB_1 receptor binding and activation of GTP-binding proteins in the basal ganglia of patients with Parkinson's disease and MPTP-treated marmosets. *European Journal of Neuroscience*, **14**, 1827–1832.

Lastres-Becker, I., Molina-Holgado, F., Ramos, J.A., Mechoulam, R., and Fernández-Ruiz, J. (2005). Cannabinoids provide neuroprotection against 6-hydroxydopamine toxicity in vivo and in vitro: relevance to Parkinson's disease. *Neurobiology of Disease*, **19**, 96–107.

Leker, R.R., Gai, N., Mechoulam, R., and Ovadia, H. (2003). Drug-induced hypothermia reduces ischemic damage: effects of the cannabinoid HU-210. *Stroke*, **34**, 2000–2006.

Lenaz, G. (2012). Mitochondria and reactive oxygen species. Which role in physiology and pathology?. *Advances in Experimental Medicine and Biology*, **942**, 93–136.

Leweke, F.M., Piomelli, D., Pahlisch, F., *et al.* (2012). Cannabidiol enhances anandamide signaling and alleviates psychotic symptoms of schizophrenia. *Translational Psychiatry*, **2**, e94.

Liscic, R.M. and Breljak, D. (2011). Molecular basis of amyotrophic lateral sclerosis. *Progress in Neuropsychopharmacology & Biological Psychiatry*, **35**, 370–372.

Liu, B. and Hong, J.S. (2003). Role of microglia in inflammation-mediated neurodegenerative diseases: mechanisms and strategies for therapeutic intervention. *Journal of Pharmacology and Experimental Therapeutics*, **304**, 1–7.

Louw, D.F., Yang, F.W., and Sutherland, G.R. (2000). The effect of Δ^9-tetrahydrocannabinol on forebrain ischemia in rat. *Brain Research*, **857**, 183–187.

Luo, S. and Rubinsztein, D.C. (2009). Huntingtin promotes cell survival by preventing Pak2 cleavage. *Journal of Cell Science*, **122**, 875–885.

Maas, A.I.R., Murray, G., Henney, H., *et al.* (2006). Efficacy and safety of dexanabinol in severe traumatic brain injury: results of a phase III randomised, placebo-controlled, clinical trial. *Lancet Neurology*, **5**, 38–45.

Madden, J.A. (2012). Role of the vascular endothelium and plaque in acute ischemic stroke. *Neurology*, **79**, S58–S62.

Malfait, A.M., Gallily, R., Sumariwalla, P.F., *et al.* (2000). The nonpsychoactive cannabis constituent cannabidiol is an oral anti-arthritic therapeutic in murine collagen-induced arthritis. *Proceedings of the National Academy of Sciences of the United States of America*, **97**, 9561–9566.

Marsicano, G., Goodenough, S., Monory, K., *et al.* (2003). CB$_1$ cannabinoid receptors and on-demand defense against excitotoxicity. *Science*, **302**, 84–88.

Marsicano, G., Moosmann, B., Hermann, H., Lutz, B., and Behl, C. (2002). Neuroprotective properties of cannabinoids against oxidative stress: role of the cannabinoid receptor CB$_1$. *Journal of Neurochemistry*, **80**, 448–456.

Martín-Moreno, A.M., Reigada, D., Ramírez, B.G., *et al.* (2011). Cannabidiol and other cannabinoids reduce microglial activation in vitro and in vivo: relevance to Alzheimer's disease. *Molecular Pharmacology*, **79**, 964–973.

Mauler, F., Hinz, V., Augstein, K.H., Fassbender, M., and Horvath, E. (2003). Neuroprotective and brain edema reducing efficacy of the novel cannabinoid receptor agonist BAY38-7271. *Brain Research*, **989**, 99–111.

Mazzoni, P., Shabbott, B., and Cortés, J.C. (2012). Motor control abnormalities in Parkinson's disease. *Cold Spring Harbor Perspectives in Medicine*, **2**, a009282.

Mechoulam, R., Spatz, M., and Shohami, E. (2002). Endocannabinoids and neuroprotection. *Science's STKE*, 2002, re5.

Medina, M., Garrido, J.J., and Wandosell, F.G. (2011). Modulation of GSK-3 as a therapeutic strategy on tau pathologies. *Frontiers in Molecular Neuroscience*, **4**, 24.

Minati, L., Edginton, T., Bruzzone, M.G., and Giaccone, G. (2009). Current concepts in Alzheimer's disease: a multidisciplinary review. *American Journal of Alzheimer's Disease and Other Dementias*, **24**, 95–121.

Molina-Holgado, E., Vela, J.M., Arévalo-Martin, A., *et al.* (2002). Cannabinoids promote oligodendrocyte progenitor survival: involvement of cannabinoid receptors and phosphatidylinositol-3 kinase/Akt signaling. *Journal of Neuroscience*, **22**, 9742–9753.

Molina-Holgado, F., Pinteaux, E., Moore, J.D., *et al.* (2003). Endogenous interleukin-1 receptor antagonist mediates anti-inflammatory and neuroprotective actions of cannabinoids in neurons and glia. *Journal of Neuroscience*, **23**, 6470–6474.

Moskowitz, M.A., Lo, E.H., and Iadecola, C. (2010). The science of stroke: mechanisms in search of treatments. *Neuron*, **67**, 181–198.

Müller-Vahl, K.R., Schneider, U., and Emrich, H.M. (1999). Nabilone increases choreatic movements in Huntington's disease. *Movement Disorders*, **14**, 1038–1040.

Nagayama, T., Sinor, A.D., Simon, R.P., *et al.* (1999). Cannabinoids and neuroprotection in global and focal cerebral ischemia and in neuronal cultures. *Journal of Neuroscience*, **19**, 2987–2995.

Nuñez, E., Benito, C., Pazos, M.R., *et al.* (2004). Cannabinoid CB$_2$ receptors are expressed by perivascular microglial cells in the human brain: an immunohistochemical study. *Synapse*, **53**, 208–213.

Oh, Y.T., Lee, J.Y., Lee, J., *et al.* (2010). Oleamide suppresses lipopolysaccharide-induced expression of iNOS and COX-2 through inhibition of NFκB activation in BV2 murine microglial cells. *Neuroscience Letters*, **474**, 148–153.

O'Sullivan, S.E. and Kendall, D.A. (2010). Cannabinoid activation of peroxisome proliferator-activated receptors: potential for modulation of inflammatory disease. *Immunobiology*, **215**, 611–616.

Pacher, P. and Mechoulam, R. (2011). Is lipid signaling through cannabinoid 2 receptors part of a protective system? *Progress in Lipid Research*, **50**, 193–211.

Palazuelos, J., Aguado, T., Pazos, M.R., *et al.* (2009). Microglial CB$_2$ cannabinoid receptors are neuroprotective in Huntington's disease excitotoxicity. *Brain*, **132**, 3152–3164.

Panikashvili, D., Simeonidou, C., Ben-Shabat, S., *et al.* (2001). An endogenous cannabinoid (2-AG) is neuroprotective after brain injury. *Nature*, **413**, 527–531.

Parmentier-Batteur, S., Jin, K., Mao, X.O., Xie, L., and Greenberg, D.A. (2002). Increased severity of stroke in CB$_1$ cannabinoid receptor knock-out mice. *Journal of Neuroscience*, **22**, 9771–9775.

Pazos, M.R., Cinquina, V., Gómez, A., *et al.* (2012). Cannabidiol administration after hypoxia-ischemia to newborn rats reduces long-term brain injury and restores neurobehavioral function. *Neuropharmacology*, **63**, 776–783.

Pérez-Rial, S., García-Gutiérrez, M.S., Molina, J.A., *et al.* (2011). Increased vulnerability to 6-hydroxydopamine lesion and reduced development of dyskinesias in mice lacking CB$_1$ cannabinoid receptors. *Neurobiology of Aging*, **32**, 631–645.

Perl, D.P. (2010). Neuropathology of Alzheimer's disease. *Mount Sinai Journal of Medicine*, **77**, 32–42.

Pintor, A., Tebano, M.T., Martire, A., *et al.* (2006). The cannabinoid receptor agonist WIN 55,212-2 attenuates the effects induced by quinolinic acid in the rat striatum. *Neuropharmacology*, **51**, 1004–1012.

Price, D.A., Martínez, A.A., Seillier, A., *et al.* (2009). WIN55,212-2, a cannabinoid receptor agonist, protects against nigrostriatal cell loss in the 1-methyl-4-phenyl-1,2,3,6-tetrahydropyridine mouse model of Parkinson's disease. *European Journal of Neuroscience*, **29**, 2177–2186.

Raman, C., McAllister, S.D., Rizvi, G., Patel, S.G., Moore, D.H., and Abood, M.E. (2004). Amyotrophic lateral sclerosis: delayed disease progression in mice by treatment with a cannabinoid. *Amyotrophic Lateral Sclerosis and Other Motor Neuron Disorders*, **5**, 33–39.

Rodríguez-Cueto, C., Benito, C., Fernández-Ruiz, J., Romero, J., Hernández-Gálvez, M., Gómez-Ruiz, M. (2014). Changes in CB1 and CB2 receptors in the post-mortem cerebellum of humans affected by spinocerebellar ataxias. *British Journal of Pharmacology* **171**, 1472–1489.

Ross, C.A. and Tabrizi, S.J. (2011). Huntington's disease: from molecular pathogenesis to clinical treatment. *Lancet Neurology*, **10**, 83–98.

Rossi, S., Bernardi, G., and Centonze, D. (2010). The endocannabinoid system in the inflammatory and neurodegenerative processes of multiple sclerosis and of amyotrophic lateral sclerosis. *Experimental Neurology*, **224**, 92–102.

Ruiz-Valdepeñas, L., Martínez-Orgado, J.A., Benito, C., Millán, A., Tolón, R.M., and Romero, J. (2011). Cannabidiol reduces lipopolysaccharide-induced vascular changes and inflammation in the mouse brain: an intravital microscopy study. *Journal of Neuroinflammation*, **8**, 5.

Sagredo, O., González, S., Aroyo, I., *et al.* (2009). Cannabinoid CB$_2$ receptor agonists protect the striatum against malonate toxicity: relevance for Huntington's disease. *Glia*, **57**, 1154–1167.

Sagredo, O., Pazos, M.R., Satta, V., Ramos, J.A., Pertwee, R.G., and Fernández-Ruiz, J. (2011). Neuroprotective effects of phytocannabinoid-based medicines in experimental models of Huntington's disease. *Journal of Neuroscience Research*, **89**, 1509–1518.

Sagredo, O., Pazos, M.R., Valdeolivas, S., and Fernandez-Ruiz, J. (2012). Cannabinoids: novel medicines for the treatment of Huntington's disease. *Recent Patents on CNS Drug Discovery*, **7**, 41–48.

Sagredo, O., Ramos, J.A., Decio, A., Mechoulam, R., and Fernández-Ruiz, J. (2007). Cannabidiol reduced the striatal atrophy caused 3-nitropropionic acid in vivo by mechanisms independent of the activation of cannabinoid, vanilloid TRPV1 and adenosine A2A receptors. *European Journal of Neuroscience*, **26**, 843–851.

Santos, C.M. (2012). New agents promote neuroprotection in Parkinson's disease models. *CNS & Neurological Disorders – Drug Targets*, **11**, 410–418.

Savonenko, A.V., Melnikova, T., Hiatt, A., *et al.* (2012). Alzheimer's therapeutics: translation of preclinical science to clinical drug development. *Neuropsychopharmacology*, **37**, 261–277.

Schinelli, S. (2002). The brain endothelin system as potential target for brain-related pathologies. *Current Drug Targets. CNS Neurological Disorders*, **1**, 543–553.

Shen, M. and Thayer, S.A. (1998). Cannabinoid receptor agonists protect cultured rat hippocampal neurons from excitotoxicity. *Molecular Pharmacology*, **54**, 459–462.

Shoemaker, J.L., Seely, K.A., Reed, R.L., Crow, J.P., and Prather, P.L. (2007). The CB_2 cannabinoid agonist AM-1241 prolongs survival in a transgenic mouse model of amyotrophic lateral sclerosis when initiated at symptom onset. *Journal of Neurochemistry*, **101**, 87–98.

Shohami, E. and Mechoulam, R. (2000). A non-psychotropic cannabinoid with neuroprotective properties. *Drug Development Research*, **50**, 211–215.

Shohami, E., Novikov, M., and Bass, R. (1995). Long-term effect of HU-211, a novel competitive NMDA antagonist, on motor and memory functions after closed head injury in the rat. *Brain Research*, **674**, 55–62.

Singh, S., Swarnkar, S., Goswami, P., and Nath, C. (2011). Astrocytes and microglia: responses to neuropathological conditions. *International Journal of Neuroscience*, **121**, 589–597.

Sinor, A.D., Irvin, S.M., and Greenberg, D.A. (2000). Endocannabinoids protect cerebral cortical neurons from in vitro ischemia in rats. *Neuroscience Letters*, **278**, 157–160.

Skaper, S.D., Buriani, A., Dal Toso, R., *et al.* (1996). The ALIAmide palmitoylethanolamide and cannabinoids, but not anandamide, are protective in a delayed postglutamate paradigm of excitotoxic death in cerebellar granule neurons. *Proceedings of the National Academy of Sciences of the United States of America*, **93**, 3984–3989.

Smith, S.R., Terminelli, C., and Denhardt, G. (2000). Effects of cannabinoid receptor agonist and antagonist ligands on production of inflammatory cytokines and anti-inflammatory interleukin-10 in endotoxemic mice. *Journal of Pharmacology and Experimental Therapeutics*, **293**, 136–150.

Stahel, P.F., Smith, W.R., Bruchis, J., and Rabb, C.H. (2008). Peroxisome proliferator-activated receptors: "key" regulators of neuroinflammation after traumatic brain injury. *PPAR Research*, **2008**, 538141.

Stella, N. (2009). Endocannabinoid signaling in microglial cells. *Neuropharmacology*, **56**, 244–253.

Stella, N. (2010). Cannabinoid and cannabinoid-like receptors in microglia, astrocytes, and astrocytomas. *Glia*, **58**, 1017–1030.

Sun, J., Fang, Y., Chen, T., *et al.* (2013b). WIN55,212-2 promotes differentiation of oligodendrocyte precursor cells and improve remyelination through regulation of the phosphorylation level of the ERK 1/2 via cannabinoid receptor 1 after stroke-induced demyelination. *Brain Research*, **1491**, 225–235.

Sun, J., Fang, Y., Ren, H., *et al.* (2013a). WIN55,212-2 protects oligodendrocyte precursor cells in stroke penumbra following permanent focal cerebral ischemia in rats. *Acta Pharmacologica Sinica*, **34**, 119–128.

Surmeier, D.J. and Sulzer, D. (2013). The pathology roadmap in Parkinson disease. *Prion*, **7**, 85–91.

Suzuki, N., Suzuki, M., Murakami, K., Hamajo, K., Tsukamoto, T., and Shimojo, M. (2012). Cerebroprotective effects of TAK-937, a cannabinoid receptor agonist, on ischemic brain damage in middle cerebral artery occluded rats and non-human primates. *Brain Research*, **1430**, 93–100.

Ternianov, A., Pérez-Ortiz, J.M., Solesio, M.E., *et al.* (2012). Overexpression of CB_2 cannabinoid receptors results in neuroprotection against behavioral and neurochemical alterations induced by intracaudate administration of 6-hydroxydopamine. *Neurobiology of Aging*, **33**, 421 e1–e16.

Valdeolivas, S., Satta, V., Pertwee, R.G., Fernández-Ruiz, J., and Sagredo, O. (2012). Sativex-like combination of phytocannabinoids is neuroprotective in malonate-lesioned rats, an inflammatory model of Huntington's disease: role of CB_1 and CB_2 receptors. *ACS Chemical Neuroscience*, **3**, 400–406.

Van der Stelt, M., Veldhuis, W.B., Bar, P.R., Veldink, G.A., Vliegenthart, J.F., and Nicolay, K. (2001). Neuroprotection by Δ^9-tetrahydrocannabinol, the main active compound in marijuana, against ouabain-induced in vivo excitotoxicity. *Journal of Neuroscience*, **21**, 6475–6579.

Venuto, C.S., McGarry, A., Ma, Q., and Kieburtz, K. (2012). Pharmacologic approaches to the treatment of Huntington's disease. *Movement Disorders*, **27**, 31–41.

Volicer, L., Stelly, M., Morris, J., McLaughlin, J., and Volicer, B.J. (1997). Effects of dronabinol on anorexia and disturbed behavior in patients with Alzheimer's disease. *International Journal of Geriatric Psychiatry*, **12**, 913–919.

Wagner, J.A., Varga, K., and Kunos, G. (1998). Cardiovascular actions of cannabinoids and their generation during shock. *Journal of Molecular Medicine*, **76**, 824–836.

Walker, F.O. (2007). Huntington's disease. *Seminars in Neurology*, **27**, 143–150.

Walter, L., Franklin, A., Witting, A., *et al.* (2003). Nonpsychotropic cannabinoid receptors regulate microglial cell migration. *Journal of Neuroscience*, **23**, 1398–1405.

Walther, S., Mahlberg, R., Eichmann, U., and Kunz, D. (2006). Δ^9-Tetrahydrocannabinol for nighttime agitation in severe dementia. *Psychopharmacology*, **185**, 524–528.

Weber, M., Goldman, B. and Truniger, S. (2010). Tetrahydrocannabinol (THC) for cramps in amyotrophic lateral sclerosis: a randomised, double-blind crossover trial. *Journal of Neurology, Neurosurgery and Psychiatry*, **81**, 1135–1140.

Wee Yong, V. (2010). Inflammation in neurological disorders: a help or a hindrance? *Neuroscientist*, **16**, 408–420.

Weydt, P., Hong, S., Witting, A., Möller, T., Stella, N., and Kliot, M. (2005). Cannabinol delays symptom onset in SOD1 (G93A) transgenic mice without affecting survival. *Amyotrophic Lateral Sclerosis and Other Motor Neuron Disorders*, **6**, 182–184.

Zani, A., Braida, D., Capurro, V., and Sala, M. (2007). Δ^9-Tetrahydrocannabinol (THC) and AM404 protect against cerebral ischaemia in gerbils through a mechanism involving cannabinoid and opioid receptors. *British Journal of Pharmacology*, **152**, 1301–1311.

Zhang, M., Adler, M.W., Abood, M.E., Ganea, D., Jallo, J., and Tuma, R.F. (2009). CB_2 receptor activation attenuates microcirculatory dysfunction during cerebral ischemic/reperfusion injury. *Microvascular Research*, **78**, 86–94.

Zuccato, C., Ciammola, A., Rigamonti, D., *et al.* (2001). Loss of huntingtin-mediated BDNF gene transcription in Huntington's disease. *Science*, **293**, 493–498.

Chapter 28

Cannabidiol/Phytocannabinoids: A New Opportunity for Schizophrenia Treatment?

Daniela Parolaro, Erica Zamberletti, and Tiziana Rubino

28.1 Introduction

Schizophrenia is a heterogeneous and severe brain disease, whose etiology and pathophysiology is still poorly understood (Broome et al. 2005), and the search for safe and effective drugs is hindered by its complex nature. A large body of evidence suggests that dysregulations in several neurotransmitter systems, such as dopaminergic, glutamatergic, gamma-aminobutyric acid (GABA)-ergic, and serotoninergic systems, play a role in the development of the typical positive symptoms (hallucination, delusions, disordered thinking, and paranoia), negative symptoms (deficit in social interaction, emotional expression, and motivation), and cognitive deficit associated with schizophrenia (Abi-Dargham and Guillin 2007). In recent years, the presence of dysregulations in the endocannabinoid system (ECS) (both in terms of cannabinoid receptors type 1 and 2 (CB_1/CB_2) and endocannabinoid levels) in animal models of psychosis as well as in schizophrenic patients suggested an involvement of the ECS in the pathophysiology of this disease. Indeed, either down-regulation, upregulation, or no change in the CB_1 receptor was found in brain regions implicated in schizophrenia, such as prefrontal cortex, basal ganglia, and hippocampus. Moreover, the presence of a negative correlation between cerebrospinal levels of the endocannabinoid anandamide (AEA) and psychopathological symptoms in acute, nonmedicated schizophrenic patients suggests the existence of an "anandamidergic dysregulation" in schizophrenia (for a review, see Zamberletti et al. 2012a). Further support for the involvement of the ECS in schizophrenia comes from the observation that high rates of cannabis consumption have been observed in patients with schizophrenia, and from prospective studies demonstrating an increased risk for schizophrenia in subjects using cannabis most frequently (Henquet et al. 2005; Kuepper et al. 2011). Indeed, cannabis consumption may induce psychotic states in normal individuals (Bhattacharyya et al. 2009), worsen psychotic symptoms in schizophrenic patients (D'Souza et al. 2005), and facilitate precipitation of schizophrenia in vulnerable individuals (Ferdinand et al. 2005). On the other hand, the self-medication hypothesis predicts that individuals may be using cannabis largely because of their predisposition to psychosis, in order to relieve negative symptoms and dysphoric states or to alleviate the side effects associated with antipsychotic therapy (Dixon et al. 1990; Krystal et al. 1999; Schneier and Siris 1987). This discrepancy at the epidemiological level may be attributed to the opposing actions on schizophrenia-related symptoms exerted by two phytocannabinoids (pCBs), cannabidiol (CBD) and delta-9-tetrahydrocannabinol (THC), that are present in some cannabis extracts. In fact, the psychotropic effects of cannabis are mainly produced by the plant cannabinoid THC, via partial agonistic effects at the central cannabinoid CB_1 receptor (Pertwee 2008). In contrast, CBD has no psychotropic activity and has been found to be a weak antagonist at the CB_1 receptor thereby inhibiting some of the pharmacological effects of THC (Thomas et al. 2007). Indeed, the use of cannabis with high CBD content is associated with significantly lower degrees of psychotic symptoms providing support for the antipsychotic potential of CBD (Di Forti et al. 2009).

This chapter focuses on the emerging potential of CBD and, possibly, other pCBs as new therapeutic agents for psychosis, in particular schizophrenia, as indicated by data obtained using preclinical in vivo animal models and by available clinical data.

28.2 Methodological considerations on rodent models of schizophrenia

Schizophrenia is a complex neurodevelopmental disorder comprising a broad spectrum of symptoms, some of which are uniquely human traits (such as disordered thoughts, verbal learning, and memory), thus it is extremely difficult to develop an animal model that mimics this psychiatric syndrome in its entirety. Therefore, research efforts have focused on the development of various animal models based on both pharmacological and nonpharmacological manipulations seeking to replicate specific symptoms observed in human patients. Accordingly, different behavioral paradigms have been considered to be translational models to assess schizophrenia symptoms in preclinical models.

The most widely used animal approaches are based on the dopaminergic or glutamatergic hypothesis of schizophrenia, and on the observation that the dopaminergic agents, amphetamine, quinpirole, cocaine, and the noncompetitive blockers of N-methyl-D-aspartate (NMDA) receptors, MK801 and phencyclidine (PCP), induce hyperlocomotion and stereotyped behaviors, resembling the positive symptoms of schizophrenia, and reduce the prepulse inhibition (PPI) of the acoustic startle reflex, modelling the impairment of sensorimotor gating observed in schizophrenics. Moreover, NMDA receptor antagonists induce negative-like symptoms such as deficits in social interaction, avolition, and cognitive impairment consistent with a schizophrenia-like effect (Bubeníková-Valesová et al. 2008).

Nonpharmacological models based on the neurodevelopmental hypothesis of schizophrenia have been developed too. Early maternal deprivation produces behavioral abnormalities resembling schizophrenia, including cognitive deficits (Ellenbroek and Riva 2003, Llorente-Berzal et al. 2011). Another neurodevelopmental model, the postweaning social isolation of rats, induces social and cognitive impairments, aggressiveness, hyperlocomotion, and reduces PPI (Fone and Porkess 2008).

Recently, genetic mouse models of schizophrenia have been developed based on candidate susceptibility genes. To date, Disrupted in Schizophrenia-1, neuregulin-1 (Nrg1), and ERbB4 mutant mice are the most widely used. These animals exhibit behavioral abnormalities relevant to schizophrenia, such as disrupted PPI and latent inhibition, as well as impaired working memory, that can be partially reversed by antipsychotic treatment (Powell et al. 2009).

In conclusion, no single animal model is able to mirror all the complex sequelae of such a complex and heterogeneous disease, and the strategy to improve our knowledge of schizophrenia and find new therapeutic tools for it is to take into account more than one model. However, often the preclinical data on pCBs have been demonstrated only in pharmacological models and thus, although positive, need to be confirmed using other experimental manipulations in order to strengthen their potential therapeutic application.

28.3 **Preclinical data**

28.3.1 **Hyperactivity and stereotypy**

Locomotor hyperactivity and stereotypy have been recognized to have some face validity as indicators of certain components of the positive symptoms of schizophrenia. The concept of testing for locomotor hyperactivity is based upon the premises that stimulation of the dopaminergic D_2 receptors (with amphetamine or apomorphine), activation of serotoninergic systems by direct 5-HT_{2A} receptor agonists (with LSD or psilocybin) and blockade of NMDA receptors by drugs such as ketamine and PCP in rodents lead to enhanced motor activity, specifically horizontal locomotor activity, rearing, or, at higher doses, stereotyped behaviors. Most of these behaviors can be measured using automated photocell cages and scored by observation. Moreover, it is possible to perform a qualitative analysis of patterns and perseverative aspects of behavior, by measuring and scoring stereotypies during the test session.

Converging lines of evidence support a potential antipsychotic activity for CBD in dopamine- and glutamate-based animal models of hyperactivity. In a pioneering study by Zuardi et al. (1991) the effect of CBD was compared with that of haloperidol in rats administered with apomorphine. These authors demonstrated that CBD was as effective as haloperidol in reducing the occurrence of stereotyped behaviors. Moreover, in contrast to the typical antipsychotic, CBD did not induce catalepsy even at the highest doses tested. The antipsychotic potential of CBD was then confirmed by the work of Moreira and Guimarães (2005) that compared the ability of CBD, haloperidol, and clozapine to prevent the hyperlocomotion induced by amphetamine or ketamine in mice. They found that CBD inhibited the hyperlocomotion induced by amphetamine in mice in a dose-related manner. In addition, the drug also attenuated the hyperlocomotion induced by ketamine, expanding its antipsychotic-like effects to a glutamate-based model. Only haloperidol induced catalepsy at doses that inhibited hyperlocomotion in mice, whereas CBD, similarly to clozapine, did not, thus suggesting a profile similar to that of atypical antipsychotics. In contrast, more recently, the antipsychotic properties of CBD were not confirmed in a glutamate-based animal model (Gururajan et al. 2011). In fact, in this study CBD failed to counteract the hyperlocomotion induced by MK801 administration in rats. Moreover, CBD per se produced hyperactivity, showing therefore some propsychotic effects. The lack of effect of CBD could be ascribed to the lower dose of CBD used in Gururajan's study compared to the one used in Zuardi's work (30 mg/kg vs. 60 mg/kg, intraperitoneally (i.p.)). It is therefore conceivable that higher doses of CBD are needed to reach a beneficial effect. However, more recently, the same group demonstrated that CBD, at very low doses (1 and 3 mg/kg, i.p.), effectively inhibited MK801-induced hyperlocomotion when tested in a novel experimental set-up that allowed the authors to assess social behavior and locomotor behavior simultaneously (Gururajan et al. 2012).

Not only acute but also chronic CBD administration has been reported to exert antipsychotic effects. Long et al. (2010) demonstrated that chronic CBD at a dose of 50 mg/kg i.p. attenuated dexamphetamine-induced hyperlocomotion without altering baseline locomotor activity in mice. Importantly, acute CBD both at low (1 mg/kg, i.p.) or high (50 mg/kg, i.p.) doses was not effective in opposing dexamphetamine-induced hyperlocomotion. This last result does not replicate the one reported by Moreira and Guimarães (2005), and the authors suggested that these discrepant findings could be due to genetic differences between the mouse strains used in the two studies. More recently, the same group demonstrated that both acute and chronic CBD did not reduce hyperlocomotion in a genetic animal model of schizophrenia, the transmembrane domain neuregulin 1 heterozygous mutant (Nrg1 TM HET) mouse (Long et al. 2012).

As a whole, the results published so far are still not conclusive but seem to support the view that CBD could exhibit a pharmacological profile similar to that of atypical antipsychotic drugs, with an even better side effect profile, since it induced no or very low side effects at its effective doses.

To date, no studies have investigated the ability of pCBs, other than CBD, in recovering hyperlocomotion and stereotypies. However, preliminary data from our group suggest that also other nonpsychoactive phytocannabinoids, specifically delta-9-tetrahydrocannabivarin (THCV) and cannabigerol (CBG), even at very low doses, are effective in reverting phencyclidine-induced hyperlocomotion and stereotyped behaviors in rats, without altering per se basal locomotion (M. Gabaglio and D. Parolaro, personal communication).

28.3.2 Prepulse inhibition

Studies of sensorimotor gating of startle responses to strong exteroceptive stimuli offer unique opportunities for cross-species explorations into information processing and attentional deficits in schizophrenia. PPI is defined as the decrease in the acoustic startle response when a nonstartling prepulse is presented 30–500 ms before the startling pulse.

It is well known that marked deficits in PPI are present in chronic schizophrenic (Braff et al. 1999) as well as nonmedicated first-episode schizophrenic patients (Ludewig et al. 2003). Similar deficits in PPI can be reproduced in rodents by pharmacological or developmental manipulations. In rodents and healthy human subjects, disruptions in PPI of startle are produced by: stimulation of D_2 dopamine receptors, with amphetamine or apomorphine; activation of serotonergic systems, produced by direct 5-HT_{2A} receptor agonists, such as LSD or psilocybin; and blockade of NMDA receptors, produced by drugs such as MK801, ketamine, or PCP. Moreover, deficits in PPI were also present in mice heterozygous for Nrg1 transmembrane domain (Falls 2003), a proposed schizophrenia-related phenotype representing a putative animal model of genetic vulnerability to schizophrenia. All these models of disrupted PPI have been applied to the identification of potential antipsychotic treatments.

Several studies have been performed in order to investigate the antipsychotic-like potential of CBD on PPI responses in different animal models of schizophrenia, whereas a CBD effect on PPI responses in healthy subjects and schizophrenic patients has not been described so far. When given alone, acute as well as chronic CBD had no effect on the startle response, but produced a significant increase of PPI in rats (Long et al. 2010). While these findings do not in themselves represent antipsychotic-like effects, it is interesting to speculate on whether such an improved baseline in sensorimotor gating, as observed with acute and chronic CBD, might interact with the effect of genetic or pharmacological challenges on PPI. CBD was able to reverse PPI deficits induced by MK801, whereas administration of CBD alone had no effect (Long et al. 2006). The same results were obtained with clozapine, suggesting once more that CBD may exhibit an atypical antipsychotic profile.

However, in a more recent study, CBD treatment alone disrupted PPI and failed to reverse MK801-induced disruption of PPI in rats (Gururajan et al. 2011), prompting the authors to suggest that CBD may exhibit propsychotic activity in this glutamatergic model of psychosis. Finally, Long et al. (2012), testing the efficacy of CBD at reversing the schizophrenic phenotype present in the Nrg1 HET mice (locomotor hyperactivity, PPI deficits and reduced 5-HT_{2A} receptor binding density in the substantia nigra), demonstrated that after 21 days of CBD treatment these phenotypes were not reversed. However, long-term CBD (50 and 100 mg/kg, i.p.) selectively enhanced social interaction in Nrg1 TM HET mice, while acute CBD (100 mg/kg, i.p.) selectively increased PPI in Nrg1 TM HET mice, although tolerance to this effect was manifest upon repeated CBD administration.

The results of these studies are conflicting and clearly suggest the need to further investigate the effect of CBD per se on PPI as well as its ability to modulate the deficit of sensorimotor gating present in animal models of schizophrenia.

28.3.3 Negative symptoms and cognitive deficits

Since currently approved therapeutics only address psychotic symptoms, with minor negative symptom treatment, the search for drugs able to manage this dimension still represents a priority. In this context, some recent papers point toward a potential positive effect of CBD. In animal models, a decrease in social interaction has been described as a behavioral parameter that mirrors the negative symptoms of schizophrenia (Castagné et al. 2009; Sams-Dodd 1999). Using experimental models, researchers demonstrated that CBD was able to reverse social withdrawal, and this was shown both in rats treated with MK801 (Gururajan et al. 2011, 2012) or in Nrg1 TM HET mice (Long et al. 2012). However, Almeida et al. (2012) reported that CBD was not able to recover the social deficit present in Spontaneously Hypertensive Rats (SHR), considered as a good animal model for studying various aspects of schizophrenia (Calzavara et al. 2009, 2011a, 2011b; Levin et al. 2011), although it did significantly increase social interaction in healthy Wistar rats. Based on this observation they suggested that CBD could be considered to be an anxiolytic drug rather than an antipsychotic one. Thus, we need further studies in other animal models of schizophrenia, such as the ones based on environmental manipulation or on the neurodevelopmental hypothesis, to thoroughly ascertain the ability of CBD to recover negative symptoms of schizophrenia.

To date, the ability of CBD to specifically recover the cognitive deficits present in animal models of schizophrenia has not been investigated. However, data present in the literature point toward the potential use of CBD for the treatment of cognitive decline associated with neurodegenerative or neuroinflammatory disorders (Avraham et al. 2011; Cassol-Jr et al. 2010; Fagherazzi et al. 2012; Magen et al. 2010). Although these experimental manipulations are not considered as animal models of schizophrenia, this finding might suggest that CBD could be effective also in reverting the cognitive deficit associated with this psychiatric disease.

Moreover, based on some reports in the literature where synthetic CB_1 antagonists were used to recover cognitive deficits present in environmental or pharmacological animal models of schizophrenia (Black et al. 2011; Guidali et al. 2011; Zamberletti et al. 2012b, 2012c), we can speculate that pCBs showing a CB_1 antagonist profile, such as, for example, THCV (Pertwee 2008), should be tested to evaluate their potential for reducing the impairment in cognition present in schizophrenia. Accordingly, preliminary data from our laboratory indicate that acute administration of THCV, and also of CBG, effectively reverted the cognitive deficits and social withdrawal induced by subchronic PCP treatment in rats (M. Gabaglio and D. Parolaro, personal communication).

28.4 Clinical studies

As already mentioned, many epidemiological studies have revealed an association between cannabis use and acute or chronic psychosis, and these effects are mainly mediated by the major psychotropic component of cannabis, THC (Bhattacharyya et al. 2009; D'Souza et al. 2005; Moore et al. 2007). Intriguingly, some studies show that CBD can attenuate the psychotomimetic effects associated with THC, depending on the measured effect, route of administration, and dose-ratio between these two cannabinoids. Dalton et al. (1976) reported that a high dose of smoked CBD slightly inhibited the psychotomimetic effects associated with smoked THC. Another group, using mismatch negativity as a measure of auditory function, found significantly greater mismatch negativity amplitude values at central electrodes following treatment with combined CBD and THC compared to THC alone, indicating that CBD may have exerted an antipsychotic effect (Juckel et al. 2007). Finally, a recent functional magnetic resonance imaging (fMRI) trial demonstrated that THC and CBD had opposite effects in terms of the activation of brain areas using different tasks (Bhattacharyya et al. 2010). Moreover, pretreatment with CBD inhibits THC-induced psychotic episodes in healthy subjects (Bhattacharyya et al. 2010; Englund et al. 2013), suggesting that CBD can oppose the psychotic effects of THC also in humans. Overall, these results are consistent with the finding that subjects smoking strains of cannabis containing higher CBD amounts are less prone to develop psychotic symptoms than subjects smoking strains of cannabis without CBD (Di Forti et al. 2009; Morgan and Curran, 2008; Morgan et al. 2011; Schubart et al. 2011).

It is well known that binocular depth inversion is significantly altered in patients with acute productive schizophrenic psychosis. Thus the assessment of this paradigm could provide a model of impaired perception during psychotic states. In this model, impairment of the perception of the illusory image induced by nabilone was attenuated by CBD, suggesting an antipsychotic-like effect of this compound (Leweke et al. 2000).

Another important model used to evaluate antipsychotic-like activity in healthy volunteers is the administration of subanesthetic doses of ketamine. In healthy individuals, CBD has been proven to be effective in reverting the psychotic symptoms induced by subanesthetic doses of ketamine as demonstrated by a significant reduction of the total scores and factors of the Clinician Administered Dissociative States Scale (CADSS) (Bosi et al. 2003). In contrast, more recently, Hallak et al. (2011) reported that oral CBD increased ketamine-induced activation as measured by the activation subscales of the Brief Psychiatric Rating Scale (BPRS) and failed to reduce ketamine-induced positive symptoms as assessed by the CADSS.

Based on the lack of toxicity associated with CBD administration in healthy subjects, its potential antipsychotic effect has been investigated also, over the last few years, in some schizophrenic patients. In 1995, Zuardi et al. reported a significant improvement during CBD treatment in a case study with a 19-year-old schizophrenic female patient who presented serious side effects after treatment with conventional antipsychotics. Interestingly, no side effects were observed following CBD treatment. However, more recently, Zuardi et al. (2006) did not find CBD monotherapy to be effective relative to placebo in a case series of treatment-resistant schizophrenia patients. These studies suggest, therefore, that CBD has an antipsychotic-like profile in healthy volunteers, and in schizophrenic patients that are not resistant to established antipsychotic medicines. Accordingly, a 4-week, randomized controlled trial of CBD versus amisulpride did not reveal any significant differences between the groups, suggesting that the former exerted an antipsychotic effect (Leweke et al. 2007). These findings were recently replicated in another double-blind, randomized clinical trial of CBD versus amisulpride in 42 acute schizophrenia patients that revealed no marked difference between the two treatments as measured by the BPRS and Positive and Negative Syndrome Scale (PANSS) scales (Leweke et al. 2012). Intriguingly, the antipsychotic effect of CBD was even better than the one induced by amisulpiride when only the negative symptoms were taken into account (Leweke et al. 2012) and was associated with marked tolerability and safety, when compared with current medications. The beneficial effect of CBD may rely on its ability to increase serum levels of AEA by inhibiting its enzymatic degradation, for example, by fatty acid amide hydrolase (FAAH) (Leweke et al. 2012), suggesting that inhibition of AEA deactivation may potentially represent a new therapeutic strategy for the treatment of schizophrenia.

Interestingly, CBD has also been demonstrated to be effective in the treatment of psychotic symptoms associated with Parkinson's disease. Moreover, besides reducing psychosis, CBD administration to those patients also alleviated motor symptoms, suggesting its possible exploitation in the treatment of this psychiatric condition (Zuardi et al. 2009).

It is more difficult to comment on the possible exploitation of pCBs to ameliorate cognitive symptoms of schizophrenia, due to the lack of literature on this. Only one paper has appeared on this issue and it addressed the effect of CBD on the cognitive performance of schizophrenic patients (Hallak et al. 2010). The authors specifically monitored selective attention through the Stroop Color Word Test and found no evidence of improvement after a single dose of CBD. However, they claimed the possibility that chronic use may lead to cognitive improvement as has been observed with clozapine.

28.5 **Conclusions**

As a whole, data published so far seem to suggest that pCBs, and more specifically CBD, may exert beneficial effects on the positive and negative symptoms of schizophrenia. Regarding its pharmacological properties, CBD seems to possess a profile similar to that of atypical antipsychotics, but its administration is associated with lower side effects. Accordingly, when its effect on neuronal activation was investigated, CBD was demonstrated to induce c-fos immunoreactivity in the prefrontal cortex and nucleus accumbens (Guimarães et al., 2004; Murillo-Rodriguez et al. 2006) in a manner similar to clozapine (Robertson and Fibiger 1992), further supporting a pharmacological profile resembling that of atypical antipsychotics. The lack of c-fos induction in the dorsal striatum, which is associated with extrapyramidal side effects induced by typical antipsychotics (Campos et al. 2012), may explain the reduced side effects associated with its administration.

The precise mechanism of action responsible for the antipsychotic effect of CBD is still unknown. However, CBD has been reported to increase serum levels of AEA by inhibiting the enzymatic degradation of this endocannabinoid, and this effect was associated with decreased psychotic symptoms in patients (Leweke et al. 2012), in line with the "anandamidergic hypothesis"

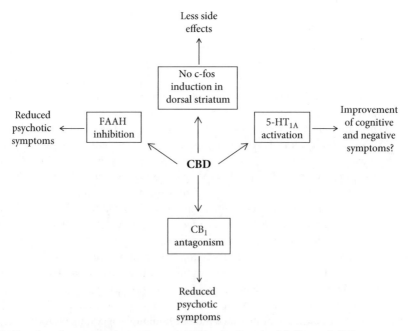

Fig. 28.1 Putative pharmacological actions underlying antipsychotic effects of CBD.

Box 28.1 Take-home messages

◆ CBD might exert an antipsychotic effect in animal models of schizophrenia.

◆ CBD might ameliorate psychotic symptoms in schizophrenic patients.

◆ CBD might exhibit a pharmacological profile similar to that of atypical antipsychotics, with lower side effects.

◆ CBD's likely antipsychotic efficacy could depend on its ability to act on multiple cellular targets (see Fig. 28.1).

◆ There is an urgent need to explore more fully whether/how CBD alleviates positive and negative symptoms of schizophrenia.

of schizophrenia. Moreover, the reported ability of CBD to activate 5-HT_{1A} receptors (Russo et al. 2005) prompts further research directed at assessing its efficacy in reverting the cognitive deficits of schizophrenia, as already demonstrated for the newest atypical antipsychotics (Sumiyoshi and Higuchi 2013). Finally, the ability of CBD to block CB_1 receptor signaling (Thomas et al. 2007) may also participate in its antipsychotic action (Roser et al. 2010). Thus, CBD can be considered as a "multitarget" drug (Fig. 28.1) whose therapeutic potential appears to be particularly interesting for the treatment of the puzzling and multifaceted disease of schizophrenia.

However, although promising, data on the antipsychotic effect of CBD are still preliminary and further investigations are needed in order to thoroughly assess its therapeutic potential for the treatment of this disorder (Box 28.1). In addition, besides CBD, other pCBs seem to possess interesting pharmacological actions that prompt us to suggest their possible exploitation for the treatment of psychosis.

References

Abi-Dargham, A. and Guillin, O. (2007). Integrating the neurobiology of schizophrenia. *International Review of Neurobiology*, **78**, xiii–xvi.

Almeida, V., Levin, R., Peres, F.F., et al. (2012). Cannabidiol exhibits anxiolytic but not antipsychotic property evaluated in the social interaction test. *Progress in Neuro-Psychopharmacology & Biological Psychiatry*, **41C**, 30–35.

Avraham, Y., Grigoriadis, N., Poutahidis, T., et al. (2011). Cannabidiol improves brain and liver function in a fulminant hepatic failure-induced model of hepatic encephalopathy in mice. *British Journal of Pharmacology*, **162**, 1650–1658.

Bhattacharyya, S., Fusar-Poli, P., Borgwardt, S., et al. (2009). Modulation of mediotemporal and ventrostriatal function in humans by Delta9-tetrahydrocannabinol: a neural basis for the effects of Cannabis sativa on learning and psychosis. *Archives of General Psychiatry*, **66**, 442–451.

Bhattacharyya, S., Morrison, P.D., Fusar-Poli, P., et al. (2010). Opposite effects of delta-9-tetrahydrocannabinol and cannabidiol on human brain function and psychopathology. *Neuropsychopharmacology*, **35**, 764–774.

Black, M.D., Stevens, R.J., Rogacki, N., et al. (2011). AVE1625, a cannabinoid CB1 receptor antagonist, as a co-treatment with antipsychotics for schizophrenia: improvement in cognitive function and reduction of antipsychotic-side effects in rodents. *Psychopharmacology (Berlin)*, **215**, 149–163.

Bosi, D.C., Hallak, J.E.C., Dursun, S.M., Deakin, J.F.W., and Zuardi, A.W. (2003). Effects of cannabidiol on (s)-ketamine-induced psychopathology in healthy volunteers. *Journal of Psychopharmacology*, **17**, A55.

Braff, D.L., Swerdlow, N.R., and Geyer, M.A. (1999). Symptom correlates of prepulse inhibition deficits in male schizophrenic patients. *American Journal of Psychiatry*, **156**, 596–602.

Broome, M.R., Woolley, J.B., Tabraham, P., *et al.* (2005). What causes the onset of psychosis? *Schizophrenia Research*, **79**, 23–34.

Bubeníková-Valesová, V., Horácek, J., Vrajová, M., and Höschl, C. (2008). Models of schizophrenia in humans and animals based on inhibition of NMDA receptors. *Neuroscience & Biobehavioral Reviews*, **32**, 1014–1023.

Calzavara, M.B., Levin, R., Medrano, W.A., *et al.* (2011a). Effects of antipsychotics and amphetamine on social behaviors in spontaneously hypertensive rats. *Behavioural Brain Research*, **225**, 15–22.

Calzavara, M.B., Medrano, W.A., Levin, R., *et al.* (2009). Neuroleptic drugs revert the contextual fear conditioning deficit presented by spontaneously hypertensive rats: a potential animal model of emotional context processing in schizophrenia? *Schizophrenia Bulletin* **35**, 748–759.

Calzavara, M.B., Medrano, W.A., Levin. R., Libânio, T.C., de Alencar Ribeiro, R., and Abílio, V.C. (2011b). The contextual fear conditioning deficit presented by spontaneously hypertensive rats (SHR) is not improved by mood stabilizers. *Progress in Neuro-Psychopharmacology and Biological Psychiatry*, **35**, 1607–1611.

Campos, A.C., Moreira, F.A., Gomes, F.V., Del Bel, E.A., and Guimarães, F.S. (2012). Multiple mechanisms involved in the large-spectrum therapeutic potential of cannabidiol in psychiatric disorders. *Philosophical Transactions of the Royal Society. Series B, Biological Sciences*, **367**, 3364–3378.

Cassol-Jr, O.J., Comim, C.M., Silva, B.R., *et al.* (2010). Treatment with cannabidiol reverses oxidative stress parameters, cognitive impairment and mortality in rats submitted to sepsis by cecal ligation and puncture. *Brain Research*, **1348**, 128–138.

Castagné, V., Moser, P.C., and Porsolt, R.D. (2009). Preclinical behavioral models for predicting antipsychotic activity. *Advances in Pharmacology*, **57**, 381–418.

D'Souza, D.C., Abi-Saab, W.M., Madonick, S., *et al.* (2005). Delta-9-tetrahydrocannabinol effects in schizophrenia: implications for cognition, psychosis, and addiction. *Biological Psychiatry*, **57**, 594–608.

Dalton, W.S., Martz, R., Lemberger, L., Rodda, B.E., and Forney, R.B. (1976). Influence of cannabidiol on delta-9-tetrahydrocannabinol effects. *Clinical Pharmacology & Therapeutics*, **19**, 300–309.

Di Forti, M., Morgan, C., Dazzan, P., *et al.* (2009). High-potency cannabis and the risk of psychosis. *British Journal of Psychiatry*, **195**, 488–491.

Dixon, L., Haas, G., Wedien, P.J., Sweeney, J., and Frances, A.J. (1990). Acute effects of drug abuse in schizophrenic patients: clinical observations and patients' self-reports. *Schizophrenia Bulletin*, **16**, 69–79.

Ellenbroek, B.A. and Riva, M.A. (2003). Early maternal deprivation as an animal model for schizophrenia. *Clinical Neuroscience Research*, **3**, 297–302.

Englund, A., Morrison, P.D. and Nottage, J., *et al.* (2013). Cannabidiol inhibits THC-elicited paranoid symptoms and hippocampal-dependent memory impairment. *Journal of Psychopharmacology*, **27**, 19–27.

Fagherazzi, E.V., Garcia, V.A., Maurmann, N., *et al.* (2012). Memory-rescuing effects of cannabidiol in an animal model of cognitive impairment relevant to neurodegenerative disorders. *Psychopharmacology (Berlin)*, **219**, 1133–1140.

Falls, D.L. (2003). Neuregulins: functions, forms, and signaling strategies. *Experimental Cell Research*, **284**, 14–30.

Ferdinand, R.F., Sondeijker, F., van der Ende, J., Selten, J.P., Huizink, A., and Verhulst, F.C. (2005). Cannabis use predicts future psychotic symptoms, and vice versa. *Addiction*, **100**, 612–618.

Fone, K.C. and Porkess, M.V. (2008). Behavioural and neurochemical effects of post-weaning social isolation in rodents-relevance to developmental neuropsychiatric disorders. *Neuroscience & Biobehavioral Reviews*, **32**, 1087–1102.

Guidali, C., Viganò, D., Petrosino S., *et al.* (2011). Cannabinoid CB$_1$ receptor antagonism prevents neurochemical and behavioural deficits induced by chronic phencyclidine. *International Journal of Neuropsychopharmacol*, **14**, 17–28.

Guimarães, V.M., Zuardi, A.W., Del Bel, E.A., and Guimarães, F.S. (2004). Cannabidiol increases Fos expression in the nucleus accumbens but not in the dorsal striatum. *Life Sciences*, 75, 633–638.

Gururajan, A., Taylor, D.A., and Malone, D.T. (2011). Effect of cannabidiol in a MK-801-rodent model of aspects of schizophrenia. *Behavioural Brain Research*, 222, 299–308.

Gururajan, A., Taylor, D.A., and Malone, D.T. (2012). Cannabidiol and clozapine reverse MK-801-induced deficits in social interaction and hyperactivity in Sprague-Dawley rats. *Journal of Psychopharmacology*, 26, 1317–1332.

Hallak, J.E., Dursun, S.M., Bosi, D.C., *et al.* (2011). The interplay of cannabinoid and NMDA glutamate receptor systems in humans: preliminary evidence of interactive effects of cannabidiol and ketamine in healthy human subjects. *Progress in Neuro-Psychopharmacology & Biological Psychiatry*, 35, 198–202.

Hallak, J.E., Machado-de-Sousa, J.P., Crippa, J.A., *et al.* (2010). Performance of schizophrenic patients in the Stroop Color Word Test and electrodermal responsiveness after acute administration of cannabidiol (CBD). *Revista Brasileira de Psiquiatria*, 32, 56–61.

Henquet, C., Krabbendam, L., Spauwen, J., *et al.* (2005). Prospective cohort study of cannabis use, predisposition for psychosis, and psychotic symptoms in young people. *British Medical Journal*, 330, 11.

Juckel, G., Roser, P., Nadulski, T., Stadelmann, A.M., and Gallinat, J. (2007). Acute effects of Delta9-tetrahydrocannabinol and standardized cannabis extract on the auditory evoked mismatch negativity. *Schizophrenia Research*, 97, 109–117.

Krystal, J.H., D'Souza, D.C., Madonick, S., and Petrakis, I.L. (1999). Toward a rational pharmacotherapy of comorbid substance abuse in schizophrenic patients. *Schizophrenia Research*, 35(Suppl), S35–S49.

Kuepper, R., van Os, J., Lieb, R., Wittchen, H.U., Höfler, M., and Henquet, C. (2011). Continued cannabis use and risk of incidence and persistence of psychotic symptoms: 10 year follow-up cohort study. *British Medical Journal*, 342, d738.

Levin, R., Calzavara, M.B., Santos, C.M., Medrano, W.A., Niigaki, S.T., and Abílio, V.C. (2011). Spontaneously Hypertensive Rats (SHR) present deficits in prepulse inhibition of startle specifically reverted by clozapine. *Progress in Neuro-Psychopharmacology & Biological Psychiatry*, 35, 1748–1752.

Leweke, F., Koethe, D., and Gerth, C.W. (2007). Double blind, controlled clinical trial of cannabidiol monotherapy versus amisulpiride in the treatment of acutely psychotic schizophrenia patients. *Schizophrenia Bulletin*, 33, 310.

Leweke, F.M., Piomelli, D., Pahlisch, F., *et al.* (2012). Cannabidiol enhances anandamide signaling and alleviates psychotic symptoms of schizophrenia. *Translational Psychiatry*, 2, e94.

Leweke, F.M., Schneider, U., Radwan, M., Schmidt, E., and Emrich, H.M. (2000). Different effects of nabilone and cannabidiol on binocular depth inversion in Man. *Pharmacology Biochemistry and Behavior*, 66, 175–181.

Llorente-Berzal, A., Fuentes, S., Gagliano, H., *et al.* (2011). Sex-dependent effects of maternal deprivation and adolescent cannabinoid treatment on adult rat behaviour. *Addiction Biology*, 16, 624–637.

Long, L.E., Chesworth, R., Huang, X.F., *et al.* (2012). Distinct neurobehavioural effects of cannabidiol in transmembrane domain neuregulin 1 mutant mice. *PLoS One*, 7, e34129.

Long, L.E., Chesworth, R., Huang, X.F., McGregor, I.S., Arnold, J.C., and Karl, T. (2010). A behavioural comparison of acute and chronic Delta9-tetrahydrocannabinol and cannabidiol in C57BL/6JArc mice. *International Journal of Neuropsychopharmacology*, 13, 861–876.

Long, L.E., Malone, D.T., and Taylor, D.A. (2006). Cannabidiol reverses MK-801-induced disruption of prepulse inhibition in mice. *Neuropsychopharmacology*, 31, 795–803.

Ludewig, K., Geyer, M.A., and Vollenweider, F.X. (2003). Deficits in prepulse inhibition and habituation in never-medicated, first-episode schizophrenia. *Biological Psychiatry*, 54,121–128.

Magen, I., Avraham, Y., Ackerman, Z., Vorobiev, L., Mechoulam, R., and Berry, E.M. (2010). Cannabidiol ameliorates cognitive and motor impairments in bile-duct ligated mice via 5-HT1A receptor activation. *British Journal of Pharmacology*, 159, 950–957.

Moore, T.H., Zammit, S., Lingford-Hughes, A., *et al.* (2007). Cannabis use and risk of psychotic or affective mental health outcomes: a systematic review. *Lancet*, **370**, 319–328.

Moreira, F.A. and Guimarães, F.S. (2005). Cannabidiol inhibits the hyperlocomotion induced by psychotomimetic drugs in mice. *European Journal of Pharmacology*, **512**, 199–205.

Morgan, C.J. and Curran, H.V. (2008). Effects of cannabidiol on schizophrenia-like symptoms in people who use cannabis. *British Journal of Psychiatry*, **192**, 306–307.

Morgan, C.J., Gardener, C., Schafer, G., *et al.* (2011). Sub-chronic impact of cannabinoids in street cannabis on cognition, psychotic-like symptoms and psychological well-being. *Psychological Medicine*, **29**, 1–10.

Murillo-Rodríguez, E., Millán-Aldaco, D., Palomero-Rivero, M., Mechoulam, R., and Drucker-Colín, R. (2006). Cannabidiol, a constituent of *Cannabis sativa*, modulates sleep in rats. *FEBS Letters*, **580**, 4337–4345.

Pertwee, R.G. (2008). The diverse CB_1 and CB_2 receptor pharmacology of three plant cannabinoids: delta-9-tetrahydrocannabinol, cannabidiol and delta-9-tetrahydrocannabivarin. *British Journal of Pharmacology*, **153**, 199–215.

Powell, S.B., Zhou, X., and Geyer, M.A. (2009). Prepulse inhibition and genetic mouse models of schizophrenia. *Behavioural Brain Research*, **204**, 282–294.

Robertson, G.S. and Fibiger, H.C. (1992). Neuroleptics increase c-fos expression in the forebrain: contrasting effects of haloperidol and clozapine. *Neuroscience*, **46**, 315–328.

Rock, E.M., Goodwin, J.M., Limebeer, C.L., *et al.* (2011). Interaction between non-psychotropic cannabinoids in marihuana: effect of cannabigerol (CBG) on the anti-nausea or anti-emetic effects of cannabidiol (CBD) in rats and shrews. *Psychopharmacology (Berlin)*, **215**, 505–512.

Roser, P., Vollenweider, F.X., and Kawohl, W. (2010). Potential antipsychotic properties of central cannabinoid (CB₁) receptor antagonists. *World Journal of Biological Psychiatry*, **11**, 208–219.

Russo, E.B., Burnett, A., Hall, B., and Parker, K.K. (2005). Agonistic properties of cannabidiol at 5-HT1a receptors. *Neurochemical Research*, **30**, 1037–1043.

Sams-Dodd, F. (1999). Phencyclidine in the social interaction test: an animal model of schizophrenia with face and predictive validity. *Reviews in the Neurosciences*, **10**, 59–90.

Schneier, F.R. and Siris, S.G. (1987). A review of psychoactive substance use and abuse in schizophrenia: patterns of drug choice. *Journal of Nervous and Mental Disorders*, **175**, 641–652.

Schubart, C.D., Sommer, I.E., van Gastel, W.A., Goetgebuer, R.L., Kahn, R.S., and Boks, M.P. (2011). Cannabis with high cannabidiol content is associated with fewer psychotic experiences. *Schizophrenia Research*, **130**, 216–221.

Sumiyoshi, T. and Higuchi, Y. (2013). Facilitative effect of serotonin1A receptor agonists on cognition in patients with schizophrenia. *Current Medicinal Chemistry*, **20**, 357–362.

Thomas, A., Baillie, G.L., Phillips, A.M., Razdan, R.K., Ross, R.A., and Pertwee, R.G. (2007). Cannabidiol displays unexpectedly high potency as an antagonist of CB_1 and CB_2 receptor agonists in vitro. *British Journal of Pharmacology*, **150**, 613–623.

Zamberletti, E., Rubino, T., and Parolaro, D. (2012a). The endocannabinoid system and schizophrenia: integration of evidence. *Current Pharmaceutical Design*, **18**, 4980–4990.

Zamberletti, E., Piscitelli, F., Cadeddu, F., *et al.* (2012b). Chronic blockade of CB(1) receptors reverses startle gating deficits and associated neurochemical alterations in rats reared in isolation. *British Journal of Pharmacology*, **167**, 1652–1664.

Zamberletti, E., Viganò, D., Guidali, C., Rubino, T., and Parolaro, D. (2012c). Long-lasting recovery of psychotic-like symptoms in isolation-reared rats after chronic but not acute treatment with the cannabinoid antagonist AM251. *International Journal of Neuropsychopharmacology*, **15**, 267–280.

Zuardi, A.W., Crippa, J.A., Hallak, J.E., *et al.* (2009). Cannabidiol for the treatment of psychosis in Parkinson's disease. *Journal of Psychopharmacology*, **23**, 979–983.

Zuardi, A.W., Hallak, J.E., Dursun, S.M., *et al.* (2006). Cannabidiol monotherapy for treatment-resistant schizophrenia. *Journal of Psychopharmacology*, **20**, 683–686.

Zuardi, A.W., Morais, S.L., Guimarães, F.S., and Mechoulam, R. (1995). Anti-psychotic effect of cannabidiol. *Journal of Clinical Psychiatry*, **56**, 485–486.

Zuardi, A.W., Rodrigues, J.A., and Cunha, J.M. (1991). Effects of cannabidiol in animal models predictive of antipsychotic activity. *Psychopharmacology (Berlin)*, **104**, 260–264.

Chapter 29

Phytocannabinoids as Novel Therapeutic Agents for Sleep Disorders

Eric Murillo-Rodríguez, Lisa Aguilar-Turton, Stephanie Mijangos-Moreno, Andrea Sarro-Ramírez, and Óscar Arias-Carrión

29.1 Introduction

Sleep may be defined using behavioral, physiological, neurochemical, and molecular criteria. For instance, behaviorally, sleep consists of a lack of mobility and an elevated arousal threshold to external stimulation. Moreover, following the rules set out by Rechtschaffen and Kales in 1968, and using physiological measurements such as electroencephalography (EEG), electrooculography (EOG), and electromyography (EMG; Fig. 29.1), the wake–sleep cycle consists of periodic alternation of three major behavioral states: waking (W), slow-wave sleep (SWS), and rapid eye movement (REM) sleep (for a comprehensive review, see Jafari and Mohsenin 2010).

Currently it is accepted that in healthy humans, EEG activity is characterized by low voltage (10–30 microvolts) as well as fast activity (16–25 Hz) whereas high amplitude is observed in EMG recordings from postural muscles. Transitions from W to sleep stages display specific polysomnographic features. For instance, during the wakefulness–sleep transition, EEG recordings show a progressive slowing of dominant frequency as well as higher-voltage activity. Once SWS is established, four stages are observed in the EEG charts: SWS1–4. The first phase of SWS (SWS1) is for approximately 5 min during the wakefulness–sleep transition. SWS1 displays EEG with low voltage and mixed-frequency activity whereas EOG shows slow rolling eye movements. The next sleep stage, SWS2, is characterized by bursts of sleep spindle sinusoidal waves (12–14 Hz) and high-voltage biphasic waves known as "K complexes." Subsequently, SWS3 displays a high-amplitude signal and slow waves (0.5–2 Hz; known as delta waves) in the EEG charts. In normal conditions (no health problems), the three phases of SWS (SWS1–3) take up 75–80% of the total sleep time. The final phase of SWS (SWS4) includes slow-wave activity and dominates the EEG recording. Under normal conditions, after SWS4, the EEG recordings register the appearance of REM sleep, a phase that was first described more than 50 years ago (Aserinsky and Kleitman 1953; Dement 1958; Jouvet and Michel 1959). REM sleep in humans as well as other mammals is characterized by the appearance of fast, desynchronized brain activity, rapid eye movements, and a loss of muscle tone. Since EEG activity during REM sleep closely resembles that of the alertness state, REM sleep is also known as "paradoxical sleep" or "active sleep."

Day after day, under normal conditions, the sleep–wake cycle in humans transits from SWS1 to SWS4 and then to periods of REM sleeps (Fig. 29.1). This progression is repeated cyclically throughout the sleep cycle at intervals of 90–100 min (Murillo-Rodríguez et al. 2009; Patil 2010). Although we have previously stated that SWS has four stages, the American Academy of Sleep Medicine (2007) further divides SWS into three stages: SWS1–3.

Circadian rhythms

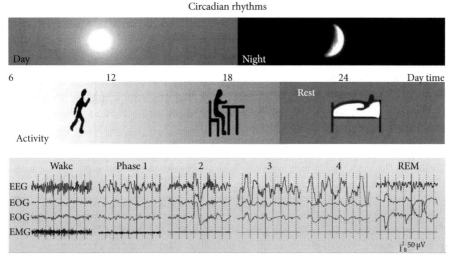

Fig. 29.1 The sleep–wake cycle in humans is characterized by different stages. In this figure, we can notice that during waking there is a low voltage activity seen in the electroencephalogram (EEG). The transition from waking to Stage 1 presents on the EEG a slower activity. Stage 2 is characterized by the presence of K complexes and sleep spindles. During Stage 3, delta waves are present in the EEG and they are present more than 50% of the time in Stage 4. During REM sleep, the EEG pattern presents once again low-voltage and phasic activity that resembles waking. The activity in the electromyogram (EMG) is higher during wakefulness and decreases across the sleep stages until virtually absent during REM sleep. EEG, electroencephalogram; EOG, electrooculogram; EMG, electromyogram; REM, rapid eye movement sleep.

The regulation of sleep involves the activity of several brain nuclei, as well as the interaction of diverse neurotransmitters (Murillo-Rodríguez et al. 2009). Different theories have been developed to explain the neurobiology of sleep. For instance, McCarley and Hobson (1975) suggested the "reciprocal interaction" model of switching circuitry regulating REM sleep generation. Briefly, this model, which is supported by a number of recent findings, proposes that neurons from brainstem nuclei, such as *locus coeruleus* (noradrenergic), *dorsal raphe* (serotoninergic), and *pontine reticular formation* (glutamatergic) are active during alertness, and that their electrophysiological activity becomes silent during SWS, and absent during REM sleep. This has prompted neurons in the locus coeruleus, dorsal raphe, and pontine reticular formation to be referred to as "REM-OFF neurons." Additional evidence, however, supports the idea that sleep is generated as a result of the inhibition of "REM-OFF neurons" by a cluster of neurons located in the laterodorsal and pedunculopontine tegmental nuclei (PPN; cholinergic) which exhibit activity exclusively during REM sleep. Neurons from PPN nuclei have been called "REM-ON neurons" (Mallick et al. 2012; Monti 2011).

While the sleep–wake cycle could be defined by polysomnographic and electrophysiological parameters, it is also possible to describe it by using neurochemical criteria. In this regard, W is generated by neurotransmitters, e.g., glutamate, norepinephrine, dopamine, serotonin, hypocretin, acetylcholine, and histamine. Neurons that release one or other of these transmitters are present in the brainstem and basal forebrain which act through the cerebral cortex to generate and maintain alertness (Murillo-Rodríguez et al. 2012). Other endogenous molecules have a key role in sleep, e.g., gamma-aminobutyric acid (GABA), peptides, cytokines and lipid sleep-inducing factors (Murillo-Rodríguez et al. 2012).

29.2 **Sleep disorders**

Sleep disturbances, that display a range of different EEG/EMG polysomnographic features, have been described, classified, and defined as *sleep disorders*. According to the *International Classification of Sleep Disorders* (ICSD; American Academy of Sleep Medicine 2001), they are classified into four categories:

1 *Dyssomnias*: problems initiating and maintaining sleep, and also excessive sleepiness.

2 *Parasomnias*: disorders of arousal, partial arousal, or sleep stage transition.

3 *Sleep disorders associated with mental, neurologic, or other medical disorders.*

4 *Other sleep disorders*: sleep disorders not included in categories 1, 2, or 3.

The ICSD was produced primarily for diagnostic and epidemiologic purposes and it provides useful and critical information. For example, to analyze sleep habits, a total of 1000 telephone interviews were conducted among a random sample of Americans between September and November 2007. Respondents had to be at least 18 years of age and working 30 h per week or more for pay. The results were included in the National Sleep Foundation Poll 2008 (US) and showed that 42% of those surveyed reported they were awake during the night, whereas 36% reported that they had fallen asleep while driving. These striking data suggest a presence of sleep disturbances and indicate the importance of exploring new therapeutic approaches to managing insomnia and sleepiness. In the following section, based on experimental evidence, we will review potential therapeutic approaches, including the use of cannabinoids, to treat and manage some sleep disorders.

29.3 **Insomnia and somnolence**

The ICSD defines *insomnia* as a dyssomnia characterized by a night complaint of an insufficient amount of sleep or not feeling rested after the habitual sleep episode. Insomnia is often associated with feelings of restlessness, irritability, anxiety, daytime fatigue, and tiredness (Pigeon and Cribbet 2012).

In contrast, *somnolence* is defined as sleep episodes that are present during the W stage that require mild to moderate attention. Somnolence might occur as a secondary health condition, For example, side effects of medication, illicit substance use, or obstructive sleep apnea (Pagel 2009).

29.3.1 **Rational therapeutic approaches to treat insomnia and somnolence**

Treatments of insomnia that are currently available include both cognitive behavioral therapy and drug therapy (Mitchell et al. 2012). In this regard, it has been suggested that benzodiazepine-receptor agonists and nonbenzodiazepine hypnotic agents (like zolpidem) are effective in the short-term management of insomnia. However, side effects (dependence and tolerance) have been reported when using these drugs (Bastien 2011; Morin and Benca 2012; Riemann and Perlis 2009).

Whereas insomnia is managed by using behavioral and/or pharmacological therapies, somnolence is treated by applying noninvasive continuous positive airway pressure (Marin et al. 2012; Sharma et al. 2011), or with drugs such as modafinil (commercially known as Provigil™) which is the first-line drug for the treatment of excessive daytime sleepiness (Darwish et al. 2011; Tembe et al. 2011). Given that somnolence could be the result of associated sleep disorders, such as sleep apnea, a differential diagnostic procedure should be used to seek out a pathognomonic sign or symptom, i.e., one that is specifically associated with a particular type of somnolence.

Promoting the use of effective treatments for insomnia or somnolence will alleviate greatly the personal burden imposed by sleep disorders. For example, the most important sleep hygiene measure is to maintain a regular sleep and wake pattern 7 days a week. However, different and novel approaches are needed to treat sleep disorders in the near future. In the next section, we present some evidence that *cannabinoids* have therapeutic potential for the treatment of insomnia and somnolence.

29.4 **Phytocannabinoids and sleep**

Marijuana is a common name given to the plant *Cannabis sativa* (*C. sativa*). This plant has been used by diverse cultures for distinct purposes, such as for mystical ceremonies, social interaction, as well as for therapeutic aims (Ameri 1999; Grant et al. 2012; Hollister 1986; Robson 2001; Zias et al. 1993).

Despite legal restriction, cannabinoids are often used for medical treatment in several countries, e.g., Canada and the UK. Moreover, changes to civil law in the US that led to the *Compassionate Use Act of 1996* (also known as Prop. 215) and the *Medical Marijuana Program* (also called SB 420), have facilitated the use of marijuana as a potential therapeutic option in sleep medicine (Reinarman et al. 2011; Swartz 2010).

The use of *C. sativa* for medical purposes is supported by experimental evidence showing that it controls and improves symptoms of several disorders, including multiple sclerosis (associated with muscle spasticity, pain, and sleep disorders), psychosis, bipolar disorder, anxiety, chronic pain, anorexia, and cancer (Arias Horcajadas 2007; Borgelt et al. 2013; Burns and Ineck 2006; Crippa et al. 2012; de Jong et al. 2005; Grant et al. 2012; Hollister, 1986; Kalant 2001; O'Sullivan et al. 2005; Robson 2001; Sarne and Mechoulam 2005; Swartz 2010).

If *C. sativa* can ameliorate sleep disorders then the question arises as to what molecule(s) from this plant would be most effective at treating these disorders? It has been demonstrated that *C. sativa* contains over 70 different chemical compounds (phytocannabinoids). Two of the most well-known examples are: delta-9- tetrahydrocannabinol (Δ^9-THC) and cannabidiol (CBD) (Gaoni and Mechoulam 1964; Mechoulam and Hanus 2002; Mechoulam et al. 2007) (Fig. 29.2). Since their discovery, the pharmacology and therapeutic potential of both these phytocannabinoids has been extensively investigated.

29.4.1 Δ^9-**THC and sleep**

It has been demonstrated that Δ^9-THC has sleep-inducing effects (Freemon 1982; Pivik et al. 1972). Daily doses of 70–210 mg of this cannabinoid induced sleep in humans (Feinberg et al. 1975, 1976) whereas in animals, the administration of Δ^9-THC (1 mg/kg) reduced the voltage of cortical activity during alertness. Moreover, the waking-associated power spectra were diminished by the administration of Δ^9-THC (Buonamici et al. 1982). Although the pharmacological effect of this cannabinoid on sleep was explored in the 1970s and 1980s, interest in this effect remains (Russo et al. 2007).

29.4.2 **CBD and sleep**

Effects of CBD on sleep are somewhat contradictory. For example, Monti (1977) reported a reduction of sleep by systemic administration of CBD whereas Carlini and Cunha (1981) reported a

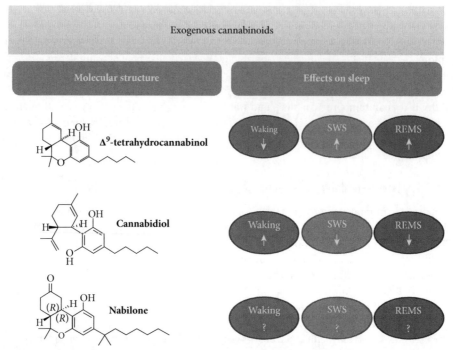

Fig. 29.2 Pharmacological effects of Δ^9-tetrahydrocannabinol, cannabidiol and nabilone on the sleep-wake cycle. REMS, rapid eye movement sleep; SWS, slow-wave sleep.

CBD-induced improvement in sleep in insomniac patients. These differences can be explained in part by differences between the methods used in these studies.

Recent data suggest that CBD might be a wake-promoting factor. For example, Nicholson et al. (2004) reported that administration of this cannabinoid increased alertness in humans, whereas our group has demonstrated that intracerebroventricular administration of CBD (10 micrograms/5 microliters) to rats at the beginning of the lights-on period increased W and decreased REM sleep. Furthermore, we have found that CBD enhanced the extracellular levels of dopamine collected from nucleus accumbens and induced an enhancement of c-Fos expression in waking-related brain areas, including hypothalamus and dorsal raphe nucleus (Murillo-Rodríguez et al. 2006). Similar results were obtained by injecting CBD into the lateral hypothalamus during the lights-on period at doses of 10 or 20 micrograms/1 microliter (Murillo-Rodríguez et al. 2008, 2011). Recently, Hsiao et al. (2012) showed that CBD efficiently blocked anxiety-induced REM sleep suppression. Taken together, these data suggest that CBD promotes alertness; however the mechanisms of action of this cannabinoid for its effect on sleep remain unclear.

29.5 Synthetic cannabinoids and sleep

Some reports have pointed out that synthetic Δ^9-THC (marinol, dronabinol), which is used clinically to suppress chemotherapy-induced nausea and vomiting and to increase appetite in patients with AIDS, can modulate sleep. Haney et al. (2007) have shown that HIV-positive marijuana smokers displayed signs of improved sleep when they received dronabinol (5 and 10 mg) four times daily over 4 days. There is also evidence that the synthetic cannabinoid, nabilone, which can also reduce chemotherapy-induced nausea and vomiting (Grotenhermen and Müller-Vahl 2012; Ware and St Arnaud-Trempe 2010), and shares the ability of Δ^9-THC to activate type 1 and 2 cannabinoid receptors (CB_1 and CB_2), can modulate sleep. It has been reported by Fraser (2009) that patients diagnosed with posttraumatic stress disorder displayed a significant improvement in sleep time and quality of sleep when treated with nabilone. Furthermore, Ware et al. (2010) showed that patients with fibromyalgia, a disease characterized by chronic pain and insomnia, who were treated with nabilone (0.5–1.0 mg before bedtime) showed a significant improvement in sleep. Despite the therapeutically-positive effects on sleep induced by dronabinol and nabilone, the mechanism of action of these drugs that underlies these effects remains unknown. No solid evidence is available regarding the manner in which nabilone affects sleep, prompting a need for further sleep research with this and other cannabinoid receptor agonists.

29.6 Potential uses of phytocannabinoids for sleep disorders

Both Δ^9-THC and CBD modulate the sleep–wake cycle by promoting sleep and alertness, respectively (Buonamici et al. 1982; Feinberg et al. 1975, 1976; Freemon 1982; Monti 1977; Murillo-Rodríguez et al. 2006, 2008, 2011; Nicholson et al. 2004; Pivik et al. 1972). Although further investigation is needed, Δ^9-THC or CBD could be of use for the prevention and management of sleep disorders in the near future. Although the effects of synthetic cannabinoids on sleep have so far been poorly described, they should be investigated as potential therapeutic options for treating sleep disorders.

29.7 Conclusions and future research directions

Modulation of the sleep–waking cycle involves the interaction of multiple neurological and neurochemical substrates (Arias-Carrión et al. 2011; Murillo-Rodríguez et al. 2009, 2012). Several endogenous and exogenous molecules, including cannabinoids, have been suggested as sleep-modulators (Buonamici et al. 1982; Carlini and Cunha 1981; Feinberg et al. 1975, 1976; Freemon 1982; Monti 1977; Murillo-Rodríguez et al. 2006, 2008, 2011; Nicholson et al. 2004; Pivik et al. 1972). There is also evidence that phytocannabinoids (Δ^9-THC and CBD) impair sleep stages, although no information about the way(s) in which nabilone improves sleep (Fig. 29.2).

Here, we have described the effects on sleep induced by two phytocannabinoids, Δ^9-THC and CBD. From these effects, it can be hypothesized that they have therapeutic potential for treating insomnia or somnolence. However, further research is imperative if the mechanisms by which Δ^9-THC and CBD modulate sleep and the way(s) in which sleep is affected by other cannabinoids are to be fully elucidated.

New treatments for sleep disorders might also reduce the risks that confront some transportation professionals. Recently, the National Sleep Foundation's (NSF) 2012 *Sleep in America*® poll reported that that pilots and train operators are most likely to report sleep-related job performance and safety problems. About 23% of pilots admitted in the poll that sleepiness had affected their job performance at least once a week, compared to nontransportation workers (17%). Curiously, a significant number of transportation professionals had reported that sleepiness had caused safety problems on the job. For example, pilots (20%) admitted that they had made a serious error. These results suggest that sleepiness has an important role in transportation accidents. This report prompts the need to explore novel rational approaches to manage and treat sleep disorders, such as insomnia or somnolence.

Finally, we must remember that however exciting their neurobiological mechanisms might be, the clinical usefulness of phytocannabinoids will be determined by their ability to provide patients with sleep disorders with safe, long-lasting, and substantial improvements in quality of life.

References

Ameri, A. (1999). The effects of cannabinoids on the brain. *Progress in Neurobiology*, **58**, 315–348.

American Academy of Sleep Medicine. (2001). *The International Classification of Sleep Disorders, Revised. Diagnostic and Coding Manual*. Westchester, IL: American Academy of Sleep Medicine.

American Academy of Sleep Medicine. (2007). *The AASM Manual 2007 for the Scoring of Sleep and Associated Events. Rules, Terminology and Technical Specifications*. Westchester, IL: American Academy of Sleep Medicine.

Arias-Carrión, O., Huitrón-Reséndiz, S., Arankowsky-Sandoval, G., and Murillo-Rodríguez, E. (2011). Biochemical modulation of the sleep-wake cycle: endogenous sleep-inducing factors. *Journal of Neuroscience Research*, **89**, 1143–1149.

Arias Horcajadas, F. (2007). Cannabinoids in eating disorders and obesity. *Molecular Neurobiology*, **36**, 113–128.

Aserinsky, E. and Kleitman, N. (1953). Regularly occurring periods of eye motility, and concomitant phenomena, during sleep. *Science*, **118**, 273–274.

Bastien, C.H. (2011). Insomnia: neurophysiological and neuropsychological approaches. *Neuropsychology Review*, **1**, 22–40.

Borgelt, L.M., Franson, K.L., Nussbaum, A.M., and Wang, G.S. (2013). The pharmacologic and clinical effects of medical cannabis. *Pharmacotherapy*, **33**, 195–209.

Buonamici, M., Young, G.A., and Khazan, N. (1982). Effects of acute delta 9-THC administration on EEG and EEG power spectra in the rat. *Neuropharmacology*, **21**, 825–829.

Burns, T.L. and Ineck, J.R. (2006). Cannabinoid analgesia as a potential new therapeutic option in the treatment of chronic pain. *The Annals of Pharmacotherapy*, **40**, 251–260.

Carlini, E.A. and Cunha, J.M. (1981). Hypnotic and antiepileptic effects of cannabidiol. *The Journal of Clinical Pharmacology*, **21**(Suppl. 8–9), 417S–427S.

Crippa, J.A., Derenusson, G.N., and Chagas, M.H. (2012). Pharmacological interventions in the treatment of the acute effects of cannabis: a systematic review of literature. *Harm Reduction Journal*, **9**, 7.

Darwish, M., Bond, M., and Ezzet, F. (2011). Armodafinil and modafinil in patients with excessive sleepiness associated with shift work disorder: a pharmacokinetic/pharmacodynamic model for predicting and comparing their concentration-effect relationships. *The Journal of Clinical Pharmacology*, **52**, 1328–1342.

Dement, W. (1958). The occurrence of low voltage, fast, electroencephalogram patterns during behavioral sleep in the cat. *Electroencephalography and Clinical Neurophysiology*, **10**, 291–296.

De Jong, B.C., Prentiss, D., McFarland, W., Machekano, R., and Israelski, D.M. (2005). Marijuana use and its association with adherence to antiretroviral therapy among HIV-infected persons with moderate to severe nausea. *Journal of Acquired Immune Deficiency Syndromes*, **38**, 43–46.

Feinberg, I., Jones, R., Walker, J., Cavness, C., and Floyd, T. (1976). Effects of marijuana extract and tetrahydrocannabinol on electroencephalographic sleep patterns. *Clinical Pharmacology & Therapeutics*, **19**, 782–794.

Feinberg, I., Jones, R., Walker, J.M., Caveness, C., and March, J. (1975). Effects of high dosage delta-9-tetrahydrocannabinol on sleep patterns in man. *Clinical Pharmacology & Therapeutics*, **17**, 458–466.

Fraser, G.A. (2009). The use of a synthetic cannabinoid in the management of treatment resistant nightmares in posttraumatic stress disorder (PTSD). *CNS Neuroscience & Therapeutics*, **15**, 84–88.

Freemon, F.R. (1982). The effect of chronically administered delta-9-tetrahydrocannabinol upon the polygraphically monitored sleep of normal volunteers. *Drug and Alcohol Dependence*, **10**, 345–353.

Gaoni, Y. and Mechoulam, R. (1964). Isolation, structure and partial synthesis of an active constituent of hashish. *Journal of the American Chemical Society*, **86**, 1646–1647.

Grotenhermen, F. and Müller-Vahl, K. (2012). The therapeutic potential of cannabis and cannabinoids. *Deutsches Ärzteblatt* International, **109**, 495–501.

Grant, I., Atkinson, J.H., Gouaux, B., and Wilsey, B. (2012). Medical marijuana: clearing away the smoke. *The Open Neurology Journal*, **6**, 18–25.

Haney, M., Gunderson, E.W., Rabkin, J., *et al.* (2007). Dronabinol and marijuana in HIV-positive marijuana smokers-caloric intake, mood, and sleep. *Journal of Acquired Immune Deficiency Syndromes*, **45**, 545–554.

Hollister, L.E. (1986). Health aspects of cannabis. *Pharmacological Reviews*, **38**, 1–20.

Hsiao, Y.T., Yi, P.L., Li, C.L., and Chang, F.C. (2012). Effect of cannabidiol on sleep disruption induced by the repeated combination tests consisting of open field and elevated plus-maze in rats. *Neuropharmacology*, **62**, 373–384 .

Jafari, B. and Mohsenin, V. (2010). Polysomnography. *Clinics in Chest Medicine*, **31**, 287–297.

Jouvet, M. and Michel, F. (1959). Electromyographic correlations of sleep in the chronic decorticate & mesencephalic cat. *Comptes Rendus des Seances de la Societe de Biologie et des ses Filiales* (Paris), **153**, 422–425.

Kalant, H. (2001). Medicinal use of cannabis: history and current status. *Pain Research & Management*, **6**, 80–91.

Mallick, B.N., Singh, A., and Khanday, M.A. (2012). Activation of inactivation process initiates rapid eye movement sleep. *Progress in Neurobiology*, **97**, 259–276.

Marin, J.M., Agusti, A., Villar, I., *et al.* (2012). Association between treated and untreated obstructive sleep apnea and risk of hypertension. *Journal of the American Medical Association*, **307**, 2169–2176.

McCarley, R.W. and Hobson, J.A. (1975). Neuronal excitability modulation over the sleep cycle: a structural and mathematical model. *Science*, **189**, 58–60.

Mechoulam, R. and Hanus, L. (2002). Cannabidiol: an overview of some chemical and pharmacological aspects. Part I: chemical aspects. *Chemistry and Physics of Lipids*, **121**, 35–43.

Mechoulam, R., Peters, M., Murillo-Rodriguez, E., and Hanus, L.O. (2007). Cannabidiol-recent advances. *Chemistry & Biodiversity*, **4**, 1678–1692.

Mitchell, M.D., Gehrman, P., Perlis, M., and Umscheid, C.A. (2012). Comparative effectiveness of cognitive behavioral therapy for insomnia: a systematic review. *BMC Family Practice*, **13**, 40.

Monti, J.M. (1977). Hypnotic-like effects of cannabidiol in the rat. *Psychopharmacology*, **55**, 263–265.

Monti, J.M. (2011). Serotonin control of sleep-wake behavior. *Sleep Medicine Reviews*, **15**, 269–281.

Morin, C.M. and Benca, R. (2012). Chronic insomnia. *Lancet*, **379**, 1129–1141.

Murillo-Rodríguez, E., Arias-Carrión, O., Sanguino-Rodríguez, K., González-Arias, M., and Haro, R. (2009). Mechanisms of sleep-wake cycle modulation. *CNS & Neurological Disorders – Drug Targets*, **8**, 245–253.

Murillo-Rodríguez, E., Arias-Carrión, O., Zavala-García, A., Sarro-Ramírez, A., Huitrón-Reséndiz, S., and Arankowsky-Sandoval, G. (2012). Basic sleep mechanisms: an integrative review. *Central Nervous System Agents in Medicinal Chemistry*, **12**, 38–54.

Murillo-Rodríguez, E., Millán-Aldaco, D., Palomero-Rivero, M., Mechoulam, R., and Drucker-Colín, R. (2006). Cannabidiol, a constituent of *Cannabis sativa*, modulates sleep in rats. *FEBS Letters*, **580**, 4337–4345.

Murillo-Rodríguez, E., Millán-Aldaco, D., Palomero-Rivero, M., Mechoulam, R., and Drucker-Colín, R. (2008). The nonpsychoactive *Cannabis* constituent cannabidiol is a wake-inducing agent. *Behavioral Neurosciences*, **122**, 1378–1382.

Murillo-Rodríguez, E., Palomero-Rivero, M., Millán-Aldaco, D., Mechoulam, R., and Drucker-Colín, R. (2011). Effects on sleep and dopamine levels of microdialysis perfusion of cannabidiol into the lateral hypothalamus of rats. *Life Sciences*, **88**, 504–511.

National Sleep Foundation. (2008). *Sleep, Performance and the Workplace*. Washington, DC: National Sleep Foundation.

National Sleep Foundation. (2012). *Transportation Workers' Sleep*. Washington, DC: National Sleep Foundation.

Nicholson, A.N., Turner, C., Stone, B.M., and Robson, P.J. (2004). Effects of Delta-9-tetrahydrocannabinol and cannabidiol on nocturnal sleep and early-morning behavior in young adults. *Clinical Psychopharmacology*, **24**, 305–313.

O'Sullivan, S.E., Kendall, D.A., and Randall, M.D. (2005). Vascular effects of delta 9-tetrahydrocannabinol (THC), anandamide and N-arachidonoyldopamine (NADA) in the rat isolated aorta. *European Journal of Pharmacology*, **507**, 211–221.

Pagel, J.F. (2009). Excessive daytime sleepiness. *American Family Physician*, **79**, 391–396.

Patil, S.P. (2010). What every clinician should know about polysomnography. *Respiratory Care*, **55**, 1179–1195.

Pigeon, W.R. and Cribbet, M.R. (2012). The pathophysiology of insomnia: from models to molecules (and back). *Current Opinion in Pulmonary Medicine*, **18**, 546–553.

Pivik, R.T., Zarcone, V., Dement, W.C., and Hollister, L.E. (1972). Delta-9-tetrahydrocannabinol and synhexl: effects on human sleep patterns. *Clinical Pharmacology & Therapeutics*, **13**, 426–435.

Rechtschaffen, A. and Kales, A. (eds.) (1968). *A manual of standardized terminology, techniques and scoring system of sleep stages in human subjects*. Los Angeles: Brain Information Service/Brain Research Institute, University of California.

Reinarman, C., Nunberg, H., Lanthier, F., and Heddleston, T. (2011). Who are medical marijuana patients? Population characteristics from nine California assessment clinics. *Journal of Psychoactive Drugs*, **43**, 128–135.

Riemann, D. and Perlis, M.L. (2009). The treatments of chronic insomnia: a review of benzodiazepine receptor agonists and psychological and behavioral therapies. *Sleep Medicine Reviews*, **13**, 205–214.

Robson, P. (2001). Therapeutic aspects of cannabis and cannabinoids. *British Journal of Psychiatry*, **178**, 107–115.

Russo, E.B., Geoffrey, W.G., and Robson, P.J. (2007). Cannabis, pain, and sleep: lessons from therapeutic clinical trials of Sativex, a cannabis-based medicine. *Chemistry & Biodiversity*, **4**, 1729–1743.

Sarne, Y. and Mechoulam, R. (2005). Cannabinoids: between neuroprotection and neurotoxicity. *Current Drug Targets. CNS and Neurological Disorders*, **4**, 677–684.

Sharma, S.K., Agrawal, S., Damodaran, D., *et al.* (2011). CPAP for the metabolic syndrome in patients with obstructive sleep apnea. *New England Journal of Medicine*, **365**, 2277–2286.

Swartz, R. (2010). Medical marijuana users in substance abuse treatment. *Harm Reduction Journal*, **7**, 3.

Tembe, D.V., Dhavale, A., Desai, H., *et al.* (2011). Armodafinil versus modafinil in patients of excessive sleepiness associated with shift work sleep disorder: a randomized double blind multicentric clinical trial. *Neurology Research International*, **2011**.

Ware, M.A., Fitzcharles, M.A., Joseph, L., and Shir, Y. (2010). The effects of nabilone on sleep in fibromyalgia: results of a randomized controlled trial. *Anesthesia and Analgesia*, **110**, 604–610.

Ware, M.A. and St Arnaud-Trempe, E. (2010). The abuse potential of the synthetic cannabinoid nabilone. *Addiction*, **105**, 494–503.

Zias, J., Stark, H., Sellgman, J., *et al.* (1993). Early medical use of cannabis. *Nature*, **363**, 215–216.

Chapter 30

Cannabis and Epilepsy

Claire M. Williams, Nicholas A. Jones,
and Benjamin J. Whalley

30.1 Epilepsy

30.1.1 Introduction

Epilepsy is a serious neurological disorder that typically manifests as recurrent, spontaneous seizures or convulsions with possible loss of consciousness as a result of disturbance to the excitatory–inhibitory equilibrium of neuronal activity (Lutz 2004) and affects approximately 1% of the world's population (Sander 2003). Epilepsy is both a life-threatening and progressive neurological disorder with patients exhibiting an average mortality rate two to three times higher compared to the general population, as well as being more likely to present with at least one learning disability such as speech and/or language disability, cognitive delay, or academic underachievement (de Boer et al. 2008; Lhatoo and Sander 2001; Seidenberg et al. 1986). Furthermore, epilepsy has numerous and significant comorbid associations with psychiatric and somatic disorders (de Boer et al. 2008; Gaitatzis et al. 2004; Téllez-Zenteno et al. 2007). However, epilepsy is not a single disease, but encompasses a diverse family of disorders, all involving an abnormally increased predisposition to seizures (Fisher et al. 2005).

30.1.2 Risk factors and development of epilepsy

Due to its complex symptomatology, many different conditions represent risk factors for developing epilepsy (de Boer et al. 2008; Duncan et al. 2006; Sander 2003). Typically, incidence is greater amongst young children and the older population (Duncan et al. 2006; Forsgren et al. 2005; MacDonald et al. 2000; Sander 2003), males are more likely to be affected than females even after accounting for gender-biased risk factors (e.g. head trauma) (Banerjee and Hauser 2008; Sander and Shorvon 1996), and the incidence rate in developing countries is typically much higher than that of developed countries. Epilepsy that develops in childhood, adolescence, or in early adulthood is most often associated with congenital, developmental, and genetic conditions (Sander 2004). Conversely, the development of epilepsy through either head trauma, infection of the central nervous system (CNS), or tumors can occur at any age (Duncan et al. 2006). In the elderly, cerebrovascular disease is the most common risk for epilepsy (Cloyd et al. 2006; Duncan et al. 2006; Sander 2003). Furthermore, geographic considerations can be important as parasitic infections such as falciparum malaria (Carter et al. 2004; Ngoungou and Preux 2008) and neurocysticercosis (Carpio 2002; Maguire 2004) are associated with epilepsy in regions where such parasites are endemic (Sander 2003).

Each of these risk factors can initiate the process of epileptogenesis; the asymptomatic process by which a normal non-epileptic brain becomes epileptic. Although the neurobiological changes occurring during epileptogenesis remain poorly understood, alterations in neuronal excitability, establishment of critical neuronal interconnections, and reorganization of such networks have all been documented before occurrence of the first spontaneous seizure (Chang and Lowenstein 2003; Engel and Pedley 2008; Pitkänen and Lukasiuk 2011). These CNS changes promote recurrent, hypersynchronous neuronal discharges that, over time, recruit other structures into the epileptogenic circuit until a sufficiently large brain area is involved to manifest clinical, epileptic seizures. In addition, changes to the functional properties of glial cells have also been described (reviewed in Steinhäuser and Seifert 2002) and abnormal patterns of neuronal migration have been seen to result in hyperexcitability of cortical networks (Chevassus-au-Louis et al. 1999; Farrell et al. 2008; Sisodiya 2004). Furthermore, genetics can play a pivotal role since approximately 40% of people with idiopathic or symptomatic epilepsies exhibit some genetic predisposition (Gardiner 2000). Importantly, nearly all genes responsible for epileptogenesis encode subunits of voltage- and ligand-gated ion channels, the majority of which can lead to channelopathies or alterations in excitatory or inhibitory neurotransmission in the CNS (reviewed in Berkovic et al. 2006; Graves 2006; Rees 2010).

30.1.3 Classification of seizures and epilepsy

Numerous seizures, epilepsies, and epileptic syndromes have been proposed in recent decades and were largely phenomenological since insufficient knowledge existed to permit a more scientific categorization. In 2010, the International League Against Epilepsy (ILAE) produced a detailed classification which will be utilized throughout the remainder of this chapter and is very briefly described here. Two broad categories of seizure have been described. Firstly, generalized seizures in which epileptiform activity originates at a specific point within the brain but rapidly distributes across the brain to affect both hemispheres. Generalized seizures can be further subdivided into three categories: (1) genetic (encompassing epilepsies with a known genetic component), (2) structural/metabolic (arising from a known structural or functional abnormality and may be acquired (e.g. structural lesion via trauma) or be of genetic origin (e.g. tuberous sclerosis complex causing nonmalignant brain tumors)), and (3) unknown (arising from an as yet unidentified genetic defect or from another undiagnosed disorder). The second broad ILAE category is focal seizures in which epileptiform activity is restricted to a discrete region of the brain or a single hemisphere. No formal subcategorization exists here, but instead a more descriptive series of categories are utilized that better describe exhibited clinical symptoms (e.g. "with/without consciousness").

30.1.4 Current pharmacological treatment

In the UK, there are now more than 20 antiepileptic drugs (AEDs) licensed for used (Kelso 2010; Martin 2013). The initial therapeutic strategy for the management of seizures typically involves prescription of a single drug ("monotherapy"; Kwan and Brodie 2000b). Approximately 50% of patients achieve remission with their first prescribed AED (Stephen and Brodie 2009) and, if this first-line treatment fails, a further 10% of patients achieve seizure control when prescribed a different AED (Kwan and Brodie 2000a; Schachter 2007). However, despite these apparently high success rates with current treatments, not only do approximately 30% of the epileptic population experience intractable seizures regardless of AED treatments used, but of all patients with epilepsy, approximately 50% will ultimately become refractory to drug treatment (Kwan and Brodie 2000a, 2007; Sander 1993). Notably, all existing AEDs are associated with numerous side effects which often negatively interact with epilepsy's comorbidities (e.g. emotional lability, cognitive dysfunction, impairment of motor function, etc.; Martin 2013). Therefore, there is still a significant clinical need for the development of new, more effective, and better tolerated AEDs and, whilst well known for the recreational exploitation of its psychoactive effects (see Curran and Morgan, Chapter 36, this volume), the extent to which cannabis's pharmacological effects and tolerability might affect its utility as an anticonvulsant are considered hereafter.

30.2 Use of cannabis in the treatment of seizures and epilepsy

Anecdotally, cannabis has been used for seizure control for many thousands of years. However, scientific evidence supporting this assertion was not presented until William O'Shaughnessy's 1840 publication describing the successful treatment of seizures in an infant by using a cannabis tincture (O'Shaughnessy 1840). Furthermore, in 1890, Queen Victoria's personal physician, J. R. Reynolds, went as far as to describe cannabis as "the most useful agent with which I am acquainted" in the treatment of "attacks or violent convulsions . . . (which) may recur two or three times in the hour . . . may be stopped with a full dose of hemp" (Reynolds 1868). In this section, we summarize the effects upon seizures either of whole cannabis herb (or extracts thereof) followed by descriptions of the effects of isolated, individual phytocannabinoids on seizures. Caution should be exercised in interpreting data obtained with herbal cannabis or unstandardized extracts since, given the diverse, emerging pharmacology of the plant cannabinoids, composition could significantly affect therapeutic effect. (For more on the composition of the herb see ElSohly and Gul, Chapter 1, this volume. For more on the molecular pharmacology of plant cannabinoids see Pertwee and Cascio, Chapter 6, and Cascio and Pertwee, Chapter 7, this volume).

30.2.1 Anticonvulsant effects of whole cannabis

At the time of writing, no full-scale clinical trials have yet been undertaken using either cannabis or cannabis extracts and so evidence of cannabis effects upon seizures comprises a small collection of individual case studies and the results of surveys of people with epilepsy who are also cannabis users. Whilst caution should be exercised if attempting to generalize effects from isolated cases or surveys whose recruitment may be subject to positive bias, a summary of the extant evidence follows.

In 1967, a single case was published detailing a proconvulsant effect of cannabis in which an epileptic patient receiving conventional anticonvulsant medication was seizure-free until engaging in a period of cannabis use during which his seizure symptoms returned (Keeler and Riefler 1967). Similarly, a 29-year-old male, diagnosed with bipolar disorder and alcoholism and admitting to chronic, daily cannabis use, reported onset of complex partial seizures following abrupt cessation of his cannabis use (Ellison et al. 1990). In contrast, Consroe et al. (1975) document the case of a 24-year-old epileptic who, in addition to receiving regularly prescribed doses of phenobarbital (30 mg four times a day) and phenytoin (100 mg four times a day), required two to five cannabis cigarettes each day to remain seizure-free (Consroe et al. 1975). Moreover, an adult cerebral palsy patient described a "marked improvement" in seizure control following cannabis use (Mortati et al. 2007).

More recently, in 1997, a critical review of the earlier-mentioned evidence also presented two new qualitative reports of successful seizure treatment with cannabis (Grinspoon and Bakalar 1997). Here, the first patient found that cannabis smoking abolished petit mal seizures previously resistant to conventional AEDs. The second patient not only reported that cannabis fully abolished his grand mal seizures and halved the incidence of petit mal seizures but permitted a reduction in the dose of conventional AED used for seizure control. Moreover and in the same year, a further 11 epileptic patients were identified as applicants to the US Compassionate Use Investigational New Drug Program that grants legal, medical exemption from prosecution for cannabis possession and use (Petro 1997).

Most recently, Hegde et al. (2012) described focal epilepsy patients whose seizures were exacerbated by cessation of cannabis consumption. In the first case, a man (43 years old) with sleep seizures (~20 per night) from 2 years old, resistant to levetiracetam and phenytoin but reduced (five to six per night) by carbamazepine, began smoking marijuana (~40 mg *Cannabis sativa* each night) and saw seizure frequency fall to one to two seizures per night. Stopping cannabis use on admission to hospital resulted in ten seizures per night which was reduced to one seizure when he consumed (orally) cannabis provided by his spouse. In the second case, a 60-year-old man with a 40-year history of marijuana smoking presented with seizure-related amnestic episodes, ceased cannabis use on admission to hospital and, within 24 h, entered status epilepticus (a persistent state of seizure) that was stopped using lorazepam and valproate. The patient ultimately discharged himself and experienced intermittent seizures partly refractory to phenytoin and continued his earlier marijuana use. Interestingly, Hegde et al. (2012) make the argument that the widespread but often intermittent use of marijuana suggests that the appearance of seizures in these individuals reflects an anticonvulsant effect of marijuana and not part of a withdrawal phenomenon.

Whilst no firm conclusions can be drawn from this small number of case studies, particularly given the diverse concomitant drug and disease states they comprise and the highly variable composition of the cannabis used, the larger number of patients reporting beneficial effects certainly justified the larger-scale survey-based studies that have been undertaken.

A detailed review of the literature in 1976 highlighted that cannabis effects upon seizure were inconclusive despite, as mentioned earlier, the majority of papers describing an attenuation of seizure activity (Feeney et al. 1976). On the basis of this review, Feeney (1978) conducted a small survey (~300 "youthful" respondents) to reveal that approximately 30% of epileptic patients smoked cannabis with no reported effect upon their seizure patterns, although one claimed that cannabis decreased his symptoms whilst another reported that it "caused his seizures" (Feeney 1978). Furthermore, a retrospective survey of 49 patients (28 male, 19 female) presenting at a San Francisco Emergency Department with "recreational drug-induced [generalized tonic–clonic] seizures" on admission revealed cannabis use in 10% of cases although, in all cases, other drugs had also been consumed (cocaine, amphetamine, or LSD) at or around the same time and all of which, alone, have been associated with seizures (Alldredge et al. 1989). However, a larger epidemiological survey of, in this case, previous heroin, marijuana, and cocaine use prior to presenting with first seizure (308 patients with seizures; 294 controls) in New York City between 1981 and 1984, revealed cannabis use as a protective factor against provoked and unprovoked first seizures in men (Brust et al. 1992; Ng et al. 1990). Finally, an interview-based study with more than 215 cannabis-using patients with active epilepsy not only showed that 90.2% of patients did not identify a relationship between cannabis use and their seizure frequency or severity but that 2.3% and 7.4% thought their seizures were more or less frequent around the time of cannabis use, respectively. Similar results were found in a telephone survey of patients treated at a tertiary care epilepsy center in Canada in 2004 where 68% of patients reported beneficial effects of cannabis upon seizure severity whilst 54% reported that cannabis reduced seizure frequency (Gross et al. 2004). Given the typically intractable nature of epilepsies referred to tertiary care centers, it is interesting to note the greater emphasis placed upon putatively beneficial effects by this patient population most resistant to conventional AEDs. Finally, in three more recent surveys, 3.6% of German medical marijuana users reported using cannabis for seizure control (Schnelle et al. 1999) whilst cannabis was used for seizure control by 4% of patients (population size: 77) supported by a medical cannabis program in the US (Corral 2001) and by 1% of patients (population size: ~2500) using medical cannabis in California, US (Gieringer 2001). Whilst this evidence clearly supports an overall anticonvulsant effect of cannabis in epilepsy, the labile nature of epilepsy, the variable composition of herbal cannabis, and its psychoactive effects argue against its widespread use beyond otherwise intractable cases.

30.2.2 Preclinical evidence of seizure-related effects of cannabis

Following on from the small number of case studies and surveys described in section 30.2.1, a variety of preclinical studies investigating the effects of cannabis upon seizure and epilepsy have been completed. In one of the earliest preclinical investigations, Ghosh and colleagues examined the effects of a cannabis resin (17% Δ^9-THC content; intraperitoneal (i.p.)), alone or in combination with a range of monoamine and catecholamine modulators (none of which affected seizure parameters alone), on maximal electroshock (MES) seizures in rats (Ghosh and Bhattacharya 1978). The MES model of generalized tonic–clonic seizures has been an important tool in the discovery of new potential AEDs for over 60 years due to its rapid throughput and clearly definable seizure endpoints although these advantages also represent limitations since it poorly discriminates between AEDs or the seizures against which a candidate AED might be effective (Bialer and White 2010; Löscher 2011; Mares and Kubova 2006; White 1997; White et al. 1995). In this model, tonic–clonic seizures are induced in healthy rodents by a brief electrical stimulation of the cornea (Löscher 2011; Mares and Kubova 2006; Swinyard 1949; Woodbury and Davenport 1952). Here, Ghosh et al. (1978) reported a monoamine involvement in the significant anticonvulsant effect of cannabis as indicated by the loss of this effect when it was coadministered with reserpine. Coadministration of 5-6-dihydroxytryptamine (DHT; selectively destroys serotonergic neurons) with cannabis, abolished the anticonvulsant effect of cannabis whilst its coadministration with 6-hydroxydopamine (6-HD; ablates adrenergic neurons) did not. Together these results suggest that the anticonvulsant effects of cannabis in MES seizures involve serotonergic signaling. However, it should be noted that the cannabinoid composition of the cannabis extract used—beyond the Δ^9-THC content assayed—was not presented such that it remains unclear which cannabinoid, noncannabinoid, or combination thereof was responsible for the serotonergically mediated anticonvulsant effect seen (Ghosh and Bhattacharya 1978).

Furthermore, Labrecque et al. (1978) examined acute and chronic effects of cannabis on seizures induced by subconvulsant penicillin (750,000 IU; intravenous (i.v.)) in mongrel dogs. Dogs "smoked" cannabis cigarettes containing 6 mg Δ^9-THC via a tracheotomy; either eight cigarettes for the acute condition or four cigarettes per day for 10 weeks in the chronic condition prior to penicillin treatment to induce seizures. In the acute condition, penicillin treatment did not produce any seizure behavior in control animals, but four out of five cannabis-treated dogs exhibited muscular jerks and one showed clonic movements. Electrocorticography (ECoG) recordings from this group showed characteristic arousal activity following application of an external stimulus that was replaced by epileptiform activity in the occipital cortex lasting 3–6 sec. In the chronic condition, penicillin treatment produced the appearance of similar epileptiform activity in both occipital and frontal cortices that was followed by generalization of the epileptiform activity and the appearance of grand mal seizures approximately 90 min after penicillin administration. The authors thus proposed that cannabis reduced the threshold for seizure, increased blood–brain barrier (BBB) permeability to penicillin, or the possibility of both contributing to the effects seen although their hypothesis of Δ^9-THC-induced changes to BBB permeability was not borne out in a study conducted around the same time (Segal et al. 1978).

Taken together, the results of these limited preclinical investigations indicate a propensity for cannabis to exert an anticonvulsant effect. However, when the highly variable and idiopathic nature of epilepsy is considered alongside the different phytocannabinoid compositions of the cannabis types used, the variable routes of administration, and the presence of complicating concomitant disease states and drugs, it is no surprise that a single conclusion regarding cannabis's effects on seizure cannot be drawn. However, in the next section we examine evidence from the more numerous preclinical investigations and small-scale clinical trials that have used individual phytocannabinoids.

30.2.3 Anticonvulsant effects of individual phytocannabinoid constituents

The identification and isolation of discrete constituents within cannabis have aided the investigation of their individual effects upon seizure. However, despite the numerous phytocannabinoids present in cannabis (for more on the constituents of cannabis please see ElSohly and Gul, Chapter 1, this volume), investigation of individual phytocannabinoid effects upon seizure remain limited to numerous studies of two of the phytocannabinoids that are usually present in smoked or heated cannabis, Δ^9-THC and cannabidiol (CBD), with a much smaller number examining, cannabinol (CBN), Δ^9-tetrahydrocannabivarin (Δ^9-THCV), and cannabidivarin (CBDV). Thus, whilst the evidence for these two principal cannabinoids and CBDV is strong, the large number of plant cannabinoids with unstudied effects on seizures represents as yet unrealized potential in drug discovery.

30.2.3.1 Tetrahydrocannabinol

One of the earliest reports from the 1940s documents that Δ^9-THC administration to a small sample of epileptic children (n = 5; orally (p.o.)) with seizures resistant to phenobarbital or phenytoin treatment, controlled seizures in two of the children although no change in seizure frequency was noted in the remaining three children (Davis et al. 1949). However, despite the promise of this preliminary finding, subsequent evidence of Δ^9-THC effects upon seizures remains limited to a number of preclinical animal studies undertaken during the 1970s and 1980s which are summarized hereafter.

Using an audiogenic seizure model, in which seizures in C57BL/6 mice are induced by a priming auditory stimulus at 19 days of age and then triggered by the same stimulus 9 days later, Δ^9-THC showed significant anticonvulsant activity (Boggan et al. 1973). Doses (i.p.) of between 2.5 and 10 mg/kg Δ^9-THC were administered 15 min prior to the seizure trigger and 10 mg/kg Δ^9-THC administered 15–45 min prior to the seizure trigger significantly reduced the number of animals exhibiting any signs of seizure. Interestingly, when treated with 10 mg/kg Δ^9-THC before the priming stimulus, only groups treated 15–45 min prior to priming showed significantly reduced seizure signs whilst Δ^9-THC administration after priming had no effect upon seizures.

Similar anticonvulsant effects have been reported using the MES model of seizure where Δ^9-THC (160–200 mg/kg) protected against hind limb extension in a QS strain of mice (Chesher and Jackson 1974) and led the authors to propose an ED_{50} of Δ^9-THC "for protection against convulsions after oral administration appears to be greater than 200 mg/kg." Interestingly, the authors also reveal administration route-dependent variation in effects since Δ^9-THC at 20 and 75 mg/kg p.o. significantly lengthened hind limb extension time, indicative of a proconvulsant effect, whilst 20 mg/kg Δ^9-THC i.v. significantly decreased hind limb extension time. This study also demonstrated that the effects of a "proconvulsant" dose of Δ^9-THC (50 mg/kg via oral gavage) could be reversed by coadministration with CBD plus CBN (both 50 mg/kg via oral gavage, doses previously shown to have no effect upon MES seizures alone; see later and Chapters 6 and 7 in this volume). Finally, this study also demonstrated a significantly reduced EC_{50} for phenytoin when coadministered with Δ^9-THC (50 mg/kg p.o.) that was even further reduced by coadministration of Δ^9-THC plus CBD (each 50 mg/kg p.o.). However, in generalized seizures induced by the administration of pentylenetetrazole (PTZ) to the same strain of mice, Δ^9-THC (1–80 mg/kg p.o. 30 min prior to seizure induction) had no significant effect.

Subsequent work by Chesher and colleagues investigated whether Δ^9-THC modulated phenobarbitone's anticonvulsant actions (Chesher et al. 1975). Here, and using the MES model of generalized seizure in QS mice, phenobarbitone (9.3–40 mg/kg; i.p.; 1 h prior to MES) was coadministered with Δ^9-THC (25–50 mg/kg) and CBD (see later; both drugs p.o. 2 h prior to MES). Δ^9-THC and CBD (each at 50 mg/kg) each significantly potentiated the beneficial effect of phenobarbitone on the presence and duration of hind limb extension although the greatest potentiation was produced by Δ^9-THC coadministration with phenobarbitone. Most notably, and in keeping with the synergism associated with phenytoin described earlier (Chesher and Jackson 1974), coadministration of Δ^9-THC plus CBD (each at 25 mg/kg) with phenobarbitone potentiated its effects to the same extent as that seen following the coadministration of phenobarbitone with 50 mg/kg Δ^9-THC only.

In a useful counterpoint to the investigation summarized earlier (Chesher and Jackson 1974), an important series of studies that compared phenobarbitone and phenytoin treatment, with Δ^9-THC and CBD (see later) treatments, in the maximal (MES), 6 Hz and 60 Hz electroshock models of generalized seizure were undertaken (Karler and Turkanis 1980). Here, animals received (all i.p.) 100 mg/kg Δ^9-THC, 120 mg/kg CBD, 9 mg/kg phenytoin, or 12 mg/kg phenobarbitone as a single dose or daily for 3–4 days. The study confirmed the anticonvulsant actions of single doses of Δ^9-THC and CBD in the 6 Hz and MES models and revealed CBD to be ineffective in the 60 Hz test whilst Δ^9-THC reduced threshold to seizure (a proconvulsant effect). Single treatments with phenytoin and phenobarbitone increased threshold to seizure in the 6 Hz and MES models although, in the 60 Hz model, this effect was not present for phenytoin. In the repeated dosing paradigm employed, tolerance to phenobarbitone appeared in the 6 Hz model but the effects of phenytoin, Δ^9-THC, and CBD were unaffected. Repeated drug treatment and use of the 60 Hz model were as seen following acute treatment except for phenytoin and phenobarbitone where increased and decreased thresholds respectively were seen. Interestingly, this study also investigated the effects of drug withdrawal after 3–4 days of administration where, in the 6 Hz model, Δ^9-THC withdrawal reduced seizure threshold, phenobarbitone and phenytoin withdrawal had no effect, whilst CBD withdrawal increased seizure thresholds. In the MES model, only phenobarbitone withdrawal decreased seizure threshold and no alterations were seen as a result of withdrawal of the other drugs used. Finally, in the 60 Hz model, Δ^9-THC and phenobarbitone withdrawal decreased threshold whilst CBD and phenytoin increased seizure threshold. Taken together, these results suggest that Δ^9-THC's anticonvulsant activity could be subject to some tolerance and withdrawal effects that are not replicated with CBD and so may reflect their differing pharmacology (Nocerino et al. 2000).

In a study that shed further light on this issue of tolerance, a spontaneously epileptic, adult gerbil strain (proposed to be a model of idiopathic human epilepsy; Loskota and Lomax 1975; Loskota et al. 1974) was employed to examine the effects of acute (single dose) and chronic (daily for 6 days) Δ^9-THC (20 or 50 mg/kg; i.p.) treatment upon seizure. Here, no significant effects were seen following acute or chronic 20 mg/kg Δ^9-THC treatment, although significant decreases in latency to seizure, duration of seizure, and seizure score were seen in animals acutely, but not chronically, treated with 50 mg/kg Δ^9-THC which could suggest a tolerance effect.

In a valuable study comparing the dose–response relationships of Δ^9-THC (up to 80 mg/kg; i.p.), phenytoin, chlordiazepoxide, and phenobarbitone upon MES-, PTZ-, nicotine-, and strychnine-induced seizures in mice (Sofia et al. 1974), the following results were reported. In MES seizures, Δ^9-THC markedly increased latency to hind limb extension, an effect mirrored by the three standard AED comparators used. In both strychnine- and PTZ-induced seizures, phenobarbitone and chlordiazepoxide exerted protective effects whilst neither phenytoin nor Δ^9-THC protected against these seizures. None of the tested compounds exerted any effect in the nicotine-induced seizure model used. The authors interpreted these effects as indicative of a specific anticonvulsant effect of phenytoin and Δ^9-THC which was in direct contrast to the generalized sedative-hypnotic, GABA-mediated actions underlying chlordiazepoxide and phenobarbitone effects in all bar one of the models used.

Whilst of dubious relevance given the uncertain etiology of the phenomenon studied, a study employing ECoG found that "polyspikes" (spike discharges induced by electrode implantation) in cortex, amygdala, and cerebellum but not hippocampus or thalamus were augmented by either acute or chronic (daily up to 140 days) 10 mg/kg p.o. Δ^9-THC (Stadnicki et al. 1974) although behavioral manifestation of seizure (jerking movement of head and paws) was seen in only one of the six treated animals. Furthermore, Δ^9-THC-induced convulsions were reported in a susceptible rabbit population (Martin and Consroe 1976) that exhibited a variety of seizure symptoms following Δ^9-THC treatments as low as 0.5 mg/kg i.v. which reduced in frequency and severity after repeated Δ^9-THC doses. The effect of a number of other plant cannabinoids (all i.v.) upon these animals was also examined (CBN (10 mg/kg), CBD (10–20 mg/kg), cannabichromene (CBC, 8 mg/kg), 11-OH-Δ^9-THC (0.5 mg/kg), and Δ^8-THC (0.5 mg/kg)) where THC forms and CBN produced similar convulsions but neither CBD nor CBC had any detectable effect. The effects of a number of conventional AEDs upon Δ^9-THC-induced (0.5 mg/kg; i.v.) convulsions in these animals were also investigated by this group (Consroe et al. 1977) where carbamazepine (EC_{50}: 2 mg/kg), diazepam (EC_{50}: 4.7 mg/kg), phenytoin (EC_{50}: 10.9 mg/kg), phenobarbital (EC_{50}: 56.9 mg/kg) and ethosuximide (EC_{50}: 306 mg/kg) inhibited seizures although the latter two drugs also produced toxic effects. Interestingly, CBD (EC_{50}: 19.7 mg/kg) inhibited these seizures but only when given prior to (c.f. concurrently) Δ^9-THC. Whilst these are very interesting reports, from a modern perspective, the lack of a defined basis for the rabbits' genetic susceptibility to Δ^9-THC-induced seizures prevents more widely generalizable conclusions from being drawn.

A number of other studies have been conducted that also used less conventional models of seizure or animal species. Two studies from the early 1970s used an electrical kindling model that targets the amygdala in cats to investigate potential antiepileptic and prophylactic actions of Δ^8-THC and Δ^9-THC (i.p.; Wada et al. 1975b). In the antiepileptic experiments, animals received Δ^8-THC or Δ^9-THC, 1 h before testing for effects upon onset of kindling, appearance of head nodding (stage 3), clonic jumping (stage 5), and at the endpoint of kindling which represents the establishment of a low-threshold generalized seizure trigger. Δ^9-THC (0.25 mg/kg), but not Δ^8-THC (0.25 mg/kg), inhibited epileptiform after-discharges at kindling onset but neither drug affected stages 3, 5, or the endpoint of kindling. In prophylaxis experiments, cats received Δ^8-THC and Δ^9-THC (i.p.; 0.5–2.5 mg/kg) daily during the kindling process (~15 days) and Δ^9-THC suppressed after-discharges at the start of kindling, effectively preventing the manifestation of spontaneous seizures although Δ^8-THC was ineffective. These results supported the assertion that Δ^9-THC effects upon seizure may be dependent upon disease progression in epilepsy.

Δ^8-THC and Δ^9-THC were also been investigated in the baboon, *Papio papio*, which exhibits a photomyoclonic response and is also susceptible to amygdaloid kindling (Wada et al. 1975a). Neither drug (each 0.25–1 mg/kg; i.p.) affected photomyclonus but both either abolished or reduced kindled seizures and inhibited epileptiform after-discharge spread; Δ^9-THC appeared to exert greater potency than Δ^8-THC. Finally, Δ^9-THC effects have been investigated in domestic chickens, some of which show a genetic susceptibility to seizure following intermittent photic stimulation (14 fps; IPS). Animals were divided into epileptic and non-epileptic groups based on IPS responsiveness and the effects of Δ^9-THC (0.25–1 mg/kg; i.v.; 0.5 or 2 h before testing) upon IPS-induced seizures (in susceptible fowl) plus PTZ-induced (i.p.) seizures in epileptic (35 mg/kg) and non-epileptic (80 mg/kg) fowl were examined (Johnson et al. 1975). Δ^9-THC (>0.25 mg/kg at 0.5 but not 2 h) significantly reduced IPS-induced seizure number and severity in epileptic fowl yet Δ^9-THC exerted no effect on PTZ-induced seizures in either population at any dose.

30.2.3.2 Cannabidiol

At the time of writing, CBD remains the only isolated, non-Δ^9-THC phytocannabinoid to have been investigated for anticonvulsant effects preclinically and clinically. Please note that some of the studies describing CBD effects upon seizure have already been summarized (section 30.2.3.1) where direct comparisons between Δ^9-THC and CBD were made; these studies will not be described again.

One of the earliest documented investigations of CBD (1.5–12 mg/kg; i.p.) effects against seizure reported significant effects in the MES model when tested 1 h after administration (Izquierdo et al. 1973) although, in a separate investigation, CBD (150 mg/kg and 50–200 mg/kg p.o.) failed to affect PTZ-induced generalized seizures or MES, respectively, in mice (Chesher and Jackson 1974). It remains uncertain whether the lack of CBD effect shown in these studies was due to inadequate CBD at the site of action or a lack of action per se. The first major study that compared the anticonvulsant effects of CBD and Δ^9-THC, in addition to a range of other cannabinoids, with the effects of phenytoin, phenobarbitone and ethosuximide in a variety of standard seizure models was undertaken by Karler and Turkanis (1978). Using the standard MES test in mice, the following cannabinoids (i.p.) showed significant anticonvulsant activity (ED_{50} values (or best estimates of these indicated by *) are shown in parentheses): CBD (120 mg/kg), Δ^9-THC (100 mg/kg), 11-OH-Δ^9-THC (14 mg/kg), 8β-, but not 8α-OH-Δ^9-THC (100 mg/kg*), Δ^9-THC acid (200–400 mg/kg), Δ^8-THC (80 mg/kg), CBN (230 mg/kg) and 9-nor-9α- or 9-nor-9β-OH-hexahydro CBN (each 100 mg/kg). This group's subsequent work showed that CBD (0.3–3 mg/kg) raised electrophysiologically recorded, epileptic after-discharge threshold in electrically kindled, limbic seizures in rats, like phenytoin but, in common with ethosuximide's effects in this model, reduced after-discharge amplitude, duration, and propagation (Turkanis et al. 1979). Notably, the authors concluded that "CBD was the most efficacious of the drugs tested against limbic ADs [after-discharges] and convulsions."

Despite the wealth of literature in support of clear anticonvulsant actions of CBD in several acute chemical models, the literature is somewhat less convincing when considering the effects of this drug in models of chronically epileptic animals. Colasanti et al. (1982) used cortical implantation of cobalt to produce a model of focal seizure with a secondary generalization and showed that 60 mg/kg CBD (i.p.) exerted no discernible effect although Δ^9-THC exerted a short-term (~1 day) anticonvulsant effect (Colasanti et al. 1982). It is noteworthy that cobalt-induced seizures share many common features with human absence seizures (Löscher 1997) and so have very little in common with the seizure models in which CBD exerts a significant anticonvulsant effect or the epilepsies in which it has been proposed to have potential clinical utility (Karler and Turkanis 1978). Such model-specific effects of CBD have also been shown by Consroe et al. (1982) where a battery of acute seizure models that included MES, 3-mercaptoproprionic acid, picrotoxin, isonicotinic acid hydrazine, bicuculline, PTZ, and strychnine-induced seizures were used. Here,

CBD (i.p.; 50–400 mg/kg) was effective as an anticonvulsant in the MES and all of the GABA inhibition-based models, but was entirely ineffective against strychnine-induced convulsions (Consroe et al. 1982).

Work from our own laboratory has shown significant antiepileptiform and anticonvulsant activity using a variety of in vitro and in vivo models (Jones et al. 2010, 2012). Using our in vitro models, spontaneous epileptiform local field potentials (LFPs) were induced, by omission of Mg^{2+} ions from, or addition of the K^+ channel blocker, 4-aminopyridine (4-AP) to the bathing solution, in acute, transverse hippocampal brain slices. In the Mg^{2+}-free model, CBD (100 µM) decreased epileptiform LFP burst amplitude and duration, whilst in the 4-AP model, CBD (100 µM) decreased LFP burst amplitude in one hippocampal region only but decreased burst duration in CA3 and dentate gyrus, and burst frequency in all regions; CBD exerted no effect upon propagation of epileptiform activity. Subsequently, we examined the anticonvulsant actions of 1, 10, and 100 mg/kg CBD (i.p., 60 min prior to convulsant challenge) in three different in vivo seizure models using Wistar Kyoto rats. In the PTZ-induced acute, generalized seizures model, 100 mg/kg CBD significantly decreased mortality and the incidence of tonic–clonic seizures (Jones et al. 2010), whilst in the acute pilocarpine model of temporal lobe seizures all doses of CBD significantly reduced the percentage of animals experiencing the most severe seizures (Jones et al. 2012). Finally, in the penicillin model of partial seizures, 10 and 100 mg/kg CBD significantly decreased the percentage of animals dying as a result of seizures and all doses of CBD also decreased the percentage of animals experiencing the most severe tonic–clonic seizures (Jones et al. 2012).

In the clinical setting, one of the first published studies documenting an anticonvulsant CBD effect was published in the early 1980s. Here, a small group of 15 patients who experienced drug-resistant partial seizures with secondary generalization received either 200–300 mg CBD or placebo daily for 4.5 months as an adjunct to their existing treatment regimen (Carlini and Cunha 1981; Cunha et al. 1980). Of the eight CBD-treated patients, four exhibited no sign of seizure at the end of the treatment period, one patient "improved markedly," one patient "improved somewhat," one showed no improvement, and one withdrew from the study. In comparison, only one of the seven patients treated with placebo showed "a little improvement" whilst the remaining six showed no change and led the authors to conclude that CBD could be of benefit to patients with secondary generalized epilepsy for whom existing medicines were ineffective. Similarly beneficial results were also found following a 10-month treatment period with doses of 900–1200 mg/day CBD (Trembly et al. 1990). However, not all clinical results have been consistent since Ames and colleagues treated 12 epileptic patients with 200–300 mg/day CBD as an adjunct to their existing treatment regimen but no change to seizure incidence was found (Ames and Cridland 1986).

30.2.3.3 Cannabidivarin

CBDV, the propyl variant of CBD, has also been reported to show significant anticonvulsant properties. Whilst only a single report has been published to date (Hill et al. 2012), the results span two in vitro models, four in vivo models of seizure, and tolerability testing which, taken together, represent a body of evidence warranting summary and comment.

Using the same in vitro models of epileptiform activity described earlier (Jones et al. 2010), CBDV significantly attenuated status epilepticus-like epileptiform LFPs at concentrations ≥10 µM in both Mg^{2+}-free and 4-AP models. In the MES model using ICR mice, 100–200 mg/kg CBDV (i.p; 60 min prior to convulsant stimulus) significantly reduced tonic hind limb extension and abolished all seizure-related deaths whilst also reducing tonic convulsions (50–200 mg/kg) and increasing the number of animals remaining seizure-free (200 mg/kg). Similar effects were seen in the PTZ model of acute generalized seizures using adult Wistar rats, where CBDV (50–200 mg/kg; i.p; 60 min prior to convulsant administration) significantly reduced seizure severity, mortality and increased the number of animals remaining seizure-free. Additional experiments using the PTZ model in which CBDV (200 mg/kg) was coadministered with either of the conventional AEDs, sodium valproate or ethosuximide, revealed that CBDV was well tolerated and, importantly, acted additively to demonstrate retention of its own anticonvulsant actions. Further experiments using the PTZ model showed that CBDV produced anticonvulsant effects when administered orally. Thus, 400 mg/kg CBDV administered by gavage 3.5 h prior to PTZ challenge significantly reduced seizure severity.

Conversely, no anticonvulsant actions of CBDV were evident in the acute, pilocarpine-induced model of temporal lobe seizures/status epilepticus; CBDV (50–200 mg/kg; i.p.; 60 min before convulsant administration) in adult Wistar rats failed to exert any statistically significant effects upon any seizure parameter measured. However, when CBDV (200 mg/kg) was coadministered with either of the conventional AEDs, sodium valproate, or phenobarbitone, in this model, CBDV itself exerted significant anticonvulsant actions, most likely as a result of the larger group sizes employed in an experimental design of this type. Importantly, CBDV acted synergistically with phenobarbitone to produce a very significant reduction in seizure behaviors.

Since little is known about the pharmacology of CBDV, it is difficult to ascribe a potential mechanism to explain these anticonvulsant actions with any confidence. However, the few studies that have investigated its pharmacology present some intriguing possibilities that require further elucidation over the coming years. Firstly, CBDV may act through transient receptor potential (TRP) channels with agonistic actions at hTRPA1, hTRPV1, and hTRPV2 channels (De Petrocellis et al. 2011, 2012), and antagonistic actions at TRPM8 channels (De Petrocellis et al. 2011) in transfected HEK-293 cells. However, not only does the role of TRP channels in epilepsy remain to be elucidated, the physiological relevance of the concentrations at which CBDV exerts these TRP channel effects remains to be demonstrated and so prevents any meaningful interpretation of putative activity at these channels. Additionally, CBDV inhibits diacylglycerol lipase-α, the primary synthetic enzyme of 2-arachidonoylglycerol in vitro (De Petrocellis et al. 2011), but, again, no role for diacylglycerol lipase-α in epilepsy has been established.

30.2.3.4 Other phytocannabinoids

Many different phytocannabinoids have been identified in cannabis (Elsohly and Slade 2005), but relatively few have undergone significant preclinical and clinical testing for their anticonvulsant actions. In this final section we briefly review the few reports that do exist which describe the effects of some of the less abundantly occurring minor cannabinoids upon seizures.

Δ^9-THCV is a propyl analogue of Δ^9-THC (Mechoulam 2005) but is an antagonist at CB_1 (Dennis et al. 2008; Thomas et al. 2005). A single study from our laboratory (Hill et al. 2010) showed that Δ^9-THCV produces significant antiepileptiform activity reducing burst incidence, amplitude, and frequency in the Mg^{2+}-free model of epileptiform activity at concentrations >20 µM. In vivo, limited anticonvulsant actions were seen at 0.25 mg/kg i.p. Δ^9-THCV which significantly reduced seizure incidence in the PTZ model of acute generalized seizures although no other measures were significantly affected.

In an investigation that also examined CBD and Δ^9-THC effects (see section 30.2.3.1 for experimental details), CBN (150 mg/kg and 50–200 mg/kg; oral gavage) had no significant effect upon chemically or electrically induced seizures respectively in mice (Chesher and Jackson 1974). CBC was also examined in the study described previously (Karler et al. 1978), although the anticonvulsant effect reported therein was tempered by the authors' observation that this effect occurred at higher doses consistent with the known toxicity of CBC and, as such, this was unlikely to be a true anticonvulsant effect.

30.3 **Summary**

The clinical evidence presented here supports the generalization that cannabis exerts an anti-convulsant effect, and rarely acts as a proconvulsant, but remains reliant on a limited and often subjective evidence base. Our limited understanding of the molecular basis for the epilepsies, the compositional variability of cannabis used, variable routes of administration, concomitant use of prescription and illicit drugs, and relevant comorbidities hinder more definitive clinical conclusions. Moreover, the psychotropic effects of Δ^9-THC will limit or prohibit widespread therapeutic use, particularly in epilepsy where regular, repeated dosing is necessary for the life of the patient. However, not only do all licensed AEDs exert significant motor and or cognitive side effects (Fisher 2012) but many epilepsy patients cannot drive or maintain employment because of drug side effects, poorly controlled seizures, or a combination of the two (Besag 2001); circumstances that might lessen concerns about Δ^9-THC's psychoactivity, particularly given its use as a licensed medicine since the early 1980s.

Conversely, CBD not only represents the most widely investigated phytocannabinoid after Δ^9-THC but, compared with Δ^9-THC, is more reliably anticonvulsant, exhibiting clinically beneficial effects in epileptic children resistant to antiepileptic medications. Moreover, in contrast to licensed AEDs, CBD was well tolerated in pediatric subjects and has not exhibited neurotoxic or motor side effects (Consroe et al. 1981; Jones et al. 2012; Martin et al. 1987). However, it is notable that repeated-dosing studies of CBD have not been undertaken in spontaneously epileptic animal disease models which are a crucial requirement for the assessment of any compound's potential for translation to clinical assessment. CBDV, CBD's naturally occurring propyl derivative, may display greater efficacy than CBD although direct comparison using a range of animal models or, ideally, in a human clinical trial, is required to categorically demonstrate this. In view of the broad anticonvulsant effects and well-tolerated nature of both drugs, such studies are clearly warranted given the unmet clinical need that has characterized epilepsy for so long.

References

Alldredge, B.K., Lowenstein, D.H., and Simon, R.P. (1989). Seizures associated with recreational drug abuse. *Neurology*, **39**(8), 1037–1039.

Ames, F.R. and Cridland, S. (1986). Anticonvulsant effect of cannabidiol. *South African Medical Journal*, **69**(1), 14.

Banerjee, P.N. and Hauser, A.W. (2008). Incidence and prevalence. In: J. Engel and T.A. Pedley (eds.). *Epilepsy: A Comprehensive Textbook*. 2nd ed. Philadelphia, PA: Lippincott Williams & Wilkins.

Berkovic, S.F., Mulley, J.C., Scheffer, I.E., and Petrou, S. (2006). Human epilepsies: interaction of genetic and acquired factors. *Trends in Neurosciences*, **29**, 391–397.

Besag, F.M. (2001). Behavioural effects of the new anticonvulsants. *Drug Safety*, **24**(7), 513–536.

Bialer, M. and White, H.S. (2010). Key factors in the discovery and development of new antiepileptic drugs. *Nature Reviews Drug Discovery*, **9**, 68–82.

Boggan, W.O., Steele, R.A., and Freedman, D.X. (1973). 9 -Tetrahydrocannabinol effect on audiogenic seizure susceptibility. *Psychopharmacologia*, **29**(2), 101–106.

Brust, J.C., Ng, S.K., Hauser, A.W., and Susser, M. (1992). Marijuana use and the risk of new onset seizures. *Transactions of American Clinical Association*, **103**, 176–181.

Carlini, E.A. and Cunha, J.M. (1981). Hypnotic and antiepileptic effects of cannabidiol. *Journal of Clinical Pharmacology*, **21**(8–9 Suppl), 417S–427S.

Carpio, A. (2002). Neurocysticercosis: an update. *The Lancet Infectious Diseases*, **2**, 751–762.

Carter, J.A., Neville, B.G.R., White, S., *et al.* (2004). Increased prevalence of epilepsy associated with severe falciparum malaria in children. *Epilepsia*, **45**, 978–981.

Chang, B.S. and Lowenstein, D.H. (2003). Mechanisms of disease: epilepsy. *New England Journal of Medicine*, **349**, 1257–1266.

Chesher, G.B. and Jackson, D.M. (1974). Anticonvulsant effects of cannabinoids in mice: drug interactions within cannabinoids and cannabinoid interactions with phenytoin. *Psychopharmacologia*, **37**(3), 255–264.

Chesher, G.B., Jackson, D.M., and Malor, R.M. (1975). Interaction of delta9-tetrahydrocannabinol and cannabidiol with phenobarbitone in protecting mice from electrically induced convulsions. *Journal of Pharmacy and Pharmacology*, **27**(8), 608–609.

Chesher, G.B., Jackson, D.M., and Starmer, G.A. (1974). Interaction of cannabis and general anaesthetic agents in mice. *British Journal of Pharmacology*, **50**(4), 593–599.

Chevassus-au-Louis, N., Baraban, S.C., Gaíarsa, J.L., and Ben-Ari, Y. (1999). Cortical malformations and epilepsy: new insights from animal models. *Epilepsia*, **40**, 811–821.

Cloyd, J., Hauser, W., Towne, A., *et al.* (2006). Epidemiological and medical aspects of epilepsy in the elderly. *Epilepsy Research*, **68**, 39–48.

Colasanti, B.K., Lindamood, C., and Craig, C.R. (1982). Effects of marihuana cannabinoids on seizure activity in cobalt-epileptic rats. *Pharmacology and Biochemistry of Behaviou*, **16**(4), 573–578.

Consroe, P., Benedito, M.A., Leite, J.R., Carlini, E.A., and Mechoulam, R. (1982). Effects of cannabidiol on behavioral seizures caused by convulsant drugs or current in mice. *European Journal of Pharmacology*, **83**(3–4), 293–298.

Consroe, P.F., Martin, P., and Eisenstein, D. (1977). Anticonvulsant drug antagonism of D9-tetrahydrocannabinol-induced seizures in rabbits *Research Communications in Chemical Pathology and Pharmacology*, **16**(1), 1–13.

Consroe, P.F., Wood, G.C., and Buchsbaum, H. (1975). Anticonvulsant nature of marihuana smoking. *Journal of the American Medical Association*, **234**(3), 306–307.

Corral, V. (2001). Differential effects of medical marijuana based on strain and route of administration: a three-year observational study. *Journal of Cannabis Therapeutics*, **1**(3), 43–59.

Cunha, J.M., Carlini, E.A., Pereira, A.E., *et al.* (1980). Chronic administration of cannabidiol to healthy volunteers and epileptic patients. *Pharmacology*, **21**(3), 175–185.

De Boer, H.M., Mula, M., and Sander, J.W. (2008). The global burden and stigma of epilepsy. *Epilepsy and Behavior*, **12**, 540–546.

De Petrocellis, L., Ligresti, A., Moriello, A.S., *et al.* (2011). Effects of cannabinoids and cannabinoid-enriched cannabis extracts on TRP channels and endocannabinoid metabolic enzymes. *British Journal of Pharmacology*, **163**, 1479–1494.

De Petrocellis, L., Orlando, P., Moriello, A.S., *et al.* (2012). Cannabinoid actions at TRPV channels: effects on TRPV3 and TRPV4 and their potential relevance to gastrointestinal inflammation. *Acta Physiology (Oxford)*, **204**(2), 255–266.

Dennis, I., Whalley, B.J., and Stephens, G.J. (2008). Effects of Delta9-tetrahydrocannabivarin on [^{35}S] GTPgammaS binding in mouse brain cerebellum and piriform cortex membranes. *British Journal of Pharmacology*, **154**(6), 1349–1358.

Duncan, J.S., Sander, J.W., Sisodiya, S.M., and Walker, M.C. (2006). Adult epilepsy. *The Lancet*, **367**, 1087–1100.

Ellison, J.M., Gelwan, E., and Ogletree, J. (1990). Complex partial seizure symptoms affected by marijuana abuse. *Journal of Clinical Psychiatry*, **51**(10), 439–440.

Elsohly, M.A. and Slade, D. (2005). Chemical constituents of marijuana: the complex mixture of natural cannabinoids. *Life Sciences*, **78**(5), 539–548.

Engel, J. and Pedley, T.A. (2008). Introduction: what is epilepsy? In: J. Engel and T.A. Pedley (eds.). *Epilepsy: A Comprehensive Textbook*. 2nd ed. Philadelphia, PA: Lippincott Williams & Wilkins.

Farrell, M.A., Blümcke, I., Khanlou, N., and Vinters, H.V. (2008). General neuropathology of epilepsy. In: J. Engel and T.A. Pedley (eds.). *Epilepsy: A Comprehensive Textbook*. 2nd ed. Philadelphia, PA: Lippincott Williams & Wilkins.

Feeney, D.M. (1976). Letter: marihuana use among epileptics. *Journal of the American Medical Association*, **235**(11), 1105.

Feeney, D.M. (1978). Marihuana and epilepsy: paradoxical anticonvulsant and convulsant effects. *Advances in Biosciences*, 22–23, 643–657.

Fisher, R.S., Boas, W.V.E., Blume, W., *et al.* (2005). Epileptic seizures and epilepsy: Definitions proposed by the International League Against Epilepsy (ILAE) and the International Bureau for Epilepsy (IBE). *Epilepsia*, **46**, 470–472.

Fisher, R.S. (2012). *Summary of Antiepileptic Drugs*. [Online]. Available at: http://www.epilepsy.com/epilepsy/newsletter/sept09/aeds (accessed May 2, 2012).

Forsgren, L., Beghi, E., Õun, A., and Sillanpää, M. (2005). The epidemiology of epilepsy in Europe – a systematic review. *European Journal of Neurology*, **12**, 245–253.

Gaitatzis, A., Carroll, K., Majeed, A., and Sander, J.W. (2004). The epidemiology of the comorbidity of epilepsy in the general population. *Epilepsia*, **45**, 1613–1622.

Gardiner, R.M. (2000). Impact of our understanding of the genetic aetiology of epilepsy. *Journal of Neurology*, **247**, 327–334.

Ghosh, P. and Bhattacharya, S.K. (1978). Anticonvulsant action of cannabis in the rat: role of brain monoamines. *Psychopharmacology (Berlin)*, **59**(3), 293–297.

Gieringer, D. (2001). Medical use of cannabis: experience in California. In: F. Grotenhermen and E. Russo (eds.). *Cannabis and Cannabinoids – Pharmacology, Toxicology and Therapeutic Potential*. New York: Haworth, pp. 153–170.

Graves, T.D. (2006). Ion channels and epilepsy. *Quarterly Journal of Medicine*, **99**, 201–217.

Grinspoon, L. and Bakalar, J.B. (1997). *Marihuana, the Forbidden Medicine*. New Haven, CT: Yale University Press.

Gross, D.W., Hamm, J., Ashworth, N.L., and Quigley, D. (2004). Marijuana use and epilepsy: prevalence in patients of a tertiary care epilepsy center. *Neurology*, **62**(11), 2095–2097.

Hegde, M., Santos-Sanchez, C., Hess, C.P., Kabir, A.A., and Garcia, P.A. (2012). Seizure exacerbation in two patients with focal epilepsy following marijuana cessation. *Epilepsy and Behavious*, **25**(4), 563–566.

Hill, A.J., Mercier, M.S., Hill, T.D., *et al.* (2012). Cannabidivarin is anticonvulsant in mouse and rat in vitro and in seizure models *British Journal of Pharmacology*, **167**(8), 1629–1642.

Hill, A.J., Weston, S.E., Jones, N.A., *et al.* (2010). Delta9-tetrahydrocannabivarin suppresses *in vitro* epileptiform and *in vivo* seizure activity in adult rats. *Epilepsia*, **51**(8), 1522–1532.

Izquierdo, I. and Tannhauser, M. (1973). Letter: the effect of cannabidiol on maximal electroshock seizures in rats. *Journal of Pharmacy and Pharmacology*, **25**(11), 916–917.

Johnson, D.D., McNeill, J.R., Crawford, R.D., and Wilcox, W.C. (1975). Epileptiform seizures in domestic fowl. V. The anticonvulsant activity of delta9-tetrahydrocannabinol. *Canadian Journal of Physiology and Pharmacology*, **53**(6), 1007–1013.

Jones, N.A., Hill, A.J., Smith, I., *et al.* (2010). Cannabidiol displays antiepileptiform and antiseizure properties in vitro and in vivo. *Journal of Pharmacology and Experimental Therapeutics*, **332**(2), 569–577.

Jones, N.A., Hill, A.J., Weston, S.E., *et al.* (2012). Cannabidiol exerts anti-convulsant effects in animal models of temporal lobe and partial seizures. *Seizure*, **21**(5), 344–352.

Karler, R. and Turkanis, S.A. (1978). Cannabis and epilepsy. *Advances in Biosciences*, 22–23, 619–641.

Karler, R. and Turkanis, S.A. (1980). Subacute cannabinoid treatment: anticonvulsant activity and withdrawal excitability in mice. *British Journal of Pharmacology*, **68**(3), 479–484.

Karler, R. and Turkanis, S.A. (1981). The cannabinoids as potential antiepileptics. *Journal of Clinical Pharmacology*, **21**(8–9 Suppl), 437S–448S.

Keeler, M.H. and Riefler, C.B. (1967). Grand mal convulsions subsequent to marijuana use. *Disorders of the Nervous System*, **28**, 474–475.

Kelso, A. (2010). The challenge of managing difficult-to-control epilepsy. *Prescriber*, **21**, 17–22.

Kwan, P. and Brodie, M.J. (2000a). Early identification of refractory epilepsy. *New England Journal of Medicine*, **342**, 314–319.

Kwan, P. and Brodie, M.J. (2000b). Epilepsy after the first drug fails: substitution or add-on? *Seizure*, **9**, 464–468.

Kwan, P. and Brodie, M.J. (2007). Emerging drugs for epilepsy. *Expert Opinion on Emerging Drugs*, **12**, 407–422.

Labrecque, G., Halle, S., Berthiaume, A., Morin, G., and Morin, P.J. (1978). Potentiation of the epileptogenic effect of penicillin G by marihuana smoking. *Canadian Journal of Physiology and Pharmacology*, **56**(1), 87–96.

Lhatoo, S.D. and Sander, J.W.A.S. (2001). The epidemiology of epilepsy and learning disability. *Epilepsia*, **42**, 6–9.

Löscher, W. (1997). Animal models of intractable epilepsy. *Progress in Neurobiology*, **53**(2), 239–258.

Löscher, W. (2011). Critical review of current animal models of seizures and epilepsy used in the discovery and development of new antiepileptic drugs. *Seizure*, **20**, 359–368.

Loskota, W.J. and Lomax, P. (1975). The Mongolian gerbil (*Meriones unguiculatus*) as a model for the study of the epilepsies: EEG records of seizures. *Electroencephalogrophy and Clinical Neurophysiology*, **38**(6), 597–604.

Loskota, W.J., Lomax, P., and Rich, S.T. (1974). The gerbil as a model for the study of the epilepsies. Seizure patterns and ontogenesis. *Epilepsia*, **15**(1), 109–119.

Lutz, B. (2004). On-demand activation of the endocannabinoid system in the control of neuronal excitability and epileptiform seizures. *Biochemistry and Pharmacology*, **68**(9), 1691–1698.

MacDonald, B.K., Cockerell, O.C., Sander, J.W.A.S, and Shorvon, S.D. (2000). The incidence and lifetime prevalence of neurological disorders in a prospective community-based study in the UK. *Brain*, **123**, 665–676.

Maguire, J.H. (2004). Tapeworms and seizures – treatment and prevention. *New England Journal of Medicine*, **350**, 215–217.

Mares, P. and Kubova, H. (2006). Electrical stimulation-induced models of seizures. In: A. Pitkanen, P.A. Schwartzkroin, and S.L. Moshe (eds.). *Models of Seizures and Epilepsy* Burlington, MA: Academic Press, pp. 153–159.

Martin, P. and Consroe, P. (1976). Cannabinoid induced behavioral convulsions in rabbits. *Science*, **194**(4268), 965–967.

Martin, J. (2013). *British National Formulary*. London: Pharmaceutical Press.

Mechoulam, R. (2005). Plant cannabinoids: a neglected pharmacological treasure trove. *British Journal of Pharmacology*, **146**(7), 913–915.

Mortati, K., Dworetzky, B., and Devinsky, O. (2007). Marijuana: an effective antiepileptic treatment in partial epilepsy? A case report and review of the literature. *Review of Neurological Disorders*, **4**(2), 103–106.

Ng, S.K., Brust, J.C., Hauser, W.A., and Susser, M. (1990). Illicit drug use and the risk of new-onset seizures. *American Journal of Epidemiology*, **132**(1), 47–57.

Ngoungou, E.B. and Preux, P.M. (2008). Cerebral malaria and epilepsy. *Epilepsia*, **49**, 19–24.

Nocerino, E., Amato, M., and Izzo, A.A. (2000). Cannabis and cannabinoid receptors. *Fitoterapia*, **71**(Suppl 1), S6–12.

O'Shaughnessy, W.B. (1840). On the preparations of the Indian hemp, or gunjah (*Cannabis indica*). *Transactions of the Medical and Physical Society of Bengal*, 71–102.

Petro, D.J. (1997). *Seizure Disorders*. Jefferson, NC: McFarland and Co.

Pitkänen, A. and Lukasiuk, K. (2011). Mechanisms of epileptogenesis and potential treatment targets. *The Lancet Neurology*, **10**, 173–186.

Ramsay, H.H. (1949). Antiepileptic action of marijuana-active substances. *Federal Proceedings of the American Society for Experimental Biology Baltimore*, **8**, 284–285.

Rees, M.I. (2010). The genetics of epilepsy – the past, the present and future. *Seizure*, **19**, 680–683.

Reynolds, J.R. (1868). Therapeutical uses and toxic effects of *Cannabis indica*. *Lancet*, **1**, 637–638.

Sander, J.W. (1993). Some aspects of prognosis in the epilepsies: a review. *Epilepsia*, **34**, 1007–1016.

Sander, J.W. (2003). The epidemiology of epilepsy revisited. *Current Opinion in Neurology*, **16**, 165–170.

Sander, J.W. (2004). Infectious agents and epilepsy. In: S. Knobler, S. O'Connor, S.M. Lemon, and M. Najafi (eds.). *The Infectious Etiology of Chronic Diseases: Defining the Relationship, Enhancing the Research and Mitigating the Effects*. Washington, DC: National Academies Press, pp. 93–99.

Sander, J.W. and Shorvon, S.D. (1996). Epidemiology of the epilepsies. *Journal of Neurology, Neurosurgery, and Psychiatry*, **61**, 433–443.

Schachter, S.C. (2007). Currently available antiepileptic drugs. *Neurotherapeutics* **4**, 4–11.

Schnelle, M., Grotenhermen, F., Reif, M., and Gorter, R.W. (1999). [Results of a standardized survey on the medical use of cannabis products in the German-speaking area]. *Forsch Komplementarmed*, **6**(Suppl 3), 28–36.

Segal, M., Edelstein, E.L., and Lerer, B. (1978). Interaction between delta-6-tetrahydrocannabinol (delta-6-THC) and lithium at the blood brain barrier in rats. *Experientia*, **34**(5), 629.

Seidenberg, M., Beck, N., Geisser, M., *et al.* (1986). Academic achievement of children with epilepsy. *Epilepsia*, **27**, 753–759.

Siemens, A.J., Kalant, H., Khanna, J.M., Marshman, J., and Ho, G. (1974). Effect of cannabis on pentobarbital-induced sleeping time and pentobarbital metabolism in the rat. *Biochemistry and Pharmacology*, **23**(3), 477–488.

Sisodiya, S.M. (2004). Malformations of cortical development: burdens and insights from important causes of human epilepsy. *The Lancet Neurology*, **3**, 29–38.

Sofia, R.D., Kubena, R.K., and Barry, H. 3rd. (1974). Comparison among four vehicles and four routes for administering delta9-tetrahydrocannabinol. *Journal of Pharmaceutical Sciences*, **63**(6), 939–941.

Stadnicki, S.W., Schaeppi, U., Rosenkrantz, H., and Braude, M.C. (1974). Delta9-tetrahydrocannabinol: subcortical spike bursts and motor manifestations in a Fischer rat treated orally for 109 days. *Life Sciences*, **14**(3), 463–472.

Steinhäuser, C. and Seifert, G. (2002). Glial membrane channels and receptors in epilepsy: impact for generation and spread of seizure activity. *European Journal of Pharmacology*, **447**, 227–237.

Stephen, L.J. and Brodie, M.J. (2009). Selection of antiepileptic drugs in adults. *Neurologic Clinics*, **27**, 967–992.

Swinyard, E.A. (1949). Laboratory assay of clinically effective antiepileptic drugs. *Journal of the American Pharmaceutical Association*, **38**, 201–204.

Téllez-Zenteno, J.F., Patten, S.B., Jetté, N., Williams, J., and Wiebe, S. (2007). Psychiatric comorbidity in epilepsy: a population-based analysis. *Epilepsia*, **48**, 2336–2344.

Thomas, A., Stevenson, L.A., Wease, K.N., *et al.* (2005). Evidence that the plant cannabinoid Delta(9)-tetrahydrocannabivarin is a cannabinoid CB_1 and CB_2 receptor antagonist. *British Journal of Pharmacology*, **146**(7), 917–926.

Trembly, B. and Sherman, M. (1990). Double-blind clinical study of cannabidiol as a secondary anticonvulsant. In: *Marijuana '90 International Conference on Cannabis and Cannabinoids*, July 8–11, Kolympari, Crete.

Turkanis, S.A., Cely, W., Olsen, D.M., and Karler, R. (1974). Anticonvulsant properties of cannabidiol. *Research Communications in Chemical Pathology and Pharmacology*, **8**(2), 231–246.

Turkanis, S.A., Smiley, K.A., Borys, H.K., Olsen, D.M., and Karler, R. (1979). An electrophysiological analysis of the anticonvulsant action of cannabidiol on limbic seizures in conscious rats. *Epilepsia*, **20**(4), 351–363.

Wada, J.A., Osawa, T., and Corcoran, M.E. (1975a). Effects of tetrahydrocannabinols on kindled amygdaloid seizures and photogenic seizures in Senegalese baboons, *Papio papio*. *Epilepsia*, **16**(3), 439–448.

Wada, J.A., Wake, A., Sato, M., and Corcoran, M.E. (1975b). Antiepileptic and prophylactic effects of tetrahydrocannabinols in amygdaloid kindled cats. *Epilepsia*, **16**(3), 503–510.

White, H.S. (1997). Clinical significance of animal seizure models and mechanism of action studies of potential antiepileptic drugs. *Epilepsia*, **38**, S9–S17.

White, H.S., Woodhead, J.H., Franklin, M.R., Swinyard, E.A., and Wolf, H.A. (1995). Experimental selection, quantification, and evaluation of antiepileptic drugs. In: R.H. Levy, R.H. Mattson, and B.S. Meldrum (eds.). *Antiepileptic Drugs*. 4th ed. New York: Raven Press, pp. 85–102.

Woodbury, L.A. and Davenport, V.D. (1952). Design and use of a new electroshock seizure apparatus, and analysis of factors altering seizure threshold and pattern. *Archives Internationales de Pharmacodynamie et de Therapie*, **92**, 97–107.

Chapter 31

Cardiovascular, Metabolic, Liver, Kidney, and Inflammatory Disorders

Pál Pacher and George Kunos

31.1 **Introduction**

There is accumulating evidence from preclinical studies that phytocannabinoids may exert beneficial effects in inflammatory, cardiovascular, metabolic, liver, and kidney disorders. For better understanding of the therapeutic effects of these compounds, it should be kept in mind that delta-9-tetrahydrocannabinol (THC) is an agonist of both cannabinoid 1 and 2 receptors (CB_1 and CB_2), delta-9-tetrahydrocannabivarin (Δ^9-THCV) is a CB_2 agonist and CB_1 receptor antagonist, and (E)-β-caryophyllene (BCP) is a CB_2 receptor agonist (Pertwee 2012). Cannabidiol (CBD) was initially considered to be devoid of effects on $CB_{1/2}$ receptors, but recent studies suggest that it may antagonize the effects of $CB_{1/2}$ receptor agonists in vitro (Thomas et al. 2007). Additionally, both CBD and THC are potent antioxidants (Hampson et al. 1998, 2000), which may underlie many of their therapeutically beneficial effects. Furthermore, at high concentrations both of these compounds have been reported to interact with a wide variety of molecular targets in in vitro systems (Izzo et al. 2009), the in vivo relevance of which remains to be established. In the following sections, we will discuss some of the most relevant in vivo effects of phytocannabinoids with potential therapeutic relevance in cardiovascular, metabolic, inflammatory, liver, and kidney diseases.

31.2 **Cardiometabolic disorders**

31.2.1 **Cardiovascular effects with clinical relevance**

THC, synthetic CB_1 receptor agonists, and endocannabinoids exert complex cardiovascular effects in rodents and humans, dominated by a decrease in blood pressure and myocardial contractility, mediated in part by CB_1 receptors located in the myocardium, vasculature, and neurons in the central and autonomic nervous systems (Pacher et al. 2005, 2006). Depending on the duration of its use, marijuana may decrease or increase heart rate and decrease blood pressure (Pacher et al. 2005). A recent controlled study at the National Institute on Drug Abuse reported on the effects of high doses of oral THC taken over a period of 6 days by 13 healthy male daily cannabis smokers. Despite the development of tolerance to the subjective intoxicating effect of THC, no tolerance was observed to its hypotensive and tachycardic effects (Gorelick et al. 2012). Increased heart rate variability in 72 young cannabis users has also been reported (Schmid et al. 2010). It should be noted that an elevated resting heart rate is a known independent risk factor for cardiovascular disease in healthy men and women (Cooney et al. 2010), and the selective CB_1 antagonist surinabant inhibited the THC-induced central nervous system and heart rate effects in humans (Klumpers et al. 2012). Furthermore, the clinical development of AstraZeneca's peripherally restricted, orally active mixed $CB_{1/2}$ agonists (AZD1940 and AZD1704) was terminated due to adverse cardiovascular effects, weight gain, and mild hepatotoxicity (Groblewski et al. 2010a, 2010b), which further highlights the cardiovascular risk caused by activation of CB_1 receptors.

In human coronary artery endothelial cells (Rajesh et al. 2010b) and cardiomyocytes tested in vitro (Mukhopadhyay et al. 2010b), or in mouse models of drug- or diabetes-induced cardiomyopathies, in vivo CB_1 activation promotes stress signaling and cell death, and decreases myocardial contractility (Mukhopadhyay et al. 2007, 2010b; Rajesh et al. 2012). CB_1 receptor signaling has also been implicated in: (1) increased cardiometabolic risk (e.g., plasma lipid alterations, hepatic steatosis, abdominal obesity, and insulin and leptin resistance), (2) obesity/metabolic syndrome (Kunos and Tam 2011; Silvestri and Di Marzo 2013) and (3) diabetes (Horvath et al. 2012b), both in rodents and humans, as well as in the pathogenesis of cardiovascular diseases, including atherosclerosis, shock, various forms of cardiomyopathies, and vascular restenosis (Pacher and Kunos 2013; see also sections 31.2.2 and 31.2.3).

In contrast, CB_2 receptor signaling exerts protective effects in rodent models of myocardial injury and atherosclerosis primarily by attenuating endothelial cell activation, the interplay of activated endothelium with inflammatory cells, and inflammatory cell chemotaxis, infiltration (Steffens and Pacher 2012).

CBD has also been reported to exert beneficial effects in rodent models of cardiovascular injury (Stanley et al. 2013) independently from CB_1/CB_2 receptors, which are highlighted later, in sections 31.2.2 and 31.2.3. Like CB_2 agonists, CBD is devoid of undesirable cardiovascular effects in healthy rodents (Rajesh et al. 2010a) or human subjects (Martin-Santos et al. 2012; Pacher and Kunos 2013).

31.2.2 Cardiovascular diseases

A study by Durst et al. investigated the potential benefits of CBD treatment in a rat model of myocardial ischemic reperfusion injury (I/R injury; a model of myocardial infarction). They found that CBD pretreatment reduced myocardial infarct size, myocardial inflammation, and attenuated the I/R-induced cardiac dysfunction, as tested 7 days following the insult (Durst et al. 2007). Another study found that acute administration of a surprisingly low dose of cannabidiol suppressed ischemia-induced cardiac arrhythmias and reduced infarct size when given at reperfusion (Walsh et al. 2010). Although these studies did not explore how the beneficial effects of CBD come about, they clearly implicated anti-inflammatory mechanisms.

The effect of CBD was also investigated in a chronic model of type 1 diabetes-induced cardiomyopathy (Rajesh et al. 2010a), the pathophysiological mechanism of which is known to involve: (1) increased oxidative/nitrative stress; (2) proinflammatory and cell death pathways such as nuclear factor NF-κB, poly(adenosine diphosphate (ADP)-ribose) polymerase (PARP), and mitogen-activated protein kinases (MAPKs); and (3) inactivation of prosurvival pathways such as Akt. These effects eventually culminate in cell death and changes in the composition of extracellular matrix with enhanced cardiac fibrosis and increased inflammation (Pacher et al. 2007). Treatment with CBD for 11 weeks following the complete destruction of pancreatic insulin-producing beta cells, attenuated myocardial oxidative-nitrative stress by decreasing myocardial reactive oxygen species (ROS) generation, and the expression of ROS generating NADPH oxidase isoforms p22(phox), p67(phox), gp91(phox). The treatment also normalized the reduced glutathione content and superoxide dismutase activity, decreased 3-nitrotyrosine formation, attenuated stress signaling (p38, p38α, JNK), and enhanced prosurvival (Akt) pathways in diabetic hearts (Rajesh et al. 2010a). CBD also attenuated NF-κB activation, expression of key

NF-κB target genes involved in orchestrating the diabetes-induced inflammation and oxidative-nitrative stress (e.g., inducible nitric oxide synthase (iNOS), tumor necrosis factor-alpha (TNF-α), and ICAM-1) in diabetic hearts, which was associated with reduced cell death and fibrosis and improved cardiac function (Rajesh et al. 2010a). Importantly, CBD treatment was also effective in attenuating/reversing some of the diabetes-induced biochemical and functional changes once diabetic cardiomyopathy with fibrosis had fully developed (Rajesh et al. 2010a). In human cardiomyocytes or endothelial cells tested in vitro, CBD attenuated the high glucose-induced ROS generation, NF-κB activation, oxidative-nitrative stress, MAPK activation, proinflammatory response, and cell death independently of $CB_{1/2}$ receptors (Rajesh et al. 2007a, 2010a).

Since oxidative stress, cardiovascular inflammation, activation of stress signaling, and cell death pathways are involved in the pathogenesis of almost all cardiovascular disorders, the results just described would predict therapeutic benefit from the use of CBD not only in myocardial infarction and diabetic cardiovascular complications, but also in other cardiovascular disorders associated with inflammation and oxidative-nitrative stress.

A recent study investigating the role of CB_1 receptor signaling in the pathogenesis of type 1 diabetic cardiomyopathy in mice has revealed novel interactions between cardiovascular CB_1 and angiotensin II receptor type 1 (AT1R) and their downstream signaling via p47(phox)/ROS-generating NADPH enzyme isoform, advanced glycation end product (AGE)-receptor (RAGE), and other proinflammatory/pro-oxidant signaling pathways in the diabetic heart, which may underlie the development of multiple diabetic complications (Rajesh et al. 2012). The diabetic cardiomyopathy was characterized by: (1) increased myocardial levels of the endocannabinoid anandamide, (2) increased oxidative/nitrative stress, (3) activation of p38/Jun MAPKs, (4) enhanced inflammation, (5) increased expression of CB_1 receptors, RAGE, AT1R, p47(phox) NADPH oxidase subunit, and β-myosin heavy chain isozyme switch, (6) accumulation of AGE, (7) fibrosis, and (8) decreased expression of sarcoplasmic/endoplasmic reticulum Ca^{2+}-ATPase. Pharmacological inhibition or genetic deletion of CB_1 receptors attenuated and/or reversed the earlier-mentioned pathological alterations and cardiac dysfunction (Rajesh et al. 2012), suggesting a detrimental role of endocannabinoid-CB_1 receptor signaling in diabetic cardiomyopathy. A recent study has demonstrated similar protective mechanisms of CB_1 receptor blockade in improving cardiac function and remodeling following myocardial infarction, as well as in an experimental model of the metabolic syndrome (Slavic et al. 2013).

Regarding THC, a recent provocative study found protective effects (reduced infarct size and attenuated neutrophil infiltration) of an "ultra-low" dose of THC (3–4 orders of magnitude lower than its conventional dose), administered 2 h, 48 h, or 3 weeks before myocardial infarction in mice (Waldman et al. 2013). However, THC was only administered as a pretreatment, and only at a single very low dose, and the role of cannabinoid receptors was not explored.

An increasing number of case reports links marijuana smoking with precipitation of acute coronary syndrome (ACS) (Singla et al. 2012). Alarmingly, this happens mostly in young healthy subjects without any prior cardiovascular disease (Leblanc et al. 2011; Pratap and Korniyenko 2012), and the risk of myocardial infarction appeared to be the highest during the first hour of marijuana exposure (Mittleman et al. 2001). In a prospective study involving 1913 adults hospitalized with myocardial infarction at 45 US hospitals between 1989 and 1994, with a median follow-up of 3.8 years, marijuana use was associated with increased risk of infarction in susceptible individuals with coronary heart disease (Mukamal et al. 2008). Habitual marijuana use among patients with acute myocardial infarction was also associated with a 29% increase in mortality over the ensuing 18 years; however, this did not reach statistical significance because of the limited sample size (Frost et al. 2013). In a series of cases, myocardial infarction was triggered in healthy children by synthetic cannabinoid use (Mir et al. 2011). Synthetic cannabinoids with high CB_1 agonist potency could also cause tachycardia, loss of consciousness, and diffuse pain in adolescents (Heath et al. 2012), raising concerns about the recreational use of these compounds. Increased plasma levels of endocannabinoids were strongly associated with coronary circulatory events in obese human subjects (Quercioli et al. 2011), as well as in individuals with impaired coronary endothelial function (Quercioli et al. 2012). Upregulation of CB_1 and downregulation of CB_2 receptors was found in samples of epicardial fat from ischemic compared to nonischemic human hearts (Cappellano et al. 2012), and CB_1 receptor density was significantly higher in atherosclerotic coronary artery sections from patients with unstable angina compared to those with stable angina (Sugamura et al. 2009).

It should be noted that THC is a relatively weak CB_1 receptor agonist compared to many synthetic ligands, is a potent antioxidant, and activates cardioprotective CB_2 receptors, which may mitigate its detrimental effects mediated by CB_1 activation. One can also surmise that long-term exposure to THC can lead to downregulation of CB_1 receptors, leading to functional CB_1 antagonism. Nevertheless, because of the lack of long-term, large-scale controlled studies in subjects with regular marijuana use, a solid conclusion on the long-term impact of cannabis or THC use on cardiovascular mortality cannot be reached. However, the described findings clearly suggest that the use of natural or synthetic ligands with CB_1 agonistic properties will likely introduce adverse cardiovascular events.

In contrast to CB_1 agonists, there is ample evidence for beneficial effects of synthetic CB_2 agonists in cardiovascular and inflammatory diseases. Therefore, one might predict that phytocannabinoids, such as Δ^9-THCV (Riedel et al. 2009), their synthetic analogs such as Δ^8-THCV (Batkai et al. 2012), or other plant-derived constituents with CB_2 agonistic properties (e.g., BCP) (Gertsch et al. 2008; Horvath et al. 2012c), would have therapeutic potential in cardiovascular and other disorders, assuming adequate bioavailability (Pertwee 2012). Consequently, the dual effects of Δ^9-THCV as CB_2 receptor agonist and CB_1 receptor antagonist (Thomas et al. 2005; Bolognini et al. 2010) if confirmed in in vivo cardiovascular disease models, could offer greater therapeutic potential than CB_2 agonists or peripherally restricted CB_1 antagonists alone, particularly if Δ^9-THCV turns out to have limited brain penetrability that would minimize CNS related side effects due to CB_1 antagonism.

31.2.3 Metabolic diseases (diabetes and diabetic complications, obesity)

Obesity is the leading risk factor for insulin resistance that can progress to type 2 diabetes. Endocannabinoids increase food intake and promote weight gain by activating central and peripheral CB_1 receptors. Consistently, treatment with brain-penetrant CB_1 receptor antagonists/ inverse agonists improved multiple cardiovascular risk factors both in preclinical models of obesity/metabolic syndrome and in clinical trials in obese/overweight subjects (Kunos and Tam 2011; Pacher and Kunos 2013). However, a small but significant number of subjects experienced increased anxiety, depression, and/or suicidal ideations, which in 2008 led to the withdrawal of rimonabant from the market in over 50 countries and discontinuation of the therapeutic development of this class of compounds (Pacher and Kunos 2013; Silvestri and Di Marzo 2013). By that time, evidence had emerged that activation of CB_1 receptors in peripheral tissues plays a key role in adipogenesis, lipogenesis, hepatic steatosis, and insulin resistance (Cota et al. 2003; Osei-Hyiaman et al. 2005). This suggested that peripherally restricted CB_1 antagonists may preserve some or most of the metabolic benefit of global CB_1 blockade while minimizing side effects resulting from blockade of CB_1 receptors in the CNS (Kunos and Tam 2011). Subsequent studies using peripherally restricted neutral CB_1 antagonists or inverse CB_1 agonists in mouse models of obesity confirmed that the therapeutic benefit of this approach is comparable to that of global CB_1 antagonists (Tam et al. 2010, 2011, 2012), and one of these compounds is being subjected to further toxicology studies for potential therapeutic development.

Δ^9-THCV, which is a neutral antagonist of CB_1 receptors and is found in marijuana, causes hypophagia in fasted and nonfasted mice (Riedel et al. 2009), and may also activate CB_2 receptors (Pertwee 2008). A recent study explored the effects of Δ^9-THCV in mice with diet-induced or genetic obesity. While Δ^9-THCV did not significantly affect food intake or body weight gain in either model studied, it produced an early and transient increase in energy expenditure while dose-dependently reducing glucose intolerance in genetically obese mice, and improving glucose tolerance and increased insulin sensitivity in diet-induced obese mice, without affecting plasma lipids (Wargent et al. 2013).

Numerous earlier preclinical studies and clinical trials with CB_1 antagonists in obesity and diabetes demonstrated improved glycemic control, suggesting that CB_1 antagonists may also exert direct effects on diabetes development, independently from their metabolic effects (Horvath et al. 2012b). However, there has been conflicting information about the presence and function of the endocannabinoid system and CB_1 and CB_2 receptors in islet cells (Horvath et al. 2012b). Some of the conflicting results might be attributable to the different species, experimental conditions, and research tools (e.g., antibodies) used in these studies. It has been recently demonstrated that CB_1 receptor inhibition may increase beta-cell proliferation by reversing CB_1-mediated inhibition of proproliferative insulin signaling in beta cells under in vitro conditions (Kim et al. 2011). However, in an in vivo rat model of type 2 diabetes, beta-cell failure in adult diabetic rats was not associated with CB_1 receptor signaling in beta cells, but rather in M1 macrophages infiltrating into pancreatic islets, where CB_1 signaling triggered activation of the Nlrp3-ASC inflammasome, leading to activation and release of IL-1β, causing apoptotic cell death in neighboring beta cells (Jourdan et al. 2013). Peripheral CB_1 receptor blockade, in vivo depletion of macrophages, or macrophage-specific knock-down of CB_1 receptors restored normoglycemia and glucose-induced insulin secretion, highlighting macrophage-expressed CB_1 receptors as therapeutic targets in type 2 diabetes mellitus (Jourdan et al. 2013).

The effect of CBD was also investigated in primary diabetes. CBD reduced the incidence of diabetes in a mouse model of type 1 autoimmune diabetes. It reduced insulitis due to a shift of the immune response from Th1 to Th2 dominance, leading to decreased levels of the proinflammatory cytokines interferon-γ and TNF-α (Weiss et al. 2006). CBD also arrested progression of the disease in nonobese diabetic mice when it was given after the development of initial symptoms of diabetes (Weiss et al. 2008).

THC also attenuated the severity of autoimmune responses in an experimental model of type 1 autoimmune diabetes induced by multiple doses of streptozotocin. It decreased lymphocyte infiltration and the expression of interferon-γ, IL-12, and TNF-α in islets, which was associated with better preservation of pancreatic insulin content and improved blood glucose levels compared to untreated diabetic animals (Li et al. 2001). In a rat model of streptozotocin-induced diabetes, THC treatment for 7 days paradoxically improved plasma lipid profile compared to vehicle-treated diabetic controls (Coskun and Bolkent 2013). Furthermore, analysis of cross-sectional data from the National Health and Nutrition Examination Survey (NHANES III, 1988–1994) indicated that marijuana use was independently associated with a lower prevalence of diabetes mellitus (Rajavashisth et al. 2012), and glucose tolerance and insulin sensitivity were found unchanged in chronic marijuana smokers (Muniyappa et al. 2013). These findings may reflect desensitization of peripheral CB_1 receptors during chronic use of marijuana in light of the demonstrated ability of acute marijuana smoking to induce insulin resistance (Hollister and Reaven 1974). A similar mechanism may account for the lower prevalence of obesity in cannabis users as compared to nonusers, an effect still present after adjusting for tobacco use, gender, and age (Le Foll et al. 2013). Likewise, repeated exposure of rats to THC in vivo leads to reduced body weight, fat pad weight, and food intake over the drug injection period (Wong et al. 2012). Interestingly, despite the reduced food intake and body weight, THC promoted adipocyte hypertrophy accompanied by a significant increase in cytosolic phosphoenolpyruvate carboxykinase expression, an enzyme involved in packaging triglycerides, and induced macrophage infiltration and increased expression of the proinflammatory cytokine TNF-α in adipose tissue (Wong et al. 2012).

The anti-inflammatory effects of THC in the islets (Li et al. 2001) may also be related to activation of CB_2 receptors or other CB receptor-independent anti-inflammatory or antioxidant mechanisms, which should be explored in future studies. Further preclinical and clinical studies should establish the potential mechanisms involved in the differential effects of acute and chronic marijuana use on glycemic control and the development and progression of diabetes.

Considerable evidence suggests that the hyperglycemia-induced increased oxidative and nitrosative stress and activation of redox-dependent proinflammatory pathways such as NF-κB play a key role in the development or progression of diabetic cardiovascular dysfunction, which also underlies the development of other diabetic complications including diabetic retinopathy, nephropathy, and neuropathy (Pacher et al. 2007). As already mentioned, previous in vitro studies suggested that CB_1 receptor activation by anandamide in human coronary endothelial cells and cardiomyocytes may amplify the ROS-MAPK activation-cell death pathway in pathological conditions where the endocannabinoid biosynthetic or metabolic pathways are dysregulated by excessive inflammation and/or oxidative/nitrosative stress, thereby contributing to the development of endothelial dysfunction and multiple cardiovascular diseases (Mukhopadhyay et al. 2010b; Rajesh et al. 2010). CB_1 receptor activation contributed to vascular inflammation and cell death in a mouse model of type 1 diabetic retinopathy and in primary retinal cells exposed to high glucose, and CB_1 receptor inhibition or deletion protected against these effects (El-Remessy et al. 2011). CB_1 inhibition or deletion also attenuated oxidative/nitrative stress, inflammation and cell death signaling, and improved cardiac function in models of type 1 and 2 diabetic cardiomyopathy (Nam et al. 2012; Rajesh et al. 2012). Furthermore, beneficial effects of CB_1 blockade were reported in rodent models of type 1 and type 2 diabetic nephropathy (Barutta et al. 2010; Nam et al. 2012), as well as in diabetic neuropathy (Comelli et al. 2010; Liu et al. 2010) and were attributed to attenuation of oxidative stress, inflammation or cell death related mechanisms (Horvath et al. 2012b).

One study also explored the role of CB_2 receptors in a type 1 diabetic nephropathy model (Barutta et al. 2011), and found that a selective CB_2 receptor agonist ameliorated albuminuria, podocyte protein downregulation and glomerular monocyte infiltration, without affecting early markers of fibrosis. They also found that the CB_2 receptor was downregulated in kidney biopsies from patients with advanced diabetic nephropathy, and renal levels of the CB_2 receptor ligand, 2-arachidonoylglycerol, were reduced in diabetic mice, suggesting impaired CB_2 receptor regulation (Barutta et al. 2011).

In vivo studies also examined the effects of CBD in experimental diabetic retinopathy. CBD attenuated the oxidative stress, inflammation, cell death, and vascular hyperpermeability associated with diabetes and inhibited p38-MAPK signaling (El-Remessy et al. 2006, 2008). The protective effects of CBD on retinal cell death were, at least in part, due to the reduction of tyrosine nitration of glutamine synthase in macroglial cells, thereby preventing the accumulation and excitotoxicity of glutamine through N-methyl-D-aspartate receptors (El-Remessy et al. 2010). CBD also attenuated high glucose–induced endothelial cell dysfunction, ROS generation, and barrier disruption in primary human coronary artery endothelial cells (Rajesh et al. 2007a), and attenuated the oxidative-nitrative stress, proinflammatory signaling, and cell death, as already described in more detail (section 31.2.2), in a model of diabetic cardiomyopathy (Rajesh et al. 2010a).

Thus, in light of the vast body of preclinical and clinical evidence suggesting that CB_1 receptor activation contributes to diabetes development and its complications (cardiovascular, neuropathic, retinopathic, and nephropathic) (Horvath et al. 2012b), the use of cannabinoids with CB_1 agonistic properties should be very carefully weighed in patients with diabetes and diabetic complications, even for neuropathic pain. In contrast, CBD appears to have a great therapeutic potential in diabetes and diabetic complications based on animal studies, which deserves to be explored in clinical trials. Since some of the beneficial effects of CBD and CB_1 receptor antagonists share similarities in diabetes and diabetic complications, and there is evidence that CBD can antagonize the effects of CB_1 receptor agonists in vitro (Thomas et al. 2007), it would be interesting to test if this antagonistic effect on CB_1 is also functional in vivo. Based on the protective effects of a CB_2 agonist in diabetic nephropathy it would also be interesting to explore the potential therapeutic effects of BCP and Δ^9-THCV; the additional interest in the latter also derives from its reported CB_1 receptor antagonism (Pertwee 2008), its hypophagic properties in fasted and nonfasted mice (Riedel et al. 2009), and its ability to ameliorate insulin sensitivity in mouse models of obesity (Wargent et al. 2013).

31.3 Inflammatory disorders (arthritis, sepsis, autoimmune disorders)

It is well documented that CB_2 receptors are primarily expressed in immune and immune-derived cells (e.g., leukocytes, various populations of T and B lymphocytes, monocytes/macrophages, dendritic cells, mast cells, microglia in the brain, Kupffer cells in the liver, etc.) and their stimulation in general attenuates proinflammatory responses (Pacher and Mechoulam 2011). Earlier studies demonstrated suppressive effects of cannabinoid ligands on B and T lymphocytes, NK cells, and macrophages, which appeared to involve both CB_1 and CB_2 receptor-dependent and independent mechanisms (Klein 2005; Klein et al. 2003). Subsequent studies also found that endocannabinoids and cannabinoids may also exert immunosuppressive effects by modulating: (1) T- and B-lymphocyte proliferation and apoptosis, (2) inflammatory cytokine production and immune cell activation by inflammatory stimuli (e.g., bacterial endotoxins), (3) macrophage-mediated killing of sensitized cells, and (4) chemotaxis and inflammatory cell migration (Klein 2005). However, many of these in vitro effects (mostly, but not always inhibitory) were largely context dependent and influenced by the endocannabinoid or synthetic agonist/antagonist, trigger/condition, and cell type used (Pacher and Mechoulam 2011). Interestingly, a recent study has also demonstrated attenuation of HIV-1 replication in macrophages by cannabinoid receptor 2 agonists (Ramirez et al. 2013). Nevertheless, the anti-inflammatory effects of CB_2 selective agonists have been confirmed in in vivo models of atherosclerosis, myocardial infarction, stroke, inflammatory pain, gastrointestinal, liver, and kidney disorders, systemic inflammation, among others (Pacher and Mechoulam 2011).

In contrast, the potential role of the CB_1 receptor in modulating inflammatory responses was largely based on the in vitro effects of very high concentrations of THC and a very few nonselective cannabinoid ligands. The interpretation of in vivo protective effects of CB_1 agonists in previous preclinical models could also be largely attributed to the direct protective effects of central

CB_1 receptor-mediated hypothermia in rodent models of tissue injury and inflammation (the hypothermic effect is absent in humans, but very powerful in rodents), as well as to antioxidant and CB receptor-independent anti-inflammatory actions. An example for the latter comes from a study demonstrating that the anti-inflammatory effects of THC in a model of allergen-induced airway inflammation was similar in $CB_{1/2}$ double knockout mice, suggesting $CB_{1/2}$ independent mechanisms (Braun et al. 2010). Recent preclinical and clinical evidence suggests that CB_1 receptor activation may in fact induce proinflammatory signaling in immune cells (e.g., macrophages (Han et al. 2009; Jourdan et al. 2013; Marquart et al. 2010; Sugamura et al. 2009)), thereby contributing to the development of diabetes, diabetic complications (retinopathy, nephropathy, cardiomyopathy), cardiomyopathies, and atherosclerosis, to mention just a few proinflammatory conditions as described in sections 31.2.2 and 31.2.3 (see also Pacher and Kunos 2013).

CBD can also exert multiple $CB_{1/2}$ receptor independent anti-inflammatory effects, including: (1) attenuation of endothelial cell activation, (2) chemotaxis of inflammatory cells and adhesion to the activated endothelium, (3) suppression of T-cell and macrophage reactivity and/or activation, (4) induction of apoptosis in T cells, and (5) decreased microglial activation. In vivo, tissue protective effects of CBD were described in models of cardiovascular diseases, stroke, brain trauma, inflammatory bowel diseases, neuroinflammatory and neurodegenerative diseases, and arthritis and sepsis, just to name a few (Fernández-Ruiz et al. 2013; Izzo et al. 2009; Stanley et al. 2013). Although primarily based on in vitro assays, a variety of potential therapeutic targets was proposed for CBD (including transient receptor potential vanilloid 1 (TRPV1), μ opioid, $5HT_{1A}$, GPR55, adenosine A_{2A} receptors, α_1-adrenoreceptors, adenosine transporter(s), the MAPK pathway, and the peroxisome proliferator activated receptor γ; Izzo et al. 2009), none of which could be convincingly validated in multiple independent in vivo studies. The most consistent effect of CBD observed across various models of tissue injury ranging from diabetic complications (Rajesh et al. 2010a) to liver (Mukhopadhyay et al. 2011b) and kidney injury (Pan et al. 2009) and neurodegeneration (Fernández-Ruiz et al. 2013), appears to be the attenuation of oxidative stress and inflammatory cell infiltration, and the expression of the redox-sensitive master proinflammatory transcription factor NF-κB and/or its related target genes, such as intracellular adhesion molecule 1, iNOS, cyclooxygenase 2 (COX-2), various ROS generating NADPH oxidases, TNF-α, among others (Fernández-Ruiz et al. 2013; Izzo et al. 2009; Stanley et al. 2013).

The therapeutic potential of CBD was also explored using a murine collagen II-induced autoimmune arthritis model. CBD was equally effective when administered orally or intraperitoneally in improving symptoms of arthritis (Malfait et al. 2000). CBD-treated mice had a diminished collagen II-specific proliferation and IFN-gamma production ex vivo, as well as a decreased release of TNF-α by knee synovial cells (Malfait et al. 2000). Preliminary assessment of the efficacy, tolerability, and safety of a cannabis-based medicine (Sativex®) in the treatment of pain caused by rheumatoid arthritis yielded favorable effects on analgesia, accompanied by only mild to moderate adverse effects (Blake et al. 2006).

CBD administration also attenuated the lipopolysaccharide (LPS)-induced rise in serum TNF-α in C57/BL6 mice (Malfait et al. 2000), indicating systemic anti-inflammatory effects. Another study investigating the effects of CBD in a mouse model of sepsis-related encephalitis that involves the intravenous administration of LPS, it was found that CBD: (1) prevented LPS-induced arteriolar and venular vasodilation and leukocyte margination; (2) abolished LPS-induced increases in TNF-α, COX-2, and iNOS expression; and (3) preserved the integrity of the blood–brain barrier (Ruiz-Valdepenas et al. 2011). CBD also attenuated the mortality of rats exposed to sepsis induced by cecal ligation and perforation, and oxidative stress in certain organs (Cassol-Jr et al. 2010). Cannabidiol also reduced the host immune response and prevented cognitive impairments in Wistar rats subjected to pneumococcal meningitis (Barichello et al. 2012). Previous studies have also documented beneficial effects of both CB_1 antagonists (Pacher et al. 2006) and CB_2 agonists (Pacher and Mechoulam 2011) in models of systemic and localized inflammation (Pacher and Kunos 2013). The potential beneficial effects of plant-derived cannabinoids in liver and kidney diseases will be discussed in sections 31.4 and 31.5, while the effects and therapeutic potential in inflammatory bowel disease, neurodegenerative, and skin disorders can be found in other chapters.

31.4 **Liver diseases**

The activation of the hepatic endocannabinoid system through CB_1 receptors contributes to various liver pathologies such as alcoholic and metabolic steatosis, liver fibrosis, and circulatory collapse associated with hepatic cirrhosis; conversely CB_1 receptor antagonism exerts beneficial effects in these conditions (Jeong et al. 2008; Mallat et al. 2011, 2013; Tam et al. 2011). In contrast, activation of CB_2 receptors predominantly in infiltrating immune cells or in immune-derived cells such as Kupffer cells, the resident macrophages of the liver, exerts beneficial effects in alcoholic fatty liver, hepatic inflammation, liver injury induced by ischemia-reperfusion (I/R), regeneration, and fibrosis. These opposing effects of CB_1 and CB_2 receptors in various liver pathologies have been extensively discussed recently, and are beyond the scope of this chapter (Mallat et al. 2011, 2013; Tam et al. 2011). Here, we will focus primarily on the liver injury models in which the beneficial effects of plant-derived cannabinoids have been recently described.

Previous studies using acute models of hepatic I/R injury demonstrated that oxidative/nitrosative/nitrative stress is involved in the activation of the endocannabinoid system during reperfusion (Batkai et al. 2007), and the modulation of peripheral CB_2 cannabinoid receptors by synthetic agonists (Batkai et al. 2007; Rajesh et al. 2007) protected against I/R-induced tissue injury and/or vascular inflammation by decreasing endothelial cell activation and inflammatory response orchestrated by activated endothelial and Kupffer cells, by infiltrating leukocytes, and by interrelated oxidative/nitrosative stress (Horvath et al. 2012). The protective effects of CB_2 receptor agonists was most pronounced when given before ischemia, but also persisted when they were administered up to 3 h following the ischemic insult (Horvath et al. 2012a). Interestingly, the effects of CB_2 agonists appeared to be synergistic with the effect of CB_1 antagonists in attenuating I/R-induced hepatic injury (Horvath et al. 2012a).

A recent study found that Δ^8-THCV, a stable synthetic analog of the plant-derived cannabinoid, Δ^9-THCV, which exerts known anti-inflammatory effects in rodents (Bolognini et al. 2010), is a potent CB_2 receptor agonist both in vitro and in vivo (Batkai et al. 2012). Δ^8-THCV, given before induction of I/R, attenuated hepatic injury (measured by serum alanine aminotransferase and aspartate aminotransferase levels), and decreased: (1) tissue protein carbonyl adducts, (2) 4-hydroxynonenal, (3) the chemokines CCL3 and CXCL2, (4) TNF-α, (5) intercellular adhesion molecule 1 (CD54) mRNA levels, (6) tissue neutrophil infiltration, (7) caspase 3/7 activity, and (8) DNA fragmentation. Protective effects of Δ^8-THCV against liver damage were still present when the compound was given at the beginning of reperfusion. Pretreatment with a CB_2 receptor antagonist attenuated the protective effects of Δ^8-THCV, while a CB_1 antagonist tended to enhance it, suggesting that the anti-inflammatory and tissue protective effects of Δ^8-THCV are mediated by CB_2 receptors (Batkai et al. 2012).

Cao et al. (2013) recently proposed a key role for monoacylglycerol lipase (MAGL), one of the main endocannabinoid degrading enzymes, in acute liver injury. They found that MAGL inhibition or its genetic deletion was associated with attenuated liver injury in several in vivo and in vitro models of liver injury. These protective effects were dependent on enhanced 2-arachidonoylglycerol-CB_2 receptor signaling and on a reduction of hepatic levels of arachidonic acid and various proinflammatory eicosanoids. These results indicated that MAGL inhibitors might be useful for treating conditions that expose the liver to acute oxidative stress and inflammatory damage (Cao et al. 2013).

Mukhopadhyay et al. (2011b) investigated the effect of CBD in the aforementioned hepatic I/R-induced injury models. They found that I/R triggered time-dependent increases in markers of: (1) liver injury (serum transaminases), (2) hepatic oxidative/nitrative stress (4-hydroxynonenal, nitrotyrosine content/staining, and gp91phox and iNOS mRNA), (3) mitochondrial dysfunction (decreased complex I activity), (4) inflammation (TNF-α), (5) COX-2, (6) macrophage inflammatory protein-1α/2, (7) intercellular adhesion molecule 1 mRNA levels, (8) tissue neutrophil infiltration, (9) NF-κB activation, (10) stress signaling (p38MAPK and JNK), and (11) cell death (DNA fragmentation, PARP activity, and TUNEL). CBD significantly reduced the extent of liver inflammation, oxidative/nitrative stress, and cell death, and also attenuated bacterial endotoxin-triggered NF-κB activation and TNF-α production in isolated Kupffer cells, as well as adhesion molecule expression in primary human liver sinusoidal endothelial cells stimulated with TNF-α, and attachment of human neutrophils to the activated endothelium. These protective effects were preserved in CB_2 knockout mice and were not prevented by $CB_{1/2}$ antagonists in vitro (Mukhopadhyay et al. 2011b). In agreement with these results a study performed in a rat model of hepatic I/R showed that the protective effects of CBD treatment extended up to 24 h following ischemic insult, and involved attenuation of liver injury, expression of iNOS, COX-2, NF-κB, and apoptosis (Fouad et al. 2012).

A recent study has also demonstrated protective effects of CBD in an experimental autoimmune hepatitis model via activation of TRPV1 receptor-dependent myeloid-derived suppressor cell activation (Hegde et al. 2011), and protective effects of CBD were also shown in thioacetamide- or bile duct ligation-induced hepatic failure/encephalopathy in mice, effects that were attributed to potential effects on central 5-HT_{1A} and adenosine A_{2A} receptors (Avraham et al. 2011; Magen et al. 2009).

Collectively, these results suggest that CBD administration may represent a promising, protective strategy against various forms of liver injury by attenuating key inflammatory pathways and oxidative/nitrative stress, independent of classical $CB_{1/2}$ receptors. In addition to synthetic selective CB_2 receptor agonists, $Δ^8$-THCV, $Δ^9$-THCV, and BCP should also be further explored as potential medicines for the treatment of liver diseases.

31.5 **Kidney diseases**

CB_1 and CB_2 receptors appear to have opposing regulatory functions not only in liver diseases (section 31.4) but also in kidney disorders. In order to explore the role of CB_1 signaling in renal inflammatory processes, Mukhopadhyay et al. (2010a) used a well-characterized model of acute nephropathy in which the antineoplastic drug cisplatin is used to induce, within 3 days, acute tubular injury that is largely dependent on inflammation and oxidative-nitrosative stress, and kidney failure. Cisplatin selectively accumulates in the proximal tubular cells via specific transport, where it triggers mitochondrial dysfunction and ROS generation (Mukhopadhyay et al. 2012; Zsengeller et al. 2012), leading to endothelial and proximal tubular cell necrosis (Mukhopadhyay et al. 2011a). This activates a cascade of secondary proinflammatory and pro-oxidant mechanisms, eventually leading to kidney dysfunction and failure. Cisplatin significantly increased anandamide content, activation of p38 and JNK mitogen-activated protein kinases (MAPKs), apoptotic and poly (ADP-ribose) polymerase-dependent cell death. It also enhanced inflammation (leukocyte infiltration, TNF-α and IL-1β) and promoted oxidative/nitrosative stress (increased expressions of superoxide-generating enzymes (NOX2(gp91phox), NOX4), inducible nitric oxide synthase and tissue 4-hydroxynonenal and nitrotyrosine levels in the kidneys of mice, effects that were accompanied by marked histopathological damage and impaired renal function (elevated creatinine and serum blood urea nitrogen) 3 days following its administration (Mukhopadhyay et al. 2010a, 2010c). Both genetic deletion and pharmacological antagonism of CB$_1$ receptors with AM281 or SR141716 (rimonabant) markedly attenuated the cisplatin-induced renal dysfunction and related oxidative/nitrosative stress, p38 and JNK MAPK activation, cell death and inflammatory response in the kidney (Mukhopadhyay et al., 2010a). These results suggest that the endocannabinoid system may, through CB$_1$ receptors, promote nephropathy by amplifying MAPK activation, cell death, and related inflammation and oxidative/nitrosative stress. These results also imply that blockade of CB$_1$ receptors may exert beneficial effects in renal (and most likely other) diseases associated with enhanced inflammation, oxidative/nitrosative stress and cell death. Consistent with these results, Barutta et al. demonstrated protective effects of CB$_1$ inhibition in a mouse model of type 1 diabetic nephropathy, in which the injury is primarily glomerular (Barutta et al. 2010). They found that CB$_1$ receptors were overexpressed within the glomeruli, predominantly by glomerular podocytes, and that blockade of CB$_1$ receptors attenuated diabetes-induced albuminuria, without exerting effects on body weight, blood glucose, or blood pressure levels in either diabetic or control mice. Furthermore, CB$_1$ blockade completely prevented diabetes-induced downregulation of nephrin, podocin, and zonula occludens-1 (Barutta et al. 2010). In obese Zucker rats, a model of obesity and type 2 diabetes, prolonged treatment with a CB$_1$ antagonist reduced mortality and markedly improved diabetes-induced kidney function, as indicated by beneficial effects on proteinuria, urinary N-acetylglucosaminidase excretion, plasma creatinine and urea nitrogen levels, and creatinine clearance. This treatment was also associated with preservation of pancreatic weight and beta-cell mass index, and marked improvements in blood glucose levels and lipid parameters (Janiak et al. 2007). It has been found as well that blockade of CB$_1$ receptors with SR141716 also improved insulin resistance, lipid metabolism, and diabetic nephropathy in a genetic mouse model of type 2 diabetes (Nam et al. 2012). Treatment with SR141716 markedly decreased urinary albumin excretion and mesangial expansion and suppressed profibrotic and proinflammatory cytokine synthesis. Furthermore, SR141716 improved renal lipid metabolism and decreased urinary 8-isoprostane levels, renal lipid hydroperoxide content, and renal lipid content (Nam et al. 2012).

Importantly, a recent study by the Centers for Disease Control and Prevention (CDC) associated multiple cases of acute kidney injury with synthetic cannabinoid use in humans, (Centers for Disease Control and Prevention 2013) raising concerns about the uncontrolled use of potent CB$_1$ agonists.

Mukhopadhyay et al. have explored the role of CB$_2$ receptors in the cisplatin-induced nephropathy model (Mukhopadhyay et al. 2010c). Cisplatin significantly increased inflammation in mice: (1) elevating proinflammatory chemokine (CXCL1/2, MCP-1) and proinflammatory cytokine (TNF-α, IL-1β) levels, (2) augmenting leukocyte infiltration and the expression of adhesion molecule ICAM-1, (3) markedly enhancing the expression of several superoxide-generating NADPH oxidase enzyme isoforms (NOX2, NOX4, and NOX1), and (4) increasing oxidative stress, iNOS expression, nitrotyrosine formation, and apoptotic and poly(ADP-ribose) polymerase-dependent kidney cell death (Mukhopadhyay et al. 2010c). These cisplatin-induced changes were associated with marked histopathological damage and impaired renal function (elevated serum blood urea nitrogen and creatinine levels) 3 days after the administration of the drug. CB$_2$ receptor agonists attenuated the cisplatin-induced inflammatory response, oxidative/nitrosative stress, and cell death in the kidney and improved renal function, whereas CB_2 knockouts developed enhanced inflammation and tissue injury. These results suggest that the endocannabinoid system, through CB_2 receptors, is protective against the development of cisplatin-induced kidney damage by attenuating inflammation and oxidative/nitrosative stress, and that selective CB_2 agonists may represent a promising novel approach to preventing this complication of chemotherapy (Mukhopadhyay et al. 2010c). In a subsequent study, Barutta et al. (2011) have reported protective effects of a CB_2 agonist using a mouse model of type 1 diabetes. CB_2 receptor agonist ameliorated albuminuria, podocyte protein downregulation, and glomerular monocyte infiltration and chemokine signaling (Barutta et al. 2011), which is consistent with the attenuated chemokine signaling observed in the cisplatin-induced nephropathy model (Mukhopadhyay et al. 2010c).

Horvath et al. have recently explored the therapeutic potential of BCP (Horvath et al. 2012c), which was identified as a CB_2 agonist both in vitro and in vivo (Gertsch et al. 2008), in the cisplatin-induced nephropathy model. BCP dose-dependently ameliorated cisplatin-induced kidney dysfunction, morphological damage, and renal inflammatory responses. It also markedly mitigated oxidative/nitrative stress and cell death. The protective effects of BCP against biochemical and histological markers of nephropathy were absent in CB_2 knockout mice, suggesting that it may be an excellent therapeutic agent for preventing cisplatin-induced nephrotoxicity through a CB_2 receptor-dependent pathway (Horvath et al. 2012c). Given the excellent safety profile of BCP in humans (US Food and Drug Administration-approved food additive) it has tremendous therapeutic potential in a multitude of diseases associated with inflammation and oxidative stress (Gertsch et al. 2008).

CBD has also been found to exert dose-dependent protective effects against cisplatin-induced histopathological and functional injury. The protective effects were attributed to attenuation of cisplatin-induced oxidative/nitrative stress, inflammatory cell infiltration and cell death (Pan et al. 2009). These findings are particularly exciting since numerous studies have demonstrated antineoplastic effects of CBD in both in vitro and in vivo models of various malignancies (Massi et al. 2013). CBD also attenuated I/R-induced kidney injury in rats, by attenuating NF-κB activation, iNOS, COX-2, and TNF-α expression, and cell death (Fouad et al. 2012).

Collectively, the described studies have revealed important opposing regulatory roles of CB_1 and CB_2 cannabinoid receptors on oxidative/nitrative stress, inflammation and tissue injury associated with nephropathy (CB_1 receptors promote oxidative/nitrosative stress, inflammation and cell death while CB_2 receptors attenuate these variables). Thus, both CB_2 agonists and CB_1 antagonists, alone or in combination, are expected to exert beneficial effects in kidney diseases, prompting a need for additional testing of BCP and Δ^9-THCV in various models of kidney injury. The therapeutic potential of CBD for the treatment of kidney diseases should also be further explored.

31.6 **Conclusions**

Recent clinical studies have provided proof of the principle that cannabinoid-based extracts with controlled doses of plant-derived cannabinoids can provide symptomatic relief in a subset of patients suffering from spasticity and pain as a consequence of multiple sclerosis. On the basis of the encouraging preclinical studies briefly summarized in this chapter there is certainly a hope that some of these natural constituents, or their combinations, together with their synthetic derivatives, would eventually contribute to our therapeutic armamentarium for easing human suffering in various cardiometabolic, inflammatory, liver, kidney, and neurodegenerative diseases.

Acknowledgments

Author's contribution to the Work was done as part of the Author's official duties as an NIH employee and is a Work of the United States Government. Therefore, copyright may not be established in the United States.

References

Avraham, Y., Grigoriadis, N., Poutahidis, T., *et al.* (2011). Cannabidiol improves brain and liver function in a fulminant hepatic failure-induced model of hepatic encephalopathy in mice. *British Journal of Pharmacology*, **162**, 1650–1658.

Barichello, T., Ceretta, R.A., Generoso, J.S., *et al.* (2012). Cannabidiol reduces host immune response and prevents cognitive impairments in Wistar rats submitted to pneumococcal meningitis. *European Journal of Pharmacology*, **697**, 158–164.

Barutta, F., Corbelli, A., Mastrocola, R., *et al.* (2010). Cannabinoid receptor 1 blockade ameliorates albuminuria in experimental diabetic nephropathy. *Diabetes*, **59**, 1046–1054.

Barutta, F., Piscitelli, F., Pinach, S., *et al.* (2011). Protective role of cannabinoid receptor type 2 in a mouse model of diabetic nephropathy. *Diabetes*, **60**, 2386–2396.

Batkai, S., Mukhopadhyay, P., Horvath, B., *et al.* (2012). Δ^8-Tetrahydrocannabivarin prevents hepatic ischaemia/reperfusion injury by decreasing oxidative stress and inflammatory responses through cannabinoid CB2 receptors. *British Journal of Pharmacology*, **165**, 2450–2461.

Batkai, S., Osei-Hyiaman, D., Pan, H., *et al.* (2007). Cannabinoid-2 receptor mediates protection against hepatic ischemia/reperfusion injury. *FASEB Journal*, **21**, 1788–1800.

Blake, D.R., Robson, P., Ho, M., Jubb, R.W., and McCabe, C.S. (2006). Preliminary assessment of the efficacy, tolerability and safety of a cannabis-based medicine (Sativex) in the treatment of pain caused by rheumatoid arthritis. *Rheumatology (Oxford)*, **45**, 50–52.

Bolognini, D., Costa, B., Maione, S., *et al.* (2010). The plant cannabinoid Δ^9-tetrahydrocannabivarin can decrease signs of inflammation and inflammatory pain in mice. *British Journal of Pharmacology*, **160**, 677–687.

Braun, A., Engel, T., Aguilar-Pimentel, J.A., *et al.* (2011). Beneficial effects of cannabinoids (CB) in a murine model of allergen-induced airway inflammation: role of CB_1/CB_2 receptors. *Immunobiology*, **216**(4), 466–476.

Cao, Z., Mulvihill, M.M., Mukhopadhyay, P., *et al.* (2013). Monoacylglycerol lipase controls endocannabinoid and eicosanoid signaling and hepatic injury in mice. *Gastroenterology*, **144**, 808–817.

Cappellano, G., Uberti, F., Caimmi, P.P., *et al.* (2013). Different expression and function of the endocannabinoid system in human epicardial adipose tissue in relation to heart disease. *Canadian Journal of Cardiology*, **29**(4), 499–509.

Cassol-Jr, O.J., Comim, C.M., Silva, B.R., *et al.* (2010). Treatment with cannabidiol reverses oxidative stress parameters, cognitive impairment and mortality in rats submitted to sepsis by cecal ligation and puncture. *Brain Research*, **1348**, 128–138.

Centers for Disease Control and Prevention. (2013). Acute kidney injury associated with synthetic cannabinoid use – multiple States (2012). *Morbidity and Mortal Weekly Report*, **62**, 93–98.

Comelli, F., Bettoni, I., Colombo, A., Fumagalli, P., Giagnoni, G., and Costa, B. (2010). Rimonabant, a cannabinoid CB1 receptor antagonist, attenuates mechanical allodynia and counteracts oxidative stress and nerve growth factor deficit in diabetic mice. *European Journal of Pharmacology*, **637**, 62–69.

Cooney, M.T., Vartiainen, E., Laatikainen, T., Juolevi, A., Dudina, A., and Graham, I.M. (2010). Elevated resting heart rate is an independent risk factor for cardiovascular disease in healthy men and women. *American Heart Journal*, **159**, 612–619.

Coskun, Z.M. and Bolkent, S. (2013). Biochemical and immunohistochemical changes in delta-9-tetrahydrocannabinol-treated type 2 diabetic rats. *Acta Histochemica*, **S0065–1281**(13), 112–118.

Cota, D., Marsicano, G., Tschop, M., *et al.* (2003). The endogenous cannabinoid system affects energy balance via central orexigenic drive and peripheral lipogenesis. *Journal of Clinical Investigation*, **112**, 423–431.

Durst, R., Danenberg, H., Gallily, R., *et al.* (2007). Cannabidiol, a nonpsychoactive *Cannabis* constituent, protects against myocardial ischemic reperfusion injury. *American Journal of Physiology Heart and Circulation Physiology*, **293**, H3602–3607.

El-Remessy, A.B., Al-Shabrawey, M., Khalifa, Y., Tsai, N.T., Caldwell, R.B., and Liou, G.I. (2006). Neuroprotective and blood-retinal barrier-preserving effects of cannabidiol in experimental diabetes. *American Journal of Pathology*, **168**, 235–244.

El-Remessy, A.B., Khalifa, Y., Ola, S., Ibrahim, A.S., and Liou, G.I. (2010). Cannabidiol protects retinal neurons by preserving glutamine synthetase activity in diabetes. *Molecular Vision*, **16**, 1487–1495.

El-Remessy, A.B., Rajesh, M., Mukhopadhyay, P., *et al.* (2011). Cannabinoid 1 receptor activation contributes to vascular inflammation and cell death in a mouse model of diabetic retinopathy and a human retinal cell line. *Diabetologia*, **54**(6), 1567–1578.

El-Remessy, A.B., Tang, Y., Zhu, G., *et al.* (2008). Neuroprotective effects of cannabidiol in endotoxin-induced uveitis: critical role of p38 MAPK activation. *Molecular Vision*, **14**, 2190–2203.

Fernández-Ruiz, J., Sagredo, O., Pazos, M.R., *et al.* (2013). Cannabidiol for neurodegenerative disorders: important new clinical applications for this phytocannabinoid? *British Journal of Clinical Pharmacology*, **75**, 323–333.

Fouad, A.A., Al-Mulhim, A.S., and Jresat, I. (2012). Cannabidiol treatment ameliorates ischemia/reperfusion renal injury in rats. *Life Sciences*, **91**, 284–292.

Frost, L., Mostofsky, E., Rosenbloom, J.I., Mukamal, K.J., and Mittleman, M.A. (2013). Marijuana use and long-term mortality among survivors of acute myocardial infarction. *American Heart Journal*, **165**, 170–175.

Gertsch, J., Leonti, M., Raduner, S., *et al.* (2008). Beta-caryophyllene is a dietary cannabinoid. *Proceedings of the National Academy of Sciences of the United States of America*, **105**, 9099–9104.

Gorelick, D.A., Goodwin, R.S., Schwilke, E., *et al.* (2013). Tolerance to effects of high-dose oral Δ^9-tetrahydrocannabinol and plasma cannabinoid concentrations in male daily cannabis smokers. *Journal of Analytical Toxicology*, **37**(1), 11–16.

Groblewski, T., Hong, X., Lessard, E., *et al.* (2010a). Pre-clinical pharmacological properties of novel peripherally-acting CB_1-CB_2 agonists. In: *20th Annual Symposium of the Cannabinoids, International Cannabinoid Research Society*. Lund: International Cannabinoid Research Society, p. 37.

Groblewski, T., Karlsten, R., Segerdhal, M., *et al.* (2010b). Peripherally-acting CB1-CB2 agonists for pain: do they still hold promise? In: *20th Annual Symposium of the Cannabinoids, International Cannabinoid Research Society*. Lund: International Cannabinoid Research Society, p. 38.

Hampson, A.J., Grimaldi, M., Axelrod, J., and Wink, D. (1998) Cannabidiol and (-)Δ^9-tetrahydrocannabinol are neuroprotective antioxidants. *Proceedings of the National Academy of Sciences of the United States of America*, **95**, 8268–8273.

Hampson, A.J., Grimaldi, M., Lolic, M., Wink, D., Rosenthal, R., and Axelrod, J. (2000). Neuroprotective antioxidants from marijuana. *Annals of New York Academy of Sciences*, **899**, 274–282.

Han, K.H., Lim, S., Ryu, J., *et al.* (2009). CB_1 and CB_2 cannabinoid receptors differentially regulate the production of reactive oxygen species by macrophages. *Cardiovascular Research*, **84**, 378–386.

Heath, T.S., Burroughs, Z., Thompson, A.J., and Tecklenburg, F.W. (2012). Acute intoxication caused by a synthetic cannabinoid in two adolescents. *Journal of Pediatric Pharmacology and Therapeutics*, **17**, 177–181.

Hegde, V.L., Nagarkatti, P.S., and Nagarkatti, M. (2011). Role of myeloid-derived suppressor cells in amelioration of experimental autoimmune hepatitis following activation of TRPV1 receptors by cannabidiol. *PLoS One*, **6**, e18281.

Hollister, L.E. and Reaven. G.M. (1974). Delta-9-tetrahydrocannabinol and glucose tolerance. *Clinical Pharmacology Therapeutics*, **16**, 297–302.

Horvath, B., Magid, L., Mukhopadhyay, P., *et al.* (2012a). A new cannabinoid CB_2 receptor agonist HU-910 attenuates oxidative stress, inflammation and cell death associated with hepatic ischaemia/reperfusion injury. *British Journal of Pharmacology*, **165**, 2462–2478.

Horvath, B., Mukhopadhyay, P., Hasko, G., and Pacher, P. (2012b). The endocannabinoid system and plant-derived cannabinoids in diabetes and diabetic complications. *American Journal of Pathology*, **180**, 432–442.

Horvath, B., Mukhopadhyay, P., Kechrid, M., *et al.* (2012c). Beta-caryophyllene ameliorates cisplatin-induced nephrotoxicity in a cannabinoid 2 receptor-dependent manner. *Free Radical Biology & Medicine*, **52**, 1325–1333.

Izzo, A.A., Borrelli, F., Capasso, R., Di Marzo, V., and Mechoulam, R. (2009). Non-psychotropic plant cannabinoids: new therapeutic opportunities from an ancient herb. *Trends Pharmacological Sciences*, **30**, 515–527.

Janiak, P., Poirier, B., Bidouard, J.P., *et al.* (2007). Blockade of cannabinoid CB_1 receptors improves renal function, metabolic profile, and increased survival of obese Zucker rats. *Kidney International*, **72**, 1345–1357.

Jeong, W.I., Osei-Hyiaman, D., Park, O., *et al.* (2008). Paracrine activation of hepatic CB_1 receptors by stellate cell-derived endocannabinoids mediates alcoholic fatty liver. *Cell Metabolism*, **7**, 227–235.

Jourdan, T., Godlewski, G., Cinar, R., *et al.* (2013). Activation of the Nlrp3 inflammasome in infiltrating macrophages by endocannabinoids mediates beta cell loss in type 2 diabetes. *Nature Medicine*, **19**, 1132–1140.

Kim, W., Doyle, M.E., Liu, Z., *et al.* (2011). Cannabinoids inhibit insulin receptor signaling in pancreatic β-cells. *Diabetes*, **60**, 1198–1209.

Klein, T.W. (2005) Cannabinoid-based drugs as anti-inflammatory therapeutics. *Nature Reviews in Immunology*, **5**, 400–411.

Klein, T.W., Newton, C., Larsen, K., *et al.* (2003). The cannabinoid system and immune modulation. *Journal of Leukocyte Biology*, **74**, 486–496.

Klumpers, L.E., Roy, C., Ferron, G., *et al.* (2013). Surinabant, a selective CB_1 antagonist, inhibits THC-induced central nervous system and heart rate effects in humans. *British Journal of Clinical Pharmacology*, **76**(1), 65–77.

Kunos, G. and Tam, J. (2011). The case for peripheral CB_1 receptor blockade in the treatment of visceral obesity and its cardiometabolic complications. *British Journal of Pharmacology*, **163**, 1423–1431.

Le Foll, B., Trigo, J.M., Sharkey, K.A., and Le Strat, Y. (2013). Cannabis and Δ^9-tetrahydrocannabinol (THC) for weight loss? *Medical Hypotheses*, **80**, 564–567.

Leblanc, A., Tirel-Badets, A., Paleiron, N., *et al.* (2011). Cannabis and myocardial infarction without angiographic stenosis in young patient: guilty or not guilty? A case report. *Annales de Cardiologie et d'Angiologie (Paris)*, **60**, 154–158.

Li, X., Kaminski, N.E., and Fischer, L.J. (2001). Examination of the immunosuppressive effect of Δ^9-tetrahydrocannabinol in streptozotocin-induced autoimmune diabetes. *International Immunopharmacology*, **1**, 699–712.

Liu, W.J., Jin, H.Y., Park, J.H., Baek, H.S., and Park, T.S. (2010). Effect of rimonabant, the cannabinoid CB_1 receptor antagonist, on peripheral nerve in streptozotocin-induced diabetic rat. *European Journal of Pharmacology*, **637**, 70–76.

Magen, I., Avraham, Y., Ackerman, Z., Vorobiev, L., Mechoulam, R., and Berry, E.M. (2009). Cannabidiol ameliorates cognitive and motor impairments in mice with bile duct ligation. *Journal of Hepatology*, **51**, 528–534.

Malfait, A.M., Gallily, R., Sumariwalla, P.F., *et al.* (2000). The nonpsychoactive cannabis constituent cannabidiol is an oral anti-arthritic therapeutic in murine collagen-induced arthritis. *Proceedings of National Academy of Sciences of the United States of America*, **97**, 9561–9566.

Mallat, A., Teixeira-Clerc, F., Deveaux, V., Manin, S., and Lotersztajn, S. (2011). The endocannabinoid system as a key mediator during liver diseases: new insights and therapeutic openings. *British Journal of Pharmacology*, **163**, 1432–1440.

Mallat, A., Teixeira-Clerc, F., and Lotersztajn, S. (2013). Cannabinoid signaling and liver therapeutics. *Journal of Hepatology*, **59**, 891–896.

Marquart, S., Zerr, P., Akhmetshina, A., *et al.* (2010). Inactivation of the cannabinoid receptor CB1 prevents leukocyte infiltration and experimental fibrosis. *Arthritis Rheumatism*, **62**(11), 3467–3476.

Martin-Santos, R., Crippa, J.A., Batalla, A., *et al.* (2012). Acute effects of a single, oral dose of Δ9-tetrahydrocannabinol (THC) and cannabidiol (CBD) administration in healthy volunteers. *Current Pharmacological Design*, **18**, 4966–4979.

Massi, P., Solinas, M., Cinquina, V., and Parolaro, D. (2013). Cannabidiol as potential anticancer drug. *British Journal of Clinical Pharmacology*, **75**, 303–312.

Mir, A., Obafemi, A., Young, A., and Kane, C. (2011). Myocardial infarction associated with use of the synthetic cannabinoid K2. *Pediatrics*, **128**, e1622–1627.

Mittleman, M.A., Lewis, R.A., Maclure, M., Sherwood, J.B., and Muller, J.E. (2001). Triggering myocardial infarction by marijuana. *Circulation*, **103**, 2805–2809.

Mukamal, K.J., Maclure, M., Muller, J.E., and Mittleman, M.A. (2008). An exploratory prospective study of marijuana use and mortality following acute myocardial infarction. *American Heart Journal*, **155**, 465–470.

Mukhopadhyay, P., Batkai, S., Rajesh, M., *et al.* (2007). Pharmacological inhibition of CB1 cannabinoid receptor protects against doxorubicin-induced cardiotoxicity. *Journal of American College of Cardiology*, **50**, 528–536.

Mukhopadhyay, P., Horvath, B., Kechrid, M., *et al.* (2011a). Poly(ADP-ribose) polymerase-1 is a key mediator of cisplatin-induced kidney inflammation and injury. *Free Radical Biology and Medicine*, **51**, 1774–1788.

Mukhopadhyay, P., Horvath, B., Zsengeller, Z., *et al.* (2012). Mitochondrial-targeted antioxidants represent a promising approach for prevention of cisplatin-induced nephropathy. *Free Radical Biology and Medicine*, **52**, 497–506.

Mukhopadhyay, P., Pan, H., Rajesh, M., *et al.* (2010a). CB_1 cannabinoid receptors promote oxidative/nitrosative stress, inflammation and cell death in a murine nephropathy model. *British Journal of Pharmacology*, **160**, 657–668.

Mukhopadhyay, P., Rajesh, M., Batkai, S., *et al.* (2010b). CB1 cannabinoid receptors promote oxidative stress and cell death in murine models of doxorubicin-induced cardiomyopathy and in human cardiomyocytes. *Cardiovascular Research*, **85**, 773–784.

Mukhopadhyay, P., Rajesh, M., Horvath, B., *et al.* (2011b). Cannabidiol protects against hepatic ischemia/reperfusion injury by attenuating inflammatory signaling and response, oxidative/nitrative stress, and cell death. *Free Radical Biology and Medicine*, **50**(10), 1368–1381.

Mukhopadhyay, P., Rajesh, M., Pan, H., *et al.* (2010c). Cannabinoid-2 receptor limits inflammation, oxidative/nitrosative stress, and cell death in nephropathy. *Free Radical Biology and Medicine*, **48**, 457–467.

Muniyappa, R., Sable, S., Ouwerkerk, R., *et al.* (2013). Metabolic effects of chronic cannabis smoking. *Diabetes Care*, **36**, 1–8.

Nam, D.H., Lee, M.H., Kim, J.E., *et al.* (2012). Blockade of cannabinoid receptor 1 improves insulin resistance, lipid metabolism, and diabetic nephropathy in db/db mice. *Endocrinology*, **153**, 1387–1396.

Osei-Hyiaman, D., DePetrillo, M., Pacher, P., *et al.* (2005). Endocannabinoid activation at hepatic CB1 receptors stimulates fatty acid synthesis and contributes to diet-induced obesity. *Journal of Clinical Investigation*, **115**, 1298–1305.

Pacher, P., Batkai, S., and Kunos, G. (2005). Cardiovascular pharmacology of cannabinoids. *Handbook of Experimental Pharmacology*, **168**, 599–625.

Pacher, P., Batkai, S., and Kunos, G. (2006). The endocannabinoid system as an emerging target of pharmacotherapy. *Pharmacological Reviews*, **58**, 389–462.

Pacher, P., Beckman, J.S., and Liaudet, L. (2007). Nitric oxide and peroxynitrite in health and disease. *Physiological Reviews*, **87**, 315–424.

Pacher, P. and Kunos, G. (2013). Modulating the endocannabinoid system in human health and disease – successes and failures. *FEBS Journal*, **280**, 1918–1943.

Pacher, P. and Mechoulam, R. (2011). Is lipid signaling through cannabinoid 2 receptors part of a protective system? *Progress in Lipid Research*, **50**, 193–211.

Pan, H., Mukhopadhyay, P., Rajesh, M., *et al.* (2009). Cannabidiol attenuates cisplatin-induced nephrotoxicity by decreasing oxidative/nitrosative stress, inflammation, and cell death. *Journal of Pharmacology and Experimental Therapeutics*, **328**, 708–714.

Pertwee, R.G. (2008). The diverse CB_1 and CB_2 receptor pharmacology of three plant cannabinoids: delta9-tetrahydrocannabinol, cannabidiol and delta9-tetrahydrocannabivarin. *British Journal of Pharmacology*, **153**, 199–215.

Pertwee, R.G. (2012). Targeting the endocannabinoid system with cannabinoid receptor agonists: pharmacological strategies and therapeutic possibilities. *Philosophical Transactions of the Royal Society. Series B, Biological Sciences*, **367**, 3353–3363.

Pratap, B. and Korniyenko, A. (2012). Toxic effects of marijuana on the cardiovascular system. *Cardiovascular Toxicology*, **12**, 143–148.

Quercioli, A., Pataky, Z., Montecucco, F., *et al.* (2012). Coronary vasomotor control in obesity and morbid obesity: contrasting flow responses with endocannabinoids, leptin, and inflammation. *Journal of American College of Cardiology Cardiovascular Imaging*, **5**, 805–815.

Quercioli, A., Pataky, Z., Vincenti, G., *et al.* (2011). Elevated endocannabinoid plasma levels are associated with coronary circulatory dysfunction in obesity. *European Heart Journal*, **32**, 1369–1378.

Rajavashisth, T.B., Shaheen, M., Norris, K.C., *et al.* (2012). Decreased prevalence of diabetes in marijuana users: cross-sectional data from the National Health and Nutrition Examination Survey (NHANES) III. *British Medical Journal Open*, **2**, e000494.

Rajesh, M., Batkai, S., Kechrid, M., *et al.* (2012). Cannabinoid 1 receptor promotes cardiac dysfunction, oxidative stress, inflammation, and fibrosis in diabetic cardiomyopathy. *Diabetes*, **61**, 716–727.

Rajesh, M., Mukhopadhyay, P., Batkai, S., *et al.* (2007). Cannabidiol attenuates high glucose-induced endothelial cell inflammatory response and barrier disruption. *Americal Journal of Physiology Heart and Circulatory Physiology*, **293**, H610–619.

Rajesh, M., Mukhopadhyay, P., Batkai, S., *et al.* (2010a). Cannabidiol attenuates cardiac dysfunction, oxidative stress, fibrosis, and inflammatory and cell death signaling pathways in diabetic cardiomyopathy. *Journal of American College of Cardiology*, **56**, 2115–2125.

Rajesh, M., Mukhopadhyay, P., Hasko, G., Liaudet, L., Mackie, K., and Pacher, P. (2010b). Cannabinoid-1 receptor activation induces reactive oxygen species-dependent and -independent mitogen-activated protein kinase activation and cell death in human coronary artery endothelial cells. *British Journal of Pharmacology*, **160**, 688–700.

Rajesh, M., Pan, H., Mukhopadhyay, P., *et al.* (2007b). Cannabinoid-2 receptor agonist HU-308 protects against hepatic ischemia/reperfusion injury by attenuating oxidative stress, inflammatory response, and apoptosis. *Journal of Leukocyte Biology*, **82**, 1382–1389.

Ramirez, S.H., Reichenbach, N.L., Fan, S., *et al.* (2013). Attenuation of HIV-1 replication in macrophages by cannabinoid receptor 2 agonists. *Journal of Leukocyte Biology*, **93**, 801–810.

Riedel, G., Fadda, P., McKillop-Smith, S., *et al.* (2009). Synthetic and plant-derived cannabinoid receptor antagonists show hypophagic properties in fasted and non-fasted mice. *British Journal of Pharmacology*, **156**, 1154–1166.

Ruiz-Valdepenas, L., Martinez-Orgado, J.A., Benito, C., *et al.* (2011). Cannabidiol reduces lipopolysaccharide-induced vascular changes and inflammation in the mouse brain: an intravital microscopy study. *Journal of Neuroinflammation*, **8**, 1–9.

Schmid, K., Schonlebe, J., Drexler, H., and Mueck-Weymann, M. (2010). The effects of cannabis on heart rate variability and well-being in young men. *Pharmacopsychiatry*, **43**, 147–150.

Silvestri, C. and Di Marzo, V. (2013). The endocannabinoid system in energy homeostasis and the etiopathology of metabolic disorders. *Cell Metabolism*, **17**, 475–490.

Singla, S., Sachdeva, R., and Mehta, J.L. (2012). Cannabinoids and atherosclerotic coronary heart disease. *Clinical Cardiology*, **35**, 329–335.

Slavic, S., Lauer, D., Sommerfeld, M., *et al.* (2013). Cannabinoid receptor 1 inhibition improves cardiac function and remodelling after myocardial infarction and in experimental metabolic syndrome. *Journal of Molecular Medicine (Berlin)*, **91**, 811–823.

Stanley, C.P., Hind, W.H., and O'Sullivan, S.E. (2013). Is the cardiovascular system a therapeutic target for cannabidiol? *British Journal of Clinical Pharmacology*, **75**, 313–322.

Steffens, S. and Pacher, P. (2012). Targeting cannabinoid receptor CB_2 in cardiovascular disorders: promises and controversies. *British Journal of Pharmacology*, **167**, 313–323.

Sugamura, K., Sugiyama, S., Nozaki, T., *et al.* (2009). Activated endocannabinoid system in coronary artery disease and antiinflammatory effects of cannabinoid 1 receptor blockade on macrophages. *Circulation*, **119**, 28–36.

Tam, J., Cinar, R., Liu, J., *et al.* (2012). Peripheral cannabinoid-1 receptor inverse agonism reduces obesity by reversing leptin resistance. *Cell Metabolism*, **16**, 167–179.

Tam, J., Liu, J., Mukhopadhyay, B., Cinar, R., Godlewski, G., and Kunos, G. (2011). Endocannabinoids in liver disease. *Hepatology*, **53**, 346–355.

Tam, J., Vemuri, V.K., Liu, J., *et al.* (2010). Peripheral CB1 cannabinoid receptor blockade improves cardiometabolic risk in mouse models of obesity. *Journal of Clinical Investigation*, **120**, 2953–2966.

Thomas, A., Baillie, G.L., Phillips, A.M., Razdan, R.K., Ross, R.A., and Pertwee, R.G. (2007). Cannabidiol displays unexpectedly high potency as an antagonist of CB_1 and CB_2 receptor agonists in vitro. *British Journal of Pharmacology*, **150**, 613–623.

Waldman, M., Hochhauser, E., Fishbein, M., Aravot, D., Shainberg, A., and Sarne, Y. (2013). An ultra-low dose of tetrahydrocannabinol provides cardioprotection. *Biochemical Pharmacology*, **85**, 1626–1633.

Walsh, S.K., Hepburn, C.Y., Kane, K.A., and Wainwright, C.L. (2010). Acute administration of cannabidiol in vivo suppresses ischaemia-induced cardiac arrhythmias and reduces infarct size when given at reperfusion. *British Journal of Pharmacology*, **160**, 1234–1242.

Wargent, E.T., Zaibi, M.S., Silvestri, C., *et al.* (2013). The cannabinoid Δ^9-tetrahydrocannabivarin (THCV) ameliorates insulin sensitivity in two mouse models of obesity. *Nutrition & Diabetes*, **3**, e68.

Weiss, L., Zeira, M., Reich, S., *et al.* (2006). Cannabidiol lowers incidence of diabetes in non-obese diabetic mice. *Autoimmunity*, **39**, 143–151.

Weiss, L., Zeira, M., Reich, S., *et al.* (2008). Cannabidiol arrests onset of autoimmune diabetes in NOD mice. *Neuropharmacology*, **54**, 244–249.

Wong, A., Gunasekaran, N., Hancock, D.P., *et al.* (2012). The major plant-derived cannabinoid Δ^9-tetrahydrocannabinol promotes hypertrophy and macrophage infiltration in adipose tissue. *Hormone Metabolism Research*, **44**, 105–113.

Zsengeller, Z.K., Ellezian, L., Brown, D., *et al.* (2012). Cisplatin nephrotoxicity involves mitochondrial injury with impaired tubular mitochondrial enzyme activity. *Journal of Histochemistry Cytochemistry*, **60**, 521–529.

Chapter 32

Phytocannabinoids and Skin Disorders

Sergio Oddi and Mauro Maccarrone

"Quid me mihi detrahis?" inquit.
"A piget, a! non est" clamabat "tibia tanti!"
("Why do you peel me from myself?", he cried.
"Oh, I repent! Oh, a flute is not worth such price!")

Publius Ovidius Naso, Metamorphoses, *VI 385–386*

32.1 Introduction

The endocannabinoid system (ECS) refers to a group of bioactive lipids, called endocannabinoids (eCBs), and their receptors that are widely expressed throughout the body and appear to be involved in the regulation of nearly all physiological functions. Indeed, the activation of this autocrine/paracrine signaling system by delta-9-tetrahydrocannabinol (THC) and other phytocannabinoids, as well as by synthetic cannabinoids and eCBs, exerts numerous pharmacological actions, including antiemetic, analgesic, anxiolytic, antidepressant, anti-inflammatory, and antineoplastic effects (Pacher et al. 2006), to mention just a few.

In recent years, the presence of a full and functional ECS in the skin and in its adnexal structures (e.g., hair follicle, sebaceous and sweat glands) has been ascertained. Substantial evidence has been also accumulated indicating a local regulatory role of the ECS in skin physiology, including the formation of the epidermal barrier, and the regulation of melanogenesis, sebum production, and of a variety of immune responses (Biro et al. 2009). In addition, therapeutic efficacy of targeting the cutaneous ECS is beginning to be documented in several dermatological conditions, thus opening a promising new front in the field of cannabis pharmacology (Biro et al. 2009; Kupczyk et al. 2009; Pasquariello et al. 2009).

This chapter describes the expression and regulation of the ECS in skin cells, and its regulatory role under physiological and pathological conditions. Further, evidence indicating that targeted manipulation of ECS signaling by cannabis medicines may represent a valuable strategy for a broad variety of skin disorders is also discussed.

32.2 Biology of the skin

32.2.1 Anatomy and histology of the skin

The skin, or the integument, is one of the largest organs, with a surface area of about 1.8 m² and accounts for approximately 7% of total body weight in the average adult. The skin consists of

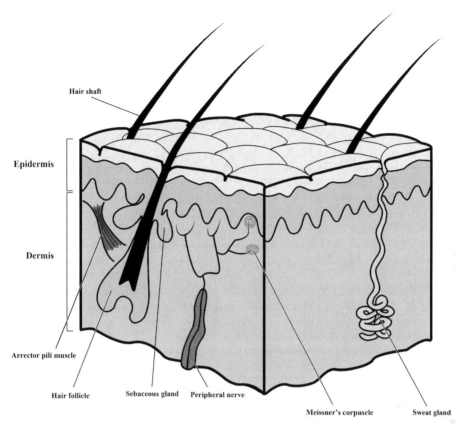

Fig. 32.1 (See also colour plate section.) Schematic representation of the skin. See text for details.

two main tissues, the epidermis and the dermis, separated by a thin sheet of fibers called the basement membrane (Fig. 32.1). Each of these layers is made of different tissues and has very different functions.

32.2.1.1 Epidermis

The epidermis is the outer layer of the skin, serving as the physical and chemical barrier between the interior body and the exterior environment. The epidermis is a multistratified squamous epithelium that is generated by specialized epithelial cells, the keratinocytes, through a tightly regulated differentiation process, called epidermal terminal differentiation or cornification (Fuchs 1990).

Topologically, the epidermis is divided into four layers, or strata, which represent the main differentiative stages of the keratinocyte: (1) the stratum germinativum or basal layer, (2) the stratum spinosum, (3) the stratum granolosum, and (4) the stratum corneum (Fig. 32.2). The innermost layer of cuboidal cells, the basal layer, represents the proliferative compartment for generation and continuous renewal of the tissue. On detachment from the basement membrane, newborn keratinocytes migrate outward through successive stages of differentiation, represented by the spinous and granular layers, toward the terminal differentiation on the surface, the stratum corneum, where they are transformed into flattened, enucleated squames, termed corneocytes. The latter cells are sloughed from the surface, and continually replaced by inner cells (Fig. 32.2).

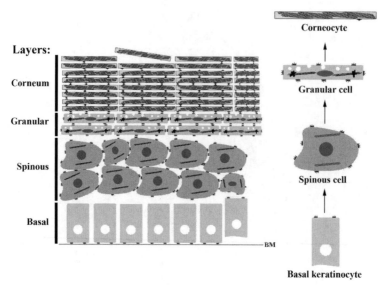

Fig. 32.2 Schematic representation showing a section of epidermis with epidermal layers labelled with different colors. During epidermal differentiation, basal keratinocytes detach from the basement membrane (BM) and start the process of keratinocyte cornification. As cells differentiate, they move up to form the different layers of the epidermis, as depicted in the right side of the figure. See text for details.

In addition to keratinocytes, the epidermis has three other cell types: melanocytes that produce a pigment called melanin, which colors the skin, and protects it against the damaging effects of solar radiation; Merkel cells that provide sensory information; and Langerhans cells that are a specialized subset of dendritic cells serving as the first line of defense against pathogens invading the skin.

32.2.1.2 Dermis

The innermost and much thicker of the two skin layers, the dermis, is a sensitive connective tissue containing most of the skin's specialized cells and structures, including nerve endings, hair roots, sweat and sebaceous glands, and blood and lymph vessels (Fig. 32.1). Therefore, most of the skin functions, such as sensory perception, immunologic surveillance, and thermoregulation, are carried out by dermis. The latter is also responsible for the mechanical properties and the trophic support of the skin.

Anatomically, the dermis is divided into two layers: the papillary region and the reticular dermis. The papillary region consists of finger-like projections just beneath the basement membrane of the epidermis. In this portion, the collagen fibers, that represent the more important structural components of the dermis, form a loose three-dimensional network that contains terminal portions of blood capillaries, free nerve endings, and tactile Meissner's corpuscles (Fig. 32.1). The reticular dermis is composed of a much denser network of thick collagenous, elastic, and reticular fibers. These fibrillar components, interdispersed in an amorphous ground substance, give the dermis its mechanical properties. Also located within the reticular region are the roots of the hair, sebaceous glands, arrectores pilorum muscles, nerve endings, and several specialized sensory receptors (Fig. 32.1).

Dermal fibroblasts are the major cell type in dermis and produce and organize the extracellular matrix of the tissue. In addition, they are involved in the production of growth factors/cytokines and in inflammatory responses. Other cellular populations of the dermis include smooth muscle cells, vascular and lymphatic endothelial cells, and various cells of hematopoietic origin. These include a constitutive population of dendritic cells and a more heterogeneous population of leukocytes, comprising mast cells, monocytes/macrophages, neutrophils, and lymphocytes.

32.2.2 Physiology of the skin

Placed at the interface between the organism and its environment, the skin is primarily a dynamic barrier against injuries, infections, water loss, and ultraviolet radiation. Further, the skin carries out important sensory functions and contributes to the homeostasis of the body, taking a crucial part in thermoregulation, hydrosaline balance, and metabolism of certain hormones and vitamins (Chu 2012).

The barrier function of the skin is mainly established through the hydrolipidic film into the top layers of the stratum corneum of the epidermis, that ensures a defense against microbial and chemical agents and prevents an excessive dehydration. The network of collagen and elastin fibers produced by the fibroblasts in the dermis, the dermo-epidermal junction (basement membrane), and the system of intercellular connections in the epidermis confer to the skin its mechanical properties of strength, extensibility, and elasticity that enable it to resist mechanical injuries. The skin immune cells (primarily Langerhans cells, dermal dendritic cells, mast cells, macrophages, and T-cell subpopulations) are involved in the local defense against chemical and/or biological insults. Finally, the melanocytes protect the skin against the damaging effects of solar ultraviolet radiation.

Through its abundant innervation, the skin is the largest sense organ in the body, that mediates the sensory perception of touch, pressure, vibration, temperature, pain, and itch associated with skin disorders. The ability of this organ to regulate body temperature depends on the presence of dermal blood vessels that, together with their arteriovenous anastomoses, are also involved in the regulation of blood pressure. Finally, the skin serves as a metabolic regulator that transforms various hormones and inactivates potentially harmful substances of exogenous or endogenous origin.

32.3 Expression of the endocannabinoid system in the skin

The biological and pharmacological effects of phytocannabinoids and their synthetic analogs are primarily attributable to their modulatory activities toward the so-called ECS (Russo 2011). This signaling system consists of at least two receptors, the G-protein coupled cannabinoid receptors 1 and 2 (CB_1 and CB_2), their endogenous ligands, the eCBs, along with their transport proteins and metabolic enzymes (De Petrocellis and Di Marzo 2009).

Arachidonoylethanolamide (AEA) and 2-arachidonoylglycerol (2-AG), the most prominent eCBs, are generally considered to be produced "on demand" in response to stressful stimuli from cell membrane components. Yet, recent evidence points toward a key role of intracellular transporters and storage organelles in controlling eCB tone (Maccarrone et al. 2010). Because of their high lipophilicity, the signaling activity of eCBs is short-lasting and limited to those cells or tissues that are subjected to stress or damage. In addition, other lipid mediators have been discovered, of which the most relevant is the antiproliferative N-palmitoylethanolamine (PEA). PEA is not considered an eCB, but rather an "eCB-like" compound, since it does not activate cannabinoid receptors, but is able to potentiate the activity of AEA or 2-AG by influencing their transport and degradation (De Petrocellis and Di Marzo 2009).

32.3.1 **CB$_1$ and CB$_2$ receptors**

Immunohistological investigations of the precise localization of CB$_1$ and CB$_2$ receptors in sections of human and rodent skin revealed their presence in virtually all the skin cell populations. In particular, both receptors were observed in epidermal keratinocytes, cutaneous nerve fibers, dermal cells, and specialized cells with adnexal structures (Table 32.1) (Casanova et al. 2003; Ibrahim et al. 2005; Stander et al. 2005). Interestingly, in one of these immunohistochemical studies on human skin, CB$_1$ and CB$_2$ were found to be distributed in a complementary fashion, in epidermis, hair follicle, and sebaceous gland, with CB$_1$ and CB$_2$ being predominantly expressed

Table 32.1 Expression of the ECS in the skin

ECS member	Epidermis	Dermis	Nerve fibers	Adnexal structures
CB$_1$	Suprabasal keratinocytes; primary melanocytes	Fibroblasts; mast cells, macrophages	Single epidermal nerve fibers, small unmyelinated subepidermal nerves, large dermal myelinated nerves	Differentiated sebocytes, differentiated epithelial cells of the infundibulum and inner root sheath of hair follicles, myoepithelial cells of eccrine sweat glands, sweat gland duct
CB$_2$	Basal keratynocytes; primary melanocytes	Fibroblasts, mast cells; vascular smooth muscle cells	Single epidermal nerve fibers, small unmyelinated subepidermal nerves, large dermal myelinated nerves	Undifferentiated sebocytes, undifferentiated infundibular hair follicle cells, myoepithelial cells of eccrine sweat glands, sweat gland duct, mast cells, macrophages
AEA	Primary keratinocytes and melanocytes	Macrophages		Human sebocytes SZ95
2-AG	Primary keratinocytes and melanocytes	Macrophages		Human sebocytes SZ95
PEA	Primary keratinocytes and melanocytes			
NAPE-PLD	Keratinocytes; melanocytes	Primary fibroblasts		
FAAH	Keratinocytes; melanocytes	Primary fibroblasts		
MAGL	Primary keratinocytes and melanocytes	Primary fibroblasts		Human sebocytes SZ95
DAGL	Primary keratinocytes and melanocytes	Primary fibroblasts		Human sebocytes SZ95

For acronyms, see the list of abbreviations at the beginning of the chapter.

in differentiated and undifferentiated cells, respectively, suggesting that the two receptors play nonredundant roles during differentiation of keratinocytes and sebocytes. In rat skin, CB_2 immunolabeling was found beyond the basal layer, but fairly uniformly distributed throughout the epidermis (Ibrahim et al. 2005).

In the dermis, abundant labeling for CB_1 and CB_2 was identified on the myoepithelial cells of the secretory portion of eccrine sweat glands, but not in secretory cells (Stander et al. 2005). Positive immunoreactivity for CB_1 and CB_2 was also found in mast cells and in most but not all CD68-positive macrophages (Stander et al. 2005; Sugawara et al. 2012). In mouse skin, positive staining of CB_2 was detected in myofibroblasts and vascular smooth muscle cells (Zheng et al. 2012). Concerning their localization on human primary sensory nerves, CB_1 and CB_2 were identified on large (myelinated) and thin (unmyelinated) calcitonin gene-related peptide positive nerve fibers (Stander et al. 2005). The available data concerning the expression of cannabinoid receptors in the skin are summarized in Table 32.1.

Additionally, these receptors were found to be expressed in cultured melanocytes (Magina et al. 2011; Pucci et al. 2012), fibroblasts (McPartland 2008), and sweat gland epithelial cells (Czifra et al. 2012).

32.3.2 Enzymes

The expression and/or activity of the main AEA-metabolizing enzymes (i.e., fatty acid amide hydrolase, FAAH, and N-acyl phosphatidylethanolamine phospholipase D, NAPE-PLD) have been documented for rodent skin (Karsak et al. 2007; Khasabova et al. 2012; Petrosino et al. 2010) (Table 32.1). On the other hand, the presence in the skin of the main enzymes involved in 2-AG biosynthesis and metabolism (i.e., diacylglycerol lipase, DAGL, and monoacylglycerol lipase, MAGL, respectively) is not yet well characterized, and has only been assessed in cultured keratinocytes (Berdyshev et al. 2000; Maccarrone et al. 2003; Oddi et al. 2005), melanocytes (Hamtiaux et al. 2012; Pucci et al. 2012), sebocytes (Dobrosi et al. 2008), and fibroblasts (McPartland 2008).

32.3.3 Endocannabinoids

The levels of the main eCBs (AEA and 2-AG) and of PEA have been measured in rodent paw skin by several laboratories (Calignano et al. 1998; Felder et al. 1996; Khasabova et al. 2008, 2011, 2012; Maione et al. 2007), and results are summarized in Table 32.2.

In vitro studies ascertained that different skin cell populations, including keratinocytes (Maccarrone et al. 2003; Magina et al. 2011; Toth et al. 2011), sebocytes (Dobrosi et al. 2008),

Table 32.2 Levels of AEA, 2-AG, and PEA in paw skin from mice or rats

Compound				
Tissue	AEA (pmol/g tissue)	2-AG (nmol/g tissue)	PEA (pmol/g tissue)	Reference
Rat paw skin	49 ± 9	6.10 ± 0.08	692 ± 119	Calignano et al. 1998
	30 ± 9		750 ± 100	Felder et al. 1996
	143 ± 14			Maione et al. 2007
Mouse paw skin	34.9 ± 2.6	1.60 ± 0.25	790 ± 89	Khasabova et al. 2012
	176 ± 35	4.1 ± 0.6	130 ± 20	Maione et al. 2007

Values are expressed as mean ± standard error of the mean.

melanocytes (Pucci et al. 2012), sweat gland epithelial cells (Czifra et al. 2012), and macrophages (Jiang et al. 2009), synthesize and release eCBs under basal and stimulated conditions.

32.4 Role of the endocannabinoid system in skin physiology

32.4.1 Biological activities of the endocannabinoid system in skin cells

Alterations in eCB levels were observed in a variety of physiological and pathophysiological conditions of the skin. For example, ultraviolet B exposure increased the levels of AEA in cultured keratinocytes, suggesting that this eCB is involved in cellular responses to stress (Berdyshev et al. 2000; Magina et al. 2011). Instead, 12-O-tetradecanoylphorbol-13-acetate and calcium, two well-established inducers of keratinocyte differentiation, markedly reduced the endogenous level of AEA, due to its enhanced degradation by FAAH (Maccarrone et al. 2003; Oddi et al. 2005).

Generally, a strong elevation of eCB levels in the skin was found to follow the application of irritant and inflammatory stimuli (Costa et al. 2010; Karsak et al. 2007; Maione et al. 2007; Oka et al. 2006; Petrosino et al. 2010). These changes are thought to represent an adaptive response aimed at reducing pain and inflammation (Di Marzo 2008). Indeed, genetic or pharmacological inactivation of eCB degradative enzymes usually counteracts pain and inflammation (Petrosino and Di Marzo 2010). However, emerging evidence suggests that AEA and 2-AG, as well as CB_1 and CB_2 receptors, may have different, sometimes even opposing, role(s) in many inflammatory conditions, with AEA and CB_1 playing immunosuppressive roles, and 2-AG and CB_2 acting as both pro- and anti-inflammatory mediators (Di Marzo and Petrosino 2007).

Growing evidence supports a functional role of eCB signaling in skin cells. For example, AEA inhibited the formation of cornified envelope, a hallmark of terminal keratinocyte differentiation, through a CB_1-dependent reduction of transglutaminase and protein kinase C activities (Maccarrone et al. 2003), suggesting an important role of eCB signaling in epidermal differentiation. This antidifferentiative action of AEA was found to be associated with the silencing of genes involved in keratinocyte differentiation (i.e., keratin 1, keratin 10, involucrin, and transglutaminase 5) by selective DNA methylation of their promoters (Paradisi et al. 2008). On the other hand, in hair follicles it was demonstrated that CB_1 activation by AEA inhibited hair shaft elongation and the proliferation of hair matrix keratinocytes, and also induced intraepithelial apoptosis and premature hair follicle regression (Telek et al. 2007). Interestingly, these cells failed to respond to 2-AG stimulation, highlighting the nonredundancy of these two prototypic eCBs (Telek et al. 2007). Consistent with an inhibitory role of AEA in keratinocyte growth, CB_1 activation by AEA was found to markedly suppress proliferation and induce cell death in both human cultured keratinocytes and skin organ-culture models (Toth et al. 2011), most probably due to an elevation of intracellular Ca^{2+} concentration via the transient receptor potential vanilloid type 1 (TRPV1). The latter is one of the most prominent members of the TRP family of ion channels that is now established as an important target for phytocannabinoids (Costa et al. 2004b; De Petrocellis et al. 2011).

In human sebocytes, AEA stimulated lipid production at low concentrations, but induced apoptosis at higher levels, in a CB_2-mediated manner (Dobrosi et al. 2008). A similar biphasic behavior of AEA was observed also in human melanocytes, where AEA had melanogenic, mitogenic, and dendritogenic effects at low doses (via CB_1) and proapoptotic effects at higher doses (via TRPV1) (Pucci et al. 2012). Finally, in human eccrine sweat gland epithelial cells both AEA and 2-AG suppressed proliferation, induced apoptosis, altered expression of various structural proteins (i.e., involucrin, filaggrin, loricrin, and keratins), and upregulated lipid synthesis; remarkably, all these effects were CB_1-, CB_2-, and TRPV1-independent (Czifra et al. 2012).

32.4.2 **Role of cannabinoid receptors in the epidermal barrier**

Important information on the role of the cannabinoid receptors in skin biology has been recently obtained from knockout mice. Previous experiments have shown that CB_1 and CB_2 deficient mice, as well as $CB_1^{-/-}/CB_2^{-/-}$ double knockout mice, do not display any obvious skin maturation defect. However, a more focused study on the role of cannabinoid receptors in mouse epidermis has recently revealed that these two receptors operate in an opposite manner to regulate epidermal structure and function (Roelandt et al. 2012). In particular, targeted disruption of CB_1 receptors caused the formation of a thicker epidermis with an increased rate of keratinocyte proliferation, accompanied by a reduced expression of some relevant markers of keratinocyte differentiation (i.e., involucrin, loricrin, and filaggrin, caspase 14 activation), as well as by altered lipid bilayer structures (Roelandt et al. 2012). Conversely, the absence of CB_2 led to the formation of a thinner epidermis with reduced proliferative rates of keratinocytes, paralleled by a strong expression of the main epidermal differentiation markers (Roelandt et al. 2012). Moreover, functional data provided from these mouse models demonstrated that the recovery of the permeability barrier function of the epidermis following acute removal of corneocytes from the stratum corneum was impaired in $CB_1^{-/-}$, whilst it was enhanced in $CB_2^{-/-}$ mice. These findings strongly suggest that CB_1 signaling is a positive regulator, whereas CB_2 signaling is a negative regulator, of epidermal differentiation.

32.4.3 **Role of cannabinoid receptors in peripheral analgesia**

Both cannabinoid receptors have been found to inhibit pain responses in models of acute, inflammatory, and neuropathic pain by acting at peripheral sites (Bridges et al. 2001; Ellington et al. 2002; Malan et al. 2002; Richardson et al. 1998; Rukwied et al. 2003). By using transgenic mice selectively lacking CB_1 in nociceptors innervating the skin, Agarwal et al. (2007) demonstrated a critical role for CB_1 expressed by skin primary sensory neurons in the tonic inhibition of pain by eCBs, as well as in exogenous cannabinoid-induced analgesia for chronic inflammatory and neuropathic pain (Agarwal et al. 2007). For CB_2-mediated antinociceptive effects, an indirect mechanism has been identified. Indeed, peripherally administered CB_2 agonists caused the release from skin keratinocytes of the endogenous opioid β-endorphin, which then acts at μ-opioid receptors on primary afferent neurons to inhibit nociception (Ibrahim et al. 2005).

32.5 **Phytocannabinoids and skin pathophysiology**

32.5.1 **Psoriasis**

Psoriasis is one of the most common inflammatory skin disorders, characterized by well-demarcated erythematous, scaly plaques appearing on the surface of the epidermis. The hallmarks of psoriasis are abnormal differentiation and hyperproliferation of keratinocytes, accompanied by an excessive inflammatory response, mainly triggered by T-helper 1 (Th1) cells (Krueger and Bowcock 2005).

In view of their prodifferentiating, antiproliferative, and immunomodulatory effects, phytocannabinoids could be useful for the development of topical therapy for psoriasis. Indeed, phytocannabinoids (THC, cannabinol (CBN), cannabidiol (CBD), and cannabigerol (CBG)), as well as synthetic cannabinoid receptor agonists (JWH-015, BML-190, and HU-210), inhibited growth of a hyperproliferating human keratinocyte cell line (HPV-16) and human epidermal keratinocytes (Wilkinson and Williamson 2007) (Table 32.3). Other investigations demonstrated that cannabinoids inhibit proliferation of epidermal (Ibrahim et al. 2005; Paradisi et al. 2008; Toth et al.

Table 32.3 Emerging functions of phytocannabinoids in cutaneous biology

Phytocannabinoid	Biological or pharmacological effects	Reference
Δ⁹-Tetrahydrocannabinol (THC)	Antipruritic effects in patients with chronic cholestatic liver disease	Neff et al. 2002
	Vasorelaxation in isolated blood vessels	O'Sullivan et al. 2005
	Inhibits carrageenan-induced edema in rats	Sofia et al. 1973
	Inhibits croton oil-induced edema in mice	Tubaro et al. 2010
	Attenuates allergic contact dermatitis in mice	Karsak et al. 2007
	Inhibits keratinocyte proliferation in vitro	Wilkinson and Williamson 2007
	Antitumoral effects in vitro (melanoma and squamous cell carcinoma cells)	Blazquez et al. 2006; Hart et al. 2004
Cannabidiol (CBD)	Inhibits TPA-induced erythema in mice	Formukong et al. 1988
	Inhibits keratinocyte proliferation in vitro	Wilkinson and Williamson 2007
	Inhibits croton oil-induced ear edema in mice	Tubaro et al. 2010
	Inhibits carrageenan-induced edema in mice and rats	Costa et al. 2004a; Lodzki et al. 2003
	Inhibits collagen-induced inflammation in mice	Malfait et al. 2000
Cannabigerol (CBG)	Inhibits keratinocyte proliferation in vitro	Wilkinson and Williamson 2007
	Antitumoral effects in vitro (human oral epitheliod carcinoma cell lines)	Baek et al. 1998
Cannabinol (CBN)	Inhibits keratinocyte proliferation in vitro	Wilkinson and Williamson 2007
Cannabichromene (CBC)	Inhibits carrageenan-induced edema in rats	Turner and Elsohly 1981

2011) and hair matrix keratinocytes (Telek et al. 2007), and induced intraepithelial apoptosis and premature regression of hair follicles (Telek et al. 2007; Toth et al. 2011).

With respect to their immunomodulatory properties, several studies showed that cannabinoids suppress the production of proinflammatory cytokines (Klein 2005). For example, the use of cannabis was associated with a decrease of proinflammatory Th1 cytokines, such as interferon-γ and interleukin (IL)-2, and an increase in anti-inflammatory Th2 cytokines, such as IL-4 and IL-10 (Pacifici et al. 2003). Consistently, THC exposure suppressed the cell-mediated Th1 response (reducing the release of IL-2, tumor necrosis factor-α, interferon-γ) and simultaneously enhanced Th2-associated cytokines (such as IL-4) in mice infected with *Legionella pneumophila* (Klein et al. 2000; Newton et al. 1994). In addition, THC showed an impressive anti-inflammatory activity in the carrageenan-induced paw edema model in rats (Sofia et al. 1973), and was also active topically in the croton oil-induced ear edema model in mice (Tubaro et al. 2010). Interestingly, as well, the nonpsychotropic cannabinoids, CBD (Costa et al. 2004a; Formukong et al. 1988; Tubaro et al. 2010) and cannabichromene (CBC) (Turner and Elsohly 1981; Wirth et al. 1980) displayed a striking potency in in vivo assays of inhibition of inflammatory responses, despite their negligible activity as ligands of cannabinoid receptors (Stern and Lambert 2007) (Table 32.3).

Although direct studies using preclinical models of psoriasis have not yet been conducted, the antiproliferative effects of cannabinoids and AEA on keratinocytes and the earlier mentioned roles of CB_1 and CB_2 in epidermal biology, suggest that the ECS could be involved in the etiology of psoriasis.

32.5.2 **Skin tumors**

Skin cancers are one of the most common malignancies in humans. There are two main types of malignant skin tumors, namely carcinomas derived from epidermal cell lineage, and melanomas derived from melanocytes.

32.5.2.1 Melanoma

Melanoma is the least common but most dangerous form of skin cancer because of its chemoresistance and propensity to metastasis. Many patients with melanoma experience loss of appetite and nausea unresponsive to conventional antiemetics. THC has been successfully used as a palliative therapy in patients with malignant melanoma, preventing chemotherapy-induced nausea and vomiting, stimulating appetite, and alleviating cancer-associated pain (Gonzalez-Rosales and Walsh 1997; Zutt et al. 2006).

In the last years, emerging evidence has been obtained that suggests that phyto-, endo-, and synthetic cannabinoids could be useful in the treatment of cancer due to their ability to regulate signaling pathways that are involved in the control of basic cell functions, such as the balance between cell death and survival (Guzman 2003). Specifically, it has been found that human melanoma cells express functional cannabinoid receptors (Blazquez et al. 2006; Magina et al. 2011; Scuderi et al. 2011). Blazquez et al. (2006) found that cannabinoid receptor agonists decreased growth, proliferation, angiogenesis, and metastasis of human melanoma both in vitro and in vivo, thus revealing the potential benefits of the ECS in the treatment of this type of cancer (Blazquez et al. 2006).

The mechanisms whereby cannabinoids exerted such antimelanoma effects are currently unclear. On the one hand, it has been suggested that cannabinoids (THC, WIN 55,212-2, JWH-133) act on melanoma cells to arrest the cell cycle at the G1–S transition stage via cannabinoid receptor-dependent stimulation of the prosurvival protein Akt and hypophosphorylation of the retinoblastoma protein tumor suppressor (Blazquez et al. 2006). In another study, the antimi-togenic effects of WIN 55,212-2 on human melanoma cells were exerted independently of can-nabinoid or vanilloid receptors, but required lipid raft integrity and were mediated by caspase activation and phosphorylation of extracellular-signal-regulated kinase (Scuderi et al. 2011). Also in line with a possible involvement of $nonCB_{1/2}$ receptors in the antiproliferative action of can-nabinoids, PEA used in association with the FAAH inhibitor URB597 considerably reduced cell viability of mouse melanoma cells, both in vitro and in vivo (Hamtiaux et al. 2012).

32.5.2.2 Skin carcinomas

Nonmelanomas are named after the type of epidermal cell from which they arise: basal cell car-cinomas which originate from the basal layer of the epidermis, and squamous cell carcinomas which derive from, or are composed of, all epidermal layers. CB_1 and CB_2 receptors have been shown to be expressed in both basal cell carcinomas and squamous cell carcinomas in mouse and humans (Casanova et al. 2003; Zhao et al. 2010).

Local treatment with the mixed CB_1/CB_2 agonist WIN 55,212-2 or the selective CB_2 agonist JWH-133 inhibited the growth of malignant tumors generated by inoculation of epidermal tumor cells into nude mice (Casanova et al. 2003). Both cannabinoids induced apoptosis of nonmela-noma tumor cells and inhibition of tumor angiogenesis (Casanova et al. 2003). Remarkably, these antitumoral effects were associated with the abrogation of epidermal growth factor receptor func-tion (Casanova et al. 2003), an important player in the development of nonmelanoma skin cancers that triggers the angiogenic switch necessary for skin tumor growth (El-Abaseri et al. 2005).

Although CB_1 and CB_2 receptors are physiologically linked with skin cancer, their functional role in cancer is not fully understood. On the one hand, the pharmacological stimulation of CB_1 and CB_2 receptors has been found to induce apoptosis in skin carcinoma and melanoma cells (Blazquez et al. 2006; Casanova et al. 2003). On the other hand, CB_1 and CB_2 deficiency has been shown to suppress skin papilloma formation in a two-stage skin carcinogenesis mouse model, indicating that CB_1 and/or CB_2 receptors could have a role in promoting skin tumorigenesis, possibly by enhancing ultraviolet light-induced inflammation (Zheng et al. 2008). Moreover, THC treatment displayed a bimodal action on squamous cell carcinoma (SCC-9) growth, with low concentrations (nM range) being protumoral and high concentrations (μM range) having antitumoral effects (Hart et al. 2004).

32.5.3 Dermatitis

32.5.3.1 Atopic dermatitis

Atopic dermatitis is a chronic, relapsing inflammatory skin disorder that involves scaly and itchy rashes. Although the mechanism underlying atopic dermatitis is still elusive, it is believed that this condition is due to an immediate hypersensitivity reaction, mediated by Th2 cells, in response to various external factors such as irritants and allergens. Activated T cells stimulate B cells to produce immunoglobulin E, which, in turn, activates mast cells, producing many inflammatory and/or pruritogenic mediators, such as histamine, serotonin, proteases, and cytokines (Leung and Bieber 2003).

Emerging evidence has revealed the ECS as a key player in controlling mast cell biology (De Filippis et al. 2008; Maccarone et al. 2000; Sugawara et al. 2012). In fact, natural and synthetic cannabinoids displayed protective effects both in acute and chronic inflammatory pathologies sustained by excessive accumulation and degranulation of these immunocompetent cells. More specifically, the selective CB_2 agonist JWH-133 reduced mast cell-dependent edema in mice

(Jonsson et al. 2006). Moreover, the other CB_2 selective agonist HU-308 reduced arachidonic acid-induced edema in mice (Hanus et al. 1999), and both the nonpsychotropic CB_2 agonist, HU-320, and CBD were shown to inhibit murine collagen-induced arthritis (Malfait et al. 2000). Furthermore, both the CB_1-selective agonist arachidonyl-2′-chloroethylamide (ACEA) and the CB_2-selective agonist JWH-015 reduced granuloma formation and related angiogenesis in rats (De Filippis et al. 2007). Finally, topical application of adelmidrol, a PEA analog, has been shown to be an effective treatment for atopic dermatitis, by downregulating mast cell activation and the subsequent inflammatory effects (Cerrato et al. 2010; Pulvirenti et al. 2007).

Pruritus is a major characteristic and one of the most debilitating symptoms in allergic and atopic diseases, and represents the diagnostic hallmark of atopic dermatitis. Repeated administration of JTE-907, a CB_2 receptor inverse agonist, significantly inhibited spontaneous scratching behavior in a mouse model of atopic dermatitis (Maekawa et al. 2006), suggesting a yet-to-be-clarified CB_2 involvement in allergic itch.

32.5.3.2 Contact allergic dermatitis

Contact dermatitis is an eczematous skin reaction caused by direct and usually repeated exposure to small allergenic molecules. Immunologically, contact dermatitis is a form of delayed type hypersensitivity that consists of two phases. In the sensitization phase, which occurs at the first contact of the skin with the hapten, the resident antigen-presenting cells (i.e., Langerhans cells and dermal dendritic cells) pick up and process the antigen. Hapten-bearing dendritic cells migrate to the draining lymph nodes, where the allergen is exposed to T lymphocytes. During the following stage, the so-called elicitation phase, after a new contact with the same antigen, memory T cells are activated and exert direct and indirect cytotoxic effects toward cells of the skin, causing edema, erythema, and induration at the site of contact in sensitized humans or animals.

The involvement of the ECS in contact dermatitis is supported by several studies performed in different preclinical models of this pathology. During the experimental allergy contact dermatitis induced by 2,4-dinitrofluorobenzene (DNFB), levels of AEA and 2-AG were found to increase, and a downregulation of CB_1 receptors was observed whereas CB_2 receptors were upregulated (Karsak et al. 2007). Petrosino et al. (2010) found that DNFB increased AEA, 2-AG, and PEA levels in ear skin, and upregulated TRPV1 and NAPE-PLD in ear keratinocytes (Petrosino et al. 2010). Finally, in another model of contact dermatitis induced by oxazolone an increase of 2-AG, but not of AEA, was demonstrated (Oka et al. 2006).

Cannabinoids exert an overall antiallergic effect, yet the mechanism of action remains elusive. Studies with animals genetically devoid of CB_1 and CB_2 receptors have generated contradictory findings about the effective contribution of these receptors to allergic dermatitis. On the one hand, using single and double CB_1/CB_2 receptor knockout, Karsak et al. (2007) demonstrated that both receptors exerted a protective role in DNFB-sensitized/challenged mice. In particular, it has been reported that $CB_2^{-/-}$ mice experienced pronounced chronic inflammation that was alleviated or exacerbated by CB_2 agonists or antagonists, respectively (Karsak et al. 2007). On the other hand, $CB_2^{-/-}$ mice were found to exhibit a significant suppression of DNFB-induced edema and acanthosis (i.e., diffuse epidermal hyperplasia), and, consistently, a CB_2-selective antagonist was found to alleviate chronic inflammation induced by DNFB in wild-type mice (Mimura et al. 2012; Ueda et al. 2005). Moreover, a CB_2-selective agonist induced ear swelling in wild-type mice (Ueda et al. 2007), suggesting that the CB_2 receptor plays a stimulatory role in the sensitization and exacerbation of allergic inflammation. A possible explanation for these conflicting results could reside in the different doses of DNFB used to induce a dermal reaction. However, in other contact dermatitis models, in which ovalbumin or oxazolone were repeatedly applied, there was a significant decrease in ear swelling and acanthosis in $CB_2^{-/-}$ mice compared with wild-type animals, strongly supporting the notion that CB_2 and its endogenous ligand 2-AG enhance dermal reactions to allergens (Mimura et al. 2012). Recently, Petrosino et al. (2010) found that systemic administration of PEA markedly inhibited DNFB-induced ear inflammation, in a manner that could be attenuated by TRPV1 antagonism, indicating that also the latter receptor is a valuable target for treating contact allergic dermatitis (Petrosino et al. 2010).

Notably, THC and CBN were found to be strong sensitizers in an animal model of contact allergic dermatitis (Watson et al. 1983), suggesting that phytocannabinoids could act as allergens and cause allergic reactions.

32.5.4 Scleroderma

Systemic sclerosis (or scleroderma) is a heterogeneous disorder which affects the dermis, as well as the connective tissue of a variety of internal organs (LeRoy and Medsger 2001). Early stages of scleroderma are characterized by an infiltration of affected skin by inflammatory cells, mostly macrophages and activated T cells. Later stages of the disease are characterized by an excessive collagen synthesis and deposition by fibroblasts, resulting in pathologic organ fibrosis.

Systemic sclerosis represents an example of how CB_1 and CB_2 receptors, activated by elevated eCB levels (Palumbo-Zerr et al. 2012), can be detrimental and beneficial, respectively, under pathological conditions. Indeed, $CB_1^{-/-}$ mice, or controls treated with CB_1 antagonists, were protected from bleomycin-induced skin fibrosis, exhibiting a reduced dermal thickening, associated with a decreased number of myofibroblasts, infiltrating T cells, and macrophages (Marquart et al. 2010). In marked contrast, $CB_2^{-/-}$ mice, or controls treated with CB_2 antagonists, were more susceptible to the same model of scleroderma, with clinical symptoms markedly worsened (Akhmetshina et al. 2009). Similarly, $CB_2^{-/-}$ mice were shown to develop a more exacerbated hypochlorite-induced fibrosis compared with wild-type animals (Servettaz et al. 2010). Experiments involving bone marrow transplantation revealed that these two receptors indirectly regulate the activation of fibroblasts by orchestrating the infiltration of leukocytes into lesional skin (Marquart et al. 2010; Servettaz et al. 2010). Finally, Palumbo-Zerr et al. (2012) found that the inhibition of CB_1 completely abrograted the profibrotic effects of FAAH inactivation, whereas the inhibition of CB_2 only modestly enhanced fibrosis, suggesting that CB_1 is the predominant receptor for eCBs in skin fibrosis, and that AEA exerts antifibrogenic activity (Palumbo-Zerr et al. 2012).

Notably, the profibrogenic and antifibrotic effects mediated by CB_1 and CB_2 receptors, respectively, were not restricted to the skin, but were also observed under other fibrotic conditions affecting liver and pancreas (Julien et al. 2005; Michalski et al. 2008; Teixeira-Clerc et al. 2006). From these preclinical data it is arguable that selective antagonism and agonism of CB_1 and CB_2 receptors, respectively, may have therapeutic potential for the treatment of early inflammatory stages of scleroderma.

32.5.5 Acne vulgaris

Acne vulgaris is one of the most common skin disorders, characterized by increased sebum production and inflammation of the sebaceous glands and hyperkeratinisation of the follicular epithelium. Acne can be induced and/or aggravated by stress, endocrine conditions (adolescence), immune/inflammatory factors, *Propionibacterium acnes* infection of the skin, and diet. Treatments for acne are directed at correcting defects in keratinocyte proliferation, reducing the bacterial population, decreasing sebaceous gland activity, and limiting the inflammatory process (Williams et al. 2012).

The role of the ECS in the biology of hair follicle and sebaceous gland biology has only recently been evaluated. Both human organ-cultured hair follicles and sebaceous gland-derived sebocytes (SZ95) have been reported to produce AEA and 2-AG (Dobrosi et al. 2008; Telek et al. 2007). Specifically, in these studies eCBs were shown to stimulate sebocyte lipid synthesis and apoptosis, hallmarks of sebocyte differentiation, and hence a model of holocrine sebum production, in a CB_2 receptor-dependent manner (Dobrosi et al. 2008). Additionally, sebocytes are known to express TRPV1, a receptor that is activated by AEA and is also involved in sebocyte lipid biosynthesis (Toth et al. 2011).

These preliminary findings suggest that the ECS may have a regulatory role in sebaceous gland lipid homeostasis, encouraging the systematic exploration of the question of whether distinct ECS components can be targeted in the management of acne, as well as of other common skin disorders characterized by sebaceous gland dysfunctions, such as seborrhea, dry skin, and sebaceous gland-derived tumors.

32.6 **Conclusions**

Few organs are as large, accessible, multifunctional, and yet underappreciated as the skin. Possibly for this reason, over the last decades, the therapeutic efficacy of phytocannabinoids in dermatology has been little investigated. However, the recent discovery that virtually all cell populations in mammalian skin generate endogenous cannabinoids, such as AEA and 2-AG, and use them to modulate multiple different functions (e.g., epidermal barrier formation, hair growth, melanin, sebum and sweat production, and dermal fibrogenesis), indicates that the ECS plays important roles in skin biology and that it is also a potential target for drugs that could be used to treat a number of skin pathologies, particularly those involving inflammation and hyperproliferation, such as skin tumors, psoriasis, and dermatitis.

Growing research in this still neglected field has revealed that cutaneously expressed CB_1 and CB_2 receptors, and their endogenous ligands AEA and 2-AG, exert divergent, and sometimes even opposing, effects on skin functions, underlying the complexity of the endocannabinergic network in the skin. Thus, it is conceivable that, depending on the particular pathological condition, either activation or blockade of cutaneous eCB signaling may have therapeutic potential for treating skin disorders (Biro et al. 2009).

However, a lot of exciting work remains to be done in order to unravel the multifaceted functions of the ECS in skin biology and pathophysiology, and to establish whether phytocannabinoids are indeed a new valuable generation of dermatological drugs.

References

Agarwal, N., Pacher, P., Tegeder, I., *et al.* (2007). Cannabinoids mediate analgesia largely via peripheral type 1 cannabinoid receptors in nociceptors. *Nature Neuroscience*, **10**, 870–879.

Akhmetshina, A., Dees, C., Busch, N., *et al.* (2009). The cannabinoid receptor CB_2 exerts antifibrotic effects in experimental dermal fibrosis. *Arthritis and Rheumatism*, **60**, 1129–1136.

Baek, S.H., Kim, Y.O., Kwag, J.S., *et al.* (1998). Boron trifluoride etherate on silica-A modified Lewis acid reagent (VII). Antitumor activity of cannabigerol against human oral epitheloid carcinoma cells. *Archives of Pharmacal Research*, **21**, 353–356.

Berdyshev, E.V., Schmid, P.C., Dong, Z., *et al.* (2000). Stress-induced generation of N-acylethanolamines in mouse epidermal JB6 P+ cells. *Biochemistry Journal*, **346**(Pt. 2), 369–374.

Biro, T., Toth, B.I., Hasko, G., *et al.* (2009). The endocannabinoid system of the skin in health and disease: novel perspectives and therapeutic opportunities. *Trends in Pharmacological Sciences*, **30**, 411–420.

Blazquez, C., Carracedo, A., Barrado, L., *et al.* (2006). Cannabinoid receptors as novel targets for the treatment of melanoma. *FASEB Journal*, **20**, 2633–2635.

Bridges, D., Ahmad, K., and Rice, A.S. (2001). The synthetic cannabinoid WIN55,212-2 attenuates hyperalgesia and allodynia in a rat model of neuropathic pain. *British Journal of Pharmacology*, **133**, 586–594.

Calignano, A., La Rana, G., Giuffrida, A., *et al.* (1998). Control of pain initiation by endogenous cannabinoids. *Nature*, **394**, 277–281.

Casanova, M.L., Blazquez, C., Martinez-Palacio, J., *et al.* (2003). Inhibition of skin tumor growth and angiogenesis in vivo by activation of cannabinoid receptors. *The Journal of Clinical Investigation*, **111**, 43–50.

Cerrato, S., Brazis, P., della Valle, M.F., *et al.* (2010). Effects of palmitoylethanolamide on immunologically induced histamine, PGD2 and TNFalpha release from canine skin mast cells. *Veterinary Immunology and Immunopathology*, **133**, 9–15.

Chu, D.H. (2012). Development and structure of skin. In: L.A. Goldsmith, S.I. Katz, B.A. Gilchrest, A.S. Paller, D.J. Leffell, and K. Wolff (eds.). *Fitzpatrick's Dermatology in General Medicine*. 8th ed. New York: McGraw-Hill, pp. 57–73.

Costa, B., Bettoni, I., Petrosino, S., *et al.* (2010). The dual fatty acid amide hydrolase/TRPV1 blocker, N-arachidonoyl-serotonin, relieves carrageenan-induced inflammation and hyperalgesia in mice. *Pharmacological Research*, **61**, 537–546.

Costa, B., Colleoni, M., Conti, S., *et al.* (2004a). Oral anti-inflammatory activity of cannabidiol, a non-psychoactive constituent of cannabis, in acute carrageenan-induced inflammation in the rat paw. *Naunyn-Schmiedeberg's Archives of Pharmacology*, **369**, 294–299.

Costa, B., Giagnoni, G., Franke, C., *et al.* (2004b). Vanilloid TRPV1 receptor mediates the antihyperalgesic effect of the nonpsychoactive cannabinoid, cannabidiol, in a rat model of acute inflammation. *British Journal of Pharmacology*, **143**, 247–250.

Czifra, G., Szollosi, A.G., Toth, B.I., *et al.* (2012). Endocannabinoids regulate growth and survival of human eccrine sweat gland-derived epithelial cells. *The Journal of Investigative Dermatology*, **132**, 1967–1976.

De Filippis, D., D'Amico, A., and Iuvone, T. (2008). Cannabinomimetic control of mast cell mediator release: new perspective in chronic inflammation. *Journal of Neuroendocrinology*, **20** Suppl 1, 20–25.

De Filippis, D., Russo, A., De Stefano, D., *et al.* (2007). Local administration of WIN 55,212-2 reduces chronic granuloma-associated angiogenesis in rat by inhibiting NF-kappaB activation. *Journal of Molecular Medicine*, **85**, 635–645.

De Petrocellis, L. and Di Marzo, V. (2009). An introduction to the endocannabinoid system: from the early to the latest concepts. *Best Practice & Research. Clinical Endocrinology & Metabolism*, **23**, 1–15.

De Petrocellis, L., Ligresti, A., Moriello, A.S., *et al.* (2011). Effects of cannabinoids and cannabinoid-enriched Cannabis extracts on TRP channels and endocannabinoid metabolic enzymes. *British Journal of Pharmacology*, **163**, 1479–1494.

Di Marzo, V. (2008). Targeting the endocannabinoid system: to enhance or reduce? *Nature Reviews. Drug Discovery*, **7**, 438–455.

Di Marzo, V. and Petrosino, S. (2007). Endocannabinoids and the regulation of their levels in health and disease. *Current Opinion in Lipidology*, **18**, 129–140.

Dobrosi, N., Toth, B.I., Nagy, G., *et al.* (2008). Endocannabinoids enhance lipid synthesis and apoptosis of human sebocytes via cannabinoid receptor-2-mediated signaling. *FASEB Journal*, **22**, 3685–3695.

El-Abaseri, T.B., Fuhrman, J., Trempus, C., *et al.* (2005). Chemoprevention of UV light-induced skin tumorigenesis by inhibition of the epidermal growth factor receptor. *Cancer Research*, **65**, 3958–3965.

Ellington, H.C., Cotter, M.A., Cameron, N.E., *et al.* (2002). The effect of cannabinoids on capsaicin-evoked calcitonin gene-related peptide (CGRP) release from the isolated paw skin of diabetic and non-diabetic rats. *Neuropharmacology*, **42**, 966–975.

Felder, C.C., Nielsen, A., Briley, E.M., *et al*. (1996). Isolation and measurement of the endogenous can-nabinoid receptor agonist, anandamide, in brain and peripheral tissues of human and rat. *FEBS Letters*, **393**, 231–235.

Formukong, E.A., Evans, A.T., and Evans, F.J. (1988). Analgesic and antiinflammatory activity of constitu-ents of *Cannabis sativa* L. *Inflammation*, **12**, 361–371.

Fuchs, E. (1990). Epidermal differentiation. *Current Opinion in Cell Biology*, **2**, 1028–1035.

Gonzalez-Rosales, F. and Walsh, D. (1997). Intractable nausea and vomiting due to gastrointestinal mucosal metastases relieved by tetrahydrocannabinol (dronabinol). *Journal of Pain and Symptom Management*, **14**, 311–314.

Guzman, M. (2003). Cannabinoids: potential anticancer agents. *Nature Reviews. Cancer*, **3**, 745–755.

Hamtiaux, L., Masquelier, J., Muccioli, G.G., *et al*. (2012). The association of N-palmitoylethanolamine with the FAAH inhibitor URB597 impairs melanoma growth through a supra-additive action. *BMC Cancer*, **12**, 92.

Hanus, L., Breuer, A., Tchilibon, S., *et al*. (1999). HU-308: a specific agonist for CB(2), a peripheral can-nabinoid receptor. *Proceedings of the National Academy of Sciences of the United States of America*, **96**, 14228–14233.

Hart, S., Fischer, O.M., and Ullrich, A. (2004). Cannabinoids induce cancer cell proliferation via tumor necrosis factor alpha-converting enzyme (TACE/ADAM17)-mediated transactivation of the epidermal growth factor receptor. *Cancer Research*, **64**, 1943–1950.

Ibrahim, M.M., Porreca, F., Lai, J., *et al*. (2005). CB2 cannabinoid receptor activation produces antinoci-ception by stimulating peripheral release of endogenous opioids. *Proceedings of the National Academy of Sciences of the United States of America*, **102**, 3093–3098.

Jiang, L.S., Pu, J., Han, Z.H., *et al*. (2009). Role of activated endocannabinoid system in regulation of cel-lular cholesterol metabolism in macrophages. *Cardiovascular Research*, **81**, 805–813.

Jonsson, K.O., Persson, E., and Fowler, C.J. (2006). The cannabinoid CB_2 receptor selective agonist JWH133 reduces mast cell oedema in response to compound 48/80 in vivo but not the release of beta-hexosaminidase from skin slices in vitro. *Life Sciences*, **78**, 598–606.

Julien, B., Grenard, P., Teixeira-Clerc, F., *et al*. (2005). Antifibrogenic role of the cannabinoid receptor CB_2 in the liver. *Gastroenterology*, **128**, 742–755.

Karsak, M., Gaffal, E., Date, R., *et al*. (2007). Attenuation of allergic contact dermatitis through the endo-cannabinoid system. *Science*, **316**, 1494–1497.

Khasabova, I.A., Khasabov, S.G., Harding-Rose, C., *et al*. (2008). A decrease in anandamide signaling con-tributes to the maintenance of cutaneous mechanical hyperalgesia in a model of bone cancer pain. *The Journal of Neuroscience*, **28**, 11141–11152.

Khasabova, I.A., Chandiramani, A., Harding-Rose, C., *et al*. (2011). Increasing 2-arachidonoyl glyc-erol signaling in the periphery attenuates mechanical hyperalgesia in a model of bone cancer pain. *Pharmacological Research*, **64**, 60–67.

Khasabova, I.A., Khasabov, S., Paz, J., *et al*. (2012). Cannabinoid type-1 receptor reduces pain and neuro-toxicity produced by chemotherapy. *The Journal of Neuroscience*, **32**, 7091–7101.

Klein, T.W. (2005). Cannabinoid-based drugs as anti-inflammatory therapeutics. *Nature Reviews. Immunology*, **5**, 400–411.

Klein, T.W., Newton, C.A., Nakachi, N., *et al*. (2000). Delta 9-tetrahydrocannabinol treatment suppresses immunity and early IFN-gamma, IL-12, and IL-12 receptor beta 2 responses to *Legionella pneumophila* infection. *Journal of Immunology*, **164**, 6461–6466.

Krueger, J.G. and Bowcock, A. (2005). Psoriasis pathophysiology: current concepts of pathogenesis. *Annals of the Rheumatic Diseases*, **64**, 30–36.

Kupczyk, P., Reich, A., and Szepietowski, J.C. (2009). Cannabinoid system in the skin – a possible target for future therapies in dermatology. *Experimental Dermatology*, **18**, 669–679.

LeRoy, E.C. and Medsger, T.A., Jr. (2001). Criteria for the classification of early systemic sclerosis. *The Journal of Rheumatology*, **28**, 1573–1576.

Leung, D.Y. and Bieber, T. (2003). Atopic dermatitis. *Lancet*, **361**, 151–160.

Lodzki, M., Godin, B., Rakou, L., *et al.* (2003). Cannabidiol-transdermal delivery and anti-inflammatory effect in a murine model. *Journal of Controlled Release*, **93**, 377–387.

Maccarrone, M., Dainese, E., Oddi, S. (2010), Intracellular trafficking of AEA: new concepts for signaling, *Trends in Biochemical Sciences*, **35** (11), 601–608.

Maccarrone, M., Di Rienzo, M., Battista, N., *et al.* (2003). The endocannabinoid system in human keratinocytes. Evidence that anandamide inhibits epidermal differentiation through CB1 receptor-dependent inhibition of protein kinase C, activation protein-1, and transglutaminase. *The Journal of Biological Chemistry*, **278**, 33896–33903.

Maccarrone, M., Fiorucci, L., Erba, F., *et al.* (2000). Human mast cells take up and hydrolyze anandamide under the control of 5-lipoxygenase and do not express cannabinoid receptors. *FEBS Letters*, **468**, 176–180.

Maekawa, T., Nojima, H., Kuraishi, Y., *et al.* (2006). The cannabinoid CB_2 receptor inverse agonist JTE-907 suppresses spontaneous itch-associated responses of NC mice, a model of atopic dermatitis. *European Journal of Pharmacology*, **542**, 179–183.

Magina, S., Esteves-Pinto, C., Moura, E., *et al.* (2011). Inhibition of basal and ultraviolet B-induced melanogenesis by cannabinoid CB_1 receptors: a keratinocyte-dependent effect. *Archives of Dermatological Research*, **303**, 201–210.

Maione, S., De Petrocellis, L., de Novellis, V., *et al.* (2007). Analgesic actions of N-arachidonoyl-serotonin, a fatty acid amide hydrolase inhibitor with antagonistic activity at vanilloid TRPV1 receptors. *British Journal of Pharmacology*, **150**, 766–781.

Malan, T.P., Jr., Ibrahim, M.M., Vanderah, T.W., *et al.* (2002). Inhibition of pain responses by activation of CB_2 cannabinoid receptors. *Chemistry and Physics of Lipids*, **121**, 191–200.

Malfait, A.M., Gallily, R., Sumariwalla, P.F., *et al.* (2000). The nonpsychoactive cannabis constituent cannabidiol is an oral anti-arthritic therapeutic in murine collagen-induced arthritis. *Proceedings of the National Academy of Sciences of the United States of America*, **97**, 9561–9566.

Marquart, S., Zerr, P., Akhmetshina, A., *et al.* (2010). Inactivation of the cannabinoid receptor CB1 prevents leukocyte infiltration and experimental fibrosis. *Arthritis and Rheumatism*, **62**, 3467–3476.

McPartland, J.M. (2008). Expression of the endocannabinoid system in fibroblasts and myofascial tissues. *Journal of Bodywork and Movement Therapies*, **12**, 169–182.

Michalski, C.W., Maier, M., Erkan, M., *et al.* (2008). Cannabinoids reduce markers of inflammation and fibrosis in pancreatic stellate cells. *PLoS One*, **3**, e1701.

Mimura, T., Ueda, Y., Watanabe, Y., *et al.* (2012). The cannabinoid receptor-2 is involved in allergic inflammation. *Life Sciences*, **90**, 862–866.

Neff, G.W., O'Brien, C.B., Reddy, K.R., *et al.* (2002). Preliminary observation with dronabinol in patients with intractable pruritus secondary to cholestatic liver disease. *The American Journal of Gastroenterology*, **97**, 2117–2119.

Newton, C.A., Klein, T.W., and Friedman, H. (1994). Secondary immunity to Legionella pneumophila and Th1 activity are suppressed by delta-9-tetrahydrocannabinol injection. *Infection and Immunity*, **62**, 4015–4020.

O'Sullivan, S.E., Tarling, E.J., Bennett, A.J., *et al.* (2005). Novel time-dependent vascular actions of Delta9-tetrahydrocannabinol mediated by peroxisome proliferator-activated receptor gamma. *Biochemical and Biophysical Research Communications*, **337**, 824–831.

Oddi, S., Bari, M., Battista, N., *et al.* (2005). Confocal microscopy and biochemical analysis reveal spatial and functional separation between anandamide uptake and hydrolysis in human keratinocytes. *Cellular and Molecular Life Sciences*, **62**, 386–395.

Oka, S., Wakui, J., Ikeda, S., *et al.* (2006). Involvement of the cannabinoid CB_2 receptor and its endogenous ligand 2-arachidonoylglycerol in oxazolone-induced contact dermatitis in mice. *Journal of Immunology*, **177**, 8796–8805.

Pacher, P., Batkai, S., and Kunos, G. (2006). The endocannabinoid system as an emerging target of pharmacotherapy. *Pharmacological Reviews*, **58**, 389–462.

Pacifici, R., Zuccaro, P., Pichini, S., *et al.* (2003). Modulation of the immune system in cannabis users. *JAMA: the Journal of the American Medical Association*, **289**, 1929–1931.

Palumbo-Zerr, K., Horn, A., Distler, A., *et al.* (2012). Inactivation of fatty acid amide hydrolase exacerbates experimental fibrosis by enhanced endocannabinoid-mediated activation of CB1. *Annals of the Rheumatic Diseases*, **71**, 2051–2054.

Paradisi, A., Pasquariello, N., Barcaroli, D., *et al.* (2008). Anandamide regulates keratinocyte differentiation by inducing DNA methylation in a CB1 receptor-dependent manner. *The Journal of Biological Chemistry*, **283**, 6005–6012.

Pasquariello, N., Oddi, S., Malaponti, M., *et al.* (2009). Regulation of gene transcription and keratinocyte differentiation by anandamide. *Vitamins and Hormones*, **81**, 441–467.

Petrosino, S., Cristino, L., Karsak, M., *et al.* (2010). Protective role of palmitoylethanolamide in contact allergic dermatitis. *Allergy*, **65**, 698–711.

Petrosino, S. and Di Marzo, V. (2010). FAAH and MAGL inhibitors: therapeutic opportunities from regulating endocannabinoid levels. *Current Opinion in Investigational Drugs*, **11**, 51–62.

Pucci, M., Pasquariello, N., Battista, N., *et al.* (2012). Endocannabinoids stimulate human melanogenesis via type-1 cannabinoid receptor. *The Journal of Biological Chemistry*, **287**, 15466–15478.

Pulvirenti, N., Nasca, M.R., and Micali, G. (2007). Topical adelmidrol 2% emulsion, a novel aliamide, in the treatment of mild atopic dermatitis in pediatric subjects: a pilot study. *Acta dermatovenerologica Croatica*, **15**, 80–83.

Richardson, J.D., Kilo, S., and Hargreaves, K.M. (1998). Cannabinoids reduce hyperalgesia and inflammation via interaction with peripheral CB_1 receptors. *Pain*, **75**, 111–119.

Roelandt, T., Heughebaert, C., Bredif, S., *et al.* (2012). Cannabinoid receptors 1 and 2 oppositely regulate epidermal permeability barrier status and differentiation. *Experimental Dermatology*, **21**, 688–693.

Rukwied, R., Watkinson, A., McGlone, F., *et al.* (2003). Cannabinoid agonists attenuate capsaicin-induced responses in human skin. *Pain*, **102**, 283–288.

Russo, E.B. (2011). Taming THC: potential cannabis synergy and phytocannabinoid-terpenoid entourage effects. *British Journal of Pharmacology*, **163**, 1344–1364.

Scuderi, M.R., Cantarella, G., Scollo, M., *et al.* (2011). The antimitogenic effect of the cannabinoid receptor agonist WIN55212-2 on human melanoma cells is mediated by the membrane lipid raft. *Cancer Letters*, **310**, 240–249.

Servettaz, A., Kavian, N., Nicco, C., *et al.* (2010). Targeting the cannabinoid pathway limits the development of fibrosis and autoimmunity in a mouse model of systemic sclerosis. *The American Journal of Pathology*, **177**, 187–196.

Sofia, R.D., Nalepa, S.D., Harakal, J.J., *et al.* (1973). Anti-edema and analgesic properties of delta9-tetrahydrocannabinol (THC). *The Journal of Pharmacology and Experimental Therapeutics*, **186**, 646–655.

Stander, S., Schmelz, M., Metze, D., *et al.* (2005). Distribution of cannabinoid receptor 1 (CB1) and 2 (CB2) on sensory nerve fibers and adnexal structures in human skin. *Journal of Dermatological Science*, **38**, 177–188.

Stern, E. and Lambert, D.M. (2007). Medicinal chemistry endeavors around the phytocannabinoids. *Chemistry & Biodiversity*, **4**, 1707–1728.

Sugawara, K., Biro, T., Tsuruta, D., *et al.* (2012). Endocannabinoids limit excessive mast cell maturation and activation in human skin. *The Journal of Allergy and Clinical Immunology*, **129**, 726–738.

Teixeira-Clerc, F., Julien, B., Grenard, P., *et al.* (2006). CB_1 cannabinoid receptor antagonism: a new strategy for the treatment of liver fibrosis. *Nature Medicine*, **12**, 671–676.

Telek, A., Biro, T., Bodo, E., *et al.* (2007). Inhibition of human hair follicle growth by endo- and exocannabinoids. *FASEB Journal*, **21**, 3534–3541.

Toth, B.I., Dobrosi, N., Dajnoki, A., *et al.* (2011). Endocannabinoids modulate human epidermal keratinocyte proliferation and survival via the sequential engagement of cannabinoid receptor-1 and transient receptor potential vanilloid-1. *The Journal of Investigative Dermatology*, **131**, 1095–1104.

Tubaro, A., Giangaspero, A., Sosa, S., *et al.* (2010). Comparative topical anti-inflammatory activity of cannabinoids and cannabivarins. *Fitoterapia*, **81**, 816–819.

Turner, C.E. and Elsohly, M.A. (1981). Biological activity of cannabichromene, its homologs and isomers. *Journal of Clinical Pharmacology*, **21**, 283S–291S.

Ueda, Y., Miyagawa, N., Matsui, T., *et al.* (2005). Involvement of cannabinoid CB$_2$ receptor-mediated response and efficacy of cannabinoid CB$_2$ receptor inverse agonist, JTE-907, in cutaneous inflammation in mice. *European Journal of Pharmacology*, **520**, 164–171.

Ueda, Y., Miyagawa, N., and Wakitani, K. (2007). Involvement of cannabinoid CB$_2$ receptors in the IgE-mediated triphasic cutaneous reaction in mice. *Life Sciences*, **80**, 414–419.

Watson, E.S., Murphy, J.C., and Turner, C.E. (1983). Allergenic properties of naturally occurring cannabinoids. *Journal of Pharmaceutical Sciences*, **72**, 954–955.

Wilkinson, J.D. and Williamson, E.M. (2007). Cannabinoids inhibit human keratinocyte proliferation through a non-CB$_1$/CB$_2$ mechanism and have a potential therapeutic value in the treatment of psoriasis. *Journal of Dermatological Science*, **45**, 87–92.

Williams, H.C., Dellavalle, R.P., and Garner, S. (2012). Acne vulgaris. *Lancet*, **379**, 361–372.

Wirth, P.W., Watson, E.S., ElSohly, M., *et al.* (1980). Anti-inflammatory properties of cannabichromene. *Life Sciences*, **26**, 1991–1995.

Zhao, Z.G., Li, Y.Y., Yang, J., *et al.* (2010). Expression of cannabinoid receptor 2 in squamous cell carcinoma. *Journal of Southern Medical University*, **30**, 593–595.

Zheng, D., Bode, A.M., Zhao, Q., *et al.* (2008). The cannabinoid receptors are required for ultraviolet-induced inflammation and skin cancer development. *Cancer Research*, **68**, 3992–3998.

Zheng, J.L., Yu, T.S., Li, X.N., *et al.* (2012). Cannabinoid receptor type 2 is time-dependently expressed during skin wound healing in mice. *International Journal of Legal Medicine*, **126**, 807–814.

Zutt, M., Hanssle, H., Emmert, S., *et al.* (2006). Dronabinol for supportive therapy in patients with malignant melanoma and liver metastases. *Der Hautarzt; Zeitschrift fur Dermatologie, Venerologie, und Verwandte Gebiete*, **57**, 423–427.

Chapter 33

Phytocannabinoids in Degenerative and Inflammatory Retinal Diseases: Glaucoma, Age-Related Macular Degeneration, Diabetic Retinopathy, and Uveoretinitis

Heping Xu and Augusto Azuara-Blanco

33.1 Introduction

The eye detects light and converts it into electrochemical impulses in neurons. Together with the brain, the eye provides us with vision. The eye acquires images in a similar manner to a camera. Light that enters the eye is focused onto the back, i.e., the retina, by the optic system. The optic system of the eye consists of cornea, lens, and vitreous. The retina is like the photographic film in a camera containing chemicals that can convert light into electrochemical impulses. There are three layers of neuronal cells in the retina that can transmit these impulses to the brain: photoreceptors, bipolar cells, and ganglion cells. Photoreceptors together with an adjacent monolayer of cells named retinal pigment epithelium (RPE) convert light signals into electrochemical impulses, which are then transmitted to bipolar cells. Ganglion cells receive signals from bipolar cells and then transmit the signals through the optic nerve to the visual cortex, which is located in the occipital lobe at the back of the brain, where visual information is formed.

The eye may lose its visual-acquiring function if pathologies occur in the optic system or the neural retinal system. Whilst vision loss related to optic system dysfunction, such as corneal opacification and cataract can be cured by surgical procedures, managing vision loss caused by neural retinal dysfunction is more challenging. A number of degenerative and inflammatory conditions may cause neural retinal dysfunction. These include glaucoma, diabetic retinopathy (DR), age-related macular degeneration (AMD), and uveoretinitis. Although different retinal diseases have different etiologies and involve different molecular pathways, these sight-threatening diseases share some similarities. For example, both inflammation and neurodegeneration appear to play a role in lesion development in these conditions. Current management strategies center predominately on either the removal of the initial triggers, or relieving symptoms, and the long-term effects are not satisfactory. Future therapies may need to bring neuroprotection and anti-inflammation into the equation.

This chapter discusses the potential of phytocannabinoids as anti-inflammatory or neuroprotective reagents in the management of glaucoma, DR, AMD, and uveoretinitis.

33.2 **Cannabinoids and the eye**

The effect of cannabinoids on the visual system has been known for a long time. Smoking marijuana can cause conjunctival vasodilation (so-called red eye) and a reduction of intraocular pressure (IOP) (Adams et al. 1978; Green 1979). Marijuana smoking can also affect visual function, including a reduction in visual acuity (VA), alterations in color discrimination, and an increase in photosensitivity (Dawson et al. 1977; Kiplinger and Manno 1971; Russo et al. 2004). There are also numerous anecdotal reports that smoking marijuana improves dim-light vision, including the famous report that Jamaican fishermen smoked marijuana to improve night vision when they went fishing (Wes 1991). The underlying mechanisms related to marijuana smoking-mediated visual effects are not fully understood.

The active component of the marijuana plant, *Cannabis sativa*, is delta-9-tetrahydrocannabinol (THC). THC mimics the action of endogenous fatty acid derivatives, referred to as endocannabinoids (eCBs). Endocannabinoids are known to have neuromodulatory roles and are present in neural and non-neural tissues throughout the body. The effects of THC and the endocannabinoids are mediated by metabotropic and ionotropic receptors that are present in the central nervous system (CNS) and peripheral organs (Diaz-Laviada and Ruiz-Llorente 2005; Pertwee 2005). There are two well-defined metabotropic cannabinoid receptors, cannabinoid receptor types 1 (CB_1) and 2 (CB_2) (Matsuda et al. 1990; Munro et al. 1993). Both CB_1 and CB_2 receptors are G protein-coupled receptors (McAllister and Glass 2002; Munro et al. 1993; Pertwee and Ross 2002). In addition, the G protein-coupled receptor 55 (GPR55) can also bind cannabinoids (Sawzdargo et al. 1999). Some eCBs such as arachidonoyl ethanolamide (anandamide, AEA) can activate the ionotropic transient receptor potential (TRP) vanilloid type-1 cation channel (TRPV1), also known as vanilloid receptor 1 (VR1) (Ross 2003; Toth et al. 2005).

CB_1 receptors and TRPV1 cation channels are expressed predominately by neuronal tissues (Toth et al. 2005; Tsou et al. 1998), whereas CB_2 receptors are expressed mainly in peripheral non-neuronal tissues (Galiegue et al. 1995). In the eye, CB_1 receptors and TRPV1 have been detected in the neural retina. CB_1 receptor but not CB_2 receptor mRNA was detected in embryonic rat retina (Buckley et al. 1998) and human retina (Porcella et al. 2000). CB_1 receptor mRNA also exists in the ciliary body of the eye (Porcella et al. 1998). Localization of the CB_1 receptor in the retina has been investigated by using immunohistochemistry by several groups. Straiker et al. (1999b) and Yazulla et al. (1999) reported CB_1 receptor expression by bipolar cells, GABAergic amacrine cells, horizontal cells, and in the inner plexiform layer. CB_1 receptors were also detected in rod and cone photoreceptor terminals (Straiker et al. 1999b). In addition, CB_1 receptor expression has also been observed in goldfish retina (Fan and Yazulla 2003; Straiker et al. 1999a). In mouse eyes, we detected CB_1 receptors in the corneal epithelia, and stroma (Fig. 33.1A), ciliary body (Fig. 33.1B), retinal ganglion cells (Fig. 33.1C), photoreceptor inner segments (the layer between outer nuclear layer (ONL) and RPE layer) (Fig. 33.1D), and the optic nerve (Fig. 33.1E).

There is only limited information about the expression of TRPV1 in the eye. Sappington and Calkins (2008) detected TRPV1 mRNA and protein expression in cultured microglia from rat retina. Leonelli et al. (2009) found that during the early phases of development, TRPV1 was expressed mainly in the neuroblastic layer of the retina and in the RPE. In the adult, TRPV1 was found in microglial cells, blood vessels, astrocytes and in neuronal structures: namely synaptic boutons of both retinal plexiform layers, as well as in cell bodies of the inner nuclear layer and the ganglion cell layer (Leonelli et al. 2009). They further showed that there was a higher TRPV1 expression in the peripheral regions than in the central regions of the retina (Leonelli et al., 2009). Zimov and Yazulla (2007) reported TRPV1 expression in retinal amacrine cells in goldfish retina.

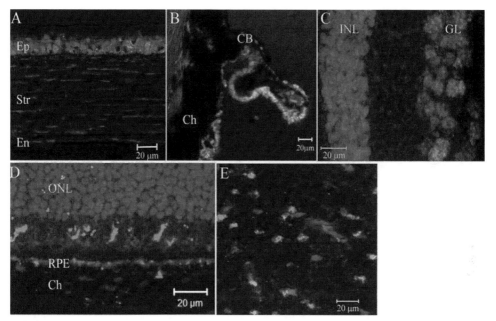

Fig. 33.1 (See also colour plate section.) CB_1 receptor expression in mouse eye. Eye sections from a 3-month-old mouse were stained for CB_1 receptor (green) and propidium iodide (red), and observed by confocal microscopy. (A) cornea, (B) ciliary body, (C) inner retina, (D) outer retina; (E) optic nerve. CB, ciliary body; Ch, choroid; En, endothelia; Ep, epithelia; GL, ganglion layer; INL, inner nuclear layer; ONL, outer nuclear layer; RPE, retinal pigment epithelia; Str, stroma.

Any expression of TRPV1 in other parts of the eye such as cornea, ciliary body, choroid, and optic nerve has yet to be detected.

In the eye, there is evidence that demonstrates CB_2 receptor expression in the trabecular meshwork. Cells cultured from porcine trabecular meshwork expressed high levels of CB_2 receptor (Zhong et al. 2005), and treatment of these cells with a CB_2 agonist, JWH-015, resulted in p42/44 MAP kinase activation (He et al. 2012; McIntosh et al. 2007; Zhong et al. 2005). The expression of CB_2 receptors in the trabecular meshwork is known to be important for cannabinoid-mediated lowering of IOP. In mouse eyes, we detected CB_2 receptors in the corneal epithelia (Fig. 33.2A) and ciliary body (Fig. 33.2B).

The expression of CB_2 receptors in the retina is controversial. Early work by Porcella et al. showed that CB_2 mRNA expression was undetectable in rat (Porcella et al. 1998) and human (Porcella et al. 2000) retina. However, Lu et al. (2000) demonstrated CB_2 mRNA expression in rat retina, particularly in the retinal ganglion cell layer, the inner nuclear layer, and the inner segment of photoreceptor cells. This observation was confirmed by Lopez and colleagues (2011). Using immunohistochemistry, Lopez et al. (2011) showed that the CB_2 receptor was localized in retinal pigment epithelium, inner photoreceptor segments, horizontal and amacrine cells, cells localized in the ganglion cell layer, and in the fibers of the inner plexiform layer. The presence of cannabinoid receptors in human retinal pigment epithelial cells was reported in primary cultures and ARPE-19 cells (Wei et al. 2009). These authors also showed that oxidative stress upregulated CB_2 receptor expression (Wei et al. 2009). The role of CB_2 receptors expressed in retinal cells under pathophysiological condition remains to be elucidated.

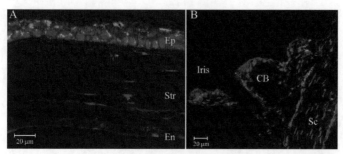

Fig. 33.2 (See also colour plate section.) CB_2 receptor expression in mouse cornea and ciliary body. Eye sections from a 3-month-old mouse were stained for CB_2 receptor (green) and propidium iodide (red), and observed by confocal microscopy. (A) cornea, (B) ciliary body. CB, ciliary body; En, endothelia; Ep, epithelia; Sc, sclera; Str, stroma.

33.3 Phytocannabinoids in glaucoma

33.3.1 What is glaucoma?

Glaucoma is an age-related chronic optic neuropathy causing progressive visual field (i.e., peripheral vision) loss and, if untreated, it may lead to blindness. The most representative pathologic finding in glaucoma is the death of retinal ganglion cells by apoptosis.

Glaucoma is the leading cause of irreversible blindness in the world (Congdon et al. 2004). In Western countries it is the second leading cause of blindness (after AMD), affecting 1–2% of the population over 40 years old (Bunce and Wormald 2006). With the ageing population the burden of glaucoma is expected to increase. Treatment (medical or surgical) is aimed at reducing IOP and helps reduce sight loss from glaucoma. However, for some individuals current treatments are either not tolerated or ineffective and thus new therapies are needed.

33.3.2 The effect of phytocannabinoids in glaucoma

In 1971, Hepler and Frank first reported a 25–30% IOP lowering effect of smoking marijuana in a small number of subjects (Hepler and Frank 1971). Other early studies confirmed this effect in glaucoma patients (Green and Roth 1982; Merritt et al. 1980). The duration of action was relatively short, about 3–4 hours, and there seemed to be a dose–response relationship. Smoking marijuana is not advisable for a chronic condition because of the side effects. In addition to the acute side effects, long-term marijuana smoking is associated with emphysema, and possible increase in the frequency of lung cancer. Although using marijuana for glaucoma may not be illegal in some countries or states, professional ophthalmological societies advise against marijuana smoking for glaucoma (Buys and Rafuse 2010; Jampel 2010). Oral, sublingual, and topical routes of administration of cannabinoids have been explored but with variable clinical success (Flach 2002; Porcella et al. 2001; Tomida et al. 2006). In a prospective, nonrandomized study in California led by Flach (2002), glaucoma patients not responding to conventional treatment were offered orally administered THC or inhaled marijuana in addition to their therapeutic regimen. Nine patients were enrolled, and although a decrease in IOP was observed in all patients, all chose to discontinue treatment within 9 months for various reasons (Flach 2002).

IOP is maintained in the eye by the balance between aqueous humor secretion and outflow. The mechanism of action of cannabinoids in the eye is not well understood, but it probably involves ocular CB receptors (Crandall et al. 2007; Tomida et al. 2004). The expression of CB_1 and CB_2

receptors has been described in the ocular tissues involved in IOP regulation, specifically in the tissues responsible for aqueous humor secretion (ciliary body epithelium), trabecular meshwork outflow (trabecular meshwork and Schlemm canal), and uveoscleral outflow (ciliary muscle). Using the synthetic cannabinoid WIN 55,212-2, Chien et al. (2003) could demonstrate an 18% reduction in aqueous humor production in monkeys but no significant change in the trabecular outflow facility. As this percentage appeared not sufficient to account for the total IOP lowering effect, other additional mechanisms were thought to be involved (Chien et al. 2003). The IOP reducing effect does not seem to be related to a systemic reduction of arterial blood pressure (Korczyn 1980). However, a direct effect on the ciliary processes, and specifically a reduction in capillary pressure, leading to changes in aqueous humor dynamics, has been proposed (McDonald et al. 1991). Green and Pederson (1973) showed that THC decreased the secretion of ciliary processes and led to a dilatation of the ocular blood vessels through a possible β-adrenergic action. Indirect sympatholytic actions in the eye have also been proposed recently (Hudson et al. 2011). In addition, Sugrue (1997) indicated that cannabinoids may inhibit calcium influx through presynaptic channels and in this way reduce norepinephrine release in the ciliary body, leading to a decrease in the production of aqueous humor. Porcella et al. (1998) proposed that cannabinoids might be acting as vasodilators on blood vessels of the anterior uvea, thus improving the aqueous humor uveoscleral outflow. Green et al. (1974, 2001) postulated that some cannabinoids may influence IOP through a prostaglandin mediated mechanism.

In addition to the IOP-lowering effect of cannabinoids, their neuroprotective properties may be potentially useful (Crandall et al. 2007; Yazulla 2008). In glaucoma, the final pathway leading to visual loss is the selective death of retinal ganglion cells through apoptosis. Numerous studies have documented the neuroprotective properties of cannabinoids in the retina (Levin 1999). There is evidence that THC can inhibit glutamic acid release by increasing K^+ and decreasing Ca^{2+} permeability and that some synthetic cannabinoids can block glutamate (NMDA) receptors (Jin et al. 2000; Marsicano et al. 2002; Pertwee 2000a; Yoles et al. 1996). These actions are mediated by presynaptic CB_1 receptors. Yoles et al. (1996) using a calibrated crush injury to adult rat optic nerve (optic nerve axotomy), showed a beneficial effect of HU-211 on injury-induced metabolic and electrophysiological deficits. However, the optic nerve crush model may not be suitable for investigating mechanisms responsible for glaucomatous nerve damage. Cannabinoids such as THC, HU-211, and cannabidiol (CBD) have antioxidant properties. As a result, they can prevent neuronal death by scavenging toxic reactive oxygen species produced by overstimulation of receptors for the excitatory neurotransmitter, glutamic acid (Hampson et al. 1998, 2000; Pertwee 2000b).

33.3.3 Topical application of cannabinoids for glaucoma

To minimize possible systemic, adverse side effects and maximize the dose at the site of action, topical application would be the ideal form of administration. However, natural cannabinoid extracts as well as synthetic forms are highly lipophilic and have low aqueous solubility, creating practical difficulties for this mode of administration.

The cornea is usually the major pathway for intraocular penetration of topical medications. The corneal epithelium is highly lipophilic and its penetration is a rate-limiting step for lipophilic drugs such as cannabinoids (Green and Roth 1982; Jarho et al. 1996; Jay and Green 1983). Aqueous solubility of the drug is another property important for efficacy of delivery, as the surface of the eye is constantly moistened by tear fluid. Additional factors affecting corneal absorption include the molecular size, charge, and degree of ionization. Previous experiments with topical cannabinoid solutions involved the use of light mineral oil as a vehicle, but proved to be irritant to the human eye (Green and Roth 1982). Recently, different microemulsions and cyclodextrins (macrocyclic oligosaccharides) have been shown to improve the corneal penetration of cannabinoids. These formulations successfully induced an IOP lowering effect (Green and Kearse 2000; Jarho et al. 1998; Laine et al. 2002; Naveh et al. 2000; Porcella et al. 2001).

33.3.4 Future directions in glaucoma

Cannabinoids have the potential of becoming a useful treatment for glaucoma, as they reduce IOP and seem to have neuroprotective properties. However, several challenges need to be overcome, including the problems associated with unwanted systemic side effects (psychotropic, reduction in systemic blood pressure), possible tolerance, and the difficulty in formulating a stable and effective topical preparation. Some cannabinoids such as cannabidiol do not have psychotropic effects, while maintaining their IOP-lowering action, so that further research on these compounds would be desirable. Tolerance may develop after repeated use of cannabinoids. However, tolerance might be beneficial if it develops only or preferentially to unwanted side effects. Research on the possible use of microemulsions and cyclodextrins or novel formulations to overcome the barriers to ocular penetration of topically applied cannabinoids should be encouraged (Hingorani et al. 2012).

33.4 Phytocannabinoids in diabetic retinopathy

33.4.1 What is diabetic retinopathy?

Diabetic patients may develop a number of eye complications, including diabetic cataract and DR, both of which can lead to vision loss. A cataract can be removed by surgery, whereas the management of DR is more problematic. DR is the leading cause of blindness among people of working age in Western countries (Aiello et al. 1998). The longer a person has diabetes, the higher the chance he/she might develop DR. After 20 years of disease, nearly all patients with type 1 diabetes will have at least some DR. For type 2 diabetes, around 80% who are insulin-dependent and 50% who are non-insulin-dependent will have DR after 20 years' disease duration (Romero-Aroca et al. 2010).

At the early stage, the disease is called nonproliferative DR. Patients may present with microaneurysms (localized dilations of the retinal microvasculature), hard exudates, superficial retinal hemorrhages, and cotton-wool spots in the fundus. Sometimes, the diseased vessels may leak fluid from the circulation. If the macula is affected by leaky fluid (i.e., diabetic macular edema), vision loss may ensue. As the disease progresses, damaged blood vessels may not be able to supply sufficient oxygen and nutrients, and new blood vessels grow (proliferative DR). The new blood vessels are fragile and can cause hemorrhage and ultimately destroy the retina.

In addition to vascular damage, retinal neural cells may also be affected even at the early stages of the disease leading to retinal neural degeneration. There is growing evidence to suggest that retinal neurodegeneration is an early event in DR pathogenesis (Lieth et al. 2000; Simo et al. 2012). Retinal ganglion cell and neural cell death is known to be responsible, at least in part, for the degenerative changes in DR (Kern and Barber 2008).

The underlying mechanisms leading to diabetic retinal vasculopathy and neuropathy are not fully understood, although oxidative stress and inflammation are known to be important detrimental factors. Increased superoxide concentration is considered as a causal link between elevated glucose and the other metabolic abnormalities important in the pathogenesis of DR (Kowluru and Chan 2007). Cyclooxygenase (COX), and inflammatory mediators, including tumor necrosis factor (TNF)-α, interleukin (IL)-1β and nitric oxide (NO), are known to be involved in increased vascular permeability, capillary degeneration, and neurodegeneration in the DR (Tang and Kern 2011).

Apart from controlling hyperglycemia, there is no specific therapy for early stages of DR. The treatments for proliferative DR include laser (e.g., panretinal photocoagulation (PRP)), vitrectomy, and intravitreal anti-vascular endothelial growth factor (VEGF) antibody or steroid injection. Although these therapies can reduce the risk of catastrophic vision loss from DR if used appropriately and in a timely manner, the beneficial effects are accomplished at the cost of sacrificing other retinal functions (e.g., PRP destroys the peripheral retina and damages peripheral vision), or of increasing the risk of developing other ocular complications (e.g., cataract formation and steroid-induced glaucoma).

Given the limitations and side effects of current treatment modalities for DR, there has been a continuing effort to explore new effective and safe therapies. Future therapies should tackle the initial trigger (oxidative stress), reduce the subsequent inflammation, and perhaps also be directed at improving the ability of host cells to deal with the stress (neuroprotection). Cannabinoids are known to possess therapeutic properties including inhibition of oxidative damage (Hampson et al. 1998; Marsicano et al. 2002) and inflammation (Buckley et al. 2000; Malfait et al. 2000). Experimental evidence suggests that cannabinoids may interact with endogenous neurotrophic factors and may have therapeutic potential for DR (Buckley et al. 2000).

33.4.2 The effect of phytocannabinoids in diabetic retinopathy

The endocannabinoid system is known to be linked to obesity and type 2 diabetes (Lipina et al. 2012). Activation of cannabinoid receptors can affect feeding behavior and energy expenditure and metabolism (Lipina et al. 2012), and blocking CB_1 receptors has been found to prevent obesity and metabolic dysfunction in various murine models and in humans (Despres, 2007). Endocannabinoid dysregulation is also involved in diabetic complications. Although the endocannabinoid system is known to exist in the eye, its pathophysiological role remains elusive (Yazulla 2008). Under diabetic conditions, the levels of AEA were increased in the retina, ciliary body, and the cornea, whereas the levels of 2-arachidonoylglycerol (2-AG) were only increased in the iris compared to age-matched healthy controls (Matias et al. 2006). The levels of palmitoylethanolamide (PEA) were slightly increased (1.3-fold) in the ciliary body, but not in other tissues of the eye when compared to age-matched healthy controls (Matias et al. 2006). A more recent study has shown that hyperglycemia can upregulate CB_1 receptor expression and induces cell death in human retinal pigment epithelia, a type of cell important for the development of DR (Lim et al. 2012). The role of the CB_1 receptor in DR was further confirmed by El-Remessy et al. (2011) who showed that depletion of CB_1 receptors or their blockade with SR141716 could prevent retinal cell death in diabetic mice. These results suggest that the endocannabinoid system is dysregulated in diabetes and may contribute to DR development, and that modulating the endocannabinoid system may have therapeutic potential.

Indeed, a beneficial effect of the marijuana-derived cannabinoid, the non-psychotropic phytocannabinoid, CBD, has been demonstrated by El-Remessy et al. (2006) in a rat model of DR. The authors showed that injection of 10 mg/kg CBD every other day in rats reduced streptozotocin (STZ)-induced diabetes, prevented blood–retinal barrier (BRB) breakdown and retinal neural cell death (El-Remessy et al. 2006). They further showed that CBD induces its beneficial effects by reducing diabetes-induced oxidative and nitrative stress and suppressing TNF-α and VEGF expression in diabetic rat retina (El-Remessy et al. 2006). In a follow-up study, this group showed that CBD can enhance the anti-inflammatory effects of adenosine in the retina (Liou 2010; Liou et al. 2008). In humans, CBD is well tolerated when chronically administered (Cunha et al. 1980), and has been approved for the treatment of inflammation, pain, and spasticity associated with multiple sclerosis since 2005 (Barnes 2006). Neither the efficacy of CBD in diabetic patients nor its limitations have been tested thus far.

33.4.3 Future directions in diabetic retinopathy

Retinal neural degeneration and vascular damage are two major features of DR, and for which there is currently no effective therapy. The endocannabinoid system appears to be disrupted in DR, and preclinical studies have shown a protective role of cannabinoids in this disorder. Whilst the mechanisms underlying the protective actions of cannabinoids should be further investigated, the clinical efficacy of cannabinoid-based medicines should also be explored. Cannabis and cannabinoids (GW42004 and GW42003) have been used in phase 1/2 clinical trials in diabetic patients to treat diabetic painful peripheral neuropathy or to control cholesterol levels (ClinicalTrials.gov 2008). It will be worth investigating how these treatments might affect the progression of DR in such patients.

33.5 Phytocannabinoids in age-related macular degeneration

33.5.1 What is age-related macular degeneration?

AMD is a disease in which retinal neurons of the macula (central part of the retina) degenerate with age, resulting in loss of visual function. AMD is the leading cause of blindness in the elderly in developed countries. In the US about 15% of people over 80 years old had AMD in 2000 (Friedman et al. 2004) and this number is estimated to increase by more than 50% by 2020, with over 2.95 million people having AMD (Friedman et al. 2004). In the UK, AMD accounts for more than 50% of all cases of registered blind or partially sighted (Bunce and Wormald 2006; Coleman et al. 2008). The prevalence of AMD is continuing to increase with the ageing population (Congdon et al. 2004).

The early stage of the disease is sometimes referred to as age-related maculopathy (ARM). ARM is linked to drusen formation and hypo- and hyperpigmentation of RPE in the macular area and at this stage is not associated with any obvious visual impairment. A significant number of patients with ARM will progress into two late stages, dry AMD (also called geographic atrophic (GA)) and wet AMD (also called neovascular AMD (nAMD)). Wet AMD accounts for two-thirds of all late-stage AMD and the remaining one-third is dry AMD. While there is symmetry of late-stage disease in the two eyes of a person, these late stages are not mutually exclusive. Patients with late stages of AMD lose their central vision.

Dry AMD is caused by macular RPE cell death and photoreceptor degeneration and currently, there is no treatment for dry AMD. Wet AMD is a condition in which abnormal blood vessels grow into the subretinal space of the macula causing visual damage. Treatment modalities for wet AMD, however, have improved dramatically over the past decade. Before photodynamic therapy (PDT) with verteporfin was introduced in 2000 (Schmidt-Erfurth and Hasan 2000), laser photo-coagulation was the only available treatment option (Custis et al. 1993). The emergence of anti-VEGF as an effective treatment for wet AMD has revolutionized the management of wet AMD. Licensed anti-VEGFs for wet AMD include pegaptanib (Macugen®), which was approved in the European Union in 2006 (European Medicines Agency 2013a) and ranibizumab (Lucentis®▼), approved in 2007 (European Medicines Agency 2013b). Ranibizumab is now considered the standard care for wet AMD. The combination of PDT and anti-VEGF may provide additional benefits to certain patients (e.g., reduce the frequency of intravitreal anti VEGF injection and better VA improvement) (Heier et al. 2006).

Although anti-VEGF therapy has revolutionized the management of wet AMD, the long-term effect is not satisfactory. Two phase 3 clinical trials have shown that only 30–38% of patients had gained greater than 15 letters VA (i.e., be able to read 15 more letters in the VA test) after 2 years of monthly injections, and around 10% of patients had lost greater than 15 letters VA (Rosenfeld et al. 2011). Vision loss was associated with an increase in lesion area and RPE atrophy (Rosenfeld et al. 2011). Further VA improvement in patients receiving anti-VEGF therapy may require protection of photoreceptors and RPE function.

33.5.2 Therapeutic potential of phytocannabinoids in age-related macular degeneration

Oxidative stress is known to be the initial trigger of AMD, and inflammation may play an important role in retinal lesion development. A combination of antioxidant and anti-inflammatory activity may offer the possibility to prevent the onset or delay AMD progression. Cannabinoids possess antioxidant, anti-inflammatory, and neuroprotective properties and may be potential candidates for future AMD therapy. There is evidence to suggest that the endocannabinoid system is disrupted in human AMD eyes (Matias et al. 2006). The levels of AEA in AMD eyes were increased compared to age-matched control eyes, although the levels of 2-AG and PEA were not affected (Matias et al. 2006). We have found that in normal mouse retina, there is an age-dependent increase in the levels of 2-AG and AEA (Fig. 33.3). In mouse models of AMD, in which the mice have a deficiency either of chemokine C-C motif ligand 2 (CCL2) or of its receptor (CCR2) and age-dependently develop retinal geographic atrophy (Ambati et al. 2003; Chen et al. 2011), there is an age-dependent decrease in the levels of 2-AG, and the basal levels of 2-AG (i.e., at the age of 3 months) are higher in the CCL2 and CCR2 knockout mice than in wild-type mice (Fig. 33.3). There is no significant difference in the levels of AEA between wild-type and knockout mice in any age group (Fig. 33.3). Our data suggest that dysregulation of the 2-AG/CB_1 pathway may be involved in retinal pathology in AMD.

RPE cell death underlies the pathology of dry AMD. A previous study by Wei et al. has shown that human RPE cells express both CB_1 and CB_2 receptors and that the CB_1/CB_2 receptor agonist, CP55,940, and the CB_2 receptor agonist, JWH-015 significantly protected RPE cells from oxidative damage (Wei et al. 2009). These authors further showed that CP55,940 significantly reduced the levels of intracellular reactive oxygen species (ROS), strengthened oxidative stress-induced activation of PI3K/Akt, and reduced activation of the ERK1/2 signal pathway in RPE cells (Wei et al. 2009). This result suggests that modulating the endocannabinoid system with appropriate synthetic compounds or phytocannabinoids in AMD may protect RPE from oxidative stress-induced cell death.

33.5.3 Future directions in age-related macular degeneration

Oxidative stress and inflammation play an important role in the pathogenesis of AMD. Cannabinoids have antioxidant, anti-inflammatory, and neuroprotective properties and should potentially be one of the future therapies for AMD. Future research in preclinical models should address important practical questions, e.g., which cannabinoids are most effective in AMD, what is the best route for delivering cannabinoids, and what are the potential side effects?

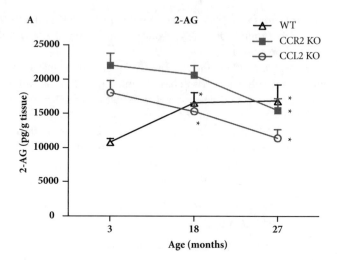

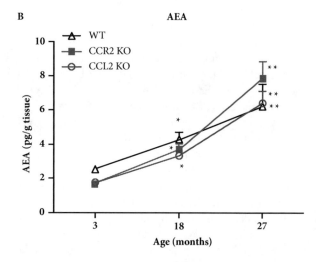

Fig. 33.3 2-AG and AEA levels in the retina from mice of different ages. The retinal tissues from mice of different ages were collected and subjected to liquid chromatography/mass spectrometry analysis for AEA and 2-AG quantification. 2-AG and AEA levels were normalized by tissue weight as well as tissue total protein content. *P < 0.05; **P < 0.01 compared to a group of 3-month old mice of the same strain (n ≥ 6). CCL KO, chemokine CCL2 knockout; CCR2 KO, chemokine receptor CCR2 knockout.

33.6 Phytocannabinoids in uveoretinitis

33.6.1 What is uveoretinitis?

Uveoretinitis is an inflammatory condition that involves the uveal tract and the retina. The disease, if left untreated, can cause devastating vision loss. This condition, which can be of infectious (e.g., bacteria, viruses, parasites, etc.) or non-infectious origin, is known as posterior segment intraocular inflammation (PSII). PSII is a major cause of visual impairment in working populations. Current treatment of PSII is through local or general suppression of the immune system and there is an urgent requirement to replace this with one that acts specifically to alleviate disease and does not raise safety concerns.

Experimental animal models are powerful tools for studying disease mechanisms and testing potential medicines. Infectious uveoretinitis is modeled by endotoxin-induced uveitis (EIU)

(Rosenbaum et al. 1980), whereas noninfectious autoimmune uveoretinitis is modeled by immunization with retinal antigens or peptides in rats or mice (i.e., experimental autoimmune uveoretinitis, EAU) (Caspi et al. 1988; 1990; Forrester et al. 1992). Although there are no clinical data on the effects of cannabinoids or endocannabinoids on uveoretinitis, studies using animal models have shown that certain cannabinoid compounds possess anti-inflammatory and neuroprotective properties, and so may have therapeutic potential for the treatment of uveoretinitis.

33.6.2 Therapeutic potential of phytocannabinoids in uveoretinitis

EAU is known to be mediated by T cells autoreactive to retinal antigen (Caspi et al. 1986; Liversidge and Forrester 1988). Using EAU as a model, we have shown that a CB_2 receptor selective agonist, JWH-133 (Pertwee 1997, 1999) can suppress retinal inflammation (Xu et al. 2007). JWH-133 suppresses inflammation at multiple points in this autoimmune disease model. Firstly, JWH-133 can suppress dendritic cell activation and antigen presentation by down-regulating the Myd88 signaling pathway (Xu et al. 2007). Secondly, JWH-133 can suppress T cell activation, proliferation, and inflammatory cytokine production, and finally, JWH-133 can prevent leukocyte trafficking into the inflamed retina (Xu et al. 2007). Since the binding affinity of JHW-133 for the CB_2 receptor is more than 200-fold higher than for the CB_1 receptor (Huffman et al. 1998), the immunosuppressant effect of JWH-133 on EAU is likely to be mediated predominately by the CB_2 receptor.

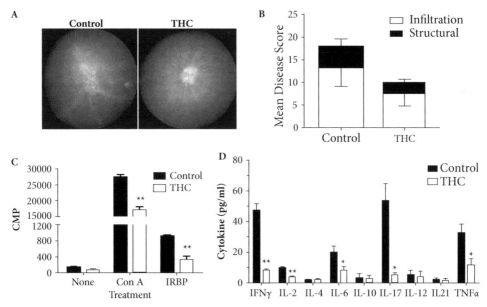

Fig. 33.4 (See also colour plate section.) The effect of THC on EAU. EAU was induced in C57BL/6 mice using interphotoreceptor retinoid binding protein (IRBP) peptide 1–20 immunization. Mice were treated with THC (i.p., daily 5 mg/kg) from day 1–20 post-immunization. Control mice were treated with the vehicle (Tween-20). (A) Fundus images from control and THC-treated EAU mice. (B) Histological investigation showing the retinal structural score and infiltration score. (C) T-lymphocyte proliferation in response to concanavalin A (Con A) or IRBP1-20 peptide stimulation. (D) Cytokine production by splenocytes from control and THC treated EAU mice. *P < 0.05; **P < 0.01 compared to control group (n ≥ 5).

The fact that JWH-133 has an immunosuppressant effect in the CNS is supported by other studies in which it has been shown that JWH-133 can suppress microglial activation (Ramirez et al. 2005), prevent leukocyte adhesion to brain endothelial cells and reduce leakage via the blood–brain barrier (BBB) under inflammatory conditions (Ramirez et al. 2012).

THC also has anti-inflammatory and neuroprotective effects in a mouse model of EAU. Mice treated with THC developed less severe retinal inflammation (Fig. 33.4A), and had a smaller amount of both structural damage and cell infiltration (Fig. 33.4B). The reduced inflammation and retinal neural damage correlate with reduced T cell proliferation (Fig. 33.4C) and inflammatory cytokine (IFN-γ, IL-2, IL-6, IL-17F, and TNF-α) production (Fig. 33.4D).

Not all cannabinoids have the same effect on endotoxin (i.e., lipopolysaccharide, LPS) induced EIU. El-Remessy et al. (2008) showed that CBD (5 mg/kg) suppressed inflammation and neuronal apoptosis in a rat model of EIU. However, AEA, an endogenous cannabinoid receptor agonist, exacerbates retinal inflammation in a rabbit model of EIU (Altinsoy et al. 2011), and the CB_1 receptor inverse agonist AM251 reverses some components of the AEA-induced exacerbation of inflammation (Altinsoy et al. 2011).

33.6.3 Future directions in uveoretinitis

Uveoretinitis is an inflammation-dominated disease with neurodegenerative components. Inflammation-induced oxidative stress is known to be the key cause of neurodegeneration. Uveoretinitis can be pathogen-induced or of autoimmune origin. Experimental studies with preclinical models have yielded inconclusive results. Future studies should clarify whether cannabinoid therapy is beneficial to both infectious and autoimmune uveoretinitis. Furthermore, understanding the role of CB_1 and CB_2 activation in retinal inflammation and neural degeneration in uveoretinitis will be important for designing a target-specific cannabinoid-based therapy.

33.7 Summary

Oxidative stress and inflammation are two major detrimental factors in sight-threatening diseases including glaucoma, DR, AMD, and uveoretinitis although the relative contribution of each factor to different diseases may differ. In glaucoma, DR, and AMD, oxidative stress is considered to be the initial trigger and inflammatory responses secondary to oxidative damage may further contribute to neural cell death, whereas uveoretinitis is an inflammation dominated disease. The generation of ROS or reactive nitrogen species is a key component of the inflammatory response and plays detrimental roles in neural cell death in uveoretinitis. Targeting oxidative stress and inflammation is a promising strategy for treating these conditions. Cannabinoids have antioxidative, anti-inflammatory, and neuroprotective properties. The nonpsychotropic cannabinoid, CBD, which has been shown to have therapeutic potential in a number of preclinical animal models, offers a promising starting point for further drug development.

References

Adams, A.J., Brown, B., Haegerstrom-Portnoy, G., Flom, M.C., and Jones, R.T. (1978). Marijuana, alcohol, and combined drug effects on the time course of glare recovery. *Psychopharmacology (Berlin)*, **56**, 81–86.

Aiello, L.P., Gardner, T.W., King, G.L., *et al.* (1998). Diabetic retinopathy. *Diabetes Care*, **21**, 143–156.

Altinsoy, A., Dilekoz, E., Kul, O., *et al.* (2011). A cannabinoid ligand, anandamide, exacerbates endotoxin-induced uveitis in rabbits. *Journal of Ocular Pharmacology and Therapetics*, **27**, 545–552.

Ambati, J., Anand, A., Fernandez, S., *et al.* (2003). An animal model of age-related macular degeneration in senescent Ccl-2- or Ccr-2-deficient mice. *Nature Medicine*, **9**, 1390–1397.

Barnes, M.P. (2006). Sativex: clinical efficacy and tolerability in the treatment of symptoms of multiple sclerosis and neuropathic pain. *Expert Opinion in Pharmacotherapy*, **7**, 607–615.

Buckley, N.E., Hansson, S., Harta, G., and Mezey, E. (1998). Expression of the CB_1 and CB_2 receptor messenger RNAs during embryonic development in the rat. *Neuroscience*, **82**, 1131–1149.

Buckley, N.E., McCoy, K.L., Mezey, E., *et al.* (2000). Immunomodulation by cannabinoids is absent in mice deficient for the cannabinoid CB_2 receptor. *European Journal of Pharmacology*, **396**, 141–149.

Bunce, C. and Wormald, R. (2006). Leading causes of certification for blindness and partial sight in England & Wales. *Biomed Central Public Health*, **6**, 58.

Buys, Y.M. and Rafuse, P.E. (2010). Canadian Ophthalmological Society policy statement on the medical use of marijuana for glaucoma. *Canadian Journal of Ophthalmology*, **45**, 324–326.

Caspi, R.R., Chan, C.C., Wiggert, B., and Chader, G.J. (1990). The mouse as a model of experimental autoimmune uveoretinitis (EAU). *Current Eye Research*, **9**(Suppl), 169–174.

Caspi, R.R., Roberge, F.G., Chan, C.C., *et al.* (1988). A new model of autoimmune disease. Experimental autoimmune uveoretinitis induced in mice with two different retinal antigens. *Journal of Immunology*, **140**, 1490–1495.

Caspi, R.R., Roberge, F.G., McAllister, C.G., *et al.* (1986). T cell lines mediating experimental autoimmune uveoretinitis (EAU) in the rat. *Journal of Immunology*, **136**, 928–933.

Chen, M., Forrester, J.V., and Xu, H. (2011). Dysregulation in retinal para-inflammation and age-related retinal degeneration in CCL2 or CCR2 deficient mice. *PLoS One*, **6**, e22818.

Chien, F.Y., Wang, R.F., Mittag, T.W., and Podos, S.M. (2003). Effect of WIN 55212-2, a cannabinoid receptor agonist, on aqueous humor dynamics in monkeys. *Archives of Ophthalmology*, **121**, 87–90.

ClinicalTrials.gov. (2008). Efficacy of inhaled cannabis in diabetic painful peripheral neuropathy. Available at: http://clinicaltrials.gov/show/NCT00781001 (accessed December 30, 2012).

Coleman, H.R., Chan, C.C., Ferris, F.L. 3rd., and Chew, E.Y. (2008). Age-related macular degeneration. *Lancet*, **372**, 1835–1845.

Congdon, N., O'Colmain, B., Klaver, C.C., *et al.* (2004). Causes and prevalence of visual impairment among adults in the United States. *Archives of Ophthalmology*, **122**, 477–485.

Crandall, J., Matragoon, S., Khalifa, Y.M., *et al.* (2007). Neuroprotective and intraocular pressure-lowering effects of (-)Delta9-tetrahydrocannabinol in a rat model of glaucoma. *Ophthalmic Research*, **39**, 69–75.

Cunha, J.M., Carlini, E.A., Pereira, A.E., *et al.* (1980). Chronic administration of cannabidiol to healthy volunteers and epileptic patients. *Pharmacology*, **21**, 175–185.

Custis, P.H., Bressler, S.B., and Bressler, N.M. (1993). Laser management of subfoveal choroidal neovascularization in age-related macular degeneration. *Current Opinion in Ophthalmology*, **4**, 7–18.

Dawson, W.W., Jimenez-Antillon, C.F., Perez, J.M., and Zeskind, J.A. (1977). Marijuana and vision – after ten years' use in Costa Rica. *Investigative Ophthalmology and Visual Science*, **16**, 689–699.

Despres, J.P. (2007). The endocannabinoid system: a new target for the regulation of energy balance and metabolism. *Critical Pathways in Cardiology*, **6**, 46–50.

Diaz-Laviada, I. and Ruiz-Llorente, L. (2005). Signal transduction activated by cannabinoid receptors. *Mini Reviews in Medical Chemistry*, **5**, 619–630.

El-Remessy, A.B., Al-Shabrawey, M., Khalifa, Y., Tsai, N.T., Caldwell, R.B., and Liou, G.I. (2006). Neuroprotective and blood-retinal barrier-preserving effects of cannabidiol in experimental diabetes. *American Journal of Pathology*, **168**, 235–244.

El-Remessy, A.B., Rajesh, M., Mukhopadhyay, P., *et al.* (2011). Cannabinoid 1 receptor activation contributes to vascular inflammation and cell death in a mouse model of diabetic retinopathy and a human retinal cell line. *Diabetologia*, **54**, 1567–1578.

El-Remessy, A.B., Tang, Y., Zhu, G., *et al.* (2008). Neuroprotective effects of cannabidiol in endotoxin-induced uveitis: critical role of p38 MAPK activation. *Molecular Vision*, **14**, 2190–2203.

European Medicines agency. (2013a). *Macugen.* [Online] Available at: http://www.ema.europa.eu/ema/index.jsp?curl=pages/medicines/human/medicines/000620/human_med_000898.jsp&mid=WC0b01ac058001d124 (accessed December 30, 2012).

European Medicines agency. (2013b). *Lucentis.* [Online] Available at: http://www.ema.europa.eu/ema/index.jsp?curl=pages/medicines/human/medicines/000715/human_med_000890.jsp&mid=WC0b01ac058001d124 (accessed December 30, 2012).

Fan, S.F. and Yazulla, S. (2003). Biphasic modulation of voltage-dependent currents of retinal cones by cannabinoid CB1 receptor agonist WIN 55212-2. *Visual Neuroscience,* **20,** 177–188.

Flach, A.J. (2002). Delta-9-tetrahydrocannabinol (THC) in the treatment of end-stage open-angle glaucoma. *Transactions of the American Ophthalmological Society,* **100,** 215–222; discussion 222–224.

Forrester, J.V., Liversidge, J., Dua, H.S., Dick, A., Harper, F., and McMenamin, P.G. (1992). Experimental autoimmune uveoretinitis: a model system for immunointervention: a review. *Current Eye Research,* **11**(Suppl), 33–40.

Friedman, D.S., O'Colmain, B.J., Munoz, B., *et al.* (2004). Prevalence of age-related macular degeneration in the United States. *Archives of Ophthalmology,* **122,** 564–572.

Galiegue, S., Mary, S., Marchand, J., *et al.* (1995). Expression of central and peripheral cannabinoid receptors in human immune tissues and leukocyte subpopulations. *European Journal of Biochemistry,* **232,** 54–61.

Green, K. (1979). Marihuana in ophthalmology-past, present and future. *Annals of Ophthalmology,* **11,** 203–205.

Green, K. and Roth, M. (1982). Ocular effects of topical administration of delta 9-tetrahydrocannabinol in man. *Archives of Ophthalmology,* **100,** 265–267.

Green, K. and Podos, S.M. (1974). Antagonism of arachidonic acid-induced ocular effects by delta1-tetrahydrocannabinol. *Investigative Ophthalmology,* **13,** 422–429.

Green, K. and Pederson, J.E. (1973). Effect of 1-tetrahydrocannabinol on aqueous dynamics and ciliary body permeability in the rabbit. *Experimental Eye Research,* **15,** 499–507.

Green, K., Kearse, E.C., and McIntyre, O.L. (2001). Interaction between delta-9-tetrahydrocannabinol and indomethacin. *Ophthalmic Research,* **33,** 217–220.

Green, K.E. and Kearse, C.E. (2000). Ocular penetration of topical delta9-tetrahydrocannabinol from rabbit corneal or cul-de-sac application site. *Current Eye Research,* **21,** 566–570.

Hampson, A.J., Grimaldi, M., Axelrod, J., and Wink, D. (1998). Cannabidiol and (-)delta9-tetrahydrocannabinol are neuroprotective antioxidants. *Proceedings of the National Academy of Sciences of the United States of America,* **95,** 8268–8273.

Hampson, A.J., Grimaldi, M., Lolic. M., Wink, D., Rosenthal, R., and Axelrod, J. (2000). Neuroprotective antioxidants from marijuana. *Annals of the New York Academy of Sciences,* **899,** 274–282.

He, F., Kumar, A., Song, Z.H. (2012). Heat shock protein 90 is an essential molecular chaperone for CB_2 cannabinoid receptor-mediated signaling in trabecular meshwork cells. *Molecular Vision,* **18,** 2839–2846.

Heier, J.S., Boyer, D.S., Ciulla, T.A., *et al.* (2006). Ranibizumab combined with verteporfin photodynamic therapy in neovascular age-related macular degeneration: year 1 results of the FOCUS Study. *Archives of Ophthalmology,* **124,** 1532–1542.

Hepler, R.S. and Frank, I.R. (1971). Marihuana smoking and intraocular pressure. *Journal of the American Medical Association,* **217,** 1392.

Hingorani, T., Gul, W., Elsohly, M., Repka, M.A., and Majumdar, S. (2012). Effect of ion pairing on in vitro transcorneal permeability of a delta9-tetrahydrocannabinol prodrug: potential in glaucoma therapy. *Journal of Pharmaceutical Sciences,* **101,** 616–626.

Hudson, B.D., Beazley, M., Szczesniak, A.M., Straiker, A., and Kelly, M.E. (2011). Indirect sympatholytic actions at beta-adrenoceptors account for the ocular hypotensive actions of cannabinoid receptor agonists. *Journal of Pharmacology and Experimental Therapeutics,* **339,** 757–767.

Huffman, J.W., Liddle, J., Duncan, S.G., Jr., Yu, S., Martin, B.R., and Wiley, J.L. (1998). Synthesis and pharmacology of the isomeric methylheptyl-delta8-tetrahydrocannabinols. *Bioorganic and Medical Chemistry*, **6**, 2383–2396.

Jampel, H. (2010). American glaucoma society position statement: marijuana and the treatment of glaucoma. *Journal of Glaucoma*, **19**, 75–76.

Jarho, P., Pate, D.W., Brenneisen, R., and Jarvinen, T. (1998). Hydroxypropyl-beta-cyclodextrin and its combination with hydroxypropyl-methylcellulose increases aqueous solubility of delta9-tetrahydrocannabinol. *Life Sciences*, **63**, PL381–384.

Jarho, P., Urtti, A., Jarvinen, K., Pate, D.W., and Jarvinen, T. (1996). Hydroxypropyl-beta-cyclodextrin increases aqueous solubility and stability of anandamide. *Life Sciences*, **58**, PL181–185.

Jay, W.M. and Green, K. (1983). Multiple-drop study of topically applied 1% delta 9-tetrahydrocannabinol in human eyes. *Archives of Ophthalmology*, **101**, 591–593.

Jin, K.L., Mao, X.O., Goldsmith, P.C., and Greenberg, D.A. (2000). CB_1 cannabinoid receptor induction in experimental stroke. *Annals of Neurology*, **48**, 257–261.

Kearse, E.C. and Green, K. (2000). Effect of vehicle upon in vitro transcorneal permeability and intracorneal content of Delta9-tetrahydrocannabinol. *Current Eye Research*, **20**, 496–501.

Kern, T.S. and Barber, A.J. (2008). Retinal ganglion cells in diabetes. *Journal of Physiology*, **586**, 4401–4408.

Kiplinger, G.F. and Manno, J.E. (1971). Dose-response relationships to cannabis in human subjects. *Pharmacology Reviews*, **23**, 339–347.

Korczyn, A.D. (1980). The ocular effects of cannabinoids. *General Pharmacology*, **11**, 419–423.

Kowluru, R.A. and Chan, P.S. (2007). Oxidative stress and diabetic retinopathy. *Experimental Diabetes Research*, **2007**, 43603.

Laine, K., Jarvinen, K., Mechoulam, R., Breuer, A., and Jarvinen, T. (2002). Comparison of the enzymatic stability and intraocular pressure effects of 2-arachidonylglycerol and noladin ether, a novel putative endocannabinoid. *Investigative Ophthalmology and Visual Science*, **43**, 3216–3222.

Leonelli, M., Martins, D.O., Kihara, A.H., and Britto, L.R. (2009). Ontogenetic expression of the vanilloid receptors TRPV1 and TRPV2 in the rat retina. *International Journal of Developmental Neuroscience*, **27**, 709–718.

Levin, L.A. (1999). Direct and indirect approaches to neuroprotective therapy of glaucomatous optic neuropathy. *Survey of Ophthalmology*, **43**(Suppl 1), S98–101.

Lieth, E., Gardner, T.W., Barber, A.J., Antonetti, D.A., Penn State Retina Research Group. (2000). Retinal neurodegeneration: early pathology in diabetes. *Clinical and Experimental Ophthalmology*, **28**, 3–8.

Lim, S.K., Park, M.J., Lim, J.C., *et al.* (2012). Hyperglycemia induces apoptosis via CB1 activation through the decrease of FAAH 1 in retinal pigment epithelial cells. *Journal of Cell Physiology*, **227**, 569–577.

Liou, G.I. (2010). Diabetic retinopathy: role of inflammation and potential therapies for anti-inflammation. *World Journal of Diabetes*, **1**, 12–18.

Liou, G.I., Auchampach, J.A., Hillard, C.J., *et al.* (2008). Mediation of cannabidiol anti-inflammation in the retina by equilibrative nucleoside transporter and A2A adenosine receptor. *Investigative Ophthalmology and Visual Science*, **49**, 5526–5531.

Lipina, C., Rastedt, W., Irving, A.J., and Hundal, H.S. (2012). New vistas for treatment of obesity and diabetes? Endocannabinoid signalling and metabolism in the modulation of energy balance. *Bioessays*, **34**, 681–691.

Liversidge, J. and Forrester, J.V. (1988). Experimental autoimmune uveitis (EAU): immunophenotypic analysis of inflammatory cells in chorio retinal lesions. *Current Eye Research*, **7**, 1231–1241.

Lopez, E.M., Tagliaferro, P., Onaivi, ES., and Lopez-Costa, J.J. (2011). Distribution of CB_2 cannabinoid receptor in adult rat retina. *Synapse*, **65**, 388–392.

Lu, Q., Straiker, A., Lu, Q., and Maguire, G. (2000). Expression of CB2 cannabinoid receptor mRNA in adult rat retina. *Visual Neuroscience*, **17**, 91–95.

Malfait, A.M., Gallily, R., Sumariwalla, P.F., *et al.* (2000). The nonpsychoactive cannabis constituent cannabidiol is an oral anti-arthritic therapeutic in murine collagen-induced arthritis. *Proceedings of the National Academy of Sciences of the United States of America*, **97**, 9561–9566.

Marsicano. G., Moosmann, B., Hermann, H., Lutz, B., and Behl, C. (2002). Neuroprotective properties of cannabinoids against oxidative stress: role of the cannabinoid receptor CB1. *Journal of Neurochemistry*, **80**, 448–456.

Matias, I., Wang, J.W., Moriello, A.S., Nieves, A., Woodward, D.F., and Di Marzo, V. (2006). Changes in endocannabinoid and palmitoylethanolamide levels in eye tissues of patients with diabetic retinopathy and age-related macular degeneration. *Prostaglandins, Leukotrienes & Essential Fatty Acids*, **75**, 413–418.

Matsuda, L.A., Lolait, S.J., Brownstein, M.J., Young, A.C., and Bonner, T.I. (1990). Structure of a cannabinoid receptor and functional expression of the cloned cDNA. *Nature*, **346**, 561–564.

McAllister, S.D. and Glass, M. (2002). CB_1 and CB_2 receptor-mediated signalling: a focus on endocannabinoids. *Prostaglandins, Leukotrienes & Essential Fatty Acids*, **66**, 161–171.

McDonald, T.F., Cheeks, L., Slagle, T., and Green, K. (1991). Marijuana-derived material-induced changes in monkey ciliary processes differ from those in rabbit ciliary processes. *Current Eye Research*, **10**, 305–312.

McIntosh, B.T., Hudson, B., Yegorova, S., Jollimore, C.A., and Kelly, M.E. (2007). Agonist-dependent cannabinoid receptor signalling in human trabecular meshwork cells. *British Journal of Pharmacology*, **152**, 1111–1120.

Mechoulam, R., Peters, M., Murillo-Rodriguez, E., and Hanus, L.O. (2007). Cannabidiol--recent advances. *Chemistry & Biodiverssity*, **4**, 1678–1692.

Merritt, J.C., Crawford, W.J., Alexander, P.C., Anduze, A.L., and Gelbart, S.S. (1980). Effect of marihuana on intraocular and blood pressure in glaucoma. *Ophthalmology*, **87**, 222–228.

Munro, S., Thomas, K.L., and Abu-Shaar, M. (1993). Molecular characterization of a peripheral receptor for cannabinoids. *Nature*, **365**, 61–65.

Naveh, N., Weissman, C., Muchtar, S., Benita, S., and Mechoulam, R. (2000). A submicron emulsion of HU-211, a synthetic cannabinoid, reduces intraocular pressure in rabbits. *Graefes Archives of Clinical and Experimental Ophthalmology*, **238**, 334–338.

Pertwee, R.G. (2005). The therapeutic potential of drugs that target cannabinoid receptors or modulate the tissue levels or actions of endocannabinoids. *The AAPS Journal*, **7**, E625–54.

Pertwee, R.G. (2000a). Cannabinoid receptor ligands: clinical and neuropharmacological considerations, relevant to future drug discovery and development. *Expert Opinion on Investigational Drugs*, **9**, 1553–1571.

Pertwee, R.G. (2000b). Neuropharmacology and therapeutic potential of cannabinoids. *Addiction Biology*, **5**, 37–46.

Pertwee, R.G. (1999). Pharmacology of cannabinoid receptor ligands. *Current Medicinal Chemistry*, **6**, 635–664.

Pertwee, R.G. (1997). Pharmacology of cannabinoid CB_1 and CB_2 receptors. *Pharmacology & Therapeutics*, **74**, 129–180.

Pertwee, R.G. and Ross, R.A. (2002). Cannabinoid receptors and their ligands. *Prostaglandins, Leukotrienes & Essential Fatty Acids*, **66**, 101–121.

Porcella, A., Maxia, C., Gessa, G.L., and Pani, L. (2001). The synthetic cannabinoid WIN55212-2 decreases the intraocular pressure in human glaucoma resistant to conventional therapies. *European Journal of Neuroscience*, **13**, 409–412.

Porcella, A., Maxia, C., Gessa, G.L., and Pani, L. (2000). The human eye expresses high levels of CB_1 cannabinoid receptor mRNA and protein. *European Journal of Neuroscience*, **12**, 1123–1127.

Porcella, A., Casellas, P., Gessa, G.L., and Pani, L. (1998). Cannabinoid receptor CB1 mRNA is highly expressed in the rat ciliary body: implications for the antiglaucoma properties of marihuana. *Molecular Brain Research*, **58**, 240–245.

Ramirez, B.G., Blazquez, C., Gomez, d.P., Guzman, M., and de Ceballos, M.L. (2005). Prevention of Alzheimer's disease pathology by cannabinoids: neuroprotection mediated by blockade of microglial activation. *Journal of Neuroscience*, **25**, 1904–1913.

Ramirez, S.H., Hasko, J., Skuba, A., *et al.* (2012). Activation of cannabinoid receptor 2 attenuates leukocyte-endothelial cell interactions and blood-brain barrier dysfunction under inflammatory conditions. *Journal of Neuroscience*, **32**, 4004–4016.

Romero-Aroca, P., Sagarra-Alamo, R., Basora-Gallisa, J., Basora-Gallisa, T., Baget-Bernaldiz, M., and Bautista-Perez, A. (2010). Prospective comparison of two methods of screening for diabetic retinopathy by nonmydriatic fundus camera. *Clinical Ophthalmology*, **4**, 1481–1488.

Rosenbaum, J.T., McDevitt, H.O., Guss, R.B., and Egbert, P.R. (1980). Endotoxin-induced uveitis in rats as a model for human disease. *Nature*, **286**, 611–613.

Rosenfeld, P.J., Shapiro, H., Tuomi, L., *et al.* (2011). Characteristics of patients losing vision after 2 years of monthly dosing in the phase III ranibizumab clinical trials. *Ophthalmology*, **118**, 523–530.

Ross, R.A. (2003). Anandamide and vanilloid TRPV1 receptors. *British Journal of Pharmacology*, **140**, 790–801.

Russo, E.B., Burnett, A., Hall, B., Parker, K.K. (2005). Agonistic properties of cannabidiol at 5-HT1a receptors. *Neurochemical Research*, **30**, 1037–1043.

Russo, E.B., Merzouki, A., Mesa, J.M., Frey, K.A., and Bach, P.J. (2004). Cannabis improves night vision: a case study of dark adaptometry and scotopic sensitivity in kif smokers of the Rif mountains of northern Morocco. *Journal of Ethnopharmacology*, **93**, 99–104.

Ryberg, E., Larsson, N., Sjogren, S., *et al.* (2007). The orphan receptor GPR55 is a novel cannabinoid receptor. *British Journal of Pharmacology*, **152**, 1092–1101.

Sappington, R.M. and Calkins, D.J. (2008). Contribution of TRPV1 to microglia-derived IL-6 and NFkappaB translocation with elevated hydrostatic pressure. *Investigative Ophthalmology and Visual Science*, **49**, 3004–3017.

Sawzdargo, M., Nguyen, T., Lee, D.K., *et al.* (1999). Identification and cloning of three novel human G protein-coupled receptor genes GPR52, PsiGPR53 and GPR55: GPR55 is extensively expressed in human brain. *Molecular Brain Research*, **64**, 193–198.

Schmidt-Erfurth, U., Hasan, T. (2000). Mechanisms of action of photodynamic therapy with verteporfin for the treatment of age-related macular degeneration. *Survey of Ophthalmology*, **45**, 195–214.

Simo, R., Hernandez, C., European Consortium for the Early Treatment of Diabetic Retinopathy (EUROCONDOR). (2012). Neurodegeneration is an early event in diabetic retinopathy: therapeutic implications. *British Journal of Ophthalmology*, **96**, 1285–1290.

Straiker, A., Stella, N., Piomelli, D., Mackie, K., Karten, H.J., and Maguire, G. (1999a). Cannabinoid CB1 receptors and ligands in vertebrate retina: localization and function of an endogenous signaling system. *Proceedings of the National Academy of Sciences of the United States of America*, **96**, 14565–14570.

Straiker, A.J., Maguire, G., Mackie, K., and Lindsey, J. (1999b). Localization of cannabinoid CB1 receptors in the human anterior eye and retina. *Investigative Ophthalmology and Visual Science*, **40**, 2442–2448.

Sugrue, M.F. (1997). New approaches to antiglaucoma therapy. *Journal of Medical Chemistry*, **40**, 2793–2809.

Tang, J., Kern, T.S. (2011). Inflammation in diabetic retinopathy. *Progress in Retinal and Eye Research*, **30**, 343–358.

Tomida, I., Pertwee, R.G., and Azuara-Blanco, A. (2004). Cannabinoids and glaucoma. *British Journal of Ophthalmology*, **88**, 708–713.

Tomida, I., Azuara-Blanco, A., House, H., Flint, M., Pertwee, R.G., and Robson, P.J. (2006). Effect of sublingual application of cannabinoids on intraocular pressure: a pilot study. *Journal of Glaucoma*, **15**, 349–353.

Toth, A., Boczan, J., Kedei, N., *et al.* (2005). Expression and distribution of vanilloid receptor 1 (TRPV1) in the adult rat brain. *Molecular Brain Research*, **135**, 162–168.

Tsou, K., Brown, S., Sanudo-Pena, M.C., Mackie, K., and Walker, J.M. (1998). Immunohistochemical distribution of cannabinoid CB1 receptors in the rat central nervous system. *Neuroscience*, **83**, 393–411.

Wei, Y., Wang, X., and Wang, L. (2009). Presence and regulation of cannabinoid receptors in human retinal pigment epithelial cells. *Molecular Vision*, **15**, 1243–1251.

West, M.E. (1991). Cannabis and night vision. *Nature*, **351**, 703–704.

Xu, H., Cheng, C.L., Chen, M., *et al.* (2007). Anti-inflammatory property of the cannabinoid receptor-2-selective agonist JWH-133 in a rodent model of autoimmune uveoretinitis. *Journal of Leukocyte Biology*, **82**, 532–541.

Yazulla, S. (2008). Endocannabinoids in the retina: from marijuana to neuroprotection. *Progress in Retinal and Eye Research*, **27**, 501–526.

Yazulla, S., Studholme, K.M., McIntosh, H.H., and Deutsch, D.G. (1999). Immunocytochemical localization of cannabinoid CB1 receptor and fatty acid amide hydrolase in rat retina. *Journal of Comparative Neurology*, **415**, 80–90.

Yoles, E., Belkin, M., and Schwartz, M. (1996). HU-211, a nonpsychotropic cannabinoid, produces short- and long-term neuroprotection after optic nerve axotomy. *Journal of Neurotrauma*, **13**, 49–57.

Zhong, L., Geng, L., Njie, Y., Feng, W., and Song, Z.H. (2005). CB_2 cannabinoid receptors in trabecular meshwork cells mediate JWH015-induced enhancement of aqueous humor outflow facility. *Investigative Ophthalmology and Visual Science*, **46**, 1988–1992.

Zimov, S. and Yazulla, S. (2007). Vanilloid receptor 1 (TRPV1/VR1) co-localizes with fatty acid amide hydrolase (FAAH) in retinal amacrine cells. *Visual Neuroscience*, **24**, 581–591.

Chapter 34

Bone As a Target for Cannabinoid Therapy

Itai Bab

34.1 Introduction

Bone consists of a mineralized extracellular matrix (MEM) and three major cell types, osteoblasts that form the MEM, osteoclasts that resorb the MEM, and osteocytes that regulate its metabolism. The osteoblasts and osteoclasts are present on MEM surfaces, whereas the osteocytes are embedded within lacunae within the MEM. By contrast to its inactive appearance, bone is a metabolically active tissue. Bone mass, the primary determinant of skeletal strength, displays sequential stages throughout life, comprising: (1) a rapid skeletal growth phase accompanied by accrual of peak bone mass, (2) a steady-state phase whereby bone mass remains constant, and (3) age-related bone loss (Bab et al. 2007). These changes are governed by bone remodeling, a continuous lifetime process that consists of resorption of the MEM by osteoclasts, and formation of new MEM by osteoblasts (Parfitt 1982). Osteoporosis is the most widespread example of a bone remodeling disease. It is the consequence of accelerated loss of bone mass and disrupted architecture, which leads to weakening of the skeleton and increased fracture risk. The case of osteoporosis highlights the pathophysiologic importance of bone remodeling. With the progressive aging of the population, osteoporosis is becoming one of the most serious epidemics in developed countries. Nearly 10 million osteoporotic bone fractures in European and North America cost the health system more than $60 billion annually; half a million elderly people are killed from related complications, a number expected to double by 2050. Presently, women are more likely to die from a hip fracture than from breast cancer (Cauley and Bulstra 2007).

It is therefore not surprising that the discovery of the skeleton as a cannabinoid target in the past decade has triggered a growing interest in the potential of cannabinoids for pharmacological treatment and genetic diagnosis of bone deficits, primarily osteoporosis. A recent Web of Science search revealed more than 700 citations of reports on the skeletal cannabinoid system (SCS) published since 2005 (Bab 2005; Idris et al. 2005; Karsak et al. 2005). This chapter focuses on the SCS as a therapeutic target for patients with osteoporosis, bone metastatic cancer, and skeletal wounds.

34.2 The skeletal cannabinoid system

Several key components of the endocannabinoid system have been identified in bone. Anandamide (AEA) and 2-arachidonoylglycerol (2-AG), are produced by osteoblasts and osteoclasts, reaching pmol/g and nmol/g concentrations, respectively, similar to their brain levels (Tam et al. 2008). In addition, a novel endocannabinoid-like, oleoyl serine (OS) has been recently discovered in bone (Smoum et al. 2010). Diacylglycerol lipases α and β, enzymes critically involved in 2-AG biosynthesis, are expressed in osteoblasts, osteocytes, bone-lining cells, and osteoclasts (Tam et al. 2008). The respective AEA biosynthetic and degrading enzymes, N-acyl phosphatidylethanolamine phospholipase D and fatty acid amide hydrolase (FAAH) are also expressed in bone cells (our unpublished results). There is a general agreement that type 2 cannabinoid receptors (CB_2) are expressed in both osteoblasts and osteoclasts as well as in their precursors (Bab 2005; Idris et al. 2005; Ofek et al. 2006; Rossi et al, 2013; Scutt and Williamson 2007). Cannabinoid CB_1 receptors are present in sympathetic nerve terminals in bone (Tam et al. 2006). Possibly, CB_1 is also expressed at low levels in osteoblasts and osteoclasts (Idris et al. 2005; Ofek et al. 2006); however, the evidence in support of these findings is still awaiting confirmation.

Although both 2-AG and AEA are considered nonselective agonists of CB_1 and CB_2, findings in bone and bone cell cultures suggest differential effects of these ligands. While 2-AG administered to mice activates CB_1 in skeletal sympathetic nerve terminals, thus stimulating bone formation (Tam et al. 2008; our unpublished results), it has no effect on osteoblasts and may even act as an inverse agonist in these cells (Tam et al. 2008). AEA stimulates in vitro osteoblast proliferation (Smoum et al. 2010). In addition, the number of osteoclasts in culture is increased by a direct challenge with AEA (Idris et al. 2005) or through the action of the FAAH inhibitor URB597 that leads to increased AEA levels endogenously. It remains to be seen whether these actions of AEA are mediated by CB_1 and/or CB_2.

Activation of CB_2 has different effects in early osteoblast progenitors and in more mature osteoblastic cells. Early precursors, represented by partially differentiated osteoblastic cells derived from bone marrow stromal (mesenchymal) stem cells, show limited CB_2 expression. Nevertheless, the selective CB_2 agonist HU–308 induces marked expansion of the preosteoblastic pool (Ofek et al. 2006). Ex vivo colony forming units osteoblastic (CFU-Ob, a surrogate of in vivo pre-osteoblast number) by bone marrow stromal CB_2-deficient cells is markedly diminished, whereas CFU-Ob formation by wild type (WT) cells is stimulated by HU-308 (Ofek et al. 2006; Scutt and Williamson 2007). In mature osteoblastic cells, represented by the MC3T3 E1 cell line, the same ligand stimulates osteoblast differentiated functions such as alkaline phosphatase activity and matrix mineralization (Bab 2005; Ofek et al. 2006). The mitogenic signaling cascade triggered by CB_2 in osteoblast precursors has been fully elucidated. It consists of Gi-protein-dependent Erk1/2 activation, followed by transcriptional activation of Mapkapk2, which in turn stimulates CREB and cyclin D1 (Ofek et al. 2011).

In mouse bone marrow-derived osteoclastogenic cultures and in the RAW 264.7 cell line, CB_2 activation inhibits osteoclast formation by restraining mitogenesis at the monocytic stage, prior to incubation with receptor activator of nuclear factor kappa-B ligand (RANKL). It also suppresses osteoclast formation by repressing RANKL expression in osteoblasts and osteoblast progenitors (Ofek et al. 2006). Likewise, it has been recently shown that the cannabinoid receptor agonist ajulemic acid also suppresses osteoclastogenesis (George et al. 2008). Formation of human osteoclasts is also inhibited by activation of CB_2 (Rossi et al. 2013). By contrast, other studies have reported the stimulation of mouse osteoclast formation and bone resorption by cannabinoid receptor agonists and their inhibition by antagonists (Idris et al. 2005, 2008) and inhibition of osteoclastogenesis by inverse agonists at CB_2 (Yang et al. 2013). These allegedly paradoxical effects may be species and/or ligand dependent or result from differences in culture conditions.

GPR55, which is antagonized by cannabidiol (CBD), is also present in osteoblasts and osteoclasts. GPR55 activation decreases both osteoclastogenesis and osteoclast function (Whyte et al. 2009). Surprisingly, treatment of mice with CBD reduced bone resorption in vivo (section 34.2.3). However, inconsistent with this attenuation of bone resorption an effect of CBD on bone mass has not been reported.

Although OS does not target CB_1 or CB_2, it does increase osteoblast number. In addition, it is apoptotic for osteoclasts, thus reducing bone resorption by shortening their life span (Smoum et al. 2010).

34.2.1 CB_1 and bone mass

Cannabinoid receptor mutant mice have been extensively used to assess the physiologic role of CB_1 and CB_2 in the control of bone mass. While the effect of constitutive CB_1 deficiency appears to depend on the mouse sex and background strain, that of CB_2 is more robust. Perhaps more importantly, the pertinence of findings in CB_2, but not CB_1 mutant mice to human skeletal health have already been demonstrated (section 34.3).

A high bone mass phenotype was reported in young, sexually mature CB_1-null mice generated on a CD1 background (Idris et al. 2005). However, this observation has been confirmed only in males (Tam et al. 2006). By contrast, both male and female CB_1-null mice generated on a C57BL/6J background have a low bone mass phenotype secondary to decreased bone formation rate and increased osteoclast number, a histomorphometric surrogate of bone resorption (Tam et al. 2006). CB_1-deficient mice on either background develop age-related osteoporosis due to a progressive decrease in bone formation (Idris et al. 2009; our unpublished findings). Regardless of whether or not CB_1 has a role in peak bone mass accrual, the consistent set of data obtained in aging mice suggests an important role for CB_1 signaling in the regulation of bone remodeling and bone mass.

We have further used CB_1-null mice to analyze the mechanism involved in CB_1-mediated effects on bone. In humans, traumatic brain injury (TBI) often stimulates bone formation and bone mass (Morley et al. 2005). Using a mouse model for TBI, we have replicated the same phenomenon in WT animals, demonstrating an increase in bone formation already 24 h after TBI. However, this increase could not be reproduced in CB_1-null mice (Tam et al. 2008). Given that (1) CB_1 is expressed in sympathetic terminals in close proximity to osetoblasts, (2) sympathetic signaling restrains bone formation, and (3) retrograde CB_1 presynaptic signals inhibit neurotransmitter release, we assumed that CB_1 super activation after TBI reduces bone norepinephrine levels, which in turn results in increased bone formation. Indeed, we showed that in WT, but not in CB_1 knockout mice, 2-AG production by osteoblasts is stimulated within hours after TBI and is followed by inhibition of norepinephrine levels and increased bone formation rate (Tam et al. 2008).

34.2.2 CB_2 and bone mass

During their first 2–3 months of life, CB_2-deficient mice accrue a normal peak trabecular bone mass, but later display a markedly enhanced age-related bone loss; their trabecular bone volume density at 1 year of age is approximately half compared to WT controls (Ofek et al. 2006; Sophocleous et al. 2011). Reminiscent of human postmenopausal osteoporosis, the CB_2-null mice have a high bone turnover with increases in both bone resorption and formation which are in a net negative balance (Ofek et al. 2006). Importantly, low bone mass is the only spontaneous phenotype so far reported in these mice. Hence, because healthy CB_2 mutant mice are otherwise normal, it appears that the main physiologic role of CB_2 is the maintenance of balanced bone remodeling.

34.2.3 GPR55 and bone mass

Consistent with the in vitro inhibition of osteoclast function by GPR55, young, sexually mature GPR55-deficient male, but not female mice have a high bone mass phenotype (Whyte et al. 2009).

However, in two independent studies administration of CBD to WT animals had no effect on their peak bone mass (Whyte et al. 2009; our unpublished results). The effect of CBD on age-related bone loss has not been studied yet.

34.3 The skeletal cannabinoid system as a therapeutic target

The discovery and characterization of the SCS in mice was soon followed by genetic association studies of polymorphisms in the human *CNR1* and *CNR2* loci to assess the cannabinoid receptors as targets for the risk assessment and treatment of osteoporosis. The *CNR1* locus is on chromosome 5q15, a site previously not implicated in osteoporosis. By contrast, the *CNR2* locus is on chromosome 1p36, a genomic region linked to bone mineral density (BMD) and osteoporosis in several independent association analyses. Its mouse ortholog on chromosome 4 is also associated with low bone mass (Devoto et al. 2001).

A genetic association analysis of *CNR1* and *CNR2* in French Caucasian cohorts of postmenopausal osteoporotic women with a low BMD and of age-matched healthy controls suggested that the *CNR1* gene did not play a major role in bone in this sample of osteoporotic women (Karsak et al. 2005). In contrast, several single nucleotide polymorphisms in the *CNR2* gene showed a significant association with the disease phenotype, suggesting that *CNR2* polymorphisms are important genetic risk factors for osteoporosis. Sequencing the CB_2 coding exon in all patients and controls identified two missense variants, Gln63Arg and His316Tyr, with the Gln63Arg variant being more common in the osteoporotic patients than in the healthy controls (Karsak et al. 2005). These findings have been confirmed in large Chinese and Japanese cohorts and in an ethnically homogeneous healthy sample of a Chuvashian family (Huang et al. 2009; Karsak et al. 2009;Yamada et al. 2007).

Potentially, CB_1 ligands could be tested for osteoporosis. However, given their central adverse effects there is one study in mice, published prior to the withdrawal of rimonabant, reporting the efficacy of a nonperipheralized CB_1 antagonist in the prevention of osteoporosis (Idris et al. 2005). Although the efficacy of peripheralized CB_1 antagonists has been demonstrated in animal models of the metabolic syndrome (Tam et al. 2010, 2012), skeletal effects of such agonists have not been reported. Overall, it seems that the uncertainties associated with the skeletal role of CB_1 has held back further assessment of CB_1-based antiosteoporotic therapies.

Unlike CB_1, CB_2 does not mediate cannabinoid-induced psychotropic, metabolic, or reproductive effects. Therefore, CB_2–specific ligands offer an opportunity to prevent and/or rescue bone loss while avoiding the adverse effects of cannabinoids. Antiosteoporotic therapies are classified as either preventive, which inhibit bone destruction, or anabolic, which rescue bone loss. Most of the drugs in use belong to the preventive category, and are generally not particularly efficacious in the millions of patients who require the addition of new bone to replace that which has already been lost. Unfortunately, there is only one approved bone anabolic drug, recombinant human parathyroid hormone (sold as Forteo®), which has limited efficacy on certain skeletal sites and can be given only by subcutaneous injection for a maximum of 2–3 years (Uihlein and Leder 2012). Synthetic CB_2 agonists like HU-308, which are orally available and have minimal side effects, if any, offer a solution for this need. Indeed, preclinical studies testing such agonists have demonstrated complete rescue of bone loss induced by estrogen depletion in ovariectomized (OVX) mice, mainly by stimulating bone formation (Bab et al. 2008; our unpublished results). These agonists only mildly attenuated OVX-induced bone loss by inhibiting bone resorption (Ofek et al. 2006). Notably, in the rescue model the drug is first given 6 weeks after OVX to allow for bone loss to occur and for the establishment of a new bone remodeling balance. In the preventive model, agonist administration commences immediately after OVX, at a time when bone presents high turnover, negatively balanced remodeling. In either protocol, the cannabinoid treatment consisted of daily intraperitoneal (i.p.) injections for 4–6 weeks. Hence, CB_2 agonists are promising candidates, particularly for anabolic therapy for osteoporosis patients.

The endocannabinoid-like OS also has bone anabolic properties. Moreover, its anabolic action not only rescues bone loss, by both stimulating bone formation and inhibiting bone resorption, but also increases bone mass in normal mice. In these normal animals it acts only to restrain resorption. A preliminary indication that other fatty acid amides may have bone anabolic activity has also been obtained (Smoum et al. 2010).

Interestingly, marijuana smoke inhalation has recently been reported to inhibit endosseous implant anchorage in rats, negatively affecting both the bone-implant contact and peri-implant bone (Nogueira-Filho Gda et al. 2008). This is not necessarily inconsistent with the bone anabolic activity displayed by well-defined cannabinoid receptor agonists, as marijuana contains a mixture of biologically active phytocannabinoids whose skeletal effects have not been tested yet. In addition, the peri-implant healing process may differ considerably from remodeling of the nontraumatized skeleton and thus responds differently to cannabinoids. Another potentially confounding issue is the nonselectivity/nonspecificity of many cannabinoid ligands either endogenous, plant derived, or synthetic. The skeletal relevance of this issue has been recently demonstrated in a study showing that, at a daily dose of 0.1 mg/kg i.p., the "so-called" CB_2 selective inverse agonist AM630 prevented OVX-induced bone loss in WT but not in CB_2-null mice, therefore indicating CB_2 selectivity at this low dose. However, the same preparation was equally effective in preventing bone loss in WT and CB_2-deficient mice at higher doses (Idris et al. 2008). Hence, in the skeleton and probably elsewhere, cannabinoid ligands may have CB_1 and/or CB_2 independent effects, depending on the concentrations or doses used.

Metastatic bone cancer has recently raised interest as a promising target for CB_2-based therapy. Although currently used chemotherapeutics prolong the life of these patients, metastases still lead to bone loss and increased fracture incidence as well as severe side effects. Opiates, used as first-line analgesics in these patients, also induce bone loss. In either case, the bone loss is treated with bisphosphonates, which in turn cause nephrotoxicity and osteonecrosis of the jaws. Using a mouse model for bone metastatic breast cancer it has been recently demonstrated that the CB_2-selective agonist JWH015, administered systemically, reduces bone pain, bone loss, and cancer cell proliferation (Lozano-Ondoua et al. 2013). However, it has not been determined whether these effects were mediated through a direct action on osteoblasts, osteoclasts, or the cancer cells, or indirectly, for example, through CB_2 activation in resident immune cells. Further studies addressing this and other mechanistic issues will hopefully identify more specific modes and sites of action.

34.4 **Summary**

With osteoporosis being the most prevalent degenerative disease in developed countries, it has attracted a lot of experimental and public attention following the discovery of the skeletal cannabinoid system. Obviously, specific CB_2 agonists hold great promise for the millions of osteoporotic patients worldwide. Questions have been frequently asked regarding whether cannabis and phytocannabinoids are "friends or foes." Studies carried out in our laboratory and by others have so far provided negative results: tetrahydrocannabinol (THC) had a small inhibitory effect on peak bone mass accrual, if any. In addition, we found no skeletal effects of CBD. These data are not conclusive as these cannabinoids could have skeletal effects in older age. In addition, inhaled cannabis seems to slow down bone wound healing. By contrast, preliminary studies in our laboratory suggest that CBD, but not THC, improves fracture healing. It would also be interesting to assess the skeletal efficacy of other plant-derived cannabinoids, like the CB_1/CB_2 ligand tetrahydrocannabivarin (Pertwee 2007) and the CB_2 agonist β-caryophyllene (Gertsch et al. 2008). Obviously, large-scale clinical and epidemiological studies should provide answers to these pending issues in spite of the logistic difficulty of conducting such trials.

References

Bab, I. (2005). The skeleton: stone bones and stoned heads? In: R. Mechoulam (ed.). *Cannabinoids as Therapeutics*. Milestones in Drug Therapy Series. Basel: Birkhäuser Verlag, pp. 201–206.

Bab, I., Hajbi-Yonissi, C., Gabet, Y., and Müller, R. (2007). Gender and age differences. In: *Micro-Tomographic Atlas of the Mouse Skeleton*. New York: Springer, pp. 195–199.

Bab, I., Ofek, O., Tam, J., Rehnelt, J., and Zimmer, A. (2008). Endocannabinoids and the regulation of bone metabolism. *Journal of Neuroendocrinology*, **20**(Suppl 1), 69–74.

Cauley, J. and Bulstra, S. (2007). Mortality greater for hip fracture than breast cancer in elderly women. In: *American Geriatrics Society Annual Scientific Meeting*, Abstract P28, May 2–6, Seattle, Washington.

Devoto, M., Specchia, C., Li, H.H., *et al.* (2001). Variance component linkage analysis indicates a QTL for femoral neck bone mineral density on chromosome 1p36. *Human Molecular Genetics*, **10**, 2447–2452.

George, K.L., Saltman, L.H., Stein, G.S., Lian, J.B., and Zurier, R.B. (2008). Ajulemic acid, a nonpsychoactive cannabinoid acid, suppresses osteoclastogenesis in mononuclear precursor cells and induces apoptosis in mature osteoclast-like cells. *Journal of Cellular Physiology*, **214**, 714–720.

Gertsch, J., Leonti, M., Raduner, S., *et al.* (2008). Beta-caryophyllene is a dietary cannabinoid. *Proceedings of the National Academy of Sciences of the United States of America*, **105**, 9099–9104.

Huang, Q.Y., Li, G.H., and Kung A.W. (2009). Multiple osteoporosis susceptibility genes on chromosome 1p36 in Chinese. *Bone*, **44**, 984–988.

Idris, A.I., Sophocleous, A., Landao-Bassonga, E., van't Hof, R.J., and Ralston, S.H. (2008). Regulation of bone mass, osteoclast function, and ovariectomy-induced bone loss by the type 2 cannabinoid receptor. *Endocrinology*, **149**, 5619–5626.

Idris, A.I., Sophocleous, A., Landao-Bassonga, E., *et al.* (2009). Cannabinoid receptor type 1 protects against age-related osteoporosis by regulating osteoblast and adipocyte differentiation in marrow stromal cells. *Cell Metabolism*, **10**, 139–147.

Idris, A.I., van't Hof, R.J., Greig, I.R., *et al.* (2005). Regulation of bone mass, bone loss and osteoclast activity by cannabinoid receptors. *Nature Medicine*, **11**, 774–779.

Karsak, M., Cohen-Solal, M., Freudenberg, J., *et al.* (2005). Cannabinoid receptor type 2 gene is associated with human osteoporosis. *Human Molecular Genetics*, **14**, 3389–3396.

Karsak, M., Malkin, I., Toliat, M.R., *et al.* (2009). The cannabinoid receptor type 2 (CNR2) gene is associated with hand bone strength phenotypes in an ethnically homogeneous family sample. *Human Genetics*, **126**, 629–636.

Lozano-Ondoua, A.N., Hanlon, K.E., Symons-Liguori, A.M., *et al.* (2013). Disease modification of breast cancer-induced bone remodeling by cannabinoid 2 receptor agonists. *Journal of Bone and Mineral Research*, **28**, 92–107.

Morley, J., Marsh, S., Drakoulakis, E., Pape, H.C., and Giannoudis, P.V. (2005). Does traumatic brain injury result in accelerated fracture healing? *Injury*, **36**, 363–368.

Nogueira-Filho Gda, R., Cadide, T., and Rosa, B.T. (2008). *Cannabis sativa* smoke inhalation decreases bone filling around titanium implants: a histomorphometric study in rats. *Implant Dentistry*, **17**, 461–470.

Ofek, O., Attar-Namdar, M., Kram, V., *et al.* (2011). CB_2 cannabinoid receptor targets mitogenic Gi protein-cyclin D1 axis in osteoblasts. *Journal of Bone and Mineral Research*, **26**, 308–316.

Ofek, O., Karsak, M., Leclerc, N., *et al.* (2006). Peripheral cannabinoid receptor, CB$_2$, regulates bone mass. *Proceedings of the National Academy of Sciences of the United States of America*, **103**, 696–701.

Parfitt, A.M. (1982). The coupling of bone formation to bone resorption: a critical analysis of the concept and of its relevance to the pathogenesis of osteoporosis. *Metabolic Bone Diseases and Related Research*, **4**, 1–6.

Pertwee, R.G. (2008). The diverse CB$_1$ and CB$_2$ receptor pharmacology of three plant cannabinoids: delta9-tetrahydrocannabinol, cannabidiol and delta9-tetrahydrocannabivarin. *British Journal of Pharmacology*, **153**, 199–215.

Rossi, F., Bellini, G., Luongo, L., *et al.* (2013). The 17-β-oestradiol inhibits osteoclast activity by increasing the cannabinoid CB$_2$ receptor expression. *Pharmacology Research*, **68**, 7–15.

Scutt, A. and Williamson, E.M. (2007). Cannabinoids stimulate fibroblastic colony formation by bone marrow cells indirectly via CB$_2$ receptors. *Calcified Tissue International*, **80**, 50–9.

Smoum, R., Bar, A., Tan, B., *et al.* (2010). Oleoyl serine, an endogenous N-acyl amide, modulates bone remodeling and mass. *Proceedings of the National Academy of Sciences of the United States of America*, **107**, 17710–17715.

Sophocleous, A., Landao-Bassonga, E., Van't Hof, R.J., Idris, A.I., and Ralston, S.H. (2011). The type 2 cannabinoid receptor regulates bone mass and ovariectomy-induced bone loss by affecting osteoblast differentiation and bone formation. *Endocrinology*, **152**, 2141–2149.

Tam, J., Cinar, R., Liu, J., *et al.* (2012). Peripheral cannabinoid-1 receptor inverse agonism reduces obesity by reversing leptin resistance. *Cell Metabolism*, **16**, 167–179.

Tam, J., Ofek, O., Fride, E., *et al.* (2006). Involvement of neuronal cannabinoid receptor CB$_1$ in regulation of bone mass and bone remodeling. *Molecular Pharmacology*, **70**, 786–792.

Tam, J., Trembovler, V., Di Marzo V., *et al.* (2008). The cannabinoid CB$_1$ receptor regulates bone formation by modulating adrenergic signaling. *FASEB Journal*, **22**, 285–294.

Tam, J., Vemuri, V.K., Liu, J., *et al.* (2010). Peripheral CB1 cannabinoid receptor blockade improves cardiometabolic risk in mouse models of obesity. *Journal of Clinical Investigation*, **120**, 2953–2966.

Uihlein, A.V. and Leder, B.Z. (2012). Anabolic therapies for osteoporosis. *Endocrinology and Metabolism Clinics of North America*, **41**, 507–525.

Yamada, Y., Ando, F., and Shimokata, H. (2007). Association of candidate gene polymorphisms with bone mineral density in community-dwelling Japanese women and men. *International Journal of Molecular Medicine*, **19**, 791–801.

Yang, P., Myint, K.Z., Tong, Q., *et al.* (2012). Lead discovery, chemistry optimization, and biological evaluation studies of novel biamide derivatives as CB$_2$ receptor inverse agonists and osteoclast inhibitors. *Journal of Medicinal Chemistry*, **55**, 9973–9987.

Whyte, L.S., Ryberg, E., Sims, N.A., *et al.* (2009). The putative cannabinoid receptor GPR55 affects osteoclast function in vitro and bone mass in vivo. *Proceedings of the National Academy of Sciences of the United States of America*, **106**, 16511–16516.

Chapter 35

Cancer

Guillermo Velasco, Cristina Sánchez,
and Manuel Guzmán

35.1 Introduction

Preparations from *Cannabis sativa* L. (marijuana) have been used for many centuries both medicinally and recreationally. However, the chemical structures of their unique active components—the cannabinoids—were not elucidated until the 1960s. Three decades later the first solid clues on cannabinoid molecular action were established, which led to an impressive expansion of basic cannabinoid research and to a renaissance in the study of the therapeutic effects of cannabinoids in various fields, including oncology. Today it is widely accepted that, out of the approximately 108 cannabinoids produced by *C. sativa*, delta-9-tetrahydrocannabinol (THC) is the most relevant owing to its high potency and abundance in plant preparations (Gaoni et al. 1964; Pertwee 2008). THC exerts a wide variety of biological effects by mimicking endogenous substances—the endocannabinoids anandamide (Devane et al. 1992) and 2-arachidonoylglycerol (2-AG) (Mechoulam et al. 1995; Sugiura et al. 1995)—that engage specific cell-surface cannabinoid receptors (Pertwee et al. 2010). So far, two major cannabinoid-specific receptors—CB_1 and CB_2—have been cloned and characterized from mammalian tissues (Matsuda et al. 1990; Munro et al. 1993). In addition, other receptors such as the transient receptor potential cation channel subfamily V member 1 (TRPV1) and the orphan G protein-coupled receptor GPR55 have been proposed to act as endocannabinoid receptors (Pertwee et al. 2010). Most of the effects produced by cannabinoids in the nervous system and in non-neural tissues rely on CB_1 receptor activation. In contrast, the CB_2 receptor was initially described to be present in the immune system (Pertwee et al. 2010), but more recently it has been shown to be expressed as well in cells from other origins (Atwood et al. 2010; Fernandez-Ruiz et al. 2007). Of note, expression of CB_1 and CB_2 receptors has been found in many types of cancer cells, which does not necessarily correlate with the expression of these receptors in the tissue type of origin (Fernandez-Ruiz et al. 2007; Guzmán et al. 2006; Sarfaraz et al. 2008).

The endocannabinoids, together with their receptors and the proteins responsible for their synthesis, transport, and degradation, constitute the endocannabinoid system. Aside from its pivotal neuromodulatory activity (Katona et al. 2008), the endocannabinoid system exerts other regulatory functions in the body such as the control of cardiovascular tone, energy metabolism, immunity, and reproduction (Pacher et al. 2006; Pertwee 2009). This miscellaneous activity makes the pharmacological manipulation of the endocannabinoid system a promising strategy for the management of many different diseases. Specifically, cannabinoids are well known to exert palliative effects in cancer patients (Pacher et al. 2006; Pertwee 2009). The best-established use is the inhibition of chemotherapy-induced nausea and vomiting (Guzmán 2003; Pertwee 2009). Today, capsules of THC (Marinol®) and its synthetic analogue nabilone (Cesamet®) are approved for this purpose. Cannabinoids also inhibit pain, and thus a standardized cannabis extract (Sativex®) has been already approved in Canada and is currently the subject of large-scale Phase 3 clinical trials for managing cancer-associated pain. Another potential palliative effect of cannabinoids in oncology, supported by Phase 3 clinical trials, includes appetite stimulation and attenuation of wasting. In relation to this, Marinol® can currently be prescribed for anorexia associated with weight loss in AIDS patients.

The therapeutic potential of cannabinoids in oncology may not be restricted to their aforementioned palliative actions. Thus, numerous studies have provided evidence that THC and other cannabinoids exhibit antitumor effects on a wide array of animal models of cancer (Guzmán 2003; Sarfaraz et al. 2008; Velasco et al. 2012). Moreover, these observations led to the development of a pilot clinical study to investigate the antitumor activity of THC in glioma patients. Nonetheless, a few studies have shown that, under certain conditions, cannabinoid treatment can stimulate cancer cell proliferation in vitro (Cudaback et al. 2010; Hart et al. 2004) and interfere with the tumor-suppressor role of the immune system (McKallip et al. 2005; Zhu et al. 2000). Likewise, there are conflicting reports regarding the role (tumor-suppressor or oncogenic) of the endocannabinoid system in cancer (Malfitano et al. 2011) (Box 35.1).

Box 35.1 Biological role of the endocannabinoid system in tumor generation and progression

To date, little is known about the biological role of the endocannabinoid system in cancer physiopathology. Although there are some exceptions that may be tumor type-specific, both cannabinoid receptors and their endogenous ligands are generally upregulated in tumor tissue compared with non-tumor tissue (Caffarel et al. 2006; Guzmán 2003; Malfitano et al. 2011; Sánchez et al. 2001). Additionally, different studies have associated the expression levels of cannabinoid receptors, endocannabinoids, and/or endocannabinoid-metabolizing enzymes with tumor aggressiveness (Malfitano et al. 2011; Nomura et al. 2010; Thors et al. 2010), which suggests that the endocannabinoid system may be overactivated in cancer and hence protumorigenic (Malfitano et al. 2011). In support of this, in mouse models of cancer, genetic ablation of CB_1 and CB_2 receptors reduces ultraviolet light-induced skin carcinogenesis (Zheng et al. 2008), and CB_2 receptor overexpression enhances the predisposition to leukemia after leukemia virus infection (Joosten et al. 2002).

Conversely, and in line with the evidence supporting the hypothesis that pharmacological activation of cannabinoid receptors reduces tumor growth (Guzmán 2003; Sarfaraz et al. 2008), the upregulation of endocannabinoid-degrading enzymes has been observed in aggressive human tumors and cancer cell lines (Nomura et al. 2010; Thors et al. 2010), indicating that endocannabinoid signaling can also have a tumor-suppressive role. In support of this, deletion of CB_1 receptors accelerates intestinal tumor growth in a genetic mouse model of colon cancer (Wang et al. 2008), increased endocannabinoid levels diminish azoxymethane-induced precancerous lesions in the mouse colon (Izzo et al. 2008), and a reduction in the expression of the endocannabinoid-degrading enzyme monoacylglycerol lipase reduces tumor growth in xenografted mice (Nomura et al. 2010).

Further studies, including those analyzing the activation of the precise signaling mechanisms involved in the regulation of cannabinoid-induced cell death or cell proliferation upon genetic or pharmacological manipulation of the endocannabinoid system, are therefore needed to clarify which are the contextual determinants for this system to act as either a guardian or an inducer of tumorigenesis or tumor progression.

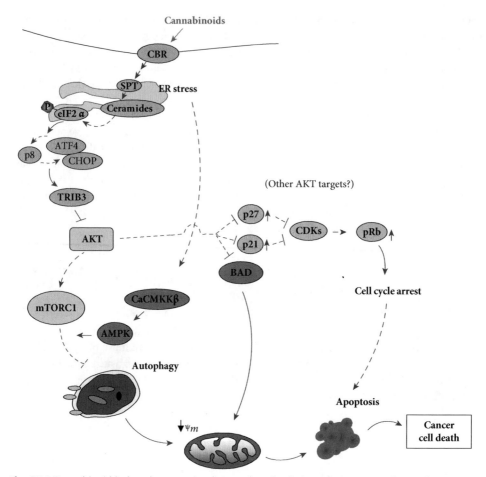

Fig. 35.1 Cannabinoid-induced apoptosis relies on the stimulation of ER stress and autophagy. Scheme depicting the mechanism of cannabinoid-induced apoptosis in glioma, pancreatic, and hepatocellular carcinoma cells. This signaling route may constitute the main mechanism of cannabinoid-induced cell death, with some variations inherent to different types of cancer cells. Cannabinoid agonists bind to CB_1 and/or CB_2 receptors (CBR) to stimulate de novo synthesis of ceramide (Carracedo et al. 2006b; Galve-Roperh et al. 2000; Gomez del Pulgar et al. 2002; Herrera et al. 2006; Salazar et al. 2009), which triggers the induction of an endoplasmic reticulum (ER) stress-related response that promotes the upregulation of the transcription factor p8 and several of its downstream targets, including the pseudokinase Tribbles 3 (TRIB3) (Carracedo et al. 2006a; Salazar et al. 2009). This favors the interaction of TRIB3 with AKT (Du et al. 2003; Salazar et al. 2009), thus leading to the inhibition of the AKT–mechanistic target of rapamycin C1 (mTORC1) axis and the subsequent induction of autophagy (Salazar et al. 2009). Autophagy is upstream of intrinsic mitochondrial apoptosis in the process of cannabinoid-induced cell death. The importance of this pathway is highlighted by the ability of different chemical and genetic manipulations to block cannabinoid-induced cell death. In hepatocellular carcinoma cells the cannabinoid-evoked and ER stress-dependent activation of calcium/calmodulin-dependent protein kinase kinase 2-beta (CaCMKKβ) and AMP-activated protein kinase (AMPK) leads, together with the p8–TRIB3 pathway, to autophagy and apoptosis (Vara et al. 2011). The cannabinoid-evoked inhibition of AKT could promote cycle arrest in breast cancer and melanoma cells, as well as apoptosis, through

This chapter summarizes these observations and provides an integrated view of the molecular mechanisms responsible for cannabinoid antitumor activity. It also discusses the experimental evidence supporting the existence of mechanisms of resistance to the cell death-promoting actions of THC in certain types of cancer cells, the possible strategies that could be undertaken to overcome such resistance, and the preclinical data supporting that the combined administration of cannabinoids and other drugs could be useful in anticancer therapies.

35.2 **Preclinical antitumor activity**

Since the late 1990s, a large body of evidence has accumulated demonstrating that various cannabinoids exert antitumor effects in a wide variety of experimental models of cancer, ranging from cancer cell lines in culture to genetically engineered mice (reviewed by Velasco et al. 2012). Multiple cannabinoids have shown this activity, including THC, the endocannabinoids 2-AG and anandamide, and different synthetic cannabinoid receptor agonists that have either comparable affinity for CB_1 and CB_2 receptors (e.g., WIN 55212-2 or HU-210), higher affinity for CB_1 (e.g., methanandamide), or higher affinity for CB_2 (e.g., JWH-133). These findings strongly support that, aside from the role played by the endogenous cannabinoid system in cancer, pharmacological stimulation of CB receptors is in most cases antitumorigenic. Nonetheless, a few reports have proposed a tumor-promoting effect of cannabinoids (Cudaback et al. 2010; Hart et al. 2004; McKallip et al. 2005; Zhu et al. 2000). These apparently conflicting observations are discussed in later sections.

Cannabinoids impair tumor progression at different levels. Their most prevalent effect is the induction of cancer cell death by apoptosis and the inhibition of cancer cell proliferation. At least one of these actions has been demonstrated in virtually all cancer cell types tested (Velasco et al. 2012). In addition, in vivo experiments have shown that cannabinoids impair tumor angiogenesis and block invasion and metastasis.

35.3 **Mechanisms of antitumor effects**

35.3.1 **Induction of cancer cell death**

A significant amount of the research conducted so far on the mechanism of cannabinoid antitumor activity has focused on glioma cells. Initial studies showed that THC and other cannabinoids induce the apoptotic death of glioma cells via CB_1- and CB_2-dependent stimulation of the de novo synthesis of the proapoptotic sphingolipid ceramide (Blazquez et al. 2004; Galve-Roperh et al. 2000; Gomez del Pulgar et al. 2002; Sánchez et al. 2001). Further studies, based on the analysis of the gene expression profile of THC-sensitive and -resistant glioma cells, gave further

---

Fig. 35.1 (continued) additional mechanisms, including the decreased phosphorylation of the proapoptotic protein BCL2-associated agonist of cell death (BAD) (Ellert-Miklaszewska et al. 2005) and the activation of the cyclin-dependent kinase (CDK) inhibitory proteins p21 and p27 (Blazquez et al. 2006; Caffarel et al. 2008; Caffarel et al. 2006). This would lead to the subsequent decreased phosphorylation of the retinoblastoma protein (pRB), which thus would be active to arrest cell cycle. ATF4: activating transcription factor 4; CHOP: C/EBP homology protein; eIF2α: eukaryotic translation initiation factor 2 alpha; SPT: serine palmitoyltransferase.

insight into the specific signaling events downstream of ceramide that are activated in cancer cells by cannabinoids (Carracedo et al. 2006b). THC acutely upregulates the expression of the stress-regulated protein p8 (also named NUPR1), a transcriptional regulator that has been implicated in the control of tumorigenesis and tumor progression (Encinar et al. 2001), together with several of its downstream targets such as the endoplasmic reticulum (ER) stress-related transcription factors ATF4 and CHOP, and the pseudokinase tribbles-homologue 3 (TRIB3) (Carracedo et al. 2006b) (Fig. 35.1).

ER stress, as induced by different anticancer agents, can also lead through different mechanisms (Verfaillie et al. 2010) to the stimulation of autophagy, an essential cellular process participating in a number of physiological functions within the cell (Mizushima et al. 2008; Verfaillie et al. 2010). During autophagy organelles and other cytoplasmic components are engulfed within double-membrane vesicles designated autophagosomes. The maturation of these vesicles involves their fusion with lysosomes, which leads in turn to the degradation of the autophagosome components by lysosomal enzymes (Mizushima et al. 2008). Autophagy is primarily a cytoprotective mechanism, although its activation can also lead to cell death (Eisenberg-Lerner et al. 2009; Mizushima et al. 2008). Indeed, THC-triggered stimulation of the p8-regulated pathway enhances the inhibitory interaction of TRIB3 with a prosurvival kinase, AKT which leads to the inhibition of the mammalian target of rapamycin complex 1 (mTORC1) and the subsequent stimulation of autophagy-mediated cell death (Salazar et al. 2009) (Fig. 35.1). Cannabinoids induce autophagy in different types of cancer cells in culture, and pharmacological or genetic inhibition of autophagy prevents cannabinoid antitumor action in different animal models of cancer (Fig. 35.1), thus demonstrating that autophagy is important for cannabinoid antineoplastic activity (Salazar et al. 2009; Vara et al. 2011). Moreover, autophagy blockade prevents cannabinoid-induced apoptosis and cell death whereas apoptosis blockade prevents cannabinoid-induced cell death but not autophagy (Salazar et al. 2009; Vara et al. 2011). This indicates that autophagy is upstream of apoptosis in the mechanism of cannabinoid-induced cell death (Fig. 35.1).

The direct participation of the p8-mediated autophagy pathway in the antitumor action of cannabinoids has been clearly demonstrated in glioma cells and pancreatic and hepatic cancer cells (Carracedo et al. 2006a, 2006b; Salazar et al. 2009; Vara et al. 2011). At least part of this signaling route has also been found to be upregulated on cannabinoid treatment in other types of cancer cells. This suggests that—with some variations—this could be a general mechanism by which activation of CB_1 and CB_2 receptors promotes cancer cell death.

Additional mechanisms may nonetheless cooperate with the p8-mediated autophagy pathway to evoke cancer cell death (Fig. 35.1). For example, in hepatocellular carcinoma cells, cannabinoids can trigger an ER stress-dependent activation of AMPK that cooperates with the TRIB3-mediated inhibition of the AKT–mTORC1 axis in the stimulation of autophagy-mediated cell death (Vara et al. 2011). In melanoma (Blazquez et al. 2006), breast carcinoma (Caffarel et al. 2006, 2012), and prostate carcinoma (Sarfaraz et al. 2006) cells cannabinoids can induce cell cycle arrest in concert with apoptosis (Blazquez et al. 2006; Caffarel et al. 2006; Sarfaraz et al. 2006). Of note, cannabinoid antiproliferative action—at least in melanoma (Blazquez et al. 2006) and breast cancer (Caffarel et al. 2006) cells—also relies on AKT inhibition.

Likewise, the effect of cannabinoids in hormone-dependent tumors may rely, at least in part, on their ability to interfere with the activation of growth factor receptors (Guzmán 2003; Sarfaraz et al. 2008). Some of these and other mechanisms (Guindon et al. 2011) may participate in the cytotoxic action of cannabinoids in different types of cancer cells together with the autophagy-mediated cell death pathway. However, further investigation is required to clarify this issue (Box 35.2).

Box 35.2 Mechanism of cannabinoid receptor-mediated cancer cell death: some important unanswered questions

Research conducted during the last few years has shed light onto the intracellular signaling mechanisms underlying cannabinoid anticancer action. However, a number of important observations—in particular ones related to the role played by cannabinoid receptors in the triggering of these signals—remain to be clarified. For example:

♦ Unlike the cell death-promoting action of cannabinoids on cancer cells, the viability of normal (non-transformed) cells is unaffected or—under certain conditions—even enhanced by cannabinoid challenge (Carracedo et al. 2006b; Galve-Roperh et al. 2000, 2008; Gomez del Pulgar et al. 2002; Salazar et al. 2009). For example, THC treatment of astrocytes (a cell type that expresses functional CB_1 receptors) does not trigger the activation of ER stress, the upregulation of the p8 pathway, the inhibition of the AKT–mTORC1 axis or the stimulation of autophagy and apoptosis, even when concentrations of THC higher than those that promote glioma cell death are used (Carracedo et al. 2006b; Salazar et al. 2009). Similar results were obtained with primary embryonic fibroblasts (Carracedo et al. 2006a; Salazar et al. 2009) and other types of nontransformed cells expressing functional cannabinoid receptors when compared with their transformed counterparts (Blazquez et al. 2006; Caffarel et al. 2006; Casanova et al. 2003; Chan et al. 1996). Thus, stimulation of cannabinoid receptors seems to be coupled to the activation of different signaling mechanisms in transformed and nontransformed cells. The precise molecular reasons for this different behavior remain as an important open question in the cannabinoid field.

♦ Another intriguing observation is that, in some types of cancer cells, such as glioma cells, pharmacological blockade of either CB_1 or CB_2 receptors prevents cannabinoid-induced cell death with similar efficacy (Galve-Roperh et al. 2000; Lorente et al. 2011), while in other types of cancer cells, for example, pancreatic (Carracedo et al. 2006b), breast (Caffarel et al. 2006), or hepatic (Vara et al. 2011) carcinoma cells, antagonists of CB_2 but not of CB_1 receptors inhibit cannabinoid antitumor actions. Why the receptor type through which cannabinoids produce their antitumor action depends on the type of cancer cell studied has yet to be established.

♦ Some cannabinoid receptor agonists promote cancer cell death more efficiently than other agonists that exhibit similar or even higher affinity for CB_1 or CB_2 receptors. For example, THC promotes cancer cell death in a CB_1- and/or CB_2-dependent manner at lower concentrations than the synthetic cannabinoid receptor agonist WIN 55,212-2, although the latter agent displays significantly higher affinity for CB_1 and CB_2 receptors in binding assays (Pertwee et al. 2010).

Further work aimed at investigating, for example, CB receptor homo or hetero-oligomerization in response to different cannabinoid agonists, their association with specific domains in the plasma membrane such as lipid rafts, changes in the subcellular location of CB receptors, and the selective coupling to different G proteins and other signaling proteins will be essential to answer these questions and precisely define the role played by each cannabinoid receptor type as an anticancer signaling platform.

Of note, cannabidiol (CBD), a phytocannabinoid with low affinity for cannabinoid receptors (Pertwee 2009), and other marijuana-derived cannabinoids (Ligresti et al. 2006) have also been proposed to promote the apoptotic death of cancer cells acting independently of CB_1 and CB_2 receptors. The mechanism by which CBD produces this effect has not been completely clarified as yet, but seems to rely—at least in part—on its ability to enhance the production of reactive oxygen species in cancer cells (Massi et al. 2008; Shrivastava et al. 2011). It has also been proposed that CBD may activate TRPV2 receptors to promote glioma cell death (Nabissi et al. 2012).

35.3.2 Inhibition of angiogenesis, invasion, and metastasis

In cancer cells, cannabinoids block the activation of the vascular endothelial growth factor (VEGF) pathway, an inducer of angiogenesis. Specifically, different elements of this cascade, such as the main ligand (VEGF) and the active forms of its main receptors (VEGFR1 and VEGFR2), are downregulated on cannabinoid treatment of skin carcinomas (Casanova et al. 2003), gliomas (Blazquez et al. 2003, 2004), and thyroid carcinomas (Portella et al. 2003). In vascular endothelial cells, cannabinoid receptor activation inhibits proliferation and migration, and induces apoptosis (Blazquez et al. 2003; Pisanti et al. 2007). These and perhaps other cannabinoid-evoked actions result in a normalized tumor vasculature; that is, smaller and/or fewer vessels that are more differentiated and less leaky.

Likewise, cannabinoids reduce the formation of distant tumor masses in animal models of both induced and spontaneous metastasis and inhibit adhesion, migration, and invasiveness of glioma (Blazquez et al. 2008), breast (Grimaldi et al. 2006; Qamri et al. 2009), lung (Preet et al. 2008; Ramer et al. 2008), and cervical (Ramer et al. 2008) cancer cells in culture. These effects depend, at least in part, on the modulation of extracellular proteases (such as matrix metalloproteinase 2 (MMP2)) (Blazquez et al. 2008) and their inhibitors (such as tissue inhibitor of matrix metalloproteinases 1 (TIMP1)) (Ramer et al. 2008).

Of note, pharmacological inhibition of ceramide biosynthesis abrogates the antitumor and antiangiogenic effect of cannabinoids in glioma xenografts, and decreases VEGF production by glioma cells in vitro and in vivo (Blazquez et al. 2004). Likewise, inhibition of MMP-2 expression and glioma cell invasion is prevented by blocking ceramide biosynthesis and by knocking-down p8 expression (Blazquez et al. 2008). Although further research is still necessary to precisely define the molecular mechanisms responsible for these actions of cannabinoids, these observations indicate that the ceramide/p8-regulated pathway plays a general role in the antitumor activity of cannabinoids targeting CB_1 and CB_2 receptors.

It is worth noting that CBD, by acting independently of CB_1 and CB_2 receptors, produces a remarkable antitumor effect—including reduction of invasiveness and metastasis—in different animal models of cancer. This effect of CBD seems to rely—at least in part—on the downregulation of the helix-loop-helix transcription factor inhibitor of DNA binding-1 (ID-1) (McAllister et al. 2011; Soroceanu et al. 2012).

35.3.3 Regulation of antitumor immunity

Of note, stimulation of cannabinoid receptors may lead to important changes in the processes that regulate antitumor immunity. Thus, for example, treatment of mice with THC triggers a shift (from Th1 to Th2) on the cytokine profile (Lu et al. 2006; McKallip et al. 2005; Newton et al. 2009; Steffens et al. 2005) and induces mobilization of myeloid-derived suppressor cells (Hegde et al. 2010), two events that play a critical role in the suppression of antitumor immunity. In agreement with this notion, stimulation of CB_2 receptors has been proposed in some reports to enhance tumorigenesis by interfering with tumor surveillance by the immune system (McKallip et al. 2005; Zhu et al. 2000). By contrast, cannabinoids may also enhance immune system-mediated tumor surveillance in some contexts: the antitumor action of WIN 55212-2 (a CB_1/CB_2-mixed agonist) or JWH-133 (a CB_2-selective agonist) was more pronounced in melanoma xenografts generated in immunocompetent mice compared with those in immunodeficient mice (Blazquez et al. 2006). This also indicates that, at least in this model, stimulation of CB_2 receptors primarily inhibits tumor growth through direct effects on cancer cells rather than necessarily through interfering with the normal antitumor function of the immune system. In line with this idea, treatment for 2 years of immunocompetent rats with very high doses (50 mg/kg/day five times a week) of THC decreased the incidence of several types of tumors and enhanced the overall survival of these animals (Chan et al. 1996). These observations might be related to the ability of THC to reduce inflammation (Burstein et al. 2009; Liu et al. 2010), an effect that may prevent certain types of cancer (Liu et al. 2010). For cannabinoid use to be clinically successful, antitumor effects will need to overcome immunosuppressive (potentially tumor-promoting) effects. Additional studies should clarify this issue. For example, it could be conceivable to study the effect of cannabinoid administration on the generation and progression of tumors exhibiting different sensitivity to cannabinoids and generated in immunocompetent or immunodeficient mice in which the expression of CB_1 and/or CB_2 receptors in cells from the immune system has been genetically manipulated.

35.4 **Resistance mechanisms**

Numerous studies have contributed to our appreciation of the heterogeneity of cancer, whereby each subtype of cancer, and even each individual tumor, exhibits a series of molecular characteristics that determines its behavior and, in particular, its responsiveness to different anticancer drugs. In agreement with this line of reasoning, a recent report investigated the molecular features associated with the resistance of a collection of human glioma cell lines and primary cultures to cannabinoid antitumor action (Lorente et al. 2011). This study showed that, although the apoptotic effect of THC on glioma cells relied on the stimulation of cannabinoid receptors and the activation the p8-mediated autophagy pathway, the differences in the sensitivity to THC-induced cell death correlated with the enhanced expression of a particular set of genes in the THC-resistant glioma cells rather than with the presence of different expression levels of CB_1 or CB_2 receptors (Lorente et al. 2011). Of interest, upregulation of one of these genes, midkine (*MDK*), that encodes a growth factor that has been previously associated with increased malignancy and resistance to anticancer therapies in several types of tumors (Kadomatsu 2005; Mirkin et al. 2005), correlates with a lower overall survival of patients with glioblastoma (Lorente et al. 2011). Moreover, MDK plays a direct role in the resistance to THC action via stimulation of the anaplastic lymphoma kinase (ALK) (Palmer et al. 2009). Thus, the stimulation of ALK by MDK inhibits the THC-evoked autophagy-mediated cell death pathway. Further research should clarify whether this mechanism could also be responsible for the resistance of cancer cells expressing high levels of MDK to other therapies. Interestingly, in vivo silencing of MDK or pharmacological inhibition of ALK in a mouse xenograft model abolishes the resistance to THC treatment of established tumors derived from cannabinoid-resistant glioma cells (Lorente et al. 2011).

Taken together, these findings support the idea that stimulation of the MDK–ALK axis promotes resistance to THC antitumor action in gliomas and could help to set the basis for the potential clinical use of THC in combination with inhibitors of this axis (Fig. 35.2). In line with this idea, ALK inhibitors have started to be used in clinical trials for the management of non-small-cell

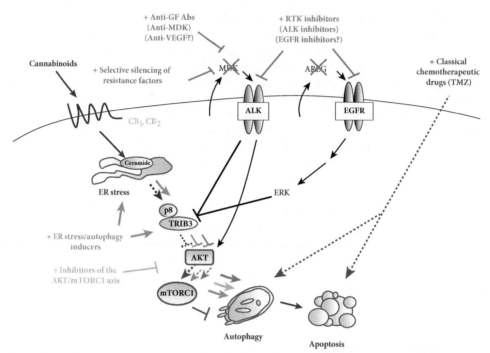

Fig. 35.2 (See also colour plate section.) Possible strategies aimed at optimizing cannabinoid-based therapies against gliomas. Glioblastoma is highly resistant to current anticancer therapies (Lonardi et al. 2005; Nieder et al. 2006; Purow et al. 2009). Specifically, resistance of glioma cells to cannabinoid-induced cell death relies, at least in part, on the enhanced expression of the growth factor midkine (MDK) and the subsequent activation of the anaplastic lymphoma receptor tyrosine kinase (ALK) (Lorente et al. 2011). Likewise, enhanced expression of the heparin-bound EGFR-ligand amphiregulin (AREG) can promote resistance to THC antitumor action via ERK stimulation (Lorente et al. 2009). Combination of THC with pharmacological inhibitors of ALK (or genetic inhibition of MDK) enhances cannabinoid action in resistant tumors, which provides the rationale for the design of targeted therapies capable of increasing cannabinoid antineoplastic activity (Lorente et al. 2011). Combinations of cannabinoids with classical chemotherapeutic drugs such as the alkylating agent temozolomide (TMZ; the benchmark agent for the management of glioblastoma (Lonardi et al. 2005; Stupp et al. 2005)) have been shown to produce a strong anticancer action in animal models (Torres et al. 2011). Combining cannabinoids and TMZ is thus a very attractive possibility for clinical studies aimed at investigating cannabinoids antitumor effects in glioblastoma. Other potentially interesting strategies to enhance cannabinoid anticancer action (still requiring additional experimental support from data obtained using preclinical models) could be combining cannabinoids with endoplasmic reticulum (ER) stress and/or autophagy inducers or with inhibitors of the AKT–mechanistic target of rapamycin C1 (mTORC1) axis. Abs: antibodies; EGFR: epidermal growth factor receptor; ERK: extracellular signal-regulated kinase; GF: growth factors; RTK: receptor tyrosine kinase; TRIB3: tribbles 3; VEGF: vascular endothelial growth factor.

lung cancer and other types of tumors (de Bono et al. 2010; Grande et al. 2011). Future research should clarify whether this mechanism of resistance to cannabinoid action operates in other types of tumors. In agreement with this possibility, MDK silencing enhanced the sensitivity of cannabinoid-resistant pancreatic cancer cells to THC-induced cell death (Lorente et al. 2011).

The release by cancer cells of other growth factors has also been implicated in the mechanism of resistance to cannabinoid antitumor action. Thus, increased expression of the heparin-bound epidermal growth factor receptor (EGFR) ligand amphiregulin is associated with enhanced resistance to THC antitumor action in glioma xenografts (Lorente et al. 2009). Of note, illustrating that the dose of cannabinoids could be crucial for their optimal therapeutic effect, low (submicromolar) concentrations of THC or other synthetic cannabinoid agonists enhance the proliferation of several cancer cell lines in vitro. This effect relies on the activation of the protease ADAM17, the shedding of heparin-bound EGFR ligands, including amphiregulin, and the subsequent stimulation of extracellular signal-regulated kinase (ERK) and AKT pathways (Hart et al. 2004). In line with this idea, a recent report has shown that treatment with the synthetic cannabinoid, CP-55,940, increases the proliferation of murine glioma cells engineered to express CB_1 or CB_2 receptors only when these receptors were coupled to AKT activation (Cudaback et al. 2010). Although a protumorigenic effect has not been observed on the growth of tumor xenografts generated with glioma cells and treated with low doses of THC (Torres et al. 2011), increased expression of amphiregulin promotes resistance to THC antitumor action through a mechanism that involves the EGFR-dependent stimulation of ERK and the subsequent inhibition of p8 and TRB3 expression. Likewise, pharmacological inhibition of EGFR, ERK (Lorente et al. 2009) or AKT (authors' unpublished observations) enhances the cell death-promoting action of THC in cultures of glioma cells. These observations suggest that targeting EGFR and the AKT and ERK pathways could enhance the antitumor effect of cannabinoids.

35.5 **Cannabinoid-based combinational therapies**

The use of combinational anticancer therapies has a number of theoretical advantages over single-agent-based strategies as they allow the simultaneous targeting of tumor growth, progression, and spreading at different levels. In line with this idea, recent observations suggest that the combined administration of cannabinoids with other anticancer drugs acts synergistically to reduce tumor growth. For example, the administration of THC and temozolomide (the benchmark agent for the management of glioblastoma) exerts a strong antitumor action in glioma xenografts, an effect that is also evident in temozolomide-resistant tumors (Torres et al. 2011). Of interest, no toxicity was observed in mice treated with combinations of THC and temozolomide (Torres et al. 2011). As most patients with glioblastoma undergo temozolomide treatment, these findings indicate that the combined administration of temozolomide and cannabinoids could be therapeutically exploited for the management of glioblastoma (Fig. 35.2).

Likewise, another study has recently shown that the combined administration of gemcitabine (the benchmark agent for the treatment of pancreatic cancer) and different cannabinoid agonists synergistically reduces the viability of pancreatic cancer cells (Donadelli et al. 2011). Other reports indicate that anandamide and HU-210 may also enhance the anticancer activity of paclitaxel (Miyato et al. 2009) and 5-fluorouracil (Gustafsson et al. 2009), respectively.

An additional approach has been to combine THC with CBD, a phytocannabinoid that reduces—although to a lower extent than THC—the growth of several types of tumor xenografts through a still poorly defined mechanism (Massi et al. 2006; McAllister et al. 2007; Shrivastava et al. 2011). Combined administration of THC and CBD enhances the anticancer activity of THC and reduces the doses of THC needed to induce its tumor growth-inhibiting activity (Marcu et al. 2010; Torres et al. 2011). Moreover, the combination of THC and CBD together with temozolomide produces a striking reduction in the growth of glioma xenografts even when low doses of THC are used (Torres et al. 2011). Of note, CBD has also been shown to alleviate some of the undesired effects of THC administration, such as convulsions, discoordination and psychotic events, and therefore improves the tolerability of cannabis-based medicines (Pertwee 2009). As mentioned earlier, *Cannabis sativa* produces approximately 108 different cannabinoids and, apart from CBD, some of the other cannabinoids present in marijuana might attenuate the psychoactive side effects of THC or even produce other therapeutic benefits (Pertwee 2009). Thus, we think that clinical studies aimed at analyzing the efficacy of cannabinoids as antitumor agents should be based on the use both of pure substances, such as THC and CBD, and of cannabis extracts containing controlled amounts of THC, CBD, and other cannabinoids.

35.6 Clinical antitumor effects of cannabinoids

Although the clinical approval of cannabinoids is largely restricted to palliative uses in various diseases, following promising preclinical data, the antitumor effects of cannabinoids are beginning to be clinically assessed. In a pilot Phase 1 clinical study, nine patients with actively growing recurrent glioblastoma that had previously failed standard therapy underwent intracranial THC administration (Guzmán et al. 2006). Under these conditions cannabinoid delivery was safe and could be achieved without significant unwanted effects. In addition, although no statistically significant conclusions can be extracted from a cohort of nine patients, the results obtained in that study suggested that some patients responded—at least partially—to THC treatment in terms of decreased tumor growth rate, as evaluated by magnetic resonance imaging (Guzmán

Box 35.3 Different pharmacological approaches to target cancer cells with cannabinoids

Cannabinoid agonists or enhancers of endocannabinoid tone?

Administration of endocannabinoids or inhibitors of endocannabinoid-degrading enzymes has been shown to reduce the growth of different types of tumor xenografts (Bifulco et al. 2001; Ligresti et al. 2003) and, therefore, could be a reasonable strategy for targeting cannabinoid receptors for anticancer purposes. However, as discussed in Box 35.1, the role of the endocannabinoid system, including the endocannabinoid-degrading enzymes, in the control of tumor generation and progression is not well understood. Since enhancing endocannabinoid tone only has mild antitumor effects in mice and since no inhibitor of endocannabinoid degradation has been approved as yet for use in humans, clinical studies aimed at analyzing the efficacy of cannabinoids as antitumor agents should be based on the use of plant-derived or synthetic agonists of cannabinoid receptors rather than on endocannabinoids or inhibitors of endocannabinoid degradation.

Cannabis extracts or pure cannabinoids?

The long-known therapeutic properties of *Cannabis sativa*—including amelioration of symptoms associated with cancer and its chemotherapy—have led to the authorization of the

> **Box 35.3 Different pharmacological approaches to target cancer cells with cannabinoids** (*continued*)
>
> medical use of this plant and its extracts in several countries. As mentioned in the text, *C. sativa* produces about 108 different cannabinoids, including THC and CBD. Some of the other cannabinoids present in marijuana may contribute to the attenuation of THC psychoactive side effects or even to the production of other therapeutic benefits (Pertwee 2009). However, pure drugs are more prone to standardization than complex molecular cocktails. Thus, it would be ideal that studies aimed at investigating the anticancer actions of cannabinoids in patients were performed comparatively with both pure substances and cannabis extracts containing controlled amounts of THC, CBD, and other cannabinoids.
>
> ## Which routes of cannabinoid administration?
>
> The most widely used route of administration of recreational and self-medicated marijuana is smoking. Although THC and other phytocannabinoids are rapidly absorbed by inhalation, smoking is an unattractive clinical option. Preclinical work in animal models has typically administered cannabinoids intra peritumorally. Likewise, in the only clinical trial in which a cannabinoid has been assayed as an antitumor agent, THC was administered locally (intracranial delivery to GBM patients) (Guzmán et al. 2006). Nevertheless, this route of administration has many obvious limitations. Currently available cannabis-based medicines are administered as capsules or using an oromucosal spray (Pertwee 2009). Preclinical animal models have yielded data indicating that systemic (oral or intraperitoneal) administration of cannabinoids effectively reduces tumor growth (authors' unpublished observations), so it seems reasonable that future clinical studies directed at determining the efficacy of cannabinoids as antitumor agents use oral or oromucosal routes of administration.

et al. 2006). Importantly, analyses of samples obtained from two patients in this study before and after THC administration indicate that the molecular mechanism of cannabinoid antitumor action delineated in the previous sections, namely p8 and TRIB3 upregulation (Carracedo et al. 2006b; Salazar et al. 2009), mTORC1 inhibition (Salazar et al. 2009), stimulation of autophagy and apoptosis (Carracedo et al. 2006a; Guzmán et al. 2006; Salazar et al. 2009), inhibition of cell proliferation(Guzmán et al. 2006), decreased VEGF signaling (Blazquez et al. 2004), and MMP-2 downregulation (Blazquez et al. 2008), also operates in cancer patients. These findings were encouraging and reinforced the interest on the potential use of cannabinoids in cancer therapies. However, they also highlighted the need for further research aimed at optimizing the use of cannabinoids in terms of patient selection, combination with other anticancer agents, and use of other routes of administration (see Box 35.3).

35.7 **Conclusions and future directions**

It is widely believed that strategies aimed at reducing mortality from cancer should consist of targeted therapies capable of providing the most efficacious and selective treatment for each individual tumor and patient. Thus, the major focus of anticancer-drug development has progressively moved from nonspecific chemotherapies to molecularly targeted inhibitors. However, despite the huge amount of preclinical literature on how these rationally designed compounds work, the advance in the use of most of these drugs in the clinical practice is still limited.

How do cannabinoid-based medicines fit into this ongoing scenario? Let us consider gliomas, the type of cancer on which the most detailed cannabinoid research has been conducted to date. As discussed earlier, engagement of a molecular target (CB receptors) by a family of selective drugs (THC and other cannabinoid agonists) inhibits tumor growth in animal models through a well-established mechanism of action that seems to operate in patients. Moreover, cannabinoids potentiate the antitumor efficacy of temozolomide and ALK inhibitors in mice harboring gliomas. These findings provide preclinical proof-of-concept that "cannabinoid sensitizers" could improve the clinical efficacy of classical cytotoxic drugs in glioblastoma (Fig. 35.2) and perhaps other highly malignant tumors such as pancreatic cancer, melanoma, and hepatocellular carcinoma. However, further research is required to define the precise molecular cross-talk between cannabinoids and chemotherapeutic drugs and to optimize the pharmacology of preclinical cannabinoid-based combinational therapies.

Regarding patient stratification, we should unequivocally determine which particular individuals are potentially responsive to cannabinoid administration. For this purpose, high-throughput approaches should be implemented to find cannabinoid therapy-associated biomarkers in tumor biopsies or, ideally, in easily-acquired fluids containing circulating cancer cells or enhanced levels of resistance factors that could have been released by cancer cells. These biomarkers would conceivably relate to cannabinoid pharmacodynamics—namely expression and activity of cannabinoid receptors and their downstream cell death-inducing effectors. This would be analogous to the biochemical evaluation of estrogen and ERBB2 receptors, which predict the benefit from endocrine therapies and trastuzumab, respectively, in breast cancer. Predictive markers to define the sensitivity of a particular tumor to cannabinoid-based therapies could also include the status of growth factors, such as MDK in gliomas, as well as their receptors and signaling partners.

In conclusion, cannabinoids induce tumor cell death and inhibit tumor angiogenesis and invasion in animal models of cancer and there are indications that they do so as well in patients with glioblastoma. As cannabinoids show an acceptable safety profile, clinical trials testing them as single drugs or, ideally, in combination therapies in glioblastoma and other types of cancer are both warranted and urgently needed.

Acknowledgments

This work was supported by grants from Spanish Ministry of Economy and Competitiveness (MINECO) (PI12/02248, FR2009-0052, and IT2009-0053 to GV; and PI11/00295 to CS), Comunidad de Madrid (S2011/BMD-2308 to MG), GW Pharmaceuticals (to GV, CS, and MG), and Fundación Mutua Madrileña (AP101042012 to GV).

Potential conflict of interest

We declare that GW Pharmaceuticals funded part of the research of our laboratory. Likewise, part of the data obtained by the authors in relation with the antitumor action of cannabinoids is included in three patent applications presented by GW Pharmaceuticals.

References

Atwood, B.K. and Mackie, K. (2010). CB$_2$: a cannabinoid receptor with an identity crisis. *British Journal of Pharmacology*, **160**, 467–479.

Bifulco, M., Laezza, C., Portella, G., *et al.* (2001). Control by the endogenous cannabinoid system of ras oncogene-dependent tumor growth. *FASEB Journal*, **15**, 2745–2747.

Blazquez, C., Carracedo, A., Barrado, L., *et al.* (2006). Cannabinoid receptors as novel targets for the treatment of melanoma. *FASEB Journal*, **20**, 2633–2635.

Blazquez, C., Casanova, M.L., Planas, A., *et al.* (2003). Inhibition of tumor angiogenesis by cannabinoids. *FASEB Journal*, **17**, 529–531.

Blazquez, C., Gonzalez-Feria, L., Alvarez, L., *et al.* (2004). Cannabinoids inhibit the vascular endothelial growth factor pathway in gliomas. *Cancer Research*, **64**, 5617–5623.

Blazquez, C., Salazar, M., Carracedo, A., *et al.* (2008). Cannabinoids inhibit glioma cell invasion by down-regulating matrix metalloproteinase-2 expression. *Cancer Research*, **68**, 1945–1952.

Burstein, S.H. and Zurier, R.B. (2009). Cannabinoids, endocannabinoids, and related analogs in inflammation. *AAPS Journal*, **11**, 109–119.

Caffarel, M.M., Andradas, C., Perez-Gomez, E., Guzmán, M., and Sánchez, C. (2012). Cannabinoids: a new hope for breast cancer therapy? *Cancer Treatment Reviews*, **38**, 911–918.

Caffarel, M.M., Moreno-Bueno, G., Cerutti, C., *et al.* (2008). JunD is involved in the antiproliferative effect of Delta9-tetrahydrocannabinol on human breast cancer cells. *Oncogene*, **27**, 5033–5044.

Caffarel, M.M., Sarrio, D., Palacios, J., Guzmán, M., and Sánchez, C. (2006). Delta9-tetrahydrocannabinol inhibits cell cycle progression in human breast cancer cells through Cdc2 regulation. *Cancer Research*, **66**, 6615–6621.

Carracedo, A., Gironella, M., Lorente, M., *et al.* (2006a). Cannabinoids induce apoptosis of pancreatic tumor cells via endoplasmic reticulum stress-related genes. *Cancer Research*, **66**, 6748–6755.

Carracedo, A., Lorente, M., Egia, A., *et al.* (2006b). The stress-regulated protein p8 mediates cannabinoid-induced apoptosis of tumor cells. *Cancer Cell*, **9**, 301–312.

Casanova, M.L., Blazquez, C., Martinez-Palacio, J., *et al.* (2003). Inhibition of skin tumor growth and angiogenesis in vivo by activation of cannabinoid receptors. *The Journal of Clinical Investigation*, **111**, 43–50.

Cudaback, E., Marrs, W., Moeller, T., and Stella, N. (2010). The expression level of CB1 and CB2 receptors determines their efficacy at inducing apoptosis in astrocytomas. *PLoS One*, **5**, e8702.

Chan, P.C., Sills, R.C., Braun, A.G., Haseman, J.K., and Bucher, J.R. (1996). Toxicity and carcinogenicity of delta 9-tetrahydrocannabinol in Fischer rats and B6C3F1 mice. *Fundamental and Applied Toxicology*, **30**, 109–117.

De Bono, J.S. and Ashworth, A. (2010). Translating cancer research into targeted therapeutics. *Nature*, **467**, 543–549.

Devane, W.A., Hanus, L., Breuer, A., *et al.* (1992). Isolation and structure of a brain constituent that binds to the cannabinoid receptor. *Science*, **258**, 1946–1949.

Donadelli, M., Dando, I., Zaniboni, T., *et al.* (2011). Gemcitabine/cannabinoid combination triggers autophagy in pancreatic cancer cells through a ROS-mediated mechanism. *Cell Death and Disease*, **2**, e152.

Du, K., Herzig, S., Kulkarni, R.N., and Montminy, M. (2003). TRB3: a tribbles homolog that inhibits Akt/PKB activation by insulin in liver. *Science*, **300**, 1574–1577.

Eisenberg-Lerner, A., Bialik, S., Simon, H.U., and Kimchi, A. (2009). Life and death partners: apoptosis, autophagy and the cross-talk between them. *Cell Death and Differentiation*, **16**, 966–975.

Ellert-Miklaszewska, A., Kaminska, B., and Konarska, L. (2005). Cannabinoids down-regulate PI3K/Akt and Erk signalling pathways and activate proapoptotic function of Bad protein. *Cell Signal*, **17**, 25–37.

Encinar, J.A., Mallo, G.V., Mizyrycki, C., *et al.* (2001). Human p8 is a HMG-I/Y-like protein with DNA binding activity enhanced by phosphorylation. *The Journal of Biological Chemistry*, **276**, 2742–2751.

Fernandez-Ruiz, J., Romero, J., Velasco, G., *et al.* (2007). Cannabinoid CB_2 receptor: a new target for controlling neural cell survival? *Trends in Pharmacological Sciences*, **28**, 39–45.

Galve-Roperh, I., Aguado, T., Palazuelos, J., and Guzmán, M. (2008). Mechanisms of control of neuron survival by the endocannabinoid system. *Current Pharmaceutical Design*, **14**, 2279–2288.

Galve-Roperh, I., Sánchez, C., Cortes, M.L., *et al.* (2000). Anti-tumoral action of cannabinoids: involvement of sustained ceramide accumulation and extracellular signal-regulated kinase activation. *Nature Medicine*, **6**, 313–319.

Gaoni, Y. and Mechoulam, R. (1964). Isolation, structure and partial synthesis of an active constituent of hashish. *Journal of the American Chemical Society*, **86**, 1646–1647.

Gomez del Pulgar, T., Velasco, G., Sánchez, C., Haro, A., and Guzmán, M. (2002). De novo-synthesized ceramide is involved in cannabinoid-induced apoptosis. *Biochemical Journal*, **363**, 183–188.

Grande, E., Bolos, M.V., and Arriola, E. (2011). Targeting oncogenic ALK: a promising strategy for cancer treatment. *Molecular Cancer Therapeutics*, **10**, 569–579.

Grimaldi, C., Pisanti, S., Laezza, C., *et al.* (2006). Anandamide inhibits adhesion and migration of breast cancer cells. *Experimental Cell Research*, **312**, 363–373.

Guindon, J. and Hohmann, A.G. (2011). The endocannabinoid system and cancer: therapeutic implication. *British Journal of Pharmacology*, **163**, 1447–1463.

Gustafsson, S.B., Lindgren, T., Jonsson, M., and Jacobsson, S.O. (2009). Cannabinoid receptor-independent cytotoxic effects of cannabinoids in human colorectal carcinoma cells: synergism with 5-fluorouracil. *Cancer Chemotherapy and Pharmacology*, **63**, 691–701.

Guzmán, M. (2003). Cannabinoids: potential anticancer agents. *Nature Reviews Cancer*, **3**, 745–755.

Guzmán, M., Duarte, M.J., Blazquez, C., *et al.* (2006). A pilot clinical study of Delta9-tetrahydrocannabinol in patients with recurrent glioblastoma multiforme. *British Journal of Cancer*, **95**, 197–203.

Hart, S., Fischer, O.M., and Ullrich, A. (2004). Cannabinoids induce cancer cell proliferation via tumor necrosis factor alpha-converting enzyme (TACE/ADAM17)-mediated transactivation of the epidermal growth factor receptor. *Cancer Research*, **64**, 1943–1950.

Hegde, V.L., Nagarkatti, M., and Nagarkatti, P.S. (2010). Cannabinoid receptor activation leads to massive mobilization of myeloid-derived suppressor cells with potent immunosuppressive properties. *European Journal of Immunology*, **40**, 3358–3371.

Herrera, B., Carracedo, A., Diez-Zaera, M., *et al.* (2006). The CB_2 cannabinoid receptor signals apoptosis via ceramide-dependent activation of the mitochondrial intrinsic pathway. *Experimental Cell Research*, **312**, 2121–2131.

Izzo, A.A., Aviello, G., Petrosino, S., *et al.* (2008). Increased endocannabinoid levels reduce the development of precancerous lesions in the mouse colon. *Journal of Molecular Medicine*, **86**, 89–98.

Joosten, M., Valk, P.J., Jorda, M.A., *et al.* (2002). Leukemic predisposition of pSca-1/Cb2 transgenic mice. *Experimental Hematology*, **30**, 142–149.

Kadomatsu, K. (2005). The midkine family in cancer, inflammation and neural development. *Nagoya Journal of Medical Science*, **67**, 71–82.

Katona, I. and Freund, T.F. (2008). Endocannabinoid signaling as a synaptic circuit breaker in neurological disease. *Nature Medicine*, **14**, 923–930.

Ligresti, A., Bisogno, T., Matias, I., *et al.* (2003). Possible endocannabinoid control of colorectal cancer growth. *Gastroenterology*, **125**, 677–687.

Ligresti, A., Moriello, A.S., Starowicz, K., *et al.* (2006). Antitumor activity of plant cannabinoids with emphasis on the effect of cannabidiol on human breast carcinoma. *Journal of Pharmacology and Experimental Therapeutics*, **318**, 1375–1387.

Liu, W.M., Fowler, D.W., and Dalgleish, A.G. (2010). Cannabis-derived substances in cancer therapy– an emerging anti-inflammatory role for the cannabinoids. *Current Clinical Pharmacology*, **5**, 281–287.

Lonardi, S., Tosoni, A., and Brandes, A.A. (2005). Adjuvant chemotherapy in the treatment of high grade gliomas. *Cancer Treatment Reviews*, **31**, 79–89.

Lorente, M., Carracedo, A., Torres, S., *et al.* (2009). Amphiregulin is a factor for resistance of glioma cells to cannabinoid-induced apoptosis. *Glia*, **57**, 1374–1385.

Lorente, M., Torres, S., Salazar, M., *et al.* (2011). Stimulation of the midkine/ALK axis renders glioma cells resistant to cannabinoid antitumoral action. *Cell Death and Differentiation*, **18**, 959–973.

Lu, T., Newton, C., Perkins, I., Friedman, H., and Klein, T.W. (2006). Cannabinoid treatment suppresses the T-helper cell-polarizing function of mouse dendritic cells stimulated with *Legionella pneumophila* infection. *Journal of Pharmacology and Experimental Therapeutics*, **319**, 269–276.

Malfitano, A.M., Ciaglia, E., Gangemi, G., *et al.* (2011). Update on the endocannabinoid system as an anti-cancer target. *Expert Opinion on Therapeutic Targets*, **15**, 297–308.

Marcu, J.P., Christian, R.T., Lau, D., *et al.* (2010). Cannabidiol enhances the inhibitory effects of delta9-tetrahydrocannabinol on human glioblastoma cell proliferation and survival. *Molecular Cancer Therapeutics*, **9**, 180–189.

Massi, P., Vaccani, A., Bianchessi, S., *et al.* (2006). The non-psychoactive cannabidiol triggers caspase activation and oxidative stress in human glioma cells. *Cellular and Molecular Life Sciences*, **63**, 2057–2066.

Massi, P., Valenti, M., Vaccani, A., *et al.* (2008). 5-Lipoxygenase and anandamide hydrolase (FAAH) mediate the antitumor activity of cannabidiol, a non-psychoactive cannabinoid. *Journal of Neurochemistry*, **104**, 1091–1100.

Matsuda, L.A., Lolait, S.J., Brownstein, M.J., Young, A.C., and Bonner, T.I. (1990). Structure of a cannabinoid receptor and functional expression of the cloned cDNA. *Nature*, **346**, 561–564.

McAllister, S.D., Christian, R.T., Horowitz, M.P., Garcia, A., and Desprez, P.Y. (2007). Cannabidiol as a novel inhibitor of Id-1 gene expression in aggressive breast cancer cells. *Molecular Cancer Therapeutics*, **6**, 2921–2927.

McAllister, S.D., Murase, R., Christian, R.T., *et al.* (2011). Pathways mediating the effects of cannabidiol on the reduction of breast cancer cell proliferation, invasion, and metastasis. *Breast Cancer Research and Treatment*, **129**, 37–47.

McKallip, R.J., Nagarkatti, M., and Nagarkatti, P.S. (2005). Delta-9-tetrahydrocannabinol enhances breast cancer growth and metastasis by suppression of the antitumor immune response. *The Journal of Immunology*, **174**, 3281–3289.

Mechoulam, R., Ben-Shabat, S., Hanus, L., *et al.* (1995). Identification of an endogenous 2-monoglyceride, present in canine gut, that binds to cannabinoid receptors. *Biochemical Pharmacology*, **50**, 83–90.

Mirkin, B.L., Clark, S., Zheng, X., *et al.* (2005). Identification of midkine as a mediator for intercellular transfer of drug resistance. *Oncogene*, **24**, 4965–4674.

Miyato, H., Kitayama, J., Yamashita, H., *et al.* (2009). Pharmacological synergism between cannabinoids and paclitaxel in gastric cancer cell lines. *Journal of Surgical Research*, **155**, 40–47.

Mizushima, N., Levine, B., Cuervo, A.M., and Klionsky, D.J. (2008). Autophagy fights disease through cellular self-digestion. *Nature*, **451**, 1069–1075.

Munro, S., Thomas, K.L., and Abu-Shaar, M. (1993). Molecular characterization of a peripheral receptor for cannabinoids. *Nature*, **365**, 61–65.

Nabissi, M., Morelli, M.B., Santoni, M., and Santoni, G. (2012). Triggering of the TRPV2 channel by cannabidiol sensitizes glioblastoma cells to cytotoxic chemotherapeutic agents. *Carcinogenesis*, **34**, 48–57.

Newton, C.A., Chou, P.J., Perkins, I., and Klein, T.W. (2009). CB_1 and CB_2 cannabinoid receptors mediate different aspects of delta-9-tetrahydrocannabinol (THC)-induced T helper cell shift following immune activation by *Legionella pneumophila* infection. *Journal of Neuroimmune Pharmacology*, **4**, 92–102.

Nieder, C., Adam, M., Molls, M., and Grosu, A.L. (2006). Therapeutic options for recurrent high-grade glioma in adult patients: recent advances. *Critical Reviews in Oncology/Hematology*, **60**, 181–193.

Nomura, D.K., Long, J.Z., Niessen, S., *et al.* (2010). Monoacylglycerol lipase regulates a fatty acid network that promotes cancer pathogenesis. *Cell*, **140**, 49–61.

Pacher, P., Batkai, S., and Kunos, G. (2006). The endocannabinoid system as an emerging target of pharmacotherapy. *Pharmacological Reviews*, **58**, 389–462.

Palmer, R.H., Vernersson, E., Grabbe, C., and Hallberg, B. (2009). Anaplastic lymphoma kinase: signalling in development and disease. *Biochemical Journal*, **420**, 345–361.

Pertwee, R.G. (2008). The diverse CB_1 and CB_2 receptor pharmacology of three plant cannabinoids: Δ^9-tetrahydrocannabinol, cannabidiol and Δ^9-tetrahydrocannabivarin. *British Journal of Pharmacology*, **153**, 199–215.

Pertwee, R.G. (2009). Emerging strategies for exploiting cannabinoid receptor agonists as medicines. *British Journal of Pharmacology*, **156**, 397–411.

Pertwee, R.G., Howlett, A.C., Abood, M.E., *et al.* (2010). International Union of Basic and Clinical Pharmacology. LXXIX. Cannabinoid receptors and their ligands: beyond CB_1 and CB_2. *Pharmacological Reviews*, **62**, 588–631.

Pisanti, S., Borselli, C., Oliviero, O., *et al.* (2007). Antiangiogenic activity of the endocannabinoid anandamide: correlation to its tumor-suppressor efficacy. *Journal of Cellular Physiology*, **211**, 495–503.

Portella, G., Laezza, C., Laccetti, P., *et al.* (2003). Inhibitory effects of cannabinoid CB_1 receptor stimulation on tumor growth and metastatic spreading: actions on signals involved in angiogenesis and metastasis. *FASEB Journal*, **17**, 1771–1773.

Preet, A., Ganju, R.K., and Groopman, J.E. (2008). Delta9-tetrahydrocannabinol inhibits epithelial growth factor-induced lung cancer cell migration in vitro as well as its growth and metastasis in vivo. *Oncogene*, **27**, 339–346.

Purow, B. and Schiff, D. (2009). Advances in the genetics of glioblastoma: are we reaching critical mass? *Nature Reviews Neurology*, **5**, 419–426.

Qamri, Z., Preet, A., Nasser, M.W., *et al.* (2009). Synthetic cannabinoid receptor agonists inhibit tumor growth and metastasis of breast cancer. *Molecular Cancer Therapeutics*, **8**, 3117–3129.

Ramer, R. and Hinz, B. (2008). Inhibition of cancer cell invasion by cannabinoids via increased expression of tissue inhibitor of matrix metalloproteinases-1. *Journal of the National Cancer Institute*, **100**, 59–69.

Salazar, M., Carracedo, A., Salanueva, I.J., *et al.* (2009). Cannabinoid action induces autophagy-mediated cell death through stimulation of ER stress in human glioma cells. *The Journal of Clinical Investigation*, **119**, 1359–1372.

Sánchez, C., de Ceballos, M.L., del Pulgar, T.G., *et al.* (2001). Inhibition of glioma growth in vivo by selective activation of the CB_2 cannabinoid receptor. *Cancer Research*, **61**, 5784–5789.

Sarfaraz, S., Adhami, V.M., Syed, D.N., Afaq, F., and Mukhtar, H. (2008). Cannabinoids for cancer treatment: progress and promise. *Cancer Research*, **68**, 339–342.

Sarfaraz, S., Afaq, F., Adhami, V.M., Malik, A., and Mukhtar, H. (2006). Cannabinoid receptor agonist-induced apoptosis of human prostate cancer cells LNCaP proceeds through sustained activation of ERK1/2 leading to G1 cell cycle arrest. *The Journal of Biological Chemistry*, **281**, 39480–39491.

Shrivastava, A., Kuzontkoski, P.M., Groopman, J.E., and Prasad, A. (2011). Cannabidiol induces programmed cell death in breast cancer cells by coordinating the cross-talk between apoptosis and autophagy. *Molecular Cancer Therapeutics*, **10**, 1161–1172.

Soroceanu, L., Murase, R., Limbad, C., *et al.* (2012). Id-1 is a key transcriptional regulator of glioblastoma aggressiveness and a novel therapeutic target. *Cancer Research*, **73**, 1559–1569.

Steffens, S., Veillard, N.R., Arnaud, C., *et al.* (2005). Low dose oral cannabinoid therapy reduces progression of atherosclerosis in mice. *Nature*, **434**, 782–786.

Stupp, R., Mason, W.P., van den Bent, M.J., *et al.* (2005). Radiotherapy plus concomitant and adjuvant temozolomide for glioblastoma. *The New England Journal of Medicine*, **352**, 987–996.

Sugiura, T., Kondo, S., Sukagawa, A., *et al.* (1995). 2-Arachidonoylglycerol: a possible endogenous cannabinoid receptor ligand in brain. *Biochemical and Biophysical Research Communication*, **215**, 89–97.

Thors, L., Bergh, A., Persson, E., *et al.* (2010). Fatty acid amide hydrolase in prostate cancer: association with disease severity and outcome, CB_1 receptor expression and regulation by IL-4. *PLoS One*, **5**, e12275.

Torres, S., Lorente, M., Rodriguez-Fornes, F., *et al.* (2011). A combined preclinical therapy of cannabinoids and temozolomide against glioma. *Molecular Cancer Therapeutics*, **10**, 90–103.

Vara, D., Salazar, M., Olea-Herrero, N., *et al.* (2011). Anti-tumoral action of cannabinoids on hepatocellular carcinoma: role of AMPK-dependent activation of autophagy. *Cell Death and Differentiation*, **18**, 1099–1111.

Velasco, G., Sánchez, C. and Guzmán, M. (2012). Towards the use of cannabinoids as antitumour agents. *Nature Reviews Cancer*, **12**, 436–444.

Verfaillie, T., Salazar, M., Velasco, G. and Agostinis, P. (2010). Linking ER stress to autophagy: potential implications for cancer therapy. *International Journal of Cell Biology*, **2010**, 930509.

Wang, D., Wang, H., Ning, W., *et al.* (2008). Loss of cannabinoid receptor 1 accelerates intestinal tumor growth. *Cancer Research*, **68**, 6468–6476.

Zheng, D., Bode, A.M., Zhao, Q., *et al.* (2008). The cannabinoid receptors are required for ultraviolet-induced inflammation and skin cancer development. *Cancer Research*, **68**, 3992–3998.

Zhu, L.X., Sharma, S., Stolina, M., *et al.* (2000). Delta-9-tetrahydrocannabinol inhibits antitumor immunity by a CB_2 receptor-mediated, cytokine-dependent pathway. *The Journal of Immunology*, **165**, 373–380.

Part 6

Recreational Cannabis: Sought-After Effects, Adverse Effects, Designer Drugs, and Harm Minimization

Wayne Hall

Part 6 Overview

The first four chapters in Part 6 deal with what we know about the risks of cannabis, mainly when it is used by young adults to produce pleasure, euphoria, relaxation, and enhance sociability. In the four decades since cannabis first began to be widely used by young people in the US, many young people now start cannabis use in their mid to late teens, an important period of psychosocial transition when misadventures arising from chronic drug intoxication and dependence can adversely affect a young person's life by reducing their chances of completing education, developing satisfactory relationships, and entering the workforce.

In Chapter 36, Curran and Morgan describe the major reasons why young people use cannabis, namely, to experience euphoria, relaxation, sociability, heightened appreciation of sensory experiences, eating, sex, and aesthetic experiences. They also review research on some undesired adverse effects of cannabis use such as dependence, psychosis, and cognitive impairment.

In Chapter 37, Morrison, Bhattacharyya, and Murray review the epidemiological and clinical evidence that cannabis use (especially when initiated in early adolescence and used regularly during young adulthood) increases the risks of developing schizophrenia. They argue that evidence from longitudinal studies of young people have ruled out reverse causation and tested competing explanations of the association. Experimental provocation studies have also shown that Δ^9-tetrahydrocannabinol (THC) produces psychotic symptoms in persons with and without schizophrenia in a dose-dependent way.

In Chapter 38, Grotenhermen reviews the non-psychological adverse health effects of cannabis. These include: the adverse acute effects of cannabis intoxication on psychomotor performance and the risks of motor vehicle accidents; the adverse effects of chronic cannabis use that arise from smoking as a route of administration, such as respiratory and cardiovascular disease, and from the development of tolerance to the physical and psychological effects of THC that may lead to dependence. He also considers the effects of chronic use on the hormonal system and fertility, pregnancy outcomes and fetal development, and on the immune, gastrointestinal, and other organ systems.

In Chapter 39, Hall and Degenhardt outline harm minimization strategies that have been adopted or could be adopted to reduce the harms of cannabis use in developed countries. These include: roadside drug testing to deter cannabis-intoxicated driving; education of cannabis users about patterns of use that increase the risks of dependence, poor mental health, and respiratory problems; and depenalization and decriminalization of cannabis use to reduce harms arising from cannabis prohibition.

In the final chapter (Chapter 40), Thomas and colleagues move away from recreational cannabis to examine the possible adverse public health effects and the regulatory challenges that are posed by the marketing of cannabinoid designer drugs over the past decade. These synthetic cannabinoids act like THC as agonists at the cannabinoid CB_1 receptor, although their other biological effects are not well understood. The desired subjective effects of these drugs resemble those of herbal cannabis but are often reported to be more intense. Human pharmacological data are sparse because these drugs were primarily used in animal research exploring mechanisms of cannabinoid action. Systematic toxicological data in humans is very sparse.

Chapter 36

Desired and Undesired Effects of Cannabis on the Human Mind and Psychological Well-Being

H. Valerie Curran and Celia J.A. Morgan

36.1 Desired effects of cannabis

A small amount consumed in a reefer, bong or pipe induces laughter, hunger, random silliness and great interest in boring items. Highly recommended for long camping trips, family reunions, first dates and gloomy Sundays.

Alfred Gingold (1982), US humorist.

For centuries cannabis has been used for various "desired" effects. Getting "stoned" as described by Gingold is an aim of many of the estimated 166 million people worldwide who use cannabis recreationally (United Nations Office on Drugs and Crime 2009). In reality, the "stoned" experience can vary enormously, depending on factors such as prior experience of cannabis (D'Souza et al. 2009), the setting, and the type of cannabis ingested (Morgan et al. 2010c). Common desired feelings include disinhibition, dreaminess, and a communion with other smokers. Desired sensations reported are heightened awareness of music, sounds, colors, textures, and tastes (Tyler 1986). Cannabis users also often report insights into new meanings, an impulse to utter profundities, to giggle, and to eat a lot (Tyler 1986). Across the centuries many writers and artists have attempted to describe the cannabis experience. For example, in 1854 the American writer Bayard Taylor tried the drug on a trip to Egypt and noted:

The sensations it then produced were . . . Mentally of a wonderfully keen perception of the ludicrous in the most simple and familiar objects . . . the objects by which I was surrounded assumed a strange whimsical expression . . . I was provoked into a long fit of laughter . . . [the effect] died away as gradually as it came, leaving me overcome with a soft and pleasant drowsiness, from which I sank into a deep and refreshing sleep. (Taylor 1854, cf. Grinspoon 1993)

Early records suggest that cannabis was first desired, not for its recreational effects, but rather its medicinal properties. Analgesic use dates to the Chinese pharmacopoeia of 2800 BC and East Indian documents in the Athera Veda of about 2000 BC (Gurley et al. 1998). In ancient Greece and Rome, both the Herbal of Dioscorides and the writings of Galen referred to the medical use of cannabis (Gurley et al. 1998). Western medicine was much slower to use the plant therapeutically although Culpepper in medieval times mentions it (cf. Carter and Ugalde 2004) and Queen Victoria was famously prescribed tincture of cannabis to relieve pain related to menstruation and childbirth.

Today, two cannabis derivatives are licensed in several countries for their desired medical effects and several more cannabinoids are under investigation (see Chapters 23–26, this volume).

The main psychoactive ingredient of cannabis which produces the effects that users seek is delta-9-tetrahydrocannabinol (THC) and this is prescribed medically, as dronabinol/Marinol®, for reduction of chemotherapy-induced nausea and for appetite stimulation in human immunodeficiency virus (HIV) patients. THC combined with the second most abundant cannabinoid in cannabis, cannabidiol (CBD), is licensed for muscle spasm in multiple sclerosis. In terms of desired psychological effects, whilst as yet unlicensed for this use, several studies have demonstrated a positive impact of CBD alone on anxiety in patients with social anxiety disorder (Bergamaschi et al. 2011; Guimares et al. 1990; Schier 2012). A further intriguing, potentially highly desirable, property of CBD appears to be the capacity to reduce psychotic symptoms in schizophrenia (Leweke et al. 2012), although this work needs replication. Recent evidence also suggests that CBD may have emerging use as a treatment to modulate memory, by either enhancing fear extinction learning (Das et al. 2013) or blocking "reconsolidation"—the process by which memories are made labile to allow them to be strengthened or updated or disrupted (Stern et al. 2012). Either of these approaches makes CBD a candidate treatment for disorders of pathological fear memory, such as posttraumatic stress disorder and phobias. We have also gathered preliminary data that suggests that CBD might reduce cigarette smoking (Morgan et al. 2013a), therefore this desired effect of this constituent of cannabis may also be a candidate for reducing addiction. A recent review has addressed the broad spectrum of, almost panacea-like, therapeutic uses of CBD, attributing them to a range of neurotransmitter actions (Campos et al. 2012).

In some parts of the US, "medical marijuana" is available on prescription for a wide range of conditions, particularly chronic pain and anxiety. In a survey of 1000 of these patients prescribed the drug for these two conditions, we found they rated cannabis as more effective and having fewer side effects than their conventional pharmaceutical medication (Lu et al. in preparation). Other less common conditions that "medical marijuana" is prescribed for include addiction management, bipolar disorder, glaucoma, anorexia, and even writer's block. Scripts for the unconventional diagnosis of writer's block may well reflect a widely held view that this drug can enhance human creativity. Despite numerous anecdotes from musicians, writers, and other artists, scientific evidence for this has proved elusive, not the least because it is extremely difficult to empirically define "creativity." In an early, highly controlled laboratory study of the dose–response effects of THC, the one positive cognitive effect of the drug was to enhance verbal fluency—the speed with which an individual could generate words that begin with the same letter (Curran et al. 2002). This effect was recently replicated in a naturalistic study of individuals smoking their own chosen variety of cannabis—again the drug acutely increased the number of words generated (Schafer et al. 2012). Importantly, several days later these users did not differ from control nonusers in fluency, indicating the enhancement was an acute effect of cannabis. A naturalistic study by Morgan et al. (2010c) suggests that one of marijuana's properties is an ability to increase semantic priming, or an individual's ability to make connections between seemingly unrelated concepts. However, other studies have found no acute enhancement on a variety of so-called "creativity" tasks (e.g., Bourasa and Vaugeois 2001) and, given the publication bias against negative findings, it is likely that many other studies have found no effect. Further, the acute positive effects of the drug on fluency and semantic priming may reflect the disinhibiting effects of cannabis rather than a direct creative enhancement.

One way to index a drug's desired effects is to ask users to rate the comparative benefits of differing recreational compounds. Using this approach, nearly 6000 participants responded to our international survey by ranking the 15 most common psychotropic drugs used recreationally (including alcohol and tobacco) on ten potential benefits (Morgan et al. 2013b). Cannabis was ranked the highest drug for enjoyment and pain relief, and as high as benzodiazepine tranquilizers on relaxation and stress relief. It also ranked amongst the top five drugs in aiding sleep, mood, and socializing. This concurs with the self-reported effects of cannabis in other studies that suggest euphoria and relaxation are the most consistently reported acute effects (see Green et al. 2003 for a review), although a wide variation in self-reported effects, even in the same individuals, has been reported. It is known that there are marked individual differences such that one person's feelings of acute relaxation may contrast with another's anxiety or paranoia. And the setting in which the drug is ingested will also influence this. Similarly the undesired effects of this drug show clear individual and contextual differences. Below we focus on the undesired psychological effects of cannabis use; unwanted effects on physical health are discussed by Franjo Grotenhermen (Chapter 38, this volume).

36.2 Undesired effects of cannabis

The undesired effects of cannabis use on the mind and psychological well-being have been much more widely studied than its desired effects. Four major areas of harm have been the focus of this research: addiction, cognitive impairment, anxiety and depression, and psychosis. Importantly, these areas interact and overlap. For example, neurocognitive impairment is a key feature of both psychosis and addiction and both clinical conditions involve abnormal salience attribution (Freeman et al. 2012). Further, many individuals with a diagnosis of a psychotic disorder are also frequent users of drugs like tobacco and cannabis. In the following sections we describe the major undesired short- and longer-term consequences of cannabis use before considering what makes an individual more or less vulnerable to those effects.

36.2.1 Cannabis and addiction

The last decade has witnessed increasing concern about a subset of about one in nine recreational users who develop clinically defined cannabis dependence (e.g., Fergusson and Horwood 2000; Hall and Degenhardt 2007; Linszen and van Amelsvoort 2007). Worldwide, around 16–17 million people will meet these clinical criteria in the current psychiatric classification system of the *Diagnostic and Statistical Manual of Mental Disorders* (DSM). This is more than the number dependent on any other illicit drug.

In Europe, about 1% of all adults and nearly 2% of 14–17-year-olds are addicted to cannabis (Wittchen et al. 2011; European Monitoring Centre for Drugs and Drug Addiction (EMCDDA) 2011). Among UK first-time drug treatment clients, the primary addiction is to cannabis in 28% of cases, second only to heroin (41%) (EMCDDA 2011). Despite evidence that numbers of cannabis users are no longer increasing in several European countries, demand for cannabis treatment has more than doubled in the UK and throughout Europe since 2001 (United Nations Office on Drugs and Crime 2010). A cannabis withdrawal syndrome is increasingly recognized in treatment studies although this is not seen as clinically significant in current DSM criteria for cannabis dependence (Budney and Hughes 2006).

As yet, cannabis dependence is a relatively under-researched area with most studies looking at "recreational" use (usually weekly or monthly). Irrespective of the drug, risk of dependency increases the more a drug is used, and daily users will be at highest risk. Acute response to cannabis itself may also dictate the risk of dependency: blunted negative and enhanced euphoric effects may predispose an individual to use the drug more regularly (Ren et al. 2009). Although various treatments of cannabis dependency have been trialed—including THC itself, gabapentin, and venlafaxine (Mason et al. 2012; Levin et al. 2013)—there is still no effective pharmacological treatment of cannabis dependency. This is an important therapeutic chasm especially given the large numbers of adolescent users whose brains are still developing. They may experience negative cognitive and motivational effects, which impact negatively on their school or college attendance and academic achievement in the longer term.

In general, the reinforcing effects of drugs of abuse in human beings are often thought to be contingent on the rate of dopamine (DA) increases in the striatum (Volkow et al. 2007). This generalization may not hold for THC/cannabis. Two positron emission tomography (PET) studies have shown no effect of acute THC on striatal DA release, when administered orally (Stokes et al. 2009) and intravenously (Barkus et al. 2011) whilst another did show significant DA release when THC was smoked (Bossong et al. 2010). Neuroimaging studies have also sought to determine differences between those who are dependent on cannabis from those who use occasionally or not at all. Reduced striatal DA synthesis capacity in heavy cannabis users relative to nonuser controls has recently been found (Bloomfield et al. 2014) and reduced DA D_2/D_3 receptor availability has been linked to cannabis use in users in some (Albrecht et al. 2013; Sevy et al. 2008) but not all (Stokes et al. 2012) studies. No relationship has been found between reduced DA synthesis/receptor availability and psychosis-like symptoms from cannabis (Barkus et al. 2011; Bloomfield et al. 2014), interestingly suggesting this biological marker is more important in addiction than psychosis in individuals using cannabis recreationally.

The endocannabinoid (eCB) system, upon which cannabis acts, is also now thought to be intrinsic to reward and reinforcement circuits by fine tuning DA neurons in the striatum (Melis and Pistis 2012; Serrano and Parsons 2011), so it is likely that this is how the dependence forming properties of cannabis are modulated, and the indirect action on DA may account for inconsistencies in the human studies. While enhancement of eCB signaling per se is not thought to produce robust addiction-related behaviors, growing evidence implicates eCB signaling in the modulation of the motivational effects produced by ethanol, nicotine, opiates (e.g., Gonzalez et al. 2002), and to a lesser degree psychostimulant drugs (Pan et al. 2008). Further, preclinical studies suggest that type 1 cannabinoid receptors (CB_1) are implicated in the relapse to drug-seeking behaviors, both from exposure to drug-conditioned cues and drug administration itself (Serrano and Parsons 2011). These finding suggest that modulating the eCB system may be a promising target in the treatment of addiction (Morgan et al. 2013c).

Clinically, a major unmet challenge is the development of a safe, effective pharmacological treatment for cannabis dependence which can be used conjointly with psychosocial therapies to boost the current low efficacy of all treatment approaches. An effective pharmacological treatment would impact significantly not only on medical and legal costs associated with addiction, but also—via neurocognitive and motivational enhancement—improve educational/vocational achievement of young cannabis users. Critically it could also reduce their risks of associated mental health problems such as psychosis and of cognitive impairment.

36.2.2 Cannabis and psychosis

Converging evidence suggests that cannabis and THC can acutely produce a wide range of transient schizophrenia-like positive, negative, and cognitive symptoms (D'Souza et al. 2004; Mason et al. 2009). Indeed, intravenous THC is one of the current pharmacological models of psychosis alongside N-methyl-D-aspartate (NMDA) receptor antagonists like ketamine and serotonergic hallucinogens like psilocybin.

Evidence for an association between long-term cannabis use and psychosis continues to accumulate with a number of longitudinal, population-based studies showing a roughly twofold increase in psychotic symptoms or psychotic diagnoses in young adults who use cannabis heavily (di Forti et al. 2007; Henquet et al. 2005; Moore et al. 2007; see Morrison et al., Chapter 37, this volume). The extent to which cannabis is causative in this association is hotly debated. The vast majority of people who use cannabis do not develop schizophrenia, and many people diagnosed with schizophrenia have never used cannabis. More agreement is found in evidence that heavy cannabis use may result in young people who are *vulnerable* to psychosis for various genetic and environmental risk factors, experiencing their first episode around 2 years earlier than they might without using the drug. Earlier initiation of use will in turn impact negatively on both their clinical and neurocognitive prognosis. People vary along a continuum of psychosis-proneness (or schizotypy) which can be assessed with valid questionnaire measures. Henquet et al. (2005), in a prospective study of 2400 young Germans, found that those who were more psychosis-prone at baseline were no more likely than others to use cannabis 4 years later. However, those psychosis-prone individuals who did use cannabis showed a 24% increased risk for psychotic symptoms at follow-up compared to an increased risk of only 6% in those who were not psychosis-prone.

Clinically, much effort is being devoted to the early diagnosis of young people who, for various genetic and environmental reasons, are at ultra-high risk (UHR) of developing schizophrenia in the future. Prior to the first psychotic episode, during what is termed the "prodromal phase," UHR individuals experience mild cognitive and mood symptoms similar to those seen in the full clinical disorder. Cannabis use in adolescence has been linked with greater prodromal symptoms (Mietunnen et al. 2008). The symptom profile of this prodromal phase has been described in various ways including Klosterkotter et al.'s (2001) framework. Using this framework we compared groups of sober individuals who were dependent on skunk (see section 36.4) with a group dependent on the NMDA antagonist ketamine, a drug also acutely associated with psychotomimetic effects (Morgan et al. 2012a) and with control groups who did not use these drugs. We then compared the daily skunk and ketamine users with the symptom profile of a group of UHR individuals who went on subsequently to develop schizophrenia. The profile of ketamine addicts was virtually indistinguishable from the UHR group. Skunk users showed very similar cognitive disturbances to both these groups but did not show the same reduced emotional responsiveness, lack of tolerance to stress, or perceptual disturbances (Morgan et al. 2012a). Given the current market dominance of skunk, it is important, if difficult, to differentiate chronic, drug-related symptoms from a clinical prodromal state. One obvious method for this is to reassess patients following 4 weeks' abstinence from skunk although many cannabis-dependent patients will find this abstinence period very challenging.

Cannabinoid research has also enhanced our clinical understanding of the significance of the human brain's endogenous cannabinoid system. Higher levels of anandamide in cerebrospinal fluid (CSF) have been associated with lower psychotic symptoms both in individuals diagnosed with schizophrenia (Giuffrida et al. 2004; Leweke et al. 1999) and in those classified as prodromal (Koethe et al. 2009). Interestingly, schizophrenics with low (<5 times) use of cannabis had 10-fold higher levels of CSF anandamide than higher users (>20 times) or healthy low or high users (Leweke et al. 2007). To investigate whether cannabis use was associated with alterations in eCB levels in recreational users of cannabis, Morgan et al. (2013c) measured CSF anandamide levels in heavy cannabis users (use 22.6 ± 7.2 days/month), light cannabis users (4.3 ± 3.4 days/month), and controls (nonusers). Anandamide levels were significantly lower in heavy than light users. Intriguingly, levels of anandamide correlated negatively with psychotic-like symptoms, paralleling results with prodromal and schizophrenic individuals. Although obtaining CSF samples from humans is not easy, these are the only current markers of central eCBs and more research in this area will help elucidate how these brain chemicals may mediate individual differences in the mental health effects of exogenous cannabinoids.

36.2.3 Cannabis and neurocognitive function

ECBs are crucial in certain forms of neuronal plasticity and THC has been shown to disrupt long-term potentiation (a model for learning and memory) and long-term depression in preclinical studies (Zhu 2006). In humans, this is reflected in the ability of acute cannabis and acute THC to robustly impair cognitive function, especially working and episodic memory (Curran et al. 2002; Gonzalez 2007). Working memory deficits are seen less in the ability to simply hold information online for brief periods (e.g., remembering a telephone number before dialing it) and more in the ability to manipulate that information whilst holding it online (e.g., doing mental arithmetic). Episodic memory refers to one's personal, contextualized autobiography—for example, your recollection of what movie you last saw, who with, where, and whether you ate popcorn or went for a meal afterwards. Both working and episodic memory deficits induced by THC or cannabis show a clear dose dependency and increase with task difficulty (for reviews see Gonzalez 2007; Solowij and Battisti 2008). These robust effects of THC and cannabis are commensurate with the high density of cannabinoid CB_1 receptors in the hippocampus and frontal cortex (Ranganathan and D'Souza 2006), areas critical in memory. Several brain imaging studies have shown that recreational cannabis users show altered regional cerebral blood flow during memory tasks (e.g., Block et al. 2002) and signs of reduced neuronal activity in the dorsolateral prefrontal cortex alongside deficits in working memory and attention (e.g., Hermann et al. 2007). Recently Solowij et al. (2013) showed that hippocampal changes were associated with long-term cannabis use and that these were most marked in psychotic individuals who also used cannabis.

Systematic reviews and meta-analyses suggest that residual impairments a day or so after cannabis use are restricted to performance on fairly artificial tasks like remembering word-lists and are very small in terms of effect size (Gonzalez 2007). A controlled study of THC (7.5, 15 mg) found no residual cognitive impairment 24 h after ingestion (Curran et al. 2002). Similarly, long-term effects after abstinence are inconsistent, with some studies showing no impairment a few weeks after abstinence (Pope et al. 2001) and others showing very subtle deficits persisting longer term in heavier users (Gonzalez 2007; Solowij and Battisti 2008). Based on the Dunedin longitudinal cohort, Meier et al. (2012) concluded that heavy cannabis use was associated with a decline of around eight intelligence quotient (IQ) points from childhood to early adulthood. This interpretation was challenged by a re-analysis of the same data (Rogeberg 2013) which suggested that the apparent link between IQ and heavy cannabis use was an artefact due to important differences such as socioeconomic status between the relatively small group of 38 heavy cannabis users and 1000 other individuals. It also seems incongruous that the heavy users in Meier et al.'s (2012) study showed impairments across the board on every neurocognitive test employed rather than the differential effects on memory expected from previous studies. One reason why findings on residual and long-term effects of this drug are inconsistent may be that, like psychotic and addictive effects, there is marked individual variation in the cognitive effects of cannabis which may also depend on the type of cannabis used.

36.2.4 Cannabis, anxiety, and depression

There is also evidence that chronic cannabis use is associated with changes in other indices of mental health and well-being. Preclinical studies have implicated the eCB system in the regulation of emotion (Moriera and Wotjak 2010). Thus it follows that long-term disruption of this system by the self-administration of exogenous cannabinoids could disrupt mood regulation. Meta-analyses have suggested a link between heavy cannabis use and depression (e.g., Moore et al. 2007). In our own studies of young, daily cannabis users, we have found that higher THC levels in hair are significantly associated with higher levels of both depression and anxiety (Morgan et al. 2012b). However, a recent epidemiological study (Degenhart et al. 2013) suggested increases in depression are not long-lasting, as they found no consistent associations between adolescent cannabis use and depression at age 29 years. The same study showed daily cannabis use and cannabis dependence in early adulthood was associated with more than double the rate of anxiety disorders at 29 years of age. The authors conclude that the association reported between cannabis use and anxiety may arise because the same factors that predispose people to use cannabis also increase their risks for common mental disorders. These common factors might include a combination of biological, personality, social, and environmental factors. This is plausible given social disadvantage is more common both among problematic drug users and among those who meet criteria for common mental disorders.

36.3 What determines individual variation in experiencing the desired and undesired effects of cannabis?

In some European countries like the UK, around 50% of 16–24-year-olds have used cannabis. Cannabis use, in a sense, is approaching "normative" behavior for this age group. Although most cannabis users will experience at least transient memory impairments, only around 10% of regular users will become dependent on the drug and only a tiny minority will ever develop psychosis. So what determines an individual's vulnerability to experiencing the undesired effects of cannabis?

Greater frequency, duration, and amount of cannabis use is one factor influencing vulnerability to both dependence *and* psychosis (di Forti et al. 2009; Moore et al. 2007). Increased use also means an individual is less likely to experience the desired effects of cannabis, as tolerance develops (D'Souza et al. 2009). Age of first cannabis use and years of use are often confounded in studies but the former appears to show an overall influence on vulnerability (McGrath et al. 2010; Solowij et al. 2011) which might be mediated in part by effects on white matter in the developing brain (Zalesky et al. 2012). Psychosis-proneness influences the psychotic-like effects of acute THC/cannabis (Barkus et al. 2006, Henquet et al. 2005; Mason et al. 2009; Verdoux et al. 2003). Finally various genetic factors have been a focus of several studies: e.g., the catechol-*O*-methyl transferase (*COMT*) gene (Caspi et al. 2005; Zammit et al. 2007, 2011) and the RAC-alpha serine/threonine-protein kinase gene, *AKT1* (di Forti et al. 2012). Although Caspi et al. (2005) suggested that cannabis use was associated with psychosis more in those with the Val/Val than Val/Met or Met/Met alleles of the *COMT* gene, subsequent larger-scale studies by Zammit and colleagues (Williams et al. 2005; Zammit et al. 2011) have not replicated this. Variations in several other genes either have been associated with cannabis abuse/dependence or are components of the eCB system tentatively associated with susceptibility to schizophrenia. These include the $GABA_A$ receptor gene, *GABRA2* (Agrawal et al. 2006), and fatty acid amide hydrolase (Tyndale et al. 2007) and cannabinoid CB_1 receptor genes (*CNR1*) (e.g., Schact et al. 2012; Ujike et al. 2002). One finding which may at first seem paradoxical is that, within those diagnosed with schizophrenia, those with a history of cannabis use are found to have superior neurocognitive functioning than those without (e.g., Yücel et al. 2012). Perhaps the most parsimonious interpretation of this at present is that the group mean effect is driven by a subgroup of cognitively less impaired and higher socially functioning individuals who only developed psychosis after a relatively early initiation into cannabis use.

One factor which recent research strongly suggests may mediate the association between cannabis and addiction, psychosis, and cognitive impairment is the type and level of cannabinoids in the cannabis an individual smokes.

36.4 **How does variation in strains of cannabis influence desired and undesired effects?**

Weed. Charis. Pot. Dagga. Ganja. Afghan Black. Purple Haze. Northern Lights. Thai Stick. Sensi. Reefer. Bhang. Skunk. Sinsemilla. Herbal. Hash. Green. These are just a few of the many names given to cannabis. Connoisseurs will discuss the pros and cons of different varieties much as a master of wine will debate grapes. Whilst these names are presumed to be partly culturally mediated, some reflect the strengths and compositions of different varieties of cannabis. What biochemically differentiates these different types is likely to be the combinations and quantities of up to around 100 cannabinoids in any strain (Pertwee 2008), perhaps the most relevant of which, as discussed earlier, are THC and CBD.

The relative THC/CBD ratio in cannabis varies greatly. Levels of CBD can range from virtually none to up to 40% (Hardwick and King 2008). Higher levels of THC and negligible levels of CBD have been found in varieties grown hydroponically under intense farming conditions. These strains known as "skunk" or sinsemilla are increasingly dominating the market in the UK, the Netherlands, and other European countries (e.g., Hardwick and King 2008).

Although high THC cannabis has become increasingly available over recent years, little is known about changes in levels of other cannabinoids as these are seldom measured. One study in the US, however, analyzed over 30,000 confiscated samples and found that between 1994 and 2004, the THC content of cannabis trebled in resin and doubled in leaf, whilst the average level of other cannabinoids, including CBD, remained unchanged (Mehmedic et al. 2005). This implies that the THC/CBD ratio has risen over recent years. However, our current knowledge of THC and CBD levels stems only from drug seizures and little is known about the ratio in "street" cannabis. Importantly, we do not know how increased THC in strains like skunk affects the individual's intake. Just as people will vary their drinking behavior according to whether a glass of colorless liquid contains water, white wine, or vodka, cannabis users may adjust their intake according to the THC content as judged by the subjective effects experienced.

In an opportunistic study, we used hair analysis to explore the impact of smoking different levels of cannabinoids on psychotic-like symptoms in a population of drug users (Morgan and Curran 2008). We hypothesized that habitual use of cannabis richer in CBD may protect people from the psychotic-like effects of THC. We found that individuals whose hair indicated that they had been habitually smoking cannabis that contained CBD (as well as THC) showed fewer psychotic-like symptoms than those whose hair showed no evidence of CBD. There are two main interpretations of this finding. First, individuals who are higher in psychosis proneness prefer and selectively choose to smoke cannabis which is higher in THC and lacking CBD. There is some tentative evidence for this interpretation (di Forti et al. 2009). Second, CBD may reduce the capacity of THC to induce psychotic-like symptoms in recreational cannabis users.

A subsequent study designed to contrast these two interpretations ruled out the former interpretation (Morgan et al. 2012b). We found differences only between daily and less than daily recreational users in preference for cannabis, with daily users preferring to smoke strains with a high THC content. This probably reflects the development of tolerance to cannabis and subsequent need to use more potent forms to maintain the same psychological effect. In fact, when asked about their preference for different strains, there were no differences between the CBD present and CBD absent groups. Further, recreational users generally showed a greater preference for strains other than the high-THC, low-CBD form of cannabis known as "skunk" or sinsemilla. We found that individuals with greater psychotic like symptoms expressed a greater preference for non-skunk strains (Morgan et al. 2012b). Of the 412 samples analyzed, 75% were skunk whereas only 34% of the 412 cannabis users assessed preferred skunk to higher CBD varieties. The dominance of skunk in our community sample is similar to that estimated from cannabis seizures in the UK which was 80% in 2008 (Hardwick and King 2009), a marked rise from 55% in 2004/2005 (Potter et al. 2008) and 30% in 2002 (King et al. 2005). Worryingly this data suggests that the market in some countries like the UK as well as the Netherlands (Pijlman et al. 2005) is increasingly dominated by skunk.

Recently we investigated the acute impact of different levels of cannabinoids by taking samples of cannabis actually smoked by users and relating these to the acute effects of the drug taken in a naturalistic environment. These studies showed that acutely smoking cannabis with higher levels of CBD protects users against the memory impairing effects of THC (Morgan et al. 2010b). Thus the presence of CBD in cannabis, at a level that did not affect cannabis-induced psychotic-like symptoms, prevented memory impairment and also reduced anxiety levels. Further we found that the presence of CBD in an individual's cannabis reduced "attentional bias" toward not only cannabis-related cues but also food stimuli (Morgan et al. 2010a). So although the presence of CBD had no effect on how stoned or "high" participants felt, it did prevent the ability of acute THC to grab the individual's attention toward drug- and food-related pictures. These findings concur with recent preclinical findings that suggest CBD may reduce the salience of drug cues (Ren et al. 2009) and findings in healthy human volunteers that suggest that CBD and THC may have opposing effects on some of the neural substrates of human memory (Bhattacharyya et al. 2010). As memory function can impact on educational and vocational achievement, it is important to determine whether these acute, protective effects of CBD on memory might also be seen longer term.

36.5 **Conclusions**

Cannabis has been used for thousands of years for its desired effects, which include a range of clinical and medicinal properties as well as the psychological and social effects valued by recreational users. This use can carry a penalty: a range of undesired effects that vary in the severity of their impact on the life of the individual. Although evidence of clear causality is lacking, these undesired effects span mild cognitive impairment, to perhaps the most disabling of all psychiatric disorders, schizophrenia. However both medical and recreational users of cannabis often seem to rate the benefits as outweighing the risks in choosing to continue their cannabis use. Both desired and undesired effects of cannabis will depend on a range of factors including an individual's level of cannabis use, personality (psychosis-proneness), mental health status, the particular cannabinoids ingested (especially THC and CBD), the relative dosages of these cannabinoids, the frequency of cannabis ingestion, and the periods over the individual's life span in which this ingestion occurs.

Young people, especially those more likely to be vulnerable to psychosis or addiction for genetic and/or environmental reasons, should be clearly warned of the greater harms of smoking high-THC, low-CBD strains of cannabis such as "skunk." The therapeutic potential of the many cannabinoids present in cannabis plants is tantalizing. Taken in the context of research on the acute and chronic effects of THC and CBD in cannabis that users smoke naturalistically, there is great promise for one or more of those cannabinoids to be potential treatments, even for some of the undesired mental health effects of cannabis itself.

Acknowledgments

This work was supported by grants to HVC and CJAM from the UK Medical Research Council and European College of Neuropsychopharmacology. The authors have no conflict of interest. The authors thank Sharinjeet Dhiman for her kind help in the preparation of this chapter. They also would like to thank all the cannabis users who took part in their studies and the UK Home Office and the ex-Forensic Science Service for their support of the aims of their research.

References

Agrawal, A., Grant, J.D., and Waldron, M. (2006). Risk for initiation of substance use as a function of age of onset of cigarette, alcohol and cannabis use: findings in a Midwestern female twin cohort. *Preventative Medicine*, **43**, 125–128.

Albrecht, D.S., Skosnik, P.D., Vollmer, J.M., *et al.* (2013). Striatal D_2/D_3 receptor availability is inversely correlated with cannabis consumption in chronic marijuana users. *Drug and Alcohol Dependence*, **128**, 52–57.

Barkus, E., Morrison, P.D., Vuletic, D., *et al.* (2011). Does intravenous Δ9-tetrahydrocannabinol increase dopamine release? A SPET study. *Journal of Psychopharmacology*, **25**, 1462–1468.

Barkus, E.J., Stirling, J., Hopkins, R.S., and Lewis, S. (2006). Cannabis-induced psychosis-like experiences are associated with high schizotypy. *Psychopathology*, **39**, 175–178.

Bergamaschi, M.M., Queiroz, R.H., Chagas, M.H., *et al.* (2011). Cannabidiol reduces the anxiety induced by simulated public speaking in treatment-naive social phobia patients. *Neuropsychopharmacology*, **36**, 1219–1226.

Bhattacharyya, S., Morrison, P.D., Fusar-Poli, P., *et al.* (2010). Opposite effects of delta-9-tetrahydrocannabinol and cannabidiol on human brain function and psychopathology. *Neuropsychopharmacology*, **35**, 764–774.

Block, R.I., O'Leary, D.S., Hichwa, R.D., *et al.* (2002). Effects of frequent marijuana use on memory related regional cerebral blood flow. *Pharmacology, Biochemistry, and Behavior*, **72**, 237–250.

Bloomfield, M.A.P, Morgan, C.J.A., Egerton, A., Kapur, S., Curran, H.V., and Howes, O.D. (2014). Dopaminergic function in cannabis users and its relationship to cannabis-induced psychotic symptoms. *Biological Psychiatry*, **75**, 470–478.

Bossong, M.G., van Berckel, B.N., Boellaard, R., *et al.* (2009). Delta-9-tetrahydrocannabinol induces dopamine release in the human striatum. *Neuropsychopharmacology*, **34**, 759–766.

Bourassa, M. and Vaugeois, P. (2001). Effects of marijuana use on divergent thinking. *Creativity Research Journal*, **13**, 411–416.

Budney, A.J. and Hughes, J.R. (2006). The cannabis withdrawal syndrome. *Current Opinion in Psychiatry*, **19**, 233–238.

Campos, A.C., Moreira, F.A., Gomes, F.V., Del Bel, E.A., and Guimarães, F.S. (2012). Multiple mechanisms involved in the large-spectrum therapeutic potential of cannabidiol in psychiatric disorders. *Philosophical Transactions of the Royal Society. Series B, Biological Sciences*, **367**, 3364–3378.

Carter, G.T. and Ugalde, V. (2004). Medical marijuana: emerging applications for the management of neurologic disorders. *Physical Medicine and Rehabilitation Clinics of North America*, **15**, 943–954.

Caspi, A., Moffitt, T.E., and Cannon, M. (2005). Moderation of the effect of adolescent-onset cannabis use on adult psychosis by a functional polymorphism in the catechol-O methyltransferase gene: longitudinal evidence of a gene X environment interaction. *Biological Psychiatry*, **15**, 1117–1127.

Curran, H.V., Brignell, C., Fletcher, S., Middleton, P., and Henry, J. (2002). Cognitive and subjective dose-response effects of acute oral Delta 9-tetrahydrocannabinol (THC) in infrequent cannabis users. *Psychopharmacology (Berlin)*, **164**, 61–70.

Das, R.K., Ramadas, M., Yogan, K., *et al.* (2013). Cannabidiol enhances consolidation of fear extinction in humans. *Psychopharmacology (Berlin)*, **226**, 781–792.

Degenhardt, L., Coffey, C., Romaniuk, H., *et al.* (2013). The persistence of the association between adolescent cannabis use and common mental disorders into young adulthood. *Addiction*, **108**, 124–133.

Di Forti, M., Iyegbe, C., Sallis H., *et al.* (2012). Confirmation that the AKT1 (rs2494732) genotype influences the risk of psychosis in cannabis users. *Biological Psychiatry*, **72**, 811–816.

Di Forti, M., Morgan, C., Dazzan, P., *et al.* (2009). High-potency cannabis and the risk of psychosis. *British Journal of Psychiatry*, **195**, 488–491.

Di Forti, M., Morrison, P.D., Butt, A., and Murray, R.M. (2007). Cannabis use and psychiatric and cognitive disorders: the chicken or the egg? *Current Opinion in Psychiatry*, **20**, 228–234.

D'Souza, D.C., Perry, E., MacDougall, L., *et al.* (2004). The psychotomimetic effects of intravenous delta-9-tetrahydrocannabinol in healthy individuals: implications for psychosis. *Neuropsychopharmacology*, **29**, 1558–1572.

D'Souza, D.C., Pittman, B., Perry, E., and Simen, A. (2009). Preliminary evidence of cannabinoid effects on brain-derived neurotrophic factor (BDNF) levels in humans. *Psychopharmacology (Berlin)*, **202**, 569–578.

D'Souza, D.C., Ranganathan, M., Braley G., *et al.* (2008). Blunted psychotomimetic and amnestic effects of Delta-9-tetrahydrocannabinol in frequent users of cannabis. *Neuropsychopharmacology*, **33**, 2505–2516.

European Monitoring Centre for Drugs and Drug Addiction. (2011). *Annual Report on the State of the Drugs Problem in Europe*. Lisbon: EMCDDA.

Fergusson, D.M. and Horwood, L.J. (2000). Does cannabis use encourage other forms of illicit drug use? *Addiction*, **95**, 505–520.

Freeman, T.P., Morgan, C.J.A.M., and Curran, H.V. (2012). Drug-cue induced overshadowing: selective disruption of natural reward processing by cigarette cues amongst abstinent but not satiated smokers. *Psychological Medicine* **42**, 161–171.

Gingold, A. (1982). *Our Own Marijuana*. New York: Avon Books.

Giuffrida, A., Leweke, M., Gerth, C.W., *et al.* (2004). Cerebrospinal anandamide levels are elevated in acute schizophrenia and are inversely correlated with psychotic symptoms. *Neuropsychopharmacology*, **29**, 2108–2114.

Gonzalez, R. (2007). Acute and non-acute effects of cannabis on brain functioning and neuropsychological performance. *Neuropsychology Review*, **17**, 347–361.

González, R., Carey, C., and Grant, I. (2002). Nonacute (residual) neuropsychological effects of cannabis use: a qualitative analysis and systematic review. *Journal of Clinical Pharmacology*, **42**(11 Suppl.), 48S–57S.

González, S., Cascio, M.G., Fernández-Ruiz, J., Fezza, F., Di Marzo, V., and Ramos, J.A. (2002). Changes in endocannabinoid contents in the brain of rats chronically exposed to nicotine, ethanol or cocaine. *Brain Research*, **954**, 73–81.

Green, B., Kavanagh, D., and Young, R. (2003). Being stoned: a review of self-reported cannabis effects. *Drug and Alcohol Review*, **22**, 453–460.

Grinspoon, L. and Bakalar, J. (1993). *Marihuana, the Forbidden Medicine*. New Haven, CT: Yale University Press.

Guimares, F.S., Chiaretti, T.M., and Graeff, F.G. (1990). Antianxiety effects of cannabidiol in the elevated plus-maze. *Psychopharmacology (Berlin)*, **100**, 558–559.

Gurley, R.J., Aranow, R., and Katz, M. (1998). Medicinal marijuana: a comprehensive review. *Journal of Psychoactive Drugs*, **30**, 137–147.

Hall, W. and Degenhardt, L. (2007). Prevalence and correlates of cannabis use in developed and developing countries. *Current Opinion in Psychiatry*, **20**, 393–397.

Hardwick, S. and King, L.A. (2008). *Home Office Cannabis Potency Study*. St Albans: Home Office Scientific Development Branch.

Henquet, C., Murray, R., Linszen, D., and van Os, J. (2005). The environment and schizophrenia: the role of cannabis use. *Schizophrenia Bulletin*, **31**, 608–612.

Hermann, D., Sartorius, A., Welzel, H., *et al.* (2007). Dorsolateral prefrontal cortex N-acetylaspartate/total creatine (NAA/tCr) loss in male recreational cannabis users. *Biological Psychiatry*, **61**, 1281–1289.

King, L.A., Carpentier, C., and Griffiths, P. (2005). Cannabis potency in Europe. *Addiction*, **100**, 884–886.

Klosterkotter, J. Hellmich, M., Steinmeyer, E.M., and Schultze-Lutter, F. (2001). Diagnosing schizophrenia in the initial prodromal phase. *Archives of General Psychiatry*, **58**, 158–164.

Koethe, D., Giuffrida, A., Schreiber, D., *et al.* (2009). Anandamide elevation in cerebrospinal fluid in initial prodromal states of psychosis. *British Journal of Psychiatry*, **194**, 371–372.

Levin, F.R., Mariani, J., Brooks, D.J., *et al.* (2013). A randomized double-blind, placebo controlled trial of venlafaxine-extended release for co-occurring cannabis dependence and depressive disorders. *Addiction*, **108**, 1084–1094.

Leweke, F.M., Giuffrida, A., Wurster, U., *et al.* (1999). Elevated endogenous cannabinoids in schizophrenia. *NeuroReport*, **10**, 1665–1669.

Leweke, F.M., Giuffrida, A., Koethe D., *et al.* (2007). Anandamide levels in cerebrospinal fluid of first-episode schizophrenic patients: impact of cannabis use. *Schizophrenia Research*, **94**, 29–36.

Leweke, F.M., Piomelli, D., Pahlisch, F., *et al.* (2012). Cannabidiol enhances anandamide signaling and alleviates psychotic symptoms of schizophrenia. *Translational Psychiatry*, **2**, e94.

Linszen, D. and van Amelsvoort, T. (2007). Cannabis and psychosis: an update on course and biological plausible mechanisms. *Current Opinion in Psychiatry*, **20**, 116–120.

Lu, L., Fielding, A., Janicheck, J., Francese, C., Curran, H.V., and Morgan, C.J.A. (in preparation). Patients' perception of the effectiveness of medical marijuana: impact of different cannabinoids.

Mason, B.J., Crean, R., Goodell, V., *et al.* (2012). A proof-of-concept randomized controlled study of gabapentin: effects on cannabis use, withdrawal and executive function deficits in cannabis-dependent adults. *Neuropsychopharmacology*, **37**, 1689–1698.

Mason, O., Morgan, C.J., Dhiman, S.K., *et al.* (2009). Acute cannabis use causes increased psychotomimetic experiences in individuals prone to psychosis. *Psychological Medicine*, **39**, 951–956.

McGrath, J., Welham, J., Scott, J., *et al.* (2010). Association between cannabis use and psychosis-related outcomes using sibling pair analysis in a cohort of young adults. *Archives of General Psychiatry*, **67**, 440–447.

Mehmedic, Z., Martin, J., Foster, S. and ElSohly, M.A. (2005). Δ9-THC and other cannabinoids content of confiscated marijuana: potency trends, 1994–2004. In: *International Association for Cannabis as Medicine (IACM) 3rd conference on Cannabinoids in Medicine*. Leiden: IACM.

Meier, M.H., Caspi, A., and Ambler, A. (2012). Persistent cannabis users show neuropsychological decline from childhood to midlife. *Proceedings of the National Academy of Sciences of the United States of America*, **109**, E2657–E2664.

Melis, M. and Pistis, M. (2012). Hub and switches: endocannabinoid signalling in midbrain dopamine neurons. *Philosophical Transactions of the Royal Society. Series B, Biological Sciences*, **367**, 3276–3285.

Miettunen, J., Törmänen, S., Murray G.K., *et al.* (2008). Association of cannabis use with prodromal symptoms of psychosis in adolescence. *British Journal of Psychiatry*, **192**, 470–471.

Moore, T.H., Zammit, S., Lingford-Hughes, A., *et al.* (2007). Cannabis use and risk of psychotic or affective mental health outcomes: a systematic review. *Lancet*, **370**, 319–328.

Moreira, F.A. and Wotjak, C.T. (2010). Cannabinoids and anxiety. *Current Topics in Behavioral Neurosciences*, **2**, 429–450.

Morgan, C.J., Duffin, S., Hunt, S., Monaghan, L., Mason, O., and Curran, H.V. (2012a). Neurocognitive function and schizophrenia-proneness in individuals dependent on ketamine, on high potency cannabis ('skunk') or on cocaine. *Pharmacopsychiatry*, **45**, 269–74.

Morgan, C.J., Freeman, T.P., Schafer, G.L., and Curran, H.V. (2010a). Cannabidiol attenuates the appetitive effects of Delta(9)-tetrahydrocannabinol in humans smoking their chosen cannabis. *Neuropsychopharmacology*, **35**, 1879–1885.

Morgan, C.J., Noronha, L.A., Muetzelfeldt, M., Fielding, A., and Curran, H.V. (2013b). Harms and benefits associated with psychoactive drugs: findings of an international survey of active drug users. *Journal of Psychopharmacology*, **27**, 497–506.

Morgan, C.J., Rothwell, E., Atkinson, H., Mason, O., and Curran, H.V. (2010c). Hyper-priming in cannabis users: a naturalistic study of the effects of cannabis on semantic memory function. *Psychiatry Research*, **176**, 213–218.

Morgan, C.J., Schafer, G., Freeman, T.P., and Curran, H.V. (2010b). Impact of cannabidiol on the acute memory and psychotomimetic effects of smoked cannabis: naturalistic study. British *Journal of Psychiatry*, **197**, 285–290.

Morgan, C.J.A. and Curran, H.V. (2008). Effects of cannabidiol on schizophrenia-like symptoms in cannabis users. *British Journal of Psychiatry*, **192**, 306–307.

Morgan, C.J.A., Das, R.K., Joye, A., Curran, H.V. and Kamboj, S.K. (2013a). Cannabidiol reduces cigarette consumption in tobacco smokers: preliminary findings. *AddictiveBehaviors*, **38**, 2433–2436

Morgan, C.J.A., Gardener, C., Schafer, G., *et al.* (2012b). Sub-chronic impact of cannabinoids in street cannabis on cognition, psychotic-like symptoms and psychological well-being. *Psychological Medicine*, **42**, 391–400.

Morgan, C.J.A., Page, E., Schaefer, C., *et al.* (2013). Cerebrospinal fluid anandamide levels, cannabis use and psychotic-like symptoms. *British Journal of Psychiatry*, **202**, 381–382.

Pan, B., Hillard, C.J., and Liu, Q.S. (2008). Endocannabinoid signaling mediates cocaine-induced inhibitory synaptic plasticity in midbrain dopamine neurons. *Journal of Neuroscience*, **28**, 1385–1397.

Pertwee, R.G. (2008). The diverse CB_1 and CB_2 receptor pharmacology of three plant cannabinoids: delta9-tetrahydrocannabinol, cannabidiol and delta9-tetrahydrocannabivarin. *British Journal of Pharmacology*, **153**, 199–215.

Pijlman, F.T., Rigter, S.M., Hoek, J., Goldschmidt, H.M., and Niesink, R.J. (2005). Strong increase in total delta-THC in cannabis preparations sold in Dutch coffee shops. *Addiction Biology*, **10**, 171–180.

Pope, H.G. Jr., Gruber, A.J., Hudson, J.I., Huestis, M.A., and Yurgelun-Todd, D. (2005). Neuropsychological performance in long-term cannabis users. *Archive of General Psychiatry*, **58**, 909–915.

Potter, D.J., Clark, P., and Brown, M.B. (2008). Potency of delta 9-THC and other cannabinoids in cannabis in England in 2005: implications for psychoactivity and pharmacology. *Journal of Forensic Sciences*, **53**, 90–94.

Ranganathan, M. and D'Souza, D.C. (2006). The acute effects of cannabinoids on memory in humans: a review. *Psychopharmacology (Berlin)*, **188**, 425–444.

Ren, Y., Whittard, J., Higuera-Matas, A., Morris, C.V., and Hurd, Y.L. (2009). Cannabidiol, a nonpsychotropic component of cannabis, inhibits cue-induced heroin seeking and normalizes discrete mesolimbic neuronal disturbances. *The Journal of Neuroscience*, **29**, 14764–14769.

Rogeberg, O. (2013). Correlations between cannabis use and IQ change in the Dunedin cohort are consistent with confounding from socioeconomic status. *Proceedings of the National Academy of Sciences of the United States of America*, **110**, 4251–4254.

Schacht, J.P., Hutchison, K.E., and Filbey, F.M. (2012). Associations between cannabinoid receptor-1 (CNR1) variation and hippocampus and amygdala volumes in heavy cannabis users. *Neuropsychopharmacology*, **37**, 2368–2376.

Schafer, G., Feilding, A., Morgan, C.J., Agathangelou, M., Freeman, T.P., and Curran H.V. (2012). Investigating the interaction between schizotypy, divergent thinking and cannabis use. *Consciousness and Cognition*, **21**, 292–298.

Schier, A.R., Ribeiro, N.P., Silva, A.C., *et al.* (2012). Cannabidiol, a *Cannabis sativa* constituent, as an anxiolytic drug. *Revista Brasileira de Psiquiatria*, **34**(Suppl.1), 104–111.

Serrano, A. and Parsons, L.H. (2011). Endocannabinoid influence in drug reinforcement, dependence and addiction-related behaviors. *Pharmacology & Therapeutics*, **132**, 215–241.

Sevy, S., Smith, G.S, Ma, Y., *et al.* (2008). Cerebral glucose metabolism and D_2/D_3 receptor availability in young adults with cannabis dependence measured with positron emission tomography. *Psychopharmacology (Berlin)*, **197**, 549–556.

Solowij, N. and Battisti, R. (2008). The chronic effects of cannabis on memory in humans: a review. *Current Drug Abuse Reviews*, **1**, 81–98.

Solowij, N., Jones, K.A., Rozman, M.E., *et al.* (2011). Verbal learning and memory in adolescent cannabis users, alcohol users and non-users. *Psychopharmacology (Berlin)*, **216**, 131–144.

Solowij, N., Walterfang, M., Lubman, D.I., *et al.* (2013). Alteration to hippocampal shape in cannabis users with and without schizophrenia. *Schizophrenia Research*, **143**, 179–184.

Stern, C.A., Gazarini, L., Takahashi, R.N., Guimarães, F.S., and Bertoglio, L.J. (2012). On disruption of fear memory by reconsolidation blockade: evidence from cannabidiol treatment. *Neuropsychopharmacology*, **37**, 2132–2142.

Stokes, P.R., Egerton, A., Watson, B., *et al.* (2012). History of cannabis use is not associated with alterations in striatal dopamine D_2/D_3 receptor availability. *Journal of Psychopharmacology*, **26**, 144–149.

Stokes, P.R., Mehta, M.A., Curran, H.V., Breen, G., and Grasby, P.M. (2009). Can recreational doses of THC produce significant dopamine release in the human striatum? *Neuroimage*, **48**, 186–190.

Taylor, B. (1854). *The Lands of the Saracen*. New York: Putnam.

Tyler, A. (1986) *Street Drugs*. London: New English Library

Tyndale, R.F., Payne, J.I., Gerber, A.L., and Sipe, J.C. (2007). The fatty acid amide hydrolase C385A (P129T) missense variant in cannabis users: studies of drug use and dependence in Caucasians. *American Journal of Medical Genetics*, **44B**, 660–666.

Ujike, H., Takaki, M., Nakata, K., *et al.* (2002). CNR1, central cannabinoid receptor gene, associated with susceptibility to hebephrenic schizophrenia. *Molecular Psychiatry*, **7**, 515–518.

United Nations Office on Drugs and Crime. (2009). *World Drug Report 2009*. New York: United Nations.

United Nations Office on Drugs and Crime. (2010). *World Drug Report 2010*. New York: United Nations.

Verdoux, H., Gindre, C., Sorbara, F., Tournier, M., and Swendsen, J.D. (2003).Effects of cannabis and psychosis vulnerability in daily life: an experience sampling test study. *Psychological Medicine*, **33**, 23–32.

Volkow, N.D., Fowler, J.S., Wang, G.J., Swanson, J.M., and Telang, F. (2007). Dopamine in drug abuse and addiction: results of imaging studies and treatment implications. *Archives of Neurology*, **64**, 1575–1579.

Williams, H.J., Glaser, B., Williams, N.M., Norton, N., and Zammit, S. (2005). No association between schizophrenia and polymorphisms in COMT in two large samples. *The American Journal of Psychiatry*, **162**, 1736–1738.

Wittchen, H.U., Jacobi, F., Rehm, J., *et al.* (2011). The size and burden of mental disorders and other disorders of the brain in Europe 2010. *European Neuropsychopharmacology*, **21**, 655–679.

Yücel, M., Bora, E., Lubman, D.I., *et al.* (2012). The impact of cannabis use on cognitive functioning in patients with schizophrenia: a meta-analysis of existing findings and new data in a first-episode sample. *Schizophrenia Bulletin*, **38**, 316–330.

Zalesky, A., Solowij, N., Yücel, M., *et al.* (2012). Effect of long-term cannabis use on axonal fibre connectivity. *Brain*, **135**, 2245–2255.

Zammit, S., Owen, M.J., Evans, J., Heron, J., and Lewis, G. (2011). Cannabis, COMT and psychotic experiences. *British Journal of Psychiatry*, **199**, 380–385.

Zammit, S., Spurlock, G., Williams, H., *et al.* (2007). Genotype effects of CHRNA7, CNR1 and COMT in schizophrenia: interactions with tobacco and cannabis use. *British Journal of Psychiatry*, **191**, 402–407.

Zhu, H.J., Wang, J.S., Markowitz, J.S., *et al.* (2006). Characterization of P-glycoprotein inhibition by major cannabinoids from marijuana. *Journal of Pharmacology and Experimental Therapeutics*, **317**, 850–857.

Chapter 37

Recreational Cannabis: The Risk of Schizophrenia

Paul D. Morrison, Sagnik Bhattacharyya, and Robin M. Murray

37.1 Introduction

Cannabis is the most widely used illicit drug in the world. Various preparations are available including traditional hash resin and marijuana as well as more potent products such as sinsemilla (often termed "skunk"). The increasing availability of the latter product caused alarm in the media although this has now been largely superseded by concern over the so-called "legal highs," a range of substances, which can be purchased online, that includes stimulants as well as synthetic cannabinoids (sometimes termed "spice") containing HU-210, JWH-018, etc. (Gunderson et al. 2012). The main worry regarding the recreational use of cannabinoids (herbal or synthetic) is the risk to users' mental health, specifically the risk of psychotic illness (Hall 2006).

37.2 Cannabis use, transient psychosis, and the onset of schizophrenia

It has long been known that, in some users, cannabis/tetrahydrocannabinol (THC) intoxication can elicit an acute paranoid psychosis (Murray et al. 2007). This is beyond doubt, appearing in the ancient Chinese and Indian medical texts, the writings of Baudelaire and Moreau from the nineteenth century, and latterly, in formal laboratory- or community-based experimental studies (D'Souza et al. 2004, 2005; Henquet et al. 2006; Morrison et al. 2009; Verdoux et al. 2003). There is also no doubt that cannabis use can worsen the course of a pre-existing chronic psychotic disorder, with a recurrence or worsening of positive symptoms (hallucinations and delusions) and further hospitalization (Bahorik et al. 2013; Degenhardt et al. 2007; Foti et al. 2010; Grech et al. 2005; Hides et al. 2006; Wobrock et al. 2013). And it is now clear from numerous studies that patients with schizophrenia who have a history of cannabis use have their first psychotic breakdown at an earlier age, compared to those who did not use the drug (Barnes et al. 2006; Barrigon et al. 2010; Buhler et al. 2002; Dekker et al. 2012; Gonzalez-Pinto et al. 2008; Myles et al. 2012; Sugranyes et al. 2009; Tosato et al. 2013; Veen et al. 2004), by 2.7 years on average (Large et al. 2011). This is not merely a statistical point because the earlier a psychosis emerges the worse is the outcome (Lauronen et al. 2007). Where there has been some controversy is around the issue of whether cannabis can actually cause schizophrenia *in the first place* (Gage et al. 2013).

37.2.1 Cannabis use and schizophrenia

Epidemiological surveys conducted in numerous countries, since the late 1980s, have been consistent in showing an association between cannabis use and psychotic symptoms/schizophrenia

(Andreasson et al. 1987; Arseneault et al. 2002; Callaghan et al. 2012; Ferdinand et al. 2005; Fergusson et al. 2005; Henquet et al. 2005b; Rossler et al. 2012; Tien and Anthony 1990; van Os et al. 2002; Weiser et al. 2002; Zammit et al. 2002). *But* an association is not the same as causation. Alternative explanations, at least in theory, are reverse causality (i.e., that people with an existing psychosis are more likely to use cannabis, *perhaps as self-medication*) and confounding (e.g. cannabis is merely a marker for a "true" causative agent, *perhaps the use of another drug such as amphetamine*) (Zammit et al. 2012).

Regarding the issue of reverse causality, in longitudinal follow-up studies, where the temporal relationship between cannabis use and schizophrenia can be assessed with some confidence, the most consistent finding is that cannabis use predates the onset of psychosis (Castle 2013; Zammit et al. 2012). Regarding confounding, all of the longitudinal studies to date have made allowances, by incorporating factors such as amphetamine use into the statistical model (Castle 2013; Zammit et al. 2012). The general finding is that the incorporation of these putative confounders reduces the strength of the association between cannabis and schizophrenia, but that the association remains (and remains statistically significant) (Zammit et al. 2012). In theory, it is possible that residual confounding persists, and that an unknown factor "drives" the relationship—but there are no suggestions as to what this unknown factor could be (Gage et al. 2013).

37.2.2 Cannabis and schizophrenia: the strength of the relationship

The strength of the association between cannabis and schizophrenia is best framed in terms of an odds ratio. Overall, taking an average of the recent studies, it has been found that cannabis use approximately doubles the odds of developing schizophrenia (Arseneault et al. 2004; Casadio et al, 2011; Henquet et al. 2005a; Moore et al. 2007). Importantly, however, there appears to be a dose–response relationship, in that the more extensive the use of cannabis, the higher the risk. The Swedish conscript study showed this clearly; for those men that reported having taken cannabis on over 50 occasions by age 18 years, the odds of developing a schizophrenic illness increased from ×2 (in those who endorsed ever having taken cannabis) to ×7 (Zammit et al. 2002). A recent study from Di Forti and colleagues also found a clear relationship between the frequency of cannabis use and the chances of developing a psychotic illness (Di Forti et al. 2009).

37.2.3 Cannabis is a risk factor for schizophrenia

It has been pointed out repeatedly, that the use of cannabis is neither necessary nor sufficient for the development of schizophrenia. *People can develop schizophrenia having never taken cannabis, and millions of people worldwide have used cannabis without developing a major mental illness.* But the same can be said for cigarettes and lung cancer (where the risk is much higher). It is perhaps more useful to consider cannabis use as a risk factor (or component cause) for major mental illness, in the same way that there are risk factors for cardiovascular disease, such as high-fat diet, cigarette smoking, etc. (Castle 2013).

37.2.3.1 Interactions between cannabis use and other risk factors for schizophrenia

A major theme has been to clarify which additional factors interact with cannabis to confer risk. Some studies have investigated the interaction between cannabis and known environmental risk factors (such as being brought up in an urban versus a rural setting, or having a history of maltreatment in childhood) (van Os et al. 2010). In general, an additive effect has been observed between cannabis use and these other risk factors, but whether it is super-additive (synergistic) remains uncertain (Harley et al. 2010; Houston et al. 2008, 2011; Konings et al. 2012; Kuepper et al. 2011).

37.2.3.2 Cannabis use and susceptibility genes

Why only a minority of cannabis users develop psychosis has attracted a lot of attention. It is suspected that particular genetic variants modulate the risk of cannabis for users in terms of psychosis outcomes. Polymorphic variations in dopamine components and in postdopamine signaling have attracted the most interest. Initial work implicated an interaction between cannabis and a functional polymorphism in the gene for catechol-O-methyltransferase (COMT) (Caspi et al. 2005), and this interaction received support in laboratory- and community-based experimental studies (Henquet et al. 2006, 2009). However, two further epidemiological studies have been negative (Zammit et al. 2007, 2011).

More recently two independent groups have observed an interaction between cannabis and polymorphic variation at rs2494732 in the gene for the intracellular enzyme AKT1. This is an intermediate between neurotrophin receptors and mRNA translation within dendritic spines, and is involved in postdopamine receptor signaling on the pathway to GSK3Beta. Both studies found that, *in conjunction with cannabis use*, people who had the CC (cytosine, cytosine) genotype at rs2494732 were twice as likely as those with the TT (thymine, thymine) genotype to develop a psychotic disorder (Di Forti et al. 2012; van Winkel et al. 2011).

37.2.4 The age of cannabis onset

The risk of cannabis in terms of adverse mental health outcomes also depends on the age when the subject begins to use cannabis. There appears to be a higher risk for use that starts in early/mid adolescence compared to use that begins in adulthood (Arseneault et al. 2002; McGrath et al. 2010; Schubart et al. 2011b). An appealing explanation is that cannabis impacts upon the developing neural networks. Some animal studies, but not all (O'Shea et al. 2006), support the idea that the sustained adverse consequences of cannabinoid receptor type 1 (CB_1) agonists on cognition and social interaction arise if the drug is administered during maturation as opposed to adulthood (O'Shea et al. 2004; Quinn et al. 2008; Schneider and Koch 2003). Certainly, and perhaps to an even greater extent in higher primates, there is a massive reorganization of the nervous system in adolescence. In humans, the reorganization of synapses occurs in parallel with the development of abstract reasoning, and the emergence of social, philosophical, political, and lifestyle attitudes (Citri and Malenka 2008). The implication is that cannabis has the ability to disrupt the unfolding of the highest faculties of the nervous system, increasing the chances of future involvement with mental health services. The long-term impact of cannabis on IQ also appears to be age dependent.

A recent longitudinal follow-up of the Dunedin birth cohort to age 38 has suggested that cannabis use has a detrimental effect on IQ and that this is also age dependent. And again it is the adolescent period that appears to constitute the window of greatest vulnerability (Meier et al. 2012). However, confirmation is required before we can accept this striking finding.

37.2.5 The type of cannabis

Recent epidemiological studies have begun to explore the nuances of the cannabis–schizophrenia relationship in more detail. One question in particular is whether sinsemilla—high THC: negligible cannabidiol (CBD) (Potter et al. 2008)—constitutes a higher risk for psychosis than traditional cannabis products. This appears to be the case. A study from South London showed that patients in the midst of their first psychotic breakdown and healthy matched controls were equally likely to endorse ever having taken cannabis, but the probability of suffering from psychotic disorder was almost seven times greater in those who had preferentially used sinsemilla (skunk) compared with those who had used resin (hash) (Di Forti et al. 2009). The higher the frequency of sinsemilla use, the higher the risk. Sinsemilla is largely devoid of CBD, which can pharmacologically antagonize some of the effects of THC (Pertwee 2008), and may have antipsychotic properties in its own right (Leweke et al. 2012), suggesting that the higher risk of sinsemilla might be partly accounted for by the absence of CBD rather than by elevated THC alone (Smith 2005). It has been argued that users of sinsemilla might self-titrate their intake of THC, much in the same way that spirit drinkers consume a lower volume of fluid than beer drinkers; however, if the critical factor is the ratio of THC:CBD, then self-titration might be less important. Two epidemiological studies have shown that the relative absence of CBD in cannabis products is associated with more positive psychotic symptoms (Morgan and Curran 2008; Schubart et al. 2011a). This is in agreement with laboratory-based studies in healthy controls in which doses of the two cannabinoids can be tightly controlled (Englund et al. 2013; Morrison et al. 2010).

37.2.6 Heavy use of cannabis and cannabis addiction

The South London study also showed that a significant proportion of the general population use cannabis (including sinsemilla) every day without obvious ill effects (Di Forti et al. 2009). Many psychiatrists in clinical practice will encounter people who freely admit to having used cannabis, all day, every day, beginning immediately on waking. Some initial reports have suggested that sinsemilla is more addictive than traditional forms of cannabis, and similar to the case with psychosis, the relative absence of CBD may be a factor (Morgan et al. 2010). Studies are now beginning to explore whether CBD has efficacy against cannabis dependence.

It is now clear that cannabis dependence exists as a phenomenon (Swift et al. 2001), and there is little doubt that a cannabis withdrawal syndrome exists, characterized by cravings, nervousness, insomnia, nightmares, irritability, and abdominal pain (Allsop et al. 2012; Hasin et al. 2008). Not surprisingly, people who experience the most severe withdrawals are much more likely to relapse and begin taking cannabis again (Allsop et al. 2012). People who are addicted to cannabis suffer poorer mental health generally *compared to nondependent users*, with elevated rates of mood disorders as well as psychotic disorders (Arias et al. 2013; van der Pol et al. 2013).

37.2.7 An acute cannabis-psychosis is a marker for the emergence of schizophrenia

People who experience an acute psychotic episode following the use of cannabis, to the extent that treatment is needed, are at high risk of going on to develop a chronic psychotic disorder (Arendt et al. 2005). In a recent study from Finland (n = 18,478), 46% (95% confidence interval (CI), 35–57%) of people who had been hospitalized for cannabis induced psychosis developed schizophrenia over the next 8 years, compared to 30% (95% CI, 14–46%) who had been hospitalized because of amphetamine-induced psychosis (Niemi-Pynttari et al. 2013). This suggests that acute psychotic experiences following cannabis are not as benign as was once believed.

37.2.8 Summary

There is little doubt that some people run into problems with cannabis, as is the case for any recreational drug. The worry in regard to cannabis is that although it is relatively safe, so many young people are consuming it that a minority end up putting their long-term mental health at risk.

Early, heavy, and dependent patterns of use clearly amplify any inherent risk of cannabis per se. Sinsemilla appears to be more habit-forming than traditional forms of cannabis, and the evidence that it constitutes an elevated risk for psychosis is now fairly robust. There may well be single nucleotide polymorphisms (SNPs) that determine how risky cannabis is (in terms of psychosis outcome) for a particular individual. Currently variation in the gene for AKT1 is the most convincing, although COMT has not been discounted. Small-scale genetic studies can be revealing but carry the danger of false positives, and at the present time, there is no genetic test that can be used clinically to estimate the risk of cannabis-addiction or cannabis-psychosis for a particular individual.

But what we can say with some confidence is that the following patterns of cannabis use put any individual at risk—particularly if the personality and mind are still maturing: (1) everyday (dependent) use and (2) the use of high-potency products. Those with a family history of psychosis or with a psychosis-prone personality appear especially at risk. Finally, a history of an acute cannabis-induced psychosis must be regarded as a "red flag" warning against further use.

37.3 Cannabis and psychosis: imaging correlates

While the evidence regarding the association between cannabis use and schizophrenia is fairly robust and the various parameters that determine this relationship are increasingly clear, delineation of the underlying mechanism is important not only for a greater degree of confidence in the nature of this relationship but also for a better understanding of the neurobiology of schizophrenia itself. The ideal approach to demonstrate this would be through naturalistic studies that prospectively delineate the effect of cannabis exposure on neural function in the substrates implicated in schizophrenia among healthy cannabis users and relate these changes to subsequent transition to psychosis. However, such studies are logistically demanding and no data currently exist that delineate the neural mechanisms underlying the increased risk for psychosis in such a precise manner. Pharmacological challenge studies involving the administration of cannabis or THC in combination with neuroimaging offer a way to reversibly model aspects of psychosis in humans and understand their neural underpinnings.

37.3.1 Electrophysiological studies

At the cellular level, animal studies have clearly shown that THC and other CB_1 agonists target glutamate and gamma-aminobutyric acid (GABA) terminals and impact upon glutamate and GABA signaling within the central nervous system (Chevaleyre et al. 2006; Katona and Freund 2012). The hippocampus has been utilized as a model system to investigate the effects of cannabinoids on fine-grained neural network behavior. Cannabinoid CB_1 agonists can disrupt the synchronization of individual neurons within the hippocampus and disrupt oscillations within the theta (4–8 Hz) and gamma (>40 Hz) range, and these effects on network electrical activity show a close correlation with functional deficits in cognitive performance (Hajos et al. 2008; Robbe et al. 2006). Electrical studies in humans are few in number, but similar findings have been observed (Bocker et al. 2010). Our group found that intravenous THC decreased the amplitude, synchronization, and consistency over time of theta oscillations in the frontal cortex with functional consequences at the level of the mind (Morrison et al. 2011; Stone et al. 2012).

37.3.2 Functional magnetic resonance imaging studies

Effects of a modest (10 mg) oral dose of THC on the blood oxygen level-dependent (BOLD) hemodynamic response have been investigated in healthy occasional cannabis users while performing verbal learning (Bhattacharyya et al. 2009) and attentional salience processing tasks (Bhattacharyya et al. 2012a). THC disrupted the normal linear decrement in medial temporal engagement while the subjects were learning new information. Furthermore, the normal relationship between medial temporal engagement and subsequent memory performance was no longer present under the influence of THC (Bhattacharyya et al. 2009). Inefficient encoding of contextual information in the parahippocampal cortex under the influence of THC appears to result in greater parahippocampal engagement in an effort to maintain subsequent memory performance. This is consistent with evidence that THC impairs medial temporal function in animals (Puighermanal et al. 2009; Robbe et al. 2006; Wise et al. 2009) and memory performance in animals and man (Curran et al. 2002; D'Souza et al. 2004; Puighermanal et al. 2009; Robbe et al. 2006; Wise et al. 2009). While the subjects were recalling learnt information, THC augmented activation in the left medial prefrontal and dorsal anterior cingulate cortex (ACC), areas that have been related to retrieval monitoring and verification (Fleck et al. 2006; Simons et al. 2005) and attenuated left rostral ACC and bilateral striatal activation. The effect of THC on striatal function was directly correlated with the severity of psychotic symptoms induced by it concurrently, suggesting that the acute induction of psychotic symptoms by THC is related to its effects on striatal function. Consistent with this, THC has been shown to attenuate activation in the right caudate during the processing of "salient" oddball stimuli relative to "nonsalient" standard stimuli (Bhattacharyya et al. 2012a). THC also reduced the response latency to standard relative to oddball stimuli, suggesting that THC may have made the nonsalient stimuli to appear relatively more salient.

In one recent study (Bhattacharyya et al. 2012b), the acute effects of THC on striatal and midbrain activation were shown to be greater in those individuals who carried the risk variants of genes modulating central dopaminergic neurotransmission, such as the AKT1 and dopamine transporter (DAT1) genes. This awaits replication.

37.3.3 **Neurochemical imaging studies**

Evidence regarding the effects of THC on central dopamine neurotransmission has been equivocal. The first human study, using positron emission tomography (PET) (Bossong et al. 2009), reported a modest increase in striatal dopamine levels as evident from an approximately 3.5% decrease in the binding of $[^{11}C]$ raclopride in the ventral striatum and precommissural dorsal putamen after THC inhalation. However, another study employing the same PET technique (Stokes et al. 2009) found no significant effect of orally administered THC on striatal $[^{11}C]$ raclopride binding; curiously, the same group (Stokes et al. 2009) reported an effect of THC on dopamine release in extrastriatal brain regions such as the lateral prefrontal cortex (Stokes et al. 2010). A more recent study using ^{123}I-iodobenzamide ($[^{123}I]$IBZM) single photon emission tomography (SPET) found no evidence of a significant effect of intravenously administered THC on indices of striatal dopamine (Barkus et al. 2011). While various factors such as different routes of administration, magnitude of previous exposure to cannabis in study participants and differing genetically moderated sensitivity to the effects of THC may account for these discrepant results, nevertheless they point towards a relatively modest effect of THC on central dopamine neurotransmission, at most, as measured using neurochemical imaging techniques. Kuepper and colleagues (personal communication) have suggested that schizophrenic patients and their relatives show a greater effect of THC on striatal dopamine, possibly reflecting their genetic vulnerability.

37.3.4 **Summary of neural mechanisms**

It is evident that THC, the phytocannabinoid that is principally linked to psychotic symptoms and disorder, has an effect on the synchronicity of neural oscillations and on brain regions such as the medial temporal and prefrontal cortex and the striatum, consistent with similar abnormalities reported in schizophrenia (Ford et al. 2007; van Os and Kapur 2009) and complementary evidence of alterations of the endocannabinoid system in schizophrenia (Marco et al. 2011). The key functional magnetic resonance imaging finding of interest regarding the neurobiological basis of the link between cannabis use and psychosis, relate to the acute effect of THC on striatal activity which were directly related to the severity of transient psychotic symptoms induced experimentally under its influence (Bhattacharyya et al. 2012a, 2012b). While the precise neurochemical mechanisms underlying these effects of THC are unclear, THC is known to alter central dopamine transmission in animals (Bossong et al. 2009; Stokes et al. 2010) and perturbed dopamine function may be a key factor in the inappropriate attribution of salience to environmental stimuli or events (Berridge 2007; Kapur et al. 2005). It is thought that striatal dopamine dysfunction leads to the development of psychotic symptoms through an effect on salience processing (Kapur 2003). Thus, one possibility is that THC present in cannabis alters the processing of salient and nonsalient stimuli and the induction of psychotic symptoms through its effects on striatal dopamine function. Another possibility, which is in agreement with animal work, is that THC disrupts the synchronized neural rhythms that depend on reciprocal glutamatergic and GABAergic connections (Ford and Mathalon 2008; Robbe et al. 2006; Uhlhaas et al. 2008) interfering with the spatiotemporal connectivity within the brain.

37.4 **Conclusions and future directions**

The majority of people who use cannabis do not develop schizophrenia. However, there is little doubt that cannabis can elicit an acute psychosis, worsens the course of pre-existing schizophrenia, and is a risk factor for the development of schizophrenia. Cannabis use beginning in adolescence, heavy use, and the use of high THC:low CBD strains are known to increase the risk whilst a transient cannabis-induced psychotic episode requiring hospitalization is a critical warning sign. Genetic variation is believed to impact on the risk of cannabis, and at present the most consistent evidence is an interaction between cannabis use and a SNP in the gene coding for the intracellular enzyme AKT1. At the synaptic cellular level and local network levels, the mechanisms of THC are well understood—disruption of glutamate and GABA signaling, and disruption of network oscillations. Disruption of oscillations has now been observed in humans using electroencephalography with functional correlates at the level of the mind. Cerebral blood flow changes in response to individual cannabinoids have been characterized under numerous cognitive demands. To date, neurochemical imaging has focused on dopamine. However, acute THC, in healthy subjects, appears to have a negligible effect on striatal dopamine release. Whether schizophrenic patients and their genetic relatives display a more sensitized dopamine system awaits demonstration.

References

Allsop, D.J., Copeland, J., Norberg, M.M., *et al.* (2012). Quantifying the clinical significance of cannabis withdrawal. *PLoS One*, **7**, e44864.

Andreasson, S., Allebeck, P., Engstrom, A., and Rydberg, U. (1987). Cannabis and schizophrenia. A longitudinal study of Swedish conscripts. *Lancet*, **2**, 1483–1486.

Arendt, M., Rosenberg, R., Foldager, L., Perto, G., and Munk-Jorgensen, P. (2005). Cannabis-induced psychosis and subsequent schizophrenia-spectrum disorders: follow-up study of 535 incident cases. *British Journal of Psychiatry*, **187**, 510–515.

Arias, F., Szerman, N., Vega, P., *et al.* (2013). Abuse or dependence on cannabis and other psychiatric disorders. Madrid study on dual pathology prevalence. *Actas Espanolas de Psiquiatria*, **41**, 122–129.

Arseneault, L., Cannon, M., Poulton, R., Murray, R., Caspi, A., and Moffitt, T.E. (2002). Cannabis use in adolescence and risk for adult psychosis: longitudinal prospective study. *British Medical Journal*, **325**, 1212–1213.

Arseneault, L., Cannon, M., Witton, J., and Murray, R.M. (2004). Causal association between cannabis and psychosis: examination of the evidence. *British Journal of Psychiatry*, **184**, 110–117.

Bahorik, A.L., Newhill, C.E., and Eack, S.M. (2013). Characterizing the longitudinal patterns of substance use among individuals diagnosed with serious mental illness after psychiatric hospitalization. *Addiction*, **108**, 1259–1269.

Barkus, E., Morrison, P.D., Vuletic, D., *et al.* (2011). Does intravenous Delta9-tetrahydrocannabinol increase dopamine release? A SPET study. *Journal of Psychopharmacology*, **25**, 1462–1468.

Barnes, T.R., Mutsatsa, S.H., Hutton, S.B., Watt, H.C., and Joyce, E.M. (2006). Comorbid substance use and age at onset of schizophrenia. *British Journal of Psychiatry*, **188**, 237–242.

Barrigon, M.L., Gurpegui, M., Ruiz-Veguilla, M., *et al.* (2010). Temporal relationship of first-episode non-affective psychosis with cannabis use: a clinical verification of an epidemiological hypothesis. *Journal of Psychiatric Research*, **44**, 413–420.

Berridge, K.C. (2007). The debate over dopamine's role in reward: the case for incentive salience. *Psychopharmacology*, **191**, 391–431.

Bhattacharyya, S., Atakan, Z., Martin-Santos, R., *et al.* (2012b). Preliminary report of biological basis of sensitivity to the effects of cannabis on psychosis: AKT1 and DAT1 genotype modulates the effects of delta-9-tetrahydrocannabinol on midbrain and striatal function. *Molecular Psychiatry*, **17**, 1152–1155.

Bhattacharyya, S., Crippa, J.A., Allen, P., *et al.* (2012a). Induction of psychosis by Delta9-tetrahydrocannabinol reflects modulation of prefrontal and striatal function during attentional salience processing. *Archives of General Psychiatry*, **69**, 27–36.

Bhattacharyya, S., Fusar-Poli, P., Borgwardt, S., *et al.* (2009). Modulation of mediotemporal and ventros-triatal function in humans by Delta9-tetrahydrocannabinol: a neural basis for the effects of *Cannabis sativa* on learning and psychosis. *Archives of General Psychiatry*, **66**, 442–451.

Bocker, K.B., Hunault, C.C., Gerritsen, J., Kruidenier, M., Mensinga, T.T., and Kenemans, J.L. (2010). Cannabinoid modulations of resting state EEG theta power and working memory are correlated in humans. *Journal of Cognitive Neuroscience*, **22**, 1906–1916.

Bossong, M.G., van Berckel, B.N., Boellaard, R., *et al.* (2009). Delta 9-tetrahydrocannabinol induces dopamine release in the human striatum. *Neuropsychopharmacology*, **34**, 759–766.

Buhler, B., Hambrecht, M., Loffler, W., an der Heiden, W., and Hafner, H. (2002). Precipitation and determination of the onset and course of schizophrenia by substance abuse – a retrospective and prospective study of 232 population-based first illness episodes. *Schizophrenia Research*, **54**, 243–251.

Callaghan, R.C., Cunningham, J.K., Allebeck, P., *et al.* (2012). Methamphetamine use and schizophrenia: a population-based cohort study in California. *American Journal of Psychiatry*, **169**, 389–396.

Casadio, P., Fernandes, C., Murray, R.M., and Di Forti M. (2011). Cannabis use in young people: the risk for schizophrenia. *Neuroscience and Biobehavioral Reviews*, **35**, 1179–1187.

Caspi, A., Moffitt, T.E., Cannon, M., *et al.* (2005). Moderation of the effect of adolescent-onset cannabis use on adult psychosis by a functional polymorphism in the catechol-O-methyltransferase gene: longitudinal evidence of a gene X environment interaction. *Biological Psychiatry*, **57**, 1117–1127.

Castle, D.J. (2013). Cannabis and psychosis: what causes what? *F1000 Med Rep*, **5**, 1.

Chevaleyre, V., Takahashi, K.A., and Castillo, P.E. (2006). Endocannabinoid-mediated synaptic plasticity in the CNS. *Annual Review of Neuroscience*, **29**, 37–76.

Citri, A. and Malenka, R. C. (2008). Synaptic plasticity: multiple forms, functions, and mechanisms. *Neuropsychopharmacology*, **33**, 18–41.

Curran, H.V., Brignell, C., Fletcher, S., Middleton, P., and Henry, J. (2002). Cognitive and subjective dose-response effects of acute oral Delta 9-tetrahydrocannabinol (THC) in infrequent cannabis users. *Psychopharmacology*, **164**, 61–70.

D'Souza, D.C., Abi-Saab, W.M., Madonick, S., *et al.* (2005). Delta-9-tetrahydrocannabinol effects in schizophrenia: implications for cognition, psychosis, and addiction. *Biological Psychiatry*, **57**, 594–608.

D'Souza, D.C., Perry, E., MacDougall, L., *et al.* (2004). The psychotomimetic effects of intravenous delta-9-tetrahydrocannabinol in healthy individuals: implications for psychosis. *Neuropsychopharmacology*, **29**, 1558–1572.

Degenhardt, L., Tennant, C., Gilmour, S., *et al.* (2007). The temporal dynamics of relationships between cannabis, psychosis and depression among young adults with psychotic disorders: findings from a 10-month prospective study. *Psychological Medicine*, **37**, 927–934.

Dekker, N., Meijer, J., Koeter, M., *et al.* (2012). Age at onset of non-affective psychosis in relation to cannabis use, other drug use and gender. *Psychological Medicine*, **42**, 1903–1911.

Di Forti, M., Iyegbe, C., Sallis, H., *et al.* (2012). Confirmation that the AKT1 (rs2494732) genotype influences the risk of psychosis in cannabis users. *Biological Psychiatry*, **72**, 811–816.

Di Forti, M., Morgan, C., Dazzan, P., *et al.* (2009). High-potency cannabis and the risk of psychosis. *British Journal of Psychiatry*, **195**, 488–491.

Englund, A., Morrison, P.D., Nottage, J., *et al.* (2013). Cannabidiol inhibits THC-elicited paranoid symptoms and hippocampal-dependent memory impairment. *Journal of Psychopharmacology*, **27**, 19–27.

Ferdinand, R.F., Sondeijker, F., van der Ende, J., Selten, J.P., Huizink, A., and Verhulst, F.C. (2005). Cannabis use predicts future psychotic symptoms, and vice versa. *Addiction*, **100**, 612–618.

Fergusson, D.M., Horwood, L.J., and Ridder, E.M. (2005). Tests of causal linkages between cannabis use and psychotic symptoms. *Addiction*, **100**, 354–366.

Fleck, M.S., Daselaar, S.M., Dobbins, I.G., and Cabeza, R. (2006). Role of prefrontal and anterior cingulate regions in decision-making processes shared by memory and nonmemory tasks. *Cerebral Cortex*, **16**, 1623–1630.

Ford, J.M., Krystal, J.H., and Mathalon, D.H. (2007). Neural synchrony in schizophrenia: from networks to new treatments. *Schizophrenia Bulletin*, **33**, 848–852.

Ford, J.M. and Mathalon, D.H. (2008). Neural synchrony in schizophrenia. *Schizophrenia Bulletin*, **34**, 904–906.

Foti, D.J., Kotov, R., Guey, L.T., and Bromet, E.J. (2010). Cannabis use and the course of schizophrenia: 10-year follow-up after first hospitalization. *American Journal of Psychiatry*, **167**, 987–993.

Gage, S.H., Zammit, S., and Hickman, M. (2013). Stronger evidence is needed before accepting that cannabis plays an important role in the aetiology of schizophrenia in the population. *F1000 Med Rep*, **5**, 2.

Gonzalez-Pinto, A., Vega, P., Ibanez, B., *et al.* (2008). Impact of cannabis and other drugs on age at onset of psychosis. *Journal of Clinical Psychiatry*, **69**, 1210–1216.

Grech, A., Van Os, J., Jones, P.B., Lewis, S.W., and Murray, R.M. (2005). Cannabis use and outcome of recent onset psychosis. *European Psychiatry*, **20**, 349–353.

Gunderson, E.W., Haughey, H.M., Ait-Daoud, N., Joshi, A.S., and Hart, C.L. (2012). "Spice" and "K2" herbal highs: a case series and systematic review of the clinical effects and biopsychosocial implications of synthetic cannabinoid use in humans. *American Journal of Addiction*, **21**, 320–326.

Hajos, M., Hoffmann, W.E., and Kocsis, B. (2008). Activation of cannabinoid-1 receptors disrupts sensory gating and neuronal oscillation: relevance to schizophrenia. *Biological Psychiatry*, **63**, 1075–1083.

Hall, W. (2006). Is cannabis use psychotogenic? *Lancet*, **367**, 193–195.

Harley, M., Kelleher, I., Clarke, M., *et al.* (2010). Cannabis use and childhood trauma interact additively to increase the risk of psychotic symptoms in adolescence. *Psychological Medicine*, **40**, 1627–1634.

Hasin, D.S., Keyes, K.M., Alderson, D., Wang, S., Aharonovich, E., and Grant, B.F. (2008). Cannabis withdrawal in the United States: results from NESARC. *Journal of Clinical Psychiatry*, **69**, 1354–1363.

Henquet, C., Krabbendam, L., Spauwen, J., *et al.* (2005b). Prospective cohort study of cannabis use, predisposition for psychosis, and psychotic symptoms in young people. *British Medical Journal*, **330**, 11–14.

Henquet, C., Murray, R., Linszen, D., and van Os, J. (2005a). The environment and schizophrenia: the role of cannabis use. *Schizophrenia Bulletin*, **31**, 608–612.

Henquet, C., Rosa, A., Delespaul, P., *et al.* (2009). COMT ValMet moderation of cannabis-induced psychosis: a momentary assessment study of 'switching on' hallucinations in the flow of daily life. *Acta Psychiatrica Scandinavica*, **119**, 156–160.

Henquet, C., Rosa, A., Krabbendam, L., *et al.* (2006). An experimental study of catechol-o-methyltransferase val(158)met moderation of delta-9-tetrahydrocannabinol-induced effects on psychosis and cognition. *Neuropsychopharmacology*, **31**, 2748–2757.

Hides, L., Dawe, S., Kavanagh, D.J., and Young, R.M. (2006). Psychotic symptom and cannabis relapse in recent-onset psychosis. Prospective study. *British Journal of Psychiatry*, **189**, 137–143.

Houston, J.E., Murphy, J., Adamson, G., Stringer, M., and Shevlin, M. (2008). Childhood sexual abuse, early cannabis use, and psychosis: testing an interaction model based on the National Comorbidity Survey. *Schizophrenia Bulletin*, **34**, 580–585.

Houston, J.E., Murphy, J., Shevlin, M., and Adamson, G. (2011). Cannabis use and psychosis: re-visiting the role of childhood trauma. *Psychological Medicine*, **41**, 2339–2348.

Kapur, S. (2003). Psychosis as a state of aberrant salience: a framework linking biology, phenomenology, and pharmacology in schizophrenia. *American Journal of Psychiatry*, **160**, 13–23.

Kapur, S., Mizrahi, R., and Li, M. (2005). From dopamine to salience to psychosis--linking biology, pharmacology and phenomenology of psychosis. *Schizophrenia Research*, **79**, 59–68.

Katona, I. and Freund, T.F. (2012). Multiple functions of endocannabinoid signaling in the brain. *Annual Review of Neuroscience*, **35**, 529–558.

Konings, M., Stefanis, N., Kuepper, R., *et al.* (2012). Replication in two independent population-based samples that childhood maltreatment and cannabis use synergistically impact on psychosis risk. *Psychological Medicine*, **42**, 149–159.

Kuepper, R., van Os, J., Lieb, R., Wittchen, H.U., and Henquet, C. (2011). Do cannabis and urbanicity co-participate in causing psychosis? Evidence from a 10-year follow-up cohort study. *Psychological Medicine*, **41**, 2121–2129.

Large, M., Sharma, S., Compton, M.T., Slade, T., and Nielssen, O. (2011). Cannabis use and earlier onset of psychosis: a systematic meta-analysis. *Archives of General Psychiatry*, **68**, 555–561.

Lauronen, E., Miettunen, J., Veijola, J., Karhu, M., Jones, P.B., and Isohanni, M. (2007). Outcome and its predictors in schizophrenia within the Northern Finland 1966 Birth Cohort. *European Psychiatry*, **22**, 129–136.

Leweke, F.M., Piomelli, D., Pahlisch, F., *et al.* (2012). Cannabidiol enhances anandamide signaling and alleviates psychotic symptoms of schizophrenia. *Translational Psychiatry*, **2**, e94.

Marco, E.M., Garcia-Gutierrez, M.S., Bermudez-Silva, F.J., *et al.* (2011). Endocannabinoid system and psychiatry: in search of a neurobiological basis for detrimental and potential therapeutic effects. *Frontiers in Behavioural Neuroscience*, **5**, 63.

McGrath, J., Welham, J., Scott, J., *et al.* (2010). Association between cannabis use and psychosis-related outcomes using sibling pair analysis in a cohort of young adults. *Archives of General Psychiatry*, **67**, 440–447.

Meier, M.H., Caspi, A., Ambler, A., *et al.* (2012). Persistent cannabis users show neuropsychological decline from childhood to midlife. *Proceedings of the National Academy of Sciences of the United States of America*, **109**, E2657–E2664.

Moore, T.H., Zammit, S., Lingford-Hughes, A., *et al.* (2007). Cannabis use and risk of psychotic or affective mental health outcomes: a systematic review. *Lancet*, **370**, 319–328.

Morgan, C.J. and Curran, H.V. (2008). Effects of cannabidiol on schizophrenia-like symptoms in people who use cannabis. *British Journal of Psychiatry*, **192**, 306–307.

Morgan, C.J., Freeman, T.P., Schafer, G.L., and Curran, H.V. (2010). Cannabidiol attenuates the appetitive effects of Delta 9-tetrahydrocannabinol in humans smoking their chosen cannabis. *Neuropsychopharmacology*, **35**, 1879–1885.

Morrison, P.D., Murray, R.M., and Kapur, S. (2010). In healthy subjects cannabidiol inhibits delta-9-tetrahydrocannabinol induced acute psychosis and tachycardia via a non-pharmacokinetic mechanism. *Journal of Psychopharmacology*, **24**, A61.

Morrison, P.D., Nottage, J., Stone, J. M., *et al.* (2011). Disruption of frontal theta coherence by Delta9-tetrahydrocannabinol is associated with positive psychotic symptoms. *Neuropsychopharmacology*, **36**, 827–836.

Morrison, P.D., Zois, V., McKeown, D.A., *et al.* (2009). The acute effects of synthetic intravenous Delta9-tetrahydrocannabinol on psychosis, mood and cognitive functioning. *Psychological Medicine*, **39**, 1607–1616.

Murray, R.M., Morrison, P.D., Henquet, C., and Di Forti, M. (2007). Cannabis, the mind and society: the hash realities. *Nature Reviews Neuroscience*, **8**, 885–895.

Myles, N., Newall, H., Nielssen, O., and Large, M. (2012). The association between cannabis use and earlier age at onset of schizophrenia and other psychoses: meta-analysis of possible confounding factors. *Current Pharmaceutical Design*, **18**, 5055–5069.

Niemi-Pynttari, J.A., Sund, R., Putkonen, H., Vorma, H., Wahlbeck, K., and Pirkola, S.P. (2013). Substance-induced psychoses converting into schizophrenia: a register-based study of 18,478 Finnish inpatient cases. *Journal of Clinical Psychiatry*, **74**, e94–e99.

O'Shea, M., McGregor, I.S., and Mallet, P.E. (2006). Repeated cannabinoid exposure during perinatal, adolescent or early adult ages produces similar longlasting deficits in object recognition and reduced social interaction in rats. *Journal of Psychopharmacology*, **20**, 611–621.

O'Shea, M., Singh, M.E., McGregor, I.S., and Mallet, P.E. (2004). Chronic cannabinoid exposure produces lasting memory impairment and increased anxiety in adolescent but not adult rats. *Journal of Psychopharmacology*, **18**, 502–508.

Pertwee, R.G. (2008). The diverse CB_1 and CB_2 receptor pharmacology of three plant cannabinoids: delta9-tetrahydrocannabinol, cannabidiol and delta9-tetrahydrocannabivarin. *British Journal of Pharmacology*, **153**, 199–215.

Potter, D.J., Clark, P., and Brown, M.B. (2008). Potency of delta 9-THC and other cannabinoids in cannabis in England in 2005: implications for psychoactivity and pharmacology. *Journal of Forensic Sciences*, **53**, 90–94.

Puighermanal, E., Marsicano, G., Busquets-Garcia, A., Lutz, B., Maldonado, R., and Ozaita, A. (2009). Cannabinoid modulation of hippocampal long-term memory is mediated by mTOR signaling. *Nature Neuroscience*, **12**, 1152–1158.

Quinn, H.R., Matsumoto, I., Callaghan, P.D., *et al.* (2008). Adolescent rats find repeated Delta(9)-THC less aversive than adult rats but display greater residual cognitive deficits and changes in hippocampal protein expression following exposure. *Neuropsychopharmacology*, **33**, 1113–1126.

Robbe, D., Montgomery, S.M., Thome, A., Rueda-Orozco, P.E., McNaughton, B.L., and Buzsaki, G. (2006). Cannabinoids reveal importance of spike timing coordination in hippocampal function. *Nature Neuroscience*, **9**, 1526–1533.

Rossler, W., Hengartner, M.P., Angst, J., and Ajdacic-Gross, V. (2012). Linking substance use with symptoms of subclinical psychosis in a community cohort over 30 years. *Addiction*, **107**, 1174–1184.

Schneider, M. and Koch, M. (2003). Chronic pubertal, but not adult chronic cannabinoid treatment impairs sensorimotor gating, recognition memory, and the performance in a progressive ratio task in adult rats. *Neuropsychopharmacology*, **28**, 1760–1769.

Schubart, C.D., Sommer, I.E., van Gastel, W.A., Goetgebuer, R.L., Kahn, R.S., and Boks, M.P. (2011a). Cannabis with high cannabidiol content is associated with fewer psychotic experiences. *Schizophrenia Research*, **130**, 216–221.

Schubart, C.D., van Gastel, W.A., Breetvelt, E.J., *et al.* (2011b). Cannabis use at a young age is associated with psychotic experiences. *Psychological Medicine*, **41**, 1301–1310.

Simons, J.S., Gilbert, S.J., Owen, A.M., Fletcher, P.C., and Burgess, P.W. (2005). Distinct roles for lateral and medial anterior prefrontal cortex in contextual recollection. *Journal of Neurophysiology*, **94**, 813–820.

Smith, N. (2005). High potency cannabis: the forgotten variable. *Addiction*, **100**, 1558–1560; author reply 1560–1561.

Stokes, P.R., Egerton, A., Watson, B., *et al.* (2010). Significant decreases in frontal and temporal [11C]-raclopride binding after THC challenge. *Neuroimage*, **52**, 1521–1527.

Stokes, P.R., Mehta, M.A., Curran, H.V., Breen, G., and Grasby, P.M. (2009). Can recreational doses of THC produce significant dopamine release in the human striatum? *Neuroimage*, **48**, 186–190.

Stone, J.M., Morrison, P.D., Brugger, S., *et al.* (2012). Communication breakdown: delta-9 tetrahydrocannabinol effects on pre-speech neural coherence. *Molecular Psychiatry*, **17**, 568–569.

Sugranyes, G., Flamarique, I., Parellada, E., *et al.* (2009). Cannabis use and age of diagnosis of schizophrenia. *European Journal of Psychiatry*, **24**, 282–286.

Swift, W., Hall, W., and Teesson, M. (2001). Characteristics of DSM-IV and ICD-10 cannabis dependence among Australian adults: results from the National Survey of Mental Health and Wellbeing. *Drug and Alcohol Dependence*, **63**, 147–153.

Tien, A.Y. and Anthony, J.C. (1990). Epidemiological analysis of alcohol and drug use as risk factors for psychotic experiences. *Journal of Nervous and Mental Disease*, **178**, 473–480.

Tosato, S., Lasalvia, A., Bonetto, C., *et al.* (2013). The impact of cannabis use on age of onset and clinical characteristics in first-episode psychotic patients. Data from the Psychosis Incident Cohort Outcome Study (PICOS). *Journal of Psychiatric Research*, **47**, 438–444.

Uhlhaas, P.J., Haenschel, C., Nikolic, D., and Singer, W. (2008). The role of oscillations and synchrony in cortical networks and their putative relevance for the pathophysiology of schizophrenia. *Schizophrenia Bulletin*, **34**, 927–943.

Van der Pol, P., Liebregts, N., de Graaf, R., *et al.* (2013). Mental health differences between frequent cannabis users with and without dependence and the general population. *Addiction*, **108**, 1459–1469.

Van Os, J., Bak, M., Hanssen, M., Bijl, R. V., de Graaf, R., and Verdoux, H. (2002). Cannabis use and psychosis: a longitudinal population-based study. *American Journal of Epidemiology*, **156**, 319–327.

Van Os, J. and Kapur, S. (2009). Schizophrenia. *Lancet*, **374**, 635–645.

Van Os, J., Kenis, G., and Rutten, B.P. (2010). The environment and schizophrenia. *Nature*, **468**, 203–212.

Van Winkel, R. (2011). Family-based analysis of genetic variation underlying psychosis-inducing effects of cannabis: sibling analysis and proband follow-up. *Archives of General Psychiatry*, **68**, 148–157.

Veen, N.D., Selten, J.P., van der Tweel, I., Feller, W.G., Hoek, H.W., and Kahn, R.S. (2004). Cannabis use and age at onset of schizophrenia. *American Journal of Psychiatry*, **161**, 501–506.

Verdoux, H., Gindre, C., Sorbara, F., Tournier, M., and Swendsen, J.D. (2003). Effects of cannabis and psychosis vulnerability in daily life: an experience sampling test study. *Psychological Medicine*, **33**, 23–32.

Weiser, M., Knobler, H.Y., Noy, S., and Kaplan, Z. (2002). Clinical characteristics of adolescents later hospitalized for schizophrenia. *American Journal of Medical Genetics*, **114**, 949–955.

Wise, L.E., Thorpe, A.J., and Lichtman, A.H. (2009). Hippocampal CB_1 receptors mediate the memory impairing effects of Δ^9-tetrahydrocannabinol. *Neuropsychopharmacology*, **34**, 2072–2080.

Wobrock, T., Falkai, P., Schneider-Axmann, T., *et al.* (2013). Comorbid substance abuse in first-episode schizophrenia: effects on cognition and psychopathology in the EUFEST study. *Schizophrenia Research*, **147**, 132–139.

Zammit, S., Allebeck, P., Andreasson, S., Lundberg, I., and Lewis, G. (2002). Self reported cannabis use as a risk factor for schizophrenia in Swedish conscripts of 1969: historical cohort study. *British Medical Journal*, **325**, 1199–1201.

Zammit, S., Arseneault, L., Cannon, M., and Murray, R.M. (2012). Does cannabis use cause schizophrenia? The epidemiological evidence. In: D. Castle, R.M. Murray, and C. D'Souza (eds.). *Marijuana and Madness*. 2nd ed. Cambridge: Cambridge University Press, pp. 169–183.

Zammit, S., Owen, M.J., Evans, J., Heron, J., and Lewis, G. (2011). Cannabis, COMT and psychotic experiences. *British Journal of Psychiatry*, **199**, 380–385.

Zammit, S., Spurlock, G., Williams, H., *et al.* (2007). Genotype effects of CHRNA7, CNR1 and COMT in schizophrenia: interactions with tobacco and cannabis use. *British Journal of Psychiatry*, **191**, 402–407.

Chapter 38

Nonpsychological Adverse Effects

Franjo Grotenhermen

38.1 Introduction

Scientists generally agree on the acute and short-lasting physical effects of cannabis products, while questions and controversy remain with regard to possible chronic and long-term effects, for example, effects on the fetus. But there are also some unanswered questions on acute physical effects, mainly with regard to severe cardiovascular consequences.

This review will concentrate on the toxicity of cannabis and its main psychoactive constituent tetrahydrocannabinol (THC, dronabinol). This restriction is justified by the fact that cannabis used recreationally usually contains high THC concentrations of 2–25% and low concentrations of other cannabinoids as well as the fact that the main problems concerning adverse effects are associated with cannabinoid receptor type 1 (CB_1) receptor activation. In recent years cannabis strains high in CBD (cannabidiol), which has a very favorable side effect profile, became available and this issue will be covered also in brief. It is not easy to draw a clear line between those effects that are sought after by the recreational user and adverse effects. Desirable effects for one user may be unwanted for another. This is not only the case for psychological effects but also for somatic effects such as increased appetite with THC and blocking of THC effects on appetite with CBD.

Most important physical adverse effects of cannabis are related to the pulmonary effects of smoking cannabis. However, these effects are not attributable to any inherent cannabis compounds but instead to combustion products generated when dried plant material is smoked rather than taken orally or through other advisable modes of administration such as vaporization. In addition, there are increasing concerns among scientists about major adverse effects of severe cannabis prohibition exerted by many governments. Detrimental consequences to the user range from poisoning by adulterants of illegal products to the death penalty. Detrimental effects to society range from a high economic burden from the prosecution of criminal activities, to the corruption and destruction of civil societies, mainly in certain countries of Africa and South America.

38.2 Overall toxicity

The acute toxicity of THC is low. Acute lethal human toxicity for cannabis has not been substantiated. The median lethal dose (LD_{50}) of oral THC in rats was 800–1900 mg/kg depending on sex and strain (Thompson et al. 1973). There were no cases of death due to toxicity following the maximum THC dose in dogs (up to 3000 mg/kg THC) and monkeys (up to 9000 mg/kg THC).

The long-term use of cannabis was not associated with an increased mortality in animals (Chan et al. 1996). Chan et al. (1996) administered 50 mg/kg THC to rats for a period of 2 years. At the end of the observation overall survival was higher in the treated animals (70%) than in the untreated controls (45%), which was attributed to the lower incidence of cancer in the

Box 38.1 Possible physical adverse effects of cannabis

- *Overall toxicity:* insufficient evidence of cannabis use on all-cause mortality.
- *Psychomotor performance:* reduced coordination of movements; altered perception of time; changes in visual perception; reduced attention; disturbances of short-term memory; reduced reaction time; reduced multitasking capacity.
- *Traffic and other accidents:* dose-dependent increase of traffic accidents by about a factor of 2; dose dependency much weaker than with alcohol; inconclusive results concerning a possible increase of other accidents (falls at home, etc.).
- *Circulation:* tachycardia; changes in blood pressure; orthostatic hypotension; syncope; heart attacks; arteritis (?); stroke (?).
- *Digestive tract:* reduced production of saliva with dried mouth; periodontitis; caries; cyclic vomiting in some chronic users; reduced pacemaker frequency of stomach motility; delayed gastric emptying; moderately reduced to no reduced bowel movements.
- *Hormonal system and fertility:* decreased sperm count in very heavy users without impairment of function; inconclusive effects on menstrual cycle length; transient decrease of prolactin and LH; inconclusive evidence on fertility in males and females; transient increase in plasma cortisol level; no influence on insulin; impaired glucose tolerance after high doses, increase in ghrelin and leptin; decrease in peptide YY.
- *Pregnancy and fetal development:* shorter duration of pregnancy; inconsistent evidence on possible reduced birth weight; subtle disturbances of cerebral development; subtle cognitive impairment in children exposed to THC in utero; lower school achievement.
- *Immune system:* shift of Th1 and Th2 lymphocytes; decrease of pro-inflammatory cytokines (IFN-γ, IL-2, tumour necrosis factor-alpha); complex effects on HIV/AIDS with unfavorable and favorable actions.
- *Liver:* possible increased risk of liver cirrhosis and fatty liver in patients with hepatitis C with heavy use.
- *Eye:* reddening of the eyes; slowed pupils' reaction to light; reduced tear flow; decreased eye blink rates.
- *Skin:* reduced pigmentation induced by ultraviolet B (UVB) radiation.

THC groups. A literature review on human studies concluded that there is currently insufficient evidence to assess whether the all-cause mortality rate is elevated among cannabis users or not (Calabria et al. 2010) (see Box 38.1).

Alcohol is generally regarded as much more dangerous by scientists than cannabis. According to a ranking published in *The Lancet*, alcohol was most harmful, with a score of 72, followed by heroin with 55. Among some of the other drugs assessed were cocaine (27), tobacco (26), cannabis (20), and benzodiazepines (15) (Nutt et al. 2010).

38.3 **Interindividual variability of adverse effects**

There is a large interindividual variation of tolerated doses, which is illustrated by the different daily doses tolerated by patients in clinical studies, which may range from 2.5 to 120 mg THC (Wade et al. 2004).

Since tolerance develops to central and peripheral effects of THC, regular cannabis users may tolerate considerably higher doses. In a study by Bowman and Phil on cognitive performance of cannabis users in Jamaica, participants reported a mean daily intake of about 24.5 g cannabis, corresponding to about 1000 mg THC (Bowman and Phil 1973). Today, many heavy regular cannabis users smoke 5 g or even 10 g of dried cannabis flowers with high THC content achieving daily doses even above 1000 mg THC (personal communications).

Genetic variations and polymorphisms of constituents of the endocannabinoid system, including cannabinoid receptors and enzymes that catalyze the production or degradation of endocannabinoids, may influence susceptibility to cannabinoids, for example, the risk of developing anxiety disorders from cannabis use (Heitland et al. 2012). Certain diseases and severe stress may be associated with changes of cannabinoid receptor density, which may alter tolerance to cannabis (Campos et al. 2012; Van Laere et al. 2010).

38.4 Psychomotor performance

Cannabis effects include disturbances of fine motor control and coordination, a reduction in psychomotor activity, and prolonged, but also unaffected, reaction times (Chait and Pierri 1989; Leweke et al. 1998). In addition, the clinically reported aberrations in visual perception (Carlin et al. 1972; Leweke et al. 1999) and the subjective overestimation of the duration of a given time period (Jones and Stone 1970) have been replicated under experimental conditions (see Box 38.1). However, frequent cannabis users estimated time correctly (Sewell et al. 2013). Multitasking capacity is reduced (Wetherell et al. 2012). Attentional inhibition is enhanced, changing the way mental tasks are performed under the influence of cannabis (Vivas et al. 2012). In regular cannabis users the drug produced only minimal effects on complex cognitive task performance, a clear indication of tolerance (Hart et al. 2001). There was an increase in functional interactions between the prefrontal cortex and the occipitoparietal cortex in regular cannabis smokers compared to nonusers, which may have a compensatory role in mitigating cannabis-related impairments (Harding et al. 2012).

38.5 Traffic and other accidents

THC impairs perception, psychomotor performance, and cognitive and affective functions, which may all contribute to a driver's increased risk of causing a traffic accident. After alcohol, cannabis and benzodiazepines are the drugs most frequently found in impaired drivers and in drivers involved in accidents (Jones et al. 2003; Tunbridge et al. 2000). In a large case–control study conducted in the US, the presence of THC or its metabolites in blood or urine was associated with an increase in potentially unsafe driving actions of 29% compared to an increase of 101% for drivers with a blood alcohol concentration of 0.05% or more (Bédard et al. 2007).

Some of the impairment caused by cannabis is mitigated since subjects appear to perceive that they are indeed impaired (Smiley 1999). Where they can compensate, they do, for example, by not overtaking, by slowing down, and by focusing their attention when they know a response will be required. Such compensation is not always possible, however, where drivers are faced with unexpected events.

The two major responsibility studies conducted so far underline the importance of alcohol as the major causal factor in traffic accidents (Drummer et al. 2004; Laumon et al. 2005). The responsibility study by Drummer et al. (2004), conducted in Australia and using information on 3398 fatally injured drivers, showed an odds ratio (OR) of 6.0 for alcohol above a blood alcohol concentration (BAC) of 0.05% with an OR of 3.7 for the BAC range of 0.1–0.15% and of 25 for a BAC of more than 0.2% (Drummer et al. 2004). THC was associated with an increased overall risk of 2.7. A THC blood concentration of less than 5 ng/mL was associated with an OR of 0.7 (Drummer 2004, personal communication), while a blood concentration above 5 ng/mL was associated with an OR of 6.6.

The French study by Laumon et al. (2005) with 9772 drivers involved in an accident, in which at least one subject was fatally injured, found an OR of 8.5 for all alcohol positive drivers and an OR of 1.8 for all THC positive drivers after adjustment for substances, age, time of accident, and vehicle type (Laumon et al. 2005). A BAC of below 0.05% was associated with an OR of 2.7 and a BAC of above 0.2% with an OR of 39.6.

Similarly, according to a review, acute cannabis use increases the risk of traffic accidents only by a factor of 2 (see Box 38.1), far below the risk caused by alcohol (Asbridge et al. 2012). Driving under the influence of cannabis was associated with a significantly increased risk of motor vehicle collisions compared with unimpaired driving (OR: 1.9). Collision risk estimates were higher in case–control studies (OR: 2.8) and studies of fatal collisions (OR: 2.1) than in culpability studies (OR: 1.65) and studies on nonfatal collisions (OR: 1.7).

Drivers who switch from alcohol to cannabis use may reduce their accident risk. The first study on the relationship between laws on the medicinal use of cannabis in the US and traffic deaths found a nearly 9% drop in traffic deaths and a 5% reduction in beer sales (Anderson and Rees 2011).

The results of studies on the correlation between cannabis use and injuries from a range of different kinds of accident requiring hospitalization are somewhat conflicting. Vinson found no increased risk for cannabis users in 2161 injured subjects requiring emergency room treatment and 1856 controls (Vinson 2006). Among the cases, 27% were injured in a fall, 19% were struck by an object, 18% were in a motor vehicle crash, and the rest were injured in a variety of other ways. Self-reported cannabis use in the previous 7 days was associated in this study with a decreased risk of injury, while the use of other illicit drugs and recent use of alcohol was associated with an increased risk. In contrast, a study by Gerberich et al. (2003) found a small increased risk of hospitalized injury in cannabis users. In their retrospective study with 64,657 subjects who completed a questionnaire about health behaviors including cannabis use, that use was independently associated in the follow-up with an increased risk for injury hospitalizations of 1.28 for men and 1.37 for women.

38.6 **Circulation**

THC produces reversible and dose-dependent tachycardia with increased cardiac output and oxygen demand and increased diastolic blood pressure (in horizontal position) associated with a decreased parasympathetic tone (Clark et al. 1974) (see Box 38.1). Due to tolerance to these effects, chronic use can lead to bradycardia (Jones et al. 1981). At higher doses, orthostatic hypotension may occur due to a dilation of blood vessels, which may result in dizziness and syncope. Myocardial infarction may be triggered by THC due to these effects on circulation (Mittleman et al. 2001). Dilation of blood vessels also causes conjunctival reddening. In a literature review on triggers of myocardial infarction cannabis use was estimated to be responsible for 0.8% of cases (Nawrot et al. 2011). In 3886 patients, who have survived myocardial infarction and were followed for up to 18 years, there was no statistically significant association between cannabis use and mortality (Frost et al. 2013).

Chronic cannabis use was not associated with cardiovascular risk factors such as changes in blood triglyceride levels and blood pressure in the longitudinal CARDIA study, which began in 1986 (Rodondi et al. 2006). In an animal model of atherosclerosis, low doses of THC inhibited disease progression (Steffens et al. 2005). This was associated with a decreased interferon-gamma (IFN-γ) secretion by lymphoid cells and reduced macrophage chemotaxis. Some groups (Hoyer et al. 2011; Zhao et al. 2010), but not all (Willecke et al. 2011) obtained evidence that these protective effects were mediated by the cannabinoid CB_2 receptor.

There are a few case reports of an association between arteriopathies such as Buerger's disease and cannabis use, but it is unclear whether this is a "cause and effect" relationship since the study subjects usually also smoked tobacco, which is the major risk factor for Buerger's disease (Grotenhermen 2010). About 60 cases of stroke related to cannabis use have been reported in the literature. Proposed mechanisms of action are orthostatic hypotension with secondary impairment of the autoregulation of cerebral blood flow, reversible cerebral vasoconstrictive syndrome, and multifocal intracranial stenosis, but the causal role of cannabis remains unclear since other confounding factors (lifestyle, genetic factors) have to be considered (Wolff et al. 2013).

38.7 **Digestive tract**

THC has a cholinergic effect on the salivary glands leading to hyposalivation and dry mouth (see Box 38.1). This effect is mediated by both CB_1 and CB_2 receptors (Kopach et al. 2012). In a longitudinal study the use of cannabis was associated with an approximately doubled risk of signs of periodontitis (Thomson et al. 2008). Cannabis users have a similar risk of caries as tobacco smokers (Ditmyer et al. 2013; Schulz-Katterbach et al. 2009).

Several case series of cannabis-induced hyperemesis have been reported. In the largest series with 98 patients with a history of recurrent vomiting with no other explanation for symptoms, most used cannabis for more than 2 years before symptom onset (Simonetto et al. 2012). Of these, 52 reported relief of symptoms with hot showers or baths.

Cannabinoids induce a reduction in pacemaker frequency of stomach motility (Percie et al. 2010). Research on colon motility is somewhat conflicting. THC reduced postprandial colonic motility and tone (Esfandyari et al. 2007) in one study and motility of the colon in patients with irritable bowel syndrome during the fasting state in another (Wong et al. 2011), while a later controlled study did not find any effects of THC on food transit in stomach, small bowel, or colon (Wong et al. 2012).

38.8 **Hormonal system and fertility**

Changes in human hormone levels due to acute cannabis or THC ingestion are minor and usually remain in the normal range (Hollister 1986). Tolerance develops to these minor effects, however, and even regular cannabis users demonstrate normal hormone levels. Reductions in male fertility by cannabis are reversible and only seen in animals at THC blood concentrations higher than those found in chronic cannabis users (see Box 38.1). After several weeks of daily smoking 8–10 cannabis cigarettes a slight decrease in sperm count was observed in humans, without impairment of their function (Hembree et al. 1978).

There is no conclusive evidence on any cannabis-associated influences on menstrual cycle length, on the number of cycles without ovulation, or on plasma concentrations of estrogens, progesterone, testosterone, prolactin, luteinizing hormone (LH) or follicle-stimulating hormone in female cannabis users. A transient cannabis-induced suppression of prolactin and LH levels was observed if the drug was inhaled during the luteal phase of the menstrual cycle (Mendelson et al. 1985). The follicular phase of the menstrual cycle may be prolonged in cannabis users (Jukic et al. 2007).

There are few epidemiological data on influences of cannabis on fertility, and these provide no definitive answers. In an Indian study, 150 married male cannabis users that initiated cannabis use shortly before marriage were compared to an equal number of opium users and nonusers of drugs; 1% of nonusers, 2% of cannabis users, and 10% of opium users were childless (Chopra and Jandu 1976). The sterility rate in bhang users (cannabis leaves) with an average daily consumption of about 150 mg THC was lower (0.4%) than in nonusers, whereas the users of ganja and charas (flowers and resin) with a daily consumption of about 300 mg THC was higher (5.7%).

Mueller et al. (1990) investigated effects on female sterility. There was a low increase of sterility risk associated with cannabis use (OR: 1.7). The risk was only increased in occasional users and not in more heavy users. Joesoef et al. (1993) investigated the period of time from "child wish" until conception in 2817 women. Regular users of cannabis became pregnant most quickly (mean time = 3.7 months). Tobacco smokers needed an average of 5.1 months and drug-free women 4.3 months.

Grotenhermen and Leson (2001) reviewed the effects of cannabis and THC on other hormones. A single oral administration did not elevate plasma cortisol in man. However, smoking two cannabis cigarettes caused a transient significant increase in plasma cortisol level (Cone et al. 1986). Chronic heavy cannabis users did not show any significant differences in their cortisol levels. Cannabis does not alter thyroid function in regular users (Bonnet et al. 2012). It does not result in measurable changes in blood glucose level, but may influence glucose tolerance (Permutt et al. 1976). However, relatively high doses are needed. In a clinical study cannabis influenced blood levels of appetite hormones in people with HIV (Riggs et al. 2011). Compared to placebo, cannabis administration was associated with significant increases in plasma levels of ghrelin and leptin, and decreases in peptide YY, but did not significantly influence insulin levels.

According to a study with 10,896 citizens, a nationally representative sample of the US population, cannabis users had a significantly lower risk of developing both types of diabetes mellitus compared to nonusers (adjusted OR: 0.36) (Rajavashisth et al. 2012).

38.9 **Pregnancy and fetal development**

The endocannabinoid system plays a crucial role in pregnancy. Successful pregnancy implantation and progression seem to require low levels of anandamide (Habayeb et al. 2004). At term, anandamide levels dramatically increase during labor and are affected by the duration of labor, which may explain a sometimes observed shorter gestation in cannabis users. In a large study with 3234 healthy pregnant women, of whom 4.9% had a preterm birth, cannabis use was associated with a slightly increased preterm birth risk (Dekker et al. 2012).

THC rapidly crosses the placenta and the time course of changes of THC levels in fetal blood coincides well with that in the maternal blood, though fetal plasma concentrations are lower than maternal levels in rats (Hutchings et al. 1989). It is unlikely that cannabis causes embryonic or fetal malformations and there are inconsistent epidemiological data on its effect on birth weight. There is evidence of subtle disturbances of cerebral development resulting in cognitive impairment in offspring of cannabis users from two longitudinal studies conducted in Canada and the US (Fried et al. 2003; Richardson et al. 2002). This impairment might not be observed before preschool or school age (see Box 38.1). In 13- to 16-year-old adolescents the strongest relationship between prenatal maternal cigarette smoking and cognitive variables was seen with overall intelligence and aspects of auditory functioning whereas prenatal exposure to cannabis was negatively associated with tasks that required visual memory, analysis, and integration

(Fried et al. 2003). School achievement at age of 14 was lower in adolescents who were exposed to cannabis during pregnancy (Goldschmidt et al. 2011). Similar to prenatal tobacco exposure, cannabis exposure was associated with deficits in visual–motor coordination at the age of 16 (Willford et al. 2010).

38.10 Immune system

It has been demonstrated that THC may cause a shift in the development of type 1 and 2 T-helper cells (Th1 and Th2) (see Box 38.1). THC treatment of cell cultures (Klein et al. 1998) and the use of cannabis (Pacifici et al. 2003) was associated with a decrease of proinflammatory Th1 cytokines, such as IFN-γ and (interleukin 2 (IL-2), and an increase in anti-inflammatory Th2 cytokines, such as IL-4 and IL-10. In clinical studies no such changes were observed (Katona et al. 2005), which may be due to the use of lower doses. These effects on the immune system may be beneficial in inflammatory diseases such as Crohn's disease and multiple sclerosis, but may have a negative impact in immunocompromised subjects such as AIDS and cancer patients. Studies investigating the effects of cannabis or THC on the course of AIDS have yielded conflicting results. In a prospective study by Kaslow et al. (1989) the use of cannabis in HIV-infected persons was not associated with the onset of AIDS. Di Franco et al. (1996) also failed to detect any association between cannabis use and AIDS onset in HIV infected men in a 6-year epidemiological study. On the other hand, Tindall et al. (1988) and Whitfield et al. (1997) did obtain evidence for such an association.

No effect of cannabis use on subpopulations of T lymphocytes in men with HIV were observed in a longitudinal study (Chao et al. 2008). This observation was confirmed in rhesus monkeys infected with SIV, the HIV equivalent in monkeys, who received different THC doses without adversely affecting viral load or other markers of disease progression during the early stages of infection (Winsauer et al. 2011). It may be possible that CB_2 receptor agonists (Costantino et al. 2012) and THC (Molina et al. 2010) inhibit the replication of the HI-virus.

The use of cannabis was not associated with the natural course of cervical human papillomavirus and cervical cancer in HIV positive and HIV negative women in a large epidemiological study (D'Souza et al. 2010).

38.11 Other organ systems

38.11.1 Liver

Daily cannabis use was a risk factor for progression of fibrosis in chronic hepatitis C in two small epidemiological studies (Hézode et al. 2005; Ishida et al. 2008), while occasional use was not (Hézode et al. 2005). Daily cannabis use was also associated with an increased risk of fatty liver in patients with hepatitis C (Hézode et al. 2008). However, a link between cannabis use and progression to liver fibrosis or cirrhosis could not be confirmed in a large longitudinal study (Brunet et al. 2013). Cannabis use improved retention and virological outcomes in patients treated for hepatitis C with interferon and ribavirin (Sylvestre et al. 2006; Costiniuk et al. 2008).

38.11.2 Ophthalmic effects

The use of cannabis may disturb accommodation, and the pupil's reaction to light is slowed. High doses of cannabis may increase eye pupil size (Merzouki et al. 2008). Tear flow is decreased (Hollister 1986). Decreased tear flow may potentially increase the risk of infections of the eye (keratitis, conjunctivitis). Regular cannabis use was shown to decrease eye blink rates in a dose-dependent manner (Kowal et al. 2011).

38.11.3 **Effects on the skin**

Activation of the CB_1 receptor reduces pigmentation of the skin induced by ultraviolet B radiation (Magina et al. 2011).

38.12 **Tolerance to physical effects**

Humans can develop tolerance to cannabis-induced cardiovascular and autonomic changes, decreased intraocular pressure, and changes in sleep, sleep electroencephalogram, and mood, and to certain cannabis-induced behavioral changes (Jones et al. 1981). In a number of studies, Jones and Benowitz (1976) orally administered daily THC doses of 210 mg to about 120 volunteers for 11–21 days. Participants developed tolerance to cognitive and psychomotor impairment and to the psychological high by the end of these studies (Jones et al. 1976). After a few days an increased heart rate was replaced by a normal or a slowed heart rate. Tolerance develops also to cannabinoid-induced orthostatic hypotension (Benowitz and Jones 1975). Speed and intensity of tolerance varies according to effect. In a short clinical study with subjects receiving high THC doses tolerance developed quickly to subjective intoxication, but not to cardiovascular effects (Gorelick et al. 2012).

Clinical long-term studies with THC and cannabis in patients suffering from multiple sclerosis (Zajicek et al. 2005), spasticity and pain (Maurer et al. 1990), and AIDS (Beal et al. 1997) did not find tolerance to the medicinal effects of moderate doses (usually 5–30 mg THC daily) within 6–12 months.

38.13 **Adverse effects of cannabidiol**

CBD is nontoxic in nontransformed cells and does not induce changes in food intake, induce catalepsy, affect physiological parameters (heart rate, blood pressure, and body temperature), affect gastrointestinal transit, or alter psychomotor or psychological functions (Bergamaschi et al. 2011). It antagonizes several effects of CB_1 receptor agonists, including increased appetite, reduced cognition, and psychological effects (Englund et al. 2012; Morgan et al. 2010; Scopinho et al. 2011). CBD may cause increased wakefulness (Nicholson et al. 2004). According to animal research (Chagas et al. 2013) and experiences of cannabis users (personal communications) CBD may also improve sleep. Perhaps the use of different doses may explain these different sleep observations.

38.14 **Harmful interactions of cannabinoids with other drugs**

Because THC is metabolized mainly in the liver by cytochrome P-450 isoenzymes (principally CYP2C9), it may interact with other medications metabolized in the same way (Grotenhermen 2005). Several phytocannabinoids (THC, CBN, CBD) reduce the degradation of warfarin and of diclofenac increasing their effect and duration of action. This cannabinoid effect was due to the inhibition of CYP2C9 in the liver (Yamaori et al. 2012). Cannabis smoking can reduce the plasma concentration of individual antipsychotics (clozapine, olanzapine). However, neither in AIDS patients nor in cancer patients were the plasma levels of various antiretroviral drugs or cytostatics altered by simultaneous treatment with cannabinoids (Engels et al. 2007; Kosel et al. 2002).

Cannabinoids interact most often with substances that produce similar effects, leading to mutual enhancement or attenuation of such effects (Hollister 1999). The principal clinically relevant interactions are increased tiredness when cannabinoids are taken together with other psychotropic agents (e.g., alcohol and benzodiazepines) or interactions with drugs that also act on the cardiovascular system (such as amphetamines).

38.15 **Risks of smoking**

One of the greatest concerns about chronic effects of recreational cannabis use pertains to the inhalation of combustion products that may damage the mucous membranes, if the drug is smoked as a cannabis cigarette ("joint") or in a pipe (see Box 38.2). The cannabis plant contains more than 500 chemical compounds including amino acids, fatty acids, etc., which generally have a very low toxic potential. Pyrolysis creates at least 200 thermal degradation products in smoke not found in cannabis, including mutagenic polycyclic hydrocarbons such as benz[α]anthracene, benzo[α]pyrene, naphthalene, and several cresols and phenols. The composition of these combustion products is at least qualitatively similar to that of tobacco smoke or that of the smoke generated from other dried plant material, despite some minor differences (British Medical Association 1997). Thus, one would expect similar damage to the mucosa by cannabis smoke as following the use of tobacco. Indeed, signs of airway inflammation (vascular hyperplasia, submucosal edema, inflammatory cell infiltrates, and goblet cell hyperplasia) were found in bronchial biopsies of cannabis smokers, all changes similar to those seen in tobacco smokers (Roth et al. 1998). Regular cannabis smoking in young adults was associated with wheezing, shortness of breath during exercise, and the production of sputum as it is in tobacco smokers (Taylor et al. 2000). Smoking of cannabis increases the risk of chronic bronchitis (Tashkin et al. 2012). However, in a long-term epidemiological study with 5115 men and women cannabis smoking did not reduce lung function and did not increase the risk for chronic obstructive pulmonary disease (COPD) (Pletcher et al. 2012). Some case studies reported an increased risk of the development of lung emphysema and spontaneous pneumothorax in young cannabis smokers (Beshay et al. 2007; Hii et al. 2008; Jakab et al. 2012).

Biopsies from cannabis smokers have also revealed a higher rate of precancerous pathological changes compared to nonsmokers (Barsky et al. 1998; Fligiel et al. 1997), which is suggestive of an increased risk of cancer in the respiratory tract or elsewhere. So far, the epidemiological data are inconclusive. A review of two cohort studies and 14 case–control studies by the International Agency for Research on Cancer (IARC) did not find a clear association between cannabis use and cancer (Hashibe et al. 2005). Authors noted that sufficient studies are not available to adequately evaluate whether cannabis smoking significantly increases the risk of developing cancer, and published studies often have limitations including too few heavy cannabis users in the study samples (see Box 38.2). The largest epidemiological study conducted so far with 1212 incident cancer cases and 1040 cancer-free controls did not find a positive association between cannabis smoking and the investigated cancer types (mouth, larynx, lung, pharynx) (Hashibe et al. 2006). There was no dose–effect relationship and even heavy use was not associated with an increased risk, which may be due to inhibition of tumor growth by THC observed in vivo (Preet et al. 2008).

Box 38.2 **Risks of cannabis smoking**

- Vascular hyperplasia, submucosal edema, inflammatory cell infiltrates, goblet cell hyperplasia, and precancerous pathological changes in bronchial biopsies of cannabis smokers.
- Chronic bronchitis.
- No reduction in lung function or COPD.
- Case reports of lung emphysema and spontaneous pneumothorax.
- No clear association between cannabis smoking and cancer.

38.16 **Harms of prohibition**

Cannabis is the world's most widely produced and used illicit substance: it is grown in almost all countries of the world, and is smoked by 130–190 million people at least once a year (press release by UNODC of June 23, 2010).

The prohibition of cannabis use may harm both cannabis users and society as a whole (see Box 38.3). In contrast to other social activities that may be harmful to the individual and/or society, the use of cannabis remains illegal in most countries. Advocates of cannabis prohibition believe that it reduces trafficking and use, thereby improving productivity and health. Critics believe that prohibition curbs trafficking and use only modestly while causing several negative side effects, such that the well-known harms of prohibition enhance the toxicity from consumption of the drug itself. In 2007, the Commission on Illegal Drugs, Communities and Public Policy of the UK Action and Research Centre (RSA) stated in a report: "The current law is out of date, unwieldy and peppered with anomalies, an agglomeration of miscellaneous provisions adopted to address situations that in many cases no longer apply. It causes some social harm while limiting others. It acknowledges no parallels and no relationships between the use of illegal drugs and the use of alcohol and tobacco" (RSA Commission on Illegal Drugs 2007, p. 284).

Cannabis prohibition may cause several undesirable social and health effects. They include an insufficient access to its medicinal benefits, the loss of the driver's license, the need for cannabis users to interact with a criminal milieu, and an erosion of the credibility of governments that created laws considered by many to be unjust and unenforceable. Cannabis prohibition also may have disrupted small-scale outdoor production, driven commercial growers indoors, and likely contributed to the observed increase in the potency of illegal cannabis, as its producers tried to maximize profits and minimize their risks (Hall and Degenhardt 2006).

These and other consequences of cannabis prohibition, such as the need to build and maintain a growing criminal system, including courts and prisons, also generate considerable costs to society. Based on a report on the economics of cannabis prohibition, the late Nobel Prize winning economist Milton Friedman and more than 500 of his colleagues released an open letter to President Bush calling for "an open and honest debate about marijuana prohibition." They added, "We believe such

---

Box 38.3 **Harms of prohibition**

- Insufficient access to its medicinal benefits.
- Poisoning with adulterants of illegal products.
- Use of more dangerous synthetic cannabinoids.
- A criminal record for otherwise law-abiding young adults, which may have negative effects on their job-related future.
- The need for cannabis users to interact with a criminal milieu.
- Erosion of the credibility of governments that created laws considered by many to be unjust.
- Increase in the potency of illegal cannabis.
- Creation of a reason for building and maintaining a growing criminal system.
- Considerable financial costs to society.
- Encouragement of organized crime.

a debate will favour a regime in which marijuana is legal but taxed and regulated like other goods" (Miron 2005). It is estimated that the Netherlands earns 400 million Euros annually in tax revenues from the sales of cannabis in coffee shops (NIS News Bulletin 2008). According to a report by the Cato Institute, US, legalizing cannabis would save the US altogether 8.7 billion dollars per year as a result of both a reduction in government expenditure on enforcement of prohibition and an increase in tax income (Miron and Waldock 2010). Currently the profits from drug trafficking only benefit the traffickers and are often used to finance criminal activities, including acts of terrorism.

There is no agreement among scientists on how decriminalization or legalization of cannabis would affect key parameters, such as the prevalence of cannabis use by adults and adolescents, price trends, and the extent of unregulated home production. Effects will vary between countries and their sociocultural settings. Decriminalization and legalization would certainly increase availability of cannabis and there is great concern that this will also increase use (Joffe et al. 2004), but available data do not support this concern (van den Brink 2008). According to a study by the World Health Organization, which describes data from 17 countries participating in the World Mental Health Survey Initiative of the World Health Organization, "drug use is not distributed evenly and is not simply related to drug policy, since countries with stringent user-level illegal drug policies did not have lower levels of use than countries with liberal ones" (Degenhardt et al. 2008). Laws that legalized the medical use of cannabis in several US states did not increase use in adolescents (Harper et al. 2012). A representative survey of 15,191 adolescents aged 15–24 years from different European countries concluded that the legal status had no effect on drug use (Vuolo et al. 2013).

Instead, several studies found that social background, emotional, and other psycho-social factors were more reliable predictors of cannabis use and generally problematic drug use than the availability of the drug or its legal status.

References

Anderson, D.M. and Rees D.I. (2011). *Medical Marijuana Laws, Traffic Fatalities, and Alcohol Consumption*. IZA, Discussion Paper No. 6112. Available at: http://ftp.iza.org/dp6112.pdf.

Asbridge, M., Hayden, J.A., and Cartwright, J.L. (2012). Acute cannabis consumption and motor vehicle collision risk: systematic review of observational studies and meta-analysis. *BMJ*, **344**, 536.

Barsky, S.H., Roth, M.D., Kleerup, E.C., Simmons, M., and Tashkin, D.P. (1998). Histopathologic and molecular alterations in bronchial epithelium in habitual smokers of marijuana, cocaine, and/or tobacco. *Journal of the National Cancer Institute*, **90**, 1198–1205.

Bátkai, S., Rajesh, M., Mukhopadhyay, P., et al. (2007). Decreased age-related cardiac dysfunction, myocardial nitrative stress, inflammatory gene expression, and apoptosis in mice lacking fatty acid amide hydrolase. *American Journal of Physiology. Heart and Circulatory Physiology*, **293**, 909–918.

Beal, J.E., Olson, R., Lefkowitz, L., et al. (1997). Long-term efficacy and safety of dronabinol for acquired immunodeficiency syndrome-associated anorexia. *Journal of Pain and Symptom Management*, **14**, 7–14.

Bédard, M., Dubois, S., and Weaver, B. (2007). The impact of cannabis on driving. *Canadian Journal of Public Health. Revue Canadienne de Sante Publique*, **98**, 6–11.

Benowitz, N.L. and Jones, R.T. (1975). Cardiovascular effects of prolonged delta-9-tetrahydrocannabinol ingestion. *Clinical Pharmacology and Therapeutics*, **18**, 287–297.

Bergamaschi, M.M., Queiroz, R.H., Zuardi, A.W., and Crippa, J.A. (2011). Safety and side effects of cannabidiol, a *Cannabis sativa* constituent. *Current Drug Safety*, **6**, 237–249.

Beshay, M., Kaiser, H., Niedhart, D., Reymond, M.A., and Schmid, R.A. (2007). Emphysema and secondary pneumothorax in young adults smoking cannabis. *European Journal of Cardio-Thoracic Surgery*, **32**, 834–838.

Bonnet, U. (2013). Chronic cannabis abuse, delta-9-tetrahydrocannabinol and thyroid function. *Pharmacopsychiatry*, **46**, 35–36.

Bowman, M. and Phil, R.O. (1973). Cannabis: psychological effects of chronic heavy use. A controlled study of intellectual functioning in chronic users of high potency cannabis. *Psychopharmacologia*, **29**, 159–170.

British Medical Association. (1997). *Therapeutic Uses of Cannabis*. Amsterdam: Harwood Academic Publishers.

Brunet, L., Moodie, E.E.M., Rollet, K., *et al.* for the Canadian Co-infection Cohort Investigators (2013). Marijuana smoking does not accelerate progression of liver disease in HIV-hepatitis C coinfection: a longitudinal cohort analysis. *Clinical Infectious Diseases*, **57**, 663–670.

Calabria, B., Degenhardt, L., Hall, W., and Lynskey, M. (2010). Does cannabis use increase the risk of death? Systematic review of epidemiological evidence on adverse effects of cannabis use. *Drug and Alcohol Review*, **29**, 318–330.

Campos, A.C., Ferreira, F.R., da Silva, W.A. Jr., and Guimarães, F.S. (2013). Predator threat stress promotes long lasting anxiety-like behaviors and modulates synaptophysin and CB1 receptors expression in brain areas associated with PTSD symptoms. *Neuroscience Letter*, **533**, 34–38.

Carlin, A.S., Bakker, C.B., Halpern, L., and Post, R.D. (1972). Social facilitation of marijuana intoxication: impact of social set and pharmacological activity. *Journal of Abnormal Psychology*, **80**, 132–140.

Chagas, M.H., Crippa, J.A., Zuardi A.W., *et al.* (2013). Effects of acute systemic administration of cannabidiol on sleep-wake cycle in rats. *Journal of Psychopharmacology*, **27**, 312–316.

Chait, L.D. and Pierri, J. (1989). Some physical characteristics of NIDA marijuana cigarettes. *Addictive Behaviors*, **14**, 61–67.

Chan, P.C., Sills, R.C., Braun, A.G., Haseman, J.K., and Bucher, J.R. (1996). Toxicity and carcinogenicity of delta 9-tetrahydrocannabinol in Fischer rats and B6C3F1 mice. *Fundamental and Applied Toxicology*, **30**, 109–117.

Chao, C., Jacobson, L.P., Tashkin, D., *et al.* (2008). Recreational drug use and T lymphocyte subpopulations in HIV-uninfected and HIV-infected men. *Drug and Alcohol Dependence*, **94**, 165–171.

Chopra, G.S. and Jandu, B.S. (1976). Psychoclinical effects of long-term marijuana use in 275 Indian chronic users. A comparative assessment of effects in Indian and USA users. *Annals of the New York Academy of Sciences*, **282**, 95–108.

Clark, S.C., Greene, C., Karr, G.W., Maccannell, K.L., and Milstein, S.L. (1974). Cardiovascular effects of marihuana in man. *Canadian Journal of Physiology and Pharmacology. Revue Canadienne de Sante Publique*, **52**, 706–719.

Cone, E.J., Johnson, R.E., Moore, J.D., and Roache, J.D. (1986). Acute effects of smoking marijuana on hormones, subjective effects and performance in male human subjects. *Pharmacology, Biochemistry, and Behavior*, **24**, 1749–1754.

Costantino, C,M., Gupta, A., Yewdall, A.W., Dale, B.M., Devi, L.A., and Chen, B.K. (2012). Cannabinoid receptor 2-mediated attenuation of CXCR4-tropic HIV infection in primary CD4+ T cells. *PLoS One*, **7**, e33961.

Costiniuk, C.T., Mills, E., and Cooper, C.L. (2008). Evaluation of oral cannabinoid-containing medications for the management of interferon and ribavirin-induced anorexia, nausea and weight loss in patients treated for chronic hepatitis C virus. *Canadian Journal of Gastroenterology. Journal Canadien de Gastroenterologie*, **22**, 376–380.

D'Souza, G., Palefsky, J.M., Zhong, Y., *et al.* (2010). Marijuana use is not associated with cervical human papillomavirus natural history or cervical neoplasia in HIV-seropositive or HIV-seronegative women. *Cancer Epidemiology, Biomarkers & Prevention*, **19**, 869–872.

Dekker, G.A., Lee, S.Y., North, R.A., McCowan, L.M., Simpson, N.A., and Roberts, C.T. (2012). Risk factors for preterm birth in an international prospective cohort of nulliparous women. *PLoS One*, **7**, e39154.

Degenhardt, L., Chiu, W.T., Sampson, N., *et al.* (2008). Toward a global view of alcohol, tobacco, cannabis, and cocaine use: findings from the WHO World Mental Health Surveys. *PLoS Medicine*, **5**, 141.

Deusch, E., Kress, H.G., Kraft, B., and Kozek-Langenecker, S.A. (2004). The procoagulatory effects of delta-9-tetrahydrocannabinol in human platelets. *Anesthesia and Analgesia*, **99**, 1127–1130.

Di Franco, M.J., Shephard, H.W, Hunter, D.J., Tosteson, T.D., and Ascher, M.S. (1996). The lack of association of marijuana and other recreational drugs with progression to AIDS in the San Francisco Men's Health Study. *Annals of Epidemiology*, **6**, 283–289.

Ditmyer, M., Demopoulos, C., McClain, M., Dounis, G., and Mobley, C. (2013). The effect of tobacco and marijuana use on dental health status in Nevada adolescents: a trend analysis. *The Journal of Adolescent Health*, **52**, 641–648.

Drummer, O.H., Gerostamoulos, J. and Batziris, H., *et al.* (2004). The involvement of drugs in drivers of motor vehicles killed in Australian road traffic crashes. *Accident Analysis and Prevention*, **36**, 239–248.

Engels, F.K., de Jong, F.A., Sparreboom, A., *et al.* (2007). Medicinal cannabis does not influence the clinical pharmacokinetics of irinotecan and docetaxel. *The Oncologist*, **12**, 291–300.

Englund, A., Morrison, P.D., Nottage, J., *et al.* (2013). Cannabidiol inhibits THC-elicited paranoid symptoms and hippocampal-dependent memory impairment. *Journal of Psychopharmacology (Oxford)*, **27**, 19–27.

Esfandyari, T., Camilleri, M., Busciglio, I., Burton, D., Baxter, K., and Zinsmeister, A.R. (2007). Effects of a cannabinoid receptor agonist on colonic motor and sensory functions in humans: a randomized, placebo-controlled study. *American Journal of Physiology. Gastrointestinal and Liver Physiology*, **293**, 137–145.

European Monitoring Centre for Drugs and Drug Addiction. (2006). *Annual Report 2006*. Available at: http://ar2006.emcdda.europa.eu/en/home-en.html.

Fligiel, S.E., Roth, M.D., Kleerup, E.C., Barsky, S.H., Simmons, M.S., and Tashkin, D.P. (1997). Tracheobronchial histopathology in habitual smokers of cocaine, marijuana, and/or tobacco. *Chest*, **112**, 319–326.

Fried, P.A., Watkinson, B., and Gray, R. (2003). Differential effects on cognitive functioning in 13- to 16-year-olds prenatally exposed to cigarettes and marihuana. *Neurotoxicology and Teratology*, **25**, 427–436.

Frost, L., Mostofsky, E., Rosenbloom, J.I., Mukamal, K.J., and Mittleman, M.A. (2013). Marijuana use and long-term mortality among survivors of acute myocardial infarction. *American Heart Journal*, **165**, 170–175.

Gerberich, S.G., Sidney, S., Braun, B.L., Tekawa, I.S., Tolan, K.K., and Quesenberry, C.P. (2003). Marijuana use and injury events resulting in hospitalization. *Annals of Epidemiology*, **13**, 230–237.

Goldschmidt, L., Richardson, G.A., Willford, J.A., Severtson, S.G., and Day, N.L. (2012). School achievement in 14-year-old youths prenatally exposed to marijuana. *Neurotoxicology and Teratology*, **34**, 161–167.

Gorelick, D.A., Goodwin, R.S., Schwilke, E., *et al.* (2013). Tolerance to effects of high-dose oral Δ9-tetrahydrocannabinol and plasma cannabinoid concentrations in male daily cannabis smokers. *Journal of Analytical Toxicology*, **37**, 11–16.

Gorman, D.M. and Charles Huber Jr., J. (2007). Do medical cannabis laws encourage cannabis use? *The International Journal on Drug Policy*, **18**, 160–167.

Grotenhermen, F. (2005). Cannabinoids. *Current Drug Targets. CNS and Neurological Disorders*, **4**, 507–530.

Grotenhermen, F. (2010). Cannabis-associated arteritis. *Vasa*, **39**, 43–53.

Grotenhermen, F., Leson, G. and Pless, P. (2001). *Assessment of Exposure to and Human Health Risk from THC and Other Cannabinoids in Hemp Foods*. Berkeley, CA: Leson Environmental Consulting.

Habayeb, O.M., Taylor, A.H., Evans, M.D., *et al.* (2004). Plasma levels of the endocannabinoid anandamide in women – a potential role in pregnancy maintenance and labor? *The Journal of Clinical Endocrinology and Metabolism*, **89**, 5482–5487.

Hall, W. and Degenhardt, L. (2006). What are the policy implications of the evidence on cannabis and psychosis? *Canadian Journal of Psychiatry. Revue Canadienne de Psychiatrie*, **51**, 566–574.

Harding, I.H., Solowij, N., Harrison, B.J., *et al.* (2012). Functional connectivity in brain networks underlying cognitive control in chronic cannabis users. *Neuropsychopharmacology*, **37**, 1923–1933.

Hart, C.L., van Gorp, W., Haney, M., Foltin, R.W., and Fischman, M. W. (2001). Effects of acute smoked marijuana on complex cognitive performance. *Neuropsychopharmacology*, **25**, 757–765.

Hashibe, M., Morgenstern, H., Cui, Y., *et al.* (2006). Marijuana use and the risk of lung and upper aerodigestive tract cancers: results of a population-based case-control study. *Cancer Epidemiology, Biomarkers & Prevention*, **15**, 1829–1834.

Hashibe, M., Straif, K., Tashkin, D.P., Morgenstern, H., Greenland, S., and Zhang, Z.F. (2005). Epidemiologic review of marijuana use and cancer risk. *Alcohol*, **35**, 265–275.

Heitland, I., Klumpers, F., Oosting, R.S., Evers, D.J., Leon Kenemans, J., and Baas, J.M. (2012). Failure to extinguish fear and genetic variability in the human cannabinoid receptor 1. *Translational Psychiatry*, **2**, 162.

Hembree, W.C., Nahas, G.G., Zeidenberg, P., and Huang, H.F. (1978). Changes in human spermatozoa associated with high dose marihuana smoking. *Advances in the Biosciences*, **22**, 429–439.

Hézode, C., Roudot-Thoraval, F., Nguyen, S., *et al.* (2005). Daily cannabis smoking as a risk factor for progression of fibrosis in chronic hepatitis C. *Hepatology (Baltimore, Md.)*, **42**, 63–71.

Hézode, C., Zafrani, E.S., Roudot-Thoraval, F., *et al.* (2008). Daily cannabis use: a novel risk factor of steatosis severity in patients with chronic hepatitis C. *Gastroenterology*, **134**, 432–439.

Hii, S.W., Tam, J.D., Thompson, B.R., and Naughton, M.T. (2008). Bullous lung disease due to marijuana. *Respirology*, **13**, 122–127.

Hollister, L.E. (1986). Health aspects of cannabis. *Pharmacological Reviews*, **38**, 1–20.

Hollister, L.E. (1999). Interactions of marihuana and 9-THC with other drugs. In: G. Nahas, K.M. Sutin, D.J. Harvey, and S. Agurell (eds.). *Marihuana and Medicine*. Totowa, NJ: Humana Press, pp. 273–277.

Hoyer, F.F., Steinmetz, M., Zimmer, S., *et al.* (2011). Atheroprotection via cannabinoid receptor-2 is mediated by circulating and vascular cells in vivo. *Journal of Molecular and Cellular Cardiology*, **51**, 1007–1014.

Hutchings, D.E., Martin, B.R., Gamagaris, Z., Miller, N., and Fico, T. (1989). Plasma concentrations of delta-9-tetrahydrocannabinol in dams and fetuses following acute or multiple prenatal dosing in rats. *Life Sciences*, **44**, 697–701.

Ishida, J.H., Peters, M.G., Jin, C., *et al.* (2008). Influence of cannabis use on severity of hepatitis C disease. *Clinical Gastroenterology and Hepatology*, **6**, 69–75.

Jakab, L., Szántó, Z., Benkő, I., Szalai, Z., Pótó, L., and Molnár, F.T. (2012). [On the ethiogenesis of spontaneus primary pneumothorax. Marijuana: a cause or blame?]. *Magyar Sebészet*, **65**, 421–425.

Joesoef, M.R., Beral, V., Aral, S.O., Rolfs, R.T., and Cramer, D.W. (1993). Fertility and use of cigarettes, alcohol, marijuana, and cocaine. *Annals of Epidemiology*, **3**, 592–594.

Joffe, A., Yancy, S., and the Committee on Substance Abuse and Committee on Adolescence. (2004). Legalization of marijuana: potential impact on youth. *Pediatrics*, **113**, 632–638.

Jones, R.K., Shinar, D., and Walsh, J.M. (2003). *State of Knowledge of Drug Impaired Driving.*. Final report, National Highway Traffic Safety Administration Report DOT HS 809 642 Washington, DC: National Highway Traffic Safety Administration.

Jones, R.T. and Benowitz, N. (1976). The 30-day trip – clinical studies of cannabis tolerance and dependence. In: M.C. Braude, S. Szara (eds.). *The Pharmacology of Marihuana*. Vol. 2. New York: Raven Press, pp. 627–642.

Jones, R.T. and Stone, G.C. (1970). Psychological studies of marijuana and alcohol in man. *Psychopharmacologia*, **18**, 108–117.

Jones, R.T., Benowitz, N., and Bachman, J. (1976). Clinical studies of cannabis tolerance and dependence. *Annals of the New York Academy of Sciences*, **282**, 221–239.

Jones, R.T., Benowitz, N., and Herning, R.I. (1981). Clinical relevance of cannabis tolerance and dependence. *Journal of Clinical Pharmacology*, **21**, 143–152.

Jukic, A.M., Weinberg, C.R., Baird, D.D., and Wilcox, A.J. (2007). Lifestyle and reproductive factors associated with follicular phase length. *Journal of Women's Health (2002)*, **16**, 1340–1347.

Julien, R.M. (1998). *A Primer of Drug Action*, New York: W.H. Freeman and Company.

Katona, S., Kaminski, E., Sanders, H., and Zajicek, J. (2005). Cannabinoid influence on cytokine profile in multiple sclerosis. *Clinical and Experimental Immunology*, **140**, 580–585.

Klein, T.W., Newton, C., and Friedman, H. (1998). Cannabinoid receptors and the cytokine network. *Advances in Experimental Medicine and Biology*, **437**, 215–222.

Kopach, O., Vats, J., Netsyk, O., Voitenko, N., Irving, A., and Fedirko, N. (2012). Cannabinoid receptors in submandibular acinar cells: functional coupling between saliva fluid and electrolytes secretion and Ca^{2+} signalling. *Journal of Cell Science*, **125**, 1884–1895.

Kosel, B.W., Aweeka, F.T., Benowitz, N.L., *et al.* (2002). The effects of cannabinoids on the pharmacokinetics of indinavir and nelfinavir. *AIDS*, **16**, 543–550.

Kowal, M.A., Colzato, L.S., and Hommel, B. (2011). Decreased spontaneous eye blink rates in chronic cannabis users: evidence for striatal cannabinoid-dopamine interactions. *PLoS One*, **6**, e26662.

Laumon, B., Gadegbeku, B., Martin, J.L., and Biecheler, M.B. (2005). Cannabis intoxication and fatal road crashes in France: population based case-control study. *British Medical Journal*, **331**, 1371.

Leweke, F.M., Kampmann, C., Radwan, M., *et al.* (1998). The effects of tetrahydrocannabinol on the recognition of emotionally charged words: an analysis using event-related brain potentials. *Neuropsychobiology*, **37**, 104–111.

Leweke, F.M., Schneider, U., Thies, M., Münte, T.F., and Emrich, H.M. (1999). Effects of synthetic delta9-tetrahydrocannabinol on binocular depth inversion of natural and artificial objects in man. *Psychopharmacology*, **142**, 230–235.

Magina, S., Esteves-Pinto, C., Moura, E., *et al.* (2011). Inhibition of basal and ultraviolet B-induced melanogenesis by cannabinoid CB_1 receptors: a keratinocyte-dependent effect. *Archives of Dermatological Research*, **303**, 201–210.

Maurer, M., Henn, V., Dittrich, A., and Hofmann, A. (1990). Delta-9-tetrahydrocannabinol shows antispastic and analgesic effects in a single case double-blind trial. *European Archives of Psychiatry and Clinical Neuroscience*, **240**, 1–4.

Mendelson, J.H., Mello, N.K., and Ellingboe, J. (1985). Acute effects of marihuana smoking on prolactin levels in human females. *The Journal of Pharmacology and Experimental Therapeutics*, **232**, 220–222.

Merzouki, A., Molero Mesa, J., Louktibi, A., Kadiri, M., and Urbano, G.V. (2008). Assessing changes in pupillary size in Rifian smokers of kif (*Cannabis sativa* L.). *Journal of Forensic and Legal Medicine*, **15**, 335–338.

Miron, J.A. (2005). *The Budgetary Implications of Marijuana Prohibition*. Available at: http://www.prohibitioncosts.org.

Miron, J.A. and Waldock, K. (2010). *The Budgetary Impact of Ending Drug Prohibition*. Washington DC: Cato Institute. Available at: http://www.cato.org/publications/white-paper/budgetary-impact-ending-drug-prohibition.

Mittleman, M.A., Lewis, R.A., Maclure, M., Sherwood, J.B., and Muller, J.E. (2001). Triggering myocardial infarction by marijuana. *Circulation*, **103**, 2805–2809.

Molina, P.E., Winsauer, P., Zhang, P., *et al.* (2011). Cannabinoid administration attenuates the progression of simian immunodeficiency virus. *AIDS Research and Human Retroviruses*, **27**, 585–592.

Morgan, C.J., Freeman, T.P., Schafer, G.L., and Curran, H.V. (2010). Cannabidiol attenuates the appetitive effects of Delta 9-tetrahydrocannabinol in humans smoking their chosen cannabis. *Neuropsychopharmacology*, **35**, 1879–1885.

Mueller, B.A., Daling, J.R., Weiss, N.S. and Moore, D.E. (1990). Recreational drug use and the risk of primary infertility. *Epidemiology*, **1**, 195–200.

Nawrot, T.S., Perez, L., Künzli, N., Munters, E., and Nemery, B. (2011). Public health importance of triggers of myocardial infarction: a comparative risk assessment. *Lancet*, **377**, 732–740.

Nicholson, A.N., Turner, C., Stone, B.M., and Robson, P.J. (2004). Effect of Delta-9-tetrahydrocannabinol and cannabidiol on nocturnal sleep and early-morning behavior in young adults. *Journal of Clinical Psychopharmacology*, **24**, 305–313.

NIS News Bulletin. (2008). *State Earns 400 Million Euros a Year from Cannabis Bars.* May 3. Available at: http://www.nisnews.nl.

Nutt, D.J., King, L.A., and Phillips, L.D. (2010). Independent Scientific Committee on Drugs. Drug harms in the UK: a multicriteria decision analysis. *Lancet*, **376**, 1558–1565.

Pacifici, R., Zuccaro, P., Pichini, S., *et al.* (2003). Modulation of the immune system in cannabis users. *Journal of the American Medical Association*, **289**, 1929–1931.

Percie du Sert, N., Ho, W.S., Rudd, J.A., Andrews, P.L. (2010). Cannabinoid-induced reduction in antral pacemaker frequency: a telemetric study in the ferret. *Neurogastroenterology and Motility*, **22**, 1257–1266.

Permutt, M.A., Goodwin, D.W., Schwin, R., and Hill, S.Y. (1976). The effect of marijuana on carbohydrate metabolism. *The American Journal of Psychiatry*, **133**, 220–224.

Pletcher, M.J., Vittinghoff, E., Kalhan, R., *et al.* (2012). Association between marijuana exposure and pulmonary function over 20 years. *Journal of the American Medical Association*, **307**, 173–181.

Preet, A., Ganju, R.K., and Groopman, J.E. (2008). Delta9-Tetrahydrocannabinol inhibits epithelial growth factor-induced lung cancer cell migration in vitro as well as its growth and metastasis in vivo. *Oncogene*, **10**, 339–346.

Prestifilippo, J.P., Fernandez-Solari, J., de la Cal, C., *et al.* (2006). Inhibition of salivary secretion by activation of cannabinoid receptors. *Experimental Biology and Medicine (Maywood, N.J.)*, **231**, 1421–1429.

Rajavashisth, T.B., Shaheen, M., and Norris, K.C., *et al.* (2012). Decreased prevalence of diabetes in marijuana users: cross-sectional data from the National Health and Nutrition Examination Survey (NHANES) III. *BMJ Open*, **2**, 494.

Richardson, G.A., Ryan, C., Willford, J., Day, N.L., and Goldschmidt, L. (2002). Prenatal alcohol and marijuana exposure: effects on neuropsychological outcomes at 10 years. *Neurotoxicology and Teratology*, **24**, 309–320.

Riggs, P.K., Vaida, F., Rossi, S.S., *et al.* (2012). A pilot study of the effects of cannabis on appetite hormones in HIV-infected adult men. *Brain Research*, **1431**, 46–52.

Rodondi, N., Pletcher, M.J., Liu, K., Hulley, S.B., and Sidney, S. (2006). Marijuana use, diet, body mass index, and cardiovascular risk factors (from the CARDIA study). *The American Journal of Cardiology*, **98**, 478–484.

Roth, M.D., Arora, A., Barsky, S.H., Kleerup, E.C., Simmons, M., and Tashkin, D.P. (1998). Airway inflammation in young marijuana and tobacco smokers. *American Journal of Respiratory and Critical Care Medicine*, **157**, 928–937.

RSA Commission on Illegal Drugs, Communities and Public Policy (2007). *Drugs – Facing Facts.* Available at: http://www.rsadrugscommission.org/.

Schulz-Katterbach, M., Imfeld, T., and Imfeld, C. (2009). Cannabis and caries – does regular cannabis use increase the risk of caries in cigarette smokers? *Schweizer Monatsschrift für Zahnmedizin = Revue Mensuelle Suisse d'odonto-stomatologie = Rivista Mensile Svizzera di Odontologia e Stomatologia/SSO*, **119**, 576–583.

Scopinho, A.A., Guimarães, F.S., Corrêa, F.M., and Resstel, L.B. (2011). Cannabidiol inhibits the hyperphagia induced by cannabinoid-1 or serotonin-1A receptor agonists. *Pharmacology, Biochemistry, and Behavior*, **98**, 268–272.

Sewell, R.A., Schnakenberg, A., Elander, J., *et al.* (2013). Acute effects of THC on time perception in frequent and infrequent cannabis users. *Psychopharmacology*, **226**, 401–413.

Simonetto, D.A., Oxentenko, A.S., Herman, M.L., and Szostek, J.H. (2012). Cannabinoid hyperemesis: a case series of 98 patients. *Mayo Clinic Proceedings*, **87**, 114–119.

Smiley, A.M. (1999). Marijuana: on road and driving simulator studies. In: H. Kalant, W. Corrigal, W. Hall, and R. Smart (eds.). *The Health Effects of Cannabis*. Toronto: Addiction Research Foundation, pp. 173–191.

Steffens, S., Veillard, N.R., Arnaud, C., *et al.* (2005). Low dose oral cannabinoid therapy reduces progression of atherosclerosis in mice. *Nature*, **434**, 782–786.

Sylvestre, D.L., Clements, B.J., and Malibu, Y. (2006). Cannabis use improves retention and virological outcomes in patients treated for hepatitis C. *European Journal of Gastroenterology & Hepatology*, **18**, 1057–1063.

Tashkin, D.P., Simmons, M.S., and Tseng, C.H. (2012). Impact of changes in regular use of marijuana and/or tobacco on chronic bronchitis. *Journal of Chronic Obstructive Pulmonary Disease*, **9**, 367–374.

Taylor, D.R., Poulton, R., Moffitt, T.E., Ramankutty, P., and Sears, M.R., (2000). The respiratory effects of cannabis dependence in young adults. *Addiction*, **95**, 1669–1677.

Thomas, H. (1993). Psychiatric symptoms in cannabis users. *British Journal of Psychiatry*, **163**, 141–149.

Thompson, G.R., Rosenkrantz, H., Schaeppi, U.H., and Braude, M.C. (1973). Comparison of acute oral toxicity of cannabinoids in rats, dogs and monkeys. *Toxicology and Applied Pharmacology*, **25**, 363–372.

Thomson, W.M., Poulton, R., Broadbent, J.M., *et al.* (2008). Cannabis smoking and periodontal disease among young adults. *JAMA*, **299**, 525–531.

Tindall, B., Philpot, C.R., Cooper, D.A., *et al.* (1988). The Sydney AIDS Project: development of acquired immunodeficiency syndrome in a group of HIV seropositive homosexual men. *Australian and New Zealand Journal of Medicine*, **18**, 8–15.

Tunbridge, R., Clark, A., Ward, B.N., Dye, L., and Berghaus, G. (2000). *Prioritising Drugs and Medicines for Development of Roadside Impairment Testing*. Project Deliverable DR1, CERTIFIED EU Research Project (Contract No RO-98-3054). Leeds: School of Psychology, University of Leeds.

Van den Brink, W. (2008). Forum: decriminalization of cannabis. *Current Opinion in Psychiatry*, **21**, 122–126.

Van Laere, K., Casteels, C and Dhollander, I., *et al.* (2010). Widespread decrease of type 1 cannabinoid receptor availability in Huntington disease in vivo. *Journal of Nuclear Medicine: Official Publication, Society of Nuclear Medicine*, **51**, 1413–1417.

Vinson, D. (2006). Marijuana and other illicit drug use and the risk of injury: A case-control study. *Missouri Medicine*, **103**, 152–156.

Vivas, A.B., Estevez, A.F., Moreno, M., Panagis, G. and Flores, P. (2012). Use of cannabis enhances attentional inhibition. *Human Psychopharmacology*, **27**, 464–469.

Vuolo, M. (2013). National-level drug policy and young people's illicit drug use: a multilevel analysis of the European Union. *Drug and Alcohol Dependence*, **131**, 149–156.

Wade, D.T., Makela, P., Robson, P., House, H. and Bateman C. (2004). Do cannabis-based medicinal extracts have general or specific effects on symptoms in multiple sclerosis? A double-blind, randomized, placebo-controlled study on 160 patients. *Multiple Sclerosis Journal*, **10**, 434–441.

Wetherell, M.A., Atherton, K., Grainger, J., Brosnan, R. and Scholey, A.B. (2012). The effects of multitasking on psychological stress reactivity in recreational users of cannabis and MDMA. *Human Psychopharmacology*, **27**, 167–176.

Whitfield, R.M., Bechtel, L.M. and Starich, G.H. (1997). The impact of ethanol and Marinol/marijuana usage on HIV+/AIDS patients undergoing azidothymidine, azidothymidine/dideoxycytidine, or dideoxyinosine therapy. *Alcoholism, Clinical and Experimental Research*, **21**, 122–127.

Willecke, F., Zeschky, K. and Ortiz Rodriguez, A., *et al.* (2011). Cannabinoid receptor 2 signaling does not modulate atherogenesis in mice. *PLoS One*, **6**, 19405.

Willford, J.A., Chandler, L.S., Goldschmidt, L. and Day, N.L. (2010). Effects of prenatal tobacco, alcohol and marijuana exposure on processing speed, visual-motor coordination, and interhemispheric transfer. *Neurotoxicology and Teratology*, **32**, 580–588.

Winsauer, P.J., Molina, P.E. and Amedee, A.M., *et al.* (2011). Tolerance to chronic delta-9-tetrahydrocannabinol (Δ⁹-THC) in rhesus macaques infected with simian immunodeficiency virus. *Experimental and Clinical Psychopharmacology*, **19**, 154–172.

Wolff, V., Armspach, J.P. and Lauer V., *et al.* (2013). Cannabis-related stroke: Myth or reality? *Stroke; A Journal of Cerebral Circulation*, **44**, 558–563.

Wong, B.S., Camilleri, M. and Busciglio, I., *et al.* (2011). Pharmacogenetic trial of a cannabinoid agonist shows reduced fasting colonic motility in patients with nonconstipated irritable bowel syndrome. *Gastroenterology*, **141**, 1638–1647.

Wong, B.S., Camilleri, M. and Eckert, D., *et al.* (2012). Randomized pharmacodynamic and pharmacogenetic trial of dronabinol effects on colon transit in irritable bowel syndrome-diarrhea. *Neurogastroenterology and Motility*, **24**, 358–e169.

Yamaori, S., Koeda, K., Kushihara, M., Hada, Y., Yamamoto, I. and Watanabe K. (2012). Comparison in the in vitro inhibitory effects of major phytocannabinoids and polycyclic aromatic hydrocarbons contained in marijuana smoke on cytochrome P450 2C9 activity. *Drug Metabolism and Pharmacokinetics*, **27**, 294–300.

Zajicek, J.P., Sanders, H.P. and Wright, D.E., *et al.* (2005). Cannabinoids in multiple sclerosis (CAMS) study: safety and efficacy data for 12 months follow up. *Journal of Neurology, Neurosurgery and Psychiatry*, **76**, 1664–1669.

Zhao, Y., Liu, Y. and Zhang, W., *et al.* (2010). WIN55212-2 ameliorates atherosclerosis associated with suppression of pro-inflammatory responses in ApoE-knockout mice. *European Journal of Pharmacology*, **649**, 285–292.

Chapter 39

Harm Reduction Policies for Cannabis

Wayne Hall and Louisa Degenhardt

39.1 Introduction

Cannabis is the most widely used recreational illicit drug globally, and its use has probably increased over the past decade. In 2011, an estimated 119–224 million adults (2.5–6.0% of the global adult population aged 15–64 years) had used cannabis in the previous year (UNODC 2012). In the World Mental Health Surveys, the lifetime use of cannabis was higher in the US and New Zealand than in Europe, which had higher rates of reported cannabis use than the Middle East, Africa, and Asia (Degenhardt et al. 2008).

In most countries cannabis use for recreational reasons begins in the mid to late teens and is most common in the early 20s (Degenhardt et al. 2008; Hall and Degenhardt 2009). Most cannabis use is intermittent and time-limited (Bachman et al. 1997), with about 10% of users becoming daily users, and another 20–30% weekly users (Hall and Pacula 2010). Cannabis use declines during the early to mid 20s as young adults enter full-time employment, marry, and have children (Anthony 2006; Bachman et al. 1997; Fergusson et al. 2012).

Cannabis is also used for medicinal reasons although this type of use is much less common than recreational use. The focus of this chapter is on policies that aim to reduce harm from recreational cannabis use.

39.2 What are harm reduction policies?

The term "harm reduction" was first used in the area of injecting drug use to describe policies to prevent the spread of HIV/AIDS among drug injectors without requiring abstinence of them e.g., advising injectors not to share injecting equipment and providing clean needles and syringes to reduce sharing (Riley et al. 2012). Harm reduction has since expanded to cover polices that aim to reduce the harmful consequences of all types of drug use without necessarily requiring drug users to stop or reduce their drug use (IHRA 2010; Lenton and Single 1998).

Advocates of harm reduction accept that some people will engage in risky patterns of illegal drug use, despite the efforts of government and civil society to discourage such use. They attach a higher priority to keeping these people alive and preventing serious damage to their health than insisting upon abstinence as the only acceptable goal. They encourage problem drug users to seek treatment, but users who are not interested in treatment are advised on how to reduce harms arising from their drug use using approaches that are practical, feasible, effective, safe, and cost-effective (Carter et al. 2012), such as: user-based education about injecting and overdose risks, providing clean needles and syringes, and distributing opioid antagonists to revive drug users who overdose (Darke and Hall 1997; Strang and Farrell 1992).

Harm reduction policies for cannabis have been underdeveloped by comparison with those for injected drugs. This seems to be for two main reasons (Hall and Pacula 2010). First, many who advocate for more liberal cannabis policies do not accept that cannabis use harms users; they claim that the harms arising from criminal records cause greater harms than cannabis use (Wodak et al. 2002). Second, those who support a continuation of current cannabis policies oppose harm reduction because they argue that this approach implicitly condones cannabis use. In their view, the only acceptable policies are criminal penalties for cannabis use and abstinence oriented-treatment for problem cannabis users (DuPont 1996).

We do not accept either of these views. There is good evidence that cannabis use harms some users (Hall and Degenhardt 2009) and given this, there is a strong ethical case for warning cannabis users about these risks. We also believe that harm reduction advice to current cannabis users need not condone use; such advice can be an effective way of communicating the risks of cannabis use to users who reject the advocacy of abstinence.

We consider approaches to reducing cannabis-related harm under the following three headings: (1) advice to cannabis users about how to reduce their risks to themselves and others; (2) specific interventions for problem cannabis users to reduce these risks; (3) policies that combine education with fines or criminal sanctions to deter people from using cannabis in ways that may harm others, e.g., driving a motor vehicle while cannabis-impaired; and (4) legislative approaches that aim to reduce the harms of cannabis prohibition by removing or reducing penalties for cannabis use and possession.

A harm reduction approach to cannabis use (Fischer and Kendall 2011; Hall 1995; Swift et al. 2000) requires a specification of the harms that cannabis use can cause and of the patterns of use most likely to produce these harms. We therefore first summarize what is known about the connection between cannabis use and various harms before considering ways in which these harms can be reduced. We begin with the harms of acute cannabis use: those that can occur after a single occasion of use, focusing on the harm that can potentially most seriously affect cannabis users and other persons, i.e., motor vehicle accidents caused by cannabis-impaired drivers. We then consider harms arising from chronic use, that is daily or near daily use over periods of months or years. These harms primarily affect cannabis users.

39.3 Harms of acute cannabis use

39.3.1 Accidental injury and death in car crashes

Cannabis and tetrahydrocannabinol (THC) produce dose-related impairments in laboratory measures of reaction time, information processing, perceptual-motor coordination, motor performance, attention, and tracking (Ramaekers et al. 2004; Solowij 1998). All these effects could increase the risk of accidents if users drive a car while acutely intoxicated.

Experimental studies of the effects of cannabis upon driving have reported more modest impairments than intoxicating doses of alcohol. Cannabis-impaired drivers appear to be more aware that they are impaired and attempt to compensate for their impairment by driving more slowly and taking fewer risks than alcohol-impaired drivers (Smiley 1999). But not all cannabis-related impairment can be compensated for: drivers' responses to simulated emergency situations are impaired by cannabis use (Robbe 1994; Smiley 1999).

Epidemiological studies (Drummer et al. 2004; Gerberich et al. 2003; Laumon et al. 2005; Mura et al. 2003) also indicate that cannabis users who drive while intoxicated are at increased risk of motor vehicle crashes. Gerberich et al. (2003) found that cannabis users had higher rates of hospitalization for injury from all causes than former cannabis users or nonusers in a cohort of 64,657 patients from a US Health Maintenance Organization. Mura et al. (2003) found a similar relationship in a study of 900 persons hospitalized for motor vehicle injuries and 900 age- and sex-matched controls admitted to French hospitals. Drummer et al. (2004), who assessed THC in blood in 1420 Australian drivers killed in accidents, found that cannabis users were more likely to be culpable (odds ratio (OR) = 2.5) and those with THC levels greater than 5 micrograms/mL had a higher accident risk (OR = 6.6) than those without THC. Laumon et al. (2005) compared blood THC levels in 6766 culpable and 3006 nonculpable drivers in France between October 2001 and September 2003. They found increased culpability among drivers with THC levels of greater than 1 microgram/ml (OR = 2.87). A dose–response relationship between THC and culpability persisted after controlling for blood alcohol concentration, age, and time of accident.

A systematic review of the epidemiological evidence by Asbridge and colleagues (2012) analyzed the role of cannabis in fatal and nonfatal accidents in nine case–control and culpability studies. Recent cannabis use approximately doubled the risk of motor vehicle crashes (OR = 1.92 95% CI: 1.35, 2.73) and the risk was higher in studies that were better designed (2.21 vs. 1.78), in case–control rather than culpability studies (2.79 vs. 1.65) and in studies of fatalities rather than injuries (2.10 vs. 1.74). The twofold increase in the risk of motor vehicle crashes after using cannabis compares with a 6–15 times higher risk for alcohol. Mura et al. (2003) estimated that 2.5% of fatal accidents in France could be attributed to cannabis compared with 29% for alcohol.

39.3.2 Reducing cannabis-impaired driving

Cannabis users should refrain from driving within several hours of using cannabis, but it is uncertain how many will act on road safety education campaigns that provide such advice. Similar campaigns to discourage alcohol-impaired driving had limited effects on their own (Homel 1988). More effective deterrence combines public education with well-publicized enforcement of laws that forbid driving while alcohol intoxicated, usually defined as driving with a blood alcohol content (BAC) above a specified level (typically 0.08% or 0.05%). The deterrent effect of these laws is enhanced by random roadside alcohol breath testing (RBT) accompanied by publicity campaigns that alert drivers to the risk of detection and loss of license if they drive while intoxicated (Homel 1988).

Cannabis users will also need to be persuaded that they are at risk of being detected if they drive while impaired (Watling et al. 2010). Governments in Australia, Western Europe, and the US have pursued such deterrence by introducing roadside drug testing (RDT) for cannabis (Butler 2007). This has been modelled on RBT but uses a saliva test to detect recent use of cannabis. RDT does not use an epidemiological rationale for a specified level of detected cannabis use to define impaired driving like that for alcohol. In the case of RBT for alcohol, there is a simple relationship between alcohol breath concentration, blood alcohol level, and impairment, with the risk of a crash doubling after 0.05%. It has been more difficult to define cannabis-impaired driving because of the lack of a simple relationship between blood levels of THC and impaired driving (Grotenhermen et al. 2007). Governments that have introduced such testing (Butler 2007) have defined any detectable level of cannabis in saliva (which is indicative of recent use) as evidence of impairment. The Australian State of Victoria introduced this type of RDT saliva testing in 2004; so have other Australian States since, and 13 US states (Butler 2007; Lacey et al. 2010).

Legislators in these countries have assumed that RDT will reduce road crash deaths in the same way that RBT reduced alcohol-related crashes (Henstridge et al. 1997; Lacey et al. 2010). This may be an optimistic assumption, because of major differences in the ways that RBT and RDT have been implemented. RBT in Australia has been accompanied by widespread publicity campaigns and high rates of roadside testing (Homel 1988). RDT, by contrast, has typically been introduced on a small scale, with much less publicity, and unknown deterrent effects (Watling et al. 2010). Nearly a decade after its introduction, political support for RDT still relies on borrowing evidence of effectiveness from RBT, because there is no direct evidence that RDT has reduced cannabis- or other drug-related fatalities or deterred drug users from driving while impaired.

A more harm reduction-focused version of RDT would use measures of cannabis use that predicted impaired driving. Such an approach has been advocated by Grotenhermen et al. (2007). This could be combined with educational campaigns to encourage cannabis users to adopt "designated driver" programs.

39.4 The harms of chronic cannabis use

In the absence of measures of the doses of THC that regular users typically consume, "chronic" cannabis use has usually been defined in epidemiological studies as near daily cannabis use over months or years. This is the pattern of use that has been most consistently associated with adverse health outcomes in adolescence and adulthood (Hall and Degenhardt 2009). The major challenge in interpreting these studies is in ruling out alternative explanations of the associations between regular cannabis use and these outcomes. Heavy cannabis use is highly correlated with regular alcohol, tobacco, and other illicit drug use, all of which can adversely affect health (Hall and Pacula 2010). Regular cannabis users also differ from nonusers (before they use cannabis) in ways that may affect their risk of experiencing these adverse outcomes (Hall and Pacula 2010). Statistical control of confounding has been used to assess these relationships, but there are epidemiologists who argue that this strategy cannot wholly exclude confounding (Hall and Pacula 2010; Macleod et al. 2004).

39.4.1 Cannabis dependence

Cannabis dependence is characterized by impaired control over cannabis use, and difficulty in ceasing use despite harms caused by it. In Australia, Canada, and the US, cannabis dependence is the most common type of drug dependence after dependence upon alcohol and tobacco (Hall and Pacula 2010). It affects 1–2% of adults in the past year, and 4–8% of adults during their lifetime. Over the past two decades, increasing numbers of persons have sought help to stop using cannabis in the US, Europe, and Australia (Hall and Pacula 2010). After tobacco and alcohol, cannabis was the most common form of drug dependence in the US in the 1990s and early 2000s (Anthony 2006). The same was true in Australia in the late 1990s (Roxburgh et al. 2010).

The lifetime risk of dependence among US cannabis users was estimated at 9% (Anthony 2006) in the early 1990s and at one in six among those who initiated in adolescence (Anthony 2006). The equivalent risks were 32% for nicotine, 23% for heroin, 17% for cocaine, 15% for alcohol and 11% for stimulant users (Anthony et al. 1994).

39.4.2 Reducing the risks of cannabis dependence

Harm reduction approaches to cannabis dependence are underdeveloped (Hall and Swift 2006). Current and potential cannabis users should be informed about the risks of developing cannabis dependence, probably a still underappreciated risk of cannabis use. Research is needed into the most persuasive ways of informing young people about the risks of dependence. The following are suggestions about the type of advice that could be given:

◆ Cannabis users can become dependent on cannabis.

◆ The risk is around 10%, a little lower than that for alcohol, nicotine, and opiates (Hall and Degenhardt 2009) but risk increases the younger the age that a person begins to use (Anthony 2006).

◆ Using cannabis more than weekly increases the risks of dependence and probably increases the risks of other adverse effects of use (Hall and Degenhardt 2009).

1 2 3

Plausible harm reduction strategies for cannabis can be modelled on strategies that have been used to reduce alcohol-related harm (Hall and Swift 2006). These could include screening and brief advice for heavy cannabis consumers seen in general practice, hospital, or nonmedical settings (Fischer et al. 2009). Research is needed to assess whether these approaches reduce consumption and problems as do similar approaches for problem alcohol use (e.g., Babor et al. 2010a; Shand et al. 2003). This approach could be used, for example, with young adults who present with respiratory problems and anxiety and depression in primary care (Degenhardt et al. 2001).

Brief interventions could also be targeted at populations in which cannabis dependence is known to be high, e.g., youth mental health services, juvenile justice centers, and college students (Fischer et al. 2009; Hall et al. 2008). A "check-up" approach modelled on the Brief Drinker Check-up (Miller and Sovereign 1989) provides a promising way of raising the health risks of cannabis use in a nonconfrontational way (see Berghuis et al. 2006; Martin and Copeland 2008; Stephens et al. 2007).

There are limited harm reduction options for those who require assistance to deal with cannabis dependence. Cognitive behavioral therapy reduces cannabis use and cannabis-related problems, but only 15% of those treated remain abstinent 6–12 months after treatment (Hall and Pacula 2010). Pharmacological treatments have been trialed to reduce severity of withdrawal syndrome, but trials have so far found modest efficacy (Danovitch and Gorelick 2012). Abstinence-based 12-step approaches (e.g., Marijuana Anonymous) that involve changing friendship networks that encourage cannabis use and using self-help support groups to sustain abstinence remain to be evaluated.

39.4.3 The respiratory risks of cannabis smoking

Regular cannabis smokers report more chronic bronchitis (wheeze, sputum production, and chronic coughs) than nonsmokers (Tetrault et al. 2007). The immunological competence of the respiratory system is also impaired, increasing cannabis users' health service use for respiratory infections (Tashkin et al. 2002).

The effects of long-term cannabis smoking on respiratory function are less certain (Howden and Naughton 2011; Lee and Hancox 2011; Tetrault et al. 2007). A longitudinal study of 1037 New Zealand youths followed until the age of 26 (Taylor et al. 2002) found impaired respiratory function in cannabis dependent users, but this was not replicated in a longer-term follow-up of US users (Tashkin et al. 2002). Chronic cannabis smoking has not been found to increase the risk of emphysema in follow-ups over 8 years in cannabis-only smokers in the US (Tashkin 2005) or New Zealand (Aldington et al. 2007).

Cannabis smoke contains many of the same carcinogens as tobacco smoke, some at higher levels (Moir et al. 2008). It is also mutagenic and carcinogenic in the mouse skin test, and chronic cannabis smokers show pathological changes in lung cells (Tashkin 1999). Epidemiological studies, however, have not so far found increased risks of upper respiratory tract cancers. Sidney et al. (1997) found no increased risk of respiratory cancer among current or former cannabis users in an 8.6 year follow-up of 64,855 members of the Kaiser Permanente Medical Care Program. Zhang et al. (1999) reported an increased risk (OR = 2) of squamous cell carcinoma of the head and neck among cannabis users in 173 cases and 176 controls that persisted after adjusting for cigarette smoking, alcohol use, and other risk factors. Three other case–control studies of these cancers, however, have failed to find any such association (Hashibe et al. 2005).

Case–control studies of lung cancer have produced more consistent associations with cannabis use, but their interpretation is complicated by confounding by cigarette smoking (Mehra et al. 2006). A pooled analysis of three Moroccan case–control studies also found an elevated risk of lung cancer among cannabis smokers but all of them also smoked tobacco (Berthiller et al. 2008). A New Zealand case–control study of lung cancer in 79 adults under the age of 55 years and 324 community controls (Aldington et al. 2008) found a dose–response relationship between frequency of cannabis use and lung cancer risk. A US case–control study found a simple association between cannabis smoking and head and neck and lung cancers but these associations were no longer significant after controlling for tobacco use (Hashibe et al. 2006). Larger cohort and better designed case–control studies are needed to clarify whether there are any such risks from chronic cannabis smoking (Hashibe et al. 2005; Howden and Naughton 2011).

39.4.4 Cardiovascular risks of cannabis smoking

Cannabis and THC increase heart rate in a dose-related way, but healthy young adults quickly develop tolerance to these effects (Jones 2002; Sidney 2002). Cannabis smoking may precipitate myocardial infarctions in older adults with cardiovascular disease (Jones 2002; Sidney 2002). A case-crossover study by Mittleman et al. (2001) of 3882 patients who had had a myocardial infarction found that cannabis use increased the risk of a myocardial infarction 4.8 times in the hour after use. A prospective study of 1913 of these adults found a dose–response relationship between cannabis use and mortality over 3.8 years (Mukamal et al. 2008), with the risk increased 2.5 times for those who used less than weekly and 4.2 times among more than weekly users. These findings are supported by laboratory findings that smoking cannabis provokes angina in patients with heart disease (Gottschalk et al. 1977). Given the low prevalence of cannabis smoking in older adults, cannabis smoking is estimated to account for a smaller proportion of myocardial infarctions than air pollution (Nawrot et al. 2011).

39.4.5 Reducing the respiratory and cardiovascular risks of cannabis smoking

The respiratory risks of cannabis smoking would be eliminated if cannabis users used the oral route of administration. This is unlikely to happen, because most regular cannabis users find smoking the most efficient way to titrate their dose of THC (Grotenhermen 2004; Iversen 2007). Putatively "safer" forms of cannabis smoking, such as water pipes, have become popular in Australia (Hall and Swift 2000), but research suggests that water pipes deliver more tar per dose of THC than joints (Gowing et al. 2000). It is unclear how much the respiratory risks of cannabis smoking might be reduced if users were to smoke a smaller amount of more potent cannabis (Melamede 2005) because it is unclear whether cannabis users can reliably titrate their dose and, if they can, whether they do so (Hall and Pacula 2010).

Vaporizers are a potentially promising way of reducing the carcinogens and toxicants inhaled in cannabis smoke (Gieringer et al. 2004; Grotenhermen 2004; Melamede 2005). They deliver inhaled THC without carcinogens and toxicants by heating rather than burning cannabis. Gieringer et al. (2004) found that a Volcano® vaporizer achieved a similar delivery of THC to a cannabis cigarette while very substantially reducing the amount of carcinogens. Hazekamp et al. (2006) found that the same device had acceptable safety properties in delivering pure THC but Bloor et al. (2008) found that levels of released ammonia were still well above recommended safe levels.

Abrams et al. (2007) compared the effects of varying doses of cannabis delivered by a Volcano® and a joint in 18 subjects under double-blind conditions. The vaporizer delivered similar amounts of THC and produced similar psychological effects, with 16/18 subjects preferring the vaporizer. They did not test for delivery of tars and carcinogens, but found lower carbon monoxide levels in blood after using a vaporizer. Earleywine and Barnwell (2007) found that vaporizer users recruited via the Internet reported fewer respiratory symptoms. The rate of respiratory symptoms (bronchitis, wheeze, breathlessness) among 150 persons who only used vaporizers was 40% of that reported by cannabis smokers (after controlling for cigarette smoking, duration of use and amount typically used). More research needs to be done to evaluate the long term safety of vaporizers in reducing the respiratory risks of cannabis use.

39.4.6 Cognitive impairment

Deficits in verbal learning, memory, and attention are reported by heavy cannabis users, but these have not been consistently related to duration and frequency of use or cumulative dose of THC (Solowij et al. 2002). Debate continues about whether these deficits are due to acute drug effects, residual drug effects, or the effects of cumulative THC exposure (Solowij et al. 2002).

A recent prospective study (Meier et al. 2012) greatly strengthened the case that regular cannabis use, starting in adolescence and continuing throughout young adulthood, can cause cognitive decline in mid adulthood. In this study the authors examined changes in overall IQ and in specific cognitive abilities from early adolescence to mid adulthood in a cohort of 1037 New Zealanders born in Dunedin in 1972/1973. A detailed neuropsychological assessment was done at age 13 (before cannabis was first used) and again at age 38. There was a dose–response relationship between cannabis use and cognitive decline that persisted after adjustment for other factors known to affect cognitive abilities (e.g., recent cannabis use, alcohol, tobacco and other drug use, and schizophrenia). The cognitive decline was largest in those who began to use cannabis in adolescence and used regularly into adulthood. The decline was not explained by the lower educational achievement among cannabis users, because the effects were also found in cannabis users who finished high school. There was limited cognitive recovery in adolescent-onset users who had only stopped using cannabis for a year or more. There was no cognitive decline in adult-onset users who ceased cannabis use 12 months prior to interview. Key informants who knew the study participants well were more likely to report that heavy persistent cannabis users had problems with memory and attention than their peers who had not used the drug in this way.

39.4.7 Educational outcomes

Regular cannabis use in adolescence is associated with poor educational attainment (Lynskey and Hall 2000) but it has been unclear whether: (1) cannabis use is a contributory cause, (2) cannabis use is a consequence of poor educational attainment, or (3) cannabis use and poor educational attainment are the result of other factors (Lynskey and Hall 2000).

Longitudinal studies have found a relationship between cannabis use before the age of 15 years and early school leaving, and this has persisted after adjustment for confounders (e.g., Ellickson et al. 1998). The most plausible hypothesis is that impaired educational outcomes reflect a combination of: a higher pre-existing risk of school failure, the effects of regular cannabis use on cognitive performance, increased affiliation with peers who reject school, and a strong desire to make an early transition to adulthood (Lynskey and Hall 2000). A recent meta-analysis of three Australasian longitudinal studies by Horwood et al. (2010) suggested that the early use of cannabis increases the rate of failure to complete high school, enroll at university, and complete a degree.

39.4.8 Other illicit drug use

In the US, Australia, and New Zealand, regular cannabis users were most likely to later use heroin and cocaine, and the earlier they begin to use cannabis, the more likely they are to do so (Kandel 2002). Three explanations have been offered for these findings: (1) cannabis users have more opportunities to use other illicit drugs because they obtain cannabis from the same black market as other illicit drugs, (2) early cannabis users are more likely to use other illicit drugs for reasons that are unrelated to their cannabis use, and (3) the pharmacological effects of cannabis increase the propensity to use other illicit drugs (Hall and Pacula 2010).

There is some support for all three: young cannabis users report more opportunities to use cocaine at an earlier age (Wagner and Anthony 2002); socially deviant young people (who are more likely to use cocaine and heroin) start using cannabis at an earlier age than their peers (Fergusson et al. 2008); a simulation study (Morral et al. 2002) has shown that if the second hypothesis were true, it would predict the relationships observed between cannabis and other illicit drug use; and animal studies suggest that cannabis, cocaine, and heroin all act on the brain's "reward center," the nucleus accumbens (Gardner 1999), and that the cannabinoid and opioid systems in the brain interact with each other (Manzanares et al. 1999).

The second hypothesis has been tested in longitudinal studies that assess whether cannabis users are more likely to report heroin and cocaine use after statistically controlling for confounders (e.g., Lessem et al. 2006). Adjustment for confounders (Fergusson et al. 2006) attenuates but does not eliminate the relationships between regular cannabis use and other illicit drug use (Hall and Lynskey 2005). Studies of twins discordant for cannabis use (Lynskey et al. 2003) found that the twin who had used cannabis was more likely to have used other illicit drugs than their co-twin who had not and the relationship persists after controlling for nonshared environmental factors.

39.4.9 **Psychosis and schizophrenia**

A 15-year follow-up of 50,465 Swedish male conscripts found that those who had tried cannabis by age 18 were 2.4 times more likely to be diagnosed with schizophrenia than those who had not (Andréasson et al. 1987). The risk increased with the frequency of cannabis use and remained significant after statistical adjustment for a limited set of confounding variables. Those who had used cannabis ten or more times by age 18 were 2.3 times more likely to be diagnosed with schizophrenia than those who had not.

Zammit et al. (2002) reported a 27-year follow-up of the same cohort which also found a dose–response relationship between frequency of cannabis use at age 18 and risk of schizophrenia during the follow-up period that persisted after statistically controlling for other confounding factors. They estimated that 13% of cases of schizophrenia could be averted if all cannabis use were prevented. Zammit et al.'s findings have been supported by longitudinal studies in the Netherlands (van Os et al. 2002), Germany (Henquet et al. 2004), and New Zealand (Arseneault et al. 2002; Fergusson et al. 2003), all of which found a similar relationship that persisted after adjustment for confounders.

A meta-analysis of these longitudinal studies reported a pooled OR of 1.4 (95% confidence interval (CI): 1.20, 1.65) of psychotic symptoms or psychotic disorder among those who had ever used cannabis (Moore et al. 2007). The risk of psychotic symptoms or psychotic disorders was higher in regular users (OR = 2.09 (95% CI: 1.54, 2.84)). Reverse causation was implausible because, in most of these studies, cases reporting psychotic symptoms at baseline were excluded or the relationship persisted after statistical adjustment for pre-existing psychotic symptoms. The hypothesis that cannabis use and psychosis are both caused by confounding factors was harder to exclude because the association between cannabis use and psychosis was attenuated after statistical adjustment for potential confounders and no study assessed all major confounders.

The evidence is conflicting on whether the incidence of schizophrenia has increased as cannabis use has increased among young adults, as would be expected if the relationship were causal. An Australian study did not find clear evidence of increased psychosis incidence despite steep increases in cannabis use during the 1980s and 1990s (Degenhardt et al. 2003). A British study (Hickman et al. 2007) suggested that it was too early to detect any increased incidence in Britain in the 1990s. Another British (Boydell et al. 2006) and a Swiss study (Ajdacic-Gross et al. 2007) reported increased incidence of psychoses in recent birth cohorts but a third British study failed to do so (Advisory Council on the Misuse of Drugs 2008).

39.4.10 Cannabis use and other mental disorders and symptoms

Less consistent and weaker relationships have been reported between regular cannabis use and depression. Fergusson and Horwood (1997), for example, found a dose–response relationship between frequency of cannabis use by age 16 and depressive disorder but the relationship was no longer statistically significant after adjusting for confounders. A meta-analysis of these studies (Moore et al. 2007) found an association between cannabis use and depressive disorders (OR = 1.49 (95% CI: 1.15, 1.94)). The authors argued, however, that these studies had not controlled for confounders, and had not convincingly excluded the possibility that depressed young people are more likely to use cannabis.

Several case–control studies have found a relationship between cannabis use and suicide in adolescents but it is unclear whether this is causal. For example, a New Zealand case control study (Beautrais et al. 1999) of serious suicide found that 16% of the 302 suicide attempters had a cannabis disorder compared with 2% of the 1028 community controls. Controlling for social disadvantage, depression, and alcohol dependence reduced but did not eliminate the association (OR = 2). The evidence from prospective studies is mixed. Fergusson and Horwood (1997), for example, found a dose–response relationship between frequency of cannabis use by age 16 and a self-reported suicide attempt but the association did not persist after controlling for confounders. Patton et al. (1997) found that cannabis was associated with self-harmful behavior among females but not males, after controlling for depression and alcohol use. A meta-analysis (Moore et al. 2007) of these studies reported that they were too heterogeneous to estimate risk, and few had excluded reverse causation or properly controlled for confounding.

39.4.11 Reducing harms from adolescent cannabis use

The epidemiological evidence on cannabis dependence and adverse effects on cognitive performance and poorer educational outcomes provides good reasons for reducing cannabis-related harm among adolescents. Even if cannabis use is not a direct cause of illicit drug use, regular cannabis use probably increases opportunities to use other drugs. The risks of psychosis may be modest, but the severity of the outcome warrants preventive attention on prudential grounds.

The undecided issue is how best to discourage early and regular cannabis use in adolescents. Educational campaigns to discourage use are of limited value, with their effectiveness ranging from modest, at best, having no impact in most cases, to in some cases, increasing experimentation (Babor et al. 2010b). We need to be realistic about the impacts of educational messages (Caulkins et al. 2004; White and Pitts 1998). Small, statistically significant reductions in cannabis use may be observed in well-conducted programs (Caulkins et al. 2004; Gorman 1995; Tobler et al. 1999; White and Pitts 1998) but the primary impact is on knowledge rather than behavior (White and Pitts 1998). Behavior change is more likely to occur among less frequent rather than heavier users (Gorman 1995). The best way to deliver the advice will depend upon good social marketing research on the views of young people (Grier and Bryant 2005).

Young people need to be made aware of the mental health risks of regular intoxication with both alcohol and cannabis. They need to be told about high-risk groups, namely, those with a family history of psychosis, and those who have had unpleasant psychological experiences when using cannabis. This education needs be directed at both cannabis users and their peers in order to increase recognition of these problems so that peers can encourage affected friends to cease using or seek help.

A challenge is framing the magnitude of the risk of psychosis for young people. The risk for any individual who uses cannabis increases from around 7 in 1000 (Saha et al. 2005) to 14 in 1000. The temptation is to argue that everyone is at risk because it is difficult to predict who is most vulnerable. We think this a doubtful strategy that may undermine the credibility of the message by being seen to exaggerate the risk.

Harm reduction approaches to cannabis may also be indirect. They could include more effective parenting education such as Positive Parenting programs that aim to improve parental responses to adolescent behavior in ways that reduce oppositional behavior and improve relations between parents and adolescents. These programs appear to be effective in reducing oppositional and conduct disorders and thereby indirectly, reducing adolescent alcohol and cannabis use (De Graaf et al. 2008; Sanders 2012).

39.4.12 Interventions with high-risk populations

Early intervention programs to reduce cannabis use in adolescents and high-risk youth are a plausible approach that is worthy of research. To date, most attention has been paid to reducing cannabis use in young people with psychoses or other symptoms of poor mental health. Results of these interventions have so far not been encouraging.

Young people who use cannabis and experience psychotic symptoms should be strongly encouraged to stop, and if they refuse to stop, counseled to reduce their frequency of use. The challenges will be persuading young persons with schizophrenia to stop doing something they enjoy and to help those who want to stop but find it difficult to do so.

Recent evaluations (see Roffman and Stephens 2006) of psychological interventions for cannabis dependence in persons *without* psychoses report modest rates of abstinence at the end of treatment (20–40%) and substantial rates of relapse thereafter (Denis et al. 2006). Many persons with schizophrenia have characteristics that predict a poor outcome, namely, they: lack social support, may be cognitively impaired, are often unemployed, and may not comply with treatment (Kavanagh 1995; Mueser et al. 1992). There are very few controlled studies of substance abuse treatment in schizophrenia (Lehman et al. 1993). A recent Cochrane review identified only six relevant studies, four of which were small (Jeffery et al. 2004) and found no evidence that supported substance abuse treatment in schizophrenia over standard care.

39.4.13 Reducing the harms of higher THC cannabis products

Concerns have been expressed over the last 20 years that increased THC content of cannabis products will increase their adverse effects (Hall and Pacula 2010). Recent studies suggest that THC content increased during the late 1990s (McLaren et al. 2008). Any health effects of increased THC dose will depend on whether users are able and willing to titrate their dose of THC. A higher THC content may increase anxiety, depression, and psychotic symptoms in naive users while increasing the risk of dependence and psychotic symptoms if regular users do not titrate their dose. Adverse effects on the respiratory and cardiovascular systems may be reduced if regular users titrate their dose of THC and reduce the amount they smoke. Increased THC content could also increase the risk of road traffic crashes if users drive while more heavily intoxicated (Hall and Pacula 2010).

There are potential policies to reduce the harms of increased THC levels in cannabis products. This could include: evaluating advice to users on the desirability of titrating the use of high THC cannabis products; imposing higher legal penalties on the cultivation and sale of cannabis products with higher THC levels; and in countries with de facto legal cannabis markers, regulating the THC (and possibly the cannabidiol) content in cannabis that is offered for sale.

39.5 Reducing the harms of cannabis prohibition

In most developed countries cannabis users can, in theory, be sentenced to prison if caught using by police. Such prison sentences are rarely imposed but a criminal conviction for using cannabis can still be acquired that may adversely affect the lives of users (Lenton 2000). Some critics argue that these social harms from an arrest or conviction are more serious than any harms that result from using cannabis (Wodak et al. 2002), e.g., by impeding employment opportunities and adversely affecting personal relationships (Room et al. 2008). Research on users prosecuted for cannabis use (Erickson 1980; Lenton et al. 1999a, 1999b) also suggests that a criminal conviction has no effect on their cannabis use.

The removal of criminal penalties for personal use is one way of reducing the adverse effects on detected users. The Netherlands was one of the first European countries to do so in 1976 and Portugal has recently done so. Studies of the impact of these changes have typically found that they have little effect on rates of population cannabis use in Australia (e.g., Donnelly et al. 1999), the US (Pacula et al. 2004), and European countries including the Netherlands (Greenwald 2009; Room et al. 2008). This suggests that this policy change has little or no effect on cannabis-related harms while reducing enforcement costs (Room et al. 2008).

An unintended consequence of depenalization via civil penalties could be an increase in numbers of persons fined by the police, an effect referred to as "net widening." This occurs because the police find it easier and less time-consuming to impose a fine than to arrest and process a criminal charge. If more fines are issued and offenders do not pay their fines, then more cannabis users may end up in prison for fine-default than would be the case if cannabis use remained a criminal offence (Room et al. 2008). The removal or the nonenforcement of any penalties for personal use (as in the Netherlands) avoids this problem (Hall and Pacula 2010; Room et al. 2008) as does enforcing payment of fines in ways that avoid imprisonment (Room et al. 2008).

39.6 Research priorities for cannabis harm reduction

Research is needed on the effectiveness of these proposed ways of reducing the harms of cannabis use. Among the priorities for future inquiry are the following questions:

- What do cannabis users believe are the harms of using cannabis?
- Are they persuaded by the type of evidence presented for these adverse effects?
- Are they prepared to act on advice about how to reduce these harms?
- Does roadside drug testing deter cannabis users from driving while intoxicated? If so, does this reduce motor vehicle accident fatalities? Does it do so at an acceptable social and economic cost? Are there better ways than deterrence policies to reduce risks related to cannabis and driving?
- Do adolescent users accept that cannabis use can be harmful? Are they prepared to act on harm reduction advice? Are brief interventions in medical or nonmedical settings effective in changing risk patterns of use or practices?
- Do vaporizers substantially reduce the respiratory risks of cannabis smoking?

◆ Do cannabis users titrate their doses of THC?

◆ Could regulation of the content of cannabinoids such as cannabidiol (Morgan et al. 2010) reduce some the adverse effects of cannabis use?

Priorities for research on the effects of harm reduction measures for legal policies such as depenalization and decriminalization include the following:

◆ Do depenalization or decriminalization policies change patterns or rates of cannabis use, or attitudes towards cannabis use, especially among vulnerable/high-risk populations?

◆ How will more tolerant policies for cannabis use affect access to or use of other illicit drugs?

◆ Do decriminalization approaches result in tangible savings of public resources (e.g., enforcement time)?

Acknowledgment

This is an extensively revised version of material originally published in: Hall, W. and Fischer, B. Harm reduction policies for cannabis. Chapter 8 pp. 257–276 in T. Rhodes and D. Hedrich (eds.). *Harm Reduction; Evidence, Impacts and Challenges*. European Monitoring Centre for Drugs and Drug Addiction Monograph 10, Lisbon, 2010.

References

Abrams, D., Vizoso, H., Shade, S., Jay, C., Kelly, M., and Benowitz, N. (2007). Vaporization as a smokeless cannabis delivery system: a pilot study. *Clinical Psychopharmacology & Therapeutics*, **82**, 572–578.

Advisory Council on the Misuse of Drugs. (2008). *Cannabis: Classification and Public Health*. London: Home Office.

Ajdacic-Gross, V., Lauber, C., Warnke, I., Haker, H., Murray, R.M., and Rossler, W. (2007). Changing incidence of psychotic disorders among the young in Zurich. *Schizophrenia Research*, **95**, 9–18.

Aldington, S., Williams, M., Nowitz, M., *et al.* (2007). Effects of cannabis on pulmonary structure, function and symptoms. *Thorax*, **62**, 1058–1063.

Aldington, S., Harwood, M., Cox, B., *et al.* (2008). Cannabis use and risk of lung cancer: a case-control study. *European Respiratory Journal*, **31**, 280–286.

Andréasson, S., Engstrom, A., Allebeck, P., and Rydberg, U. (1987). Cannabis and schizophrenia: a longitudinal study of Swedish conscripts. *Lancet*, **2**, 1483–1486.

Anthony, J.C., Warner, L., and Kessler, R. (1994). Comparative epidemiology of dependence on tobacco, alcohol, controlled substances and inhalants: basic findings from the National Comorbidity Survey. *Experimental and Clinical Psychopharmacology*, **2**, 244–268.

Anthony, J.C. (2006). The epidemiology of cannabis dependence. In: R.A. Roffman and R.S. Stephens (eds.). *Cannabis Dependence: Its Nature, Consequences and Treatment*. Cambridge: Cambridge University Press, pp. 58–105.

Arseneault, L., Cannon, M., Poulton, R., Murray, R., Caspi, A., and Moffitt, T.E. (2002). Cannabis use in adolescence and risk for adult psychosis: Longitudinal prospective study. *British Medical Journal*, **325**, 1212–1213.

Asbridge, M., Hayden, J.A., and Cartwright, J.L. (2012). Acute cannabis consumption and motor vehicle collision risk: systematic review of observational studies and meta-analysis. *BMJ*, **344**, e536.

Babor, T., Caetano, R., Casswell, S., *et al.* (2010a). *Alcohol: No Ordinary Commodity: Research and Public Policy*. 2nd ed. Oxford: Oxford University Press.

Babor, T., Caulkins, J.P., Edwards, G., *et al.* (2010b). *Drug Policy and the Public Good*. Oxford: Oxford University Press.

Bachman, J.G., Wadsworth, K.N., O'Malley, P.M., Johnston, L.D., and Schulenberg, J. (1997). *Smoking, Drinking, and Drug Use in Young Adulthood: The Impacts of New Freedoms and New Responsibilities.* Mahwah, NJ: Lawrence Erlbaum.

Beautrais, A.L., Joyce, P.R., and Mulder, R.T. (1999). Cannabis abuse and serious suicide attempts. *Addiction*, **94**, 1155–1164.

Berghuis, J.P., Swift, W., Roffman, R., Stephens, R., and Copeland, J. (2006). The teen cannabis check-up: Exploring strategies for reaching young cannabis users. In: R.A. Roffman and R.S. Stephens (eds.). *Cannabis Dependence: Its Nature, Consequences and Treatment*. Cambridge: Cambridge University Press, pp. 275–292.

Berthiller, J., Straif, K., Boniol, M., *et al.* (2008). Cannabis smoking and risk of lung cancer in men: a pooled analysis of three studies in Maghreb. *Journal of Thoracic Oncology*, **3**, 1398–1403.

Bloor, R.N., Wang, T.S., Spanel, P., and Smith, D. (2008). Ammonia release from heated 'street' cannabis leaf and its potential toxic effects on cannabis users. *Addiction*, **103**, 1671–1677.

Boydell, J., van Os, J., Caspi, A., *et al.* (2006). Trends in cannabis use prior to first presentation with schizophrenia, in South-East London between 1965 and 1999. *Psychological Medicine*, **36**, 1441–1446.

Butler, M. (2007). Australia's approach to drugs and driving. *Of Substance: The National Magazine on Alcohol, Tobacco, and Other Drugs*, **5**, 24–26.

Carter, A., Miller, P.G., and Hall, W. (2012). The ethics of harm reduction. In: R. Pates and D. Riley (eds.). *Harm Reduction in Substance Use and High Risk Behaviour: International Policy and Practice*. Chichester: Wiley-Blackwell, pp. 111–123.

Caulkins, J.P., Pacula, R.L., Paddock, S., and Chiesa, J. (2004). What we can – and cannot –expect from school-based drug prevention. *Drug and Alcohol Review*, **23**, 79–87.

Danovitch, I. and Gorelick, D.A. (2012). State of the art treatments for cannabis dependence. *Psychiatric Clinics of North America*, **35**, 309–326.

Darke, S. and Hall, W.D. (1997). The distribution of naloxone to heroin users. *Addiction*, **92**, 1195–1199.

De Graaf, I., Speetjens, P., Smit, F., de Wolff, M., and Tavecchio, L. (2008). Effectiveness of Triple P Positive Parenting program on behavioural problems in children: a meta-analysis. *Behavior Modification*, **23**, 714–735.

Degenhardt, L., Chiu, W., Sampson, N., *et al.* (2008). Toward a global view of alcohol, tobacco, cannabis and cocaine use: findings from the WHO World Mental Health Surveys. *PLoS Medicine*, **5**, e141.

Degenhardt, L., Hall, W., and Lynskey, M.T. (2001). The relationship between cannabis use, depression and anxiety among Australian adults: findings from the National Survey of Mental Health and Well-being. *Social Psychiatry and Psychiatric Epidemiology*, **36**, 219–227.

Degenhardt, L., Hall, W.D., and Lynskey, M.T. (2003). Testing hypotheses about the relationship between cannabis use and psychosis. *Drug and Alcohol Dependence*, **71**, 37–48.

Donnelly, N., Hall, W.D., and Christie, P. (1999). *Effects of the Cannabis Expiation Notice Scheme on Levels and Patterns of Cannabis Use in South Australia: Evidence from the National Drug Strategy Household Surveys 1985–1995* (Vol. 37). Canberra: Australian Government Publishing Service.

Drummer, O.H., Gerostamoulos, J., Batziris, H., *et al.* (2004). The involvement of drugs in drivers of motor vehicles killed in Australian road traffic crashes. *Accident Analysis and Prevention*, **36**, 239–248.

DuPont, R.L. (1996). Harm reduction and decriminalization in the United States: a personal perspective. *Substance Use and Misuse*, **31**, 1929–1945; discussion 1947–1972.

Earleywine, M. and Barnwell, S.S. (2007). Decreased respiratory symptoms in cannabis users who vaporize. *Harm Reduction Journal*, **4**, 11.

Ellickson, P., Bui, K., Bell, R., and McGuigan, K.A. (1998). Does early drug use increase the risk of dropping out of high school? *Journal of Drug Issues*, **28**, 357–380.

Erickson, P.G. (1980). *Cannabis Criminals: The Social Effects of Punishment on Drug Users*. Toronto: Addiction Research Foundation.

Fergusson, D.M., Boden, J.M., and Horwood, L.J. (2006). Cannabis use and other illicit drug use: testing the cannabis gateway hypothesis. *Addiction*, **101**, 556–569.

Fergusson, D.M., Boden, J.M., and Horwood, L.J. (2008). The developmental antecedents of illicit drug use: evidence from a 25-year longitudinal study. *Drug and Alcohol Dependence*, **96**, 165–177.

Fergusson, D.M., Boden, J.M., and John, H.L. (2012). Transition to parenthood and substance use disorders: findings from a 30-year longitudinal study. *Drug and Alcohol Dependence*, **125**, 295–300.

Fergusson, D.M. and Horwood, L.J. (1997). Early onset cannabis use and psychosocial adjustment in young adults. *Addiction*, **92**, 279–296.

Fergusson, D.M., Horwood, L.J., and Swain-Campbell, N.R. (2003). Cannabis dependence and psychotic symptoms in young people. *Psychological Medicine*, **33**, 15–21.

Fischer, B., Rehm, J., and Hall, W. (2009). Cannabis use in Canada: the need for a 'public health' approach. *Canadian Journal of Public Health*, **100**, 101–103.

Fischer, B. and Kendall, P. (2011). Nutt *et al.*'s harm scales for drugs: room for improvement but better policy based on science with limitations than no science at all. *Addiction*, **106**, 1891–1892; discussion 1896–1898.

Gardner, E. (1999). Cannabinoid interaction with brain reward systems. In: G.G. Nahas, K. Sutin, D. Harvey, and S. Agurell (eds.). *Marihuana and Medicine*. Towa, NJ: Humana Press, pp. 187–205.

Gerberich, S.G., Sidney, S., Braun, B.L., Tekawa, I.S., Tolan, K.K., and Quesenberry, C.P. (2003). Marijuana use and injury events resulting in hospitalization. *Annals of Epidemiology*, **13**, 230–237.

Gieringer, D., St Laurent, J., and Goodrich, S. (2004). Cannabis vaporizer combines efficient delivery of THC with effective suppression of pyrolytic compounds. *Journal of Cannabis Therapeutics*, **4**, 7–27.

Gorman, D.M. (1995). On the difference between statistical and practical significance in school-based drug abuse prevention. *Drugs-Education Prevention and Policy*, **2**, 275–283.

Gottschalk, L., Aronow, W., and Prakash, R. (1977). Effect of marijuana and placebo-marijuana smoking on psychological state and on psychophysiological and cardiovascular functioning in angina patients. *Biological Psychiatry*, **12**, 255–266.

Gowing, L.R., Ali, R.L., and White, J.M. (2000). *Respiratory Harms of Smoked Cannabis* (DASC Monograph No. 8). Parkside, SA: Drug and Alcohol Services Council South Australia.

Greenwald, G. (2009). *Drug Decriminalization in Portugal: Lessons for Creating Fair and Successful Drug Policies*. Washington, DC: Cato Institute.

Grier, S. and Bryant, C.A. (2005). Social marketing in public health. *Annual Review of Public Health*, **26**, 319–339.

Grotenhermen, F. (2004). Cannabinoids for therapeutic use: Designing systems to increase efficacy and reliability. *American Journal of Drug Delivery*, **2**, 229–240.

Grotenhermen, F., Leson, G., Berghaus, G., et al. (2007). Developing limits for driving under cannabis. *Addiction*, **102**, 1910–1917.

Hall, W.D. (1995). The public health significance of cannabis use in Australia. *Australian Journal of Public Health*, **19**, 235–242.

Hall, W.D. and Degenhardt, L. (2009). The adverse health effects of nonmedical cannabis use. *Lancet*, **374**, 1383–1391.

Hall, W.D., Degenhardt, L., and Patton, G.C. (2008). Cannabis abuse and dependence. In: C.A. Essau (ed.). *Adolescent Addiction: Epidemiology, Treatment and Assessment*. London: Academic Press, pp. 117–148.

Hall, W.D. and Lynskey, M.T. (2005). Is cannabis a gateway drug? Testing hypotheses about the relationship between cannabis use and the use of other illicit drugs. *Drug and Alcohol Review*, **24**, 39–48.

Hall, W.D. and Pacula, R.L. (2010). *Cannabis Use and Dependence: Public Health and Public Policy* (reissue of 2003 1st ed.). Cambridge: Cambridge University Press.

Hall, W.D. and Swift, W. (2000). The THC content of cannabis in Australia: evidence and implications. *Australian and New Zealand Journal of Public Health*, **24**, 503–508.

Hall, W.D. and Swift, W. (2006). The policy implications of cannabis dependence. In: R.A. Roffman and R.S. Stephens (eds.), *Cannabis Dependence: Its Nature, Consequences and Treatment.* Cambridge: Cambridge University Press, pp. 315–339.

Hashibe, M., Morgenstern, H., Cui, Y., *et al.* (2006). Marijuana use and the risk of lung and upper aerodigestive tract cancers: Results of a population-based case-control study. *Cancer Epidemiology, Biomarkers and Prevention,* **15**, 1829–1834.

Hashibe, M., Straif, K., Tashkin, D.P., Morgenstern, H., Greenland, S., and Zhang, Z.F. (2005). Epidemiologic review of marijuana use and cancer risk. *Alcohol,* **35**, 265–275.

Hazekamp, A., Ruhaak, R., Zuurman, L., van Gerven, J., and Verpoorte, R. (2006). Evaluation of a vaporizing device (Volcano) for the pulmonary administration of tetrahydrocannabinol. *Journal of Pharmaceutical Sciences,* **95**, 1308–1317.

Henquet, C., Krabbendam, L., Spauwen, J., *et al.* (2004). Prospective cohort study of cannabis use, predisposition for psychosis, and psychotic symptoms in young people. *British Medical Journal,* **330**, 11.

Henstridge, J., Homel, R., and Mackay, P. (1997). *The Long-Term Effects of Random Breath Testing in Four Australian States: A Time Series Analysis.* Canberra: Federal Office of Road Safety.

Hickman, M., Vickerman, P., Macleod, J., Kirkbride, J., and Jones, P.B. (2007). Cannabis and schizophrenia: model projections of the impact of the rise in cannabis use on historical and future trends in schizophrenia in England and Wales. *Addiction,* **102**, 597–606.

Homel, R. (1988). *Policing and Punishing the Drinking Driver: A Study of General and Specific Deterrence.* New York: Springer.

Horwood, L.J., Fergusson, D.M., Hayatbakhsh, M.R., *et al.* (2010). Cannabis use and educational achievement: findings from three Australasian cohort studies. *Drug and Alcohol Dependence,* **110**, 247–253.

Howden, M.L. and Naughton, M.T. (2011). Pulmonary effects of marijuana inhalation. *Expert Reviews,* **5**, 87–92.

IHRA. (2010). *What is Harm Reduction? A Position Statement from the International Harm Reduction Association* (IHRA Briefing). London: IHRA.

Iversen, L. (2007). *The Science of Marijuana.* 2nd ed. Oxford: Oxford University Press.

Jeffery, D., Ley, A., McLaren, S., and Siegfried, N. (2004). Psychosocial treatment programmes for people with both severe mental illness and substance misuse. *Cochrane Database of Systematic Reviews,* 2000, Issue 2.

Jones, R.T. (2002). Cardiovascular system effects of marijuana. *Journal of Clinical Pharmacology,* **42**, 58S–63S.

Kandel, D.B. (2002). *Stages and Pathways of Drug Involvement: Examining the Gateway Hypothesis.* New York: Cambridge University Press.

Kavanagh, D.J. (1995). An intervention for substance abuse in schizophrenia. *Behaviour Change,* **12**, 20–30.

Lacey, J., Brainard, K., and Snitow, S. (2010). *Drug Per Se Laws: Review of Their Use in States.* (DOT HS). Washington, DC: National Highway Traffic Safety Administration, Department of Transportation.

Laumon, B., Gadegbeku, B., Martin, J.L., and Biecheler, M.B. (2005). Cannabis intoxication and fatal road crashes in France: population based case-control study. *British Medical Journal,* **331**, 1371.

Lee, M.H.S. and Hancox, R.J. (2011). Effects of smoking cannabis on lung function. *Expert Reviews,* **5**, 537–546.

Lehman, A.F., Herron, J.D., Schwartz, R.P., and Myers, C.P. (1993). Rehabilitation for adults with severe mental illness and substance use disorders: a clinical trial. *Journal of Nervous and Mental Disease,* **181**, 86–90.

Lenton, S. (2000). Cannabis policy and the burden of proof: is it now beyond reasonable doubt that cannabis prohibition is not working? *Drug and Alcohol Review,* **19**, 95–100.

Lenton, S., Bennett, M., and Heale, P. (1999a). *The Social Impact of a Minor Cannabis Offence Under Strict Prohibition: The Case of Western Australia.* Perth: National Centre for Research into the Prevention of Drug Abuse.

Lenton, S., Christie, P., Humeniuk, R., Brooks, A., Bennet, M., and Heale, P. (1999b). *Infringement versus Conviction: The Social Impact of a Minor Cannabis Offence Under a Civil Penalties System and Strict Prohibition in two Australian States* (Vol. 36). Canberra: Commonwealth Department of Health and Aged Care.

Lenton, S. and Single, E. (1998). The definition of harm reduction. *Drug and Alcohol Review*, **17**, 213–219.

Lessem, J.M., Hopfer, C.J., Haberstick, B.C., *et al.* (2006). Relationship between adolescent marijuana use and young adult illicit drug use. *Behavior Genetics*, **36**, 498–506.

Lynskey, M.T. and Hall, W.D. (2000). The effects of adolescent cannabis use on educational attainment: a review. *Addiction*, **96**, 433–443.

Lynskey, M.T., Heath, A.C., Bucholz, K.K., and Slutske, W.S. (2003). Escalation of drug use in early-onset cannabis users vs co-twin controls. *JAMA*, **289**, 427–433.

Macleod, J., Oakes, R., Copello, A., *et al.* (2004). Psychological and social sequelae of cannabis and other illicit drug use by young people: A systematic review of longitudinal, general population studies. *Lancet*, **363**, 1579–1588.

Manzanares, J., Corchero, J., Romero, J., Fernandez-Ruiz, J.J., Ramos, J.A., and Fuentes, J.A. (1999). Pharmacological and biochemical interactions between opioids and cannabinoids. *Trends in Pharmacological Sciences*, **20**, 287–294.

Martin, G. and Copeland, J. (2008). The adolescent cannabis check-up: randomized trial of a brief intervention for young cannabis users. *Journal of Substance Abuse Treatment*, **34**, 407–414.

McLaren, J., Swift, W., Dillon, P., and Allsop, S. (2008). Cannabis potency and contamination: A review of the literature. *Addiction*, **103**, 1100–1109.

Mehra, R., Moore, B.A., Crothers, K., Tetrault, J., and Fiellin, D.A. (2006). The association between marijuana smoking and lung cancer: a systematic review. *Archives of Internal Medicine*, **166**, 1359–1367.

Meier, M.H., Caspi, A., Ambler, A., *et al.* (2012). Persistent cannabis users show neuropsychological decline from childhood to midlife. *Proceedings of the National Academy of Sciences of the United States of America*, **109**, E2657–E2664.

Melamede, R. (2005). Harm reduction: the cannabis paradox. *Harm Reduction Journal*, **2**, 17.

Miller, W.R. and Sovereign, R.G. (1989). The check-up: A model for early intervention in addictive behaviors. In: T. Leberg, W. Miller, G. Nathan, and G. Marlatt (eds.). *Addictive Behaviors: Prevention and Early Intervention*. Amsterdam: Swets and Zeitlinger, pp. 219–231.

Mittleman, M.A., Lewis, R.A., Maclure, M., Sherwood, J.B., and Muller, J.E. (2001). Triggering myocardial infarction by marijuana. *Circulation*, **103**, 2805–2809.

Moir, D., Rickert, W.S., Levasseur, G., *et al.* (2008). A comparison of mainstream and sidestream marijuana and tobacco cigarette smoke produced under two machine smoking conditions. *Chemical Research in Toxicology*, **21**, 494–502.

Moore, T.H., Zammit, S., Lingford-Hughes, A., *et al.* (2007). Cannabis use and risk of psychotic or affective mental health outcomes: a systematic review. *Lancet*, **370**, 319–328.

Morgan, C.J., Schafer, G., Freeman, T.P., and Curran, H.V. (2010). Impact of cannabidiol on the acute memory and psychotomimetic effects of smoked cannabis: naturalistic study. *British Journal of Psychiatry*, **197**, 285–290.

Morral, A.R., McCaffrey, D.F., and Paddock, S.M. (2002). Reassessing the marijuana gateway effect. *Addiction*, **97**, 1493–1504.

Mueser, K.T., Bellack, A.S., and Blanchard, J.J. (1992). Comorbidity of schizophrenia and substance abuse: implications for treatment. *Journal of Consulting and Clinical Psychology*, **60**, 845–856.

Mukamal, K.J., Maclure, M., Muller, J.E., and Mittleman, M.A. (2008). An exploratory prospective study of marijuana use and mortality following acute myocardial infarction. *American Heart Journal*, **155**, 465–470.

Mura, P., Kintz, P., Ludes, B., *et al.* (2003). Comparison of the prevalence of alcohol, cannabis and other drugs between 900 injured drivers and 900 control subjects: results of a French collaborative study. *Forensic Science International*, **133**, 79–85.

Nawrot, T.S., Perez, L., Kunzli, N., Munters, E., and Nemery, B. (2011). Public health importance of triggers of myocardial infarction: a comparative risk assessment. *Lancet*, **377**, 732–740.

Pacula, R.L., Chriqui, J.F., and King, J. (2004). *Marijuana Decriminalization: What Does it Mean in the United States?* (Working Paper No. WR-126). Santa Monica, CA: RAND.

Patton, G.C., Harris, J.B., Schwartz, M., and Bowes, G. (1997). Adolescent suicidal behaviors: a population-based study of risk. *Psychological Medicine*, **27**, 715–724.

Ramaekers, J.G., Berghaus, G., van Laar, M., and Drummer, O.H. (2004). Dose related risk of motor vehicle crashes after cannabis use. *Drug and Alcohol Dependence*, **73**, 109–119.

Riley, D., Pates, R., Monaghan, G., and O'Hare, P. (2012). A brief history of harm reduction. In: R. Pates and D. Riley (eds.). *Harm Reduction in Substance Use and High Risk Behaviour: International Policy and Practice*. Chichester: Wiley-Blackwell, pp. 5–16.

Robbe, H.W.J. (1994). *Influence of Marijuana on Driving*. Maastricht: Institute for Human Psychopharmacology.

Roffman, R.A. and Stephens, R.S. (eds.). (2006). *Cannabis Dependence: Its Nature, Consequences and Treatment*. Cambridge: Cambridge University Press.

Room, R., Fischer, B., Hall, W.D., Lenton, S., and Reuter, P. (2008). *Cannabis Policy: Moving Beyond Stalemate* (Global Cannabis Commission Report). Oxford: Beckley Foundation.

Roxburgh, A., Hall, W.D., Degenhardt, L., McLaren, J., Black, E., Copeland, J., et al. (2010). The epidemiology of cannabis use and cannabis-related harm in Australia 1993-2007. *Addiction*, **105**, 1071–1079.

Saha, S., Chant, D., Welham, J., and McGrath, J. (2005). A systematic review of the prevalence of schizophrenia. *PLoS Medicine*, **2**, e141.

Sanders, M.R. (2012). Development, evaluation, and multinational dissemination of the triple P-Positive Parenting Program. *Annual review of clinical psychology*, **8**, 345–379.

Shand, F., Gates, J., Fawcett, J., and Mattick, R. (2003). *The Treatment of Alcohol Problems: A Review of the Evidence*. Canberra: Commonwealth Department of Health and Ageing.

Sidney, S., Quesenberry, C.P., Jr., Friedman, G.D., and Tekawa, I.S. (1997). Marijuana use and cancer incidence (California, United States). *Cancer Causes and Control*, **8**, 722–728.

Sidney, S. (2002). Cardiovascular consequences of marijuana use. *Journal of Clinical Pharmacology*, **42**, 64S–70S.

Smiley, A. (1999). Marijuana: on road and driving simulator studies. In: H. Kalant, W. Corrigall, W.D. Hall, and R. Smart (eds.). *The Health Effects of Cannabis*. Toronto: Centre for Addiction and Mental Health, pp. 171–191.

Solowij, N. (1998). *Cannabis and Cognitive Functioning*. Cambridge: Cambridge University Press.

Solowij, N., Stephens, R.S., Roffman, R.A., et al. (2002). Cognitive functioning of long-term heavy cannabis users seeking treatment. *JAMA*, **287**, 1123–1131.

Stephens, R.S., Roffman, R.A., Fearer, S.A., Williams, C., and Burke, R.S. (2007). The marijuana check-up: promoting change in ambivalent marijuana users. *Addiction*, **102**, 947–957.

Strang, J. and Farrell, M. (1992). Harm minimisation for drug misusers. *British Medical Journal*, **304**, 1127–1128.

Swift, W., Copeland, J., and Lenton, S. (2000). Cannabis and harm reduction. *Drug and Alcohol Review*, **19**, 101–112.

Tashkin, D.P. (1999). Effects of cannabis on the respiratory system. In: H. Kalant, W. Corrigall, W.D. Hall, and R. Smart (eds.). *The Health Effects of Cannabis*. Toronto: Centre for Addiction and Mental Health, pp. 311–345.

Tashkin, D.P. (2005). Smoked marijuana as a cause of lung injury. *Monaldi Archives for Chest Disease*, **63**, 93–100.

Tashkin, D.P., Baldwin, G.C., Sarafian, T., Dubinett, S., and Roth, M.D. (2002). Respiratory and immunologic consequences of marijuana smoking. *Journal of Clinical Pharmacology*, **42**, 71S–81S.

Taylor, D.R., Fergusson, D.M., Milne, B.J., et al. (2002). A longitudinal study of the effects of tobacco and cannabis exposure on lung function in young adults. *Addiction*, **97**, 1055–1061.

Tetrault, J.M., Crothers, K., Moore, B.A., Mehra, R., Concato, J., and Fiellin, D.A. (2007). Effects of marijuana smoking on pulmonary function and respiratory complications: a systematic review. *Archives of Internal Medicine*, **167**, 221–228.

Tobler, N.S., Lessard, T., Marshall, D., Ochshorn, P., and Roona, M. (1999). Effectiveness of school-based drug prevention programs for marijuana use. *School Psychology International*, **20**, 105–137.

UNODC. (2012). *World Drug Report 2012*. Vienna: United Nations Office on Drugs and Crime.

Van Os, J., Bak, M., Hanssen, M., Bijl, R.V., de Graaf, R., and Verdoux, H. (2002). Cannabis use and psychosis: a longitudinal population-based study. *American Journal of Epidemiology*, **156**, 319–327.

Wagner, F.A., and Anthony, J.C. (2002). Into the world of illegal drug use: exposure opportunity and other mechanisms linking the use of alcohol, tobacco, marijuana, and cocaine. *American Journal of Epidemiology*, **155**, 918–925.

Watling, C.N., Palk, G.R., Freeman, J.E., and Davey, J.D. (2010). Applying Stafford and Warr's reconceptualization of deterrence theory to drug driving: can it predict those likely to offend? *Accident Analysis and Prevention*, **42**, 452–458.

White, D., and Pitts, M. (1998). Educating young people about drugs: a systematic review. *Addiction*, **93**, 1475–1487.

Wodak, A., Reinarman, C., and Cohen, P. (2002). Cannabis control: costs outweigh benefits. *BMJ*, **324**, 105–106.

Zammit, S., Allebeck, P., Andréasson, S., Lundberg, I., and Lewis, G. (2002). Self reported cannabis use as a risk factor for schizophrenia in Swedish conscripts of 1969: historical cohort study. *BMJ*, **325**, 1199–1201.

Zhang, Z.F., Morgenstern, H., Spitz, M.R., *et al.* (1999). Marijuana use and increased risk of squamous cell carcinoma of the head and neck. *Cancer Epidemiology, Biomarkers and Prevention*, **8**, 1071–1078.

Chapter 40

Cannabinoid Designer Drugs: Effects and Forensics

Brian F. Thomas, Jenny L. Wiley, Gerald T. Pollard, and Megan Grabenauer

40.1 Introduction

Cannabinoid designer drugs are defined here as clandestinely synthesized structures that function as agonists at cannabinoid (CB) receptors and are used to produce marijuana-like intoxication. Most such drugs are previously known structures or their derivatives, notably those synthesized by Huffman for research purposes in the past two decades. They are formulated as additives in smokable herbal mixtures with benign labels such as "incense" and "not for human consumption" but with names and package graphics that leave no doubt of their psychotropic purpose. Appearing about 2004 and proliferating by 2008 (Seely et al. 2012a), they have been sold under dozens of product names such as Spice and K2. They are readily available on the Internet and can still be found in head shops and other convenient outlets. Legal controls are circumvented by rapid substitution of similar structures not yet controlled. This chapter will summarize the general chemistry, pharmacology, epidemiology, legal status, and methods of detection of cannabinoid designer drugs, and will suggest possible future developments in their control.

40.2 General chemistry

40.2.1 Analogs of phytocannabinoids in basic research and medicinal chemistry

Following the chemical isolation of cannabis constituents in the 1940s, a variety of novel cannabinol, cannabidiol, and tetrahydrocannabinol analogs were synthesized and tested. These early efforts culminated in the discovery of extremely potent and long-acting dimethylheptylpyran (DMHP) analogs (Adams et al. 1949) which were quite similar in structure to the principal psychoactive component in cannabis, delta-9 (Δ^9)-tetrahydrocannabinol (THC) (Gaoni and Mechoulam 1964; Wollner et al. 1942), differing only in the position of one double bond (from Δ^{9-10} in Δ^9-THC to Δ^{6a-10a} in DMHP) and the extension of the 3-pentyl chain to 3-(1,2-dimethylheptyl) (Table 40.1). This evolving knowledge culminated in the 1970s with the first synthetic cannabinoid to be approved for oral administration by the FDA, nabilone (Cesamet®), which has both a 1,1,-dimethylheptyl side chain at the 3-position and a 9-keto hexahydrocannabinol ring system (Table 40.1).

In the 1980s, researchers at Pfizer integrated the available information into a medicinal chemistry campaign to identify and develop cannabinoid-based, nondependence-producing analgesics. Focusing on the 9-nor-9-OH-hexahydrocannabinol framework described by Wilson and May

Table 40.1 A selection of cannabinoid receptor agonists[a]

Structure	Name	R	R′
	Δ^9-THC		
	DMHP		
	Nabilone		
	Levonantradol		
	CP-47,497		
	Cannabicyclohexanol (CP-47,497 – C8 analog)		
	CP-55,940		

Table 40.1 (continued) A selection of cannabinoid receptor agonists[a]

Structure	Name	R	R′
	CP-55,244		
	HU-210		
	WIN 55,212-2		
	WIN 48,098 or Pravadoline	4-MeO-Phenyl	Me
	WIN 55,225 or JWH-200	1-Naphthyl	H
	JW -018	n-Pentyl	H
	JWH-073	n-Butyl	H

[a] For a comprehensive list of synthetic cannabinoids as reported by the National Forensic Laboratory Information System (NFLIS), a Drug Enforcement Administration program that systematically collects drug chemistry analysis results, as well as other related information, from cases analyzed by state, local and federal forensic laboratories, see https://www.nflis. deadiversion.usdoj.gov/.

(Wilson et al. 1976) and the 3-position side chain, these investigators proposed a pharmaco-phore model that led to the identification of an entirely new structural class of potent compounds (Howlett et al. 1988; Johnson et al. 1981a, 1981b) described as nonclassical cannabinoids, and to the unequivocal identification of pharmacologically relevant G-protein coupled cannabinoid receptors in the central nervous system (CNS) (Devane et al. 1988; Herkenham et al. 1990, 1991; Howlett et al. 1990). At the time of the discovery of the type 1 cannabinoid receptor (CB_1) in the late 1980s, there were two main chemical classes of psychotropic agonists, the "classical" consisting of the ABC-tricyclic dibenzopyrans such as THC and of a variety of synthetic ABC-tricyclic analogs such as DMHP, nabilone, and desacetyl-levonantradol, and the "nonclassical" such as CP-47,497, CP-55,940, and CP-55,244 (Table 40.1).

The availability of high-affinity, high-efficacy, potent ligands facilitated the delineation of cannabinoid receptors and signal transduction pathways and enabled the development of high-throughput radioligand binding assays for screening. Other chemical classes were soon described, such as the aminoalkylindoles (e.g., WIN 55,212-2 (Table 40.1) discovered by the Sterling Research Group (D'Ambra et al. 1992)). The CB_1 and CB_2 receptors were cloned (Matsuda et al. 1990 and Munro et al. 1993, respectively), and the first endogenous endocannabinoid agonists, arachidonoyl ethanolamide (anandamide) and 2-arachidonoylglycerol (2-AG), were described (Devane et al. 1992). The endocannabinoid system was further defined through the discovery of substrate specific enzymes catalyzing degradation, including fatty acid amide hydrolases, monoacylglycerol lipase (MAGL), the serine hydrolases α/β-hydrolase 6 and 12, and N-acylethanolamine-hydrolyzing acid amidase (for review, see Feledziak et al. 2012).

The exact nature of the molecular interactions of cannabinoid agonists with receptors remained unknown, and it was not clear whether all of the various structural classes of agonists, particularly the aminoalkylindoles and the endocannabinoids, shared structural elements or structure–activity relationship (SAR) with classical or nonclassical cannabinoids, or interacted within the same recognition site. So Dr. John W. Huffman designed and developed the JWH-series of alkylindoles to test a pharmacophore overlay theory for WIN 55,212-2 and classical cannabinoids. These and other efforts demonstrated that activity is retained when the aminoalkyl substituent is replaced by N-alkyl chains (Huffman et al. 1994), and that the indole nucleus can be replaced with other ring systems including indene (Kumar et al. 1995) and pyrrole (Lainton et al. 1995; Wiley et al. 1998), which led to new agonists with significant selectivity for the CB_2 receptor such as JWH-015, AM-630 (Pertwee et al. 1995), L-768,242 (also known as GW-405,833) (Gallant et al. 1996), and BAY 38-7271 (Mauler et al. 2002). In addition, efforts to combine structural elements of fatty acid ethanolamides with elements derived from olivetol (the biosynthetic precursor of THC in cannabis) or substituted resorcinol again led to high affinity ligands at CB_1 and CB_2 (Brizzi et al. 2005, 2009), including CB-25 and CB-52, which are partial agonists at CB_1 and neutral antagonists at CB_2 (Cascio et al. 2006).

As additional classes were discovered, the structural requirements for pharmacological affinity, selectivity, efficacy, and potency were further described, often with a common goal of delineating mechanisms of action or maximizing desirable therapeutic properties (e.g., analgesia, antiemesis) while minimizing or eliminating side effects (e.g., lethargy, sedation, psychoactivity). Much of this information was made publically available through publications or patents, as is typical for such efforts. This availability facilitates advances in understanding the molecular basis of activity and enables the translation of research findings into advances in health sciences and therapeutics. However, it can also be used by people with alternative ideas about how to capitalize on such findings.

40.2.2 Synthetic cannabinoids for recreational use

In 2004, "herbal products" and "incense" appeared in Europe under a variety of trade names and were alleged to produce cannabinoid effects. Analysis showed that they were intentionally adulterated with synthetic agonists. The first reported were the octyl analog of Pfizer's potent non-classical cannabinoid CP-47,497 and an alkylindole analog from Huffman's research, JWH-018 (Auwarter et al. 2009). Unregulated and misleadingly labeled formulations became increasingly prevalent across the globe. The variety of plant material and the number of synthetics increased at an alarming rate, such that by the end of 2010 herbal products being openly marketed in stores and on the Internet commonly included at least one class of synthetic agonist: naphthoylindoles (e.g.,

JWH-018, JWH-073, and JWH-200), naphthylmethylindoles (e.g., JWH-007), naphthoylpyrroles (e.g., JWH-147), phenylacetylindoles (e.g., JWH-250), cyclohexylphenols (e.g., CP-47,497), and classical cannabinoids (e.g., HU-210).

The molecules most commonly found in these products were from the published literature. As regulations progressed, previously undescribed compounds appeared. For example, XLR-11, identified in smoking blends in 2012, seems to have been invented by chemical suppliers specifically for recreational use. It is a simple 5'-fluorinated pentyl side chain derivative of 3-(tetramethylcyclopropylmethanoyl)indole compounds such as UR-144, A-796,260, and A-834,735; but it is not listed in the patent or the scientific literature alongside these compounds (Frost et al. 2010), and appears to have not previously been made by Abbott Laboratories, despite falling within the claims of patent WO 2006/069196. While often not fully disclosing active ingredients, product packaging may state that the material does not contain any US Drug Enforcement Agency (DEA) banned substances, or that it is legal in particular states.

As further regulations and enforcement actions take effect, manufacturers are forced to identify alternative molecules or structural classes. As a result, an increasing variety of unusual chemicals and unproven pharmacological approaches have been reported. Oleamide, for example, is an endocannabinoid-like molecule that binds to and modulates cannabinoid receptors and has been detected in herbal products. It induces sleep and, like anandamide, is also involved in the regulation of memory processes, body temperature, and locomotor activity. However, intuitively this compound's low volatility makes smoking or vaporizing a relatively poor choice for delivery. Alternative approaches that increase endocannabinoid tone by using chemicals to inhibit the degradation of endocannabinoids, such as the MAGL inhibitor URB-754 (Makara et al. 2005), are also appearing (Uchiyama et al. 2012a). However, the ability to increase anandamide or 2-AG levels and induce psychotomimetic effects in man after inhalation is uncertain, and the dose–response relationship is not well defined. Indeed, recent studies have shown that URB-754 failed to inhibit MAGL (Saario et al. 2006), and there is controversy about its pharmacological activity (Saario et al. 2006; Vandevoorde et al. 2007). Herbal smoking products with no cannabinoid content and acting through other mechanisms are appearing as well, such as *Salvia* and kratom.

40.2.3 Perspective

From its beginnings in basic research and therapeutic drug development, chemical synthesis of cannabinoid ligands has morphed into an illicit enterprise that serves recreational drug users worldwide while keeping a step ahead of regulations and detection methods, with scant regard for social and medical consequences.

40.3 General pharmacology and physiology

40.3.1 Mechanism of action

The most common screening strategy for SAR analysis of synthetic cannabinoids has been a two-prong approach of assessment of binding affinity at CB_1 and CB_2 receptors followed by evaluation in a tetrad of tests in which cannabinoid agonists produce a characteristic profile of effects in mice: suppression of motor activity, antinociception, hypothermia, and catalepsy (Martin et al. 1991). In these assays, THC and prototypic synthetic cannabinoid agonists (e.g., WIN 55,212-2, CP-55,940) bind to CB_1 and CB_2 and are active in the tetrad battery with potencies that are strongly correlated with their affinities for CB_1 (Compton et al. 1993). While THC and CP-55,940 bind with approximately equal affinity to both identified cannabinoid receptors (THC: CB_1 K_i = 41 nM, CB_2 K_i = 36 nM;

CP-55,940: CB$_1$ K$_i$ = 0.6 nM, CB$_2$ K$_i$ = 0.7 nM), WIN 55,212-2 has better affinity for CB$_2$ (K$_i$ = 0.28 nM) vs. CB$_1$ (K$_i$ = 1.89 nM) (Showalter et al. 1996). The three compounds also differ in their in vitro efficacy at CB$_1$. Whereas THC acts as a partial agonist in functional assays such as [^{35}S]GTPγS binding, CP-55,940 and WIN 55,212-2 are full agonists (Breivogel and Childers 2000), although all three compounds show approximately equal efficacy in the mouse tetrad. Uniquely, however, the binding site of WIN 55,212-2 at the CB$_1$ receptor only partially overlaps that of THC (Song and Bonner 1996). In addition, WIN 55,212-2 possesses effects that are not shared by either THC or CP-55,940 and that are mediated via a non-CB$_1$, non-CB$_2$ mechanism (Breivogel et al. 2001; Hajos et al. 2001; Monory et al. 2002), suggesting the possibility of other cannabinoid receptors. Because structural analogs of THC have long been illegal (e.g., due to analog provisions of DEA regulations), most of the novel synthetic cannabinoids currently being abused are derived from the aminoalkylindole template, or less commonly are bicyclic analogs related to CP-55,940. Hence, this section focuses primarily on discussion of the SAR of indole-derived structures.

Indole-derived cannabinoids were originally developed as research tools designed to probe the structural properties of CB$_1$ and CB$_2$ receptors. Despite the good CB$_2$ affinity shared by many of the abused cannabinoids, the primary mechanism of action for their marijuana-like CNS effects appears to be activation of CB$_1$. Notably, however, this hypothesis has not been confirmed for all structural templates. Many of the hundreds of synthetic cannabinoids synthesized for research were evaluated in binding assays (Aung et al. 2000; Huffman et al. 2003, 2005b, 2006, 2008, 2010; Lainton et al. 1995) but were never tested in animals before they were discovered in products confiscated from human users. Nevertheless, for the compounds that have been tested in vivo, CB$_1$ affinity was highly associated with potency for producing each pharmacological effect in the mouse tetrad (Wiley et al. 1998, 2012a, 2012b) and for eliciting THC-like discriminative stimulus effects (see section 40.3.3). Further, the CB$_1$ antagonist rimonabant, but not the CB$_2$ antagonist SR 144528, reversed agonist-induced effects in the tetrad (Wiley et al. 2002). Like WIN 55,212-2, indole-derived cannabinoids are full agonists at CB$_1$ in vitro, although only a few compounds have been assessed (Atwood et al. 2010, 2011; Huffman et al. 2005a). Of importance to the current legal and forensic issues associated with synthetic cannabinoid abuse is the observation that good CB$_1$ affinity is retained across a wide array of structural manipulations (reviewed in Huffman and Padgett 2005; Manera et al. 2008). The excellent CB$_1$ affinity of several compounds that have been detected in street samples (e.g., K$_i$ = 9 nM for JWH-018 and JWH-073) (Wiley et al. 1998) suggests that these compounds would be more potent than THC, which may account for anecdotal reports that the high they produce is more intense. The affinities of abused cannabinoids for novel cannabinoid or noncannabinoid receptors and the role that these receptors may play in mediating or modulating their pharmacological effects are largely unknown. Conceivably, some of the peripheral effects could be mediated via activation of CB$_2$, as CB$_2$-selective analogs have shown anti-inflammatory and immunosuppressive activity (Arevalo-Martin et al. 2003; Lombard et al. 2007).

40.3.2 **Pharmacokinetics**

Systematic studies examining pharmacokinetics of synthetic cannabinoids have not been performed, primarily due to the vast array of compounds. However, several key points can be derived from extant data. First, the compounds are lipophilic. Consequently, absorption readily occurs via injection (intravenous, intraperitoneal, subcutaneous), as indicated by CNS-mediated activity following each route of administration (Vann et al. 2009; Wiley et al. 1998). Further, distribution of significant concentrations of JWH-018 to the brain and to most organs and tissues was reported up to 60 min after pyrolysis and inhalation (Wiebelhaus et al. 2012). Ex vivo autoradiography with the indole-derived psychoactive cannabinoid [^{131}I]AM-2233 verifies that distribution within the brain is consistent with localization of CB_1 receptors and is rimonabant reversible (Dhawan et al. 2006). Beyond these two studies, however, the majority of pharmacokinetic work has focused on identification of urinary metabolites that can be used as forensic markers (see section 40.5.2). Similar to THC, Phase 1 metabolism of synthetics is accomplished by cytochrome P450 (Chimalakonda et al. 2012). Whereas THC has one major psychoactive metabolite (11-OH-THC) (Huestis et al. 1992), metabolism of synthetic cannabinoids can proceed via several pathways (e.g., hydroxylation, glucuronidation), resulting in several metabolites, some of which retain in vivo and in vitro activity as CB_1 agonists or antagonists (Brents et al. 2011, 2012; Chimalakonda et al. 2011a, 2011b; Seely et al. 2012b). Primary elimination is assumed to be through the urine (Moran et al. 2011; Sobolevsky et al. 2010).

40.3.3 Preclinical pharmacology

The preclinical pharmacology of indole-derived synthetic cannabinoids is poorly character-ized. Besides the handful of studies in the mouse tetrad (see section 40.3.1), a few others have examined their effects in a THC drug discrimination assay, a pharmacologically selective animal model of marijuana intoxication (Balster and Prescott 1992). In this procedure, animals learn to use interoceptive cues produced by THC to discriminate which of two levers to press to receive a food reward (e.g., if THC injection was received, press right lever, and if not THC, press left lever). Once the animals are trained in this task, compounds other than THC are injected to determine whether they are "THC-like." CP-55,940 and WIN 55,212-2 dose-dependently substitute for THC in rats, monkeys, and mice (McMahon et al. 2008; Wiley 1999). Replacement of the morpholino-ethyl group of WIN 55,212-2 with a carbon chain of varying length from butyl to hexyl resulted in compounds that dose-dependently substituted in THC-trained rats and rhesus monkeys at potencies consistent with their CB_1 affinity, whereas the heptyl compound did not substitute, nor did it bind to CB_1 (Wiley et al. 1998). Later studies showed that JWH-018, JWH-073, AM-2233, and AM-5983 also substituted for THC in rats and/or rhesus monkeys (Ginsburg et al. 2012; Järbe et al. 2010, 2011). Rank order potencies were consistent with CB_1 affinities, and the substitution dose-effect curves were shifted to the right by rimonabant, suggesting CB_1 mediation. Duration of action appeared to be shorter than that of THC, particularly for JWH-073 (Ginsburg et al. 2012). WIN 55,212-2 and JWH-018 also substituted in rats trained to discriminate methanandamide from vehicle (Järbe et al. 2010). In THC-trained mice, two phenylacetylindoles (JWH-204 and JWH-205) with good CB_1 affinity substituted, whereas another phenylacetylindole (JWH-202) with poor CB_1 affinity did not (Vann et al. 2009).

As described in the preceding paragraph, sparse (but increasing) research attention has been focused on the effects of acute treatment with indole-derived cannabinoids. Although stud-ies investigating the effects of repeated dosing are lacking, cross-tolerance of three compounds (CP-55,940, JWH-018, and JWH-073) has been examined in rhesus monkeys chronically treated with THC in the context of a THC discrimination procedure (Hruba et al. 2012). Monkeys exhib-ited ninefold tolerance to THC, but only three- to sixfold cross-tolerance when injected with one of the synthetics. Further, the duration of cross-tolerance was shorter than for THC. A possible translational implication is that experienced cannabis users may show more sensitivity (i.e., less cross-tolerance) to synthetics than might be expected based upon their tolerance to THC. On the other hand, JWH-018 and JWH-073 have also been shown to reverse rimonabant-induced with-drawal in THC-dependent monkeys in a rimonabant discrimination procedure (Ginsburg et al.

2012). Together, these results suggest that the effects of synthetic cannabinoid use may differ in cannabis users and nonusers.

40.3.4 Toxicology

Aside from the preclinical pharmacological data cited earlier and the clinical data cited in later sections, only two published toxicological reports were found. WIN 55,212-2 at 2 mg/kg twice daily for 21 days produced morphological changes in the hippocampus in rats, including reduction of dendrites in CA1, a structure involved in learning and memory (Lawston et al. 2000). CP-55,940, CP-47,497, and CP-47,497-C8 produced concentration-dependent cytotoxicity in the NG 108-15 (neuroblastoma-glioma hybrid) cell line; administration of a CB_1 or a CB_2 antagonist showed that the effect was CB_1 mediated (Tomiyama and Funada 2011). One other report demonstrated that CP-47,497 and JWH-018 induced more profound changes in electroencephalogram patterns in rats than did THC (Uchiyama et al. 2012b).

40.3.5 Perspective

The weight of the evidence suggests CB_1 agonism as the proximate mechanism by which synthetic cannabinoids produce their effects. Limited data show that indole-derived cannabinoids have pharmacological effects similar to those of THC; however, few studies have examined their effects in behavioral assays that are not selective for CB_1 agonists. Many of these compounds bind to CB_2 receptors and may have activity at noncannabinoid receptors, suggesting an avenue for future research.

40.4 Abuse and control

40.4.1 Prevalence

The published evidence is primarily from three types of sources: surveys, medical reports, and monitoring of drug chat rooms and other Internet sites. Each has its limitations.

- The United Nations Office on Drugs and Crime (2011) reported a pilot study which found that "about 6% of pupils in Frankfurt, Germany, aged between 15 and 18 had used 'Spice' products at least once by the end of 2008."

- The U.S. National Forensic Laboratory Information System reported an increase in cases of synthetic cannabinoids submitted to state and local forensic laboratories from 13 to 2977 between 2009 to 2010 (US Department of Justice, Drug Enforcement Administration 2011).

- The European Monitoring Center for Drugs and Drug Addiction (2012) Europol 2011 Annual Report concluded from "representative studies" that "prevalence levels are not substantial but there is a potential for rapid rise of use in certain sub-populations." The Center monitors the Internet with "snapshots" of limited scope and duration. Among its findings: online drug shops offering at least one psychoactive substance increased from 170 in January 2010 to 690 in January 2012; 23 new cannabinoids were reported by the European Union Early Warning System in 2011, at least two of which were derivatives of JWH compounds, not the compounds themselves; incidence of synthetic cannabinoid use from surveys, while quite variable, is typically in the single digits; "the extent to which these products are used is largely unknown."

- Of 20 Idaho hospitals surveyed, 11 had knowledge of Spice and more than 80 cases of suspected overdose occurred between February and August 2010 (Hurst 2010).

- An anonymous Internet survey of 391 persons identified online as users of synthetic cannabinoids in 42 US states and 12 other countries produced the following demographics: 83% were male, 90% were Caucasian, 47% were employed full time, and 48% had college degrees (Vandrey et al. 2012).

- University of Florida students were surveyed by email in September 2010 about "spice," "K2," and "legal weed." Of 852 who responded, 8% reported ever use (that is, at least once), which was "higher than ever use of many other drugs of abuse that are commonly monitored in adolescents and young adults" (Hu et al. 2011).

- The six centers of the Texas Poison Center Network, serving a state population of 25 million, reported three calls about synthetic cannabinoids in 2008, nine in 2009, and 572 in 2010 (Forrester et al. 2011).

- The American Association of Poison Control Centers (2012) reported the following numbers for "closed human exposure calls to poison centers" about synthetic cannabinoids: 53 in 2009 (cited by Hu et al. 2011), 2906 in 2010, 6959 in 2011, and 4710 in the first 10 months of 2012.

- Of 14,966 participants in a global Internet survey in late 2011, 17% reported ever use of synthetics. They showed "a strong preference for natural over synthetic cannabis"—a more pleasant high and fewer negative effects (Winstock and Barratt 2013).

"The at-risk demographics are difficult to identify, as this 'virtual' community of drug users is generally discovered only when adverse effects compel individuals to seek care from emergency departments and poison control centers" (Rosenbaum et al. 2012).

40.4.2 Adverse effects

Smokers of Spice typically report a cannabis-like high. Reasons cited for preference over herbal cannabis include legality, non-detectability by conventional screens such as urinalysis, ease of access on the Internet, in some cases superiority of subjective effects, and a perception of safety (Fattore and Fratta 2011). The literature is replete with evidence contrary to that perception. Effects include agitation, anxiety, bradycardia, cardiotoxicity, confusion, chest pain, dizziness, drowsiness, hallucinations, hypertension, irritability, memory deficits, nausea, sedation, seizures, tachycardia, vomiting, and withdrawal symptoms (Fattore and Fratta 2011; Hoyte et al. 2012; Table 1 of Seely et al. 2012a).

The most common serious complaint in surveys and case reports is tachycardia, cited in 40% of the 1353 single-agent exposures reported to the National Poison Data System of the US in the first 9 months of 2010 (Hoyte et al. 2012). Cardiovascular effects may extend to hypertension (e.g., Schneir and Baumbacher 2012) and myocardial infarction (in three 16-year-old boys after smoking K2) (Mir et al. 2011).

The incidence of psychotic symptoms is high enough to be of concern. In the National Poison Data System report, it was 9.4% (Hoyte et al. 2012). Cannabis smoking has long been associated with schizophrenia, though cause and effect have not been established (Fattore and Fratta 2011). Synthetic cannabinoids have been implicated in relapse (69% of 15 patients) (Every-Palmer 2011) and with induction of symptoms in persons with no clinical history (Bebarta et al. 2012; Benford and Caplan 2011). Of ten patients admitted to a US Navy hospital with a history of smoking synthetic cannabinoids, a diagnosis of psychosis, and no prior history of psychosis, symptoms resolved within 8 days for seven but persisted more than 5 months in the other three (Hurst et al. 2011).

Seizure seems to be rare (3.8% of the cases in Hoyte et al. (2012)) but appears in several reports (Simmons et al. (2011) and Schneir and Baumbacher (2012) from smoking; Lapoint et al. (2011)

from ingestion of powder). "The absence of anticonvulsant phytocannabinoids in spice products could potentially be one of the multiple unknown mechanisms contributing to convulsions" (Schneir and Baumbacher 2012).

Survey and case report information on long-term use is meager. Usage by the 10 patients with acute psychosis cited earlier (Hurst et al. 2011) ranged from four times over 3 weeks to daily for 1.5 years. In a group of 11 teenagers with variable durations of use at an addiction treatment center (36% used the drugs multiple times a day), all reported memory changes and 35% reported paranoid thoughts (Castellanos et al. 2011). Craving and other withdrawal signs were reported in a patient who had used daily for 8 months (Zimmerman et al. 2009; this patient had a complex medical history). Because these products come in multiple forms with various ingredients, and many or most subjects may use other potentially toxic substances, isolating the chronic effects of a single structure or class of structures will require a massive database.

Of the few deaths reported in connection with synthetic cannabinoids, none was unequivocally ascribed to direct toxicity. The immediate cause in one case was coronary ischemia and in another was suicide. The nine fatalities in Europe cited by Fattore and Fratta (2011) in the context of "a Spice-like blend called 'Krypton'" apparently did not involve synthetic cannabinoids (Kronstrand et al. 2011).

40.4.3 Legal status

The Spice phenomenon developed rapidly and was by nature unusual—legal products sold openly and claiming to be not for human consumption. Statutes varied in basis and implementation. Governments required time to formulate policy and enact regulatory measures.

Beginning in 2009, all products containing synthetic cannabinoids were placed under control in several European countries, making them inaccessible in head shops and, theoretically, on the Internet (Seely et al. 2012a). By 2011, they were controlled in Austria, Denmark, Estonia, France, Germany, Ireland, Italy, Latvia, Lithuania, Luxembourg, Poland, Romania, Sweden, and the UK (Fattore and Fratta 2011). They are now controlled in Finland, Russia, and Switzerland (Cox et al. 2012).

The US DEA identifies drugs by chemical structure for scheduling purposes. To get around the problem that abused synthetic cannabinoids are structurally distinct from THC, in November 2010 the DEA used an emergency edict to place JWH-018, JWH-200, JWH-073, CP-47,497, and cannabicyclohexanol on Schedule I for 1 year effective March 2011 (Fattore and Fratta 2011). States began to make their own regulations about this time (Fattore and Fratta 2011; United Nations Office on Drugs and Crime 2011). Canada and Chile also have instituted controls (Cox et al. 2012).

In the Asia-Pacific region, five synthetic cannabinoids were controlled under the Japanese Pharmaceutical Affairs Law in 2010. As in other countries, banned structures were quickly replaced (Kikura-Hanajiri et al. 2011). In Japan, "it is a very difficult task to change the legal status of these substances. New compounds cannot be controlled unless the pharmacological activity is proven. This requires acquisition of reference materials which in turn may slow down the process. Furthermore, assessing pharmacological activity of every single compound is time-consuming and hence hampering initiatives to control these substances" (United Nations Office on Drugs and Crime 2011). In August 2011, the New Zealand Parliament placed a 1-year ban on 16 synthetic cannabinoids found in Spice-like products (Brown 2011). South Korea, too, has instituted controls (Cox et al. 2012).

The report "Synthetic Cannabinoids in Herbal Products" by the United Nations Office on Drugs and Crime (2011), which covers developments through the end of 2010, states: "None of the synthetic cannabinoids found so far in 'Spice' and 'Spice'-like products are internationally controlled under the 1961 or 1971 UN Drug control conventions." Despite regulatory action by individual authorities, cooperative initiatives, and widespread concern (Fattore and Fratta 2011), access to these products via the Internet poses a daunting challenge.

40.4.4 Perspective

Although prevalence numbers are far from definitive, existing evidence indicates that recreational use and abuse of synthetic cannabinoids is a significant public health concern. Demand is robust despite the known dangers, the supply side is nimble, and legislation has been in some cases too ponderous to cope. The result is a pernicious problem, especially among youth.

40.5 Forensic and analytical chemistry

40.5.1 Identification of product

Synthetic cannabinoids are most often formulated for smoking by addition to non-cannabis plant material. Damiana (*Turnera diffusa*), mugwort (*Artemisia vulgaris*), coltsfoot (*Tussilago farfara*), mullein (*Verbascum thapsus*), and marshmallow (*Althaea officinalis*) are examples seen on product packaging. Plant material varies widely between branded products and may vary within a brand over time and place. The subject has received relatively little attention in the literature. Synthetics detected by forensic laboratories likewise vary widely by brand, time, and place. Recently, compounds have become more available as powder, rather than mixed with plant material, and so can be taken orally or vaporized for inhalation.

Table 40.2 shows assays used to identify synthetics in seized samples. Thin-layer chromatography (TLC) has long been used to identify phytocannabinoids and synthetics in raw products. Immunoassays are useful though limited. Assays based on mass spectrometry (MS) have advantages for both detection in raw product and analysis of parent and metabolites ex vivo (see section 40.5.3).

Many Internet websites (e.g., http://www.erowid.org and http://www.drugs-forum.com) describe products and their effects and give user-submitted suggestions on optimal dosing. This information, treated with suitable precautions, can enhance current awareness and guide selection of forensic and analytical research areas.

Table 40.2 Forensic and analytical assays for synthetic cannabinoids

Assay	Type of sample		Can identify		Good for[a]		Notes
	Raw product	Body fluid	Parent	Metabolites	Screen	Confirm	
TLC	✓		✓		✓		
Immunoassay	✓	✓	✓	✓	✓		Primarily ELISA
Full scan MS alone	✓		✓		✓		Includes DART and MALDI-TOF
Full scan GC-MS	✓	✓	✓	✓	✓	✓	
Full scan LC-MS	✓	✓	✓	✓	✓	✓	
MS/MS	✓	✓	✓	✓		✓	Includes SIM, SRM, MRM

[a] A screening assay can identify the likely presence of a compound or a member of a class of compounds. A confirmatory assay can identify a specific compound in the class.

40.5.2 **Markers of synthetic cannabinoid use**

Intact synthetic cannabinoids can be detected post consumption in saliva (Coulter et al. 2011), blood (Kacinko et al. 2011), and hair (Salomone et al. 2012). While testing hair is of limited use in emergency and medical situations, it is scientifically interesting and may be useful in longer-term treatment and forensics. An ideal noninvasive test uses urine, but intact parent compounds of synthetic cannabinoids are not usually found in urine of known users (Moller et al. 2011; Sobolevsky et al. 2010). Therefore, a system that detects metabolites is desirable. Little is known about the metabolism of most synthetic cannabinoids. The best studied are those first popularly abused, notably JWH-018 and related alkylindoles. Their common metabolites are products of mono-, di-, and tri-hydroxylation, resulting from combinations of hydroxylation on the naphthalene ring, the indole ring, and the N-alkyl group. Other commonly reported metabolic transformations are carboxylation, dealkylation, and dihydrodiol formation (Hutter et al. 2012; Kacinko et al. 2011; Zhang et al. 2006).

One complication in detection of parent or metabolite arises from the usual method of administration, smoking, which produces changes through pyrolysis. For example, the N-alkyl group of AM-2201 loses a fluorine atom to become JWH-018 and is desaturated, completing its conversion to JWH-022 (Donohue and Steiner 2012), and UR-144 and XLR11 undergo cyclopropyl rearrangements (Forendex Forum 2012). Additional research in this area is needed to determine exactly what enters the body in order to know what components are responsible for adverse effects.

40.5.3 **Analytical techniques**

40.5.3.1 Immunoassay

The first step for many commercial and forensic laboratories is a series of immunoassay screens. Immunoassays are based on the interaction between an antigen and its antibodies. A sample is mixed with a solution containing antibodies specific to a particular drug or class of drugs. If the sample contains that drug, it will react with the antibodies and produce a measurable signal such as a color change. Such screens are commonplace for most drugs of abuse, but first became widely available for synthetic cannabinoids only in early 2012 (Logan 2012). They can detect dozens of synthetic cannabinoids and their metabolites but are not comprehensive for the vast number with potential for abuse. Therefore, their main weakness is high potential for false negatives.

40.5.3.2 Mass spectrometry

Many laboratories skip immunoassays as problematic and go directly to confirmatory tests using gas chromatography (GC)-mass spectrometry (GC-MS) or liquid chromatography (LC)-MS. GC-MS (Dresen et al. 2010; Cox et al. 2012), LC-MS, LC-MS/MS (Dresen et al. 2011; Grabenauer et al. 2012; Kacinko et al. 2011; Uchiyama et al. 2010), and matrix-assisted laser desorption/ionization-time of flight (MALDI-TOF) (Gottardo et al. 2012) assays for synthetic cannabinoids have been recently published.

The most common MS technique in forensic testing is full scan GC-MS with library matching. The sample is subjected to electron ionization at 70 eV, creating a characteristic and reproducible mass spectrum of fragment ions, which is searched against a library of mass spectra of known compounds. There is no preselection of output, so the procedure is unbiased, but a match can be made only if the synthetic is already in the library. Library matching is less common with LC-MS because of non-uniformity in fragmentation patterns between LC-MS instruments, although some laboratories have created internal libraries for data acquired on the same instrument (Mueller et al. 2005).

Higher sensitivity can be attained by targeted MS analyses such as single ion monitoring (SIM), single reaction monitoring (SRM), and multiple reaction monitoring (MRM). In SIM, the detector of a mass spectrometer is fixed at the specific mass-to-charge ratio (m/z) for the compound of interest. SRM is similar to SIM in that the instrument detects only a single m/z, but the analysis is more specific because rather than detecting the parent m/z for a compound, the parent m/z is isolated then fragmented and a specific fragment ion is detected. MRM combines several parent-fragment combinations into a single analysis. While these techniques are more sensitive than full scan data acquisitions, the trade-off is that data acquisition is biased: the instrument operator must decide before a sample is run which ions to monitor, and no other data are stored.

As high-resolution MS instruments become affordable, more laboratories are using them. They are ideal for nontargeted screening and confirmatory testing. TOF and orbitrap instruments are the most common. Both can collect and store data for all ions in a sample, enabling retrospective analysis. Data can be compared against a library of molecular weights (Gottardo et al. 2012), but molecular weight alone is not enough to distinguish between isomers.

Beyond accurate mass information, high-resolution MS can be used with fractional mass filtering (also known as mass defect filtering) to detect both previously reported and new compounds. The fractional mass of a compound is the difference between its calculated exact mass and the closest integer value. For example, JWH-018 has a calculated exact mass of 341.1780. The closest integer value is 341, therefore the fractional mass of JWH-018 is 0.1780. Fractional mass filtering has been used for years to identify metabolites (Zhu et al. 2006) and has only recently been applied to detection of synthetic cannabinoids (Grabenauer et al. 2012). This technique capitalizes on the fact that families of synthetic cannabinoids have similar core structures and therefore similar fractional masses. By searching for all ions with fractional masses close to those of known compounds, the approach becomes a screening tool. It can be applied to intact parent ions and fragment ions.

40.5.4 Challenges

The number of possible chemical constituents of a Spice sample is enormous. Every step of sample preparation potentially biases the analysis, so techniques with minimal sample preparation are advantageous to detect the widest possible array. Solid phase micro extraction (SPME) headspace sampling GC-MS requires minimal preparation and is effective for rapid analysis of bulk drug substances and herbal formulations (Cox et al. 2012). Direct analysis in real time (DART) ionization (Musah et al. 2012) has also been successful and requires no sample preparation. Analysis of bodily fluids such as blood and urine generally requires a more thorough sample cleanup, but liquid-liquid extraction is sufficient for most applications (Moller et al. 2011; Sobolevsky et al. 2010). For herbal formulations, a simple ethanol or methanol extraction works well (Grabenauer et al. 2012; Uchiyama et al. 2010).

As one synthetic cannabinoid is banned, suppliers rapidly substitute an analog to evade targeted detection. Manufacturers of reference standards are quick to synthesize these new entities, but the process is still too slow. Forensic laboratories must rely on library matches to spectra of independently synthesized material; this is not ideal for casework and goes against the Scientific Working Group for the Analysis of Seized Drugs guidelines, which require confirmation by comparison to a concurrently run reference standard. An option is structural elucidation with infrared spectroscopy, MS/MS, or nuclear magnetic resonance analysis, but such a thorough characterization is very time-consuming. Furthermore, the compounds are usually not in a pure state but are present as mixtures requiring purification before final assay, and there might not be enough sample present for the analysis. Reference standards for metabolites take even longer to become available, because metabolic studies must be done to determine what to synthesize as standards.

Techniques that can unambiguously identify isomers are needed, and that means most likely a chromatographic separation prior to detection, either by LC-MS, GC-MS, or GC-IR (infrared). Techniques that can act as broad-spectrum screening tools such as IR or MS using full scan data acquisition need to be employed more routinely to catch new compounds undetectable by targeted methods. Bench chemists need to be armed with tools for structural elucidation via infrared or MS/MS fragment ion spectra to lessen dependence on commercial suppliers of reference material.

40.6 **Conclusions**

This chapter is by no means exhaustive. Designer cannabinoids have been ably reviewed elsewhere (Fattore and Fratta 2011; Seely et al. 2012a). We have tried to provide an overview of the field as reflected in the literature at the end of 2012. Neurochemically there is general agreement that, like THC, most of these drugs are agonists at the CB_1 receptor, though the downstream mechanisms are not well understood. The desired subjective effects are cannabis-like but more intense. Pharmacological data are sparse; systematic toxicological data, very sparse. Since 2008, a self-selected group numbering perhaps in the tens of thousands has been conducting what amounts to an ad hoc, uncontrolled Phase 1 clinical trial. These subjects represent a broad spectrum ranging from hardcore drug abusers to casual experimenters. The data that emerge from surveys, online chat rooms, hospital emergency rooms, and poison centers suggest that synthetic cannabinoids are more dangerous than marijuana and might even be lethal in some cases. Legal controls, where any exist, have limited effect, for three reasons: clandestine chemists can replace banned structures within weeks, Internet vendors are highly resourceful, and the demand is there. Methods of detection are improving, though the cost is still too great for widespread deployment where rapid results are needed, as in medical and enforcement settings. Thus, presently the trajectory of designer cannabinoid use seems to be continuing upward.

References

Adams, R., Harfenist, M., and Loewe, S. (1949). New analogs of tetrahydrocannabinol. XIX. *Journal of the American Chemical Society*, **71**, 1624–1628.

American Association of Poison Control Centers (2012). *Synthetic Marijuana Data*. [Online] Available at: http://www.aapcc.org/dnn/Portals/0/Synthetic%20Marijuana%20Data%20for%20Website%2012.12.2011. pdf (accessed January 16, 2013).

Arevalo-Martin, A., Vela, J.M., Molina-Holgado, E., Borrell, J., and Guaza, C. (2003). Therapeutic action of cannabinoids in a murine model of multiple sclerosis. *Journal of Neuroscience*, **23**, 2511–2516.

Atwood, B.K., Huffman, J., Straiker, A., and Mackie, K. (2010). JWH018, a common constituent of 'Spice' herbal blends, is a potent and efficacious cannabinoid CB receptor agonist. *British Journal of Pharmacology*, **160**, 585–593.

Atwood, B.K., Lee, D., Straiker, A., Widlanski, T.S., and Mackie, K. (2011). CP47,497-C8 and JWH073, commonly found in 'Spice' herbal blends, are potent and efficacious CB_1 cannabinoid receptor agonists. *European Journal of Pharmacology*, **659**, 139–145.

Aung, M.M., Griffin, G., Huffman, J.W., *et al.* (2000). Influence of the N-1 alkyl chain length of cannabimimetic indoles upon CB_1 and CB_2 receptor binding. *Drug and Alcohol Dependence*, **60**, 133–140.

Auwarter, V., Dresen, S., Weinmann, W., Muller, M., Putz, M., and Ferreiros, N. (2009). 'Spice' and other herbal blends: harmless incense or cannabinoid designer drugs? *Journal of Mass Spectrometry*, **44**, 832–837.

Balster, R.L. and Prescott, W.R. (1992). Δ^9-Tetrahydrocannabinol discrimination in rats as a model for cannabis intoxication. *Neuroscience & Biobehavioral Reviews*, **16**, 55–62.

Bebarta, V.S., Ramirez, S., and Varney, S.M. (2012). Spice: a new "legal" herbal mixture abused by young active duty military personnel. *Substance Abuse*, **33**, 191–194.

Benford, D.M. and Caplan, J.P. (2011). Psychiatric sequelae of Spice, K2, and synthetic cannabinoid receptor agonists. *Psychosomatics*, **52**, 295.

Breivogel, C.S. and Childers, S.R. (2000). Cannabinoid agonist signal transduction in rat brain: comparison of cannabinoid agonists in receptor binding, G-protein activation, and adenylyl cyclase inhibition. *Journal of Pharmacology and Experimental Therapeutics*, **295**, 328–336.

Breivogel, C.S., Griffin, G., Di Marzo, V., and Martin, B.R. (2001). Evidence for a new G protein-coupled cannabinoid receptor in mouse brain. *Molecular Pharmacology*, **60**, 155–163.

Brents, L.K., Reichard, E.E., Zimmerman, S.M., Moran, J.H., Fantegrossi, W.E., and Prather, P.L. (2011). Phase I hydroxylated metabolites of the K2 synthetic cannabinoid JWH-018 retain *in vitro* and *in vivo* cannabinoid 1 receptor affinity and activity. *PLoS One*, **6**, e21917.

Brizzi, A., Brizzi, V., Cascio, M.G., Bisogno, T., Sirianni, R. and Di Marzo, V. (2005). Design, synthesis, and binding studies of new potent ligands of cannabinoid receptors. *Journal of Medicinal Chemistry*, **48**, 7343–7350.

Brizzi, A., Brizzi, V., Cascio, M. G., *et al.* (2009). New resorcinol–anandamide "hybrids" as potent cannabinoid receptor ligands endowed with antinociceptive activity in vivo. *Journal of Medicinal Chemistry*, **52**, 2506–2514.

Brown, K. (2011). New Zealand bans synthetic cannabinoids. *BMJ*, **343**, d5395.

Cascio, M.G., Bisogno, T., Palazzo, E., *et al.* (2006). *In vitro* and in *vivo* pharmacology of synthetic olivetol- or resorcinol-derived cannabinoid receptor ligands. *British Journal of Pharmacology*, **149**, 431–440.

Castellanos, D., Singh, S., Thornton, G., Avila, M., and Moreno, A. (2011). Synthetic cannabinoid use: a case series of adolescents. *Journal of Adolescent Health*, **49**, 347–349.

Chimalakonda, K.C., Bratton, S.M., Le, V.H., *et al.* (2011a). Conjugation of synthetic cannabinoids JWH-018 and JWH-073, metabolites by human UDP-glucuronosyltransferases. *Drug Metabolism and Disposition*, **39**, 1967–1976.

Chimalakonda, K.C., Moran, C.L., Kennedy, P.D., *et al.* (2011b). Solid-phase extraction and quantitative measurement of omega and omega-1 metabolites of JWH-018 and JWH-073 in human urine. *Analytical Chemistry*, **83**, 6381–6388.

Chimalakonda, K.C., Seely, K.A., Bratton, S.M., *et al.* (2012). Cytochrome P450-mediated oxidative metabolism of abused synthetic cannabinoids found in K2/Spice: identification of novel cannabinoid receptor ligands. *Drug Metabolism and Disposition*, **40**, 2174–2184.

Compton, D.R., Rice, K.C., De Costa, B.R., *et al.* (1993). Cannabinoid structure-activity relationships: correlation of receptor binding and in vivo activities. *Journal of Pharmacology and Experimental Therapeutics*, **265**, 218–226.

Coulter, C., Garnier, M., and Moore, C. (2011). Synthetic cannabinoids in oral fluid. *Journal of Analytical Toxicology*, **35**, 424–430.

Cox, A.O., Daw, R.C., Mason, M.D., *et al.* (2012). Use of SPME-HS-GC-MS for the analysis of herbal products containing synthetic cannabinoids. *Journal of Analytical Toxicology*, **36**, 293–302.

D'Ambra, T.E., Estep, K.G., Bell, M.R., *et al.* (1992). Conformationally restrained analogues of pravadoline: nanomolar potent, enantioselective, (aminoalkyl)indole agonists of the cannabinoid receptor. *Journal of Medicinal Chemistry*, **35**, 124–135.

Devane, W.A., Dysarz, F.A. 3rd, Johnson, M.R., Melvin, L.S., and Howlett, A.C. (1988). Determination and characterization of a cannabinoid receptor in rat brain. *Molecular Pharmacology*, **34**, 605–613.

Devane, W.A., Hanus, L., Breuer, A., *et al.* (1992). Isolation and structure of a brain constituent that binds to the cannabinoid receptor. *Science*, **258**, 1946–1949.

Dhawan, J., Deng, H., Gatley, S.J., *et al.* (2006). Evaluation of the in vivo receptor occupancy for the behavioral effects of cannabinoids using a radiolabeled cannabinoid receptor agonist, R-[$^{125/131}$I]AM2233. *Synapse*, **60**, 93–101.

Donohue, K.M. and Steiner, R.R. (2012). JWH-018 and JWH-022 as combustion products of AM-2201. *Microgram Journal*, **9**, 52–56.

Dresen, S., Ferreiros, N., Putz, M., Westphal, F., Zimmermann, R., and Auwarter, V. (2010). Monitoring of herbal mixtures potentially containing synthetic cannabinoids as psychoactive compounds. *Journal of Mass Spectrometry*, **45**, 1186–1194.

Dresen, S., Kneisel, S., Weinmann, W., Zimmermann, R., and Auwarter, V. (2011). Development and validation of a liquid chromatography-tandem mass spectrometry method for the quantitation of synthetic cannabinoids of the aminoalkylindole type and methanandamide in serum and its application to forensic samples. *Journal of Mass Spectrometry*, **46**, 163–171.

European Monitoring Center for Drugs and Drug Addiction. (2012). *EMCDDA–Europol 2011 Annual Report on the implementation of Council Decision 2005/387/JHA.* [Online] Available at: http://www.emcdda.europa.eu/publications/implementation-reports/2011.

Every-Palmer, S. (2011). Synthetic cannabinoid JWH-018 and psychosis: an explorative study. *Drug and Alcohol Dependence*, **117**, 152–157.

Fattore, L. and Fratta, W. (2011). Beyond THC: the new generation of cannabinoid designer drugs. *Frontiers in Behavioural Neuroscience*, **5**, 60.

Feledziak, M., Lambert, D.M., Marchand-Brynaert, J., and Muccioli, G.G. (2012). Inhibitors of the endocannabinoid-degrading enzymes, or how to increase endocannabinoid's activity by preventing their hydrolysis. *Recent Patents on CNS Drug Discovery*, **7**, 49–70.

Forendex Forum. (2012). *Discussion Board for Forensic Chemists.* [Online] Available at: http://forendexforum.southernforensic.org/viewtopic.php?f=4&t=86&hilit=144&start=10#p650 (accessed November 20, 2012).

Forrester, M.B., Kleinschmidt, K., Schwarz, E., and Young, A. (2011). Synthetic cannabinoid exposures reported to Texas poison centers. *Journal of Addictive Diseases*, **30**, 351–358.

Frost, J.M., Dart, M.J., Tietje, K.R., et al. (2010). Indol-3-ylcycloalkyl ketones: effects of N1 substituted indole side chain variations on CB_2 cannabinoid receptor activity. *Journal of Medicinal Chemistry*, **53**, 295–315.

Gallant, M., Dufresne, C., Gareau, Y., et al. (1996). New class of potent ligands for the human peripheral cannabinoid receptor. *Bioorganic & Medicinal Chemistry Letters*, **6**, 2263–2268.

Gaoni, Y. and Mechoulam, R. (1964). Isolation, structure, and partial synthesis of an active constituent of hashish. *Journal of the American Chemical Society*, **86**, 1646–1647.

Ginsburg, B.C., Schulze, D.R., Hruba, L., and McMahon, L.R. (2012). JWH-018 and JWH-073: Δ^9-tetrahydrocannabinol-like discriminative stimulus effects in monkeys. *Journal of Pharmacology and Experimental Therapeutics*, **340**, 37–45.

Gottardo, R., Chiarini, A., Dal Pra, I., et al. (2012). Direct screening of herbal blends for new synthetic cannabinoids by MALDI-TOF MS. *Journal of Mass Spectrometry*, **47**, 141–146.

Grabenauer, M., Krol, W.L., Wiley, J.L., and Thomas, B.F. (2012). Analysis of synthetic cannabinoids using high-resolution mass spectrometry and mass defect filtering: Implications for non-targeted screening of designer drugs. *Analytical Chemistry*, **84**, 5574–5581.

Hajos, N., Ledent, C., and Freund, T.F. (2001). Novel cannabinoid-sensitive receptor mediates inhibition of glutamatergic synaptic transmission in the hippocampus. *Neuroscience*, **106**, 1–4.

Herkenham, M., Lynn, A.B., Johnson, M.R., Melvin, L.S., de Costa, B.R., and Rice, K.C. (1991). Characterization and localization of cannabinoid receptors in rat brain: a quantitative *in vitro* autoradiographic study. *Journal of Neuroscience*, **11**, 563–583.

Herkenham, M., Lynn, A.B., Little, M.D., Johnson, M.R., Melvin, L.S., de Costa, B.R. and Rice, K.C. (1990). Cannabinoid receptor localization in brain. *Proceedings of the National Academy of Sciences of the United States of America*, **87**, 1932–1936.

Howlett, A.C., Johnson, M.R., Melvin, L.S., and Milne, G.M. (1988). Nonclassical cannabinoid analgetics inhibit adenylate cyclase: development of a cannabinoid receptor model. *Molecular Pharmacology*, **33**, 297–302.

Howlett, A.C., Bidaut-Russell, M., Devane, W.A., Melvin, L.S., Johnson, M.R., and Herkenham, M. (1990). The cannabinoid receptor: biochemical, anatomical and behavioral characterization. *Trends in Neurosciences*, **13**, 420–423.

Hoyte, C.O., Jacob, J., Monte, A.A., Al-Jumaan, M., Bronstein, A.C., and Heard, K.J. (2012). A characterization of synthetic cannabinoid exposures reported to the national poison data system in 2010. *Annals of Emergency Medicine*, **60**, 435–438.

Hruba, L., Ginsburg, B., and McMahon, L.R. (2012). Apparent inverse relationship between cannabinoid agonist efficacy and tolerance/cross-tolerance produced by Δ^9-tetrahydrocannabinol treatment in rhesus monkeys. *Journal of Pharmacology and Experimental Therapeutics*, **342**, 843–849.

Hu, X., Primack, B.A., Barnett, T.E., and Cook, R.L. (2011). College students and use of K2: an emerging drug of abuse in young persons. *Substance Abuse Treatment, Prevention, and Policy*, **6**, 16.

Huestis, M.A., Henningfield, J.E., and Cone, E.J. (1992). Blood cannabinoids: I. Absorption of THC and formation of 11-OH-THC and THCCOOH during and after smoking marijuana. *Journal of Analytical Toxicology*, **16**, 276–282.

Huffman, J.W. and Padgett, L.W. (2005). Recent developments in the medicinal chemistry of cannabimimetic indoles, pyrroles and indenes. *Current Medicinal Chemistry*, **12**, 1395–1411.

Huffman, J.W., Dai, D., Martin, B.R., and Compton, D.R. (1994). Design, synthesis and pharmacology of cannabimimetic indoles. *Bioorganic & Medicinal Chemistry Letters*, **4**, 563–566.

Huffman, J.W., Hepburn, S.A., Reggio, P.H., Hurst, D.P., Wiley, J.L., and Martin, B.R. (2010). Synthesis and pharmacology of 1-methoxy analogs of CP-47,497. *Bioorganic & Medicinal Chemistry*, **18**, 5475–5482.

Huffman, J.W., Mabon, R., Wu, M.-J., *et al.* (2003). 3-Indolyl-1-naphthylmethanes: new cannabimimetic indoles provide evidence for aromatic stacking interactions with the CB_1 cannabinoid receptor. *Bioorganic & Medicinal Chemistry*, **11**, 539–549.

Huffman, J.W., Padgett, L.W., Isherwood, M.L., Wiley, J.L., and Martin, B.R. (2006). 1-Alkyl-2-aryl-4-(1-naphthoyl)pyrroles: New high affinity ligands for the cannabinoid CB_1 and CB_2 receptors. *Bioorganic & Medicinal Chemistry Letters*, **16**, 5432–5435.

Huffman, J.W., Szklennik, P.V., Almond, A., *et al.* (2005a). 1-Pentyl-3-phenylacetylindoles, a new class of cannabimimetic indoles. *Bioorganic & Medicinal Chemistry Letters*, **15**, 4110–4113.

Huffman, J.W., Thompson, A.L.S., Wiley, J.L., and Martin, B.R. (2008). Synthesis and pharmacology of 1-deoxy analogs of CP-47,497 and CP-55,940. *Bioorganic & Medicinal Chemistry*, **16**, 322–335.

Huffman, J.W., Zengin, G., Wu, M.-J., *et al.* (2005b). Structure-activity relationships for 1-alkyl-3-(1-naphthoyl)indoles at the cannabinoid CB_1 and CB_2 receptors: steric and electronic effects of naphthoyl substituents. New highly selective CB_2 receptor agonists. *Bioorganic & Medicinal Chemistry*, **13**, 89–112.

Hurst, D. (2010). Hospital survey shows more than 80 suspected cases of Spice overdose in past six months. *Idaho Reporter*, September 16. [Online] Available at: http://www.idahoreporter.com/2010/hospital-survey-shows-more-than-80-suspected-cases-of-spice-overdose-in-past-six-months/.

Hurst, D., Loeffler, G., and Mclay, R. (2011). Psychosis associated with synthetic cannabinoid agonists: a case series. *American Journal of Psychiatry*, **168**, 1119.

Hutter, M., Broecker, S., Kneisel, S., and Auwarter, V. (2012). Identification of the major urinary metabolites in man of seven synthetic cannabinoids of the aminoalkylindole type present as adulterants in 'herbal mixtures' using LC-MS/MS techniques. *Journal of Mass Spectrometry*, **47**, 54–65.

Järbe, T.U.C., Deng, H., Vadivel, S.K., and Makriyannis, A. (2011). Cannabinergic aminoalkylindoles, including AM678=JWH018 found in 'Spice', examined using drug (Δ^9-tetrahydrocannabinol) discrimination for rats. *Behavioural Pharmacology*, **22**, 498–507.

Järbe, T.U.C., Li, C., Vadivel, S.K., and Makriyannis, A. (2010). Discriminative stimulus functions of methanandamide and Δ^9-THC in rats: tests with aminoalkylindoles (WIN55,212-2 and AM678) and ethanol. *Psychopharmacology (Berlin)*, **208**, 87–98.

Johnson, M.R., Althuis, T.H., Bindra, J.S., Harbert, C.A., Melvin, L.S., and Milne, G.M. (1981a). Potent analgetics derived from 9-nor-9 beta-hydroxyhexahydrocannabinol. *NIDA Research Monographs*, **34**, 68–74.

Johnson, M.R., Melvin, L.S., Althuis, T.H., *et al.* (1981b). Selective and potent analgetics derived from cannabinoids. *Journal of Clinical Pharmacology*, **21**, 271S–82S.

Kacinko, S.L., Xu, A., Homan, J.W., McMullin, M.M., Warrington, D.M., and Logan, B.K. (2011). Development and validation of a liquid chromatography-tandem mass spectrometry method for the identification and quantification of JWH-018, JWH-073, JWH-019, and JWH-250 in human whole blood. *Journal of Analytical Toxicology*, **35**, 386–393.

Kikura-Hanajiri, R., Uchiyama, N., and Goda, Y. (2011). Survey of current trends in the abuse of psychotropic substances and plants in Japan. *Legal Medicine (Tokyo)*, **13**, 109–115.

Kronstrand, R., Roman, M., Thelander, G., and Eriksson, A. (2011). Unintentional fatal intoxications with mitragynine and O-desmethyltramadol from the herbal blend Krypton. *Journal of Analytical Toxicology*, **35**, 242–247.

Kumar, V., Alexander, M.D., Bell, M.R., *et al.* (1995). Morpholinoalkylindenes as antinociceptive agents: novel cannabinoid receptor agonists. *Bioorganic & Medicinal Chemistry Letters*, **5**, 381–386.

Lainton, J.A.H., Huffman, J.W., Martin, B.R., and Compton, D.R. (1995). 1-Alkyl-3-(1-naphthoyl)pyrroles: a new class of cannabinoid. *Tetrahedron Letters*, **36**, 1401–1404.

Lapoint, J., James, L.P., Moran, C.L., Nelson, L.S., Hoffman, R.S., and Moran, J.H. (2011). Severe toxicity following synthetic cannabinoid ingestion. *Clinical Toxicology*, **49**, 760–764.

Lawston, J., Borella, A., Robinson, J.K., and Whitaker-Azmitia, P.M. (2000). Changes in hippocampal morphology following chronic treatment with the synthetic cannabinoid WIN 55,212-2. *Brain Research*, **877**, 407–410.

Logan, B.K. (2012). *NMS Labs Trends Report: Changes in the Designer Drug Market Spring 2012* [Online] Available at: http://www.nmslabs.com/uploads/PDF/Designer%20Drug%20Spring%20Update_BKL%20 Webinar_May%202012.pdf (accessed November 28, 2012).

Lombard, C., Nagarkatti, M., and Nagarkatti, P. (2007). CB_2 cannabinoid receptor agonist, JWH-015, triggers apoptosis in immune cells: potential role for CB2-selective ligands as immunosuppressive agents. *Clinical Immunology*, **122**, 259–270.

Makara, J.K., Mor, M., Fegley, D., *et al.* (2005). Selective inhibition of 2-AG hydrolysis enhances endocannabinoid signaling in hippocampus. *Nature Neuroscience*, 8, 1139–1141. Corrigendum *Nature Neuroscience*, **10**, 137 (2007).

Manera, C., Tuccinardi, T., and Martinelli, A. (2008). Indoles and related compounds as cannabinoid ligands. *Mini-Reviews in Medicinal Chemistry*, **8**, 370–387.

Martin, B.R., Compton, D.R., Thomas, B.F., *et al.* (1991). Behavioral, biochemical, and molecular modeling evaluations of cannabinoid analogs. *Pharmacology Biochemistry and Behavior*, **40**, 471–478.

Matsuda, L.A., Lolait, S.J., Brownstein, M.J., Young, A.C., and Bonner, T.I. (1990). Structure of a cannabinoid receptor and functional expression of the cloned cDNA. *Nature*, **346**, 561–564.

Mauler, F., Mittendorf, J., Horvath, E., and De Vry, J. (2002). Characterization of the diarylether sulfonylester (−)-(R)-3-(2-hydroxymethylindanyl-4-oxy) phenyl-4,4,4-trifluoro-1-sulfonate (BAY 38-7271) as a potent cannabinoid receptor agonist with neuroprotective properties. *Journal of Pharmacology and Experimental Therapeutics*, **302**, 359–368.

McMahon, L.R., Ginsburg, B.C., and Lamb, R.J. (2008). Cannabinoid agonists differentially substitute for the discriminative stimulus effects of Δ^9-tetrahydrocannabinol in C57BL/6J mice. *Psychopharmacology (Berlin)*, **198**, 487–495.

Mir, A., Obafemi, A., Young, A., and Kane, C. (2011). Myocardial infarction associated with use of the synthetic cannabinoid K2. *Pediatrics*, **128**, e1622–e1627.

Moller, I., Wintermeyer, A., Bender, K., *et al.* (2011). Screening for the synthetic cannabinoid JWH-018 and its major metabolites in human doping controls. *Drug Testing and Analysis*, **3**, 609–620.

Monory, K., Tzavara, E.T., Lexime, J., *et al.* (2002). Novel, not adenylyl cyclase-coupled cannabinoid binding site in cerebellum of mice. *Biochemical and Biophysical Research Communications*, **292**, 231–235.

Moran, C.L., Le, V.H., Chimalakonda, K.C., *et al.* (2011). Quantitative measurement of JWH-018 and JWH-073 metabolites excreted in human urine. *Analytical Chemistry*, **83**, 4228–4236.

Mueller, C.A., Weinmann, W., Dresen, S., Schreiber, A., and Gergov, M. (2005). Development of a multi-target screening analysis for 301 drugs using a QTrap liquid chromatography/tandem mass spectrometry system and automated library searching. *Rapid Communications in Mass Spectrometry*, **19**, 1332–1338.

Munro, S., Thomas, K.L., and Abu-Shaar, M. (1993). Molecular characterization of a peripheral receptor for cannabinoids. *Nature*, **365**, 61–65.

Musah, R.A., Domin, M.A., Walling, M.A., and Shepard, J.R. (2012). Rapid identification of synthetic cannabinoids in herbal samples via direct analysis in real time mass spectrometry. *Rapid Communications in Mass Spectrometry*, **26**, 1109–1114.

Pertwee, R., Griffin, G., Fernando, S., Li, X., Hill, A., and Makriyannis, A. (1995). AM630, a competitive cannabinoid receptor antagonist. *Life Sciences*, **56**, 1949–1955.

Rosenbaum, C.D., Carreiro, S.P. and Babu, K.M. (2012). Here today, gone tomorrow . . . And back again? A review of herbal marijuana alternatives (K2, Spice), synthetic cathinones (bath salts), kratom, Salvia divinorum, methoxetamine, and piperazines. *Journal of Medical Toxicology*, **8**, 15–32.

Saario, S.M., Palomaki, V., Lehtonen, M., Nevalainen, T., Jarvinen, T., and Laitinen, J.T. (2006). URB754 has no effect on the hydrolysis or signaling capacity of 2-AG in the rat brain. *Chemistry & Biology*, **13**, 811–814.

Salomone, A., Gerace, E., D'Urso, F., Di Corcia, D., and Vincenti, M. (2012). Simultaneous analysis of several synthetic cannabinoids, THC, CBD and CBN, in hair by ultra-high performance liquid chromatography tandem mass spectrometry. Method validation and application to real samples. *Journal of Mass Spectrometry*, **47**, 604–610.

Schneir, A.B. and Baumbacher, T. (2012). Convulsions associated with the use of a synthetic cannabinoid product. *Journal of Medical Toxicology*, **8**, 62–64.

Seely, K.A., Lapoint, J., Moran, J.H., and Fattore, L. (2012a). Spice drugs are more than harmless herbal blends: a review of the pharmacology and toxicology of synthetic cannabinoids. *Progress in Neuro-Psychopharmacology and Biological Psychiatry*, **39**, 234–243.

Seely, K.A., Brents, L.K., Radominska-Pandya, A., *et al.* (2012b). A major glucuronidated metabolite of JWH-018 is a neutral antagonist at CB1 receptors. *Chemical Research in Toxicology*, **25**, 825–827.

Showalter, V.M., Compton, D.R., Martin, B.R., and Abood, M.E. (1996). Evaluation of binding in a transfected cell line expressing a peripheral cannabinoid receptor (CB2): identification of cannabinoid receptor subtype selective ligands. *Journal of Pharmacology and Experimental Therapeutics*, **278**, 989–999.

Simmons, J.R., Skinner, C.G., Williams, J., Kang, C.S., Schwartz, M.D., and Wills, B.K. (2011). Intoxication from smoking "spice." *Annals of Emergency Medicine*, **57**, 187–188.

Sobolevsky, T., Prasolov, I., and Rodchenkov, G. (2010). Detection of JWH-018 metabolites in smoking mixture post-administration urine. *Forensic Science International*, **200**, 141–147.

Song, Z.H. and Bonner, T.I. (1996). A lysine residue of the cannabinoid receptor is critical for receptor recognition by several agonists but not WIN55212-2. *Molecular Pharmacology*, **49**, 891–186.

Tomiyama, K. and Funada, M. (2011). Cytotoxicity of synthetic cannabinoids found in "Spice" products: the role of cannabinoid receptors and the caspase cascade in the NG 108-15 cell line. *Toxicology Letters*, **207**, 12–17.

U.S. Department of Justice, Drug Enforcement Administration (2011). *Special Report: Synthetic Cannabinoids and Synthetic Cathinones Reported in NFLIS, 2009-2010* [Online] Available at: http://www.deadiversion.usdoj.gov/nflis/2010rx_synth.pdf.

Uchiyama, N., Kawamura, M., Kikura-Hanajiri, R., and Goda, Y. (2012a). URB-754: A new class of designer drug and 12 synthetic cannabinoids detected in illegal products. *Forensic Science International* [Online] Available at: http://www.sciencedirect.com/science/article/pii/S0379073812004343.

Uchiyama, N., Kikura-Hanajiri, R., Matsumoto, N., Huang, Z.L., Goda, Y., and Urade, Y. (2012b). Effects of synthetic cannabinoids on electroencephalogram power spectra in rats. *Forensic Science International*, **215**, 179–183.

Uchiyama, N., Kikura-Hanajiri, R., Ogata, J., and Goda, Y. (2010). Chemical analysis of synthetic cannabinoids as designer drugs in herbal products. *Forensic Science International*, **198**, 31–38.

United Nations Office on Drugs and Crime (2011). *Synthetic Cannabinoids in Herbal Products*. [Online] Available at: http://www.unodc.org/documents/scientific/Synthetic_Cannabinoids.pdf.

Vandevoorde, S., Jonsson, K.O., Labar, G., Persson, E., Lambert, D.M. and Fowler, C.J. (2007). Lack of selectivity of URB602 for 2-oleoylglycerol compared to anandamide hydrolysis *in vitro*. *British Journal of Pharmacology*, **150**, 186–191.

Vandrey, R., Dunn, K.E., Fry, J.A., and Girling, E.R. (2012). A survey study to characterize use of Spice products (synthetic cannabinoids). *Drug and Alcohol Dependence*, **120**, 238–241.

Vann, R.E., Warner, J.A., Bushell, K., Huffman, J.W., Martin, B.R., and Wiley, J.L. (2009). Discriminative stimulus properties of Δ^9-Tetrahydrocannabinol (THC) in C57Bl/6J mice. *European Journal of Pharmacology*, **615**, 102–107.

Wiebelhaus, J.M., Poklis, J.L., Poklis, A., Vann, R.E., Lichtman, A.H., and Wise, L.E. (2012). Inhalation exposure to smoke from synthetic "marijuana" produces potent cannabimimetic effects in mice. *Drug and Alcohol Dependence*, **126**, 316–323.

Wiley, J.L. (1999). Cannabis: discrimination of "internal bliss"? *Pharmacology Biochemistry and Behavior*, **64**, 257–260.

Wiley, J.L., Compton, D.R., Dai, D., *et al.* (1998). Structure-activity relationships of indole- and pyrrole-derived cannabinoids. *Journal of Pharmacology and Experimental Therapeutics*, **285**, 995–1004.

Wiley, J.L., Jefferson, R.G., Griffin, G., *et al.* (2002). Paradoxical pharmacological effects of deoxy-tetrahydrocannabinol analogs lacking high CB_1 receptor affinity. *Pharmacology*, **66**, 89–99.

Wiley, J.L., Marusich, J.A., Martin, B.R., and Huffman, J.W. (2012a). 1-Pentyl-3-phenylacetylindoles and JWH-018 share *in vivo* cannabinoid profiles in mice. *Drug and Alcohol Dependence*, **123**, 148–153.

Wiley, J.L., Smith, V.J., Chen, J., Martin, B.R., and Huffman, J.W. (2012b). Synthesis and pharmacology of 1-alkyl-3-(1-naphthoyl)indoles: steric and electronic effects of 4- and 8-halogenated naphthoyl substituents. *Bioorganic & Medicinal Chemistry*, **20**, 2067–2081.

Wilson, R.S., May, E.L., Martin, B.R., and Dewey, W.L. (1976). 9-Nor-9-hydroxyhexahydrocannabinols. Synthesis, some behavioral and analgesic properties, and comparison with the tetrahydrocannabinols. *Journal of Medicinal Chemistry*, **19**, 1165–1167.

Winstock, A.R. and Barratt, M.J. (2013). Synthetic cannabis: a comparison of patterns of use and effect profile with natural cannabis in a large global sample. *Drug and Alcohol Dependence*. [Online] Available at: http://www.sciencedirect.com/science/article/pii/S0376871612004875.

Wollner, H. J., Matchett, J. R., Levine, J., and Loewe, S. (1942). Isolation of a physiologically active tetrahydrocannabinol from *Cannabis sativa* resin. *Journal of the American Chemical Society*, **64**, 26–29.

Zhang, Q., Ma, P., Cole, R.B., and Wang, G. (2006). Identification of in vitro metabolites of JWH-015, an aminoalkylindole agonist for the peripheral cannabinoid receptor (CB_2) by HPLC-MS/MS. *Analytical and Bioanalytical Chemistry*, **386**, 1345–1355.

Zhu, M., Ma, L., Zhang, D., *et al.* (2006). Detection and characterization of metabolites in biological matrices using mass defect filtering of liquid chromatography/high resolution mass spectrometry data. *Drug Metabolism and Disposition*, **34**, 1722–1733.

Zimmermann, U.S., Winkelmann, P.R., Pilhatsch, M., Nees, J.A., Spanagel, R., and Schulz, K. (2009). Withdrawal phenomena and dependence syndrome after the consumption of "Spice Gold." *Deutsches Ärzteblatt International*, **106**, 464–467.

Index

uveoretinitis 610–12
  clinical features 610–11
  future directions 612
  phytocannabinoids in 611–12

V
vaporization 329–30, 416–17, 697–8
vascular effects 213–19
  cell lines 220
  time-dependent responses 216–17
  vasoconstriction 217–18
  vasorelaxation 213–16
vascular endothelial growth factor (VEGF) 632
vasoconstriction 217–18
vasorelaxation 213–16
  cannabinoid receptors 215–16
  endothelium 215
  ion channel modulation 216
  metabolism 213–14
  sensory nerves 214–15
vegetative growth 75
ventral tegmental area (VTA) 173
vertical integration 348–9
viral infections, resistance to 269–70
visceral sensation 233, 236–7
Volcano vaporizer 323, 697

vomiting, cannabis-induced 678
VTA *see* ventral tegmental area
VTA-MFB-NAc reward encoding neural axis 176
VTA-NAc core reward encoding neural axis 175

W
weed 654
weight gain 424
White Widow 98, 325
Whittle, Brian 288
WIN 48,098 712
WIN 55,212-2 712
  see also R-(+)-WIN55212; WIN 55212-2;
    WIN55212-2
WIN 55212-2 629, 633
WIN 55,225 712
WIN 55212-2 160
Wo/men's Alliance for Medical Marijuana
    (WAMM) 346
women, cannabis effects
  reproductive system 251–6
  sexuality 251–2
World Health Organization 47

X
xanthones 18

Printed and bound by CPI Group (UK) Ltd, Croydon, CR0 4YY